ALEXANDER'S

SURGICAL PROCEDURES

JANE C. ROTHROCK, PhD, RN, CNOR, FAAN

Professor and Director, Perioperative Programs
Delaware County Community College
Media, Pennsylvania

SHERRI M. ALEXANDER, CST

Clinical Educator
Franciscan St. Francis Hospital
Indianapolis, Indiana

3251 Riverport Lane
St. Louis, Missouri 63043

ALEXANDER'S SURGICAL PROCEDURES

ISBN: 978-0-323-07555-8

Notices

Library of Congress Cataloging-in-Publication Data or Control Number

Alexander's surgical procedures / [edited by] Jane C. Rothrock, Sherri M. Alexander.
    p. ; cm.
  Surgical procedures
  "Derived from the 14th edition of Alexander's care of the patient in surgery"--Pref.
  Includes bibliographical references and index.
  ISBN 978-0-323-07555-8 (hardcover : alk. paper) 1. Surgical nursing. 2. Therapeutics, Surgical. I. Alexander, Edythe Louise. II. Rothrock, Jane C., 1948- III. Alexander, Sherri M. IV. Alexander's care of the patient in surgery V. Title: Surgical procedures.
  [DNLM: 1. Operating Room Technicians. 2. Surgical Procedures, Operative--methods. WY 162]
  RD99.A44 2012
  617'.0231--dc23

2011022432

Publisher: Andrew Allen
Acquisitions Editor: Jennifer Janson
Developmental Editor: Kelly Brinkman
Publishing Services Manager: Catherine Jackson
Project Manager: Carol O'Connell

Design Direction: Ashley Eberts
Cover Designer: Ashley Eberts
Text Designer: Ashley Eberts

Contributors

ROTHROCK: *ALEXANDER'S CARE OF THE PATIENT IN SURGERY*, 14th EDITION CONTRIBUTORS

Gregory J. Artz, MD

Assistant Professor
Department of Otolaryngology—Head and Neck Surgery
Thomas Jefferson University
Philadelphia, Pennsylvania
Chapter 10: Otorhinolaryngologic Surgery

Brian Blanchard, MSN, CRNP

Cardiothoracic Nurse Practitioner
Pennsylvania Hospital
Philadelphia, Pennsylvania
Chapter 14: Thoracic Surgery

Barbara A. Bowen, RN, MSN, CRNP, CRNFA

President
Perioperative Consulting & Surgical Services, LLC
Collegeville, Pennsylvania
Chapter 11: Orthopedic Surgery

Maya N. Clark, ACNP-BC

General Surgery Nurse Practitioner
Pennsylvania Hospital
Philadelphia, Pennsylvania
Chapter 4: Repair of Hernias

Troy J. DeRose, CRNP, RNFA

Certified Registered Nurse Practitioner, RN First Assistant
Department of Otolaryngology
Thomas Jefferson University Hospital
Philadelphia, Pennsylvania
Chapter 10: Otorhinolaryngologic Surgery

Leigh Ann DiFusco, MSN, RN, CNOR

Clinical Nurse Specialist
The Children's Hospital of Philadelphia
Philadelphia, Pennsylvania
Chapter 17: Pediatric Surgery

Victoria Dreger, MSN, RN, MA, CNOR

Staff Nurse/Nurse Clinician III, Surgery Department
Advocate Christ Medical Center
Oak Lawn, Illinois
Chapter 9: Ophthalmic Surgery
Chapter 13: Plastic and Reconstructive Surgery

Diane L. Ferrara-Hoffman, MSN, CRNP, RNFA, APRN, BC

Nurse Practitioner, RN First Assistant for Neurosurgery
Thomas Jefferson University Hospital
Philadelphia, Pennsylvania
Chapter 12: Neurosurgery

Sarah J. Krizman, RN, BSN, CNOR

OR Staff Nurse
Thomas Jefferson University Hospital
Philadelphia, Pennsylvania
Chapter 12: Neurosurgery

Helene Korey Marley, RN, CNOR, CRNFA

Clinical Service Coordinator, Urology
Pennsylvania Hospital
Philadelphia, Pennsylvania
Chapter 6: Genitourinary Surgery

Donna R. McEwen, RN, BSN, CNOR

Senior Educational Instructional Designer
OptumHealth Care Solutions
UnitedHealthcare
San Antonio, Texas
Chapter 5: Gynecologic and Obstetric Surgery

Janice A. Neil, RN, PhD

Associate Professor
East Carolina University
Greenville, North Carolina
Chapter 3: Surgery of the Liver, Biliary Tract, Pancreas, and Spleen

Elizabeth B. Pearsall, RN, BSN, CNOR, RNFA

Staff Nurse
Taylor Hospital
Ridley Park, Pennsylvania
Chapter 8: Breast Surgery

Jane C. Rothrock, PhD, RN, CNOR, FAAN

Professor and Director, Perioperative Programs
Delaware County Community College
Media, Pennsylvania
Chapter 4: Repair of Hernias

Diane Catherine Saullo, RN, MSN, CNOR, BC

Manager Professional Development
New Hanover Regional Medical Center
Wilmington, North Carolina
Chapter 18: Trauma Surgery

Patricia C. Seifert, RN, MSN, CNOR, CRNFA, FAAN

Education Coordinator, Cardiovascular Operating Room
Inova Heart and Vascular Institute
Editor-in-Chief, *AORN Journal*
Falls Church, Virginia
Chapter 16: Cardiac Surgery

Christine E. Smith, RN, MSN, CNOR

Perioperative Clinical Nurse Specialist
Lucile Packard Children's Hospital at Stanford
Palo Alto, California
Chapter 2: Gastrointestinal Surgery

Victoria M. Steelman, PhD, RN, CNOR, FAAN

Advanced Practice Nurse, Department of Nursing
University of Iowa Hospitals & Clinics
Iowa City, Iowa
Chapter 1: Concepts Basic to Perioperative Nursing

Joanne C. Wentzell, RN, MSN, CNOR, CRNFA

Certified RN First Assistant
Gibbsboro, New Jersey
Chapter 7: Thyroid and Parathyroid Surgery

Patricia Wieczorek, MSN, RN, CNOR

Nurse Manager
The Johns Hopkins Hospital
Baltimore, Maryland
Chapter 15: Vascular Surgery

ROTHROCK AND ALEXANDER: *ALEXANDER'S SURGICAL PROCEDURES* CONTRIBUTORS

Sherri M. Alexander, CST

Clinical Educator
Franciscan St. Francis Hospital
Indianapolis, Indiana
Chapter 1: Importance of the Surgical Technologist on the Surgical Team
Chapter 2: Gastrointestinal Surgery
Chapter 7: Thyroid and Parathyroid Surgery
Chapter 17: Pediatric Surgery
Chapter 18: Trauma Surgery

Betsy Boatwright, CST

Surgical Technologist/Preceptor
Indiana Heart Hospital
Indianapolis, Indiana
Chapter 14: Thoracic Surgery
Chapter 15: Vascular Surgery
Chapter 16: Cardiac Surgery

Jeff Feix, LVN, CST/CSFA, FAST

Surgical Technology Program Coodinator/Instructor
Vernon College
Wichita Falls, Texas
Chapter 13: Plastic and Reconstructive Surgery

Dana M. Fields, CST

OB/GYN, Maternal Fetal Medicine
Indiana University Health, University Hospital
Indianapolis, Indiana
Chapter 5: Gynecologic and Obstetric Surgery

Crit Fisher, BS, CST, FAST

National Field Training and Logistics Manager
KARL STORZ Endoscopy-America, Inc.
El Segundo, California
Chapter 4: Repair of the Hernia

Barbara Krukemeier, CST

Surgical Technologist
Wishard Hospital
Indianapolis, Indiana
Chapter 10: Otorhinolaryngologic

Christopher Lee, CST, AAS

OR Liason/Surgical Technologist, Department of Urology
Northwestern Memorial Hospital
Chicago, Illinois
Chapter 6: Genitourinary Surgery

James S. Miazga, Jr., CST, BS-Psy

Surgical Technology Instructor
Miller-Motte College
Cary, North Carolina
Chapter 8: Breast Surgery
Chapter 9: Ophthalmic Surgery

Margaret Rodriguez, BS, CSFA, FAST

Associate Professor
El Paso Community College
El Paso, Texas
Chapter 1: Importance of the Surgical Technologist on the Surgical Team
Chapter 12: Neurosurgery

Michelle Whitlow, CST, BS

Clinical Coordinator, Surgical Technology Program
IU Health
Indianapolis, Indiana
Chapter 11: Orthopedic Surgery

Michelle Williams-Callahan, CST, AAS

Surgical Technologist/General Surgery Team
University Hospital – IU Health
Indianapolis, Indiana
Chapter 3: Surgery of the Liver, Biliary Tract, Pancreas, and Spleen

Clinical Consultants

ROTHROCK: *ALEXANDER'S CARE OF THE PATIENT IN SURGERY*, 14th EDITION CLINICAL CONSULTANTS

D. Greg Anderson, MD

Associate Professor of Orthopaedic Surgery
Thomas Jefferson University
Philadelphia, Pennsylvania

Nicole Armstrong, RN, BSN, CMSRN

Registered Nurse
Thomas Jefferson University Hospital
Philadelphia, Pennsylvania

Larry L. Asplin, RN, MSN, CNOR

Clinical Director, Surgery and Sterile Processing
St. Cloud Hospital
St. Cloud, Minnesota

Kristine Biggie, RN, MSN, CRNP, CCRN

Pediatric Trauma Nurse Practitioner, Pediatric Trauma Program
The Children's Hospital of Philadelphia
Philadelphia, Pennsylvania

James W. Collins, PhD, MSME

Associate Director for Science
Division of Safety Research, National Institute for Occupational Safety and Health
Centers for Disease Control and Prevention
Morgantown, West Virginia

Debra Coston, RN, CCRN

Coordinator AHA Program, Staff Nurse STICU
New Hanover Regional Medical Center
Wilmington, North Carolina

Cynthia L. Danko, RN, MSN

Director, Surgical Services
Hillcrest Hospital
Mayfield Heights, Ohio

Beth Fitzgerald, RN, MSN, CNOR

Perioperative Nurse Internship Manager
Christiana Care Health System
Wilmington, Delaware

Allen S. Gabroy, MD, FACS

Chairman, Department of Surgery
Taylor Hospital
Ridley Park, Pennsylvania

Jerome B. Goldstein, MD, FACOG

Senior Attending, OB/GYN Department
Crozer-Keystone Health System
Upland, Pennsylvania

Ahmed Gomad, MD, ScD, MSPH

Medical Officer, Surveillance Branch
Division of Surveillance Hazard Evaluation and Health Studies
National Institute for Occupational Safety and Health
Centers for Disease Control and Prevention
Cincinnati, Ohio

Paula Graling, RN, MSN, CNS, CNOR

Clinical Nurse Specialist, Perioperative Services
Inova Fairfax Hospital
Past President of Association of periOperative Registered Nurses
Falls Church, Virginia

Joseph F. Harryhill, MD, FACS

Assistant Clinical Professor of Urology
Penn Urology at Pennsylvania Hospital
Philadelphia, Pennsylvania

Nancy L. Hughes, MS, RN

Director, Center for Occupational and Environmental Health
American Nurses Association
Silver Spring, Maryland

Rama D. Jager, MD

Assistant Professor, Department of Surgery
University of Illinois Chicago
Chicago, Illinois

Janine Jagger, MPH, PhD

Professor of Medicine
Director, International Healthcare Worker Safety Center
University of Virginia Health System
Charlottesville, Virginia

Ramasamy Kalimuthu, MD, FACS

Visiting Professor and Section Chief, Microsurgery Plastic Division
University of Illinois Chicago
Chicago, Illinois
Chief, Division of Plastic Surgery
Advocate Christ Medical Center
Oak Lawn, Illinois

Susan N. Kamerling, RN, MSN, BC

Family Services Coordinator, Perioperative Services
The Children's Hospital of Philadelphia
Philadelphia, Pennsylvania

Amy L. Kennedy, RN, MSN, CNOR

Surgical Technology Program Director
Harrisburg Area Community College
Harrisburg, Pennsylvania

Joy C. Kerr, RNFA, BSN, CNOR

RNFA—Division of Urology
The Children's Hospital of Philadelphia
Philadelphia, Pennsylvania

Mary Lou Kubu, RN, BSN, CNOR

Perioperative Education Coordinator
University Hospitals Case Medical Center
Cleveland, Ohio

Ivy Fenton Kuhn, PNP-BC, CNOR

Nurse Practitioner, Division of Ophthalmology
The Children's Hospital of Pennsylvania
Philadelphia, Pennsylvania

Linda Cunningham Lawler, RN, BSN

Family Services Coordinator
The Children's Hospital of Philadelphia
Philadelphia, Pennsylvania

Maureen Lewis, RN, BSN, CNOR, RNFA

RN First Assistant for Orthopedics
Riddle Memorial Hospital
Media, Pennsylvania
Adjunct Faculty
Delaware County Community College
Media, Pennsylvania

Patrick J. Loynd, DNP, CRNA

Associate Program Director, School of Nurse Anesthesiology
Nazareth Hospital
Philadelphia, Pennsylvania

Maureen Murphy, RN

Perioperative RN
Thomas Jefferson University Hospital
Philadelphia, Pennsylvania

Audrey L. Nelson, PhD, RN, FAAN

Director, HSR&D REAP
James A. Haley VA Medical Center
Tampa, Florida

Cheryl Osmian, CCLS

Child Life Specialist
The Children's Hospital of Philadelphia
Philadelphia, Pennsylvania

Roni L. Robinson, RN, MSN, CRNP

Nurse Practitioner
Philadelphia, Pennsylvania

Thomas R. Saullo, MD

Third Year Resident, Physical Medical Rehab
Cornell/Columbia Presbyterian Hospital
New York, New York

Beverly B. Schuler, RN, BSN

Patient Care Manager
Lucile Packard Children's Hospital
Palo Alto, California

Mary Jean Schumann, MSN, MBA, RN, CPNP

Chief Programs Officer
American Nurses Association
Silver Spring, Maryland

Susan Scully, RN, BSN, CNOR

General, Thoracic, and Fetal Surgery Specialty Nurse, Clinical Level IV
Children's Hospital of Philadelphia
Philadelphia, Pennsylvania

Katie Elaine Slavin, MS, RN

Senior Staff Specialist, Center for Occupational and Environmental Health
American Nurses Association
Silver Spring, Maryland

Benjamin H. Ticho, MD

Eye & Ear Infirmary
University of Illinois
Chicago, Illinois

Thomas R. Waters, PhD, CPE

Research Safety Engineer
National Institute for Occupational Safety and Health
Cincinnati, Ohio

Mitchell Winter, RN, BSN

Operating Room Staff Nurse, Neurosurgery
Thomas Jefferson University Hospital
Philadelphia, Pennsylvania

Reviewers

ROTHROCK: *ALEXANDER'S CARE OF THE PATIENT IN SURGERY*, 14th EDITION REVIEWERS

Mike Aldridge, MSN, RN, CCRN, CNS

Instructor of Clinical Nursing, School of Nursing
The University of Texas
Austin, Texas

Alice Erskine, RN, MSN, CNOR

Professor, Surgical Technology Program
Science, Math & Technology Department
Skyline Community College
San Bruno, California

Rachel Hottel, MSN, RN, CNOR

Advanced Practice Nurse, Perioperative Division
University of Iowa Hospitals & Clinics
Iowa City, Iowa

Christina Keels, CST, RN

Surgical Technology Program Director
Central Carolina Technical College
Sumter, South Carolina

Tom Lescarbeau, BS, CFA, CST

Program Coordinator, Surgical Technology
McCann Technical School
North Adams, Massachusetts

Elizabeth A. Matos, PhD, MSN, BSN, CNE

Assistant Professor, Department of Nursing
West Texas A & M University
Canyon, Texas

Jill E. Roofner, CST, RN, CNOR

Clinical Coordinator, Surgical Technology Program
Durham Community Technical College
Durham, North Carolina

Herman Young, BS, BM, CST/CFA

Program Director Surgical Technology, Health Professions
Oakland Community College
Southfield, Michigan

ROTHROCK AND ALEXANDER: *ALEXANDER'S SURGICAL PROCEDURES* REVIEWERS

Julia Hinkle, RN, MHA, CNOR

Professor/Program Chair, Surgical Technology
Ivy Tech Community College
Evansville, Indiana

John D. Ratliff, B.S., CST, FAST

Department Chair, Surgical Technology
York Technical College
Rock Hill, South Carolina

Elizabeth Slagle, MS, RN, CST

Associate Professor and Chair
Department of Surgical Technology
University of Saint Francis
Fort Wayne, Indiana

About the Authors

JANE C. ROTHROCK, PhD, RN, CNOR, FAAN

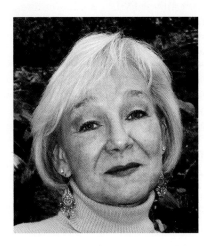

To my surgical technology students, past and current, who serve as such excellent members of the surgical team in a variety of settings. It has been my joy to watch, over the years, as you go and grow, stretch and learn, and take such pride in your work. It is my humble hope that I have taught you at least as much as you have taught me.

Dr. Jane C. Rothrock has practiced and taught perioperative nursing since 1969. In 1979 she joined the faculty of Delaware County Community College, where she is now Professor and Director of Perioperative Programs. Her responsibilities include directing the surgical technology program, entry-level, postbasic RN education programs for perioperative nursing, and advanced skill programs that prepare RN first assistants. These courses have been offered both in Pennsylvania and at various sites nationally, within host institutions. During her 32-year tenure at the college, Jane has helped to educate more than 4000 students who now practice in the field of perioperative patient care.

Jane's decades of experience include being a faculty member, author, and speaker. She has taught at the University of Pennsylvania, been an OR director, and served as the preceptor for many graduate students. She has authored 5 perioperative nursing textbooks, published more than 50 articles, and presented a host of topics to nursing audiences across the United States and internationally. Jane is an AORN past president, chaired the AORN Project Team on Professional Practice Issues, chaired the AORN Project Team on a Professional Practice Model for Perioperative Nursing in 1998-1999, and chaired the Perioperative Academic Curriculum Task Force in 2006. She has received a number of distinguished awards and is very active in both nursing and community organizations. Jane is a past member of the ANCC Magnet Commission, a past president of the ASPAN Foundation, and a past president of the AORN Foundation Board of Trustees. She served on ASPAN's first National Clinical Guideline Panel to develop the Guideline on Prevention of Unplanned Hypothermia in Adult Surgical Patients. In 2000 Jane became a Fellow of the American Academy of Nursing (FAAN). She currently serves as an "Ask the Expert" for Medscape Nursing and is a co-editor of *Tea & Toast for the Perioperative Nurse's Spirit*, a book of inspirational stories published in 2006.

Jane began her nursing education with a diploma from Bryn Mawr School of Nursing. She received her BSN and MSN from the University of Pennsylvania and was the first recipient of a doctoral degree from Widener University in suburban Philadelphia, earning her PhD in nursing in 1987.

SHERRI M. ALEXANDER, CST

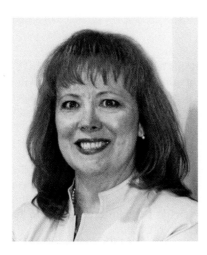

I would like to start by thanking Jane for this wonderful opportunity.
To all surgical technologists, embrace who you are and what you bring to patient care.
To Lucy and Dick, thank you for being proud of everything I have ever done, big or small.
Sydni, you have taught me patience, perseverance, and how important it is for every patient to have an "Aunt Sherri."
To David and Amanda, thank you for completing our family; and to my Abigail and Adam, the way you believe in yourselves continues to inspire me. Thank you for sharing me and for your love and support. The two of you are truly the best work I have ever done.
To my husband Phil, in this complex and ambiguous world, thank you for finally teaching me the most important lesson . . . it really is simple.
I love you all very much.

Certified Surgical Technologist Sherri M. Alexander has practiced and taught surgical technology since 1991. After excelling in orthopaedics and trauma surgery at Wishard Memorial Hospital for five years, Sherri served as a faculty member at Ivy State Tech College where she taught aseptic technique and performed mock surgeries. In 1995, Sherri assisted surgeons in outpatient surgical procedures at Surgery Center Plus before becoming a Clinical Education Specialist at Clarian Health. As a Clinical Educator in Perioperative Services at Franciscan St. Francis Hospital, Sherri currently monitors the orientation process and coordinates continuing education.

Sherri's contribution to surgical technology extends beyond her work experience. She has been involved with the Association of Surgical Technologists since 1997, becoming the president in 2007. Sherri is also an affiliate member of the American College of Surgeons, a member of the Advisory Board for the Pharmacy Technician Program, and a committee member of the Association of periOperative Registered Nurses. Such a thorough background has made Sherri a valuable speaker at a variety of events, including many AST assemblies and International Association of Healthcare Central Service Material Management meetings.

In 1991, Sherri received a technical certificate in surgical technology from Ivy Tech State College, as well as a national certification in surgical technology through the National Board for Surgical Technology and Surgical Assisting.

Preface

The first edition of *Alexander's Surgical Procedures* is derived from the trusted content of the 14th edition of *Alexander's Care of the Patient in Surgery*. This text has been revised to enhance the knowledge of the surgical technologist in the perioperative setting.

Who Will Benefit from This Book?

The surgical procedures in the book have been revised by practicing surgical technologists and surgical technology instructors, ensuring its relevance for surgical technology students.

Why Is This Book Important to the Profession?

This comprehensive textbook on surgical procedures is from the surgical technologist's point of view. All the chapters in the book have been revised by surgical technology instructors or practicing surgical technologist to provide an in-depth coverage of surgical specialties.

Organization

Alexander's Surgical Procedures is divided into 18 chapters that follow the same the organization as the 14th edition of *Alexander's Care of the Patient in Surgery*. This text opens with an introductory chapter discussing the role of the surgical technologist in the operating room, as well as basic information about the profession. Chapters 2 through 18 cover the surgical procedures by body system.

Each chapter begins with surgical anatomy and physiology, then progresses though diagnostic testing and surgical intervention. A Surgical Technologist Considerations section discusses important aspects the surgical technologist will need to keep in mind when participating in procedures for a specific body system. This section includes such topics as instrumentation and positioning information, as well as other pertinent information. After the Surgical Technologist Considerations section, surgical interventions are detailed in a comprehensive, often step-by-step, fashion.

Distinctive Features of the Book

Alexander's Surgical Procedures offers the student a Surgical Technologist Preference card for each specialty, Surgical Technologist Considerations, and a Geriatric Considerations box for each specialty.

The Surgical Technologist Preference Card outlines the materials a surgical technologist should have ready or available for a procedure within the surgical specialty. Items found on this card include necessary instrumentation, usual skin prep agents, sutures, catheters, drains, and other accessory items and equipment used in the surgical specialty. The Surgical Technologist Preference Card is intended to serve as a checklist, or guideline overview, of how to prepare for procedures in the particular surgical specialty.

Geriatric Considerations boxes highlight information about care of geriatric patients in the surgical specialties. These boxes assist the surgical technologist in recognizing important aspects of the aging process on various body systems.

Also noteworthy in this text is the addition of over 75 photographs of instruments that surgical technologists will most likely use in surgery. Instrument photos sorted by specialty allow the student to become familiar with the equipment needed for procedures, leading to successful surgical outcomes.

Learning Aids

Chapter objectives and chapter outlines introduce each chapter. These provide the student with an overview of the content to be covered. Every chapter concludes with a brief summary, review questions, and critical thinking questions to further enhance the learning of the student.

Other useful features from the 14th edition of *Alexander's Care of the Patient in Surgery* that have been repurposed for the surgical technologist include Risk Reduction Strategies, Research Highlights, Surgical Pharmacology, Ambulatory Surgery Considerations, Evidence for Practice, and Patient Safety and History boxes.

Online Ancillaries

Ancillaries for *Alexander's Surgical Procedures* can be found on the text's accompanying Evolve web site at: http://evolve .elsevier.com/Rothrock/surgical/. On this web site you will find the following assets for the student:

- Anatomy Animations
- OR Live Links and Case Studies
- Surgical Instrumentation Photos
- Surgical Pharmacology Tables

Each asset is intended to serve as supplemental material that will reinforce important concepts for the surgical technologist.

Ancillary assets available for the instructor are the following:

- Image Collection
- TEACH Lecture Outline
- TEACH Lesson Plan
- TEACH PowerPoint Slides
- Examview Test Bank

The instructor ancillaries assist the instructor in planning lessons and reducing prep time for class.

Note to the Student

You will gain a wealth of knowledge from the surgical procedures presented in this book. The Surgical Technologist Preference Cards and their broad overview will facilitate your anticipation of role responsibilities in the scrub role. Use the review questions at the end of the chapters to test your knowledge of the procedures and relevant anatomy and physiology. The history boxes will aid in understanding how far surgery has progressed. This book will serve you in the student role and in your career as surgical technologist. As a practitioner, use this book as a reference when you need to refresh for a procedure or prepare to scrub a procedure for the first time. As surgery is ever changing, you will need to continually enhance your education.

Contents

Importance of the Surgical Technologist on the Surgical Team

LEARNING OBJECTIVES

After studying this chapter the reader will be able to:
- Identify the three types of surgical technologists
- Discuss the professional settings for the surgical technologist
- Correlate education, certification, and accreditation
- Discuss surgical case management
- Explore personal characteristics of successful surgical technologists
- Demonstrate a working knowledge of the practice of anticipation
- Explain teamwork and patient safety
- Discuss other professional organizations with relevance to perioperative care

CHAPTER OUTLINE

This chapter was written by Sherri M. Alexander, CST, and Margaret Rodriguez, BS, CSFA, FAST.

SURGICAL TECHNOLOGY: BEGINNINGS

In the past, when people thought of a surgical team, the old model consisted of the surgeon as head of a team, with a specialized operating room (OR) nurse and other team members called *operating room technicians,* whose duties were delegated to them by the OR nurse. However, the past several decades have seen great strides in new responsibilities for these technicians, requiring both a new title and increased regulation to go with this expanded role on the surgical team. With the formation of the Association of Surgical Technologists (AST) in 1969 have come ever-evolving Standards of Practice and increasingly stringent education and training for the emergence of a highly respected member of the surgical team: the **Surgical Technologist** (Romig, 1997).

THREE TYPES OF SURGICAL TECHNOLOGISTS

What, then, is a surgical technologist (ST)? At its most basic, according to the AST, the role of the surgical technologist is to "ensure that the operative procedure is conducted under optimal conditions" (AST, 2010). Entry-level surgical technologists can fill any of three major roles on a surgical team: (1) scrub surgical technologist, (2) the circulating surgical technologist, and (3) the second assisting technologist.

Scrub Surgical Technologist

The first type of ST, the scrub surgical technologist, is sometimes called the **surgical technologist in the scrub role**. In this scrub role, the surgical technologist is a member of the "sterile team," working collaboratively with the registered nurse (RN), who functions in the **circulator** role. This circulating nurse coordinates the activities of the surgical team. To provide optimal care to the patient, the circulating nurse maintains mobility outside the sterile field to monitor the patient's condition throughout the surgical experience, from pre-op to post-op, and thus provides invaluable direction to the surgical technologist.

In the scrub role, the surgical technologist will assemble the instruments and supplies needed to facilitate a safe and efficient surgery and maintain the sterility of the surgical field throughout the procedure. Basic working knowledge of a wide variety of supplies, sterile techniques, and equipment is crucial for patient safety. With experience over time, each tenured surgical technologist comes to rely on a mental checklist when preparing to set up for a procedure; this is built over time and with each new experience. The fundamentals do not change with surgical specialties; they are instead uniform to each procedure.

Circulating Surgical Technologist

Sometimes the surgical technologist assists in circulating, by retrieving additional supplies, equipment, or instruments during the surgical procedure itself. In contrast to the scrub role, circulating requires working outside the sterile field. The circulating surgical technologist also monitors OR conditions and anticipates patient and surgical team needs. In the circulating role, the surgical technologist can assist in transporting and positioning the patient, assisting anesthesia personnel, securing dressings, keeping accurate records throughout the entire operation, and a variety of other duties outside the sterile field.

Second Assisting Technologist

In this more advanced role, the surgical technologist still performs in the scrub role but is also able to perform additional tasks to assist the first assistant or surgeon. These additional tasks may include any of the following, among other responsibilities: holding instruments as directed by the surgeon, performing suctioning or sponging at the operative site, applying dressings, helping to provide aid in exposure and hemostasis, connecting drains to suction apparatus, and cutting suture material as directed by the surgeon.

PROFESSIONAL SETTINGS FOR THE SURGICAL TECHNOLOGIST

The surgical technologist can work in a variety of different surgical settings. Each of these offer unique responsibilities, environmental variation, and opportunities to develop a specialized set of skills. The following are a few examples to demonstrate the varying opportunities in the growing field.

Hospital Surgical Suites

Surgical technologists are most commonly utilized in main operating rooms in large and small hospitals. They may function as part of a specialized team for a specific surgical service or function in all procedures the operating room performs. In some facilities there is a career advancement ladder for the surgical technologist, usually ranging from two to four different levels based on the needs of the facility and the education and training of the surgical technology staff. This advancement model encourages the surgical technologist to achieve additional training and education for additional recognition.

Labor and Delivery Departments

Surgical technologists are well equipped to specialize in this demanding department, both as the scrub in a cesarean section and as an assistant to the team in a vaginal delivery.

Ambulatory Surgical Centers

Less complex surgeries are being performed more often in ambulatory surgical centers. These outpatient centers offer the surgical technologist the opportunity to work in a facility specializing in minimally invasive surgery as well as short-term–stay patients. Most often these patients arrive the day of surgery and leave within 23 hours. As modern surgery has become more specialized with the advancement of minimal incision techniques and the implementation of robotic surgery, the perioperative team needs to increase their level of training. Thus, in these ambulatory surgery settings, the surgical technologist has the opportunity to expand skill sets to function in multiple specialties and highly advanced procedural changes, without the call and shift requirements of a hospital setting.

Private Surgeon's Scrub

Functioning as a private scrub technologist for a specific surgeon or group of surgeons provides the surgical technologist the ability to gain expert knowledge in a surgical specialty and function at a higher level. This career choice will present the opportunity for the surgical technologist to have more hands-on, direct patient care than working as part of a traditional hospital staff and often requires advancement to the position of surgical first assistant. Additional education and advanced knowledge of knot tying and suturing techniques are required to function as a first assistant. The private scrub may interact with the patient preoperatively and do rounds with the surgeon postoperatively. They may be involved in procedures done in the surgeon's office, and will work with the surgeon in several hospitals, requiring the surgical technologist to be credentialed in several facilities.

Sterile Processing and Decontamination Department

The experience and expertise the surgical technologist brings to surgical patient care settings can also be utilized in the sterile processing and decontamination departments. In addition to focusing on sterilization techniques, an advanced understanding of specific surgical instruments and their functionality plays an important role in the safe and efficient processing of specialized sets. Some facilities utilize surgical technologists as group leaders or coordinators in this department.

CAREER EXPANSION OPPORTUNITIES

Surgical technologists have a number of options for career paths. For instance, they might choose to pursue any of the following:

◆ Specialize in a particular area of surgery that interests them
◆ Become a private scrub for a surgeon or group of surgeons
◆ Go into medical/surgical sales
◆ Teach within the field of surgical technology education
◆ Work exclusively in central sterile processing
◆ Pursue additional training to become a surgical first assistant and experience broader surgical responsibility

Obtaining a career as a surgical technologist is the first step to a rewarding profession in healthcare.

EDUCATION AND ACCREDITATION

The educational pathway for surgical technology is through an accredited program through any of the following venues: community college, hospital setting, proprietary (private or technical) school, or the armed services. The time frame varies from an 11-month certificate or diploma program to a 2-year associate degree program. Accredited programs are designed and structured around the Core Curriculum for Surgical Technology developed by the Association of Surgical Technologists' (AST) Education and Professional Standards Committee.

In addition, all accredited programs must also meet the stringent accreditation standards developed by the Commission on Accreditation of Allied Health Programs (CAAHEP) or the Accrediting Bureau of Health Education Schools (ABHES) and verified by the Accreditation Review Council on Education in Surgical Technology and Surgical Assisting (ARC/STSA).

The Core Curriculum for Surgical Technology has been developed as an outline for instructors throughout the United States to ensure a standardized programmatic design. There is room for some degree of variability in clinical sites, class-time and lab hours, school-specific core courses, textbook selection, physical classroom facilities, and tuition. But while allowing for these variations, the goal of every surgical technology program is to graduate knowledgeable individuals with an entry-level competency appropriate to any operating room in any state in the country. With this nation-wide educational standardization, success in passing the certification (CST) exam is more likely and levels the playing field for candidates.

Course and subject areas in surgical technology curricula include the following:

◆ Basic sciences
  • Anatomy and physiology
  • Microbiology
  • Pathophysiology
  • Medical terminology
  • Pharmacology and anesthesia
◆ Legal doctrines and ethical issues
◆ Preoperative patient care
◆ Preoperative case management
  • Aseptic and sterile techniques
  • Surgical instrumentation and equipment
  • Physical environment
  • Disinfection and sterilization
  • Scrubbing, gowning, and gloving
  • Skin preparation and draping
  • Surgical count procedures
◆ Intraoperative case management
  • Safe medication practices
  • Methods of hemostasis
  • Wound closure techniques
  • Catheters, drain, tubes
  • Tissue handling
  • Specimen care
  • Emergency response
  • Protection and maintenance of the sterile field
◆ Postoperative case management
  • Surgical dressings
  • Confinement of hazardous waste
  • Decontamination procedures
  • Economy of time and resources
◆ Surgical specialties: anatomy and procedures
  • General surgery
  • Obstetrics and gynecology
  • Orthopedics
  • Genitourinary
  • Ophthalmology
  • Otorhinolaryngology
  • Plastics and reconstruction
  • Maxillofacial
  • Cardiothoracic
  • Peripheral vascular
  • Neurosurgery
◆ Special patient populations
  • Pediatric
  • Geriatric
  • Bariatric/obese
  • Trauma
◆ Technology
  • Computers
  • Ionizing and nonionizing radiation
  • Robotics
  • Guided imagery
  • Microsurgery
◆ Safety measures
  • Time-outs
  • Safety checklists

- Personal protective equipment
- Fire prevention and response
- Malignant hyperthermia treatment
- Cardiopulmonary resuscitation
- Bioterrorism
- Disease transmission
- Sharps safety techniques

Certification

The most widely accepted certification for surgical technologists is offered through the National Board for Surgical Technology and Surgical Assisting (NBSTSA). The title of Certified Surgical Technologist (CST) is a registered trademark of the NBSTSA. The outcomes-indicator for surgical technology programs is the CST exam, which can be taken before graduation or any time after graduation from an accredited program. Students are not denied graduation if they are unsuccessful at passing the exam and may retake it twice more in a year's time in an effort to attain certification. Once certified, the Certified Surgical Technologist will have 4 years to complete 60 continuing education (CE) credits to maintain certification or retest; however, the preferred method of maintaining currency and professional competency is through continuing education. These credits can be obtained in a number of ways: through meetings at the state or national level, hospital educational in-services, journal article post-tests, and qualifying college courses.

SURGICAL CASE MANAGEMENT: THE THREE PHASES OF SURGICAL TECHNOLOGIST RESPONSIBILITIES

The important thing to stress is the surgical technologist's need to understand—and even anticipate—all steps in a surgical procedure. Surgery often requires critical, quick action to protect or save a patient's life, and each surgeon requires specific instrumentation and techniques to be applied very quickly. The surgical technologist is responsible for fully understanding the procedure and, when possible, the surgeon's preferences ahead of time to anticipate the surgeon's—and ultimately the patient's—greatest needs. We'll talk more about anticipation as a special skill a little later in this chapter.

Multidisciplinary teamwork is essential for a successful outcome for the patient in surgery. Naturally, then, the primary role of the surgical technologist is always tied to being a strong team member and involves not only the practice of sterile techniques and principles of asepsis in the surgical environment, but, as we have seen, also embraces nonsterile phases of patient care (or circulating) as required, from preoperative to postoperative care. This three-phase involvement—preoperative, intraoperative, and postoperative care—is called surgical case management. Descriptions of these three phases from the point of view of the surgical technologist are explained below.

Preoperative Phase

Before surgery, the surgical team relies on the surgical technologist to prepare the OR, create a sterile field, and gather and count all necessary equipment and supplies. This last responsibility is no small matter: checking to be sure all the correct supplies, equipment, and instruments are available is paramount to achieving quality outcomes for the patient. It is impossible to anticipate every aspect of the surgical procedure; however, the more prepared you are for the unexpected, the better the flow of the surgical procedure.

Once aseptic technique has been applied in preparing the surgical environment, the surgical technologist also assists the rest of the team as they enter the sterile field. Then, the surgical technologist creates the sterile field around the patient's surgical site with the appropriate sterile drapes. More specifically, some of these presurgery responsibilities include the following:

- Opening sterile supplies with the circulator
- Performing a surgical hand scrub
- Gowning and gloving
- Performing an initial count with the circulator to establish a baseline count of sterile sharps, sponges and other soft goods, and instruments
- Receiving medication from the circulator onto the sterile field and preparing and labeling each medication appropriately
- Preparing and organizing the back table, Mayo stand, ring basin, and any additional sterile equipment
- Gowning and gloving the surgeon and other sterile team members
- Assisting the surgeon with draping of the patient and any other surgical equipment that will be part of the sterile field
- Assisting with securing the electrosurgical device, suction, and any additional items needed on the surgical field

In addition, when assisting the circulating nurse, the surgical technologist may be required to perform or assist with the following:

- Help position the patient on the surgical bed
- Open supplies for the scrubbed person
- Perform a surgical skin prep of the patient
- Insert an indwelling urinary catheter
- Provide irrigation solutions to the scrubbed person
- Facilitate an efficient and safe surgical procedure for the patient

Intraoperative Phase

During surgery, the surgical technologist ensures that a sterile field is maintained at all times, while anticipating the surgeon's and patient's needs during the procedure, including passing instrumentation and supplies to the surgeon, keeping count of those instruments and supplies to prevent retained surgical items, handling medication and specimens as needed, and applying dressings. Once the procedure begins, duties may include any or all of the following, depending on whether the surgical technologist is strictly working as the first scrub or second assisting with scrub duties:

- Handing the appropriate instruments and supplies to the surgeon
- Observing for any breaks in sterile technique
- Assisting with retracting, sponging or suctioning, and cutting suture as directed by the surgeon
- Retrieving any specimen and communicating with the circulating nurse regarding identity, proper handling, and test requirements
- Anticipating the need for additional supplies and communicating efficiently with the circulating nurse
- Providing medication and irrigation totals to the circulating nurse

- Performing sponge, sharps, and instrument counts with the circulating nurse, ensuring that all items have been retrieved from the patient
- Requesting dressing materials and assisting with sterile dressing application

Postoperative Phase

Once a surgery is completed, it remains crucial that a sterile field be maintained until the patient has been removed from the surgical setting. This responsibility naturally falls to the surgical technologist, along with removal of used instruments, equipment, and supplies. Counting supplies again becomes crucial because the surgical technologist is frequently the team member responsible for ensuring that all instruments and soft goods, such as sponges, are removed from the operative site in the patient's body. Finally, after the patient is transported from the OR, it is the surgical technologist who takes care of all instruments, equipment, and supplies and prepares the OR for the next patient. More specifically, postprocedure, the surgical technologist is usually responsible for:

- Preparing the instrument trays for decontamination
- Appropriately disposing of all sharps
- Confining and containing all biohazardous material in the appropriate containers
- Assisting with preparation of the room for the next patient (often referred to as "turn-over")
- Cleaning the room

PERSONAL CHARACTERISTICS OF SUCCESSFUL SURGICAL TECHNOLOGISTS

Surgery is a fascinating field to work in, and the challenges go beyond intellectual acumen and specialized skill set mastery. Besides education in the critical technical skills summarized above, the surgical technologist needs to possess good communication skills, both written and verbal, as well as a calming attitude when dealing with stressful situations. Respect for the entire perioperative team is paramount for achieving the common goals of preeminent patient care and safety. Certain personal traits and core values enable the surgical technologist to achieve success:

- *Respect for the entire team:* A desire to be part of a cohesive interdisciplinary team; keen understanding of the relevance of each team member to the successful outcome for the patient. This includes impeccable communication and attention to the roles and responsibilities of each surgical team member.
- *Good manual dexterity:* The ability to work effectively and quickly.
- *Organizational skills:* An affinity for prioritizing tasks, organizing and operating equipment, and handling supplies in a timely and efficient manner.
- *Surgical conscience:* The pledge to admit and own one's mistakes and the ability to provide for corrective actions.
- *Concentration and maturity:* Leaving one's personal life at home and one's professional life at work to stay focused on the tasks at hand in the operating room. Any type of distraction—hunger, stress, exhaustion, illness, or lack of sleep—can have a detrimental effect on the outcome of the surgical procedure. A seasoned practitioner knows when he/she is unable to provide optimal care and must address this issue with the proper supervisor for resolution.

- *Good sense of humor:* The ability to discern when laughter can be therapeutic and help to put things in perspective. The surgical environment can be intense at times, and knowing how and when a little appropriate levity can help is a great gift to the rest of one's team.

THE PRACTICE OF ANTICIPATION

In addition to ongoing education and training, and in addition to the personal characteristics just described, an additional essential trait is developing the *practice of anticipation*. What anticipation means in this context is that the surgical technologist must develop the ability to anticipate the needs of the surgical team. This is achieved by:

- Understanding the relevant anatomy and physiology for the surgical procedure being performed
- A strong foundation in recognition and use of surgical instruments and supplies
- A fundamental and extensive knowledge of aseptic and sterile technique

Constant changes in technology and surgeon preferences mean continuing flexibility and the ongoing study, communication, and assessment of surgical needs to be ready ahead of time for any challenge.

Anticipating Technological Advances

Surgical procedures have become extremely complex with the advent of ever-evolving technology. Surgical teams are continually adapting to innovations in a myriad of applications such as methods of hemostasis, joint replacement systems, minimally invasive surgery (MIS) equipment and applications, guidance systems, and intraoperative diagnostics.

The ability to anticipate sets the expert apart from the novice surgical technologist and is largely a result of previous experiences. However, the real expert leaves little to chance and reviews or researches surgical procedures before beginning the surgical procedure. Reference materials in the form of textbooks, anatomy atlases, or product brochures can provide invaluable clarification of procedural steps likely to be encountered.

In the case of new or complex mechanical devices, hands-on in-service training allows for practice in advance of real-time procedural use and must be provided to team members responsible for the care, handling, and setting up of such devices. In addition, surgical technologists may utilize the knowledge and assistance of industry representatives in the OR, but should not rely solely on their guidance. Situations may arise in which there may not be any available representative; for that reason, a working knowledge of instrumentation, equipment, and procedural steps will be required for positive patient outcomes.

Anticipating Surgeon Preferences and Expectations

The surgeon's preference card is another form of reference that is crucial to being prepared for the requirements of each surgical procedure. The surgeon expects to have the appropriate equipment, sutures, drapes, and instruments for his or her procedure regardless of staff assignments. Surgical technologists and circulating RNs should update the preference cards to prevent waste and intraoperative delays that could result from having to search for overlooked or unanticipated items. Many surgical technologists keep their own notes regarding surgeons' preferences. While this is an excellent habit, it should not replace information sharing and updating of preference cards for use by co-workers. Professionals work as team members who openly share valuable insights for efficiency and optimal patient care.

The skill of anticipation can seem daunting to students, but with patience and practice it can be mastered and even become second nature. Understanding the flow of the procedure and the sequential order of use of the instruments and supplies will help the surgical technologist contribute effectively and provide optimal care for every surgical patient.

TEAMWORK AND PATIENT SAFETY

We have seen how the surgical technologist supports and assists the rest of the surgical team; these responsibilities have evolved over the past several decades. The past decade in particular has demonstrated a fundamental paradigm shift regarding the roles and responsibilities of not only the surgical technologist, but of all the various healthcare practitioners working in the operating room. The old concept of the surgeon being the "captain of the ship" has been replaced by personal and professional accountability of each team member. The surgeon cannot be held accountable for failures in standards of care by the other members of the surgical team.

Suppose, for example, that a circulating nurse and surgical technologist conduct a surgical sponge count and then at a later date the patient returns with a retained sponge. The nurse and surgical technologist will be held accountable, rather than the surgeon, because they are the team members who took responsibility for the sponge count during this procedure.

This sort of error—failure to recover a sponge from a patient—is just one example of an error that affects patient safety, also called a **sentinel event**. The Joint Commission, a not-for-profit organization that establishes and operates accreditation standards for healthcare organizations, defines a sentinel event as follows:

> *A sentinel event is an unexpected occurrence involving death or serious physical or psychological injury, or the risk thereof. Serious injury specifically includes loss of limb or function. The phrase, "or the risk thereof" includes any process variation for which a recurrence would carry a significant chance of a serious adverse outcome. Such events are called "sentinel" because they signal the need for immediate investigation and response.*

(The Joint Commission, 2010)

Patient Safety Guideline Initiatives

The enhanced focus on surgical patient safety has prompted most professional associations to research methods of training healthcare providers to reduce patient injury and sentinel events.

American College of Surgeons Initiative. The American College of Surgeons (ACS) has been very active in exploring various methods of team training such as the airline model of team training, better known as crew resource management. The premise of this training as it pertains to every airline flight is that the airplane does not leave the ground until every member of the flight crew and ground crew agrees that all systems

are "go" (Science Daily, 2010). Similarly, surgical teams have learned that use of standardized checklists and deliberate and focused individual participation in carefully placed **time-outs**—safety-check pauses before and during the procedure to verify readiness and accuracy—reduces sentinel events in the operating room, improves communication, and ultimately reduces surgical patient morbidity and mortality.

World Health Organization (WHO). WHO designed a campaign titled "Safe Surgery Saves Lives," which includes a Surgical Safety Checklist to be used by any and all operating room teams to aid in the time-out process. More specifically, this checklist breaks up these safety checks into three phases of surgery: the moment of anesthesia induction, just before the first incision, and the last moment before the patient leaves the operating room. Implementing safety checks at these three phases of the surgical process has been found useful in reducing avoidable errors that could otherwise endanger a patient's safety and well-being (WHO, 2010).

Council on Surgical and Perioperative Safety. The Council on Surgical and Perioperative Safety (CSPS) is a unique coalition of seven member organizations representing 250,000 perioperative practitioners. The members of the CSPS are:
- American Association of Nurse Anesthetists (AANA)
- American Association of Surgical Physician Assistants (AASPA)
- American College of Surgeons (ACS)
- American Society of Anesthesiologists (ASA)
- American Society of PeriAnesthesia Nurses (ASPAN)
- Association of periOperative Registered Nurses (AORN)
- Association of Surgical Technologists (AST)

The CSPS's motto is "One Team. One Goal. Surgical Patient Safety." Its vision statement asserts that "The CSPS envisions a world in which all patients receive the safest surgical care provided by an integrated team of dedicated professionals." Progressing away from old issues of hierarchy and entitlement, CSPS members recognize the value, perspective, and practice parameters of every member of the surgical team in their delivery of quality surgical patient care. Their mission is thus to work together to "promote excellence in patient safety in the surgical and perioperative environment" (CSPS, 2010).

AHRQ Safety Training Guidelines. The U.S. Department of Health and Human Services' Agency for Healthcare Research and Quality (AHRQ) provides information to healthcare workers and the public regarding a wide range of patient safety issues. AHRQ's evidence-based strategies are outlined and evaluated for use by healthcare professionals. The AHRQ embraces the reality that teams "operate in complex and dynamic environments characterized by multi-component decisions, rapidly evolving and ambiguous situations, information overload, severe time constraints, and harsh consequences for mistakes." But, the agency guidelines emphasize, these same difficulties demonstrate the great value of team training, asserting that:

> *Well-organized and high-performing teams exhibit a sense of collective efficacy. Their members recognize a dependence upon one another, and share the belief that they can solve complex problems by working together.*
>
> *Moreover, effective teams are dynamic: the members optimize their resources, engage in self-correction, com-*

pensate for one another with back-up behaviors, and reallocate functions as necessary. Because they often can coordinate without overt communication, effective teams can respond efficiently in high-stress, time-restricted environments. Finally, effective teams possess the means to recognize potential difficulties or dangerous circumstances and adjust their strategies accordingly. . . . team training is charged with improving trainee competencies (e.g., knowledge, skills, and attitudes) and achieving desirable performance outcomes (e.g., timely and accurate response, reduced patient safety risks, improved quality of care) under these demanding conditions.

(AHRQ, 2010)

The surgical technologist plays an important part in the working dynamic of the surgical team and must remain vigilant in his or her efforts to provide optimal patient care to every surgical patient. As the AST motto states, *Aeger Primo,* which means "The Patient First."

PROFESSIONAL ORGANIZATION: THE ASSOCIATION OF SURGICAL TECHNOLOGISTS (AST)

The Association of Surgical Technologists (AST) is dedicated to serving the needs of certified practitioners. AST publishes a monthly journal, *The Surgical Technologist,* which offers information on current topics, events, research, and legislative initiatives in the profession on both the national and state levels. Educational articles written by CSTs for CSTs provide continuing education credit opportunities and the most current professional practice parameters and information available. In addition, the website (www.ast.org) and journal both provide classified job listings for members and nonmembers alike.

Establishing AST Position Statements, Guidelines, and Recommended Standards of Practice

In medicine, nursing, and related allied health professions, surgical patient outcomes are assessed using recommended standards of practice (RSOPs), which outline the steps for performing key procedures. In our profession's infancy, surgical technologists had only other professionals' standards available to them for guidance. However, these widely accepted RSOPs rarely addressed the specific tasks, functions, duties, and responsibilities of nonphysician and nonnursing allied health practitioners. Despite the critically important teamwork dynamic of the surgical team, there is no one-size-fits-all standardization of work practices applicable to the entire team as a unit.

Customizing Professional Standards of Practice. To fill in this gap and provide more specialized guidance, the Association of Surgical Technologists has researched, developed, and published numerous position statements, resolutions, and guidelines regarding the unique roles and responsibilities of surgical technologists. This research has resulted in the creation of a unique, profession-specific set of RSOPs, which are available on its website. The list of RSOPs is revised and updated by the Education and Professional Standards Committee members as research, job descriptions, and practice guidelines change, and

the AST Board of Directors approves their publication for use as valuable practice parameters (AST, 2010).

A First Look at Key Sections of the AST Recommended Standards of Practice. Every surgical technology student should begin to familiarize themselves as soon as possible with the *Association of Surgical Technologists' Standards of Practice,* which can be accessed on the AST website. While not all of these standards can be covered in this chapter, a brief overview will offer a glimpse into the usefulness of becoming familiar with these standards before becoming a practitioner in the field.

SECTION I: AST AND THE PROFESSIONS OF SURGICAL TECHNOLOGY AND SURGICAL ASSISTING.

Educational Standards for CSTs and Certified Surgical First Assistants. In addition to publishing the *Core Curriculum for Surgical Technology* (discussed earlier) to establish an expected base of knowledge for certification for entry-level STs, the AST also publishes the *Core Curriculum for Surgical First Assisting,* delineating the certified surgical first assistant (CSFA) role as a CST with additional education and training to "provide aid in exposure hemostasis and other technical functions." Embracing the American College of Surgeons' definitions for the qualifications of first assistants, the AST Standards also provides detailed requirements and certification requirements to delineate CSTs into varied levels of qualification and responsibilities:

- CST Level I
- CST Level II (Advanced)
- CST Level III (Specialist in one or two specialty areas)
- First Assistant (Generalist)
- First Assistant (Specialist)

AST Clinical Ladder. The clinical ladder is a tool for encouraging surgical technologists to pursue continuing education and competency in their field. A clinical ladder program improves job satisfaction by providing guidelines for professional advancement and recognition within the institution or department through the use of an AST-established set of performance-based evaluation and advancement criteria. Proving competencies in one level helps promote the practitioner to the next level, by demonstrating accomplishment based on the *Core Curriculum for Surgical Technology* standards.

Code of Ethics. Particularly in professions that serve medical and surgical patients, establishment of high standards of professional conduct are essential. The AST Code of Ethics focuses on protecting the patient foremost in areas of personal respect, legal rights, patient safety, and asepsis, but also expands to protecting the Code itself to ensure that it is not violated, so that the standards—and thus the profession's integrity—are also protected. This integrity is protected under the Code by the expectation of a commitment to teamwork, efficiency, and continuing professional improvement.

Updated Position Statements and Resolutions. As every medical journal can attest, new issues and challenges arise constantly in the field of surgery, both in general surgical arenas and specialty fields. For this reason, Section I of the *AST's Recommended Standards and Practices* provides specific guidelines that respond to topical concerns as medicine and allied health fields change and progress. While specific recommendations for standard procedures, titles, and roles are found later, in Sections II and III, position statements in Section I answer highly specific issues as they arise. As these are continually updated, the AST's position statements, recommended standards, and resolutions have expanded to include such topics as:

- Surgical technology care of patients with HIV
- Organ donor issues
- Teamwork challenges
- Preoperative procedures
- Aseptic technique
- Witnessing informed consent
- Intraoperative endoscopy
- Performance of venipuncture
- Wound closure
- Electrosurgery
- Performing dual roles intraoperatively

These are only a few of the many position statements that continually address pertinent new challenges facing the surgical technology profession. For this reason, it is vital for the professional to continually refer to the *Association of Surgical Technologists' Standards of Practice* for updated statements.

SECTIONS II AND III: GUIDELINES AND RECOMMENDED STANDARDS OF PRACTICE. An essential for not only entry-level but advanced and specialized surgical technologists is the ability to refer continually to the AST's established guidelines and recommended standards of practice for all aspects of surgical technology procedure. The Recommended Standards of Practice (Section III) covers issues of surgical attire, surgical technologist responsibilities, sterilization and disinfection, and aseptic technique. The constancy of these standards gives the practitioner a base to return to for reference before any procedure. By contrast, the Guidelines section (Section II) covers more unique events, such as protecting the patient who is allergic to latex, responding to anaphylactic reactions in the surgical patient, maintenance of normothermia in the perioperative patient, and placement of a suture bag in the sterile field, to name just a few.

SECTION IV: STATEMENTS BY THE COUNCIL ON SURGICAL AND PERIOPERATIVE SAFETY. In addition to AST position statements, the *Association of Surgical Technologists' Standards of Practice* also includes statements made by the Council on Surgical and Perioperative Safety because these frequently pertain to surgical technologists' responsibilities. These include such topics as safe handling of suture needles and other sharp items and preventing retained surgical items during surgery.

Accommodation of Specialties. There are myriad ways in which the same types of procedure can be performed, factoring in the patient as a unique individual, the surgeon's training and preferences, hospital equipment, and supply availability. In view of this array of influences on surgical situations, the *Association of Surgical Technologists' Standards of Practice* serve as a highly useful foundation from which a surgical technologist can approach any surgical procedure with a broad focus on what would be considered the nationally accepted "standard" of surgical technology practice. In some instances, such as a specialty field within the profession (and when there is evidence-based data to support them), far more narrowly defined guidelines and recommendations that apply to that specialty are added to the broader RSOP list.

Legal Protection in Standardization. In addition to helping the surgical technologist perform according to established guidelines, these official standards of practice can provide a certain degree of legal protection for the surgical technologist. For instance, in surgical procedures when patient safety is put in jeopardy, legal professionals exploring quality-of-care issues and prosecuting patient injury surgical procedures will do extensive research into standards of professional practice for all members of the healthcare team. Therefore, it is in the best interest of all parties to work within their defined roles and accepted standards.

Without continuity of care and routines, untoward events are more likely as a result of miscommunication and inconsistency. Standardization of care through application of specific RSOPs reduces errors and sentinel events, increases efficiency, and reduces procedure and anesthesia time.

CONCLUSION

The field of surgical technology is rapidly growing. This intriguing profession offers not only an entry into a healthcare career, but rich variety in work settings as well as a wide array of options for the professional career path of the tenured surgical technologist. Understanding accreditation and certification are essential for the success of the practitioner. Maintaining a professional attitude and demeanor are expected of all healthcare providers by patients and their families. Collaborative teamwork with every professional in the operating room is the only way to ensure patients receive quality care.

The pinnacle of success for every surgical technologist is an extensive knowledge of surgical procedures. The fundamental reason for the surgical technologist is to facilitate the surgeon's operative techniques through preparedness and attention to detail in every procedure. Surgical technologists must be able to build on the foundation of sterile technique and principles of asepsis to create a solid framework of technical theory and professional practice. Surgical technology is, as the name suggests, a study of techniques utilized in surgical interventions. No other member of the surgical team's educational preparation is as intensely focused on surgical anatomy, pathophysiology, instrumentation, equipment, supplies, techniques, and surgical procedural steps for every specialty. This textbook provides a clear focus on the procedural aspects of that pathway to professional success.

REVIEW QUESTIONS

1. Noah and Carmiel are in different professions, yet both have acted as a circulator. A circulator is:
   a. a member of the sterile team in the operating room
   b. a registered nurse or surgical technologist who assists the surgical team from outside the sterile field
   c. a scrub surgical technologist who maintains mobility outside the sterile field to monitor the patient from pre-op to post-op
   d. a and c
   e. b and c

2. Responsibilities of the surgical technologist in the preoperative phase include:
   a. assisting with sterile dressing application
   b. gowning and gloving personnel
   c. cutting suture as directed by the surgeon
   d. handing the appropriate instruments and supplies to the surgeon
   e. none of the above

3. Imani is preparing the instrument trays for decontamination and assisting with case turn-over. Imani is performing duties consistent with the _____ phase of surgical case management.
   a. preoperative
   b. intraoperative
   c. perioperative
   d. postoperative
   e. none of the above

4. In the middle of surgery, Min is asked to leave the OR to retrieve additional equipment needed to complete the surgical procedure. Min is most likely to be acting as a(n) _____ .
   a. scrub surgical technologist
   b. surgical technologist
   c. circulating surgical technologist
   d. second assisting surgical technologist
   e. none of the above

5. For a surgical technologist, the "practice of anticipation" involves _____.
   a. adapting to technological innovations
   b. updating and consulting the surgeon's preference card
   c. understanding the relevant anatomy and physiology for the surgical procedure being performed
   d. a and b only
   e. all of the above

6. A circulating nurse and surgical technologist conduct a surgical sponge count at the end of a surgical procedure, but then at a later date the patient returns with a retained sponge. Who is responsible for this error?
   a. As "captain of the ship," the surgeon is always responsible.
   b. The circulating nurse, as supervisor over the surgical technologist, is the one ultimately responsible for this error.
   c. The surgical technologist is the primary individual charged with accurate counts; the circulating nurse's participation does not change the fact that it is the surgical technologist who alone is ultimately responsible.
   d. The nurse and surgical technologist are responsible; this wasn't the surgeon's responsibility.
   e. All three are responsible; surgeon, nurse, and surgical technologist must share responsibility.

7. In the surgical setting, the phrase "sentinel event" means _____ .
   a. a safety check or "time-out"
   b. the individual act of monitoring for asepsis
   c. the individual act of monitoring patient care in all three phases of case management
   d. any event that demonstrates adherence to "the patient first" motto
   e. an error that affects patient safety

8. What section of the *Association of Surgical Technologists' Standards of Practice* document should Michael consult to review how to place a suture bag in the sterile field?
   a. Section II: Guidelines
   b. Section III: Recommended Standards of Practice
   c. Section I: subsection on the Clinical Ladder
   d. Section IV: Statements by the Council on Surgical and Perioperative Safety
   e. Section I: subsection on updated Position Statements and Resolutions

9. The _____ offers guidelines for professional advancement within the institution or department through the use of an AST-established set of performance-based evaluation criteria.
   a. "time-out"
   b. sentinel
   c. clinical ladder
   d. code of ethics
   e. none of the above

10. "Intraoperative" describes activities _____ the procedure.

11. The three-phase involvement in a patient's care before, during, and after surgery is referred to as _____ .

12. A number of organizations are discussed in this chapter, but only one is the official professional organization for surgical technologists, namely the _____ .

Critical Thinking Questions

1. Marjke, Dan, and Kenesha are three surgical technologists who work in three different types of roles: one works as a scrub surgical technologist, one works as a circulating surgical technologist, and one is a second assisting technologist. Today at work Marjke held a retractor for the surgeon and suctioned the operative site. Dan is the only one who works as a nonsterile member of his team. What role does each surgical technologist fill at work?

2. Two operating rooms standing side by side are both in use. In Room A, the surgical technologist is performing sponge, sharps, and instrument counts with the circulating nurse, ensuring that all items have been retrieved from the patient. In Room B, the surgical technologist is confining and con- taining all biohazardous material in the appropriate contain- ers. What phase of surgical case management is each surgical technologist involved in?

3. Juan and Elena are new surgical technologists who sit down together to study the *Association of Surgical Technologists' Standards of Practice* in preparation for work tomorrow. Juan wants to review aseptic technique one more time, while Elena wants to make sure she does everything correctly in tomorrow's surgery on a patient with AIDS. Their friend Alexandra pops in and asks them to look up a question she has about responding to anaphylactic reactions. Which sec- tions of the document might prove most helpful to each?

REFERENCES

Accreditation Review Council on Education in Surgical Technology and Surgical Assisting (ARCSTSA), available at www.arcstsa.org. Accessed March 25, 2011.

Agency for Healthcare Research and Quality (AHRQ): Medical teamwork and patient safety, available at www.ahrq.gov/qual/medteam/medteam2.htm. Accessed November 17, 2010.

Association of Surgical Technologists (AST) Standards of Practice, available at www.ast.org. Accessed October 26, 2010.

Association of Surgical Technologists (AST). Surgical technology: a grow- ing career, available at www.ast.org/professionals/about_prof.aspx. Accessed December 6, 2010.

Council on Surgical & Perioperative Safety (CSPS): Mission, vision, and values, available at www.cspsteam.org/missionvisionvalues/missionvi- sionvalues.html. Accessed November 17, 2010.

National Board of Surgical Technology and Surgical Assisting (NBSTSA), available at www.nbstsa.org. Accessed March 25, 2011.

Romig CL: Surgical technologists on the move, *AORN J* 65(2):419–421, 1997.

Science Daily: Hospitals apply lessons learned in the airline industry to improve operating room safety, available at www.sciencedaily.com/releases/2009/02/090217104447.htm. Accessed November 17, 2010.

The Joint Commission (TJC), available at www.jointcommission.org/Senti- nelEvents. Accessed November 17, 2010.

World Health Organization (WHO): Safe surgery saves lives, available at http://www.who.int/patientsafety/safesurgery/en/. Accessed December 11, 2010.

CHAPTER 2

Gastrointestinal Surgery

LEARNING OBJECTIVES

After studying this chapter the reader will be able to:
- Identify relevant anatomy of the gastrointestinal tract
- Correlate physiology to conditions requiring surgical intervention
- Discuss procedural considerations
- Identify tissue layers involved in opening and closing the gastrointestinal tract
- Compare diagnostic methods for determining surgical interventions and/or approaches
- Identify surgical incisions used in gastrointestinal surgery
- Identify instruments and equipment used in open and laparoscopic gastrointestinal procedures
- List the pharmacologic/hemostatic agents utilized during gastrointestinal surgery
- Review specific procedural steps as a guide for clinical procedure consideration
- Apply broad gastrointestinal concepts and knowledge to clinical practice for enhanced surgical patient care

CHAPTER OUTLINE

Overview
Surgical Anatomy
Surgical Technologist
    Considerations
Surgical Interventions
    Abdominal Incisions

Laparotomy
Laparoscopy
Intraoperative Intraperitoneal
    Chemotherapy
Endoscopic Procedures
Surgery of the Esophagus

Surgery of the Stomach
Bariatric Surgery
Surgery of the Small Bowel
Surgery of the Colon
Surgery of the Rectum

Overview

Surgery of the gastrointestinal (GI) system may be indicated to establish a diagnosis, to prevent or cure disease, to relieve symptoms or restore function, or to afford palliative measures that provide comfort or nutrition and promote quality of life. Advances in scientific knowledge, research, pharmacology, and technologic developments in the interventional disciplines as well as successful outcomes based on clinical evidence continue to broaden the spectrum of modalities and approaches to managing patients with GI disorders.

This chapter was originally written by Christine E. Smith, RN, MSN, CNOR, for the 14th edition of Alexander's Care of the Patient in Surgery and has been revised by Sherri M. Alexander, CST, for this text.

GI surgery, a subspecialty within the domain of general surgery, traditionally concerns itself with surgical management of the esophagus, stomach, small intestine, large intestine, and rectum. Gastroenterology is a medical specialty that diagnoses and manages GI disorders and conditions through endoscopic and pharmacologic approaches. Many surgical procedures that once entailed laparotomy and extensive postoperative recovery have been replaced or duplicated by endoscopic access and intervention. Endoscopic examination, enhanced with fluoroscopy, ultrasound, and video magnification in conjunction with interventional radiology, is a critical component of surgical diagnosis and postoperative evaluation. Laparoscopy, a minimally invasive approach to the intraabdominal compartment, has revolutionized GI surgery. Medical and surgical specialties have evolved to embrace and facilitate these advancements. Although clinicians may specialize in the disciplines of laparoscopy, gastroenterology, general surgery, bariatrics, GI surgical oncology, or colorectal surgery, the perioperative nurse and surgical technologist must know the fundamentals of GI surgery, interventional options available to patients, and care requirements common to all GI patients.

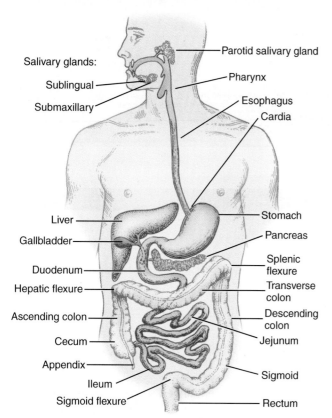

FIGURE 2-1 Alimentary canal and its appendages.

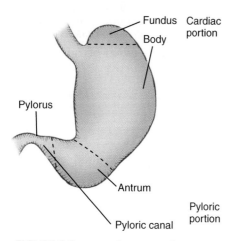

FIGURE 2-2 Regional anatomy of stomach.

Surgical Anatomy

The GI tract, or alimentary canal, is a continuous tubelike structure that extends the entire length of the trunk (Figure 2-1). The tract includes the mouth; pharynx; esophagus; stomach; small intestine, consisting of the duodenum, jejunum, and ileum; and large intestine, which comprises the cecum, ascending colon, transverse colon, descending colon, sigmoid colon, rectum, and anus. The length of the GI tract in a cadaver is about 9 meters, or 30 feet. In a living person it is shorter because of sustained muscle contraction and tone. The six

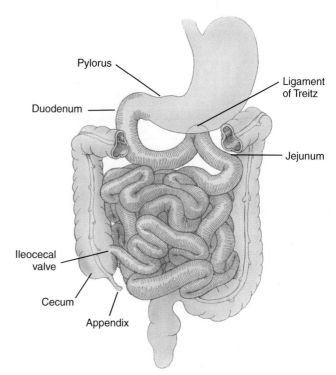

FIGURE 2-3 Illustration of the small bowel; the duodenum originates at the pylorus and flexes at the ligament of Treitz where the jejunum begins. The jejunum extends into the ileum, which terminates at the ileocecal valve at the cecum.

basic functions of the GI tract are ingestion, secretion, mixing and propulsion, digestion, absorption, and defecation.

The esophagus extends from the pharynx, at the level of the sixth cervical vertebra, and passes through the neck, posterior to the trachea and heart, and anterior to the vertebral column. The lower portion of the esophagus passes in front of the aorta and through the diaphragm, slightly to the left of the midline, to join the cardia of the stomach. Blood is supplied to the esophagus from branches of the inferior thyroid arteries, bronchial arteries, thoracic aorta, and branches of the left gastric and inferior phrenic arteries. The nerve supply comes from branches of the vagus and sympathetic nervous system. The length of the esophagus in an adult is about 25 cm, or 10 inches. The esophagus is a collapsible musculomembranous tube that functions primarily to transport ingested material, by peristalsis, from the pharynx to the stomach.

The stomach is an expanded J-shaped organ situated between the esophagus and the duodenum. It lies in the upper left abdominal cavity, slightly to the left of the midline and beneath the diaphragm. The stomach is divided into three parts: the fundus, the body, and the antrum (Figure 2-2). The fundus lies below the left dome of the diaphragm, behind the apex of the heart. The body and antrum lie in an oblique direction within the abdominal cavity. The stomach is stabilized indirectly by the lower portion of the esophagus and directly by its attachment to the duodenum, which is anchored to the posterior parietal peritoneum. The omentum, the peritoneal ligaments, and branches of the celiac vessel provide additional support to the stomach.

The convex, or lower, margin of the stomach is known as the *greater curvature;* the concave, or upper, margin is the *lesser curvature.* Attached to the greater curvature is the greater

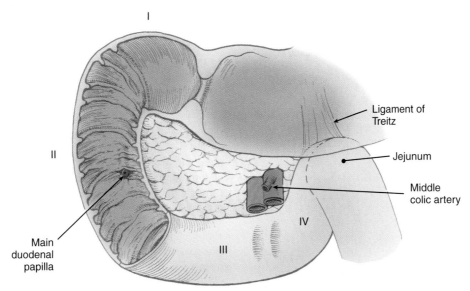

FIGURE 2-4 The duodenum consists of four portions, as illustrated.

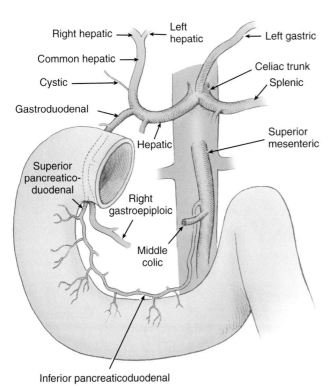

FIGURE 2-5 Blood supply of the duodenum.

omentum, which is a double fold of peritoneum containing fat. It covers the intestines loosely and is not to be confused with the mesentery, which connects the intestines with the posterior abdominal wall. The left gastroepiploic branch of the splenic artery and the right gastroepiploic branch of the hepatic artery run through the greater omentum. The lesser omentum, attached to the lesser curvature of the stomach, contains the left gastric artery, a branch of the celiac axis, and the right gastric branch of the hepatic artery.

Stomach functions include acceptance and storage of ingested material; chemical and mechanical digestion through the production of gastric lipase, pepsinogen, hydrochloric acid, gastrin, and intrinsic factor, responsibility for the absorption of vitamin B_{12}; and peristaltic waves, which both mix and propel stomach contents, or chyme, into the duodenum.

The small intestine, the longest part of the digestive tract, begins at the pylorus and ends at the ileocecal valve (Figure 2-3). The small intestine varies in size with the degree of contraction but is usually about 3 meters in length and 2.5 cm in diameter in the adult. It is divided into three parts: the duodenum, about 25 cm long; the jejunum, which is about two fifths of the length of the entire small intestine; and the ileum, which makes up the remaining length in an adult. The duodenum, which is the proximal portion of the small intestine, begins at the pylorus, is contiguous with the jejunum, and is stabilized by a fusion between the pancreas and the posterior parietal peritoneum. The duodenum is divided into four portions: superior (I), descending (II), transverse (III), and ascending (IV) (Figure 2-4). Nearly all of the superior portion mucosa is characterized by the lack of folds; it appears slightly dilated and is referred to as the *duodenal bulb*. The characteristic circular folds of the small intestinal mucosa begin proximal to the end of the superior portion of the duodenum and extend through the jejunum. They become less prominent in the ileum. The purpose of the circular mucosal folds, called *plicae circulares of Kerckring* or *valvulae conniventes,* is to provide greater mucosal surface area.

The common bile duct and the main pancreatic duct enter the medial wall of the middle of the second portion of the duodenum at the ampulla of Vater. The first, second, and third portions of the duodenum curve in a C-loop concavity in which the head of the pancreas is located. The fourth portion of the duodenum ascends to the duodenojejunal flexure. The duodenojejunal flexure is stabilized by the ligament of Treitz, which suspends the duodenum from the posterior body wall. The ligament of Treitz serves as a landmark during any abdominal exploration because it provides the surgeon with a reliable orientation of the patient's anatomy.

The blood supply of the duodenum comes from the arterial branches of the celiac axis (Figure 2-5). The gastroduodenal

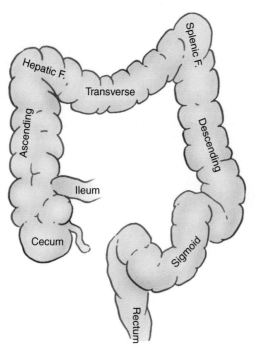

FIGURE 2-6 Anatomic division of large intestine, showing locations of hepatic flexure and splenic flexure. *F,* Flexure.

artery branches off the hepatic artery and is located behind the duodenal bulb. At the inferior margin of the bulb, the gastroduodenal artery divides into the right gastroepiploic artery and a superior pancreaticoduodenal branch. The superior pancreaticoduodenal artery supplies blood to the proximal duodenum and head of the pancreas. The inferior pancreaticoduodenal artery branch of the superior mesenteric artery supplies blood to the third and fourth portions of the duodenum as well as to the head and body of the pancreas.

The jejunum, situated in the upper portion of the abdomen, joins with the ileum, situated in the lower portion of the abdominal cavity. The ileum empties into the large intestine through the ileocecal valve. The jejunum and ileum are suspended by the mesentery, which is attached to the posterior abdominal wall. The free border of the mesentery, which is about 5.5 meters (18 feet) long, contains branches of the superior mesenteric artery, many veins, lymph nodes, and nerve fibers. The blood supply to the jejunum and ileum comes entirely from the superior mesenteric artery. The small bowel contains major deposits of lymphatic tissue, known as *Peyer's patches,* in the ileum. The rich lymphatic drainage of the small bowel plays a major role in fat absorption. Lymphatic drainage from the mucosa proceeds through the wall of the small intestine to lymph nodes adjacent to the mesentery. Lymphatic

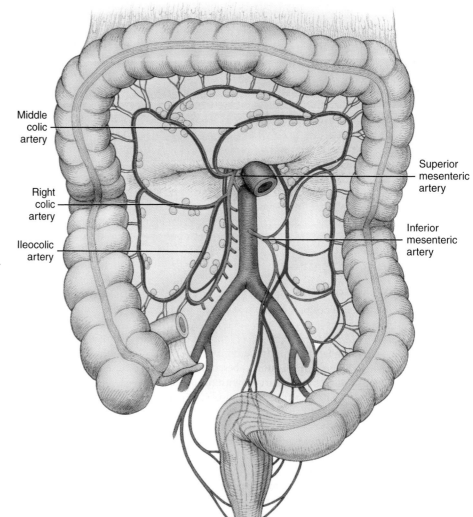

FIGURE 2-7 Blood supply of the colon.

drainage then proceeds to larger lymphatics that communicate with the retroperitoneal cisterna chyli and from there to the thoracic duct. The lymphatics of the intestine play a major role in the body's immune defense as well as in the distribution of cells arising from intestinal neoplasms.

Compared to the ileum, the jejunum has a larger circumference and thickness. The mesenteric vessels usually form only one or two arcades, a series of anastomosing arterial arches, compared with the multiple vascular arcades of the ileum. The jejunal mucosa is thick and has prominent *plicae circulares.* The ileum mucosa is thinner with few plicae.

The small intestine serves two important, but opposite, functions simultaneously. It absorbs essential nutrients at 95% efficiency while it provides an effective barrier from harmful ingested environmental elements. The remarkably large surface area of the combined small and large intestinal mucosa is estimated to be 200 square meters, about the size of a doubles' tennis court.

The large intestine begins at the ileocecal valve and ends at the anus. It is divided into the cecum, colon, and rectum. The cecum attaches to the ileum and extends about 7 cm below it. The cecum in an adult usually adheres to the posterior wall of the peritoneal cavity and has a serosal covering on its anterior wall only. The cecum forms a blind pouch from which the appendix projects.

The colon, about 1.5 meters long, is divided into four parts: the ascending colon, the transverse colon, the descending colon, and the sigmoid colon (Figure 2-6). The *ascending colon* extends upward from the ileocecal valve to the hepatic flexure. The upper portion of the ascending colon lies behind the right lobe of the liver and in front of the anterior surface of the right kidney. The *transverse colon* begins at the hepatic flexure and ends at the splenic flexure. It lies below the stomach and is attached to the transverse mesocolon. The *descending colon* extends downward from the splenic flexure to just below the iliac crest. The iliac portion of the sigmoid colon lies on the inner surface of the left iliac muscle. The remaining portion of the colon passes over the pelvic rim into the pelvic cavity and lies partly in the abdomen and partly in the pelvis. It then forms an S-shaped curve in the pelvis and terminates in the rectum at the level of the third segment of the sacral vertebrae. The blood supply to the ascending colon, hepatic flexure, and transverse colon comes from the superior mesenteric artery, whereas the blood supply to the descending colon and rectum comes from the inferior mesenteric artery (Figure 2-7).

The wall of the colon consists of taeniae coli, epiploic appendices, and haustra. The taeniae coli are three longitudinal, or axial, strips of muscles distributed around the circumference of the colon. They represent the longitudinal muscle layer, which is not complete in the colon (the small intestine and rectum have both circular and complete longitudinal muscle layers). The epiploic appendices are fatty appendages along the bowel that have no particular function. The haustra are sacculations that outpouch from the bowel wall among the taeniae coli. The diameter of the colon varies in size from about 9 cm (3½ inches) in the cecum to an average of about 1.25 cm (½ inch) in the sigmoid colon.

The rectum begins at the sigmoid colon and ends in the anus. This slightly curved passage is surrounded by the pelvic fascia as it lies on the anterior surface of the sacrum and coccyx. In the male, the rectum lies behind the prostate gland, seminal vesicles, and bladder. In the female, the rectum lies behind the uterus and the vagina. A septum rectovesical, also called *Denonvilliers' fascia,* separates the rectum from the urogenital structures. The rectum is suspended in the pelvis by fascia extending from the right and left pelvic sidewalls. Rectosacral fascia extends from the sacrum to the anorectal junction and suspends the rectum posteriorly. The rectum dilates just before it becomes the anal canal. This dilation, or ampulla, presents folds called *Houston's valves.* The wall of the rectum consists of four layers, similar to those of the small intestine.

The anal canal is a narrow passage that passes downward and slightly posteriorly. It is surrounded and controlled by two circular muscle groups, which form the external and internal anal sphincters. The internal sphincter is a continuation of the longitudinal muscle layer.

The primary function of the large intestine is to reabsorb water and electrolytes, to form solid waste into feces, to synthesize vitamin K and B-complex vitamins, and to propel and eliminate solid food residue and waste through defecation.

The GI tract constitutes a complex microbiologic ecosystem that supports and maintains essential digestive and protective functions vital to life, yet it presents significant risks and challenges during diagnostic and surgical interventions. Substantial populations of microorganisms, both obligate anaerobes and facultative bacterial spores, exist in the intestinal lumen. The organisms of the upper tract differ from those of the lower tract, with the highest concentration in the distal bowel. These organisms can contribute to contamination and disease processes within the intestinal tract and throughout the body. Gastric and intestinal pH, while necessary for digestive benefit and protection from selected organisms, can compromise peritoneal tissues and structures when unplanned spillage or leakage occurs. The pH of the stomach ranges from 1.5 to 3, whereas the pH of the intestines can range from 7 to 8.5.

Surgical Technologist Considerations

GI surgery and endoscopic procedures present special considerations related to the planned procedure, instrumentation, approach, anatomic structures involved, health status of the patient, surgeon and patient preferences, and availability of special institutional resources. Special institutional resources may include a bariatric program, an oncology program with research protocols, a transplant program, a trauma center, or a technologically advanced OR with computer-integrated imaging display and robotics.

Optimum care of the patient undergoing GI surgery and other invasive GI procedures relies on sound knowledge and experience, along with a good understanding of the complex setups in the operating room. The experienced surgical technologist will be able to anticipate the need for specialized equipment based on the surgical procedure scheduled. An expert and attentive surgical technologist will hand the surgeon the appropriate instrumentation without being asked, based on an understanding of the procedural steps and anatomy involved. GI surgery can require a sterile and a nonsterile setup for the same patient. The surgical technologist should have a good understanding of *bowel technique* and the flexibil-

SURGICAL TECHNOLOGY PREFERENCE CARD

This serves as a tool to assist the surgical technologist in the scrub role when preparing for gastrointestinal surgery. The weight of your patient will direct you in gathering additional positioning supplies for optimal patient safety.

Gastrointestinal surgery can require a sterile and a nonsterile setup for the patient. Having the correct instrumentation and supplies will facilitate appropriate aseptic technique is followed throughout the procedure. Knowing that in gastrointestinal surgery you may have other healthcare personnel in the operating room, arriving to the room early to get a feel for the room layout and room stored supplies and equipment will be beneficial. Discuss the OR bed position with the perioperative team, taking into consideration additional equipment that may be needed for gastrointestinal surgery.

Understanding the room layout before setting up for the procedure allows the traffic pattern in the room to be maximized. This step can help insure sterility of the field and facilitate effective communication of additional supplies from the circulator to the scrub, as well as provide efficient space for other healthcare providers involved in the gastrointestinal procedure.

Room Prep: Basic operating room furniture in place, thermoregulatory devices, extra blankets, padding and other positioning supplies to achieve optimal patient safety

Prep Solution: In room
- Chlorhexidine gluconate
- Iodine and iodophors

Catheters: In room and correct size
- Urinary catheter insertion tray with appropriate urinary catheter type
  - Latex/rubber
  - PVC
  - Silicone
- Sizing
  - French
- Nonretaining
  - Red rubber (Robinson)
- Retaining
  - Foley
    - 2-way
    - 3-way
  - Mushroom/Pezzer/Malecot
  - T-tube
- Other urine collection devices

PROCEDURE CHECKLIST

Instruments
- Standard sets
- Open instruments if needed to convert from laparoscopic to open
- Anticipated additional instruments
  - Bowel clamps
  - Bookwalter or other self-retaining retractor
  - Anastomotic stapling devices

Specialty Suture
- As per surgeon's preference

Hemostatic Agents
- Mechanical
  - Staplers
  - Clip appliers and clips
  - Ligatures
- Chemical
  - Absorbable gelatin
  - Collagen
  - Oxidized cellulose
  - Silver nitrate
  - Epinephrine
  - Thrombin
- Thermal
  - Electrosurgical unit
  - Harmonic scalpel
  - Argon beam coagulator
  - Laser

Additional Supplies
- If the physician is requesting supplies, instruments, or equipment not normally used, check to be sure all have arrived to the room before opening
- Bowel bag
- Wound protector
- Sponges

SURGICAL TECHNOLOGY PREFERENCE CARD—cont'd

- ◆ Drapes
- ◆ Gowns and gloves for team members
- ◆ "Have ready" or "hold" supplies

Medications and Irrigation Solutions
- ◆ Devices for warming irrigating solution as applicable
- ◆ Appropriate-sized syringes and hypodermic needles
- ◆ Marking pens and labels

Drains and Dressings
- ◆ Correct size and type for planned surgery
  - • Open—Not attached to a drainage system
    - • Penrose
    - • Cigarette
  - • Closed—Attached to a closed reservoir for fluid collection
    - • Hemovac
    - • Jackson-Pratt
    - • Autologous blood retrieval drainage system
- ◆ Anchoring methods
  - • Suture
    - • Nonabsorbable
    - • Cutting needle
  - • Tape

Specimen Care
- ◆ Proper container for each specimen
  - • Frozen
  - • Fresh
  - • Permanent
  - • Stones
  - • Body fluids or washings
  - • Cultures
- ◆ Labels for each specimen
- ◆ Proper solution for specimen type

Before opening for the procedure, the surgical technologist should:
- ◆ Arrange furniture
- ◆ Gather positioning devices
- ◆ Damp dust lights, furniture, and surfaces
- ◆ Verify functionality of equipment
- ◆ Place items to be opened in their appropriate places

When opening sterile supplies:
- ◆ Verify exposure to sterilization
- ◆ Use sterile technique
- ◆ Open bundles in appropriate locations
- ◆ Open additional supplies onto sterile field
- ◆ Open the room as close to the surgical start time as possible

ity to move swiftly from the laparoscopic approach to an open approach should the need arise. The risks for injury or failure to achieve the intended outcome are equally present in GI surgery as in any surgical or invasive procedure. No procedure is routine, and unexpected outcomes can occur even when planning and preventive measures have been employed under the most optimal circumstances.

Laboratory studies might include a complete blood count (CBC) with differential, serum electrolytes, platelet count, cholesterol level, vitamin and mineral levels, liver function, serum proteins, coagulation profile, pancreatic function, and indices of nutritional status (Table 2-1).

Diagnostic endoscopic examinations, radiologic studies with or without contrast markers, abdominal ultrasound, endoscopic ultrasound (EUS), magnetic resonance imaging (MRI), positron emission tomography (PET), and computed tomography (CT) imaging scans plus GI secretion studies add further information about the patient's health or disease process to help formulate the surgical plan. Advances in endoscopic technology provide enhanced details of GI anatomy and pathology. EUS combines endoscopy and ultrasound, using sound waves to generate an image of the histologic layers of the esophageal, gastric, and intestinal walls. The frequencies used, higher than those used in traditional ultrasound, provide high-level accuracy of depth of mucosal invasion (Birn, 2005). EUS is of critical importance in staging GI malignancies and determining surgical options and potential for therapeutic resection. Endoscopic image-enhancement techniques include high-resolution endoscopes with narrow-band imaging and magnification to identify mucosal surface details; narrow-band

TABLE 2-1

Common Serum Studies with Relevance to GI Surgery

Test	Normal Adult Values	Significance of Abnormal Values
COMPLETE BLOOD COUNT WITH DIFFERENTIAL (CBC WITH DIFF)		
Red blood cell count (RBC)	*Men:* 4.7-6.1 million/mm^3 *Women:* 4.2-5.4 million/mm^3	Low value indicates anemia from blood loss, hemolysis, dietary deficiency, drug ingestion, bone marrow failure, or chronic illness. High value indicates compensation for high altitudes, chronic anoxia, or polycythemia vera.
Hemoglobin (Hb) concentration	*Men:* 14-18 g/dl *Women:* 12-16 g/dl	Low and high values tend to be caused by same processes that cause low or high values for RBCs. Artificially high values seen in dehydration.
Hematocrit (Hct)	*Men:* 42%-52% *Women:* 37%-47%	Low and high values are same as above.
Mean corpuscular volume (MCV)	*Adults:* 80-95/mm^3	High values found in megaloblastic anemias (vitamin B_{12} deficiency). Low values seen in iron-deficiency anemia or thalassemia.
Mean corpuscular hemoglobin (MCH)	*Adults:* 27-31 pg	Low and high values tend to be caused by same processes that cause low or high values for MCV.
Mean corpuscular hemoglobin concentration (MCHC)	*Adults:* 32-36 g/dl	Low value indicates hemoglobin deficiency seen in iron-deficiency anemia or thalassemia.
White blood cell count (WBC) differential	*Adults:* 5000-10,000/mm^3	Elevated WBC level indicates infection or leukemia, trauma, or stress. Decreased WBC level may indicate bone marrow failure, overwhelming infection, dietary deficiency, drug toxicity, or autoimmune disease.
Neutrophils	55%-70%	Elevated neutrophil count may indicate acute suppurative infection.
Lymphocytes, monocytes	20%-40%, 2%-8%	Decreased neutrophil count may indicate overwhelming bacterial infection (especially in elderly) or dietary deficiency.
Eosinophils	1%-4%	Elevated lymphocyte count may indicate chronic bacterial or viral infection.
Basophils	0.5%-1%	Decreased lymphocytes may indicate sepsis. Elevated eosinophils may indicate parasitic infestation, allergic reactions, or autoimmune diseases. A "shift to the left" means percentage of neutrophils and immature leukocytes is increased, which occurs with infection.
Platelet count	150,000-400,000/mm^3	Reduced levels of platelets may result from decreased platelet production, increased sequestration (as seen in hypersplenism), increased platelet destruction or consumption (e.g., disseminated intravascular coagulation [DIC]), or loss of platelets through hemorrhage. Elevated levels may indicate severe hemorrhage, polycythemia vera, postsplenectomy syndromes, and some malignant disorders.
SERUM ELECTROLYTES		
Sodium (Na$^+$)	136-145 mEq/L	Elevated levels may be seen with excessive sweating, extensive burns, osmotic diuresis, and excessive sodium intake or reduced sodium excretion. Reduced levels may be seen with inadequate sodium intake, increased sodium losses (e.g., vomiting, nasogastric suction, diarrhea, renal disease, third-space losses of sodium).
Phosphate (PO$_4^{2-}$)	3-4 mg/dl	Decreased levels seen in long-term antacid ingestion.
Potassium (K$^+$)	3.5-5 mEq/L	Elevated levels may indicate excessive intake or reduced excretion of potassium (e.g., renal failure). Crush injuries cause release of intracellular potassium, or metabolic acidosis. Reduced levels may indicate inadequate intake or excessive losses (e.g., diarrhea, vomiting, use of diuretics, hyperaldosteronism) or result of metabolic alkalosis or administration of glucose, insulin, or calcium (which causes a shift of potassium from bloodstream into cells).
Chloride (Cl$^-$)	98-106 mEq/L	Changes in chloride concentration usually parallel changes in sodium concentration. Decreased levels seen in patients who undergo long-term gastric suctioning.
Carbon dioxide (CO$_2$)	23-30 mEq/L	Elevated levels are seen with acidosis. Reduced levels are seen with alkalosis.

TABLE 2-1

Common Serum Studies with Relevance to GI Surgery—cont'd

Test	Normal Adult Values	Significance of Abnormal Values
ARTERIAL BLOOD GASES		
pH	7.35-7.45	High levels indicate alkalosis. Low levels reflect acidosis.
Partial pressure of carbon dioxide (P_{CO_2})	35-45 mm Hg	High levels indicate carbon dioxide retention caused by respiratory depression or pulmonary disease (respiratory acidosis). Low levels reflect excessive loss of carbon dioxide through hyperventilation (respiratory alkalosis from overventilation or emotional trauma; may also be seen as compensatory response in metabolic acidosis).
Bicarbonate (HCO_3^-)	21-28 mEq/L	Low levels indicate metabolic acidosis caused by excessive acid production, resulting in depletion of HCO_3^- (e.g., diabetic acidosis); failure to eliminate H^+ ions, resulting in depletion of HCO_3^- (e.g., renal failure); or excessive loss of HCO_3^- (e.g., intestinal losses through diarrhea, fistula drainage). Low levels may also be seen with insulin overdose, insulinoma, hypothyroidism, hypopituitarism, Addison's disease, and extensive liver disease. High levels indicate metabolic alkalosis resulting from bicarbonate overdose or excessive gastric losses. May also be seen as compensatory response in patients with prolonged respiratory acidosis, pancreatic disorders (e.g., adenoma, pancreatitis), corticosteroid therapy, diuretics, Cushing's disease, and hyperthyroidism.
COAGULATION STUDIES		
Prothrombin time (PT)	85%-100% or 11-12.5 sec	Elevated times with anticoagulant, acetylsalicylic acid (ASA), and nonsteroidal antiinflammatory drug (NSAID) use. Decreased times may be seen in malignant disease caused by unidentified hypercoagulability factors.
Partial prothrombin time (PTT)	60-70 sec	Increased in acquired or congenital clotting factor deficiencies, cirrhosis, vitamin K deficiency, leukemia, DIC, heparin administration, hypofibrinogenemia, von Willebrand's disease, hemophilia. Decreased in early stages of DIC, extensive cancer.
Activated partial prothrombin time (APTT)	30-40 sec	Same as for PTT.
OTHER SERUM STUDIES		
Albumin	3.5-5.5 mg/day	Decreased levels seen in protein malnutrition and hepatocellular injury.
Alkaline phosphatase (ALP)	30-120 units/L	Slightly elevated in elderly. Elevated in intestinal ischemia. Decreased with excess vitamin B ingestion.
Amylase	60-120 Somogyi units/dl	Increased in penetrating or perforated peptic ulcer, perforated or necrotic bowel, or duodenal obstruction.
Ammonia	10-80 mcg/dl	Increased in gastrointestinal (GI) bleeding, GI obstruction, or liver disease.
Carcinoembryonic antigen (CEA)	<5 ng/ml	Elevated in GI cancer, colitis, diverticulitis, cirrhosis, peptic ulcer, hepatobiliary and pancreatic cancers.
Complement assay (C3 and C4)	C3: 55-120 mg/dl C4: 20-50 mg/dl Total complement: 75-160 mg/dl	Elevated in ulcerative colitis and cancer.
Cortisol (hydrocortisone)	8 AM: 5-23 mcg/dl 4 PM: 3-13 mcg/dl	Elevated in obesity.
C-reactive protein	<1 mg/dl	Elevated in Crohn's disease, postoperative wound infection, malignant disease.
Transferrin (serum)	250-300 mg/dl	Decreased levels may indicate protein malnutrition; transferrin levels may be used to monitor a patient's response to nutritional support therapy since half-life of transferrin is 8-10 days, whereas half-life of albumin is 19-20 days (this means that, compared to albumin levels, transferrin levels reflect changes in patient's visceral protein status much faster).

Continued

TABLE 2-1

Common Serum Studies with Relevance to GI Surgery—cont'd

Test	Normal Adult Values	Significance of Abnormal Values
Prealbumin (serum)	15-32 mg/dl	Decreased levels seen in protein malnutrition. Because half-life of prealbumin is 2-3 days, these values, compared to transferrin levels, reflect changes in patient's visceral protein status even faster.
Total lymphocyte count (serum)	>150,000/mm³	Decreased levels may be seen in protein malnutrition; however, many other conditions affect total lymphocyte count (e.g., infections, conditions affecting WBC production).

Data from Pagana KD, Pagana TJ: *Mosby's diagnostic and laboratory test reference*, ed 9, St Louis, 2009, Mosby.

filters to see capillary patterns, pits, and villi; and chromoendoscopy (staining techniques) and fluorescence to differentiate between normal and dysplastic tissue (Kwon et al, 2005).

Capsule endoscopy is an emerging technology and non-invasive diagnostic test that uses a small wireless camera in the shape of a capsule about the size of a large vitamin. It is swallowed with a few sips of water and propelled along the GI tract by normal peristalsis. The capsule glides down the esophagus taking two color digital pictures per second, which are transmitted to a data recording device worn by the patient. This device is suitable for imaging the mucosal surface of the esophagus, stomach, and small intestine. The battery power of the capsule lasts about 8 hours. The capsule is eventually passed naturally within 24 to 72 hours. The wireless capsule has dramatically enhanced the ability to visualize the mucosal surface of the small intestine. The small bowel makes up 90% of the mucosal surface of the entire GI tract and had formerly been constrained by the limits of traditional diagnostic modalities. The only preprocedure preparation is an 8-hour fast. Contraindications to capsule endoscopy include inability to swallow a large capsule; small bowel strictures, narrowing, or fistulas; swallowing disorders; suspected intestinal obstruction; and pacemakers. The patient is instructed not to undergo MRI imaging for at least 30 days to ensure that the capsule has been passed and will not cause internal thermal injury. Reports and images of capsule endoscopy results should be available at the time of surgery.

Implementation

Implementation includes activities involved with the preparation of the surgical environment; procurement of the supplies, equipment, materials, and devices; and team communication based on materials and processes typical for this particular procedure and team, along with data gathered from the patient, family, and medical record.

Both open laparotomy and laparoscopic approaches are usually performed with general endotracheal or spinal anesthesia. The choice of anesthetic depends on the patient's health status, planned surgical or laparoscopic approach, length of surgery, the patient's preference, and the collaborative judgment of the anesthesia provider and surgeon. Procedures done endoscopically, such as esophagogastroduodenoscopy (EGD) (upper endoscopy) or colonoscopy, typically use intravenous (IV) moderate sedation. Monitoring devices and parameters typical to those anesthesia plans will be used. Patients at risk for fluid and electrolyte shifts, or significant blood loss, require arterial monitoring and frequent intraoperative sampling of hemoglobin and hematocrit, arterial blood gases, electrolytes, and coagulation studies. Preoperative fasting and bowel cleansing, combined with alterations in nutrition, may severely deplete fluids and electrolytes. These must be measured, replaced, and balanced throughout and after the procedure. A nasogastric tube may be inserted to decompress the stomach and to suction gastric secretions. A urinary catheter may be inserted to decompress the bladder and provide accurate measurement of urinary output and renal function.

Preoperatively, the physician may order blood for open laparotomy or laparoscopic GI surgery patients whose blood replacement is predictable. Elective surgery patients may choose to donate 1 or 2 units of autologous blood; friends and family may also donate donor-directed blood. Autotransfusion (or cell salvage) of the patient's blood during surgery may not be appropriate, given potential contamination from bowel contents such as organisms or malignant GI neoplasm cells. Blood replacement is augmented, managed, and balanced with IV colloids and crystalloids, albumin, platelets, fresh frozen plasma, and electrolytes.

IV antibiotics are given before the incision is made and throughout the procedure (Surgical Pharmacology). Antibiotic irrigation solutions may be used intraabdominally during the procedure and before closure. Additional intraoperative medications may be indicated per institutional standard or surgeon preference. Hemostatic agents, anticoagulants, steroid preparations, and local anesthetics may be utilized. The best guide is a comprehensive and frequently updated plan of care, pick list, or surgeon/procedure preference sheet.

For laparotomy and laparoscopic approaches, the patient typically is placed in the supine position. Arms are placed on padded armboards with the palms up and fingers extended. Armboards are maintained at less than a 90-degree angle to prevent brachial plexus stretch. If there are surgical reasons to tuck the arms at the side, the elbows are padded to protect the ulnar nerve, the palms face inward, and the wrist is maintained in a neutral position (Denholm, 2009). A drape secures the arms. It should be tucked snugly under the patient, not under the mattress. This prevents the arm from shifting downward intraoperatively and resting against the OR bed rail. Modifications may include flexion of the knees to a modified lithotomy position with the legs in self-balancing stirrups (Allen or Yellofin) for procedures where access to the rectum is necessary. Check for the presence of bilateral posterior popliteal, posterior tibial, and dorsalis pedis pulses, and document. Monitor and document circulation throughout the procedure. Intraoperative access and exposure may require frequent alterations of patient position with side-to-side tilt, elevation of the kidney rest, and shifts to Trendelenburg's or reverse Trendelenburg's position to permit gravity displacement of abdominal organs for surgical exposure. Entry into the thoracic and abdominal space is often approached via thoracoabdominal access; the patient is placed and immobilized in a lateral or side-lying position. EGD is typically done with the patient in slight semi-Fowler position, whereas colonoscopy is accomplished with the patient in left lateral position with the knees flexed.

Morbidly obese patients pose a positioning challenge as to safety, exposure, and access, as well as for the safety of staff that must transfer and position the patient. These patients require a surgical bed that accommodates their weight and size, protects them from falls, and supports their frame while preventing skin and musculoskeletal injury. More than four staff persons are often needed to transfer and position the patient safely. Transfer aids, such as rollers, sliders, lift sheets, air-filled transfer mattresses, and hydraulic lifts, are used when available. Encourage patients to assist in their transfer. Determine the patient's level of comfort, and make appropriate adjustments before anesthesia induction. Meticulous assessment and continued evaluation of skin and tissue are critical to recognize compromise early and to prevent injury.

GI surgery patients will have a sequential compression device (SCD) ordered for use during surgery. SCDs are applied as soon as possible before anesthesia induction to prevent deep vein thrombosis (DVT) (Hageman et al, 2008). Wrap the sleeves around the legs smoothly, to prevent folds when the legs are positioned in stirrups. The unit is hung on the OR bed or an IV pole or is placed on the floor under the OR bed in an area away from team members' feet and areas that may be wet. The vibration noise can be buffered with a blanket or mat placed under the unit.

Positioning requires attention to body alignment; access and exposure to the intended incision site; positioning of the surgical light and instrument accessories and equipment, which may be attached to the OR bed; and padding and protection of potential pressure sites.

The large amount of skin exposure required for either a laparotomy or a laparoscopic approach presents a risk for hypothermia. Prewarming the patient for at least 15 minutes before anesthesia induction is recommended (AORN, 2009a). A forced-air warming blanket may be positioned under the sterile drapes. Temperature settings range from "low" at 32° C (89.6° F) to "high" at 43° C (109.4° F). Keep the ambient room temperature warm (between 20° C [68° F] and 26° C [78° F]) until after the patient is prepped and draped. Keep the patient covered with warm bath blankets until the skin prep is begun. Expose only the areas to be prepped. Warm all irrigation fluids to a temperature not greater than 40.5° C (105° F). Consult with the anesthesia provider for an assessment of the patient's body temperature during the procedure. Raise the room temperature before the conclusion of the procedure. IV fluids and blood products are administered by way of a fluid warming system with blood warmed to 37° C (98.6° F) and IV fluids between 37° C (98.6° F) and 40° C (104° F). Surgical skin prep solutions are not warmed unless recommended. The manufacturer of the prep solution must provide clear directions for solution warming (AORN, 2009b).

SURGICAL PHARMACOLOGY

GI-Specific Prophylactic Systemic Antibiotics

Although prophylactic systemic antibiotics are not indicated for patients undergoing low-risk, "clean" surgical procedures, there are clinical situations where their administration is beneficial. High-risk GI procedures are an example of a situation when prophylactic systemic antibiotics reduce infection and clinically benefit the patient. These procedures include surgery for gastric cancer, ulcer, obstruction, or bleeding. Antibiotics are also useful in patients whose gastric acid secretion has been suppressed and in patients undergoing gastric surgery for morbid obesity. Oral antibiotics before procedures on the colon suppress both aerobic and anaerobic flora (Anaya and Dellinger, 2008).

GASTROINTESTINAL-SPECIFIC ANTIBIOTICS

- Ampicillin—prophylaxis against gram-positive cocci such as *Enterococcus faecalis* and gram-negative bacilli such as *Salmonella* and *Shigella*
- Cephalosporin—prophylaxis against aerobes and anaerobes
- Clindamycin—prophylaxis against aerobes and anaerobes
- Ertapenem—broad-spectrum prophylaxis for colorectal surgery
- Fluoroquinolone—prophylaxis in combination with metronidazole or clindamycin
- Gentamicin—prophylaxis against gram-negative rods and enterococci
- Metronidazole HCl—prophylaxis in Crohn's disease, pseudomembranous colitis
- Tetracycline HCl—prophylaxis against shigellosis, cholera, *Helicobacter pylori*
- Tobramycin—prophylaxis against aerobic gram-negative bacilli, *Pseudomonas aeruginosa*
- Vancomycin—prophylaxis in penicillin allergy, pseudomembranous colitis, staphylococcal enterocolitis

Anaya DA, Dellinger EP et al: Surgical infection and choice of antibiotics. In Townsend CM et al, editors: *Sabiston textbook of surgery*, ed 18, Philadelphia, 2008, Saunders.

If prescribed, hair removal at the operative site is done as close as possible to the time of incision. Hair should be removed according to institutional protocol; many institutions require a physician's order for this procedure. Direct special attention to existing or intended ostomy sites, avoiding further skin injury. Existing ostomy stomas may be covered and protected with an occlusive sterile plastic dressing or a collection appliance, or be isolated with a plastic drape with adhesive strip. Antimicrobial skin preparation follows general protocol for laparotomy, with generous borders in the event that the surgeon extends the incision. Precautions are taken to prevent accumulated fluid at or under the bed line, skin injury, and surgical fires. Sites within the prep area that provide concentrated microorganisms, such as an existing ostomy, draining fistula, or the rectum, are prepped last.

Intraoperative draping follows standard draping for patients undergoing laparotomy or laparoscopy. Extra drapes are needed when the patient is placed in a modified lithotomy position and where bowel isolation precautions are taken. The patient may be redraped or the existing drapes reinforced before incision closure.

All surgical team members pause for a "time out briefing" before the incision is made. Participation is required by all team members, who engage in a comprehensive review and consensus that includes the following: an introduction of all present team members, patient identification, intended surgical procedure or procedures, marked site (and laterality if appropriate, which must be visible when the patient is draped), patient position, pertinent medical conditions or concerns, availability of implants or any special equipment or devices, potential threats to good outcome, fire risk score, and verification that prep solutions have dried.

GI surgery instrumentation, for both the laparotomy and laparoscopic approach, requires a basic laparotomy instrument set. Sharp cutting instruments include #3 and #4 knife handles (#11 or #15 knife handles are required for laparoscopic port stab incisions), curved tissue dissection scissors, and curved and straight utility scissors. Clamps include curved and straight hemostats; Kelly clamps; Kocher, right angle, and Crile (tonsil) hemostats; Babcock and Allis clamps; towel clamps; ring or sponge forceps; and assorted needle holders. Tissue-grasping forceps include short-, medium-, and long-toothed, plain, DeBakey, Adson, and Russian forceps. Handheld retractors include Army-Navy, Richardson, Deaver, malleable, or rake, and selected self-retaining retractors. Accessory instruments may include but are not limited to various grooved and nontraumatic curved, straight, and angled bowel clamps. Suction tips may include Yankauer tonsil suction, Frazier tip, cardiac suction tip, or a Poole, intestinal sump suction. Protective nontraumatic covers or shods may be slipped over the jaws of selected clamps to protect and stabilize tissue during dissection or suturing. Longer versions of many of the basic instruments will be required for low abdominal procedures, obese patients, and thoracoabdominal approaches. Examples of instruments commonly used in GI surgery are shown in Figures 2-8 through 2-19.

Laparoscopic surgery of the GI tract requires laparoscopic instruments intended for abdominal surgery. These instruments may be disposable, reusable, hybrid "reposables" (reusable instruments with disposable cutting or coagulation tips),

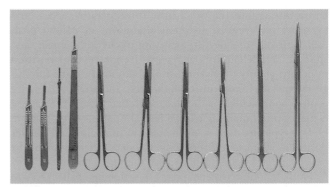

FIGURE 2-9 *Left to right:* 2 Bard-Parker knife handles #4; 1 Bard-Parker knife handle #7; 1 Bard-Parker knife handle #3, long; 1 Mayo dissecting scissors, curved; 2 Mayo dissecting scissors, straight; 1 Metzenbaum dissecting scissors, 7 inch; 1 Snowden-Pencer dissecting scissors, curved; 1 Snowden-Pencer dissecting scissors, straight.

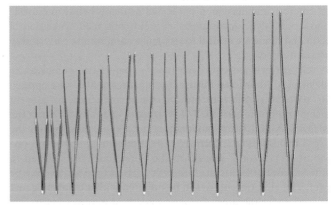

FIGURE 2-10 *Left to right:* 2 Adson tissue forceps with teeth (1 × 2 teeth); 2 Ferris Smith tissue forceps; 2 Russian tissue forceps, medium; 2 DeBakey vascular Autragrip tissue forceps, medium; 2 DeBakey vascular Autragrip tissue forceps, long; 2 Russian tissue forceps, long.

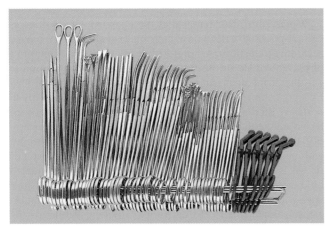

FIGURE 2-8 *Left to right:* 2 Mayo-Hegar needle holders, 7 inch; 2 Ayers needle holders, 8 inch; 3 Foerster sponge forceps; 2 Mixter hemostatic forceps, long, fine-point; 2 Babcock tissue forceps, long; 2 Allis tissue forceps, long; 6 Ochsner hemostatic forceps, long, straight; 4 Mayo-Péan hemostatic forceps, long, curved; 6 hemostatic tonsil forceps; 2 Westphal hemostatic forceps; 4 Babcock tissue forceps, short; 4 Allis tissue forceps, short; 8 Crile hemostatic forceps, curved, 6½ inch; 1 Halsted mosquito hemostatic forceps, straight; 6 paper drape clips.

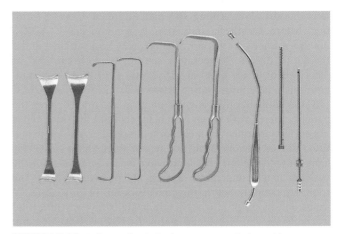

FIGURE 2-11 *Left to right:* 2 Goelet retractors; 2 Army-Navy retractors; 1 Richardson retractor, medium; 1 Richardson retractor, large; 1 Yankauer suction tube and tip; 1 Poole abdominal shield and suction tube.

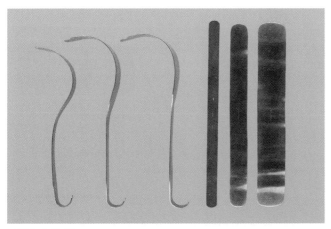

FIGURE 2-12 *Left to right:* Deaver retractors, small, medium, and large; Ochsner malleable retractors, narrow, medium, wide.

or a combination. Laparoscopic instruments have operating tips that function similarly to the basic laparotomy instruments but are designed to fit through a narrow trocar and extend into all quadrants of the abdominal cavity from the skin surface. Several laparoscopic dissectors and scissors have electrosurgical capability. Bipolar or monopolar electrosurgery may be used, with bipolar considered the safer alternative (Risk Reduction Strategies). Accessories for laparoscopic instruments, telescopes, and trocars include a light cord, insufflation tubing, camera and cord, suction-irrigation tubing, ultrasonic dissection handpiece with cord, and thermal plasma coagulation devices. Examples of laparoscopic instruments are shown in Figures 2-20 through 2-25. Safe practices when using devices that generate surgical smoke require the use of a smoke evacuation system and accessories in both open and laparoscopic procedures. When laparoscopic procedures necessitate extracorporeal (outside the abdomen) assistance for inspection, dissection, anastomosis, or specimen manipulation, a

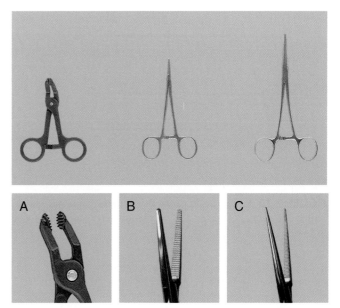

FIGURE 2-14 *Left to right:* **A,** Paper drape clip and tip; **B,** Halsted mosquito hemostatic forceps, straight, and tip; **C,** Halsted hemostatic forceps and tip.

hand-assisted port may be used to offer the surgeon a sterile, protected entry into the abdomen for his or her nondominant hand, while maintaining pneumoperitoneum. Referred to as hand-assisted laparoscopic surgery (HALS), the hand-assisted port is suitable for laparoscopic surgeries that require a mini-laparotomy to remove an organ or specimen or for extracorporeal anastomoses. A primary advantage with HALS is tactile sensation. These devices have an adhesive base to attach the sleeve and a protractor to expose the wound and to protect against contamination. Additional small incisions, or port sites, are made to introduce standard laparoscopic instruments.

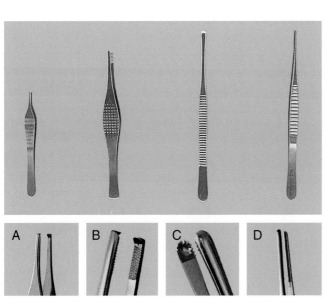

FIGURE 2-13 *Left to right:* **A,** Adson tissue forceps and tip; **B,** Ferris Smith tissue forceps and tip; **C,** Russian tissue forceps and tip; **D,** DeBakey vascular Autragrip tissue forceps and tip.

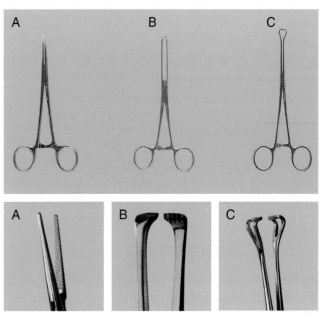

FIGURE 2-15 *Left to right:* **A,** Crile hemostatic forceps and tip; **B,** Allis tissue forceps and tip; **C,** Babcock tissue forceps.

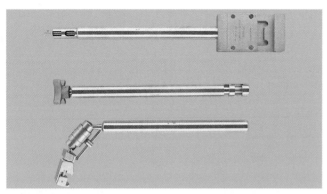

FIGURE 2-16 *Top to bottom:* Bookwalter retractor table post; Bookwalter retractor horizontal bar; Bookwalter retractor horizontal flex bar.

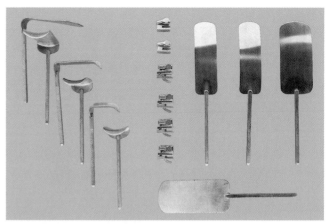

FIGURE 2-19 *Left to right:* 1 Harrington retractor blade; 1 Kelly retractor blade (2 × 6 inch); 1 Kelly retractor blade (2 × 4 inch); 1 Kelly retractor blade (2 × 3 inch); 2 Kelly retractor blades (2 × 2½ inch); 6 ratchet mechanisms; 2 malleable retractor blades (2 × 6 inch); 2 malleable retractor blades (3 × 6 inch).

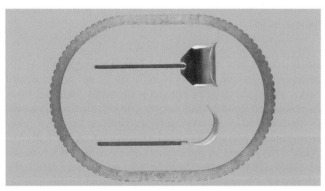

FIGURE 2-17 *Top to bottom:* Bookwalter retractor oval ring, medium; Bookwalter retractor: Balfour blades, second blade, side view.

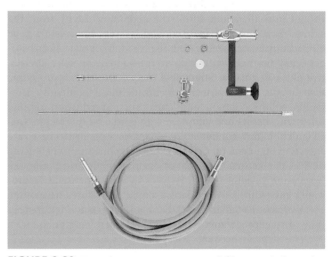

FIGURE 2-20 *Top to bottom:* Laparoscope and fiberoptic light cord.

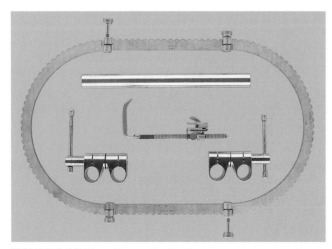

FIGURE 2-18 *Top to bottom:* Bookwalter retractor: segmented parts (2 segmented half circles, medium; 2 segmented straight extensions) placed together with 4 locking screws; 1 vertical extension bar; 1 Kelly retractor blade with ratchet mechanism attached; 2 post couplings.

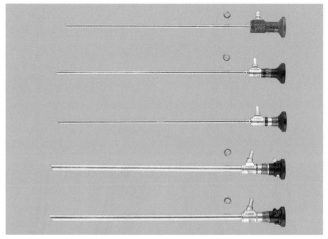

FIGURE 2-21 *Top to bottom:* Nondisposable laparoscopic lens: 0 degree, 5 mm; 25 degree, 5 mm; 50 degree, 5 mm; 25 degree, 10 mm; and 50 degree, 10 mm.

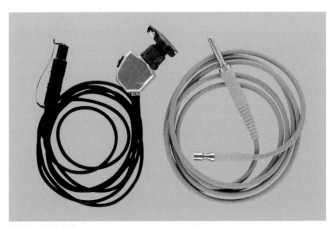

FIGURE 2-22 *Left to right:* Camera and light cord.

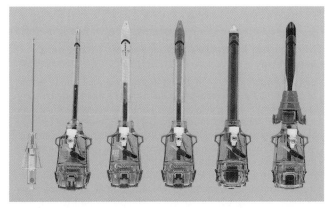

FIGURE 2-24 *Left to right:* 1 Verres needle, disposable; 3 dilating-tipped trocars, disposable, 5 mm, 10/11 mm, and 12 mm; 1 optical trocar, disposable, 10 mm; 1 blunt-tipped trocar (Hasson type), disposable, 10 mm.

Robotic or telerobotic surgical systems have advanced laparoscopic surgery, enhancing the surgeon's performance and precision by promoting an ergonomically comfortable hand position, visualizing a three-dimensional virtual field, replacing the camera holder with a stable platform, and providing unlimited motion of instrumentation (Ewing et al, 2004). Magnification and full-field lighting enhance the surgeon's orientation. Since 1997 robotic systems have been successfully employed in a broad range of GI procedures of the esophagus, stomach, and bowel, including fundoplication and bariatric procedures.

A tall, multishelf video cart, primary tower, or ceiling-mounted boom contains the primary video monitor, light source, video camera, DVD, printer, insufflator, and directed energy generators. The tower may also contain a bipolar electrosurgical unit (ESU), pulsed irrigation system, or ultrasonic dissection unit. A second tower, cart, or boom displays a second monitor, allowing the surgical team on the other side to view the procedure. The surgeon may prefer to use one monitor, placed between the patient's legs, when lithotomy position is used.

Meticulous planning ensures that all equipment is in working order. Equipment may have to be positioned after the patient is transferred to the OR bed; it is done quickly and quietly to expedite the procedure, without provoking anxiety in the patient. Place the insufflator unit on a tower shelf above the level of the patient's abdomen. This precaution prevents backflow of gas, fluid, and organic debris if the unit is turned off before the tubing is disconnected from the patient. Run electrical cords and tubing from all equipment to the nearest outlet, with consideration for staff and patient safety. Avoid areas that may be wet. Secure cords to the floor to prevent falls. Do not overload an outlet with plugs from several units that each draws considerable current, such as units that produce heat. Be prepared to connect all equipment cords and tubing after the patient is draped, and white-balance the camera. Provide a source of light for the anesthesia provider and the scrub person when the overhead room lights are turned off.

It is prudent to have an open laparotomy set with instruments and accessories available, should conversion to an open laparotomy or laparoscopic-assisted procedure be necessary. The laparotomy instruments may be opened and counted on the laparoscopy back table or a separate sterile table as per institutional protocol. All sharps must be counted or invento-

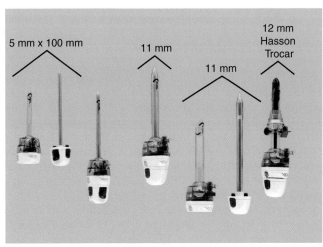

FIGURE 2-23 *Left to right:* 1 port and 1 trocar, 5 mm × 100 mm, separated, then together; port and trocar together and then separated, 11 mm × 100 mm; 1 Hasson trocar 12 mm.

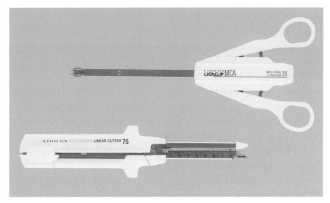

FIGURE 2-25 *Top to bottom:* Medium/large ligating and dividing Ligaclip applier; linear cutter with reloadable head.

▶▶▶ RISK REDUCTION STRATEGIES

Monitoring Integrity of Laparoscopic Instrument Insulation

Laparoscopic injury can result from electrical and thermal burns when the integrity of an instrument's insulation coating is defective. Electrosurgery has been a standard surgical tool since the 1930s and most laparoscopic procedures employ electrosurgical energy for tissue cutting and coagulation. Minimally invasive surgery provides a moist environment and limited access for visualization. Current leakage while using monopolar laparoscopic electrosurgery can occur within the trocar cannula or outside the trocar cannula, and capacitive leakage can occur from the active electrode shaft to the cannula. Significant injury can result from such stray current. Even a slight tear in the insulation can produce a power density of current and high-voltage waveform to create a larger opening in the insulation. The surgeon may not notice the change in current and the patient may not present with symptoms for several days after the procedure. Perioperative team members must continually monitor the functioning of equipment and instruments to prevent hazards and injury. The following are recommendations for care and handling of laparoscopic instruments and accessories:

◆ Use active electrode monitoring (AEM) devices with electrosurgery during patient care.
◆ Use active electrode insulation integrity testing devices before transfer to the surgeon at the sterile field and/or during instrument processing.
◆ Inspect instruments for small visible breaks in the insulation before use.
◆ Handle instruments so as to protect them from sharp objects during use, transport, and processing.
◆ Inspect insulation with a magnifying lens after decontamination.
◆ Conduct stray leakage testing with an insulation testing device after each decontamination.
◆ Remove damaged instruments from service for repair or replacement.
◆ Comply with all manufacturer care and handling instructions.

Modified from Association of PeriOperative Registered Nurses (AORN): Recommended practice for cleaning and care of surgical instruments and powered equipment. In *Perioperative standards and recommended practices,* Denver, 2009, The Association; Dennis A: Laparoscopic electrosurgical complications: stay informed, *Endonurse* 46-56, 2008; ECRI Institute: Safety technologies for laparoscopic monopolar electrosurgery: device for managing burn risks, *Health Devices* 34:259-271, 2005.

ried before the incision is made regardless of approach or size of incision (AORN, 2009c).

The surgeon may request ureteral catheters to be placed by a urologist before a GI procedure is begun. The catheters enable the surgeon to see and palpate the ureters during the procedure. A basic cystoscopy setup with sterile ureteral catheters, two of each size, will be needed.

Intraluminal examination of the bowel may be necessary during the procedure. The surgeon may request a sterile colonoscope or sigmoidoscope to insert into an opening made through the bowel wall, after the abdomen is open. Set up the scopes and accessories on a separate sterile table. This table will be considered contaminated after the scope is removed. Team

members who have directly participated in the endoscopic procedure must change gown and gloves before proceeding with the remainder of the surgical intervention.

Additional accessory instruments or devices may include a sterile plastic drawstring intestinal bag to confine loops of normal bowel from the operative segment, sterile counted radiopaque surgical towels, combination suction-irrigator, or irrigator-bipolar coagulation. Ultrasound-guided probes and ultrasonic dissection instruments are commonly used in GI surgery. Automatic stapling devices streamline the processes of ligating tissue, cross-clamping, and creating anastomoses and reservoir pouches. These instruments deliver single staples and single or double rows of closely staggered linear and circular rows of inert staples. The staple appliers may be single-fire or accept multiple cartridges for successive use. They may be designed for open laparotomy or endoscopic use. The B-shaped design of the implanted staple does not compromise the vascularity of the approximated tissue edges. These devices are available in reusable and disposable units. Personnel must be familiar with the types of available stapling equipment, applications, assembly if indicated, and proper loading.

Electrosurgery is critical to achieve and maintain hemostasis. Optimal dispersive pad sites include the thigh, flank, shoulder, upper arm, and buttocks. The pad is placed over a fleshy muscular site as close as possible to the incision, yet out of the prep area. Avoid dependent areas that may have a bony prominence or affinity for pooled solution. Choose power settings that achieve the best tissue response at the lowest setting. The smoke evacuation apparatus should be utilized. Provide long and angled ESU tips. Other hemostatic and dissection equipment and devices may include the argon beam coagulator, ultrasonic tissue dissector, radiofrequency ablation, and laser.

Suture materials used on GI tissue were traditionally chromic gut and silk. With the increased number of synthetic absorbable and nonabsorbable suture materials available, surgeons have a variety of materials from which to choose. Polyester fiber sutures and polyglycolic acid sutures are frequently employed on GI tissue. Generally, 3-0 and 4-0 sutures on a semicircular taper needle are used on intestinal tissues. Ligatures for small vessels usually require a 3-0 or 4-0 braided material, whereas 0 or 2-0 braided ligatures are used for larger vessel occlusion. For closure or anastomosis of GI layers, 3-0 or 4-0 synthetic absorbable suture with a curved intestinal needle is commonly used on the mucosa. A 3-0 or 2-0 continuous synthetic absorbable suture and 4-0 or 3-0 nonabsorbable suture with curved or straight intestinal needles may be used for the seromuscular layer. Some surgeons may prefer interrupted silk sutures on intestinal (semicircular taper) needles for anastomosis procedures. For abdominal closure 1 or 0 braided or monofilament suture is commonly used. Retention sutures may be indicated when there is potential for compromised tissue or wound healing. Checking the surgeon's preference/procedure card or pick list for appropriate suture materials not only ensures the availability of necessary supplies but also is cost-effective.

Sponges used in open laparotomy procedures include large packs (18 × 18 inches), large laps (12 × 12 inches), or small elongated tape sponges (4 × 18 inches). Sponges vary in size according to product availability. Gauze dissectors (referred to variously as "Kittners," "peanuts," or "pushers") on a Kelly clamp or right angle clamp may be used for blunt tis-

25

sue dissection. Meticulous vigilance prevents the incidental misplacement of these items. Larger gauze sponges are not recommended for use in the abdominal cavity. In the case of significant bleeding or isolation of bowel during anastomosis, lint-free radiopaque cloth towels can be used. Towels are counted, as are all sponges.

Bowel technique, also referred to as *contamination* or *isolation* technique, prevents cross-contamination of the wound or abdomen with bowel organisms. This technique is also employed during cancer procedures to prevent mechanical metastasis, or "seeding" of malignant cells throughout the abdomen. Bowel technique begins as soon as the GI tract is clamped and transected, and proceeds through wound irrigation, before wound closure. The wound edges and surrounding drapes are protected with extra drapes, while instruments used for GI tract resection and anastomosis are sequestered and used only for this part of the procedure. The rest of the sterile back table remains untouched throughout the anastomosis. Separate instruments and drapes are used for the closure. Gowns, gloves, and drapes are changed before closure. The contaminated GI tract instruments are handed off or left on a separate Mayo stand. Preplanning during preoperative setup includes extra and separate instruments ready for anastomosis and closure. These must all be included in the instrument count with provision for a closing count of the contaminated set. There is also a provision for containment and display of needles used for the anastomosis. Surgeon preference and institutional protocol determine details of bowel technique.

Specimens are handled carefully and prepared for examination by the pathologist. The specimen may be contaminated with microorganisms or malignant cells and no contamination of the sterile field and instruments can occur. The surgeon usually determines how the specimen is handled before examination. It may be sent to the pathology department fresh, in saline, or in a preservative solution. Tissue also may be sent for frozen-section examination to verify pathologic condition and to determine if tissue margins are free of malignant cells. Specimens may also be entered into research protocols, which will require further special handling, storage, and transport.

The surgical department has procedures for correct patient and specimen identification that are followed each time a specimen is collected. Accuracy is verified with the surgeon by reading back (referred to as "write down, read back") the label and pathology form before removing the specimen from the room or before the surgeon leaves the room, and documented according to institutional protocol.

Drains may be used to evacuate gastric secretions or serosanguineous fluid. A closed suction wound drain may be used. A Malecot, Pezzer, or Foley catheter in desired size may be inserted as a gastrostomy tube for drainage until normal bowel peristalsis returns. A jejunostomy tube may be placed in the jejunum after gastric resection to provide access for enteral nutrition.

Determination and documentation of wound classification are done at the end of the procedure. If the GI tract has been entered or transected, the wound class will be considered "clean-contaminated" as long as no breaks in technique have occurred or signs of infection have been discovered in the surgical wound.

Risk Factors for Postoperative Ileus

◆ Intraabdominal infection
◆ Intraabdominal inflammation
◆ Lengthy surgical procedure
◆ Prolonged exposure of abdominal organs
◆ Opioid and psychotropic drugs
◆ Inhaled anesthetics
◆ Electrolyte imbalance
◆ Retroperitoneal hemorrhage
◆ Pancreatitis

RESEARCH HIGHLIGHT

Early Feeding After Abdominal Surgery

Traditionally, postoperative fluid and food intake was delayed until evidence of bowel function returned; early feeding, however, may stimulate GI activity and return of motility, decreasing length of stay (LOS). Oral intake of nutrition as early as 4 to 12 hours postoperatively may stimulate reflexes that produce coordinated propulsion activity and release of GI hormones (Bisanz, 2008). Several recent studies investigated if a routine of permitting patients to eat normal food after major abdominal surgery would affect the return of GI motility. In one randomized controlled study (N = 447), one group of patients (227) was assigned to "nil per os" (NPO) and enteral tube feeding, while another group (220) was permitted to eat-at-will from their first day after surgery. A total of 76 NPO patients had complications compared with 62 of the eat-at-will group. Return of motility, LOS, total number of complications, and post discharge complications significantly favored the eat-at-will group (Lassen et al, 2008).

A smaller study of 128 patients separated into 2 equal groups compared the traditional progression from clear liquids to full diet over 4 days to early eat-at-will feeding. The endpoint indicators were the need to reinsert an NG tube, LOS, and postoperative complications. This study also included pain scale ratings and several quality of life criteria. There were no differences in outcomes between the two groups, including pain and quality of life indicators (Han-Geurts et al, 2007).

Gum chewing following surgery has been associated with enhanced recovery of GI function. A study of 158 patients who chewed gum had return of motility evidenced by passing of flatus and bowel movement sooner than the average of 1.10 days. It is possible that gum chewing represents a type of sham feeding that stimulates the digestive nerves and GI hormones (Purkayastha et al, 2008).

Early nutrition increases wound healing, enhances return of GI motility, shortens LOS, and decreases some postsurgical complications. For most patients, progressive feeding according to the GI tract's capability to tolerate food immediately after surgery is likely to result in significant positive outcomes.

Modified from Han-Geurts et al: Randomized clinical trial of the impact of early enteral feeding on postoperative ileus and recovery, *Br J Surg* 94: 555-561, 2007; Lassen et al: Allowing normal food at will after major upper gastrointestinal surgery does not increase morbidity: a randomized multicenter trial, *Ann Surg* 247:721-1140, 2008; Purkayastha S et al: Chewing gum associated with enhanced bowel recovery after colon surgery, *Arch Surg* 143(8):788-793, 2008.

Surgical Interventions

ABDOMINAL INCISIONS

The abdominal cavity is surgically entered more than any other anatomic region. The site of the incision (Figure 2-26) is chosen to gain quick, easy access and exposure to underlying pathology; to minimize trauma, bleeding, and postoperative discomfort; to maximize wound strength; and to afford ample room to accomplish the surgery. Each incision has advantages and disadvantages as to adequacy of exposure, length of time required for closure, disruption of surrounding blood and nerve supply, underlying muscles that must be cut or split, incidence of postoperative wound hernia, effect on pulmonary function, and cosmesis. Abdominal incisions permanently change the blood supply of the anterior abdominal wall and impact future surgeries and reconstructive options available to the patient. Any compromise of the skin, muscle, or blood supply by prior incision may preclude the use of an otherwise optimal tissue flap for reconstruction after radical thoracic, breast, or GI surgery. Minimally invasive approaches decrease the use and extent of abdominal incisions and preserve the integrity of the abdominal wall.

The abdominal wall consists of various tissue layers (Figure 2-27). Beneath the skin and subcutaneous fat are the fascia, muscles (internal and external oblique, rectus abdominis, transverse abdominis), preperitoneal fat, and peritoneum. The fascia, consisting of bands of tough fibrous connective tissue, surrounds the muscle anteriorly and posteriorly (Figure 2-28). The peritoneum is a serous membrane that lines the abdominal cavity (parietal peritoneum) and surfaces of the abdominal organs (visceral peritoneum).

Vertical Midline Incisions

The vertical midline incision is the simplest abdominal incision to perform. It is an excellent primary incision and offers good exposure to any part of the abdominal cavity. Hemostasis is easily achieved, and fewer layers are traversed. The incision can be extended from just below the sternal notch, distally around the umbilicus (which is avascular, tough connective tissue), back to the midline, and down to the symphysis pubis. The peritoneum is incised, and the round ligament of the liver may be divided. Postoperative hernias are more common above the umbilicus than below it. The midline crossover vasculature is permanently altered with this incision.

The paramedian incision, also called a *rectus* incision, is a vertical incision placed approximately 4 cm (2 inches) lateral to the midline on either side of the upper or lower abdomen. This incision is used infrequently because it adds little to the exposure obtained by way of a midline vertical incision. Paramedian incisions take longer to create and close and are more prone to herniation; this is especially true when they are more lateral.

Closure of the paramedian and midline incisions begins with the peritoneum. The peritoneum and posterior fascia may be sutured as a single layer in a continuous stitch with an absorbable suture material. The suture line may be supported with retention sutures when outward abdominal pressure on the suture line is anticipated, which raises the risk for herniation, dehiscence, or evisceration. Retention sutures are placed through all layers of the wound, using a heavy #2-gauge nylon, polypropylene, or wire suture material. Wound dehiscence, a risk of abdominal surgery, is separation of the unhealed incision. When dehiscence is severe, bowel or other abdominal structures may protrude (evisceration). Dehiscence and evisceration are most common with midline vertical incisions. Risk factors include serious nutritional deficiencies, diabetes, steroid use, obesity, infection, and improper surgical closure.

Anterior fascia, subcutaneous tissue, and skin are closed as separate layers. Anterior fascia and muscle are closed with interrupted nonabsorbable synthetic sutures. The subcutaneous layer may be closed with an absorbable interrupted suture. Skin edges are approximated and secured with interrupted nonabsorbable sutures, skin staples, subcuticular continuous closure with an absorbable suture material, skin-bonding adhesive, or sterile skin tape strips. There are many alternatives and variations to abdominal incision closure, based on the individual patient's need and surgeon preference.

Oblique Incisions

McBurney Incision. The McBurney muscle-splitting incision is commonly used for open appendectomy. It is an 8-cm oblique incision that begins well below the umbilicus, goes through McBurney point (two thirds of the distance from the umbilicus to the anterior iliac spine in the right lower quadrant), and extends upward toward the right flank. The external oblique muscle and fascia are divided bluntly (split in the direction of their fibers) and are retracted. The internal oblique muscle, transverse muscle, and fascia are also split and retracted. When muscles are divided in line with their direction of pull, as is the case with muscle-splitting incisions, there is less chance of postoperative herniation or disruption. The peritoneum is incised transversely. This incision is quick and easy to close and allows a firm wound closure. However, it does not permit good exposure and is difficult to extend. To extend the incision medially, the inferior epigastric vessels are ligated and the rectus sheath incised transversely.

Lower Oblique Inguinal Incision. An oblique right or left inguinal incision extends from the pubic tubercle to the anterior iliac crest, slightly above and parallel to the inguinal crease.

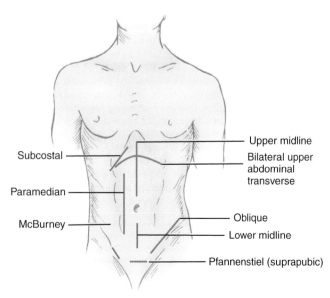

Subcostal

Paramedian

McBurney

Upper midline

Bilateral upper abdominal transverse

Oblique

Lower midline

Pfannenstiel (suprapubic)

FIGURE 2-26 Incisions made through the abdominal wall.

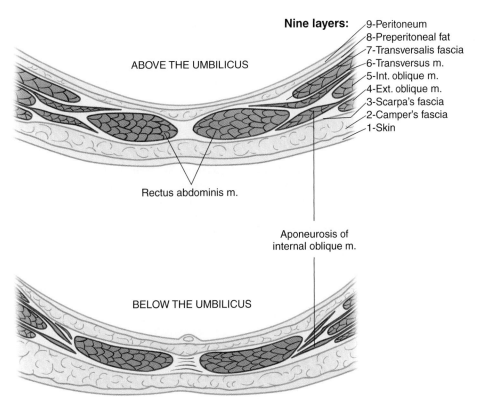

Nine layers:
9-Peritoneum
8-Preperitoneal fat
7-Transversalis fascia
6-Transversus m.
5-Int. oblique m.
4-Ext. oblique m.
3-Scarpa's fascia
2-Camper's fascia
1-Skin

ABOVE THE UMBILICUS

Rectus abdominis m.

Aponeurosis of
internal oblique m.

BELOW THE UMBILICUS

FIGURE 2-27 Horizontal section of abdominal wall. Aponeurosis of internal oblique muscle splits into two sections, one lying anterior and the other posterior to rectus abdominis muscle, thereby forming an encasing sheath around muscle above umbilicus. Below umbilicus, aponeuroses of all muscles pass anterior to rectus. *m.*, Muscle; *Int.*, internal; *Ext.*, external.

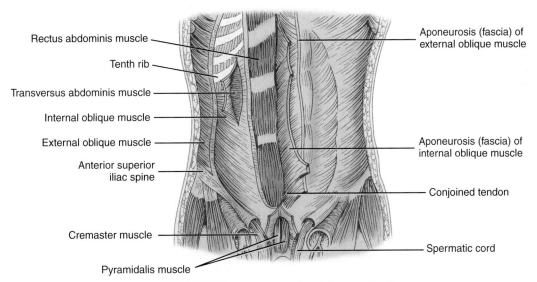

Rectus abdominis muscle

Tenth rib

Transversus abdominis muscle

Internal oblique muscle

External oblique muscle

Anterior superior
iliac spine

Cremaster muscle

Pyramidalis muscle

Aponeurosis (fascia) of
external oblique muscle

Aponeurosis (fascia) of
internal oblique muscle

Conjoined tendon

Spermatic cord

FIGURE 2-28 Superior muscles of abdominal wall.

This is the standard incision for open inguinal herniorrhaphy. Incision through the external oblique muscle provides access to the cremaster muscle, inguinal canal, and cord structures. This incision does not typically interrupt major abdominal arteries.

Long, lower abdominal oblique incisions are used for transplant, urologic, and vascular procedures. These incisions require transection of the abdominal wall and flank musculature. They may require ligation of the deep inferior epigastric artery.

Subcostal Incision. The subcostal incision is made on the right side (Kocher incision) when used for open procedures of the gallbladder, biliary system, and pancreas (Figure 2-29). A left subcostal incision is used for surgery of the spleen.

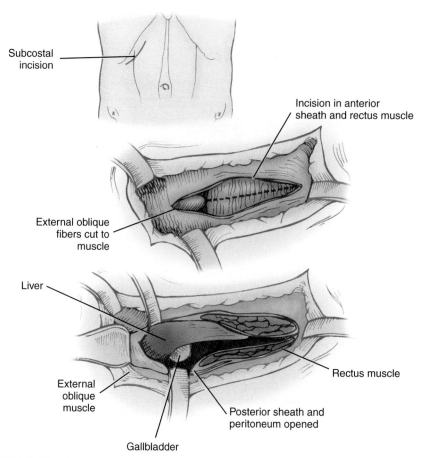

FIGURE 2-29 Subcostal incision in upper right quadrant. Anterior sheath has been divided transversely, and muscle is exposed. Posterior sheath and peritoneum have been opened transversely.

This incision provides limited exposure unless the patient is short with a wide abdomen and wide costal margins. It provides good cosmetic results because it follows the skin lines and nerve damage is minimal. Tension on the skin edges is less than that of a vertical incision, permitting wider retraction and exposure with less respiratory impairment during the procedure.

This oblique incision begins in the epigastrium and extends laterally and obliquely downward to just below the costal margin. It continues through the rectus muscle, which is retracted or transversely divided. The superior epigastric artery is occasionally sacrificed. A chevron incision (joined right and left subcostal incisions) provides excellent exposure for gastric, duodenal, pancreatic, and portal system procedures. This incision, however, interrupts lateral blood supply and innervation to the rectus muscle and postoperative muscle atrophy may occur.

Closure of this incision includes approximation of the falciform ligament, peritoneum, posterior rectus sheath, and anterior rectus sheath. Postoperatively, this is a strong but painful incision.

Transverse Incisions

Pfannenstiel Incision. The Pfannenstiel incision is used for pelvic surgery. It is a curved transverse incision across the lower abdomen through the skin, subcutaneous layer, and rectus sheath, approximately 1 cm (½ inch) above the symphysis pubis, usually within the pubic hairline (Figure 2-30). This is the standard incision for open obstetric and gynecologic procedures. The rectus muscles are separated along the midline, and the peritoneum is entered through a midline vertical incision. This incision does not alter vascular supply to the abdominal wall if the deep inferior epigastric artery is left intact. It provides good exposure and a strong postoperative scar that is cosmetically acceptable.

Midabdominal Transverse Incision. The midabdominal transverse incision is used on the right or left for a retroperitoneal approach. The incision begins slightly above or below the umbilicus on either side, extends laterally to the lumbar region at an angle between the ribs and the iliac crest, follows Langer's lines of tension of the abdominal wall, and runs parallel to vessels and nerves, rarely causing permanent damage. It is a standard incision for transverse colectomy or colostomy and choledochojejunostomy. The skin and subcutaneous tissue are incised, the anterior sheath split, the rectus muscle divided, and vessels within the rectus clamped and ligated. The posterior rectus sheath and peritoneum are cut in the direction of the fibers, preserving intercostal nerves. The peritoneum is incised along the midline, and the incision extended laterally to the oblique muscle.

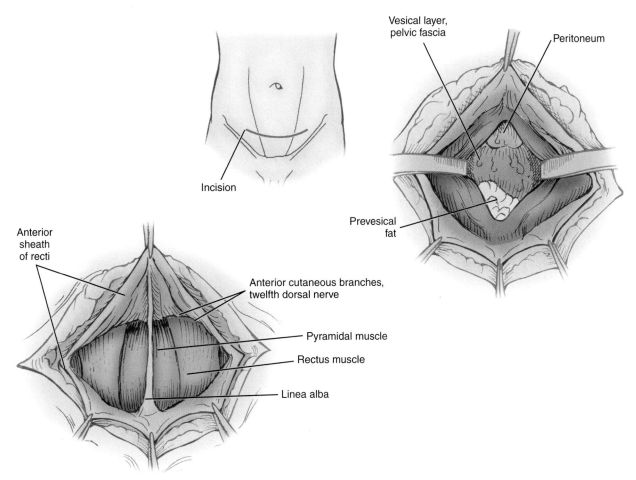

FIGURE 2-30 Pfannenstiel incision (suprapubic).

Thoracoabdominal Incision. The thoracoabdominal incision is the standard incision for surgery of the proximal stomach, distal esophagus, and anterior spine. The patient is placed in a lateral position. The incision begins at a midpoint between the xiphoid and umbilicus and extends posteriorly, across the seventh or eighth interspace and the midscapular line into the chest. The rectus, oblique, serratus, and intercostal muscles are divided down to peritoneum and pleura. The costal cartilage and diaphragm are then divided (Figure 2-31). This incision sacrifices the superior epigastric artery.

Wound closure occurs in layers with an interrupted suture technique. The peritoneum and pleura may be closed with an absorbable suture material, whereas the muscle and fascia layer may be closed with either an absorbable or a nonabsorbable synthetic suture material. Skin edges are approximated and secured with suture, staples, skin bonding adhesive, or skin tape strips.

LAPAROTOMY

An opening made through the abdominal wall into the peritoneal cavity is called a *laparotomy*. Surgical intervention may be necessary to repair or remove traumatized tissue, to cure disease processes by organ removal, or to examine by biopsy or otherwise visualize internal organs for diagnosis. Surgery may be indicated for diagnostic, therapeutic, palliative, or prophylactic reasons. Most procedures requiring a laparotomy involve the organs of the GI tract.

Procedural Considerations

A basic laparotomy set with long and short soft tissue instruments and various shallow and deep retractors is used. An ESU, smoke evacuator, and suction are basic to performing laparotomy. The patient is positioned supine with arms extended on locked armboards at less than a 90-degree angle. General anesthesia with endotracheal intubation is usual, although spinal or epidural anesthesia may be used. An indwelling urinary catheter may be inserted before the abdominal prep, which extends from above the nipple line to above the symphysis pubis. A forced-air warming blanket may be applied over or under the patient's upper body, arms, and head for thermoregulation. SCDs are applied before induction to prevent deep venous blood pooling in the lower extremities.

In select patients, laparotomy leads to the formation of adhesions and the consequent likelihood of chronic pain, infertility, painful intercourse, and small bowel obstruction. Adhesions are fibrous bands of filamentous protein tissue that form a network of fibers, causing separate tissues and organs

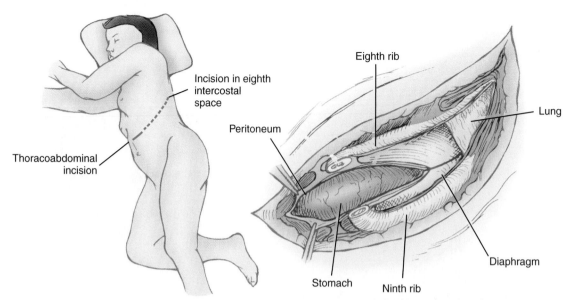

FIGURE 2-31 Thoracoabdominal incision. Patient is placed on unaffected side. Incision is usually made from point midway between xiphoid process and umbilicus to costal margin at site of eighth costal cartilage. Dissection is carried down to peritoneum and pleura. Costal cartilage and diaphragm are divided, and stomach is exposed.

to adhere to one another in the abdominal cavity (Porth and Gaspard, 2004; The Surgical and Clinical Adhesions Research [SCAR]-3 study, 2005). Adhesions are caused by a defect in the process of normal tissue healing, prompted by tissue injury, inflammation, infection, or ischemia. The peritoneum is most associated with abdominal and pelvic adhesions. Introduction of microscopic particles, such as glove powder talc or starch, gauze fibers, and suture materials, seems to promote adhesion development.

Surgical separation of individual adhesions, called *adhesiolysis*, is not always effective, with adhesions re-forming, causing a cycle of symptoms and recurrent adhesive disease. Adhesive tissues have increased levels of growth factors, which suggest a greater probability of re-formation. Adhesions may also develop as a result of radiation-induced endarteritis, endometriosis, pelvic inflammatory disease (PID), or Crohn's disease.

Adhesion-related disorder (ARD) is a chronic condition of pain, constipation, and cramping. Patients often describe substantial psychologic burdens and disability. Because adhesions are not evident on x-ray unless they present with bowel obstruction, torsion, or volvulus, many patients are misdiagnosed initially.

Pharmacologic agent interventions aimed at treating adhesions are limited. Systemic administration is essentially ineffective since surgical sites typically interrupt blood supply. Further, rapid absorption via the peritoneal membranes removes most of the agent within 24 hours after surgery. Most of the promising lytic-acting agents that interfere with production of hyperplastic adhesive fibrous tissue also interfere with normal wound healing. Historically, surgeons have tried many experimental substances and methods to delay adhesion development, such as mineral oil, animal biomembranes, silk, rubber, Teflon, gold foil, and amniotic membranes. Adhesions are best divided with sharp dissection.

Preventive measures include the following:
- Minimizing tissue trauma and inflammation with meticulous surgical technique
- Utilizing laparoscopic approach when indicated
- Reducing the time that the abdomen is open
- Minimizing use of electrosurgery
- Applying meticulous hemostasis
- Minimizing infection risk
- Avoiding gastrointestinal contamination
- Irrigating the abdomen with copious amounts of warmed solution before closure
- Administering antiinflammatory drugs such as corticosteroids and nonsteroidal antiinflammatory drugs (NSAIDs)
- Limiting suture use and using fine, nonreactive suture materials
- Mechanically separating the organs before closure with physical barriers such as omentum, polytetrafluoroethylene (PTFE), cellulose, sodium hyaluronate membrane, bioresorbable polymer films, gels, and water-soluble glucose polymer or polyethylene glycol (PEG) solution
- Using hydroflotation with saline, lactated Ringer's, or Hartmann's solution
- Using alternative therapies such as deep tissue massage, biofeedback, acupuncture, and hypnosis

Operative Procedure

Laparotomy Opening

1. The skin incision is made and carried to the fascia (Figure 2-32, *A*).
2. Bleeding is controlled with hemostats and vessels ligated with fine nonabsorbable ligatures (ties), or electrocoagulated.
3. The wound edges are retracted with small retractors.
4. With tissue forceps and scalpel, the external fascia is incised (Figure 2-32, *B*).

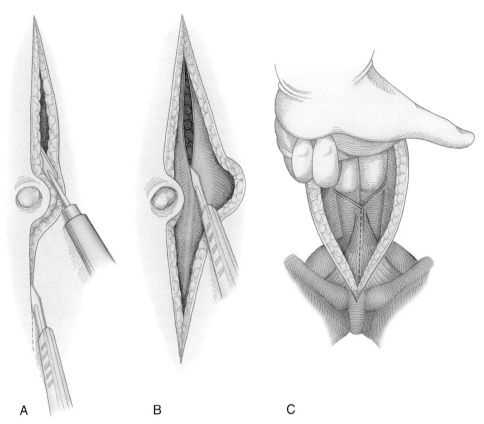

FIGURE 2-32 A, Midline laparotomy incision around the umbilicus. B, External fascia is incised. C, Entry into the peritoneal cavity.

5. With Metzenbaum, curved Mayo scissors, electrosurgery, or a knife, the external oblique muscle is split the length of the incision. Bleeding vessels are controlled with hemostats, ligating clips, medium or fine ligatures, or electrocoagulating current.

6. The external oblique muscle is retracted.

7. The internal oblique and transverse muscles are split, parallel to the fibers, up to the rectus sheath with a scalpel or scissors. These muscles are then retracted.

8. The peritoneum is exposed, grasped with smooth tissue forceps, and nicked with a #10 blade.

9. Sponges, laparotomy pads, and suction are used as needed. Culture samples may be taken at this time.

10. The peritoneal incision is extended the length of the wound with Metzenbaum or Mayo scissors (Figure 2-32, *C*).

11. The peritoneum is retracted with large Richardson retractors for initial exploration.

12. Once the affected organs are identified, a self-retaining retractor, such as a Balfour or Bookwalter retractor system, may be used to establish hands-free exposure.

Laparotomy Closure

1. Two tissue forceps or clamps are used to approximate peritoneal edges, and the peritoneum closed with a continuous synthetic absorbable suture or interrupted nonabsorbable sutures. The internal oblique fascia is usually closed with the peritoneum. Muscle tissue is approximated and may or may not be sutured.

2. The external oblique fascia is closed with interrupted sutures, staples, or both. Retraction is necessary as the various layers are closed. Richardson retractors are commonly used.

3. Fine (3-0 or 4-0) absorbable sutures are usually employed to close the subcutaneous or subcuticular tissue. Retraction is provided with laparotomy pads or small retractors.

4. Skin edges are held with Adson, Russian, or medium-toothed forceps and approximated with interrupted 3-0 or 4-0 silk, nylon, or other nonabsorbable sutures on a cutting needle. A cosmetically aesthetic wound closure is achieved in patients with limited tension on the incision by using a subcuticular closure with a 3-0 or 4-0 nonabsorbable suture. Skin staples or clips, sterile adhesive strips, or skin-bonding adhesive is often used to approximate skin edges. Retention sutures of #1 or #2 nonabsorbable suture material may be used. Prepackaged retention bridges or flexible tubing bolsters are used to protect the incision site.

LAPAROSCOPY

Laparoscopy is an approach to abdominal surgery for minimal access into the abdomen to achieve the same surgical result as open laparotomy. Laparoscopic surgery is often referred to as minimally invasive surgery (MIS), wherein the surgery is performed with instruments (rather than the surgeon's hands) inside the body, yet manipulated from outside the body (Box 2-1 describes terms used in laparoscopic gastrointestinal sur-

BOX 2-1

Laparoscopic Terminology

MAS/MIS—Minimal Access Surgery/Minimally Invasive Surgery
SPA—Single Puncture Access
SPS—Single Port Surgery
SILS—Single Incision Laparoscopic Surgery
OPUS—One Port Umbilical Surgery
NOTES—Natural Orifice Transluminal Endoscopic Surgery
NOSCAR—Natural Orifice Surgery Consortium for Assessment and Research
TOGA—Trans Oral GAstroplasty

BOX 2-2

Advantages and Disadvantages of Laparoscopic Surgery

BENEFITS FOR THE PATIENT
- Minimal blood loss
- Reduced risk for infection
- Rapid return of GI function
- Less small bowel obstruction
- Less risk for incisional hernia with smaller incisions
- Less immune suppression than open techniques
- Less postoperative pain and reduced analgesia use
- Adjunct to preoperative staging
- Application of chemotherapy and brachytherapy

DRAWBACKS FOR THE PATIENT
- Less capacity for intraabdominal inspection and large specimen removal
- Potential for port-site recurrence
- Potential for DVT
- Decreased venous return
- Decreased vital capacity
- Increased peak airway pressure, cardiac volume, systemic vascular resistance (SVR) (50%), systolic pressure
- Risk for pleural or peritoneal seeding of malignant cells

BENEFITS FOR THE SURGEON
- Enhanced imaging resolution
- Image/video-recording option
- All team members see same image
- Abundant light
- Magnification

DRAWBACKS FOR THE SURGEON
- Ergonomically challenging
- Instruments move in opposition—fulcrum effect
- Loss of haptic sensation and tactile feedback
- Critical moves necessary with nondominant hand
- Sees two dimensionally but must perceive three dimensionally
- Significant learning curve to competence

gery). The first generation of modern laparoscopic surgery began in the early 1970s in the GYN specialty; it was used primarily for diagnostic direct (eye on the telescope eye piece) visualization of endometriosis, ectopic pregnancy, and uterine fibroids, and later, laparoscopic tubal ligation with electrosurgery was performed. These procedures were originally called Band-Aid, keyhole, or belly button procedures.

Traditional laparoscopic port placement, via triangulation, is the fundamental concept of laparoscopic surgery. It places the instruments on planes where they meet to effectively support dissection with adequate visualization and identification of anatomy and pathology. Incorrectly placed ports can cause sword-fighting instruments and indirect access to the operative target. Challenges also exist in delivering intact specimens through small ports. The increased intra-abdominal pressure from the insufflation of CO_2 into the peritoneal cavity applies pressure on the diaphragm and femoral vessels. This can compromise patients with cardiac and respiratory disease and cause deep vein thrombosis. The venting of CO_2 at the end of the procedure is believed to have the potential of "blowing" cancer cells into the layers of the port site, causing later cancer recurrence of the skin and subcutaneous layers of the abdomen. This is a very rare event and probably not a concern that should eliminate laparoscopic approaches for cancer patients. Less invasive approaches to surgery are less stressful to the patient. Traditional laparoscopic surgery has many other advantages over traditional open surgical approaches (Box 2-2). These advantages, however, do not exist without technical challenges and cost concerns.

Procedures described as "laparoscopically assisted" combine laparoscopic surgical manipulation of tissue with enlargement of one of the port incisions, permitting the surgeon direct access, or hand contact, on the operative tissue. The surgeon may transfer a portion of the surgical tissue onto the abdominal surface to achieve repair outside the body (*extracorporeal repair*). *Intracorporeal* refers to inside the abdomen. Laparoscopically assisted surgery may also refer to laparoscopic dissection and resection with an open approach to remove the surgical specimen.

Laparoscopy is usually contraindicated in patients with extensive adhesions from prior surgeries. Patients with bleeding disorders or pregnancy also pose a risk. Advanced cardiac or pulmonary disease may preclude the option of a minimal access approach. Potential complications include trocar site bleeding (Patient Safety), vascular injury, hemorrhage, perforation or laceration of organs, infection, anastomotic leaks, ileus,

strictures, accidental electrosurgical injury, and pulmonary problems. The surgeon may have to convert to an open procedure in the presence of adhesions, hemorrhage, fixed small bowel, unusual anatomy, unexpected findings, or instrument failure. The potential for conversion to an open approach is discussed with the patient before surgery and documented on the consent form by the surgeon.

Single port access laparoscopy entails entry through the abdominal cavity via one port placed through the umbilicus. This approach is also called "radical endoscopy" or "stealth surgery" (surgery that takes place without leaving a trace that it occurred, since there is no scar). Access is gained through the Hasson cutdown technique with a small scalpel and bladeless dissecting-tip trocar. The port maintains pneumoperitoneum and retracts the incision. Instruments are curved and flexible to accommodate space restrictions and afford range of motion that follows the surgeon's hand movements. Multiple instruments can be used via one port with standard digital technology (video systems and processors).

Single port/puncture laparoscopy offers considerable advantages over traditional laparoscopy. The high-dexterity instrumentation that is used bends and flexes to provide manipulative options not available with traditional laparoscopy. It does so essentially with three or four instruments: a combined telescopic light/camera and two working tools. At the end of the procedure, the port is removed and the umbilicus is gently folded back into its original shape. Many procedures that can be accomplished via laparoscopic access are now approached via single puncture as well. Contraindications include multiple prior abdominal surgeries because of adhesions or altered anatomy, and morbid obesity because of decreased visibility and difficult movement inside the cavity (Curcillo, 2007; Fowler, 2008; Pasricha, 2005).

Because the umbilicus has no muscle or fascia layer, umbilical incisions are safe and less painful than other incision sites. With only one incision site, there is less risk of penetration injuries, infection, and hernia. The growing capabilities of therapeutic flexible endoscopy have ushered in a new era in treatment of GI conditions. Refinements in laparoscopic surgery have progressed to the point that complex surgical procedures, such as gastric bypass, are performed in a minimally invasive fashion.

These trends have set the stage for the development of even less invasive methods to treat conditions both in the gut lumen and in the peritoneal cavity. Major intraperitoneal surgery is being performed without skin incisions. The natural orifices may provide the entry point for surgical interventions in the peritoneal cavity, thereby avoiding abdominal wall incisions. Natural orifice transluminal endoscopic surgery (NOTES) is performed by a team that has the skills of an advanced therapeutic endoscopist and a laparoscopic surgeon. Advantages for the patient include decreased pain, blood loss, and morbidity; absence of a scar; and earlier return to activities of daily living (ADLs). Advantages for the surgeon include increased visibility with light and magnification, larger field of view, flexible tips that eliminate the need to change instruments frequently, and easy transition to traditional laparoscopy (Lucile Packard Children's Hospital, 2008). Operative costs are similar to those for traditional laparoscopy.

While single port laparoscopy was developed from the platform of traditional laparoscopic surgery, new instrumentation is advancing the ergonomics and precision of dissection (Barclay et al, 2008; Cleveland Clinic, 2008; Raman et al, 2008). Laparoscopy offers advantages over the conventional open approach in many GI procedures. Success of surgical repair, postoperative recurrence of disease, and overall survival are similar between open and laparoscopic approaches for the same surgery. Operative times vary according to many variables, including unusual occurrences, the surgeon's skill and technique, and instrumentation. Postoperative analgesia needs are the same or may be less than in the open laparotomy approach. Patients typically report less postoperative discomfort because of the absence of a large abdominal incision. Nonetheless, many do report muscle discomfort in the area of a working-port incision where significant manipulation of instruments occurred. Postoperative flatus and first bowel movement may occur a day sooner than for conventional surgery patients. Resumption of oral intake may also be sooner in this group. Minimal access approaches also result in faster recovery of pulmonary function, fewer postoperative complications, less potential for surgical site infections, improved cosmesis, shorter recovery period, and quicker return to former activities of daily living.

Procedural Considerations

Minimal access surgery requires specially designed instruments, telescopes, trocars with cannulae, suction and irrigation devices, retractors, electrosurgery, CO_2 introduction devices, stapling instruments and appliers, and video image equipment. The video camera, light source, and monitors provide indirect visualization of the surgical site, enhanced with magnification and bright illumination.

Operative Procedure

1. Initial entry is made in the periumbilical region with percutaneous puncture with an insufflation (Veress) needle (closed technique) or a sharp trocar in a sheath (direct technique). A cutdown technique (Hasson technique) may be used with a small incision through to the fascia with a #15 blade. The trocar is then introduced through and into the peritoneal cavity. In the direct technique, an optical trocar is inserted to visualize trocar placement before insufflation.
2. Pneumoperitoneum is established with insufflation of 3 to 4 liters of CO_2 into the peritoneal cavity to achieve an intraabdominal pressure of 12 to 15 mm Hg.
3. The needle is removed and replaced with a 10-mm or 11-mm trocar. The rigid laparoscope, with video camera and cord coupled to the telescope eyepiece end, is inserted into the port for visualization. Two to six more ports may be created to facilitate use of an endoscopic fan retractor; various grasping, dissection, cutting, and electrosurgery instruments; ultrasonic scalpel dissector; suction-irrigation devices; laser fibers; endoscopic clip and staple appliers; and specimen retrieval graspers. Port sites are selected to permit all instrument tips to converge at the primary surgical work site.
4. Surgical exploration, dissection, resection, anastomosis, inspection, and irrigation then follow.
5. CO_2 is exhausted and ports removed. The umbilical incision is closed with 3-0 or 4-0 nonabsorbable synthetic suture. Remaining port incisions are closed with the same suture, adhesive strips, or skin-bonding adhesive. A small dressing or bandage is applied.

INTRAOPERATIVE INTRAPERITONEAL CHEMOTHERAPY

Patients who undergo abdominal surgery for GI and peritoneal cancers may benefit from intraoperative hyperthermic intraperitoneal chemotherapy (HIPEC) to remove or to reduce the burden of tumor or diseased organs, often called cytoreductive (removing as much tumor tissue as possible) (also referred to as "debulking") surgery. HIPEC may take place while the abdomen is still open or after it is closed (referred to as the "closed" technique). The abdominal cavity is connected to an extracorporeal fluid circuit for instillation and continual perfusion of heated chemotherapeutic agents (Pappas et al, 2008). Access may be created with a peritoneal port such as a Tenckhoff catheter or with separate inflow and outflow catheters. Tissue contact can be maintained with perfusion pump–directed flow or by manually rocking the abdominal cavity (by a sterile team member) to agitate fluid around and about the abdominal organs. The procedure may take up to 2 hours. This therapy allows for a high concentration of chemotherapy to have direct contact with the tumor, surrounding organs, and visceral and parietal peritoneum. Heating the fluid increases topical absorption. Contraindications to intraperitoneal chemotherapy include adhesive disease, hypovolemia, massive ascites, malnutrition, GI dysfunction, or postoperative infection (Marin et al, 2007). Complications may include wound infection, abdominal wound dehiscence, anastomotic leak sepsis, and enterocutaneous fistula (Marin et al, 2007).

Proper personal protective equipment (PPE) must be worn and safe medication handling practices must be employed to protect all team members and the patient from accidental injury from hazardous cytotoxic drugs (Risk Reduction Strategies). HIPEC has been shown to increase survival in select patients when combined with cytoreductive surgery (Pappas et al, 2008).

ENDOSCOPIC PROCEDURES

GI endoscopy has transformed the diagnosis and treatment of patients with GI diseases. Endoscopic procedures permit direct or video visual inspection of the contents and walls of the esophagus, stomach, duodenum, and colon. Endoscopy provides significant tools for routine screening of individuals at risk for GI disease (Ransohoff, 2005), for establishing a diagnosis, for determining preferred treatment of a disease process, and for follow-up after a treatment regimen or surgery. GI endoscopy, enhanced by advances in imaging, instrumentation, and accessory devices, has evolved into an interventional discipline, offering nonsurgical approaches to cure and palliation of symptoms of selected GI diseases and conditions. Common GI endoscopy procedures include esophagogastroduodenoscopy (EGD) (also referred to as gastroscopy or upper endoscopy), small bowel endoscopy (also referred to as push enteroscopy or double-balloon enteroscopy), colonoscopy (also referred to as lower endoscopy), and sigmoidoscopy (also referred to as a "flex sig").

Endoscopic procedures are performed with local anesthetics, IV moderate sedation/analgesia, or general anesthetics, all of which ensure a safe and complete examination. Smaller caliber flexible endoscopes have evolved so that they can be passed easily without the need for sedation (Research Highlight). IV moderate sedation provides a depressed level of consciousness and tolerance of a potentially uncomfortable procedure, yet patients retain their ability to maintain their airway and respond appropriately to physical and verbal stimuli. It is administered by the attending physician/interventionalist, anesthesia provider, or a registered nurse competent to monitor the patient's heart rate and rhythm, oxygen saturation, blood pressure, respirations, level of consciousness, and comfort during and immediately after the procedure until the patient is stable and ready for discharge or transfer. Preprocedure preparation for elective procedures limits ingestion of solid foods and liquids for a prescribed period. Bowel preparation with diet limitation, bowel cleansing preparations, and sometimes enemas is prescribed before lower endoscopy procedures.

Flexible endoscopes are semicritical patient care devices that must undergo high-level disinfection before each use. They are easily damaged by misuse and should be handled according to the manufacturer's recommendations. They must be leak-tested, decontaminated, reprocessed, and dried

►► RISK REDUCTION STRATEGIES

Safe Care and Handling of Cytotoxic Drugs

Safe work practices, engineering controls, and proper use of approved protective equipment can minimize potential health effects from occupational exposure to cytotoxic, antineoplastic drugs, and other hazardous drugs. Cytotoxic drugs are pharmaceutical compounds that are destructive to cells within the body. Antineoplastic agents control or kill cancer cells. They are cytotoxic but generally more damaging to dividing cells than to resting cells. Safe work practices include:

◆ Personal protective equipment (PPE) must be used whenever there is a risk of exposure to cytotoxic or other hazardous drugs; PPE includes nonpermeable gowns, latex or nitrile chemo gloves changed every 30 minutes or when torn, masks, and eye protection whenever there is risk for splash or eye exposure.
◆ PPE is worn whenever preparing, transferring, spiking, changing, priming, and disposing of chemotherapeutic agents (chemo).
◆ Always work below eye level.
◆ Have a chemo spill kit available wherever chemo is prepared, administered, stored, or disposed.
◆ Have yellow chemo waste containers available in the work area for contaminated sharps, linen, and trash.
◆ PPE is worn during chemo spill cleaning and when handling and disposing of patient body fluids. Wear the N95 NIOSH certified respirator mask when cleaning cytotoxic spills.
◆ Unused medication vials, bags, or syringes must be returned to the pharmacy or placed in chemo waste containers in the work area.
◆ Place needles, syringes, broken glass, empty vials, and tubing in the sharps containers labeled for chemotherapy waste.
◆ Place used PPE in yellow chemo waste container. Wash hands.
◆ If exposed, wash affected area with soap and water for 15 minutes. Flush eyes with normal saline for 15 minutes. Report to employee health or appropriate healthcare provider.

Modified from National Institute for Occupational Safety and Health: *Preventing occupational exposure to antineoplastic and other hazardous drugs in the health care setting,* available at www.cdc.gov/niosh/docs/2004-165. Accessed June 14, 2009.

after each use. They must be stored in an appropriate secure and ventilated endoscope closet. Endoscopic accessories, such as biopsy forceps, snares, cytology brushes, and fine-needle aspiration (FNA) catheters, must be sterile because they are considered critical devices that invade the mucosal barrier.

Esophagogastroduodenoscopy (EGD) (Upper Endoscopy)

EGD visualizes the esophagus, stomach, and proximal duodenum. It is used for diagnosis, treatment, and documentation of abnormalities with biopsy, brush cytology, polypectomy, electrosurgery, thermal coagulation, laser therapy, dilation, banding or sclerosing of esophageal varices, removal of foreign bodies, insertion of an esophageal prosthesis, and other interventional procedures for gastroesophageal reflux disease (GERD), Barrett's esophagus, and percutaneous endoscopic gastrostomy (PEG) tubes. When an EGD is performed with a local anesthetic or sedation, the patient is usually permitted no solid food for 6 to 8 hours before the procedure but may drink liquids up to 2 hours before the procedure.

Procedural Considerations. The patient's position for EGD depends on the areas to be visualized, but a left lateral supine or low Fowler's position is commonly used. For inspection of lesions in the gastric fundus and cardia, an upright sitting position may be used. A protective bite-block is placed in the patient's mouth to protect the scope and the patient's teeth from injury. Instrumentation includes a gastroscope and video system (optional), biopsy forceps, suction, water-soluble lubricant, saline and water for irrigation, and electrosurgery capability.

A topical local anesthetic (applied to the posterior pharynx) along with IV moderate sedation is the most common technique. A perioperative or endoscopy nurse skilled and credentialed in moderate sedation and advanced cardiac life support (ACLS) or an anesthesia provider monitors the airway, vital signs, and oxygenation.

A light source with air and water infusion capability and a water bottle for irrigation are required. Suction, aspiration tubes, and a cup of saline for the biopsy specimen should be available. Lubricating jelly is placed over the sheath of the gastroscope for ease in placement. An ESU and cord are available for fulgurating a lesion or coagulating a bleeding site.

Operative Procedure

1. The gastroscope tip is completely covered with a thin coat of water-soluble lubricating jelly.
2. During introduction of the gastroscope, the patient's head and neck must remain in the sagittal plane of the spine so that the axis of the mouth is in line with the esophagus.
3. The gastroscope is slowly passed through the nasopharynx into the esophagus, stomach, and duodenum.
4. The mucosal surface is inspected and contents may be aspirated for cytologic analysis. A biopsy may be performed.
5. After the procedure, the patient is monitored and must have a gag reflex before fluids are offered.

Small Bowel Enteroscopy

The small bowel has traditionally been a difficult segment of the GI tract to reach for endoscopic visualization. Enteroscopy can be approached orally or through the anus using an adult or pediatric colonoscope, or a push enteroscope that measures 200 to 250 cm in length. Push enteroscopy advances the scope far into the small bowel. A balloon on the tip of the scope permits it to be held in place. The patient receives IV metoclopramide (Reglan), promoting peristaltic advancement of the scope. The small bowel is examined as the scope is slowly withdrawn. This procedure may take 6 to 8 hours (Society of Gastroenterology Nurses and Associates [SGNA], 2004). Push enteroscopy is useful for examining areas of bleeding and strictures.

Double-balloon enteroscopy employs an enteroscope with a balloon on its end and on the end of the overtube, which creates a traction system that permits the small bowel to pleat itself onto the overtube, and prevents overstretching of the small intestine. This technique also permits visualization and therapeutic measures such as biopsies, coagulation of small bleeders, and lysis of strictures (Lewis, 2005; Sunada et al, 2005).

Colonoscopy and Sigmoidoscopy (Lower Endoscopy)

Colonoscopy is endoscopic examination of the colon from the rectum to the ileocecal valve. The bowel wall is inspected for abnormalities such as bleeding, polyps, inflammation, ulceration, or tumors during both insertion and withdrawal of the colonoscope. Colonoscopy facilitates biopsy, removal of polyps, electrocoagulation or laser treatment of tumors or bleeders, dilation, decompression, and provision for a video and photographic record of the procedure and findings. Sigmoidoscopy, both flexible and rigid, provides access and visualization of the sigmoid or descending colon to the level of the splenic flexure. Colonoscopy or sigmoidoscopy may be performed before colon or sigmoid resection for surgical localization of the tumor site with india ink tattooing or clip placement. This permits the surgeon to identify the tumor site, viewing the marked site from the serosal side of the colon by laparotomy or laparoscopy access.

Endoscopy can also be performed through an ostomy stoma to inspect an anastomosis site or identify recurrence of disease or bleeding. Reservoir pouches can also be inspected after surgical healing for anastomosis integrity, inflammation, bleeding, and other abnormalities. The patient must receive a clear liquid diet the day before colonoscopy and sigmoidoscopy and may receive bowel-cleansing agents such as citrate of magnesia or a commercial bowel prep solution. Enemas may be necessary before the procedure.

Procedural Considerations. The instruments and equipment that must be available to perform colonoscopy and sigmoidoscopy include a colonoscope or flexible sigmoidoscope, video camera and monitors (optional), a light source, an air-insufflation device with water bottle for irrigation, a biopsy forceps, snares, cytology brush, electrosurgical-fulguration-desiccation unit and appropriate accessories, lubricating jelly, and suction.

Operative Procedure

1. The patient is positioned on the left side with knees bent.
2. The well-lubricated colonoscope is passed slowly into the anal canal and advanced continuously until it reaches the cecum in colonoscopy. The endoscopist or surgeon may ask the nurse or surgical technologist to apply gentle abdominal pressure to assist advancement of the scope around the splenic or hepatic flexures. With sigmoidoscopy, only the left colon is examined. Flexible sigmoidoscopy may be accomplished in a cooperative patient without sedation.
3. After the endoscopic examination, the patient is observed for postprocedural bleeding, pain (Rapid Response Team box), signs of perforation, or reaction to medications.

Procedures for Gastroesophageal Reflux Disease (GERD)

GERD is described as a condition of backflow of gastric or duodenal contents into the distal esophagus, causing pain, heartburn, coughing, and respiratory distress. GERD may also present with incompetence of the distal esophageal valve to the stomach or lower esophageal sphincter (LES). Chronic GERD can lead to erosive esophagitis, asthma, dysphagia, aspiration pneumonia, and Barrett's esophagus. Several innovative, nonsurgical interventional endoscopic techniques now can minimize or prevent the reflux of stomach acid into the esophagus, controlling GERD symptoms by enhancing the competency of the LES. These procedures, accomplished through an EGD, or upper endoscopy, reinforce the LES by plicating and sewing the inner lumen of the esophageal junction to re-fashion the valve, tightening the tissue above the LES to create a stricture, or implanting devices to narrow the LES lumen. The American Gastroenterological Association's guidelines address management and treatment of GERD according to evidence-based medical literature. Recommended practice includes the use of proton pump inhibitor (PPI) medications as the first line of therapy followed by antireflux surgery only when the patient can no longer tolerate acid suppression therapy (Barclay et al, 2008).

Several antireflux procedures can be performed endoscopically in an endoscopy procedure room using moderate sedation or general anesthesia. The Stretta (Curon Medical) procedure is radiofrequency heat energy delivered through an endoscopically introduced balloon catheter to the distal esophagus, creating thermal lesions that tighten the tissue.

The EndoCinch (Bard Medical) technique dilates the lumen of the esophagus before passing the EndoCinch device through an EGD scope. The device is a sewing capsule that pinches or pleats mucosal folds and anchors them in place with a suture. Several plications are placed in a circumferential or staggered vertical pattern.

The Wilson-Cook sewing system (Wilson-Cook Medical) is another submucosal plication device that suctions a small fold of tissue into the lumen of the scope accessory, and then plicates, sutures, and knots the tissue pleat.

Procedures for Barrett's Esophagus

Cellular changes, or dysplasia, of the mucosa of the distal esophagus is called Barrett's esophagus, a precursor for cancer of the esophagus. A significant percentage of patients with

GERD may develop Barrett's. Patients who show progressive dysplasia in spite of medical therapies, such as histamine blockers and proton pump inhibitors, may be treated with one of several endoscopic techniques targeted to eliminate dysplastic tissue, prevent or eliminate strictures, and promote regrowth of normal esophageal mucosa.

Endoscopic mucosal resection (EMR) is an interventional technique to remove submucosal flat or depressed lesions. EUS is used to determine depth of invasion into the esophageal wall, and the lesion or dysplastic tissue is then injected with isotonic saline, hypertonic saline, or saline with epinephrine to lift the lesion away from the muscle layer, creating a polyp-like lesion. This tissue bulge is then suctioned into a cap secured to the end of the scope, resected with a rigid wire snare, and removed. The saline creates a cushion to protect the muscle wall from perforation and facilitates snare resection. This technique also provides a tissue specimen for histologic examination. Areas of bleeding can be endoscopically electrocoagulated (Ransohoff, 2005).

Photodynamic therapy (PDT) is a technique using laser light ablation. Dysplastic tissue uptakes a photosensitizer drug, Photofrin II (sodium porfimer), which is activated by the laser. The drug is administered 48 hours before the procedure to allow for tissue uptake. Normal tissue excretes the drug sooner than abnormal or dysplastic tissues. The drug is retained in the mucosal layer, which limits the depth of the laser effect. After 48 hours, the patient returns for the endoscopic procedure. The laser fiber is introduced through the scope channel and laser light is directed toward the mucosa, causing tissue destruction and cell death of those areas identified by the uptake of the photosensitizer drug. The patient may continue to be sensitive to light for 60 to 90 days following the injection and must take precautions to prevent cutaneous burns (Wang, 2005). Unlike EMR, PDT does not provide a tissue specimen. PDT is often combined with endoscopic mucosal resection. PDT and EMR can also be used to treat the gastric and colonic mucosa.

RAPID RESPONSE TEAM

In phase II PACU, while recovering from colonoscopy under moderate sedation, the patient described vague generalized abdominal pain, increasing in intensity. He had nausea and vomiting, low-grade fever, abdominal tenderness, guarding, and muscle rigidity on palpation. Respirations were shallow and he was tachycardic and anxious. The gastroenterologist had left the building. The nurse, concerned about his increasing distress and delay in normal recovery after colonoscopy, summoned the hospital rapid response team, using the SBAR format in her call for assistance:

Situation—"I have a patient with increasing abdominal distress, tachycardia, and shallow respirations."

Background—"The patient is a 53-year-old normally healthy man post screening colonoscopy. The procedure was unremarkable; however, he has complained of increasing vague abdominal pain, nausea, and vomiting."

Assessment—"He has abdominal tenderness, guarding, and rigidity on palpation. He is tachycardic with shallow

respirations and a low-grade fever, which he did not have before the procedure. He states that he has never felt like this before and is afraid something is seriously wrong. His wife is very concerned. He has emerged from the moderate sedation; however, this is not a normal recovery from a routine colonoscopy."

Recommendation—"His condition is deteriorating and he must be seen now. I am concerned he may have a perforation of the colon. He is in Endoscopy recovery bed 4."

The rapid response team consisted of an ICU nurse, respiratory therapist, and critical care hospitalist. They performed a focused assessment and review of the medical record, placed an additional IV line and administered fluids, ordered a stat abdominal CT scan and pain medication, and called the surgeon on-call. The CT revealed free air in the abdomen and perforation at the splenic flexure of the colon. The patient had emergency surgery for repair of the perforation and recovered without incident.

Adapted from O'Brien D: Postanesthesia complications. In Drain CB, Odom-Ferren J, editors: *Perianesthesia nursing: a critical care approach*, ed 5, St Louis, 2009, Saunders.

Self-Expanding Metal Stents

Self-expanding metal stents (SEMSs) expand within a lumen to maintain patency in an area constrained by stricture or tumor. They are used in the esophagus or colon, advanced across the obstruction, and released to remain in place. They are preloaded in a closed position on a delivery catheter, introduced through an endoscope with fluoroscopy guidance, and deployed, applying radial force that holds them in place. Stents may also be made of silicone. Although initial complications are low, stents may migrate, perforate, become impacted with food, cause bleeding or fistula development, or become obstructed with tumor overgrowth. Stent placement is frequently a palliative procedure.

SURGERY OF THE ESOPHAGUS

Esophagectomy

Esophageal cancer is the sixth most common cancer worldwide and is notorious for aggressive progression of intramural invasion of the esophageal wall and lymphatic metastasis (Edmondson and Schiech, 2008). Esophageal cancer may be adenocarcinoma or squamous cell, each with an equally poor prognosis when treated in late stages. As many as 50% of patients with esophageal cancer are ineligible for surgery because of late-stage diagnosis, debilitating multisystem conditions, infection, or malnutrition.

Esophagectomy can be performed by several different approaches and procedures: transthoracic, transhiatal, video-assisted thoracotomy surgery (VATS), or laparoscopic-assisted approach. A segment of the colon or jejunum may be used as a reconstructive conduit in the patient with prior partial or total gastrectomy.

Procedural Considerations. Instrumentation includes a basic thoracotomy set, basic laparotomy set, vascular instruments, and a GI instrument set. Long versions of basic instruments, deep retractors, linear stapling devices, and vascular ligating clips should also be available. Laparoscopic and thoracoscopic instrumentation and video equipment is used in the VATS approach. The surgeon may perform an EGD before the surgical prep. The patient is positioned and secured in the preferred position for the intended surgical approach after induction of general anesthesia. A double-lumen endotracheal tube is placed in order to deflate the lung for a thoracotomy approach. Critical monitoring devices, such as arterial lines and pulmonary artery catheters, are placed. An indwelling urinary catheter is inserted. Measures are taken to ensure that the patient's body temperature is maintained in normothermia. Any of these procedures may be modified with laparoscopic, thoracoscopic, mini-laparotomy, or mini-thoracotomy access. Postoperative pain management may be augmented with interscalene perineural blockade for shoulder pain. Patients undergoing esophagectomy usually are transferred to the intensive care unit (ICU).

Transhiatal Esophagectomy

1. Transhiatal esophagectomy removes from 67% to 100% of the thoracic esophagus through an upper midline abdominal incision and an incision in the neck above the left clavicle. The abdominal component may be approached laparoscopically. Thoracotomy is avoided.

2. Accessible lymph nodes are removed for staging purposes. Not all lymph nodes can be accessed.

3. The stomach is mobilized and fashioned into a tubular shape at the greater curvature with surgical staples.

4. The tubular stomach segment is tunneled up through the posterior mediastinum to the left cervical incision. This procedure is often called a gastric pull-up.

5. The stomach is reconstructed with the fundus attached to the remaining cervical portion of the proximal esophagus using an end-to-side anastomosis. The fundus is also sutured to the cervical prevertebral fascia.

6. A pyloromyotomy or pyloroplasty then follows to increase stomach emptying. This often results in postoperative "dumping syndrome" and reflux.

7. A jejunostomy tube is placed for postoperative enteral nutrition.

8. Postoperative hoarseness and dysphagia are common because of ipsilateral nerve damage.

Transthoracic Esophagectomy

Transthoracic esophagectomy is indicated for disease of the middle third of the esophagus and high-grade dysplasia in Barrett's esophagus. This approach permits complete lymph node dissection under direct vision and combines a left-sided thoracoabdominal incision or separate right posterior lateral thoracotomy and midline abdominal incision. The latter describes the traditional Ivor Lewis approach. Another variation, sometimes called the "three-hole esophagectomy," combines a cervical, right thoracotomy, and midline laparotomy approach for proximal tumors. The single incision thoracoabdominal incision provides the best exposure for low gastroesophageal junction tumors and is indicated for patients with cardiac and pulmonary disease.

Operative Procedure
1. The skin incision is carried downward, midway between the vertebral border of the scapula and the spinous processes to the eighth rib and then forward along this rib to the costochondral junction. The extent of the vertical portion of the incision depends on the tumor's location.

2. The wound is retracted, and bleeding vessels are ligated or coagulated.

3. The chest cavity is opened, and the rib spreader is placed. Moist packs are placed, and the lung is retracted with a Deaver or Harrington retractor.

4. The mediastinal pleura is incised with long Metzenbaum scissors and long plain forceps in line with the esophagus and the lesion.

5. The esophagus is dissected free from the aorta with dry gauze dissectors.

6. Suture ligatures of 2-0 and 3-0 nonabsorbable material are used to control bleeding vessels.

7. The diaphragm is opened, and a series of traction sutures are placed.

8. The stomach is mobilized by dissection of its ligamental attachment with long scissors and curved thoracic clamps.

9. The left gastric artery is clamped, cut, and doubly ligated with 2-0 nonabsorbable suture and a suture ligature of 3-0 nonabsorbable material. The sterile field is prepared for the open method of anastomosis.

10. The stomach is transected well below the lesion with selected resection instruments.
11. Closure of the stomach is completed with two rows of intestinal sutures of 2-0 synthetic absorbable suture and sometimes with an additional row of 3-0 nonabsorbable sutures for reinforcement. A linear stapling device may be used as well.
12. A separate circular opening is usually made in the upper portion of the stomach for anastomosis to the esophagus.
13. Two Allen clamps or a stapler type of clamp is applied above the stricture, and the freed esophagus is divided.
14. The circular opening in the stomach and the transected end of the esophagus are anastomosed. The mucosal layers are approximated. The muscular layers of the esophagus and stomach are closed by two rows of interrupted sutures. A mechanical end-to-end anastomosing (EEA) surgical stapling device may also be used to accomplish the gastro-esophageal anastomosis.
15. The stomach is anchored to the pleura, and the edges of the diaphragm are sutured to the wall of the stomach with interrupted sutures of 3-0 or 2-0 nonabsorbable material.
16. The pleura is cleansed with warm normal saline irrigation, which is then removed by suctioning.
17. A thoracic catheter is inserted for closed drainage. The chest wall is closed as described for thoracotomy.

Video-Assisted Thoracotomy Surgery (VATS)

1. VATS is accomplished in three stages beginning with thoracoscopic dissection and mobilization of the esophagus.
2. The second stage is the laparoscopic dissection, mobilization, and tubular construction of the stomach. Pyloroplasty is also performed laparoscopically.
3. The third stage is the open cervical incision anastomosis.

Excision of Esophageal Diverticulum

Excision of an esophageal diverticulum, sometimes called *Zenker's diverticulum,* is removal of a weakening in the wall of the esophagus that collects small amounts of food and causes a sensation of fullness in the neck. Diverticula usually occur in the cervical portion of the esophagus, and excision usually relieves symptoms completely.

Procedural Considerations. Instrumentation includes a thyroid set with the addition of Pennington clamps, curved mosquito hemostats, 5-inch Adson forceps, and lateral retractors. The patient is positioned supine with a shoulder roll placed to assist with hyperextension of the neck. The head may be turned to the side and supported with a padded headrest. This procedure may be done endoscopically.

Operative Procedure
1. An incision is made over the inner border of the sternocleidomastoid muscle and is extended from the level of the hyoid bone to a point 2 cm above the clavicle.
2. The sac of the diverticulum is freed and ligated.
3. The pharyngeal muscle and surrounding tissues are closed.
4. In conjunction with this procedure, an esophageal myotomy is often performed distal to the diverticulum to minimize likelihood of recurrence.

Esophageal Hiatal Hernia Repair and Antireflux Procedure

Hiatal herniorrhaphy restores the LES to its correct anatomic position in the abdomen, secures it firmly in place, and corrects GERD. A hiatal hernia (also called a *diaphragmatic hernia*) is a defect, either congenital or acquired, in the diaphragm through which a portion of the stomach protrudes up into the thoracic cavity.

Hiatal hernias are usually of two types—paraesophageal and sliding. Symptoms vary from none to severe heartburn, reflux (backward flow), regurgitation, and dysphagia. When symptoms are severe, a repair of the hernia is done, usually through a transabdominal approach. A transthoracic approach is used for patients with prior left upper quadrant surgery and for those who are extremely obese.

An antireflux procedure, to prevent reflux of gastric juices into the esophagus, is also done when the hernia is repaired. The three most frequently performed antireflux procedures are the Nissen, Hill, and Belsey Mark IV.

Procedural Considerations. The patient is positioned supine but may need to be repositioned to lateral if the gastroesophageal sphincter cannot be accessed through a high midline position. An indwelling urinary catheter is inserted after induction of general anesthesia.

Instrumentation includes a basic laparotomy set, Maloney or Hurst dilators in sizes 32 French (32F) to 42F, a self-retaining retractor system, and a 1-inch Penrose drain. If a transthoracic approach is planned, a basic thoracic set is required.

Operative Procedure
1. Through a transabdominal incision, the hernia is located and a crural repair is done.
2. The fundus of the stomach is wrapped around the lower 4 to 6 cm of the esophagus and is sutured in place (Nissen fundoplication); the upper part of the lesser curvature of the stomach and the cardioesophageal junction are sutured to the median arcuate ligament (Hill procedure); or the stomach is plicated approximately 270 degrees around the esophageal circumference (Belsey Mark IV procedure). The Nissen fundoplication procedure is illustrated in Figure 2-33.
3. Vagotomy, pyloroplasty, or both may be performed at the same time.
4. The wound is closed.

Laparoscopic Nissen Fundoplication

The Nissen-Rossetti fundoplication and several other laparoscopic procedures have been developed for GERD management. Nissen fundoplication is also used in the following ways: to reduce the hernia, to eliminate the hernia sac, and to repair the large defect in the diaphragm hiatus. GERD may also be treated with a silicone prosthetic implant placed around the distal esophagus under the diaphragm and above the stomach. The prosthesis, a small donut-shaped device with an open end that is sutured to be continuous, allows food to pass but prevents the stomach from sliding into the chest cavity. This procedure may also be performed as an open laparotomy.

The patient undergoing a laparoscopic Nissen fundoplication is usually admitted the day of surgery. Surgery is performed through five trocar sites in the abdomen, which greatly reduces postoperative recovery. The patient is typically discharged by the second postoperative day if there are no complications. A postoperative upper GI series verifies functioning of the newly constructed antireflux valve.

Procedural Considerations. Surgery is performed using a general anesthetic to anesthetize the patient. A nasogastric (NG) tube and urinary drainage catheter are placed after induction and intubation. The patient is positioned supine or in the modified lithotomy position.

Instrumentation and supplies include a basic laparotomy set, laparoscope, laparoscopic camera, five trocars (trocar size or sizes depend on the surgeons' preference), a light cord, filtered insufflation tubing, and an ESU cord. Laparoscopic instruments commonly used include grasping forceps, endoscissors, endo-Babcock forceps, endodissecting forceps, endoclip appliers, an endosuturing device, and endoretractors, such as the fan retractor. Suction and a suction-irrigator are commonly used. A Penrose drain or a 12F red Robinson catheter is used to assist in isolating and retracting the distal esophagus. Bougie dilators (large sizes, such as 40F to 60F) may be used as an esophageal stent by which to secure the fundoplication. A water-based lubricating jelly is used to assist the anesthesia provider in placing the bougie. Equipment needed for the procedure includes an ESU, an insufflation unit with CO_2 gas, and two video monitors (one placed on each side of the patient).

Operative Procedure

1. A stab wound is made with a #11 blade for insertion of the first trocar.
2. The trocar is placed, and insufflation achieved. This may be performed before placing the trocar by inserting a *Veress* needle for insufflation.
3. The laparoscope is placed through the port, and the camera attached to the laparoscope.
4. Two trocars are placed below the xiphoid process, in the right upper quadrant of the abdomen, high in the costal margin, about 5 to 6 mm to the right and left of the midline. Another trocar is placed on the lateral plane to the midline in the left abdomen (left midclavicular). The last trocar is placed in the lateral abdominal wall for use by the assistant.
5. A fan-shaped endoretractor is inserted through the right midclavicular port site and used to retract the left lobe of the liver to expose the gastroesophageal junction.
6. An endo-Babcock forceps is inserted through the left midclavicular port and is used to grasp the upper aspect of the fundus of the stomach. The stomach is retracted laterally and downward. This port site is also used for insertion of a grasper to hold the Penrose drain, clip applier, and ultrasonic coagulating shears.
7. The surgeon mobilizes the distal esophagus by opening the hiatus and employs an endodissector forceps to bluntly dissect the tissue along the right and left crura.
8. Endoclips are used to ligate the most distal portion of the pericardiophrenic vessel before it is divided.
9. The posterior vagus is identified but left intact.
10. Dissection is continued to expose the posterior esophagus.
11. The upper aspect of the greater curvature of the stomach is mobilized, and dissection continues to the posterior esophagus.

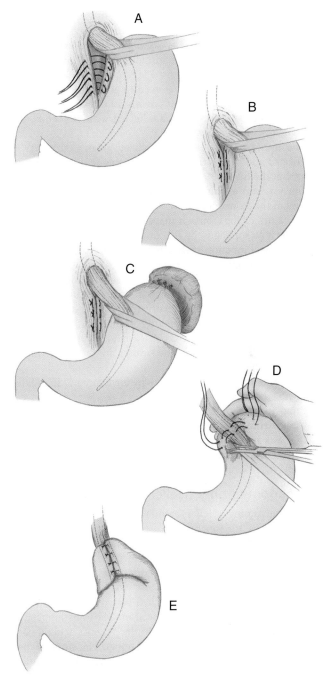

FIGURE 2-33 The Nissen fundoplication procedure begins with oral passage of a Maloney dilator (40F to 48F) into the lumen of the stomach. **A,** The esophagus is then mobilized. A Penrose drain is placed around the gastroesophageal junction to pull the esophagus down and out of the hernia. **B,** Shown are three heavy sutures (#0 braided absorbable) placed to narrow the hiatal aperture but not so tight as to constrict the esophagus, thus the purpose of stenting the esophagus with the Maloney dilator. **C,** Further traction is applied to the distal esophagus while the proximal stomach and fundus are freed from all peritoneal attachments. **D,** The posterior wall of the stomach is relocated around the distal esophagus. **E,** The stomach walls are wrapped and sutured around the intraabdominal esophagus, with the Maloney stent in place.

12. The Penrose or Robinson catheter is inserted through a sheath and is passed behind the gastroesophageal junction. The ends are united and secured with an endoclamp that is then locked and used as a traction retractor during the procedure.
13. Another grasping forceps is used to grasp the apex of the gastric fundus and retract it downward to expose the short gastric vessels. The vessels are ligated with endoclips and divided with endoscissors.
14. The upper portion of the mobilized greater curvature is grasped and passed through the opening that has been created at the hiatus.
15. Tension and adequate mobilization of the greater curvature of the stomach are assessed. The portion of the greater curvature of the stomach that has been moved around the posterior esophagus at the proximal part of the gastroesophageal junction is then manipulated over the anterior distal esophagus.
16. A nonabsorbable endosuture is passed through a 5-mm port and used to place a row of interrupted sutures to join the aspects of the greater curvature of the stomach in a 2-cm to 3-cm "wrap" around the esophagus.
17. The anesthesia provider passes a large bougie down the lumen of the esophagus. The sutures are secured with the bougie in place.
18. The catheter (or drain) and bougie are removed. The abdomen is deflated.
19. Final inspection is completed, hemostasis obtained, and the instruments and ports removed under direct vision so that any bleeding from the abdominal wall can be readily detected. The trocar sites are then closed and dressings applied.

Esophagomyotomy (Heller Procedure)

Esophagomyotomy (Heller cardiomyotomy) is myotomy of the esophagogastric junction to correct esophageal obstruction resulting from achalasia, a motility disorder of aperistalsis of the esophagus and elevated LES pressure. These patients have dysphagia, esophageal fullness, regurgitation, and weight loss (SGNA, 2004).

Procedural Considerations. Selection of a transthoracic or transabdominal incision depends on the patient's general condition and other existing pathologic factors. The surgeon may elect to perform a pyloroplasty to prevent reflux by promoting stomach emptying. Instrumentation includes a basic laparotomy set and instruments to enter and retract the thorax if necessary. Laparoscopic and VATS approaches are safe and effective alternatives to the open procedure. The laparoscopic approach offers the advantage of adding fundoplication (Lee et al, 2004). Potential postoperative complications include esophageal perforation and reflux.

Operative Procedure
1. A midline abdominal incision is made from the xiphoid process to the umbilicus.
2. After exposure of the esophagogastric junction, a Maloney dilator is inserted through the patient's oral cavity to distend the esophagus.

3. A scalpel with a #15 blade is used to make a longitudinal incision through the muscular wall of the distal esophagus and proximal stomach, leaving the mucosa intact.
4. A small portion of the fundus of the stomach may be plicated to the lateral wall of the esophagus.
5. The wound is closed.
6. VATS is approached with the patient positioned and secured in a right lateral position.
7. A 30-degree thoracoscope is inserted in the left eighth intercostal space along the left posterior axillary line.
8. The lung is retracted through a working port placed in the left anterior axillary line of the fifth space.
9. Dissection is done through a mini-thoracotomy in the left ninth intercostal space to sweep the muscular layer from the mucosa from 6 cm above and 1 cm below the gastroesophageal junction. This dissection is made halfway around the circumference of the esophagus.
10. A chest tube is placed and the incision and port sites closed.

Esophageal Dilation

Esophageal dilation may be indicated in patients who have an esophageal stricture related to past surgery, chemical or thermal injury, or anatomic anomalies. An upper GI series is required before the procedure to locate the stricture.

Procedural Considerations. Esophageal dilation is a clean procedure performed in the OR or endoscopy unit. General anesthesia or moderate sedation is usually indicated. An esophageal perforation is a complication that could require open repair. The patient is positioned supine.

A flexible gastroscope and light source with video camera and monitor, bougie dilators (Hurst or Maloney dilators are commonly used) in graduated sizes, water-soluble lubricant, gauze sponges, and gloves are required to perform the procedure. An esophageal stent that can be inserted through a large-channel gastroscope or along a guidewire may be requested. The surgeon may use fluoroscopy to demonstrate that the dilation site is accurate by combining esophagoscopy with fluoroscopy and marking the site of stricture distally and proximally with radiopaque markers taped to the patient's skin.

Operative Procedure
1. The bougies are arranged in graduated order beginning with the smallest size (24F) and progressing to the largest size (60F).
2. The surgeon may first perform gastroscopy and pass a guidewire through the esophageal stricture.
3. The bougies are then passed one at a time gently but firmly through the stricture in an attempt to dilate the esophageal lumen.
4. Continuation of the dilation to the largest bougie depends on ease of passage and the patient's tolerance.
5. Laser therapy may be indicated for palliation if a tumor mass is causing the stricture. The neodymium:yttrium-aluminum-garnet (Nd:YAG) laser energy may be delivered to the mass or stricture by way of a flexible quartz fiber passed through the operative channel of the gastroscope.
6. An esophageal stent may be placed at the stricture site to decrease the chance of recurrence.

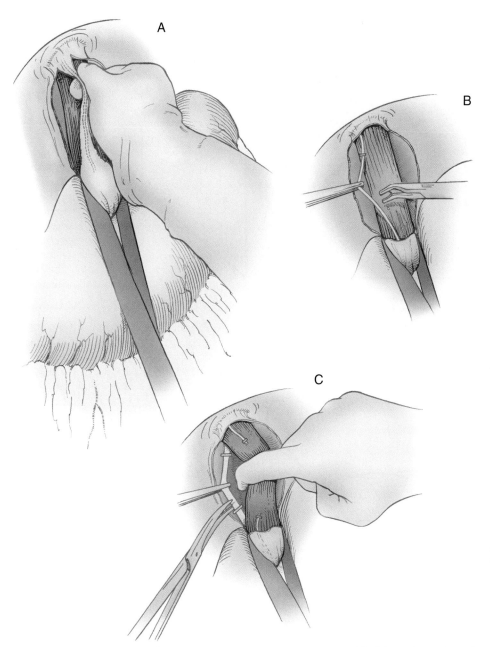

FIGURE 2-34 Truncal vagotomy. **A,** The phrenoesophageal ligament is lifted from the surface of the esophagus, and the vagal trunks are identified. **B,** Ligating clips are applied to the vagus nerve. **C,** Ligating clips have been applied to the larger posterior nerve in preparation for resecting a 2-cm segment between the clips.

SURGERY OF THE STOMACH

Vagotomy

Truncal vagotomy is identification of the two vagal trunks on the distal esophagus and resection of a segment of each, including any additional nerve fibers running separately from the trunks. By interrupting parasympathetic innervation, this procedure reduces gastric acid secretion in patients with duodenal ulcers. When truncal vagotomy was initially performed alone, a high incidence of gastric stasis resulted from the loss of cholinergic innervation to the smooth muscle of the stomach;

thus pyloroplasty or another gastric drainage procedure almost always accompanies truncal vagotomy. Truncal vagotomy deprives not only the stomach but also the liver, gallbladder, bile duct, pancreas, small intestine, and half of the large intestine of parasympathetic nerve supply (Figure 2-34). Truncal vagotomy with antrectomy or a drainage procedure is the most common operation for duodenal ulcers.

Selective vagotomy is transection of each abdominal vagus at a point just beyond its bifurcation into gastric and extragastric divisions. Thus the hepatic branch of the anterior vagus and the celiac branch of the posterior vagus are preserved.

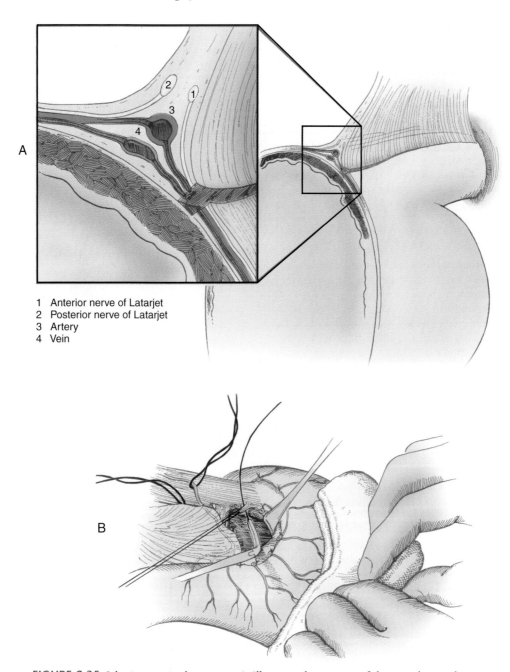

1 Anterior nerve of Latarjet
2 Posterior nerve of Latarjet
3 Artery
4 Vein

FIGURE 2-35 Selective proximal vagotomy. **A,** Illustrates the junction of the gastrohepatic ligament with the lesser curve of the stomach and demonstrates the anterior (*1*) and posterior (*2*) nerves of Latarjet, along with the artery (*3*) and vein (*4*). **B,** The lesser curve is lifted with a vein retractor to facilitate serial ligation of the intermediate and posterior neurovascular attachments.

Selective vagotomy has theoretical advantages over truncal vagotomy because vagal innervation of the viscera other than the stomach is preserved. However, selective vagotomy also denervates the entire stomach, so that addition of a drainage procedure is still necessary. Selective vagotomy may cause less postvagotomy diarrhea than truncal vagotomy does, but the incidence of dumping syndrome is probably the same or even higher. Both procedures are about equally effective in controlling duodenal ulcers.

Parietal cell vagotomy is the vagal denervation of only the parietal cell area of the stomach. The technique spares the main nerves of Latarjet, but divides all vagal branches that terminate on the proximal two thirds of the stomach. The operation has also been called *proximal gastric vagotomy* (Figure 2-35) and highly selective vagotomy. Because antral innervation is preserved, gastric emptying is unimpaired and a drainage procedure is unnecessary. The incidence of dumping and diarrhea after *parietal cell vagotomy* is much lower than that after truncal or selective vagotomy.

Procedural Considerations. Instrumentation for vagotomy includes a basic thoracotomy set (if a thoracoabdominal incision is to be used), a laparotomy set, a GI instrument set, blunt nerve hooks (Smith-Wick), 10-inch vessel clip appliers with clips, and 10-inch Metzenbaum dissecting scissors. A 1-inch Penrose drain is used to retract the esophagus. After receiving a general anesthetic, the patient is positioned supine. A laparoscopic approach may also be used.

Operative Procedure

1. A midline incision is made, and the esophagus identified and retracted with a 1-inch wide Penrose drain.
2. The vagus nerves or their branches, depending on which type of vagotomy is being done, are identified, clamped with either a ligature or a hemostatic clip, and resected.
3. The wound is closed in layers.

Pyloroplasty (Pyloromyotomy)

Pyloroplasty is the formation of a larger passageway between the prepyloric region of the stomach and the first or second portion of the duodenum. A pyloroplasty may be performed for treatment of a peptic ulcer under selected conditions but is more frequently employed to remove cicatricial bands in the pyloric ring, thus relieving spasm and permitting rapid emptying of the stomach. In adults, a vagotomy is usually performed with a pyloroplasty.

Procedural Considerations. A laparotomy set and GI instrument set are required. The patient is positioned supine, and a general anesthetic is administered. An NG tube is placed and an indwelling urinary catheter inserted.

Operative Procedure

1. The abdominal cavity is opened through a midline incision.
2. The pylorus of the stomach is isolated.
3. An incision is made through the stomach and the duodenum.
4. The pyloroplasty is closed with nonabsorbable or synthetic absorbable intestinal sutures.
5. The abdominal wound is closed in layers, and a dressing is applied.

Percutaneous Endoscopic Gastrostomy (PEG)

PEG is now the most popular gastrostomy tube placement approach. After administration of a local anesthetic or induction of moderate sedation/analgesia, the tube is placed endoscopically. It can be used for gastric decompression and enteral feedings. PEG uses a flexible gastroscope and a uniquely designed gastrostomy tube for placement through the abdominal wall; it requires a push-pull technique to insert. This procedure may be done in the endoscopy suite, in the OR, or at the bedside in a critical care unit if necessary.

Procedural Considerations. A PEG tube kit containing the following is required: a percutaneous needle, a long silk suture with one end strengthened for feeding it down the lumen of the needle, a percutaneous gastrostomy tube, and a bolster. A flexible gastroscopy system is also required as well as snare forceps.

The patient is positioned supine after being anesthetized with IV moderate sedation. A bite-block is inserted into the patient's mouth.

Operative Procedure

1. The gastroscope is passed.
2. The end of the scope is angled anteriorly to the left anterolateral wall of the stomach's fundus so that the light from the gastroscope can be seen through the abdominal wall.
3. The stomach is insufflated with air through the gastroscope.
4. A local anesthetic is injected at the site of the intended gastrostomy if the patient is awake.
5. A small stab wound is made with a #11 blade.
6. The percutaneous needle is inserted into the abdominal wall and into the stomach lumen under direct visualization of the gastroscope.
7. The long silk suture is threaded into the lumen of the needle and passed into the stomach, where it is snared with the forceps.
8. A clamp is applied to the exterior distal end of the suture after the needle is removed.
9. The gastroscope is removed, and the suture extends out of the patient's oral cavity.
10. The suture is then attached to the tapered end of the gastrostomy tube.
11. The gastrostomy tube is gently guided into the patient's oral cavity, down the esophagus, and into the lumen of the stomach and pulled through the abdominal wall ("push-pull" technique).
12. The tube is secured with an internal bolster by reinserting the gastroscope and snugging it close to the gastric wall under direct visualization.
13. An external bolster is applied over the tube and snugged to the abdominal wall. Care is taken to ensure the bolsters do not compress the tissues because such compression might compromise tissue integrity and perfusion.
14. The distal end of the tube is cut, and a connector is applied.
15. The patient's stomach is deflated, and the procedure is complete.

Closure of Perforated Gastric or Duodenal Ulcer

Closure of a perforation in the stomach or duodenum is performed through a high right rectus or midline abdominal incision.

Procedural Considerations. A perforated gastric or duodenal ulcer is treated as a surgical emergency, and the operation is performed as soon as the diagnosis is made. The patient is typed and crossmatched so that an adequate supply of blood is available. A gastric lavage is not performed, but continuous suction is used. A laparotomy set and a GI instrument set are required. Linear stapling instruments should be available.

Operative Procedure

1. Through a right rectus or midline abdominal incision, the perforation is located.
2. Suction is used to remove exudate in the peritoneal cavity.
3. The perforation is closed with a purse-string suture by inverting the raw edges and suturing a piece of omentum over the closure.
4. The ulcerated area may be resected using linear stapling devices.
5. The abdomen is copiously irrigated with warm saline, which may contain a broad-spectrum antibiotic.

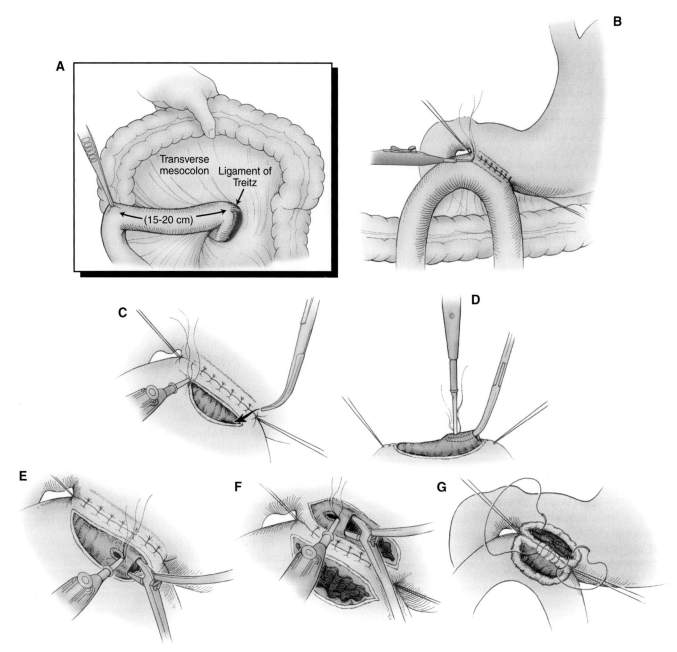

FIGURE 2-36 Gastrojejunostomy. **A,** Illustrates the selection of a segment of jejunum that will be anastomosed to the stomach; the distance between the ligament of Treitz and the anastomosis should not be excessively long or under any tension. **B,** A posterior row of interrupted sutures is placed between the gastric and jejunal serosae, and the sites of the gastric and jejunal stomas are scored with the electrosurgical pencil. **C,** The jejunal stoma is created by dissecting through the serosa and muscularis with the electrosurgical pencil. An opening is made in the mucosa, and a right-angled clamp is inserted into the lumen. **D,** The clamp is opened and elevated. **E,** Electrosurgery is applied between the two jaws of the clamp. **F,** The procedure is repeated for creating the gastric stoma. **G,** Full-thickness anastomosis is begun posteriorly.

6. The abdominal wound is closed in layers, and a dressing applied.

Gastrojejunostomy

Gastrojejunostomy establishes a permanent communication between the proximal jejunum and either the anterior or the posterior stomach, without removing any segment of the GI tract (Figure 2-36). It is accomplished through a midline or paramedian abdominal incision.

Gastrojejunostomy is performed to treat a benign obstruction at the pyloric end of the stomach or an inoperable lesion of the pylorus when a partial gastrectomy is not feasible. It also provides a large opening without sphincter obstruction.

Procedural Considerations. Laparotomy and GI instrument sets are required. Linear stapling instruments should be available. The patient is positioned supine after induction of general anesthesia. The anesthesia provider inserts an NG tube after intubation. An indwelling catheter is placed into the urinary bladder before the abdominal skin prep.

Operative Procedure

1. Through an upper midline or paramedian abdominal incision, exploration of the peritoneal cavity is completed, as described for routine laparotomy.
2. The pathologic condition is confirmed.
3. Warm, moist packs are placed, and a self-retaining retractor is positioned.
4. A loop of proximal jejunum is grasped with a Babcock forceps and freed from the mesentery.
5. The loop of jejunum is approximated to either the anterior or the posterior stomach wall several centimeters from the greater curvature of the stomach.
6. Nonabsorbable 2-0 traction sutures are placed through the serosal layers at each end of the selected portion of the jejunum and stomach.
7. Gastroenterostomy clamps may be placed before insertion of the posterior interrupted 3-0 or 2-0 nonabsorbable serosal sutures.
8. The field is draped for open anastomosis (bowel technique).
9. The jejunum and stomach are opened.
10. Bleeding points are clamped with mosquito or Crile hemostats and ligated with 3-0 synthetic absorbable sutures.
11. The inner posterior row of sutures is placed, using atraumatic intestinal needles with 2-0 or 3-0 synthetic absorbable suture, and continued for the first anterior row.
12. The anastomosis is completed with anterior serosal sutures of 3-0 or 2-0 nonabsorbable material.
13. Traction sutures are removed.
14. Interrupted 4-0 nonabsorbable sutures may be used for reinforcement.
15. Contaminated instruments are discarded into a basin.
16. The abdominal wound is closed in layers, and a dressing applied.

Partial Gastrectomy—Billroth I and Billroth II

A Billroth I gastrectomy is resection of a diseased portion of the stomach through a right paramedian or midline abdominal incision and establishment of an anastomosis between the stomach and duodenum. It is performed to remove a benign or malignant lesion located in the pylorus, or upper half of the stomach. One of several techniques may be followed to establish GI continuity, including the Schoemaker, the von Haberer-Finney, and other modifications of the Billroth I procedure (Figure 2-37).

Procedural Considerations. Laparotomy and GI instrument sets are required. Linear stapling instruments should be available. The patient is positioned supine after induction of general anesthesia. The anesthesia provider inserts an NG tube after intubation. An indwelling urinary catheter is inserted before the abdominal skin prep.

Operative Procedure

1. The abdominal wall is incised, and the peritoneal cavity is opened and explored.

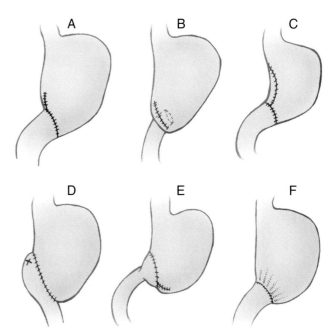

FIGURE 2-37 Diagrams illustrating resections of stomach with anastomosis of stomach and duodenum (gastroduodenal anastomosis). All are modifications of the Billroth I technique, in which the stomach is moved to the duodenum. **A**, Billroth I: after pylorus is removed, lesser curvature is partially closed and duodenum is sutured to open end of stomach at its lower margin. **B**, Kocher: distal end of stomach is closed, and duodenum is transferred up to posterior margin of closed stomach. **C**, Schoemaker: lesser curvature of stomach is sutured closed and brought down to same size as duodenum, and end-to-end anastomosis is done. **D**, von Haberer-Finney: side of duodenum is transferred up to end of stomach so that entire end of stomach is open for direct anastomosis. **E**, Horsley: lesser curvature end of stomach is used to suture to duodenum and closes greater curvature end. **F**, von Haberer: modification of operation shown in D. Stomach is, so to speak, narrowed or puckered so that it fits end of duodenum. Modification of this is done by some surgeons as follows: duodenum is split longitudinally, and its ends are flared open so that opening is large enough to fit open end of stomach.

2. Bleeding vessels are clamped and ligated or coagulated.
3. The abdominal wound is retracted, and the surrounding organs are protected with warm, moist packs.
4. The gastrocolic omentum is freed from the colon mesentery to prevent injury to the middle colic artery.
5. With hemostats and Metzenbaum scissors, the right and left gastroepiploic arteries and veins are clamped, divided, and ligated with 2-0 nonabsorbable sutures and 2-0 and 3-0 suture ligatures, thereby freeing the greater curvature of the stomach.
6. The gastric vessels are clamped, divided, and ligated to free the diseased portion of the stomach.
7. The operative field is prepared for open anastomosis (bowel technique).
8. After sectioning the stomach from the greater to lesser curvature, two Allen intestinal anastomosis clamps or other suitable clamps, or linear stapling device, are placed on the upper portion of the duodenum just distal to the pylorus.

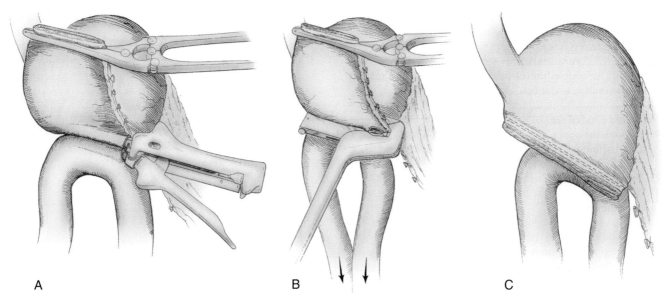

FIGURE 2-38 Subtotal gastrectomy with stapled Billroth II anastomosis. **A,** The distal stomach has been dissected free and resected just distal to the pylorus. A proximal limb of jejunum is transferred up to anastomose to the posterior wall of the stomach with a linear stapling instrument that transects between two parallel staple lines. **B,** The stomach is elevated, and a 90-degree mechanical stapling device is placed across the distal stomach. **C,** Illustration of the completed subtotal gastrectomy with stapled antecolic gastrojejunostomy.

9. The duodenum is divided by scalpel, electrosurgery, or a linear cutting and stapling device (e.g., gastrointestinal anastomosis [GIA]).
10. Additional moist packs are placed for protection, and two sets of anastomosis clamps are placed across the stomach.
11. Division of the stomach is completed.
12. At the lower margin, the opened stomach is approximated to the duodenum by a series of interrupted sutures placed in the serosal layers. An atraumatic intestinal needle with 3-0 nonabsorbable suture is used. Suture ends are held with hemostats, and the intestinal clamps are removed.
13. Stumps of the stomach and duodenum are cleansed with moist sponges, and bleeding vessels are ligated with fine suture or coagulated.
14. During anastomosis of the stomach and remaining duodenum, the involved segments may be held with rubber-shod clamps. The excess of the lesser curvature of the stomach is closed on completion of the anastomosis.
15. Instruments used in the open portion of the GI tract are discarded into a separate basin.
16. Routine laparotomy closure is completed.

A Billroth II gastrectomy is resection of the distal portion of the stomach through an abdominal incision and establishment of an anastomosis between the stomach and jejunum. It is performed to remove a benign or malignant lesion in the stomach or duodenum. This technique and modifications are selected because the volume of acidic gastric juice will be reduced and the anastomosis can be made along the greater curvature or at any point along the stump of the stomach. Modifications of the Billroth II procedure include the Polya and Hofmeister operations, which also establish GI continuity by duodenal bypass.

After surgery, duodenal and jejunal secretions empty into the remaining gastric pouch.

Procedural Considerations. Laparotomy and GI instrument sets are required. Linear stapling instruments should be available. The patient is positioned supine after induction of general anesthesia. The anesthesia provider inserts an NG tube after intubation. An indwelling urinary catheter is inserted before the abdominal skin prep.

Operative Procedure
1. The abdominal wall is incised and the peritoneal cavity opened and explored.
2. Bleeding vessels are clamped and ligated or coagulated.
3. The abdominal wound is retracted, and the surrounding organs are protected with warm, moist packs.
4. The gastrocolic omentum is freed from the colon mesentery to prevent injury to the middle colic artery.
5. With hemostats and Metzenbaum scissors, the right and left gastroepiploic arteries and veins are clamped, divided, and ligated with 2-0 nonabsorbable suture and 2-0 and 3-0 suture ligatures, thereby freeing the greater curvature of the stomach.
6. The distal portion of the stomach is isolated.
7. Moist packs are placed for protection of the viscera, and two sets of anastomosis clamps are placed across the distal stomach.
8. The stomach is resected just distal to the pylorus using a scalpel, electrosurgery, or a linear stapling and cutting device (GIA) (Figure 2-38, *A*).
9. A proximal loop of jejunum is positioned for anastomosis to the posterior wall of the remaining stomach.
10. An anastomosis is established between the stomach and jejunum using mechanical linear stapling devices (GIA and thoracoabdominal [TA] instruments) (Figure 2-38, *B, C*).
11. The abdomen is closed.

Total Gastrectomy

Total gastrectomy is complete removal of the stomach and establishment of an anastomosis between the jejunum and esophagus (esophagojejunostomy) (Figure 2-39). It includes an enteroenterostomy if indicated. Total gastrectomy is done with curative intent or as a palliative procedure to remove a malignant lesion of the stomach and metastases in the adjacent lymph nodes.

Procedural Considerations. The incision may be bilateral subcostal, long transrectus, long midline, or thoracoabdominal. Thoracotomy, GI, and laparotomy sets are necessary. Mechanical linear stapling devices should be available. In addition, two long, blunt nerve hooks and two 10-inch needle holders are required. The patient is positioned supine after induction of general anesthesia. The anesthesia provider inserts an NG tube after intubation. An indwelling urinary catheter is inserted before the abdominal skin prep.

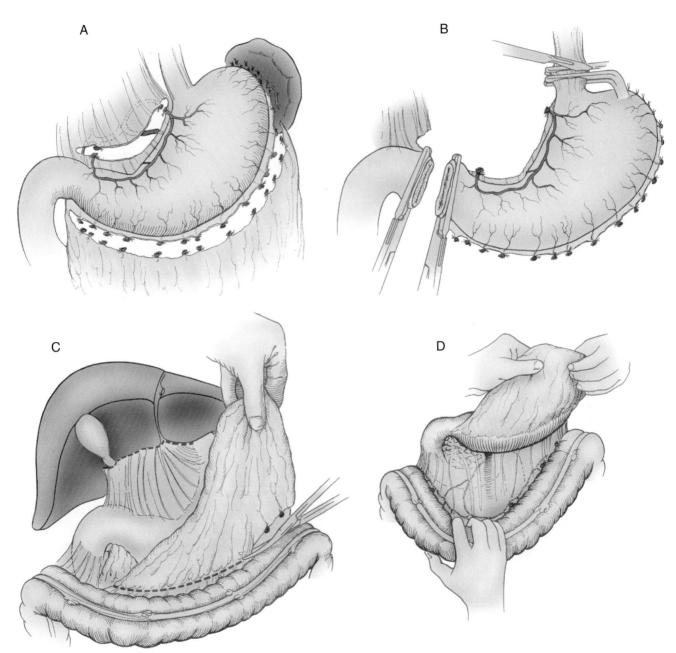

FIGURE 2-39 Total gastrectomy may be performed for benign or malignant disease. **A,** Demonstrates the mobilization of the stomach for benign disease. Serial division of the vessels in the gastrocolic ligament and gastrohepatic ligament is performed to free the greater and lesser omentum. The short gastric vessels connecting the stomach to the spleen are divided, and the spleen is preserved. **B,** The duodenum is divided distally to the pylorus, and the proximal line of division is at the distal intraabdominal esophagus. **C,** For malignancies, the line of resection includes both the lesser and the greater omentum. **D,** The retrogastric area is inspected for tumor involvement. The spleen and tail of the pancreas may be included in the resection.

Continued

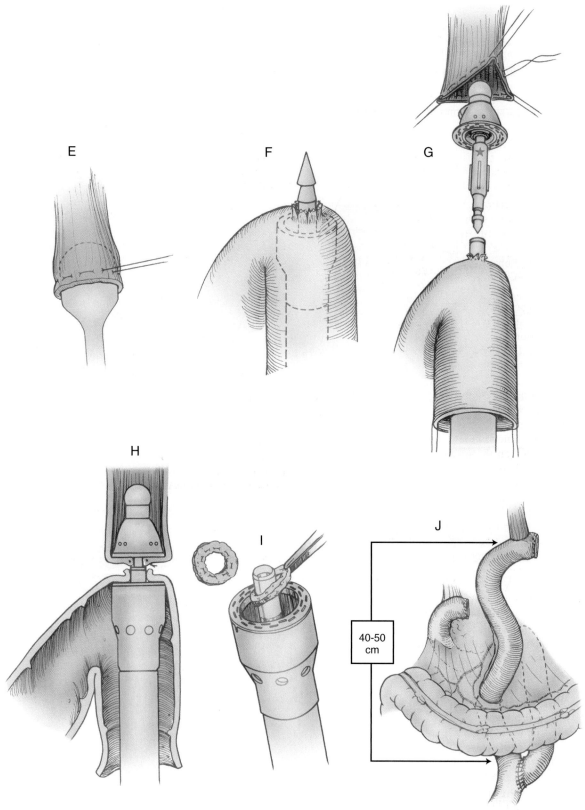

FIGURE 2-39, cont'd **E,** A sizer is inserted into the lumen of the distal esophagus. **F,** The EEA or intraluminal anastomosis (ILA) is inserted into the lumen of the jejunum to facilitate esophagojejunostomy. **G,** The anvil is inserted into the distal esophagus where purse-string sutures will be snugged around the protruding arm of the anvil. **H,** The distal esophagus and the jejunum are united by the mechanism of the stapling device, and the interluminal anastomosis will be performed. **I,** The "donuts," distal esophagus and jejunal tissues, are examined for integrity and completeness. **J,** Illustration of the esophagojejunostomy completed.

Operative Procedure

1. The abdomen is opened through an incision of choice.
2. The wound edges are protected and retracted.
3. Complete exploration for metastasis is performed.
4. The omentum is freed from the colon, using sharp dissection; vessels are ligated with 2-0 nonabsorbable suture.
5. The splenic vessels are ligated and transfixed with 2-0 and 3-0 nonabsorbable suture at the tail of the pancreas; the spleen is left attached to the omentum.
6. The duodenum is mobilized, intestinal clamps or linear stapler is applied, and the operative field is protected for transection and closure of the distal duodenum (bowel technique).
7. The right gastric artery is ligated and transfixed with 2-0 and 3-0 nonabsorbable suture, and the gastrohepatic omentum is separated from the liver.
8. After ligation of the left gastric artery, the mobilized stomach, spleen, omentum, and lesser and greater curvature ligamentous attachments are delivered into the wound.
9. The coronary ligament of the left lobe of the liver is divided, exposing the diaphragmatic peritoneum over the esophagogastric junction.
10. The liver is protected by moist packs, and gentle retraction is maintained with a Harrington, Deaver, or malleable retractor.
11. A flap of peritoneum is freed from the diaphragm, and branches of the vagus nerves are divided.
12. A loop of jejunum is selected and delivered antecolic to the esophagogastric junction for anastomosis.
13. Traction is placed on the specimen, and the posterior row of interrupted 3-0 nonabsorbable sutures is placed, or a stapling device is used.
14. As the jejunum and esophagus are incised, mosquito or Crile hemostats and ligatures of 3-0 synthetic absorbable suture control bleeding.
15. The posterior row is reinforced with 3-0 intestinal synthetic absorbable sutures or a linear staple line.
16. Division of the esophagus is completed, and the entire specimen is removed.
17. The mucosal anterior wall of the anastomosis is approximated with 4-0 interrupted synthetic absorbable sutures; an end-to-end anastomosis circular stapling device may be used to anastomose the esophagus and jejunum.
18. A second layer of sutures, 3-0 nonabsorbable or synthetic absorbable, is placed anteriorly in the seromuscular and muscular coat of the intestine.
19. A flap of the peritoneum is attached to the jejunum with interrupted 3-0 nonabsorbable sutures to relieve traction on the anastomosis.
20. A lateral jejunojejunal anastomosis is completed to permit irritating bile and pancreatic fluids to bypass the anastomosis line, thereby preventing esophageal regurgitation.
21. The abdominal wound is closed in layers. If retention sutures are used, they must be placed extraperitoneally because of the absence of omentum to protect the small bowel.

An alternative to using suture materials is the use of mechanical stapling devices. Another method of establishing continuity is a combination of a Roux-en-Y jejunojejunostomy and a jejunoesophagostomy. A Roux-en-Y, also written RNY, is any Y-shaped anastomosis in which small bowel is included.

BARIATRIC SURGERY

Bariatric surgery, also termed *weight loss or weight reduction surgery,* is surgical treatment of obesity (History box). Morbid obesity is a disease affecting more than 20 million people in the United States. Morbid obesity (also referred to as clinically

HISTORY

Bariatric Surgery

Year	Breakthrough
1950s	J. Kremen, MD, performs jejunoileal bypass. It is recognized that patients with short-bowel syndrome lose weight because of impaired absorption. Similar procedure is performed in Sweden, excising redundant portion of intestine.
1960s	Ten jejunocolic shunt procedures are reported. Shunts are eventually converted to jejunoileostomies to control diarrhea, electrolyte imbalance, and dehydration. Patients continue to experience postoperative anemia, cholelithiasis, vitamin depletion, and renal and liver disease. E. Mason, MD, performs partial gastrectomy with staples, creating a pouch anastomosed to small intestine. Early complications promote refinement of gastroplasty.
1970s	E. Mason, MD, develops vertical-banded gastroplasty (VBG). L. Wilkinson, MD, uses mesh strip for the band to reduce size of gastric reservoir. Biliopancreatic diversion is developed in Italy.
1980s	Gastric banding is refined to limit food intake. L. Kuzmak, MD, develops first adjustable gastric band and later a hollow band with inflatable ring. American Society for Bariatric Surgery (ASBS) is formed in 1983.
1990s	Laparoscopic access becomes approach of choice. Some procedures move to ambulatory surgery units.
2000s	Bariatric becomes common medical terminology. Many institutions develop interdisciplinary programs specifically for weight loss surgery. Bariatric boutique surgery centers enter surgical market. Long-term studies begin to evaluate surgery results over time. Insurance reimbursement continues to evolve as studies evaluate risks, complications, rehospitalization rates, and costs. Laparoscopic-adjustable gastric band (LAGB) approved by the Food and Drug Administration. Sleeve gastrectomy evolves as primary alternative for those not candidates for other procedures. Gastric and vagal pacing developed. Endoscopically accessed interventions evolve with implanted balloon and stapling delivery devices. Bariatric surgery viewed as significant treatment and resolution for type 2 diabetes.

Modified from Association of periOperative Registered Nurses: Bariatric surgery guideline. In *Perioperative standards and recommended practices,* Denver, 2009, The Association; Ide P et al: Perioperative nursing care of the bariatric surgical patient, *AORN J* 88(1):30-54, 2008; Adams TD et al: Long term mortality after gastric bypass surgery, cardiosource 2007, *Am Coll Cardiol,* available at www.medscape.com/viewarticle/562298. Accessed June 14, 2009; Study shows potential for resolving type 2 diabetes with bariatric surgery, *Back to EurekAlert 2009,* http://eurekalert.org/pub_releases/2009-03/ehs-ssp022709.php. Accessed June 14, 2009.

severe obesity or extreme obesity) is defined as a body mass index (BMI) of 40 kg/m² or more, the equivalent of about 45 kg (100 lb) over ideal body weight (AORN, 2009d) (Box 2-3). Obese patients typically present with serious co-existing health conditions, such as diabetes, cardiopulmonary disease, obstructive sleep apnea (OSA), gallstone disease, hypertension, hyperlipidemia, respiratory problems, or joint disease.

Eligibility criteria for patients seeking bariatric surgery include morbid obesity complicated by medical conditions secondary to obesity, history of failed dietary therapy, psychologic stability and motivation, acceptable operative risks, and a patient who is well-informed about the procedure, recovery, and postsurgical lifestyle modifications.

Contraindications are not easily generalized because morbidly obese patients are typically at greater risk for surgery. Patients at greatest risk are those with end-stage heart and lung function, inability to ambulate, weight more than 272 kg (600 lb), age younger than late teens or older than 65 years, and presence of Prader-Willi syndrome (SGNA, 2004).

There are three categories of bariatric procedures: restrictive, malabsorptive, or a combination of both. Restrictive procedures reduce the size of the stomach. When the patient eats, food is digested and absorbed normally, but the smaller capacity of the stomach gives the feeling of fullness, and the patient eats less. In malabsorptive procedures, surgery reduces the absorptive capacity of the small intestine with a bypass of a segment or segments of the proximal small bowel.

Adjustable gastric banding is a restrictive procedure. Adjustable band surgery uses a silicone strip and elastic ring called the adjustable *LAP-BAND* (INAMED Health). The band is placed laparoscopically around the top of the stomach. A fold of stomach is sutured around the band to secure it in place (Figure 2-40). The band has a port that is inflated with saline 4 weeks postoperatively. The constriction created by the inflated band restricts the amount of ingested food that can enter the stomach, preventing overeating. This procedure is adjustable and reversible (laparoscopic adjustable gastric banding, or LAGB) (Research Highlight).

Bariatric procedures have been shown to improve long-term health, including reducing the risks of cardiovascular disease

and type 2 diabetes (Adams et al, 2007; Beauchamp-Johnson, 2007; Hager, 2007).

Laparoscopic Roux-en-Y Gastric Bypass

Roux-en-Y gastric bypass (RYGB) is a largely restrictive and mildly malabsorptive procedure that reroutes the passage of ingested food and fluid from a small pouch created with surgical staples or sutures in the proximal stomach to a segment of the proximal small bowel. The jejunum or ileum is used as described under Gastrojejunosotomy. Laparoscopic RYGB is commonly performed in the United States. Postoperatively, changes in lifestyle are required for fully successful weight loss (Chambers, 2009).

Procedural Considerations. All patients undergoing bariatric surgery need special consideration, because they usually have associated serious co-morbidities that place them at risk during the procedure. A special OR bed is required that can accommodate patients who weigh more than 350 lb (159 kg). In addition to laparoscopic instrumentation and accessory supplies, extralarge blood pressure cuffs and extra-long trocars are required. Positioning requires additional padded safety restraints, pressure-reduction devices to reduce the risk of pressure injury, and properly fitting SCDs. The perioperative nurse should anticipate the potential for anesthesia assistance during intubation and airway management.

Operative Procedure

1. Five trocars are placed above the umbilicus: two on the midline, two in the left upper quadrant, and one in the right

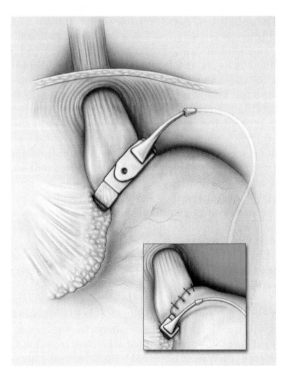

FIGURE 2-40 Proper position of the LAP-BAND. The silicone band around the fundus of the stomach creates a small gastric pouch. The inner lining of the band contains an inflatable balloon that is connected to a subcutaneous port on the patient's abdomen (not shown). The band can be inflated or deflated, adjusting the stomach size as needed.

BOX 2-3

Calculating a Patient's Body Mass Index

Obesity is defined in terms of body mass index (BMI), which is a measure of the weight-to-height ratio to gauge total body fat. BMI is expressed as kilograms per square meter and calculated by the following formula: BMI = (weight in pounds ÷ height in inches²) × 703. Obesity levels are characterized as follows:

◆ Obese: BMI of 30-39.9 kg/m²
◆ Extremely (also referred to as "morbidly") obese: BMI of 40-49 kg/m²
◆ Super obese: BMI greater than 50 kg/m²

Modified from Association of periOperative Registered Nurses: Bariatric surgery guideline. In *Perioperative standards and recommended practices*, Denver, 2009, The Association; Pelczarski KM: Take a proactive approach to bariatric patient needs, *Mater Manag Health Care* 16(6), 2007, available at www.ecri.org/Documents/News/20070601_MaterialsManagementin HealthCare_Bariatric.pdf.

RESEARCH HIGHLIGHT

Bariatric Surgery Outcomes

In this study, researchers from the Department of Health and Human Services' Agency for Healthcare Research and Quality (AHRQ) reviewed insurance claims for 9582 bariatric surgeries at 652 hospitals to determine how 6-month complication rates after bariatric surgery improved between 2001 and 2006. The 6-month complication rate for bariatric surgery in 2001 was 40%. However, surgical advances, including laparoscopic approaches, contributed to a 21% drop in complication rates for bariatric surgery by 2006. Readmissions with complications declined 31%, and surgical infection rates dropped 58%. Improvements in complication rates and readmission rates were associated with increases in surgical volume (within-hospital volume), which accounted for more surgical experience in performing bariatric procedures. Interestingly, the use of laparoscopy reduced costs by 12%, and gastric banding decreased costs by 20%. Although laparoscopy had no impact on readmissions, gastric banding did reduce readmissions.

Modified from Encinosa WE et al: Recent improvements in bariatric surgery outcomes, *Med Care* 47:531-535, 2009.

upper quadrant; an incision is made for the liver retractor (Figure 2-41).

2. The omentum is mobilized and the ligament of Treitz identified.
3. The jejunum is divided 40 cm distal to the ligament of Treitz with a vascular stapler (Figure 2-42). The proximal jejunum is left to lie in the patient's right side and the Roux limb lifted superiorly and passed through the transverse colon mesentery (Figure 2-43).
4. A gastric pouch is created with several loads of a linear stapler.
5. The Roux limb is anastomosed to the proximal gastric pouch. Methylene blue is used to check for leaks. The gastrojejunostomy may be accomplished with either traditional suturing technique or a circular EEA stapler.
6. Mesenteric defects are closed, the abdomen is inspected, and the port sites are closed.

With RYGB, a critical segment of the calorie- and nutrition-absorbing mucosal surface is avoided. The gastric pouch is generally less than 30 ml in volume. This procedure results in considerable weight loss for the patient. Serious complications may include hemorrhage, anastomotic leaks, pulmonary embolism, pneumonia, infection, small bowel obstructions or stenosis, and incisional hernia. Nutritional deficits, nausea, flatus, diarrhea, and dumping syndrome are other common complications.

Biliopancreatic diversion (Figure 2-44) and duodenal switch (Figure 2-45) procedures are largely malabsorptive and mildly restrictive. In both procedures, both the Roux limb and the biliopancreatic limb are long in length, leaving a shortened common channel where digestion and absorption of proteins, fats, and carbohydrates can occur. These procedures present more risk of complications, nutritional deficiencies, liver abnormalities, anemia, and lactose intolerance.

SURGERY OF THE SMALL BOWEL

Meckel's Diverticulectomy

Meckel's diverticulum is removed to prevent inflammation and obstruction from intussusception of the diverticulum, which consists of an unobliterated congenital duct at the umbilicus that is attached to the distal ileum. The diverticulum may contain gastric mucosa, which can ulcerate, perforate, or bleed.

Procedural Considerations. Laparotomy and GI sets are required. Linear stapling devices should be available. The patient is positioned supine after induction of general anesthesia. The anesthesia provider inserts an NG tube after intubation. An

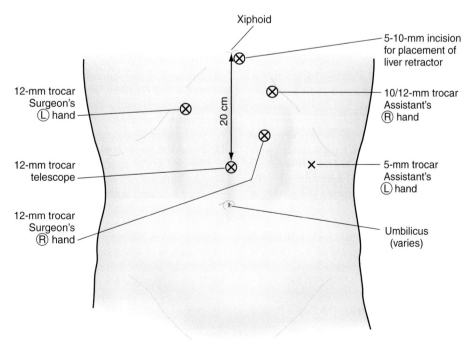

FIGURE 2-41 Trocar configuration for laparoscopic Roux-en-Y gastric bypass.

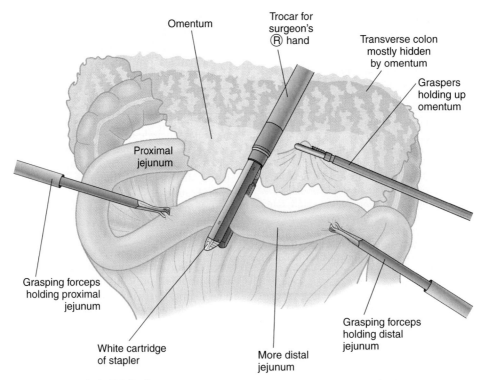

FIGURE 2-42 Placing stapler to divide jejunum to create Roux limb.

indwelling urinary catheter is inserted before the abdominal skin prep.

Operative Procedure

1. The abdomen is opened through a midline incision or laparoscopically accessed, and the diverticulum is identified.
2. If the diverticulum is long and narrow with a narrow base, the procedure is similar to that of an appendectomy (see the following discussion). If the base is broad, the loop of bowel containing the diverticulum is isolated from the mesentery and a limited small bowel resection is performed.
3. An anastomosis of the divided ends is completed with an inner continuous layer of 3-0 synthetic absorbable suture and an interrupted outer layer of 4-0 nonabsorbable sutures.
4. The abdominal wound is closed.

Appendectomy (Open Approach)

Appendectomy is severance and removal of the appendix from its attachment to the cecum through a right lower quadrant muscle-splitting incision (McBurney). This procedure is performed to remove an acutely inflamed appendix, thereby controlling the spread of infection and reducing the danger of peritonitis (Research Highlight).

Procedural Considerations. A basic laparotomy instrument set is used. The patient is positioned supine after induction of general anesthesia. Culture tubes should be available.

Operative Procedure

1. A right lower quadrant muscle-splitting (McBurney) incision is usually made.
2. Muscles are retracted with Richardson or Parker retractors to expose the peritoneum.

3. The peritoneum is grasped with tissue forceps or Allis forceps, and a small incision is made with a #15 blade.
4. A culture sample is taken.
5. The incision is completed with Metzenbaum scissors.
6. The mesoappendix is grasped near the tip with Babcock forceps or a hemostat for gentle traction.
7. The mesoappendix is dissected from the appendiceal wall and ligated with 3-0 nonabsorbable suture. If a suture ligature is required, 2-0 synthetic absorbable suture on an atraumatic GI needle is preferred.
8. The appendix is elevated as a purse-string suture of 2-0 synthetic absorbable suture is placed in the cecal wall at the appendiceal base.
9. The base of the appendix is crushed with a straight hemostat, a 3-0 synthetic absorbable suture tie placed over the crushed area, and a hemostat placed above the ligature.
10. A basin is provided for the specimen and instruments that contact the GI mucosa (bowel technique).
11. Protective gauze sponges are placed over the cecum around the base of the appendix.
12. The appendix is amputated with a scalpel. The stump is often swabbed with alcohol or povidone-iodine (Betadine) solution to reduce bacterial flora.
13. The appendiceal stump is usually inverted into the lumen of the cecum as the purse-string suture is tightened and tied by means of a fine straight hemostat and a small sponge on a holder. Soiled instruments are discarded into the basin.
14. If the appendix has ruptured, copious amounts of warm fluids are used to irrigate the peritoneal cavity. A drain may be inserted in the appendiceal bed to allow continuous drainage. Deeper layers are closed; the subcutaneous tissue and skin may be left open. The wound is then packed with moist fine-mesh gauze to heal by secondary inten-

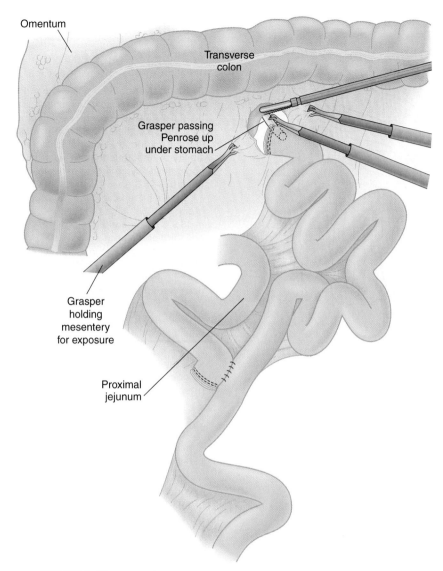

Omentum

Transverse
colon

Grasper passing
Penrose up
under stomach

Grasper
holding
mesentery
for exposure

Proximal
jejunum

FIGURE 2-43 Passing the Roux limb into a retrocolic and retrogastric position.

tion. (This method may be used in any procedure in which bowel contamination or abscess formation is present. It allows clean healing and prevents pocketing of pus.)

Laparoscopic Appendectomy

The laparoscopic approach to appendectomy may be used for uncomplicated appendicitis. In the presence of perforation, conversion to an open procedure may be necessary.

Procedural Considerations. The procedure involves the placement of three trocars with standard laparoscopic instrumentation, equipment, and supplies available. The patient is positioned supine after induction of general anesthesia. An indwelling urinary catheter may be placed before the abdominal skin prep.

Operative Procedure
1. Pneumoperitoneum is obtained by a Veress needle or through the periumbilical trocar.

2. An 11-mm or 12-mm trocar is placed in the umbilicus for insertion of the laparoscope.
3. An 11-mm or 12-mm trocar is placed in the right upper quadrant (RUQ) to serve as the working port.
4. A 5-mm trocar placed in the midline suprapubic site serves as the traction trocar.
5. A laparoscopic Babcock forceps is inserted into the RUQ trocar to grasp the cecum and retract it toward the liver.
6. The appendix is grasped at its tip by a grasping forceps that has been inserted through the suprapubic trocar and is held in an upward position.
7. The Babcock forceps is removed, and a dissecting instrument is inserted through the RUQ trocar to create a mesenteric window in the mesoappendix.
8. Dissection is performed in proximity to the appendix, beginning directly under the base and progressing to a 1-cm to 2-cm length.
9. Depending on surgeon preference, the appendix may be transected in several different ways: (a) with an endoscopic

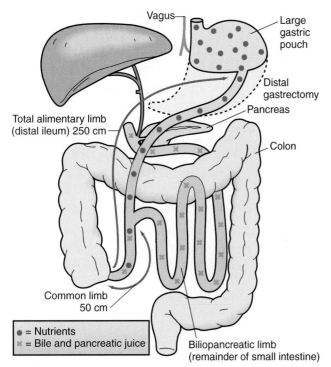

FIGURE 2-44 Configuration of the biliopancreatic diversion (BPD), which is transection of the stomach with anastomosis of the duodenum to the distal ileum. In this malabsorptive procedure, the pancreatic enzymes and bile enter near the ileum, allowing nutrients to pass from the stomach to the distal ileum without being digested. Weight loss occurs because of the partial gastrectomy, which restricts intake, and because of the shortened alimentary canal, which causes malabsorption.

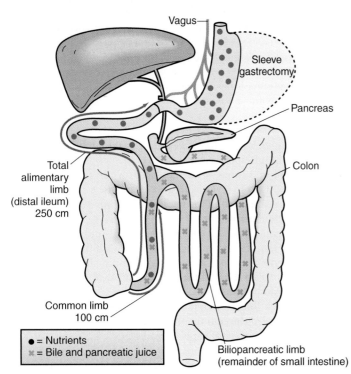

FIGURE 2-45 Configuration of the duodenal switch, which leaves a larger portion of the stomach intact, including the pyloric valve. This helps in alleviating dumping syndrome.

RESEARCH HIGHLIGHT

Antibiotic Therapy versus Appendectomy as Primary Treatment of Acute Appendicitis

Standard treatment for acute appendicitis is appendectomy to avoid perforation. However, appendectomy is associated with postoperative risks, such as small bowel obstruction. Because of such risks, there has been increased interest in antibiotic therapy as primary treatment. This study investigated the feasibility of antibiotic therapy as a first-line treatment for acute appendicitis by assigning patients (N = 369) to antibiotic treatment (n = 202) or surgery (n = 167).

Treatment efficacy was 90.8% for the antibiotic therapy group and 89.2% for the surgery group. Appendicitis recurred in 13.9% of the antibiotic group after a median of 1 year with one third of recurrences within 10 days after discharge. Eleven of the antibiotic group required an appendectomy because of clinical progression within 24 to 36 hours. Although minor complications were similar between groups, major complications were threefold higher in surgery patients.

The researchers concluded that antibiotic treatment appears to be a safe first-line therapy in patients with acute appendicitis.

Modified from Hansson J et al: Randomized clinical trial of antibiotic therapy versus appendectomy as primary treatment of acute appendicitis in unselected patients, *Br J Surg* 96:473-481, 2009.

linear stapling instrument, (b) with a ligating loop instrument, or (c) with a suturing instrument.

10. If an endoscopic linear stapling instrument is used, the lower jaw of the stapling device is passed through the mesenteric window previously created by way of the RUQ trocar.
11. The grasping forceps are used to rotate the tip of the appendix so that the stapling device can be snugged to the base of the appendix and closed.
12. The stapling instrument is fired and withdrawn, and the staple line is inspected.
13. The remainder of the mesoappendix is dissected, hemostasis achieved, and the appendix removed through the RUQ port.
14. If the appendix is too thick, a specimen pouch may be necessary for its extraction.
15. The abdomen is irrigated, irrigation fluid is aspirated with a suction and irrigation device, and the abdomen is deflated.
16. Trocar sites are closed and dressed or closed with skin-bonding sealer.

Resection of the Small Intestine

Resection of the small intestine involves excision of diseased intestine through an abdominal incision followed by reanastomosis. It is performed to remove tumors, a gangrenous portion of intestine caused by strangulation from bands of adhesions, intestinal obstruction, areas of ulceration and bleeding as in Crohn's disease, herniation of the intestine, or volvulus.

Procedural Considerations. Laparotomy and GI sets are required. Linear stapling instruments should be available. The patient is positioned supine after induction of general anesthesia. The anesthesia provider inserts an NG tube after intubation. An indwelling urinary catheter is inserted before the abdominal skin prep. The procedure may be performed laparoscopically.

Operative Procedure

1. The abdominal wall is incised through a midline incision and retracted.
2. The peritoneal cavity is explored and protected with moist, warm saline packs.
3. Intestinal clamps are placed above and below the diseased segment of small bowel and mesentery.
4. The involved area is removed with a linear stapling instrument such as a GIA, an electrosurgical blade, or a scalpel.
5. Continuity of the GI tract is established by an end-to-end, end-to-side, or side-to-side anastomosis.
6. The wound is closed and dressed.

An alternative approach to suture anastomosis is use of a mechanical stapling device to perform an end-to-end, end-to-side, or side-to-side anastomosis. An enterotomy is made close to the anastomosis site. The stapler is inserted, and the distal bowel secured between the anvil and the head of the stapler. The anvil is then inserted into the proximal loop of bowel and secured to the center rod. The gap is closed, and the stapler fired. The stapler is removed through the enterotomy. The integrity of the anastomosis is verified, and the enterotomy closed with sutures.

Ileostomy

Ileostomy is formation of a temporary or permanent opening into the ileum. This procedure is indicated in the presence of an extensive lesion to reduce large bowel activity, often called *bowel rest,* by creating a temporary fecal diversion to the outside of the body, or as permanent fecal diversion in total colectomy. The patient is site-marked before surgery and anesthesia by the WOCN.

Procedural Considerations. Laparotomy and GI sets along with linear stapling instruments are required. The patient is positioned supine after induction of general anesthesia. The anesthesia provider inserts an NG tube after intubation. An indwelling urinary catheter is inserted before the abdominal skin prep. An ostomy appliance for the stoma is available.

Operative Procedure

1. Through a midline incision, the peritoneal cavity is explored and the pathologic condition determined.
2. The ileum is mobilized with Metzenbaum scissors and hemostatic clamps.
3. The mesentery is clamped, divided, and ligated with 3-0 nonabsorbable sutures at the proposed site, usually about 15 cm from the ileocecal junction.
4. Two intestinal clamps are placed on the bowel, and the ileum is divided with a scalpel or linear stapling instrument (GIA) between the two clamps.
5. The distal end of the ileum is closed with 2-0 synthetic absorbable suture on a taper needle if a stapling device has not been used.
6. The proximal end is relocated to the skin through an opening on the right side and is held in place by clamps, making sure that the ileum is not overstretched or its blood supply compromised.

7. The mesentery of the ileum is sutured to the parietal wall to eliminate a potential internal hernia.
8. The abdomen is closed.
9. The stoma is sutured to the skin after the ileum is everted to form a protective cover over the exposed ileal serosa.
10. A disposable ostomy appliance is placed over the stoma to collect small bowel contents.

An alternative to conventional ileostomy for selected patients is the Kock pouch, or continent ileostomy. The internal pouch is created from a segment of small intestine with an outlet to the skin. When functioning properly, the stoma and pouch are continent and do not continually drain stool. A catheter is inserted into the stoma three or four times daily to evacuate the contents, eliminating the need for an external appliance.

Intestinal Transplantation

Small bowel transplantation may be indicated for patients with intestinal failure caused by short-gut syndrome as a result of extensive resections necessitated by Crohn's disease, necrotizing enterocolitis, mesenteric thrombosis, atresias, volvulus, trauma, dysmotility, or congenital enteropathy (Shortridge et al, 2004). Intestinal failure leads to malabsorption and malnutrition, preventing the bowel from meeting the body's nutrient and fluid requirements. Approximately 10 to 20 cm of small intestine with an ileocecal valve, or 40 cm without an ileocecal valve, is minimally required to maintain nutritional status. Patients with short-gut syndrome require TPN to sustain life. A critical indication for intestinal transplant arises when patients can no longer receive TPN because of clotting of major veins, frequent IV line sepsis, episodes of dehydration despite TPN and IV fluids, and TPN-induced liver failure (Markmann et al, 2008). Intestinal transplantation may also include the liver in the presence of impending progressive end-stage liver disease. The perioperative time frame, beginning with immunosuppression, surgery, transition from parenteral to enteral feedings, and the long recovery process, may be 6 months and poses many physical and emotional challenges to the patient and family. Despite these challenges, refinements in surgical technique and patient selection and advances in immunosuppression protocols have contributed to significant improvements in patient survival rates.

Procedural Considerations. The transplant surgeon does the final visual inspection and assessment of the donor organ. The allowable cold ischemic time of the donor intestine (allograft intestine) is approximately 12 hours. The patient is positioned supine and anesthetized with general endotracheal anesthesia. Arterial and multiple venous lines are inserted. An NG tube, urinary catheter, and physiologic monitoring are indicated.

Operative Procedure

1. The incision is made along previous incision lines, or a vertical midline approach is used.
2. The superior mesenteric artery of the donor organ is anastomosed to the recipient's infrarenal aorta.
3. Venous drainage of the donor organ is established by connecting the donor superior mesenteric vein to the recipient portal vein if the patient has no liver disease or signs of portal hypertension.
4. Reperfusion begins with release of venous flow when the clamps are opened.

5. Bleeding sites are identified and ligated or coagulated.
6. The arterial clamp is released.
7. Continuity of the intestine is restored after vascular supply is established.
8. Proximal anastomosis joins the donor jejunum to the recipient stomach, duodenum, or proximal jejunum.
9. The distal ileum is anastomosed side-to-side with the remaining colon.
10. A distal loop ileostomy is created for later endoscopic evaluation and intestinal biopsies.
11. The intact intestine is inspected, hemostasis verified, and the abdomen closed.

SURGERY OF THE COLON

Laparoscopic Colectomy

Resection of a segment of bowel and reanastomosis can be accomplished laparoscopically. Advantages of laparoscopic colectomy include reduction of morbidity associated with open techniques (e.g., postoperative ileus), less postoperative pain, faster return to normal activities, shorter length of stay, and improved cosmesis (Evidence for Practice). Laparoscopic colectomy is indicated for obstruction and benign tumors of the large bowel.

Procedural Considerations. Depending on the intended segment of bowel to be resected, the patient is initially positioned supine or in modified lithotomy for access to the rectum for end-to-end anastomosis. The surgeon may stand on the patient's left or between the patient's legs (modified lithotomy). SCDs are applied to minimize the risk of DVT. The patient is secured with restraining straps to support and maintain position during steep position changes. A beanbag device may be used. An NG tube and urinary catheter are inserted before the abdominal skin prep. Laparotomy instrumentation, mechanical stapling devices, and endostapling devices are required. To assist the surgeon in accurately identifying the segment of bowel to be resected, a colonoscope may be used preoperatively or during the laparoscopic procedure to tattoo the lesion with india ink. Right hemicolectomy, described below, is performed to treat disease of the cecum, ascending colon, or hepatic flexure. Extended right hemicolectomy is done to treat tumors located in the transverse colon, particularly those located to the right of the midline (Sonoda and Milsom, 2007).

Operative Procedure (Right Hemicolectomy)

1. Pneumoperitoneum is established at 10 to 12 mm Hg, and the 10-mm umbilical trocar is placed after a supraumbilical cutdown. Alternatively, a 12-mm Hasson trocar may be inserted through the rectus muscle and into the abdominal cavity by way of a small incision in the left upper quadrant, 3 to 4 cm below the costal margin.
2. Additional ports (usually 5 mm) are placed in locations dependent on the anatomic segment of colon to be resected.
3. After the patient is moved into Trendelenburg's position, with right side tilted up, dissecting scissors and a grasper are inserted. The peritoneum along the cecum is incised as are the appendiceal and terminal ileal attachments. The bowel is then bluntly dissected from the retroperitoneum, the ureter identified, and the colon mobilized as necessary for resection of the diseased segment. A mesenteric window

is created, and the mesenteric artery and vein and right colic vessels are identified and clipped.

4. A multifire endoscopic linear stapling device (GIA) is positioned over the segment of bowel and fired to both transect and staple the segment.
5. Unless an end-to-end anastomosis can be performed, as in a low sigmoid or rectal resection, a small incision is made over the area of the abdomen that will provide access to the segments for anastomosis.
6. The segment of bowel to be resected is grasped, transferred through the small incision, and transected, and anastomosis is performed in the surgeon's preferred manner (with staples or with sutures).
7. The anastomosed bowel is returned to the peritoneal cavity, and the cavity is irrigated and inspected for hemostasis and drained by suction. The cannulae are removed, port sites closed, and skin closed with subcuticular absorbable suture. Skin tapes (Steri-Strips) are applied.

Colostomy

Colostomy is mobilization of a loop of colon through a right rectus incision to expose the transverse colon. A left rectus incision can also be made to expose the descending sigmoid colon. The layers of the wound beneath or around the colostomy are subsequently closed. Colostomy is performed to treat obstruction in the sigmoid colon resulting from a malignant lesion or advanced inflammation or trauma that has caused distention or obstruction of the proximal portion of the colon. A temporary colostomy is often done to decompress the bowel or to divert bowel contents to promote healing (bowel rest) (Figure 2-46).

EVIDENCE FOR PRACTICE

Laparoscopic versus Open Colectomy

Laparoscopic-assisted colectomy is a safe alternative to traditional open colectomy. Recent research comparing open laparotomy for colectomy with laparoscopic-assisted colectomy reveals better outcomes for the laparoscopic approach for both benign and malignant disease of the colon. The laparoscopic approach has also been shown to be equivalent to open colectomy in cancer-related survival for curable cancer. A large prospective, randomized, multi-institution trial compared laparoscopic-assisted to open colectomy for colon cancer. It involved 863 patients, 66 surgeons, and 48 institutions. The primary endpoint was time-to-tumor recurrence; the secondary endpoints were disease-free and overall survival, minimal complications, and increased quality of life. At the median follow-up of 4.5 years, there was no significant difference in oncologic outcome between the two groups. A higher 5-year survival rate for patients with the laparoscopic approach was shown in a retrospective cohort study of 11,038 patients compared with 231,381 patients who had the open approach for nonmetastatic colon cancer between 1998 and 2002. Laparoscopic-assisted colectomy is a technically demanding procedure with a significant learning curve for the surgeon; the advantages for the patient, however, make this approach the treatment of choice.

From Clinical Outcomes of Surgical Therapy Study Group (COST Trial): *NEJM* 350(20):2050-2059, 2004; Hageman D et al: Laparoscopic-assisted colon surgery, *AORN J* 88:403-416, 2008; Bilimoria KY et al: Use and outcomes of laparoscopic-assisted colectomy for cancer in the United States, *Arch Surg* 143(9):832-840, 2008.

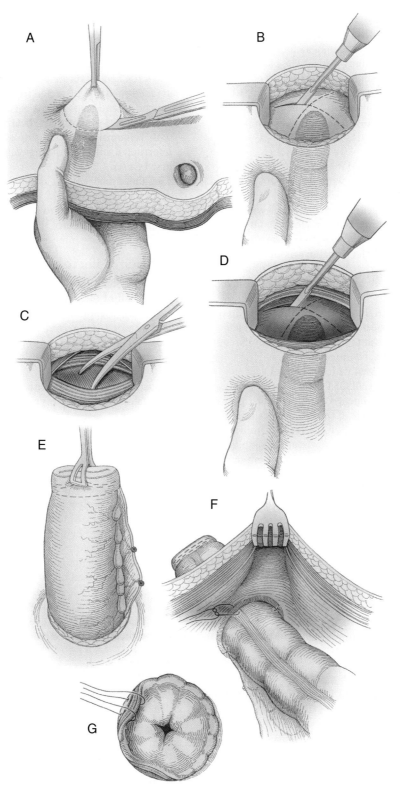

FIGURE 2-46 Construction of a colostomy through the anterior abdominal wall. **A,** A core of subcutaneous tissue is removed after making a circular skin incision with a #10 blade and using an electrosurgical pencil to dissect down to the anterior fascia. **B,** Muscle fibers are split. **C,** Tissues are dissected to the posterior layers, and, **D,** the peritoneum is opened. **E,** The colon is delivered through the abdominal wall so that it extends 2 to 3 cm beyond the skin surface. **F,** The bowel is tacked internally to the peritoneal defect. **G,** Four sutures are placed in each quadrant, incorporating the full-thickness cut end of the colon, the serosal surface approximately 1 to 2 cm below the open end of the colon, and up to the dermis. Additional sutures are used to mature the stoma, which refers to the procedure of everting the mucosa to create a stable opening through which feces can be evacuated.

Procedural Considerations. Laparotomy and GI sets are required. Linear stapling instruments may be used. Stoma appliances are required. These items may include a colostomy rod, rubber tubing, or a loop ostomy bridge. The patient is site-marked by the WOCN before surgery. The patient is positioned supine after induction of general anesthesia. The anesthesia provider inserts an NG tube after intubation. An indwelling urinary catheter is inserted before the abdominal skin prep.

Operative Procedure
FIRST-STAGE LOOP COLOSTOMY
1. The abdomen is opened, and the wound edges are protected and retracted.
2. The peritoneal cavity is opened and walled off with moist laparotomy packs, and appropriate retractors are inserted.
3. A small opening is made in the mesentery near the bowel with curved hemostats and Metzenbaum scissors.
4. A piece of tubing or Penrose drain is passed around the colon, and the two ends are held with a hemostat to maintain gentle traction.
5. The loop of colon is moved through an incision made on the left side of the midline. The abdominal incision is closed.
6. A loop ostomy bridge is used to support and retain the loop of colon in position on the abdominal wall.
7. The loop of intestine is dressed with petrolatum gauze.
    SECOND-STAGE LOOP COLOSTOMY. After 48 hours the loop of colon is completely opened with the blade tip of an electrosurgical pencil. By this time, if there is no tension, healing has advanced sufficiently to allow protection from feces contamination onto the wound. This procedure is simple and painless and is usually performed in the patient's room or in a treatment room. An ostomy appliance is applied.
TRANSVERSE COLOSTOMY
1. A short transverse or vertical incision is made to reach the transverse colon.
2. A loop of transverse colon, freed of omentum, is withdrawn (Figure 2-47).
3. A loop ostomy bridge is passed through an avascular area of the mesocolon, preventing the loop from returning to the peritoneal cavity.
4. A mushroom catheter, held in place with a purse-string suture, results in immediate decompression.
    The bowel is opened 24 to 36 hours later, and the bridge is removed in about 7 to 10 days.

Closure of a Colostomy

Closure of a colostomy reestablishes internal intestinal continuity and repairs the abdominal wall.

Procedural Considerations. When the loop has been completely divided, a closed or open anastomosis may be performed. Laparotomy and GI sets are required. Linear stapling instruments may be used. The patient is positioned supine after induction of general anesthesia. The anesthesia provider inserts a nasogastric tube after intubation. An indwelling urinary catheter is inserted before the abdominal skin prep. Depending on location of the bowel to be reanastomosed, the patient may be placed in low lithotomy position to facilitate transanal access for a circular stapling device. An end-to-end anastomosis of the left colon or ileal pouch to the rectal stump can then be achieved.

Operative Procedure
1. A circumferential incision is made around the colostomy to free the skin margin.
2. Moist packs, a scalpel with #10 blade, Metzenbaum scissors, and Crile hemostats are used as layers of the abdominal wall are identified and dissected free.
3. An end-to-end anastomosis is completed in two layers—the inner with 3-0 synthetic absorbable suture and the outer with 3-0 nonabsorbable suture on an intestinal needle, using interrupted sutures. Alternatively, a surgical stapling device may be used.
4. The abdominal wound is closed in layers and a dressing applied.
    The surgeon may elect to leave the subcutaneous tissue and skin open. In this instance the wound is packed and permitted to heal by secondary intention.

Right Hemicolectomy and Ileocolostomy

Right hemicolectomy and ileocolostomy involve resection of the right half of the colon—including a portion of the transverse colon, ascending colon, and cecum—and a segment of the terminal ileum and mesentery (Figure 2-48, *A*). An end-to-end, side-to-side, or end-to-side anastomosis is done between the transverse colon and ileum. A right hemicolectomy and ileocolostomy are performed to remove a malignant lesion of the right colon or, in some cases, to remove inflammatory lesions involving the ileum, cecum, or ascending colon.

Procedural Considerations. When a side-to-side anastomosis is carried out, the transected stumps of the ileum and transverse colon are closed before the anastomosis is done. A side-to-side anastomosis can also be performed by inserting the GIA stapler into both colon segments and firing the device. The stumps are then closed using a TA linear stapling device.

    When an end-to-end anastomosis is performed, the layers of the transected stumps of the ileum and transverse colon are sutured together. Circular linear stapling devices, such as an EEA, may also be used for anastomosis.

    Laparotomy and GI sets are required. The patient is positioned supine after induction of general anesthesia. The anesthesia provider inserts an NG tube after intubation. An indwelling urinary catheter is inserted before the abdominal skin prep.

Operative Procedure
1. The abdomen is opened, and the peritoneal cavity retracted and packed with warm, moist sponges.
2. The mesentery of the transverse colon and terminal ileum is incised at the points where the resection is to be done.
3. Moist packs are placed to isolate viscera to be resected. Metzenbaum scissors, hemostats, and 3-0 nonabsorbable ligatures are used to clamp, cut, and ligate mesentery vessels.
4. The lateral peritoneal fold along the lateral side of the right colon is incised, and the right colon is mobilized medially. Metzenbaum scissors, hemostats, and sponges on holders are used.
5. The ureter and duodenum are identified.
6. The same procedure is carried out on the terminal ileum. The mesenteric vessels are clamped and ligated with 2-0 nonabsorbable ligatures.

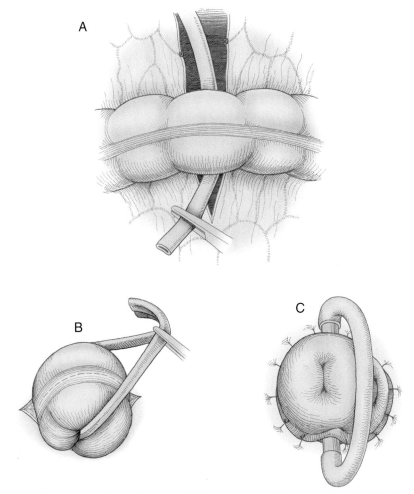

FIGURE 2-47 Transverse loop colostomy. **A,** The mesentery adjacent to the colon is taken down so that a Penrose drain may be passed beneath the colon. **B,** The colon is pulled through the transverse incision and opened longitudinally along the taeniae. **C,** An apparatus or rod is placed underneath the stoma; sutures are used to mature the colostomy. The rod can be removed after the seventh postoperative day.

7. The operative field is prepared for anastomosis (bowel technique).
8. Intestinal clamps are placed on the transverse colon and ileum.
9. Division is completed with a scalpel, and the specimen removed.
10. An end-to-end anastomosis is completed between the severed ends of the terminal ileum and transverse colon.
11. Instruments and supplies that have contacted bowel mucosa are discarded.
12. The mesentery and posterior peritoneum are closed with interrupted 3-0 nonabsorbable sutures.
13. The abdominal wound is closed and a dressing applied.

Transverse Colectomy

Transverse colectomy is excision of the transverse colon through an upper midline or transverse incision (Figure 2-48, *C* and *D*). Bowel integrity is reestablished by an end-to-end anastomosis. Transverse colectomy is performed to remove malignant lesions of the transverse colon. A more radical pro-

cedure may be required when the lesion has perforated the greater curvature of the stomach. If the entire lesion is resectable, a partial gastrectomy may also be performed.

Procedural Considerations. Laparotomy and GI sets are required. Linear stapling instruments and a self-retaining retractor system should be available. The patient is positioned supine after induction of general anesthesia. The anesthesia provider inserts an NG tube after intubation. An indwelling urinary catheter is inserted before the abdominal skin prep.

Operative Procedure
1. The abdomen is opened, and the peritoneal cavity explored to determine the pathologic area.
2. Moist packs are used to wall off surrounding structures to expose the hepatic and splenic flexures of the colon.
3. The colon is mobilized by incising the lateral peritoneum on either side and transecting the transverse mesocolon. Hemostats, Metzenbaum scissors, and 3-0 nonabsorbable ligatures are used.

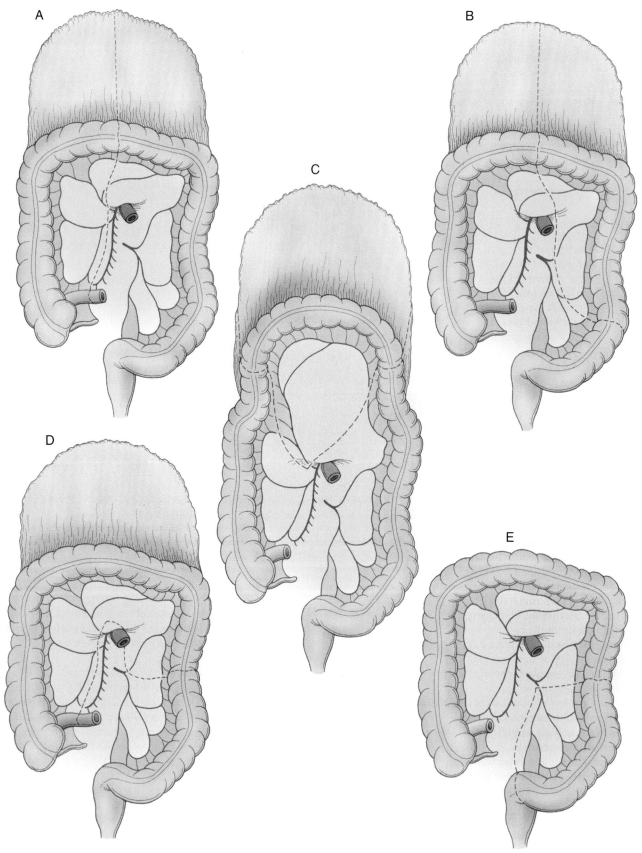

FIGURE 2-48 The resection lines for various types of colon resection. **A,** Right hemicolectomy and ileocolostomy. **B,** Left hemicolectomy. **C** and **D,** Transverse colectomy. **E,** Anterior resection of sigmoid colon and rectosigmoidostomy.

4. The operative field is prepared for resection by placing towels or laparotomy sponges around the colon to isolate any contamination from the lumen of the bowel.
5. Two intestinal resection clamps are applied.
6. Transection is completed with a scalpel or mechanical linear stapling device.
7. An end-to-end or side-to-side anastomosis is completed.
8. Contaminated articles are isolated (bowel technique).
9. Approximation of mesentery and lateral peritoneum is completed with 3-0 nonabsorbable sutures.
10. The abdominal wound is closed. Retention sutures may be used.
11. The wound is dressed.

Anterior Resection of the Sigmoid Colon and Rectosigmoidostomy

Anterior resection of the sigmoid colon and rectosigmoidostomy involve removal of the lower sigmoid and rectosigmoid portions of the rectum (Figure 2-48, *E*). This is usually done through a laparotomy incision, and an end-to-end anastomosis is completed. This procedure treats lesions in the lower portion of the sigmoid and rectum that can be excised with a wide margin of safety and still retain sufficient tissues with adequate blood supply for a viable rectosigmoid end-to-end anastomosis.

Procedural Considerations. Laparotomy and GI sets are required. Linear stapling instruments as well as the end-to-end curved mechanical stapling instruments (EEA) are used. Long instruments for dissecting into the pelvis may be necessary. A rigid sigmoidoscope is used before patient preparation and after anastomosis. A self-retaining retractor set is required. After induction of general anesthesia, the patient is placed in a modified lithotomy position with legs extended in stirrups. An indwelling urinary catheter is inserted before the abdominal and perineal preps.

If there is an assisting surgeon, a table with a basic minor set and rectal instruments should be available to facilitate end-to-end stapling of the anastomosis. Cross-contamination from the table of instruments used on the patient's rectum to the table with the laparotomy instruments is prevented. A table with laparotomy closure instruments may be the surgeon's preference. In this case, only laparotomy instruments are required.

Identification of the ureters during extensive deep abdominal procedures is achieved by preoperative placement of ureteral catheters by a transurethral approach. If the tumor is believed to involve the ureters, a urologist will place ureteral stents cystoscopically before the abdominal prep begins.

Operative Procedure
1. The abdomen is entered through a laparotomy incision.
2. The peritoneal cavity is explored for metastasis and resectability of the lesion.
3. Before the colon is mobilized, the tumor-bearing segment is isolated by ligatures to the lymphovenous drainage, provided that these structures are accessible.
4. A loop of sigmoid colon is elevated as the small intestines are walled off with moist packs; retractors are placed.
5. The peritoneum on the left side of the colon is incised with a long scalpel, scissors, hemostats, and sponge forceps.
6. Traction sutures (2-0 nonabsorbable) may be used as the peritoneum is reflected.

7. Bleeding vessels are ligated with 2-0 or 3-0 nonabsorbable ligatures.
8. The pelvic peritoneum is exposed and dissected free to form the left side of the reconstructed pelvic floor. Long dissecting instruments are used.
9. Vessels are ligated with 30-inch nonabsorbable ligatures.
10. Extreme care is exercised throughout to protect the ureters from injury.
11. The sigmoid colon is turned leftward; incision and dissection of the peritoneum are then performed on the right side of the pelvis.
12. The two incisions are then curved and joined in front of the rectum.
13. The rectum is freed anteriorly and posteriorly from adjacent structures.
14. The sigmoid colon is clamped with intestinal clamps after mobilization of the proximal portion. A right-angled intestinal clamp or a reticulating linear stapling device may be used to clamp the distal portion of the rectosigmoid colon.
15. As the sigmoid colon is divided distally to the clamp, the transected rectal edges are grasped with Allis or Ochsner forceps and the rectal opening is exposed.
16. The diseased portion is removed, and the soiled instruments are discarded into a separate basin (bowel technique).
17. Continuity is established by an end-to-end anastomosis of the proximal colon and the rectum using a curved mechanical stapling instrument (EEA) (Figure 2-49).
18. "Donuts" of tissue are removed from the EEA stapling device, examined closely for thickness and continuity, and then sent as separate specimens to the pathology laboratory.
19. The assisting surgeon passes a rigid sigmoidoscope into the lumen of the bowel transanally.
20. Warm irrigating solution is poured into the peritoneal cavity, and the lumen of the bowel is insufflated.
21. The surgeon looks for air leaks from the anastomosis and oversews the site if indicated.
22. The pelvic floor is reperitonealized, and drains may be placed.
23. The abdominal wound is closed and a dressing applied.

Abdominoperineal Resection

Abdominoperineal resection (APR), also called *Miles' resection,* is the mobilization and division of a diseased segment of the lower bowel through a midline incision. The proximal end of bowel is exteriorized through a separate stab wound as a colostomy. The distal end is pushed into the hollow of the sacrum and removed through the perineal route (Figure 2-50). APR is performed to remove malignant lesions and to treat inflammatory diseases of the lower sigmoid colon, rectum, and anus that are too low for the use of EEA stapling devices.

Procedural Considerations. The choice of patient position depends on the surgeon. Some surgeons prefer to start with the patient in supine position and move the patient into lithotomy for the perineal portion of the operation. Others initially position the patient in modified lithotomy. Thus surgery may be performed simultaneously by two teams, which may require two scrub persons with two different setups. An indwelling catheter is inserted into the urinary bladder after induction of anesthesia. The anesthesia provider inserts an NG tube after

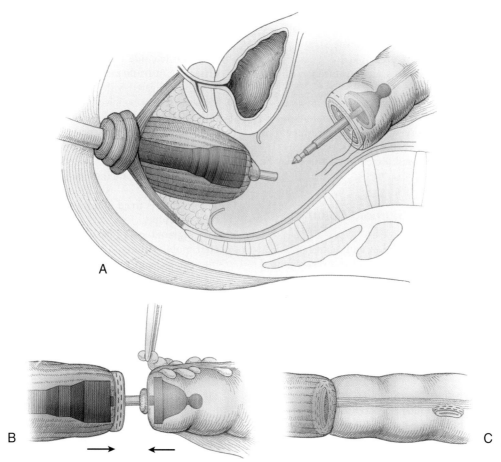

FIGURE 2-49 EEA stapling device, used to perform low anterior anastomosis. **A,** Stapler is introduced into anus, and the anvil is placed into the proximal colon loop. **B,** EEA is advanced to level of the anvil, and the EEA is closed and fired. **C,** Circular double-staggered row of staples joins bowel; simultaneously, circular blade in instrument cuts stoma. Instrument is gently removed. The resulting anastomosis is illustrated with bowel wall transparent to depict reconstruction.

intubation. A GI instrument set and an ostomy appliance are required for the abdominal portion of the procedure. A perineal set is used for the rectal portion of the procedure. Identification of the ureters during extensive deep abdominal procedures may be achieved by the preoperative placement of ureteral stents using the transurethral approach.

Operative Procedure
1. A midline incision is made.
2. After thorough exploration of the abdominal cavity and inspection of the colon, the surgeon determines the extent of the lesion and probable surgical outcome. If a resection is indicated, the sigmoid colon is retracted to the right side.
3. The peritoneum on the left of the mesocolon is divided.
4. The incision into the peritoneum is made opposite the main branches of the inferior mesenteric vessels and extended into the pelvis and around, anterior to the rectum.
5. The pelvic peritoneum is mobilized by blunt dissection to form the left side of the new pelvic floor and permit visualization of the left ureter.
6. The peritoneum is incised on the right side until the incision connects with that made on the left.
7. The right ureter is identified and protected.

8. The blood supply of the portion of intestine to be removed is isolated and ligated. Care is taken not to damage the left colic artery, which will supply blood to the colostomy.
9. The mesentery is tied to permit greater exposure in the operative field.
10. The surgeon frees the rectum, usually as low as the sacrococcygeal junction. Care is taken to avoid injury to the presacral nerves, which could result in sexual and bladder dysfunction.
11. After the bowel is freed, the distal segment is transected with a linear stapling instrument (Figure 2-50, *B*).
12. The proximal margin of resection is examined and transected. The bowel and mesentery are removed from the abdominal cavity.
13. The surgeon prepares the permanent colostomy by extending the stump through the abdominal wall. The colostomy will be "matured" (sutured externally to the abdominal wall tissues so that the mucosa is everted into a raised and secured ostomy) after abdominal closure.
14. The combined excision and perineal dissection are initiated when the lesion is determined to be resectable.
15. To prevent contamination, the anus is often closed with a purse-string suture.

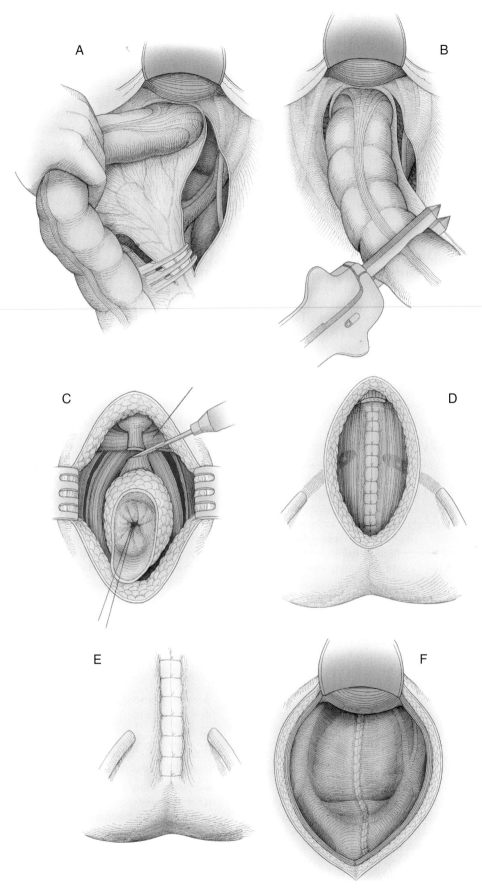

FIGURE 2-50 Abdominoperineal resection for cancer of the rectum. **A,** The sigmoid colon is deflected to the right to complete the rectosigmoid peritoneal detachment. **B,** The distal sigmoid is transected to allow for better access to mobilize the rectum from the sacrum. **C,** The rectal stump is excised from the perineal approach. **D,** Drains are placed and moved through stab wounds; the levator tissues are reapproximated with 2-0 synthetic absorbable sutures. **E,** The perineal skin is closed. **F,** The pelvic peritoneal floor is closed from the abdominal approach.

16. An incision is made around the anus in an elliptic manner outside the sphincter muscles with a generous margin of perianal skin.
17. The anus is grasped with an Allis or Ochsner forceps and tipped upward to enable its attachment to the coccyx to be severed more readily.
18. Electrodissection is used. The levator ani muscle is exposed; while the finger of the surgeon is held beneath it, it is divided as far from the rectum as possible.
19. All bleeding points are clamped and tied. The Foley catheter allows the surgeon to get as close to the bladder as possible without damaging it.
20. After the anococcygeal raphe is divided, the surgeon's hand is thrust up into the hollow sacrum to free the rectum by blunt dissection, grasp the upper end of the distal fragment, and deliver the stump through the perineum.
21. Drains may be placed into the pelvic cavity and exteriorized through stab wounds in the buttocks (Figure 2-50, *D*).
22. The surgeon is regowned and regloved before returning to the abdominal wound. When all bleeding is controlled, the incision is closed.

If two teams are not available for synchronous excision of the perineum, the perineal portion of the operation is performed after the abdominal resection is complete. In this case, the abdomen is closed and the remaining rectosigmoid stump is excised perineally.

Ileoanal Endorectal Pull-through

Ileoanal endorectal pull-through is removal of the entire colon and the proximal two thirds of the rectum. It includes a mucosectomy of the remaining distal rectum, creation of a pouch from the distal small bowel, and anastomosis of the pouch to the anus. The operation is performed to relieve ulcerative colitis and familial polyposis (e.g., diarrhea, pain, cramping, bleeding) and to prevent colon cancer in high-risk individuals. This procedure is an anal sphincter–saving operation that is done to avoid the need for ileostomy.

Procedural Considerations. The patient is usually positioned in modified lithotomy. Some surgeons prefer to perform the mucosectomy with the patient in jackknife position and then place the patient in modified lithotomy position for the remainder of the procedure. The anesthesia provider inserts an NG tube after intubation. An indwelling urinary catheter is inserted before the abdominal skin prep.

A GI instrument set, a perineal set, rectal instrumentation, and a self-retaining retractor system are used. Separate instrument tables are prepared for the rectal and abdominal approaches. Additional draping and gowning are needed because redraping and regowning occur after the mucosectomy and after the ileoanal anastomosis. An epinephrine solution should be available for injection into the submucosal tissue, proximal to the anus, to separate the mucosa from the muscularis layer. A proctoscope is available as it may be used at the conclusion of the procedure to check for leaks. Air is pumped into the scope, which is inserted into the anus. The surgeon at the abdominal site looks for air bubbles. If there are none, the anastomosis has no leaks. An ileostomy appliance is applied immediately postoperatively.

Operative Procedure
1. The anal canal is dilated and inspected through an anoscope.
2. Starting at the dentate line (the anorectal junction), epinephrine solution is injected circumferentially, separating the mucosa from the muscularis layer.
3. The mucosectomy is then performed by making a circular incision at the dentate line, cutting only through mucosa.
4. The mucosa is peeled off the muscularis tissue for a distance of 2 to 8 cm and resected.
5. When all bleeding is controlled, the patient is repositioned, if necessary, for the abdominal approach.
6. A midline incision is made, and the abdomen is explored.
7. The entire large intestine from the ileocecal junction through the upper two thirds of the rectum is freed and immobilized. All vessels are ligated.
8. The terminal ileum is separated from the cecum using a mechanical cutting and stapling device (GIA).
9. The mesocolon is ligated using suture ligatures or a ligating, dividing, and stapling (LDS) instrument.
10. The rectum is resected down to the level of the mucosectomy. The colon and resected portion of the rectum are removed en bloc.
11. The pouch is created. Most surgeons use either the J pouch or the S pouch.
12. The J pouch (Figure 2-51) is created at the terminal ileum by folding two adjacent loops of small bowel, approximately 10 to 15 cm each, parallel with each other and anastomosing them using a GIA. An opening is made at the bottom of the pouch, and the pouch is pulled through the rectal stump. The bottom of the pouch is anastomosed to the anus with interrupted absorbable sutures.
13. A Y pouch (Figure 2-52) is created by aligning the distal ileum in an S configuration with each of the three limbs approximately 10 cm in length. The most distal 2 cm of the ileum is not incorporated into the pouch but is preserved for the anastomosis to the anus. The three limbs are manually incised and anastomosed to create a pouch. Mucosal tissue is approximated with absorbable suture; nonabsorbable suture is used for the serosal layer. The preserved distal end of the ileum and the pouch are pulled through the rectal stump and anastomosed to the anus. This completes the anal portion of the procedure.
14. The scrub team changes gowns and gloves, redrapes, and completes the abdominal procedure by creating a loop ileostomy through the abdominal wall, on a previously designated site.

SURGERY OF THE RECTUM

Hemorrhoidectomy

Hemorrhoidectomy is excision and ligation of dilated veins in the anal region to relieve discomfort and to control bleeding. Hemorrhoidectomy is an ambulatory surgery procedure undertaken with the application of sclerotherapy, heater probe coagulation, monopolar or bipolar coagulation, laser, infrared energy coagulation, or Doppler-guided hemorrhoidal artery ligation (Acheson and Scholefield, 2008). Rubber band ligation is done through an anoscope without sedation in an office or endoscopy set-

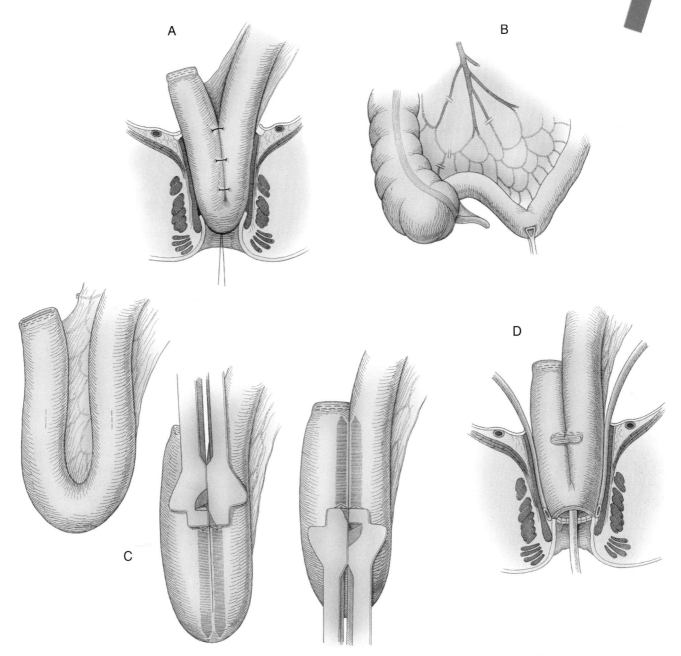

FIGURE 2-51 J pouch for ileoanal endorectal pull-through. **A,** The J pouch is created at terminal ileum by folding two adjacent loops of small bowel, approximately 10 to 15 cm each, parallel to each other. **B,** Mesenteric vascular arcades may need to be divided to provide adequate length for anal anastomosis. **C,** The two loops are anastomosed using a mechanical cutting and stapling device (GIA). **D,** Opening is made at bottom of pouch, and pouch is pulled through rectal stump. Bottom of pouch is anastomosed to anus.

ting. Larger symptomatic external and internal hemorrhoids that do not respond to conservative medical treatment are managed with surgery. This patient is at risk for hemorrhoid prolapse, strangulation, thrombosis, and possible ulceration and fistula formation. Surgical treatment aims to coagulate, seal, and excise the hemorrhoid, leaving sufficient anal mucosa surface to minimize pain and prevent stenosis or stricture. Various coagulation, vaporization, and tissue-welding technologies offer successful outcomes. Radiofrequency tissue/fusion energy (LigaSure, Valleylab, Inc.) is a unique form of electrocoagulation that provides hemostasis and sealing by fusing collagen in vessel walls. A specific stapling device may also be used (stapled hemorrhoidectomy; stapled anopexy).

Procedural Considerations. Preoperative anal dilation aids in exposing the vessels and contributes to the patient's comfort in the immediate postoperative period. Many surgeons prefer to precede the operation with a sigmoidoscopy. Spinal, caudal, epidural, or local anesthesia may be used. The patient is usu-

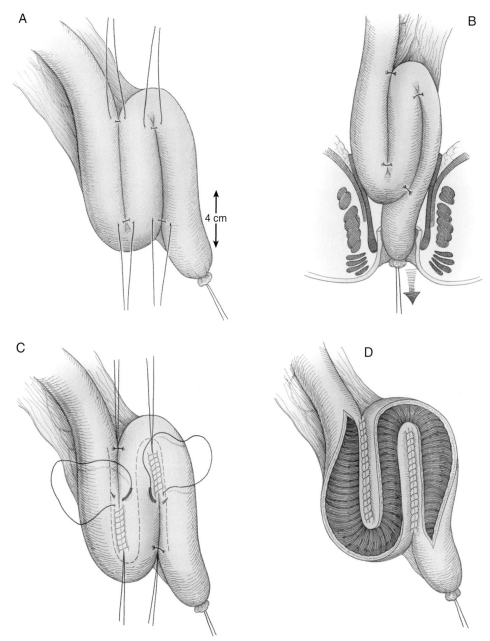

FIGURE 2-52 S pouch for ileoanal endorectal pull-through. **A,** Pouch is created by aligning distal ileum in S configuration with each limb (three in total) approximately 12 cm in length. **B,** The length is measured before anastomosis begins. **C,** Three limbs are incised and anastomosed to create pouch. **D,** Incision is made as illustrated.

ally placed in lithotomy or jackknife position. Postoperative complications include hemorrhage, pain, constipation, fecal impaction, infection, and urinary retention.

Operative Procedure

1. The anal canal is dilated and inspected through an anoscope.
2. Four Allis forceps are applied several centimeters from the anal margin to expose the anus.
3. The base of the hemorrhoid and tissue are grasped with Allis forceps and held.
4. A 2-0 synthetic absorbable intestinal suture is placed and tied at the proximal end of the hemorrhoid, and a Buie Pile forceps is applied across the base and above the proposed incision line.
5. Excision is completed with a scalpel. Coagulation and excision may also be done with monopolar or bipolar electrosurgery, laser vaporization, infrared energy, radiofrequency fusion/ligation, cryotherapy, or even heater probe coagulation. Care is directed toward preserving the rectal sphincter.
6. Loosely placed continuous sutures are placed over the Buie Pile forceps. The suture is tightened as the forceps are removed, and the suture ends are then tied.

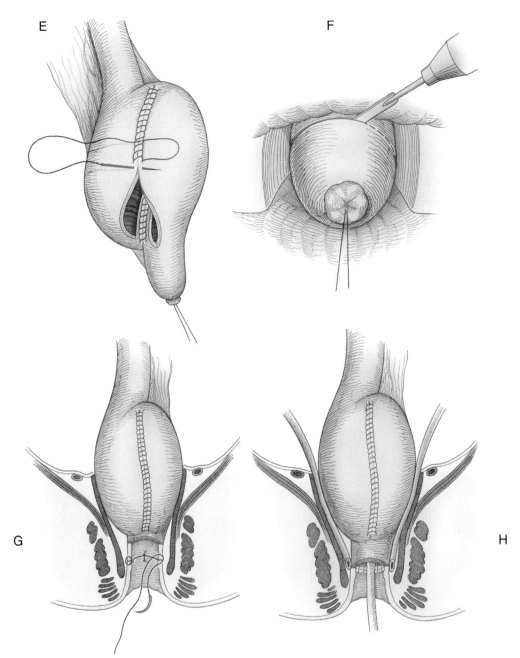

FIGURE 2-52, cont'd E, The pouch is closed using suture for the formation of the reservoir. F, Distal ends of ileum and pouch are pulled through the rectal stump, and the lower outflow tract is trimmed. G, With 3-0 absorbable sutures, the outflow tract is anastomosed to the anus at the dentate line. H, Drain in place in the lumen of the newly created ileoanal-rectal canal.

7. Traction may be maintained as hemostatic forceps are applied and dissection is completed segmentally.
8. 2-0 synthetic absorbable suture ligatures are used as each hemostat is removed.
9. Remaining hemorrhoids are excised in a similar manner.
10. Petrolatum gauze packing may be placed in the anal canal.

Excision of Pilonidal Cyst and Sinus

Excision of a pilonidal cyst and sinus is removal of the cyst with sinus tracts from the intergluteal fold on the posterior surface of the lower sacrum (Figure 2-53). A pilonidal cyst and sinus, which may be congenital in origin, rarely become symptomatic until the individual reaches adulthood, most commonly in young men. Inflammatory reaction varies from a mild, irritating, draining sinus tract to a painful, acute abscess with secondary recurrences. Treatment consists of drainage in the acute stage and total surgical excision during remission.

Excision of the cyst and sinus tracts must be complete to prevent recurrence. The defect resulting from recurrences may become too large for primary closure. In this case the wound is left open to heal by granulation.

Procedural Considerations. A minor set and rectal instruments are required, as well as methylene blue, a 10- or 20-ml syringe, and a blunt-tipped needle. The patient is placed in jackknife position with the buttocks taped open laterally and secured to the sides of the OR bed.

Operative Procedure

1. The sinus tracts are identified with probes and an incision made over the probe.
2. The tract is marked by injecting methylene blue with a blunt needle.
3. An elliptic incision is made down to the fascia.
4. A curette is used to remove granulation tissue.
5. Excision of cyst and sinus tracts is completed. Bleeding is controlled.

6. If the wound is to be left open, it is packed and a pressure dressing applied.
7. If the wound is closed, 2-0 nonabsorbable sutures are used for stay sutures on the deeper tissue and fine nonabsorbable suture is used on skin.

GASTROINTESTINAL SURGERY SUMMARY

As with any surgical specialty, in gastrointestinal surgery it is imperative to know the anatomy and physiology of the surgical area. A prepared surgical technologist needs to anticipate the unforeseen as well as be prepared for the scheduled operation. Planning ahead will greatly help the surgical team work cohesively to provide the best care possible for the patient. It is important to know and fully understand all the aspects of

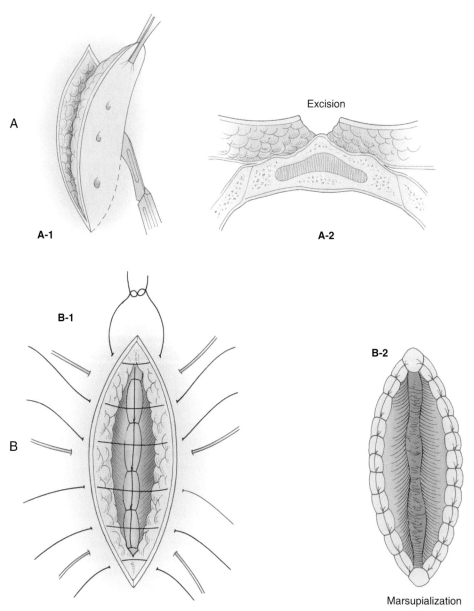

FIGURE 2-53 Pilonidal cyst. The pilonidal sinus tract is identified with injection of methylene blue into the tract. **A,** Wide elliptic incision (*A-1*) is made to include all the subcutaneous tracts and tissue that are part of the fascia overlying the sacrum and coccyx (*A-2*). **B,** Closure of the wound can be primary (*B-1*) or secondary (*B-2*).

positioning, surgical equipment, supplies, and instrumentation. The surgical technologist should understand procedural considerations of the operative procedure and should also have a good understanding of bowel technique and the flexibility to move swiftly from the laparoscopic approach to an open approach should the need arise. The risks for injury or failure to achieve the intended outcome are equally present in gastrointestinal surgery as in any surgical or invasive procedure.

GERIATRIC CONSIDERATIONS

The Elderly Patient—Gastrointestinal Surgery

It is not uncommon for older patients to mention or discuss symptoms of gastrointestinal disorders during visits with their physicians. Loss of teeth or poorly fitted dentures make chewing difficult, resulting in digestion problems. Foods that are difficult to eat are avoided, and such avoidance can affect overall nutrition. In the upper GI tract, patients may complain of dysphagia (digestive glands decrease the amount of secretions and mucus becomes thicker), heartburn, esophageal spasm, or they may have medication-induced esophageal injury; there is an increased risk of gastroesophageal reflux disease (GERD) (Geriatric Nursing Resources, 2010). Aging is also associated with alterations in the motor function of the stomach, because it takes longer for liquids, but not solids, to empty. Changes in gastric secretion also occur; there may be an increase in gastric acid secretion (Fillit et al, 2010). Atrophy of the gastric mucosa may result in decreased absorption of vitamin B_{12} and iron (Ignatavicius and Workman, 2011). In patients with decreased hydrochloric levels, bacteria may proliferate and result in atrophic gastritis. Complications of NSAID use are prevalent in elderly patients with arthritis, and those with a history of peptic ulcer or previous GI bleeding should be identified.

Malabsorption of lactose, carbohydrates, calcium, vitamin D, B_{12} and folic acid also occur in the elderly. Both celiac disease and small bowel bacterial overgrowth lead to malabsorption. Elderly patients may also have a higher incidence of Crohn's disease and ulcerative colitis. Capsule endoscopy and double-balloon enteroscopy are common diagnostic tests for small bowel disease.

The large intestine experiences decreases in peristalsis, and dulled nerve impulses. This may lead to a postponement of bowel movements and constipation. When aging is associated with diminished anal sphincter tone, patients may be susceptible to fecal incontinence. Elderly patients are also at risk of developing *Clostridium difficile* (C. diff) infections when they are hospitalized; surgery is an additional possible risk factor. Lower GI bleeding is often associated with diverticulosis.

Because the percentage of body fat increases and the lean body mass decreases, the storage of lipophilic drugs, such as diazepam and lidocaine, is enhanced. These factors are of particular importance for assessing the patient's response to preoperative and local anesthetic medications.

Modified from Fillit HM et al: *Textbook of geriatric medicine and gerontology*, ed 7, Philadelphia, 2010, Saunders; Hartford Institute for Geriatric Nursing: Geriatric nursing resources for care of older adults, available at consultgerirn.org/topics/normal_aging_changes/want_to_know_more#item_7. Accessed September 5, 2010; Ignatavicius DD, Workman ML: *Medical-surgical nursing: patient-centered collaborative care*, ed 6, Philadelphia, 2010, Saunders.

REVIEW QUESTIONS

1. The Nissen fundoplication is performed to:
   a. reduce a hernia
   b. treat GERD
   c. repair a defect in the diaphragm
   d. all of the above

2. A percutaneous endoscopic gastrostomy is used to:
   a. reduce a hernia
   b. reduce weight
   c. treat GERD
   d. enteral feedings

3. Establishes a permanent communication between the proximal jejunum and either the anterior or the posterior stomach:
   a. Billroth I
   b. gastrojejunostomy
   c. Billroth II
   d. gastric bypass

4. The formation of a temporary or permanent opening into the ileum:
   a. colostomy
   b. gastrojejunostomy
   c. ileostomy
   d. PEG

5. Resection of the right half of the colon, including a portion of the transverse colon, ascending colon, and cecum:
   a. hemicolectomy
   b. Nissen
   c. Billroth II
   d. transverse colectomy

6. Mobilization and division of a diseased segment of the lower bowel though a midline incision:
   a. ileostomy
   b. abdominoperineal resection
   c. Roux-en-Y
   d. hemorrhoidectomy

7. Incision and ligation of dilated veins in the anal region:
   a. colectomy
   b. abdominoperineal resection
   c. hemorrhoidectomy
   d. appendectomy

8. A Billroth I is the resection of a diseased portion of the stomach and the establishment of an anastomosis between:
   a. stomach and jejunum
   b. duodenum and jejunum
   c. stomach and duodenum
   d. duodenum and pyloric sphincter

9. A McBurney incision is commonly used for:
   a. femoral hernia
   b. appendectomy
   c. inguinal hernia
   d. Billroth I

10. A Billroth I is the resection of a diseased portion of the stomach and the establishment of an anastomosis between:
   a. stomach and jejunum
   b. duodenum and jejunum
   c. stomach and duodenum
   d. duodenum and pyloric sphincter

11. Define and briefly describe the following surgical procedures:
   Laparotomy
   Esophagectomy
   Transverse colectomy

Critical Thinking Question

What are the challenges you will face when positioning a morbidly obese patient, and how can you ensure the patient is positioned safely?

REFERENCES

Acheson AG, Scholefield JH: Management of haemorrhoids, *BMJ* 336: 380–383, 2008.

Adams RE et al: Long-term mortality after gastric bypass surgery, *N Engl J Med* 357:753–761, 2007.

Anaya DA, Dellinger EP et al: Surgical infection and choice of antibiotics. In Townsend CM et al, editors: *Sabiston textbook of surgery*, ed 18, Philadelphia, 2008, Saunders.

Association of periOperative Registered Nurses: Recommended practice for prevention of hypothermia. In *Perioperative standards and recommended practices,* Denver, 2009a, The Association.

Association of periOperative Registered Nurses: Recommended practice for environment of care. In *Perioperative standards and recommended practices,* Denver, 2009b, The Association.

Association of periOperative Registered Nurses: Recommended practice for sponge, sharp and instrument counts. In *Perioperative standards and recommended practices,* Denver, 2009c, The Association.

Association of periOperative Registered Nurses: Bariatric surgery guideline. In *Perioperative standards and recommended practices,* Denver, 2009d, The Association.

Barclay L: Natural orifice transluminal endoscopic surgery may allow incisionless operations, Medscape Medical News, 2008, available at www.medscape.com/viewarticle/578108. Accessed June 12, 2009.

Barclay L et al: Guidelines issued for the management of GERD, Medscape Medical News, 2008, available at cme.medscape.com/viewarticle/582673. Accessed October 9, 2009.

Beauchamp-Johnson BM: Scale down bariatric surgery risks, *OR Nurse* 48–54, January/February 2007.

Birn CS: Endoscopic ultrasound reveals GI tract secrets, *Nurs Spectr* 17:5–17, 2005.

Bisanz A et al: Characterizing postoperative paralytic ileus as evidence for future research and clinical practice, *Gastroenterol Nurs* 31(5):336–344, 2008.

Blackwood HS: Help your patient downsize with bariatric surgery, *Med Surg Insider*, Fall 2005.

Chambers KL: Obesity: an American epidemic, *Surg Technol* 41(5):213–220, 2009.

Cleveland Clinic: Cleveland Clinic First to Perform Successful Live Kidney Donation Through Single Belly Button Incision, 2008, available at http://healthorbit.ca/NewsDetail.asp?opt=1&nltid=140150708. Accessed June 12, 2009.

Curcillo PG: Drexel University College of Medicine Department of Surgery, Oral absract from SAGES Emerging Technology 2007.

Denholm B: Tucking patient's arms and general positioning, *AORN J* 89(4):755–757, 2009.

Edmondson D, Schiech L: Esophageal cancer—a tough pill to swallow, *Nursing* 38(4):44–50, 2008.

Ewing DR et al: Robots in the operating room—the history, *Seminars in laparoscopic surgery* 11(2):63–72, 2004.

Fowler D: Single Port Laparoscopy or NOTES: A Form of Image Guided Therapy? CISST ERC Seminar, 2008, available at http://cisst.org/wiki/seminar_2008_06_25_NOTES. Accessed June 12, 2006.

Hageman D et al: Laparoscopic-assisted colon surgery, *AORN J* 88:403–416, 2008.

Hager C: Quality of life after Roux-en-Y gastric bypass surgry, *AORN J* 85(4):768–778, 2007.

Kulaylat MN, Dayton MT: Surgical complications. In Townsend CM et al, editors: *Sabiston textbook of surgery*, ed 18, St Louis, 2008, Mosby.

Kwon RS et al: Gastrointestinal cancer imaging: deeper than the eye can see, *Gastroenterology* 128:1538–1553, 2005.

Lee JM et al: Enduring effects of thorascopic Heller myotomy for treating achalasia, *World J Surg* 28:55–58, 2004.

Lewis BS: Obscure gastrointestinal bleeding. In Ginsberg GG et al, editors: *Clinical gastrointestinal endoscopy*, Philadelphia, 2005, Saunders.

Lucile Packard Children's Hospital: News Release: Pediatric surgeon pushes envelope (and belly button) to remove diseased organs. July 28, 2008, available at www.lpch.org/newsEvents/NewsReleases/2008/surgeonPushesEnvelope.html. Accessed July 28, 2008.

Marin K et al: Intraperitoneal chemotherapy: implications beyond ovarian cancer, *Clin J Oncol Nurs* 11(6):881–889, 2007.

Markmann JF et al: Transplantation of abdominal ogans. In Townsend CM et al, editors: *Sabiston textbook of surgery*, ed 18, St Louis, 2008, Mosby.

Pappas SG et al: Malignant peritoneal mesothelioma, In Townsend CM et al: editors: *Sabiston textbook of surgery*, ed 18, St Louis, 2008, Mosby.

Pasricha PJ: Endoluminal surgery. In Ginsberg GG et al: *Clinical gastrointestinal endoscopy*, St Louis, 2005, Saunders, pp 841–843.

Porth CM, Gaspard KJ: *Essentials of pathophysiology: concepts of altered health states*, Philadelphia, 2004, Lippincott Williams & Wilkins.

Raman JD et al: Single incision laparoscopic surgery: initial urological experience and comparison with natural-orifice transluminal endoscopic surgery, BJU Online article, 2008, available at www.advancedsurgical.ie/BJU_Online_Article/Default.245.html. Accessed June 14, 2009.

Ransohoff DF: Colon cancer screening in 2005—status and challenges, *Gastroenterology* 128:1685–1695, 2005.

Regenbogen SE et al: Utility of the surgical Apgar score, *Arch Surg* 144(1):30–36, 2009.

Shortridge K et al: Intestinal transplantation, In Colwell JC et al: *Fecal and urinary diversions: management principles*, St Louis, 2004, Mosby.

Society of Gastroenterology Nurses and Associates: *Manual of gastrointestinal procedures*, ed 5, Philadelphia, 2004, Lippincott Williams & Wilkins.

Sonoda T, Milsom JW: Segmental colon resection. In Souba WW et al: *ACS surgery—principles and practice*, New York, 2007, WebMD.

Sunada K et al: Clinical outcomes of enteroscopy using the double balloon method for strictures of the small intestine, *World J Gastroenterol* 11(7):1087–1089, 2005.

The Surgical and Clinical Adhesions Research (SCAR)-3 study, *Colorectal Dis,* 7:551–558, 2005.

Wang KK: Endoscopic therapy for superficial esophageal carcinomas. In Ginsberg GG et al, editors: *Clinical gastrointestinal endoscopy*, St Louis, 2005, Saunders.

CHAPTER 3

Surgery of the Liver, Biliary Tract, Pancreas, and Spleen

Overview

A pathologic condition in the liver, biliary tract, pancreas, or spleen often requires surgical intervention. These organs are highly vascular and control many metabolic and immune functions of the body. Surgical intervention may be indicated for infection, cystic anomalies, congenital anomalies, metabolic

This chapter was originally written by Janice A. Neil, RN, PhD, for the 14th edition of Alexander's Care of the Patient in Surgery and has been revised by Michelle Williams-Callahan, CST, AAS, for this text.

diseases, trauma (see Chapter 18), or malignancy. Many new cases of malignancy of the pancreas, gallbladder, or extrahepatic biliary tract are diagnosed each year and the prognosis for these is often poor (Steer, 2008; Chari and Shah, 2008). Pancreatic cancer remains the fourth leading cause of death in the United States (McPhee et al, 2007). In the past decade, surgeries of the liver and biliary tract have become more advanced as research and new technology permit more complete diagnoses of pathologic conditions. A resection of the liver for carcinoma has achieved a recognized role for cure or substantial palliation with safety and low morbidity.

Cholecystectomy is the most common, nonemergency abdominal operation performed. In the United States more than 750,000 cholecystectomies are performed each year. It is

HISTORY

Solid Organ Transplant

In the eighteenth century, researchers experimented with solid organ transplants on animals and humans. Transplant science evolved after many trials and failures. Important medical breakthroughs, such as surgical technique, tissue typing, immunology, immuno-suppressant drugs, and organ preservation, have permitted more success in the viability of organs and longer survival rates for transplant recipients. The following is a summarized timeline of significant "firsts" and milestones in the evolution of solid organ transplant surgery, an often clinically effective and life-saving strategy for patients with end-stage organ failure.

Year	Breakthrough
1954	The first successful kidney transplant
	Dr. Joseph E. Murray, Brigham & Women's Hospital, Boston, Massachusetts
1963	The first lung transplant
	Dr. James Hardy, University of Mississippi, Oxford, Mississippi
1966	The first simultaneous pancreas/kidney transplant
	Dr. Richard Lillehei, William Kelly, University of Minnesota, Minneapolis, Minnesota
1967	The first successful liver transplant
	Dr. Thomas Starzl, University of Colorado Health Sciences Center, Denver, Colorado
1968	The first isolated pancreas transplant
	Dr. Richard Lillehei, University of Minnesota, Minneapolis, Minnesota
1968	The first successful heart transplant in the United States
	Dr. Norman Shumway, Stanford University Hospital, Stanford, California
1981	The first successful heart/lung transplant
	Dr. Bruce Reitz, Stanford University Hospital, Stanford, California
1983	The first successful lung transplant
	Dr. Joel Cooper, Toronto Lung Transplant Group, Toronto General Hospital, Toronto, Canada
1986	The first successful double-lung transplant
	Dr. Joel Cooper, Toronto Lung Transplant Group, Toronto General Hospital, Toronto, Canada
1989	The first living-related liver transplant
	Dr. Christoph Broelsch, University of Chicago Medical Center, Chicago, Illinois
1990	The first successful living-related lung transplant
	Dr. Vaughn A. Starnes, Stanford University Medical Center, Stanford, California
1992	The first baboon-to-human liver transplant
	The University of Pittsburgh Medical Center, Pittsburgh, Pennsylvania
1992	The first pig-to-human liver transplant
	Cedars-Sinai Medical Center, Los Angeles, California
1993	The first successful living-related lung lobes transplant (one from each of the recipient's parents)
	University of Southern California, Los Angeles, California
2002	The first uterus transplant took place in Saudi Arabia. The transplanted organ remained viable for 99 days. The intent of the transplant is to make childbirth possible for women who have undergone hysterectomies; the transplant would be temporary—the uterus would be removed once the baby was born to prevent ongoing administration of antirejection drugs
2005	The first partial face transplant, Amiens, France
2008	First partial face transplant in United States, The Cleveland Clinic, Cleveland, Ohio
2009	First simultaneous face-and-hand transplant, Paris, France. The upper half of the face, including the scalp, forehead, nose, ears, and upper and lower eyelids, was transplanted

Boston doctors perform face transplant, available at www.cbsnews.com/stories/2009/04/10/health/main4934319.shtml?source=RSSattr=HOME_4934319. Accessed April 15, 2009; *History of transplantation timeline,* available at www.organtransplants.org/understanding/history. Accessed April 1, 2009; Linden PK: History of solid organ transplantation and organ donation, *Crit Care Clin* 25(1), 2009; *Milestones in transplantation data,* available at www.unos.org/data/default.asp?display=liver&displayType=internationalData. Accessed April 1, 2009; *Saudi surgeons perform first uterus transplant,* 2002, available at www.nytimes.com/2002/03/07/world/medical-first-a-transplant-of-a-uterus.html?sec=health - 42k. Accessed April 1, 2009.

one of the most frequently performed inpatient procedures in the United States (Afdhal and Vollmer, 2008; Chari and Shah, 2008). Laparoscopic cholecystectomy has become the gold standard surgical intervention for the treatment of cholecystitis. Since the early 1990s, laparoscopic cholecystectomy, as compared with open-incision cholecystectomy, has resulted in reduced trauma to tissues as well as shorter postoperative recoveries, both distinct advantages. About 94% of cholecystectomies are elective surgeries while the remainder are emergencies (Afdhal and Vollmer, 2008). Laparoscopic cholecystectomies were the precursor to numerous abdominal

procedures now performed or assisted with the laparoscope. Current innovations in cholecystectomy are focusing on removal of the gallbladder through a natural orifice (referred to as NOTES, or natural-orifice transluminal endoscopic surgery) (Ramos et al, 2008).

New diagnostic technology and the intraoperative use of ultrasonography, biliary endoscopy, and radiography have enabled surgeons to better treat diseases of the biliary tract. Solid organ transplantation (History box), such as for the liver, pancreas, and kidneys, has become common as a means to treat

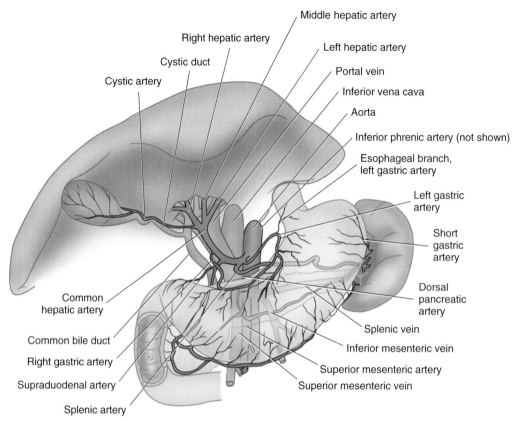

FIGURE 3-1 Intricate relationships of the arterial and venous blood supply of the liver, gallbladder, pancreas, spleen, and the biliary ductal system.

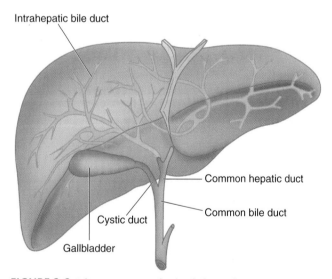

FIGURE 3-2 Biliary system can be divided into three anatomic areas: the intrahepatic bile duct, the extrahepatic bile duct (common hepatic and common bile ducts), and the gallbladder and cystic duct

primary hepatic tumors, end-stage liver disease, and insulin-deficient diabetes. Liver transplant procedures have advanced to include entire organ transplants as well as living-related organ donations.

This chapter explores the most common open and minimally invasive procedures performed on the liver, biliary tract, pancreas, and spleen.

Surgical Anatomy

The liver is in the right upper quadrant of the abdominal cavity, beneath the dome of the diaphragm and directly above the stomach, duodenum, and hepatic flexure of the colon. The external covering, known as *Glisson's capsule,* is composed of dense connective tissue. The visceral peritoneum extends over the entire surface of the liver, except at the point of posterior attachment to the diaphragm. This connective tissue branches at the porta hepatis into a network of septa that extends into an intrahepatic network of support for the more than 1 million hepatic lobules. The porta hepatis is located on the inferior surface of the liver and provides entry and exit for the major vessels, ducts, and nerves. The hepatic artery maintains the arterial blood supply, while venous blood from the stomach, intestines, spleen, and pancreas travels to the liver by the portal vein and its branches (Figure 3-1). The hepatic venous system returns blood to the heart via the inferior vena cava.

Lobules are the functional units of the liver. Each lobule contains a portal triad that consists of a hepatic duct, a hepatic portal vein branch, and a branch of the hepatic artery, nerves, and lymphatics. A central vein is located in the center of each lobule and provides venous drainage into the hepatic veins.

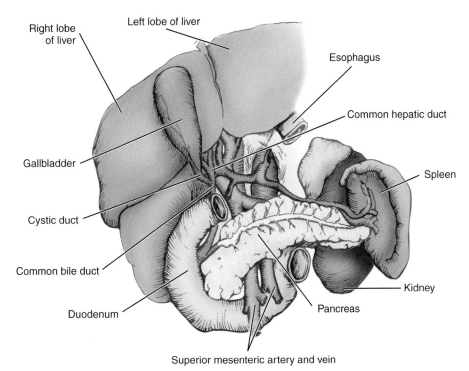

FIGURE 3-3 Gallbladder and surrounding anatomy.

Lobules also contain hepatic cords, hepatic sinusoids, and bile canaliculi. The hepatic cords consist of numerous columns of hepatocytes—the functional cells of the liver. The hepatic sinusoids are the blood channels that communicate among the columns of hepatocytes. The sinusoids have a thin epithelial lining composed primarily of Kupffer cells—phagocytic cells that engulf bacteria and toxins. The sinusoids drain into the central vein.

Bile is manufactured by the hepatocytes. The bile canaliculi are tiny bile capillary vessels that communicate among the columns of hepatocytes. The bile canaliculi collect and transport bile to the bile ducts in the portal triad of each lobule, from which bile then flows into the hepatic ducts at the porta hepatis. These ducts join immediately to form one common hepatic duct that merges with the cystic duct from the gallbladder to form the common bile duct (Figure 3-2). The common bile duct opens into the duodenum in an area called the *ampulla,* or *papilla of Vater,* located about 7.5 cm below the pyloric opening from the stomach.

Bile contains bile salts, which facilitate digestion and absorption, and various waste products. The liver is essential in the metabolism of carbohydrates, proteins, and fats. It metabolizes nutrients into stores of glycogen, used for regulation of blood glucose levels and as energy sources for the brain and body functions.

The liver plays several important roles in the blood-clotting mechanism. It is the organ that synthesizes plasma proteins, excluding gamma globulins but including prothrombin and fibrinogen. Vitamin K, a co-factor to the synthesis of prothrombin, is absorbed by the metabolism of fats in the intestinal tract as a result of bile formation by the liver. Patients with liver disease may have altered blood-coagulation abilities.

The liver also synthesizes lipoproteins and cholesterol. Cholesterol is an essential component of the blood plasma. It serves as a precursor for bile salts, steroid hormones, plasma membranes, and other specialized molecules. A diet high in cholesterol reduces the amount that must be synthesized by the liver. When the diet is deficient in cholesterol, the liver increases synthesis to maintain levels necessary for production of vital chemical molecules.

The liver also serves in the metabolic alteration of foreign molecules or biotransformation of chemicals. The microsomal enzyme system (MES) plays a major role in the body's response to foreign chemicals, such as pollutants, drugs, and alcohol. Patients with liver disease may have an altered response to chemical substances. This consideration is important in the induction and management of general anesthesia for patients with liver disorders.

The gallbladder, which lies in a sulcus on the undersurface of the right lobe of the liver, terminates in the cystic duct (Figure 3-3). This ductal system provides a channel for the flow of bile to the gallbladder, where it becomes highly concentrated during storage. The liver produces about 600 to 1000 ml of bile each day. The gallbladder's average storage capacity is 40 to 70 ml. As foods, especially fats, are ingested, the duodenal cells release cholecystokinin. As the musculature of the gallbladder contracts, bile is forced into the cystic duct and through the common duct. As the sphincter of Oddi in the ampulla of Vater relaxes, bile is released, flowing into the duodenum to aid in digestion by emulsification of fats. The gallbladder receives its blood supply from the cystic artery, a branch of the hepatic artery. The triangle of Calot contains the cystic artery (and possibly the right hepatic

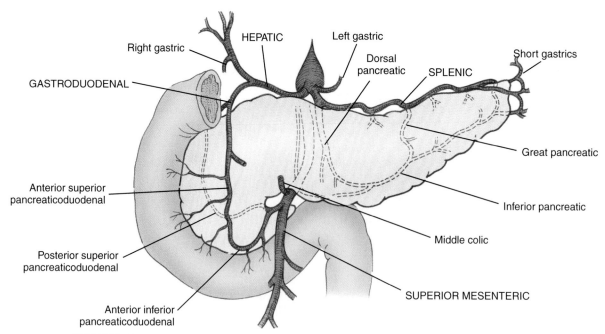

FIGURE 3-4 Arterial supply to the pancreas arises from the celiac axis (hepatic and splenic arteries) and the superior mesenteric artery. The blood supply to the head of the gland is by way of the pancreaticoduodenal (anterior and posterior) arcades, which arise from the gastroduodenal artery (superior) and superior mesenteric arteries (inferior).

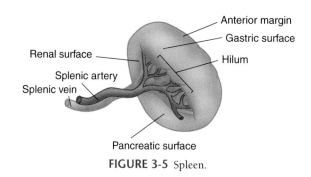

FIGURE 3-5 Spleen.

artery); it is an anatomic landmark in surgical removal of the gallbladder. Its boundaries may be remembered as "the *3 Cs*": Cystic duct, Common hepatic duct, and Cystic artery (Chari and Shah, 2008). Innervation for the gallbladder and biliary tree is controlled by the autonomic nervous system. Parasympathetic innervation stimulates contraction, whereas sympathetic innervation inhibits contraction.

The pancreas (see Figure 3-3) is a fixed structure lying transversely behind the stomach in the upper abdomen. The head of the pancreas is fixed to the curve of the duodenum. Blood is supplied to the pancreas and the duodenum from the celiac axis and superior mesenteric artery (Figure 3-4). The body of the pancreas lies across the vertebrae and over

the superior mesenteric artery and vein. The tail of the pancreas extends to the hilum of the spleen. In total, the pancreas extends about 25 cm. Pancreatic secretions containing digestive enzymes are collected in the pancreatic duct, or duct of Wirsung, which joins with the common bile duct to enter the duodenum about 7.5 cm below the pylorus. The dilated junction of the two ducts at the point of entry forms the ampulla of Vater.

The pancreas also contains groups of cells, called *islets,* or *islands, of Langerhans,* that secrete hormones into the blood capillaries instead of into the duct. These hormones are insulin and glucagon, and both are involved in carbohydrate metabolism.

The spleen (Figure 3-5) is in the upper left abdominal cavity, with full protection provided by the tenth, eleventh, and twelfth ribs; its lateral surface is directly beneath the dome of the diaphragm. The anterior medial surface is in proximity to the cardiac end of the stomach and the splenic flexure of the colon. The spleen is covered with peritoneum that forms supporting ligaments. The splenic artery, a branch of the celiac axis, furnishes the arterial blood supply. The splenic vein drains into the portal system.

The spleen has many functions. Among them are defense of the body by phagocytosis of microorganisms, formation of nongranular leukocytes and plasma cells, and phagocytosis of damaged red blood cells. It also acts as a blood reservoir.

Surgical Technologist Considerations

Hepatobiliary surgery is a demanding surgical specialty. The anatomic structures are delicate and surrounded by major blood vessels. It is important the surgical technologist be aware of the procedure, anatomy involved, surgeon's preferences, and any unique items that may be needed for each patient. Special care needs to be paid to the potential for significant blood loss. It is imperative the surgical technologist have the required items at the ready. In the event of major blood loss, vascular instruments, sutures, and hemostatic agents may be required in rapid succession.

Laparoscopic surgery and the emerging field of robotic procedures can bring a sense of simplicity to the surgery. However, the risk of bleeding or a bile duct injury can still occur. In these instances, it is vital the surgical technologist be able to rapidly convert the procedure to an open procedure. In this event maintaining the sterile field, counting multiple instrument pans, receiving medications onto the sterile field, and communicating with the surgical team must be done with the utmost accuracy. The surgical technologist needs to be aware of any patient allergies, because this may affect the medications received onto the sterile field. It is also important to keep an accurate record of irrigation used. This will help the surgical team determine the estimated blood loss.

Another vital area of importance is specimen labeling. In any large abdominal procedure multiple specimens may be received for pathology. Verification of the surgical specimen, the medium that it should be placed in, and how it will be sent to pathology are critical to obtaining a correct pathology result. Some specimens will be sent to pathology for freezing to determine if margins are clear. The surgical technologist plays a key role in this process. Specimens that are mislabeled or mishandled could affect the patient's treatment during surgery, as well as postoperatively.

Interventions

- Implement aseptic technique; communicate and correct breaks in asepsis.
- Ensure, along with the perioperative nurse and anesthesia provider, that preoperative antibiotics are administered as ordered; prophylactic antibiotics should be administered 1 hour before surgical incision is made. Follow guidelines for safe medication practices.
- Contain and confine contaminants appropriately.
- Ensure that all sterilization procedures have been properly observed.
- Ensure that the integrity of sterile supply packaging is intact before dispensing items to the sterile field.

Implementation

Patients having surgery of the liver, biliary tract, pancreas, or spleen are usually given a general anesthetic. The following pertinent factors should be considered in caring for these patients.

Universal Protocol. The Joint Commission (TJC) requires that the "wrong site, wrong procedure, wrong person" prevention protocol be carried out before each surgical procedure (TJC, 2009). This protocol involves the following principles:

- Wrong site, wrong procedure, wrong person surgery can and must be prevented.
- Active involvement and effective communication among all members of the surgical team are required.
- The patient (to the extent possible) should be involved in the process.

SURGICAL TECHNOLOGY PREFERENCE CARD

This serves as a tool to assist the surgical technologist in the scrub role when preparing for hepatobiliary surgery. Most surgeries will be done in the supine position. Occasionally an approach may require a lateral position. Be sure to account for the patient's height, weight, and age when gathering positioning supplies. Since these surgeries can be lengthy, ensure that adequate padding is available for positioning the patient and that thermoregulation measures are employed.

Hepatobiliary surgery may sometimes call for additional unexpected procedures. Unanticipated blood loss may occur requiring vascular repair or reconstruction. You may need to direct room personnel to gather extra instrumentation, supplies, and medications or even obtain phone numbers of vascular surgeons on-call. Having the necessary supplies and information readily available can make an urgent situation run smoothly.

Room Prep: Basic operating room furniture in place, thermoregulatory devices, extra blankets, padding positioning supplies to achieve optimal patient safety

Prep Solution: In room
- Chlorhexidine gluconate (CHG)
- Iodine and iodophors

Catheters: In room and correct size
- Catheter set and tray
  - Latex/rubber
  - Silicone
  - Temperature sensing
- Sizing
  - French
- Retaining
  - Foley
    - 2-way
    - 3-way
  - Mushroom/Pezzer/Malecot
  - T-tube
- Other urine collection devices

PROCEDURE CHECKLIST

Instruments
- Standard sets
- Open instruments if needed to convert from laparoscopic to open
- Anticipated additional instruments
  - Bowel clamps
  - Bookwalter or other self-retaining retractor
  - Anastomotic stapling devices
  - Pedicle clamp
  - Laser
  - Smoke evacuator

Specialty Suture
- As per surgeon's preference

Hemostatic Agents
- Mechanical
  - Staplers
  - Clip appliers and clips
  - Pressure
  - Ligatures
  - Pledgets
- Chemical
  - Absorbable gelatin
  - Collagen
  - Oxidized cellulose
  - Epinephrine
  - Thrombin
  - Dermabond
- Thermal
  - Electrosurgical unit (monopolar and/or bipolar)
  - Harmonic scalpel
  - Argon beam coagulator
  - Smoke evacuator

Additional Supplies: both sterile and nonsterile
- If the physician is requesting supplies, instruments, or equipment not normally used, check to be sure all have arrived to the room before opening any other supplies
- Bowel bag

SURGICAL TECHNOLOGY PREFERENCE CARD—cont'd

- Wound protector
- Sponges
- Drapes
- Gowns and gloves for team members
- "Have ready" or "hold" supplies

Medications and Irrigation Solutions

- Devices for warming irrigating solutions as applicable
- Appropriate-sized syringes, hypodermic needles, labels, and marking pen

Drains and Dressings

- Correct size and type for planned surgery
- Dressings as per surgeon's preference
- Drains
  - Open—Not attached to a drainage system
    - Penrose
    - Cigarette
    - T-tubes
  - Closed—Attached to a closed reservoir for fluid collection
    - Hemovac
    - Jackson-Pratt
    - Autologous blood retrieval drainage system
- Anchoring methods
  - Suture
    - Nonabsorbable
    - Cutting needle
  - Tape

Specimen Care

- Proper container for each specimen
  - Frozen
  - Fresh
  - Permanent
  - Stones
  - Body fluids or washings
  - Cultures
- Labels for each specimen
- Proper solution for specimen type

Before opening for the procedure, the surgical technologist should:

- Arrange furniture
- Gather positioning devices
- Damp dust lights, furniture, and surfaces
- Verify functionality of equipment
- Place items to be opened in their appropriate places

When opening sterile supplies:

- Verify exposure to sterilization
- Use sterile technique
- Open bundles in appropriate locations
- Open additional supplies onto sterile field
- Open the room as close to the surgical start time as possible

---

- Consistent implementation is necessary.
- The protocol is flexible to allow for implementation with adaptation to patient needs.
- Site marking should focus on operative and other invasive procedures involving right/left distinction (laterality) and multiple structures or multiple levels.
- The protocol is adaptable to all procedures that expose patients to the risk for harm.

Proper implementation of the Universal Protocol should use the following steps:

1. Preoperative verification
   - Relevant documents and studies should be available before the start of the procedure and must be consistent with each other, with the patient's expectations, and with the team's understanding of the intended patient, procedure, and site. As applicable, any implants, special equipment or positioning devices, and availability of ordered blood/blood products must be verified. Missing information or discrepancies must be addressed before starting the procedure. This begins an ongoing process of information gathering, verification, and open team communication.
   - The signed consent should have the correct site and specific procedure documented.
   - The surgical posting should match the procedure.
   - Before receiving sedation the patient (or the patient's representative) should know and be able to state in his or

Common Hepatotoxic Agents and Type of Liver Damage

Toxic Agent	Source	Liver Damage
Aflatoxin B	Moldy foods, rice, corn, cassava, oil, grain dust (during bin clean out and animal feeding in enclosed buildings)	Jaundice, fatty liver, hepatocellular carcinoma, thromboses
Amanita phalloides	Poisonous mushrooms	Centrilobular and massive necrosis
Benzene	Chemical industry, to make plastics, resins, and nylon and synthetic fibers	Fatty liver, cirrhosis
Beryllium	From x-ray tube and fluorescent lamp manufacture; alloys are used in automobiles, computers, sports equipment (golf clubs and bicycle frames)	Necrosis and granulomas
Boron, cadmium, nickel, chromium, copper	From gold smelting, plating	Liver damage, rise in levels of liver enzymes
Carbon tetrachloride	Propellants for aerosol cans, as a pesticide, cleaning fluid, degreasing agent, fire extinguishers, spot removers (now banned)	Centrilobular necrosis
Kerosene	From fuel handling	Liver damage, rise in levels of liver enzymes
Lead	Environment	Steatosis, hepatitis
Pesticides	Polyvinyl chloride, farming industry	Steatosis, angiosarcoma (liver tumors)
Phosphorus	From poisons and firecrackers	Fatty liver, necrosis, fibrosis
Toluene, xylene	Occurs naturally in crude oil	Fatty liver, fibrosis
Vinyl chloride	Used to make polyvinyl chloride (plastics; also named PVC)	Angiosarcoma (liver tumors), fibrosis

Modified from Orfei L: Toxic liver injury, 2005, available at www.meddean.luc.edu/lumen/MedEd/orfpath/toxicinjury.htm. Accessed April 1, 2009; Levels and distribution of aflatoxin B1 in grain dust, 2002, available at www.cdc.gov/nasd/docs/d001301-d001400/d001376/d001376.html. Accessed April 1, 2009; ToxFaqs for benzene, 2004, available at www.atsdr.cdc.gov/tfacts3.html. Accessed April 1, 2009; ToxFaqs for beryllium, 2004, available at www.atsdr.cdc.gov/tfacts4.html. Accessed April 1, 2009; ToxFaqs for carbon tetrachloride, 2004, available at www.atsdr.cdc.gov/tfacts30.html; ToxFaqs for toluene, 2004, available at www.atsdr.cdc.gov/tfacts56.html; ToxFaqs for vinyl chloride, 2004, available at www.atsdr.cdc.gov/tfacts20.html. Accessed April 1, 2009.

her own words the name of the procedure and the site of surgery.

2. Marking the operative site
   - This is intended to identify unambiguously the intended site of incision/insertion. For procedures with right/left, multiple structures, or multiple levels, the site must show a mark that is visible after the patient has been prepped and draped. Special marking pens are available for this process. Marking pens should only be used for a single patient and then discarded.
   - The surgeon (or another licensed independent practitioner who will be present during the procedure and is ultimately accountable for the procedure) marks the site with "yes" or his or her initials. Check marks or Xs are not appropriate.
3. "Time-out" immediately before starting the procedure (the final verification of the correct patient, procedure, and site).
   - The surgical position, and, if applicable, implants and other required special items may also be verified before the incision is made. At this time, it should also be verified that any flammable prep solutions have dried.
   - Active communication among all members of the surgical/procedure team must be consistently initiated by a designated member of the team (usually the registered nurse). This must be conducted in a "fail-safe" mode: that is, the procedure may not be started before any questions or concerns are resolved (this is also referred to as a *hard stop*).

Positioning the Patient. For biliary surgery, the patient is placed in supine position. Arms are placed on padded armboards with the palms up and fingers extended. Armboards are maintained at less than a 90-degree angle to prevent brachial plexus stretch. If there are surgical reasons to tuck the arms at the side, the elbows are padded to protect the ulnar nerve, the palms face inward, and the wrist is maintained in a neutral position (Denholm, 2009). A drape secures the arms. It should be tucked snugly, but not tightly, under the patient, not under the mattress. This prevents the arm from shifting downward intraoperatively and resting against the OR bed rail. A small positioning aid may be placed under the lower right side of the thorax to elevate the lower rib cage, providing better exposure and access to the viscera in the right upper quadrant of the abdomen. Alternatively, a lateral tilt of the OR bed may be used in combination with reverse Trendelenburg for procedures such as laparoscopic cholecystectomy.

Positioning for laparoscopic procedures requires caution when applying safety straps. Given that the patient may be placed in a severe side tilt or reverse Trendelenburg position, safety or restraining straps must be placed securely, but not too tightly. Attention is given to proper alignment of the patient's body and extremities, and padded footboards are applied to prevent the patient from slipping. Areas of pressure in the selected surgical position and bony prominences are padded well to prevent interruption of circulation and pressure injury to tissues and neurovascular structures. These precautions are especially important for diabetic, circulatory-impaired, immu-

Liver Battery (Liver Function Studies)

Test Name	Normal Values
SERUM ENZYMES	
Alkaline phosphatase (ALP)	30-120 units/L. Elevated levels with biliary obstruction, cholestatic hepatitis, liver disease.
Aspartate aminotransferase (AST; previously SGOT)	0-35 units/L. Elevated levels with hepatocellular injury, necrosis.
Alanine aminotransferase (ALT; previously SGPT)	4-36 units/L. Elevated levels with liver damage, acute hepatitis; AST/ALT ratio usually is higher in liver necrosis and acute hepatitis and lower in cirrhosis, chronic hepatitis, cancer of liver.
Lactate dehydrogenase (LDH)	100-190 units/L (normal value may differ with method). Elevated levels in liver disease, untreated pernicious anemia, acute myocardial infarction, renal disease, muscle disease, malignant tumors.
5-Nucleotidase	0-1.6 units at 37° C. Elevated levels may indicate hepatobiliary disease.
Leucine aminopeptidase (LAP)	Males: 80-200 units/ml. Females: 75-185 units/ml. Elevated in liver necrosis and cancer, extrahepatic biliary obstruction (stones), viral hepatitis.
γ-Glutamyltransferase (GGT), γ-glutamictranspeptidase (GGTP)	Adults ≥45 yr: 8-38 units/L; <45 yr: 5-27 units/L. Newborns: 5× higher than in adults. Elevated levels in cirrhosis, acute and chronic liver necrosis, alcoholism, acute and chronic hepatitis, liver cancer.
	Enzyme produced by bile ducts. Reflects rare forms of liver disease. Medications commonly cause GGTP level to be elevated. Liver toxins such as alcohol can cause increases in GGTP level.
Alpha fetoprotein	<15 ng/ml. Elevated in cirrhosis, hepatitis. May indicate liver metastases from another cancer source.
Mitochondrial antibodies	Presence of these antibodies can indicate primary biliary cirrhosis, chronic active hepatitis, certain other autoimmune disorders.
BILIRUBIN METABOLISM	
Serum Bilirubin	
Indirect (unconjugated)	0.2-0.8 mg/dl. Elevated levels with hemolysis (lysis of red blood cells) and severe liver damage.
Direct and total (conjugated)	Total: 0.3-1.0 mg/dl. Direct: 0.1-0.3 mg/dl. Newborn: 1.0-12.0 mg/dl. Elevated levels seen with intrahepatic or extrahepatic obstruction.
Urine bilirubin	Negative: 0.02 mg/dl. Bilirubin in urine may be seen with hepatic disease or biliary obstruction; only conjugated bilirubin spills into urine because unconjugated bilirubin is bound to albumin in serum and thus cannot pass glomerular membrane.
Urine urobilinogen	Random: negative or <1.0 Ehrlich unit. 2 hr: 0.3-1.0 Ehrlich unit.
	24 hr: 0.5-4.0 Ehrlich units. Increased levels seen with hemolytic processes, shunting of portal blood flow.
Fecal urobilinogen	50-300 mg/24 hr. Reduced levels cause clay-colored stools and are seen in biliary obstruction.
Ammonia	Adults: 10-80 mcg/dl. Elevated levels may be seen with liver dysfunction, hepatic failure, or heart failure.
SERUM PROTEINS	
Albumin	3.5-5.0 g/dl. Decreased levels seen in liver disease.
Globulin	Reduced levels seen with hepatocellular injury test of specific proteins:
	Serum globulin: 2.3-3.4 g/dl
	Immunoglobulin M (IgM) component: 75-300 mg/dl
	IgG component: 650-1850 mg/dl
	IgA component: 90-350 mg/dl
Total	Albumin + globulin: 6.4-8.3 g/dl. Decreased levels may be seen with hepatocellular injury.
Albumin/globulin (A/G) ratio	>1.0 (albumin ÷ globulin). Low ratio in liver disease.
Transferrin	215-365 mg/dl. Reduced levels may be seen with liver damage; increased levels may be seen with iron deficiency.
BLOOD-CLOTTING FUNCTIONS	
Prothrombin time (PT)	11-12.5 sec, or 90-100% of control. Increased levels may be seen with chronic liver disease (e.g., cirrhosis) or vitamin K deficiency.
Partial thromboplastin time (PTT)	Activated partial thromboplastin time (APTT): 30-40 sec. PTT: 60-70 sec. Increased levels may be seen with severe liver disease or heparin therapy.
International Normalized Ratio (INR)	Oral coagulant therapy: 1.5-3.5 INR. Test used to monitor therapy for patients receiving warfarin sodium (Coumadin) therapy. More consistent measure than PT.

Modified from Liver disease: common liver function tests, 2005, available at www.umm.edu/liver/tests.htm. Accessed April 1, 2009; Pagana KD, Pagana TJ: Mosby's diagnostic and laboratory test reference, St Louis, 2009, Mosby; Serum globulin electrophoresis, 2005, available at www.nlm.nih.gov/medlineplus/ency/article/003544.htm. Accessed April 1, 2009.

Tests of Pancreatic Function

Test Name	Normal Values
Serum amylase	60-120 units/dl (Somogyi method). Elevated levels are seen with acute exacerbation of chronic pancreatitis, ampulla of Vater obstruction, pancreatic duct obstruction, pancreatic cancer, acute pancreatitis, and pancreatic trauma.
Serum lipase	0-160 units/L. Elevated levels are seen with pancreatitis, renal failure, and intestinal infarction or obstruction.
Urine amylase	0-5000 Somogyi units/24 hr; 6.5-48.1 units/hr (SI units). Elevated levels are the same as for serum amylase.
Secretin-pancreozymin test	Volume: 2-4 ml/kg body weight. Assessment of exocrine secretory ability of pancreas for carcinoma, ductal obstruction, or chronic pancreatitis. Low volume may indicate obstruction.

Modified from Pagana KD, Pagana TJ: Mosby's diagnostic and laboratory test reference, St Louis, 2009, Mosby.

nocompromised, and elderly patients. Close monitoring of the patient is essential during positional changes, especially in laparoscopic procedures with decreased lighting in the room.

When anticipating an operative cholangiogram, the surgical technologist must ensure that the OR bed has been equipped and positioned so that C-arm image intensification can be accomplished efficiently. Radiation-protection devices for the surgical team and patient should be available.

Thermoregulation. The risks of intraoperative hypothermia have been well documented. When laparotomy is performed, patients are at further risk for hypothermia. To prevent unplanned hypothermia, the surgical technologist takes affirmative measures to maintain body temperature in the OR (Insler and Sessler, 2006). The environmental temperature and humidity are set to prevent body heat loss caused by evaporation and convection. A forced-air warming blanket placed over the patient's upper body, head, and neck assists in maintenance of body temperature. Minimizing body exposure to ambient air and the use of warm irrigating solutions also support thermoregulation. The temperature of irrigating fluids should be no higher than body temperature (37° C; 98.6° F) (AORN, 2009). A blood- and fluid-warming device may be used by the anesthesia provider to deliver intravenous (IV) fluids at a temperature higher than room air temperature. The anesthesia provider commonly monitors the patient's core temperature by use of an esophageal temperature probe when the duration and complexity of the surgical procedure place the patient at risk for hypothermia. Additional comfort measures include using warm blankets before and after surgery.

Application of Sequential Compression Device. Patients undergoing lengthy surgical procedures are at risk for venous dilation and blood pooling in the lower extremities. This may predispose the surgical patient to develop venous thromboembolism (VTE) in the postoperative period. Sequential compression devices (SCDs) are frequently applied in the OR before commencing lengthy surgical procedures in order to prevent or minimize VTE risks.

Draping the Patient. After the abdominal prep, time must be allowed for the prep solution to dry and vapors to dissipate. This is an essential patient safety precaution when flammable prep solutions are used in conjunction with electrosurgery (or other ignition sources, such as a laser). Sterile towels are then arranged to accommodate the intended incision. A sterile drape sheet may be placed over the patient's lower torso and a laparotomy sheet is then placed to provide a wide sterile field and to cover all exposed body surfaces except the incision site.

Instrumentation. Instrumentation for open (i.e., performed via a laparotomy incision) surgeries of the liver, biliary tract, spleen, and pancreas includes a basic laparotomy set, biliary probes and forceps for dilating and exploring the ducts of the pancreas and biliary tract, vascular clamps, gastrointestinal (GI) clamps, and ligating clips and appliers of all sizes. Linear stapling instruments also should be available. A self-retaining system such as the Bookwalter retractor set (Figure 3-6) provides excellent exposure of the abdominal viscera. In addition, a flexible choledochoscope, Cavitron ultrasound suction aspirator (CUSA), intraoperative ultrasound, laser, argon beam coagulator, harmonic scalpel, and electrosurgical unit (ESU) may be required to perform certain procedures on the hepatobiliary system. Safe practices when using devices that generate surgical smoke require the use of a smoke evacuation system and accessories in both open and laparoscopic procedures (AORN, 2009). See Figures 3-7 through 3-14 for common instruments used in procedures of the liver, biliary tract, and spleen.

The basic equipment for minimally invasive surgical (MIS) procedures consists of two high-density monitors, an insufflation unit, ESU, light source, camera, and 0-degree and 30-degree telescopes in 10-mm and 5-mm sizes. A printer is optional. An ultrasonic dissecting unit is often used with MIS procedures. Trocars and sleeves are available in reusable, disposable, and resposable designs. Trocars and sleeves are commonly designed to accommodate 10-mm to 5-mm instruments and 12-mm to 5-mm accessories and instruments. MIS instruments include scissors and shears, dissecting forceps, atraumatic grasping forceps, hooks, Babcock clamps, retractors, needles, suturing devices, pouches, suction-irrigating devices, and mechanical stapling devices.

Thrombin, Gelfoam, Surgicel, Avitene, and other chemical hemostatic agents (Surgical Pharmacology) should be available in the OR suite. Radiographic dye, supplies, and radiation-protection devices will be required if intraoperative radiography or angiography is planned as part of the procedure.

Drainage Materials. Tubes and catheters are selected for the areas to be drained. If a defective drain is used, a free fragment

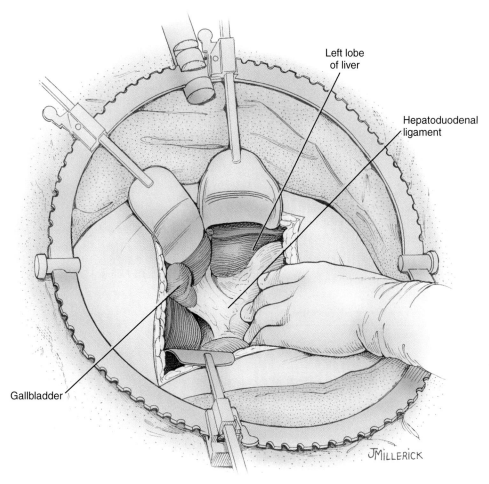

FIGURE 3-6 Bookwalter self-retaining retractor in place to provide optimal exposure to the abdominal viscera.

may remain in the wound on removal of the tube. Thus the surgical technologist should note the condition of all drainage materials and should test them for patency before they are placed in the patient.

Soft rubber or latex tissue drains may be used after an open cholecystectomy or a choledochostomy. Verify that the patient

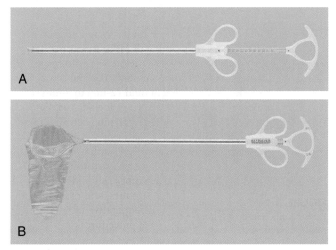

FIGURE 3-7 **A**, Endo catch with the tip closed; **B**, Endo tip with the tip expanded.

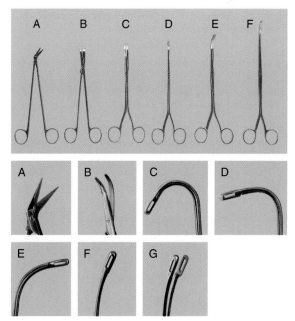

FIGURE 3-8 *Left to right:* **A**, 1 Potts-Smith cardiovascular scissors, 45 degree angle and tip; **B**, 1 Thorek scissors and tip C-G. 4 Randall stone forceps and tips; **C**, full curved; **D**, ¾ curved; **E**, ½ curved; **F**, ¼ curved, closed; **G**, ¼ open.

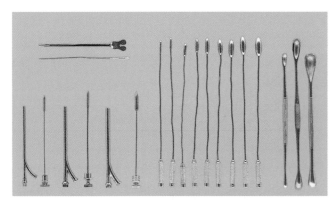

FIGURE 3-9 *Top, left:* 1 grooved director; 1 probe dilator. *Bottom, left to right:* 3 gallbladder trocars with inserts, small, medium, and large; 9 Bakes common duct dilators, #3 through #11; 3 Ferguson gallstone scoops, small, medium, and large.

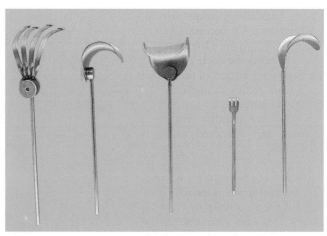

FIGURE 3-12 *Left to right:* Thompson retractor rotatable blades: 1 finger malleable; 2 Balfour, side view and back view; 1 rake Murphy, sharp, 3 prong; and 1 Balfour-Mayo center (2¾ × 5 inch), side view.

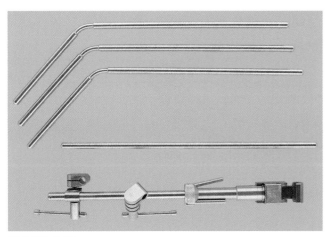

FIGURE 3-10 *Top to bottom:* Thompson retractor arms: 3 crossbar Thompson elite, angular; 1 Thompson extension, straight, 20 inch; and 1 rail clamp Thompson elite with 2 joints.

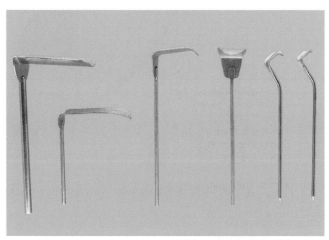

FIGURE 3-13 *Left to right:* Thompson retractor rotatable blades: Weinberg (3¼ × 5¼ inch), side view; Richardson (2 × 5 inch), side view; Kelly (2½ × 3 inch), side view; Kelly (2 × 2½), front view; and 2 Richardson carotid (1 × ¼ inch and ¾ × 1 inch), side view.

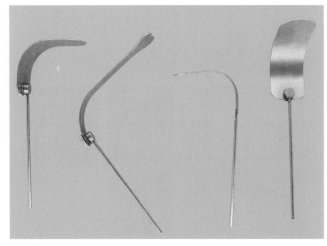

FIGURE 3-11 *Left to right:* Thompson retractor rotatable blades: 1 Deaver, medium, side view; 1 Harrington, side view; 1 Deaver, medium (2½ × 5 inch), side view; and 1 Deaver, large, front view.

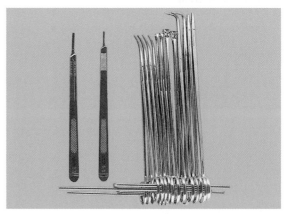

FIGURE 3-14 *Left to right:* 1 Bard-Parker knife handle #4; 1 Bard-Parker knife handle #3, long; 4 tonsil hemostatic forceps, long; 2 Allis tissue forceps, extra long; 2 Babcock tissue forceps, long; 2 Mixter hemostatic forceps, fine tip, extra long; 2 Crile-Wood needle holders, 11 inch.

has no latex allergy before using these devices and substitute nonlatex drains if necessary (Risk Reduction Strategies). The surgeon will prepare a latex rubber T-tube drain of suitable size after exploring the duct. The center of the crossbar is notched opposite the junction of the vertical limb so that its ends will bend more readily during removal. The ends are beveled and tailored to fit the duct.

Drains are usually exteriorized through separate stab wounds and anchored to skin edges to prevent their retraction.

Aseptic Considerations. When the common duct is opened or an anastomosis is established between a duct and other parts of the alimentary tract, it may be the institution's policy or the surgeon's preference to isolate contaminated instruments and materials from the remainder of the operative field, as described for GI surgery (Chapter 2). The wound is classified according to a standard system: any procedure in which the alimentary tract is entered under controlled conditions and without unusual contamination is considered a *clean contaminated wound*; if there is gross spillage, however, the wound is classified as *contaminated*. Proper wound classification is considered an important predictor of postoperative SSI (Phillips, 2007; Meakins and Masterson, 2007).

Blood Products. During the preoperative verification process, the surgical team should ascertain the type and amount of blood and blood products, both requested and available, as well as ensure the patient has a signed consent for transfusion. Constant, ongoing evaluation of blood loss is communicated to the anesthesia provider and surgical team during the procedure. When additional blood or blood products are required, the perioperative nurse communicates with blood bank personnel so that products are readily available and carries out the required steps to verify blood/blood products with the anesthesia provider before transfusion.

Autologous blood or donor-directed blood products may be used in elective procedures involving the liver, pancreas,

SURGICAL PHARMACOLOGY

Chemical Hemostatic Agents

Agent	Chemical Composition	Actions	Perioperative Precautions
Absorbable gelatin: powder or compressed forms (Gelfoam)	Purified porcine gelatin, beaten, dried, and heat sterilized	On areas of capillary bleeding, deposits fibrin, forming a clot. Absorbs 45× its own weight.	Dipped in warm saline or soaked in thrombin. Must be squeezed to remove air.
Absorbable collagen (Collastat, Superstat, Helistat, Lyostypt)	Bovine collagen origin	Collagen activates coagulation mechanism, aggregation of platelets.	Must be kept dry and applied with dry gloves. Do not use in infected areas or in pooled blood.
Microfibrillar collagen (Avitene, INSTAT)	Hydrochloric acid salt of purified bovine corium collagen	Promotes adhesion of platelets and prompt fibrin deposition.	Applied dry. Use firm pressure against bleeding surface.
Oxidized cellulose (Surgicel, Surgicel Nu-Knit)	Absorbable oxidation product of cellulose	On contact with blood, clot forms. Increases in size and forms gel. Absorbs 10× its own weight.	Applied dry. May be sutured in place.
Phenol and alcohol	Chemical compounds used to electrocoagulate tissue across lumen of appendix	Phenol coagulates proteins, and 95% alcohol neutralizes phenol.	Phenol is caustic and may cause severe burns.
Epinephrine (Adrenalin)	Adrenal hormone	Powerful vasoconstrictor—prolongs action of local anesthetics to decrease bleeding.	Gelatin sponges may be soaked in 1:1000 epinephrine; especially useful in ear and microsurgical procedures.
Silver nitrate	Crystals of silver nitrate compound mixed with silver chloride and molded onto applicator sticks	Astringent and antimicrobial. Seals areas of surgical incisions.	May also be used in treatment of burns.
Thrombin	Enzyme extracted from bovine blood	Accelerates coagulation of blood. Unites rapidly with fibrin to form clot.	May be used topically as a dry powder or as a solution in which gelatin sponges are dipped. May also be sprayed onto site. Topical use only. Loses potency after 3 hr.
Zeolite beads (QuikClot)	Derived from form of volcanic pumice	Beads cause hemostasis by absorbing water from blood.	Used for emergency hemostasis in uncontrollable bleeding or evisceration, especially in trauma. Causes an exothermic reaction. Must be removed, not biodegradable.

Modified from Phillips NF: Berry and Kohn's operating room technique, ed 11, St Louis, 2007, Mosby.

▶▶▶ RISK REDUCTION STRATEGIES

Latex Sensitivity and Allergy Guidelines

Natural rubber latex allergy can be a serious and life-threatening condition. Healthcare workers and others who have experienced repeated exposure to latex can develop latex sensitivity or allergy. The following is a list of guidelines that should be instituted in persons with suspected or known latex sensitivity or allergy:

- ◆ Identify the patient's risk factors and report them to the OR team. Those at high risk include persons with the following:
  - Myelomeningocele
  - Multiple surgeries, particularly if begun in early infancy
  - A positive serum latex antibody test
  - Occupational exposure to latex products, particularly powdered products
  - Allergy to bananas, kiwi, avocado, stone fruits, raw potato, tomato, papaya, chestnuts
  - History of hives or pruritus after incidental exposure (such as condom use, dental or other procedures)
- ◆ Schedule patients with known latex sensitivity as the first procedure of the day if facility is not latex-safe or latex-free.
- ◆ Notify the anesthesia department and OR 24 to 48 hours in advance.
- ◆ Notify healthcare providers in other perioperative areas of the patient's latex sensitivity status.
- ◆ Plan for a latex-safe environment of care:
  - Remove all latex products from the room unless no alternative exists.
  - Obtain a latex-free cart from the designated area.
  - Place a latex precaution card on the OR door.
  - Look for the signs and symptoms of latex reaction: contact rash, wheezing, bronchospasm, chest pain or tightness.

Modified from Association of periOperative Registered Nurses (AORN): *Perioperative standards and recommended practices,* Denver, 2009, The Association; Brown RH et al: The final steps in converting a health care organization to a latex-safe environment, *Jt Comm J Qual Patient Saf* 35(4):224-228, 2009; Phillips N: *Berry and Kohn's operating room technique,* ed 11, St Louis, 2007, Mosby.

spleen, and biliary tract. Cell-saver devices may be used when potential contamination of the blood from bile or bowel does not exist.

Surgical Interventions

SURGERY OF THE BILIARY TRACT

Cholecystectomy (Open Approach)

Cholecystectomy is removal of the gallbladder. It is performed for the treatment of diseases such as acute or chronic inflammation (cholecystitis) or stones (cholelithiasis) (Box 3-1). Most of these procedures are done laparoscopically. The few contraindications to the laparoscopic approach include suspected or diagnosed cancer of the gallbladder, third trimester of pregnancy, cirrhosis with portal hypertension, or poor pulmonary or cardiac reserve (Chari and Shah, 2008); these patients may not be able to tolerate the pneumoperi-

toneum required in laparoscopy. Further, if the surgeon is unable to identify all the anatomic structures during a laparoscopic approach, conversion to an open procedure becomes necessary.

Procedural Considerations. A basic laparotomy set and biliary instruments are used when cholecystectomy is performed through an open abdominal incision. The patient is positioned supine and receives a general anesthetic. After the patient is intubated, the anesthesia provider inserts an NG tube. Antibiotic prophylaxis may be administered. When an operative cholangiogram is anticipated, the OR bed should be equipped and positioned so that C-arm image intensification can be efficiently accomplished. Radiation-protection devices for the surgical team and patient are used during image intensification.

Operative Procedure

1. The abdominal cavity is opened through a right subcostal or upper midline incision.
2. Hemostasis of capillary vessels is achieved with electrocoagulation. Larger vessels are clamped with hemostats and ligated with suture material.
3. Retractors and laparotomy packs are placed as the abdominal cavity is carefully examined.
4. The common duct is palpated for evidence of stones and pathologic conditions are determined.
5. Harrington, Deaver, or self-retaining retractors, such as an upper-hand or Gomez retractor, are placed to provide exposure. Long tissue forceps and suction are used to manipulate tissues. The surrounding organs are isolated from the gallbladder region by moistened laparotomy packs and deep retractors.
6. To facilitate gentle traction, Péan forceps are usually placed on the body of the gallbladder (Figure 3-15, *A*).
7. The peritoneal fold overlying the junction of the cystic and common duct is incised with a #7 knife handle and a #15 blade, long Metzenbaum scissors, and forceps. Suction is available, and bleeding vessels are clamped and ligated or electrocoagulated.
8. Adhesions are separated by blunt dissection with small, round, dry dissector sponges; sponges on holders; and blunt right-angled clamps.
9. Dissection is continued to expose the neck of the gallbladder, the cystic artery, and the cystic duct. Lateral traction on the gallbladder neck allows incision of the peritoneum overlying the triangle of Calot.
10. Dissection is continued to expose the cystic artery as it enters the wall of the gallbladder.
11. On complete exposure and visualization of the branches, the cystic artery is doubly ligated with silk or clamped with ligating clips and divided (Figure 3-15, *B*).
12. Occasionally a third ligature or clip may be used. If the cystic artery has more than one branch, each is ligated and divided separately.
13. Abnormalities of the arterial and ductal anatomy are common (Figure 3-16), and the surgeon and assistant work with meticulous care to identify these structures.
14. The true junction of the cystic duct with the common bile duct is visualized.

BOX 3-1

Overview of Cholelithiasis and Cholecystitis

The two most common diseases of the biliary tree are *cholelithiasis* (stone formation in the gallbladder) and *cholecystitis* (inflammation of the gallbladder). These conditions may occur alone but usually occur simultaneously. Gallstones are becoming more common in the United States, affecting an estimated 8% to 10% of adults. Cholecystectomy is one of the most common surgeries performed. Gallstones are usually found in individuals older than 40 years, with a high incidence in people of Pima and Chippewa descent, white women, and African Americans.

Clinical conditions that may predispose one to gallstones include diabetes, obesity, cirrhosis, ileal disease or resection, cancer of the gallbladder, and pancreatitis. Cholecystitis usually results from obstruction of the cystic duct from gallstones (acute calculous cholecystitis); in a few patients, however, it results from stasis, bacteria, or sepsis (acute acalculous cholecystitis).

PATHOPHYSIOLOGY

The pathophysiology of gallstones depends largely on the following factors: the type of stone, the stone's location within the ductal system, and the nature of its occurrence (i.e., acute or chronic). Gallstones are formed as a result of the imbalance of cholesterol, bile salts, and calcium. The metabolism of cholesterol is often altered so that the bile is supersaturated, leading to precipitation and formation of stones. Cholesterol stones are the most common type and occur most often in women. Mixed stones are a combination of pigment and cholesterol stones. The exact cause of gallstone formation is unclear. Contributing factors may include the following:

◆ *Supersaturation of bile with cholesterol.* Bile is composed mainly of water, with other components including cholesterol, bile salts, and pigments. Cholesterol alone is insoluble in water; it must be combined with other components (e.g., bile salts) to remain in solution. When bile salts are insufficient to maintain cholesterol in solution, cholesterol crystals form.

◆ *Bile stasis.* This occurs when the gallbladder has not contracted normally in response to a meal and the bile is stagnant and then becomes thick and concentrated. This occurs in patients receiving total parenteral nutrition (TPN) for a prolonged period. Approximately 50% of these patients develop "sludge" (a mucous gel composed of calcium bilirubinate and cholesterol

crystals) in the gallbladder by week 6 of TPN therapy. Gallstones frequently occur during periods of fasting or dieting, during which there is a lack of stimulus for the gallbladder to contract.

◆ *Nucleation.* A nucleus (nidus) is formed of agents such as bacteria, bile, pigments, cellular debris, and calcium salts. Additional substances aggregate around this nucleus, forming a stone.

◆ *Genetics* may be a factor, as evidenced by increased prevalence in people of Pima and Chippewa descent.

Some stones may form and pass through the ducts without causing clinical manifestations (asymptomatic cholelithiasis). Symptomatic cholelithiasis occurs when stones intermittently become lodged in the cystic duct, causing biliary colic (episodic pain in the right upper quadrant or epigastric area). The pain usually occurs after meals, especially high-fat meals, as a result of increased intraluminal pressure when the gallbladder attempts to contract to release bile (a normal response to food entering the duodenum) against the obstructing stone.

Cholecystitis develops as stones become impacted within the cystic duct, causing unyielding obstruction, edema, distention, and inflammation of the gallbladder. In chronic cholecystitis, gallstones remain, causing recurrent obstructions and producing changes in the gallbladder wall from recurrent edema and inflammation. The muscular coat becomes fibrous, and the gallbladder functions less effectively.

COMPLICATIONS

Edema and distention of the gallbladder walls decrease blood supply, resulting in patchy areas of necrosis and gangrene. Perforation of these areas can then occur. Bile leakage through these perforations into the peritoneum results in peritonitis. Abscess formation may occur if secretions from the ruptured gallbladder are confined by the omentum or other adjacent organs (e.g., colon, stomach, duodenum, pancreas).

Stone migration from the gallbladder to the common bile duct (CBD) may cause cholangitis (acute CBD inflammation). The presence of gallstones in the CBD is called choledocholithiasis. CBD stones are a major source of morbidity in patients with symptomatic gallstone disease. Stone migration to the ampulla of Vater can cause pancreatitis.

From Lewis SL et al, editors: *Medical-surgical nursing: assessment and management of clinical problems,* ed 7, St Louis, 2007, Mosby.

---

15. The cystic duct is identified and carefully dissected down to its junction with the hepatic duct.

16. Any stones in the cystic duct are "milked" back into the gallbladder, and a tie is placed around the proximal part of the cystic duct.

17. If necessary, a cholangiogram is performed at this time (see following procedure: Intraoperative Cholangiogram). If a cholangiogram is not done, the cystic duct is doubly ligated and divided (Figure 3-15, *C*). A fine, absorbable transfixion suture may be used on the stump of the cystic duct near the common bile duct.

18. The gallbladder is then dissected from the liver bed and removed (Figure 3-15, *D*).

19. All bleeding is controlled; reperitonealization of the liver bed, if indicated, is accomplished with interrupted or continuous fine absorbable intestinal sutures.

20. A closed suction drain may be inserted near the cystic duct stump. The free end of the drain is exteriorized through a stab wound in the lateral abdominal wall.

21. The wound is closed in layers and a dressing applied.

Intraoperative Cholangiogram

An intraoperative cholangiogram is usually performed with both open and laparoscopic cholecystectomy to visualize the common bile duct and the hepatic ductal branches, and to assess the patency of the common bile duct.

Procedural Considerations. An intraoperative cholangiogram requires fluoroscopy to visualize the filling of the ducts. Before the patient's arrival in the OR, the surgical team ensures that a radiolucent bed is available or prepares the OR bed with an image-intensification attachment. The surgical technolo-

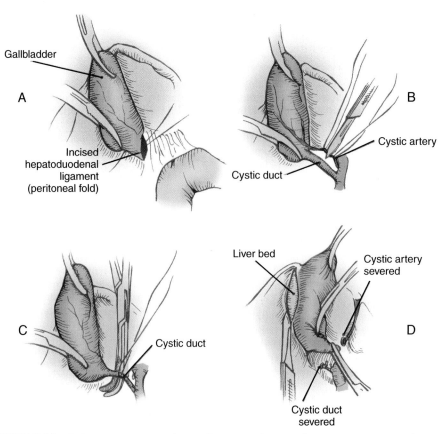

FIGURE 3-15 Cholecystectomy. **A,** With Péan forceps in place, gentle traction is maintained as peritoneum over the triangle of Calot is incised. **B,** Cystic artery is clearly visualized, doubly ligated, and divided. **C,** Cystic duct is carefully dissected and identified before forceps and ligatures are applied. **D,** Dissection of gallbladder from liver bed is completed.

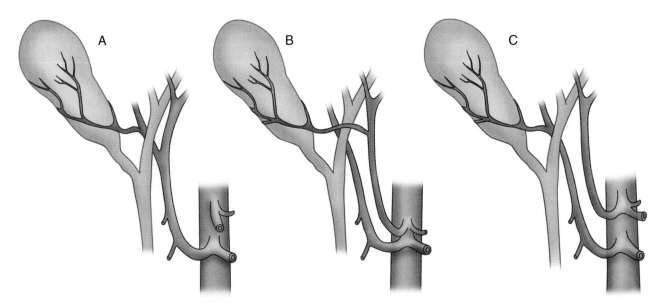

FIGURE 3-16 Arterial blood supply of the liver and biliary system is quite variable. **A,** The most common anatomic arrangement is a cystic artery arising from the right hepatic artery. **B,** A dual hepatic blood supply is found in 15% to 20% of patients, with the right hepatic artery arising from the superior mesenteric artery in a significant number of patients, as in **C.**

gist and perioperative nurse should verify all patient allergies before accepting medication onto the sterile field. Medication safety practices should be followed for labeling and dispensing all medications on the sterile field. Protection such as x-ray aprons or leaded shields is used for all members of the surgical team and the patient. As the patient's abdomen remains open while the x-ray equipment is positioned directly over the operative site, appropriate draping to maintain asepsis is necessary. Radiopaque sponges and any unnecessary instrumentation are removed from the abdominal site to avoid obscuring the view of the contrast medium filling the ducts.

The surgical technologist prepares a cholangiocatheter by attaching a stopcock with a 20-ml syringe of saline and a 20-ml syringe of contrast medium to the Luer-Lok ports. All air bubbles are removed because they might be misinterpreted as gall duct stones on the x-ray film.

Intraoperative Procedure

1. The cholangiocath is irrigated with saline before and during its insertion into the cystic and common bile ducts.
2. The cholangiocath is inserted into the duct using atraumatic grasping forceps. Irrigation during insertion facilitates dilation and reduces trauma to the ductal lumen.
3. The cholangiocath is anchored in the lumen of the common bile duct by the surgeon's preferred method. The more common methods are applying a ligaclip proximal to the insertion site; tying or suturing the catheter in place; or using a ring-jawed holding clamp, such as a Swenson clamp, that has been designed specifically for this purpose.
4. With placement of the cholangiocath confirmed and anchored, all radiopaque sponges, instruments, and obstructing equipment are removed from the field.
5. The surgical field is draped with a sterile drape sheet to maintain asepsis of the wound and field. The image-intensifier equipment (C-arm) is positioned, as the surgeon redirects the stopcock to allow for injection of the contrast medium. If stones are found, the surgeon removes them under fluoroscopic guidance.

Laparoscopic Cholecystectomy

Laparoscopic cholecystectomy is the surgical treatment of choice for patients with gallbladder disease who meet the appropriate criteria for safe laparoscopic intervention. Preoperative evaluation of patients having laparoscopic cholecystectomy differs little from that for patients scheduled for open cholecystectomy. For patients with a history of peptic ulcer disease, a flexible esophagogastroduodenoscopy (EGD) may be performed to rule out existing disease. For patients with suspected ductal stones, a preliminary ERCP or other diagnostic evaluation is often done. A laparoscopic procedure always has the potential to be converted to a laparotomy—a potential the patient should be informed about before the surgical procedure (Research Highlight). Laparotomy instrumentation and supplies should be available in the OR.

Procedural Considerations. Patients are generally admitted to the ambulatory surgery center (ASC) on the morning of surgery and will commonly require less than a 24-hour stay or admission to an extended recovery unit (ERU). A general anesthetic is used, and antibiotic prophylaxis may

---

RESEARCH HIGHLIGHT

Identifying Risk Factors for Complications of Laparoscopic Cholecystectomy

Even though laparoscopic cholecystectomy (LC) is the treatment of choice for cholecystitis, perioperative nurses anticipate possible conversion to an open procedure and have the necessary equipment and supplies available for a "difficult cholecystectomy." In this study, researchers used a large, prospective database to attempt to accomplish two objectives: (1) identify perioperative risk factors that might be used to predict a difficult cholecystectomy and (2) determine the relationship of the risk factors to perioperative complications for LC. These complications were divided into two categories: (1) local intraoperative and postoperative complications (such as bleeding or bowel injury) and (2) systemic complications (such as myocardial infarction or pulmonary embolism).

There were 22,953 patients in the study database. Their mean age was 54.5 years, there were twice as many males as females, and the majority underwent LC for chronic cholecystitis. While the overall complication rate was 7%, the rate was higher for patients with acute cholecystitis. Using multivariate analysis, the researchers identified the following associated factors for increased local intraoperative complications:

- Male gender
- Duration of the procedure
- Increased body weight
- Surgeon experience

Postoperative local complications were associated with the following factors:

- Male gender
- Patient age
- Intraoperative complication
- ASA class III or IV
- Increased body weight
- Emergency surgery
- Duration of the procedure

Systemic postoperative complications were associated with the following factors:

- Conversion to an open procedure
- ASA class III or IV
- Emergency surgery
- Duration of the procedure

During the OR briefing, the surgical team can use this information to review and communicate possible risks based on assessment findings. Physical characteristics (gender, age, body weight), ASA class, and clinical reason for the procedure (acute or chronic cholecystitis) can be used to estimate the risk of complications. A well-prepared team can mitigate against extending the duration of the surgery by good planning; complication rates in this study were 4 times higher for procedures lasting more than 2 hours.

Adapted from Giger UF et al: Risk factors for perioperative complications in patients undergoing laparoscopic cholecystectomy: analysis of 22,953 consecutive cases from the Swiss Association of Laparoscopic and Thoracoscopic Surgery database, *J Am Coll Surg* 203:723-728, 2006.

---

be administered in the immediate preoperative period. The following instrumentation, supplies, and equipment are required for laparoscopic cholecystectomy: laparoscope, two 5-mm trocars and sheaths, two 10-mm or 11-mm trocars and sheaths (trocar size depends on surgeon preference and may vary), a #7 knife handle with a #11 blade, multiple clip appliers, blunt grasping forceps (an assortment of alligator, Babcock, and spatula), and laparoscopic scissors. A laparoscopic video unit and secondary monitor, laparoscopic camera and control unit, light source, CO_2 source and insufflation unit, ESU, suction-irrigator (disposable), filtered insufflation tubing (disposable), and a pressure bag for IV saline 0.9% are commonly used. Instrumentation and supplies for laparoscopic common bile duct exploration should be available in the room. This may include a balloon-tipped Fogarty catheter, wire baskets, dilators, a T-tube, and a small, flexible choledochoscope. The patient is positioned supine with the usual comfort and safety measures observed. A Foley catheter (for bladder decompression) and an NG tube (for decompression of the stomach) will be inserted. Anesthesia is administered, the time-out completed, and the patient then placed in reverse Trendelenburg's position of 10 to 20 degrees. See Figure 3-17 for an example of the room setup for this procedure.

Pneumoperitoneum may be accomplished using the closed or open technique. In the closed technique, a special hollow insufflation needle (Veress) with a retractable cutting sheath is inserted into the peritoneal cavity through a supraumbilical incision and used for insufflation. In the open technique, sometimes termed the *Hasson technique*, a small incision is made above or below the umbilicus into the peritoneal cavity. A blunt-tipped cannula (Hasson) with a gas-tight sleeve is inserted, and then insufflation takes place. This approach is used for patients who have had a prior abdominal incision near the umbilicus or for those who have the potential for intraperitoneal adhesions. The Hasson technique may also use sutures,

placed on either side of the sleeve, to anchor and hold the sleeve in place.

CO_2 is the gas of choice for pneumoperitoneum. Gas flow is initiated at 1 to 2 L/min. Elevated CO_2 levels and respiratory acidosis may occur because CO_2 diffuses into the patient's bloodstream during laparoscopy. Intraabdominal pressure is normally between 8 and 10 mm Hg and is commonly used as an indicator for proper Veress needle placement by the surgeon. If the pressure gauge indicates a higher pressure, the needle may be in a closed space (such as fat), be buried in omentum, or be in the lumen of the intestine. The perioperative nurse should set the insufflation unit to a maximum pressure of 15 mm Hg. When intraabdominal pressure reaches 15 mm Hg, the flow will stop. Pressure higher than 15 mm Hg may result in bradycardia or a change in blood pressure, or may force a gas embolus into an exposed blood vessel during the operative procedure. Most insufflation units are equipped with an alarm mechanism to alert the operative team if the intraabdominal pressure is exceeded. Alarm systems on clinical equipment should be activated and sufficiently audible with respect to competing noise in the OR. The surgeon may frequently ask what the pressure reading is, as may the anesthesia provider.

Operative Procedure

1. A small skin incision is made in the folds of the umbilicus with a #11 blade on a #7 knife handle.
2. Pneumoperitoneum is created using either the open or the closed technique.
3. An 11-mm trocar is inserted through the supraumbilical incision; this becomes the umbilical port.
4. The laparoscope with attached video camera is inserted through the umbilical port and the peritoneal cavity is examined. The surgeon usually stands on the left side of the patient while the first assistant stands on the right. Video

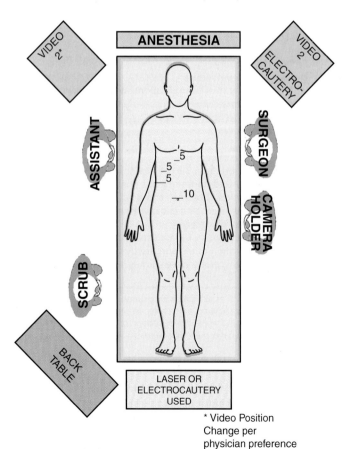

FIGURE 3-17 Position for laparoscopic cholecystectomy.

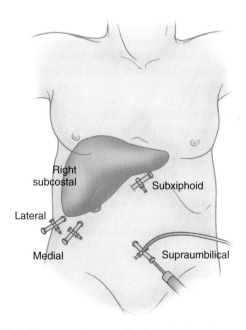

FIGURE 3-18 Trocar placement for laparoscopic cholecystectomy.

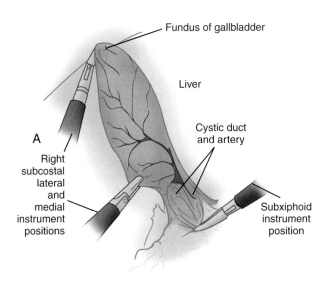

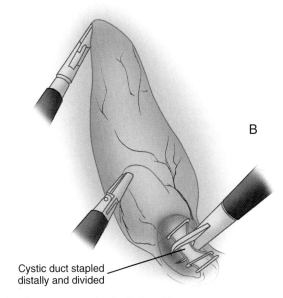

FIGURE 3-19 A, The gallbladder is retracted cephalad (using the grasper on the fundus) and laterally at the infundibulum. The peritoneum overlying the gallbladder infundibulum and neck and cystic duct is divided bluntly, exposing the cystic duct. **B,** Once the gallbladder–cystic duct junction has been clearly identified, clips are placed proximally and distally on the duct and it is sharply divided.

monitors are positioned at eye level at both the right and left sides of the operative field. The patient is then placed in a 30-degree reverse Trendelenburg's position and tilted slightly to the left.

5. Three additional trocars are inserted into the peritoneal cavity under direct visualization of the laparoscopic view (Figure 3-18).

6. Blunt grasping forceps are inserted through the medial 5-mm port to grasp the gallbladder.

7. The gallbladder is retracted laterally (Figure 3-19, *A*), exposing the triangle of Calot. The junction of the gallbladder and cystic duct is then identified. The endoscopic dissector, hook, and scissors are used to partially dissect the base of the gallbladder off the liver bed. Electrosurgery is also used. The electrosurgical instrument (active electrode) may have a channel through which suction can be applied to evacuate smoke plume. Some disposable instruments permit suction, electrocoagulation, and irrigation through the same instrument.

8. Hemoclips are placed proximally and distally on the cystic artery and the artery is divided. The use of a disposable, preloaded, multiple-clip applier assists in the placement of ligating clips in a more efficient manner than a singly loaded, reusable applier.

9. An intraoperative cholangiogram may be performed by placing a hemoclip proximally on the cystic duct, incising its anterior surface, and passing the cholangiogram catheter into the duct. Once the cholangiogram is completed, two clips are placed distally on the cystic duct and it is divided (Figure 3-19, *B*). A pretied loop ligature may be used if the duct is large.

10. Attention is then given to dissecting the gallbladder out of its fossa.

11. The surgical site is inspected for hemostasis and the gallbladder dissected off the liver.

12. The gallbladder is then removed through the umbilical port (Figure 3-20). An Endo-Bag or similar specimen-retrieval accessory may be used to secure the gallbladder for extraction.

13. The peritoneal cavity is decompressed. The port sites are closed and dressed with surgical adhesive.

Robotic-Assisted Laparoscopic Cholecystectomy

Procedural Considerations. Robotic surgery enables surgeons to perform more advanced and complex procedures. For this surgery, the surgeon controls two robotic arms with laparoscopic instruments and cameras while sitting at a console. Surgical assistants are positioned at the field. Many laparoscopic instruments have been developed to facilitate abdominal procedures. These include a bladeless trocar to minimize injury on entry and the ultrasonic shear to facilitate laparoscopic dissection with hemostasis. An endoscopic stapler and suture device may be used to facilitate intracorporeal anastomosis and knot-tying techniques (Nguyen et al, 2004). Laparoscopic cholecystectomy was one of the first procedures to demonstrate the utility of surgical robots in general surgery (Bodner et al, 2005a) (Research Highlight). For cholecystectomies, robotic operative times may be slightly longer because of equipment setup, but clinical outcomes are equivalent. The view of the ductal anatomy is subjectively superior with robotic surgery because of the magnified three-dimensional picture, which may reduce bile duct injuries (Hanley and Talamini, 2004).

The da Vinci Surgical System (Intuitive Surgical Inc., Sunnyvale, Calif) and the Zeus Robotic Surgical System (Computer Motion, Inc., Goleta, Calif) are two robotic systems used for minimally invasive laparoscopic surgery. The Automated Endoscopic System for Optimal Positioning (AESOP) can be "trained" to recognize the surgeon's voice (Jacobsen et al, 2004). A CT scan can also be imported into the console so that the surgeon can perform preoperative planning and surgical pro-

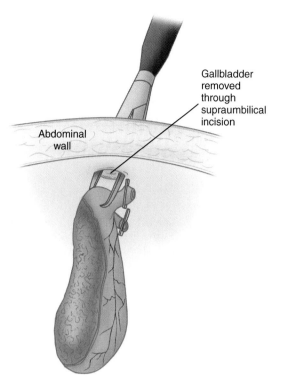

Gallbladder removed through supraumbilical incision

Abdominal wall

FIGURE 3-20 The gallbladder being removed through the supraumbilical incision.

cedure rehearsal (Hanley and Talamini, 2004). It is even possible to perform telesurgery—the complete separation of the surgeon from the operative field. Transcontinental cholecystectomies have occurred successfully between Strasbourg, France, and New York City (Bodner et al, 2005a). For advantages and myths about robotic surgery see Box 3-2 and Table 3-1.

Cholecystostomy (Open Procedure)

Cholecystostomy establishes an opening into the gallbladder to drain the organ and remove stones. The open approach is usually selected for patients with advanced medical problems who cannot tolerate general anesthesia or more extensive surgery. Ultrasound-guided percutaneous cholecystostomy has become an accepted procedure for patients who are not otherwise good candidates for surgery. In the rare situation where interventional radiology is not available, an open procedure may be done, as is described here.

Procedural Considerations. A large Toomey syringe (50 ml) or an Asepto syringe may be needed for irrigation purposes. If a local anesthetic is used, the anesthetic agent, syringes, and needles are assembled. Protocols for safe administration and labeling of all medications/solutions on and off the sterile field must be followed. Specified drainage tubes or catheters should be available. The patient is positioned supine. Although many surgeons prefer a right subcostal incision, when cholecystostomy procedures are performed as emergencies a quicker midline or transverse incision may be used. Instrumentation includes a basic laparotomy set plus a gallbladder set.

RESEARCH HIGHLIGHT

Robot-Assisted Laparoscopic Cholecystectomy

Laparoscopic cholecystectomy has been the gold standard since 1987. Robots were first used in surgery in the mid-1990s. With current robotic systems, the surgeon sits at an operative console with three-dimensional imaging and handheld controls. Movement of the controls follows the movement of the instrument's tip.

The Mayo Clinic in Scottsdale, Arizona, reviewed all robotically assisted laparoscopic cholecystectomies from October 2002 to July 2003. The Zeus Robotic Surgical System was used to dissect the cystic duct and artery, and the surgical assistant at the OR bed placed the clips on the cystic duct and artery. The robot was used to dissect the gallbladder from the liver. Cholangiocatheters were inserted into the cystic duct with the robotic instruments. Nineteen patients underwent the procedure. Sixteen were completed robotically. Conversions to laparoscopic techniques took place as a result of malfunctioning instruments; however, open procedures were not necessary. The mean setup time was 28.1 minutes (range 7 to 51 minutes). The mean hospital stay was 0.9 day (range: same-day release to 2 days postop). There were no complications or injuries related to use of the robot.

Often cholecystectomy is the initial robotically-assisted procedure to test surgical robots because the operation is technically straightforward and reproducible. Advantages of surgical robots are elimination of the surgeon's tremor, scaling of movements, increased degrees of freedom, three-dimensional visualization, and a comfortable working position for the surgeon, who sits at a console. The scaling of movements makes delicate dissection more exact, and the increased degrees of freedom make dissections simpler. Sitting at the console is ergonomically beneficial. The surgeon does not have to assume awkward positions or reach over assistants.

Telesurgery, the performance of surgery from a distant site using robotics, offers the potential of procedures being performed worldwide from remote sites.

Modified from Gomez G: Emerging technology in surgery: informatics, electronics, robotics. In Townsend CM et al, editors: *Sabiston textbook of surgery,* ed 18, Philadelphia, 2008, Saunders; Miller DW et al: Robot-assisted laparoscopic cholecystectomy: initial Mayo Clinic Scottsdale experience, *Mayo Clin Proc* 79(9):1132-1136, 2004.

Operative Procedure
1. After incision into the abdominal cavity, the gallbladder is isolated by retraction of the surrounding viscera.
2. The fundus of the gallbladder is grasped with an Allis or Babcock forceps and, if needed, the proposed opening is encircled by means of an absorbable purse-string suture, leaving the ends long.
3. If the gallbladder is distended or tense, it may be isolated with moistened laparotomy packs to protect the abdominal cavity from contamination.
4. If decompression of the gallbladder is required, a large-bore needle (e.g., 18 gauge) may be inserted with suction attached. Gallbladder contents are aspirated and the site closed using surgical clips on a clip applier.
5. If a trocar is used within the purse-string suture, suction tubing is attached to the trocar sheath.

BOX 3-2

Advantages of Robot-Assisted Surgery for the Patient and Surgeon

ADVANTAGES FOR THE PATIENT
Smaller incisions
Decreased postoperative pain
Shorter length of hospital stay
Reduced blood loss
Reduced tissue trauma and inflammatory response to surgery
Improved cosmetic result
Faster return to work

ADVANTAGES FOR THE SURGEON
Better visualization (higher magnification)
Hand tremor eliminated, allowing great precision
Three-dimensional video image of the operative field; view of ductal anatomy enhanced
Robotic "wrist" more flexible than human wrist, improving maneuverability around organs and vessels
Movements can be reduced, allowing complex technical tasks
Better ergonomic environment (sitting at a console), better levels of concentration

From Purkayastha S, Athanasiou T, Casula R, Darzi A: Robotic surgery: A review. *British Journal of Hospital Medicine* 65(3):153-159, 2004.

6. As the contents are aspirated, culture specimens may be taken. The contaminated trocar and sheath are removed and isolated in a discard basin.
7. The opening into the gallbladder can be enlarged with Metzenbaum scissors. Gallstones are removed with malleable scoops and stone forceps.
8. Irrigating the gallbladder with isotonic saline solution may be necessary to remove small stones, grit, or paste-like material. A syringe with a catheter or an Asepto syringe is sometimes used for irrigation.
9. Remaining contaminated instruments are placed in a discard basin.

10. A drainage tube is inserted into the gallbladder opening. The purse-string suture is tightened around the catheter, with care taken not to occlude it.
11. The free end of the catheter or tube is exteriorized through a stab wound and then anchored to the skin edges, as described for open cholecystectomy.
12. Drainage of the abdominal cavity is established with the exterior ends of each drain secured.
13. The wound is closed in layers, as described for laparotomy, and dressings applied at the incision and drain sites.

Open Common Bile Duct Exploration

With the advent of endoscopic, percutaneous, and laparoscopic techniques (Figure 3-21), open exploration of the common bile duct is rarely performed. When these newer methods are not available, when they are not possible because of prior surgery, or when an open procedure is otherwise necessary, open common bile duct exploration is performed.

Procedural Considerations. The patient is positioned supine after administration of a general anesthetic. The anesthesia provider inserts an NG tube after intubation. An indwelling urinary catheter may be inserted before the abdominal skin prep. Instrumentation includes a basic laparotomy set with the addition of gallbladder instruments. T-tubes of assorted sizes should be available. Intraoperative cholangiography will most likely be used to confirm that all stones have been removed; radiation-protection devices for the patient and surgical team are required. Culture tubes are needed. Soft rubber catheters for irrigation, balloon-tipped catheters such as the biliary Fogarty catheter, stone baskets, and the surgeon's preferred cholangiocath should be available, as well as both flexible and rigid choledochoscopes. A choledochoscope requires the following:

- Choledochoscope with accessories: biopsy forceps, stone-grasping forceps, and a sheath that can be used to direct other instruments into various portions of the biliary tract
- Video camera and viewing screen
- Light cord
- 0.9% normal saline (1000-ml bag)

TABLE 3-1

Myths about Robotic Surgery

Myth	Reality
Robots do all the work.	The surgeon manages the robot system from a console away from the operative field.
Robotic surgery is better than conventional surgery.	Current surgical outcomes are comparable.
Robotic arms function just like a surgeon's hands.	Robotic arms are better than human hands—steadier and more precise, with no tremor and smaller hand movements, and able to work in a very small space. However, hand dexterity is missing—a human hand can move 20 ways; robotic arm has good but not exactly replicable range of motion.
Robots make surgery simpler, faster, or less expensive.	System setup time can be lengthy. Some surgeries take longer to perform with a robotic system.
Robotic surgery has been a big disappointment.	Robotic surgery is constantly improving. This technology has significant implications for the future of surgery, with its near-perfect visualization and sophisticated camera system that provides a three-dimensional view of the heart.

Modified from 5 Myths about robotic surgery, Cleveland Clin Heart Advis 7(5):4-5, 2004; Robotics extend surgeon's reach, Cleveland Clin Heart Advis 11(3), 2008, available at www.heart-advisor.com/cgi-bin/texis/scripts/heartadvisor-search/search.html?query=robotic+heart+surgery. Accessed April 1, 2009.

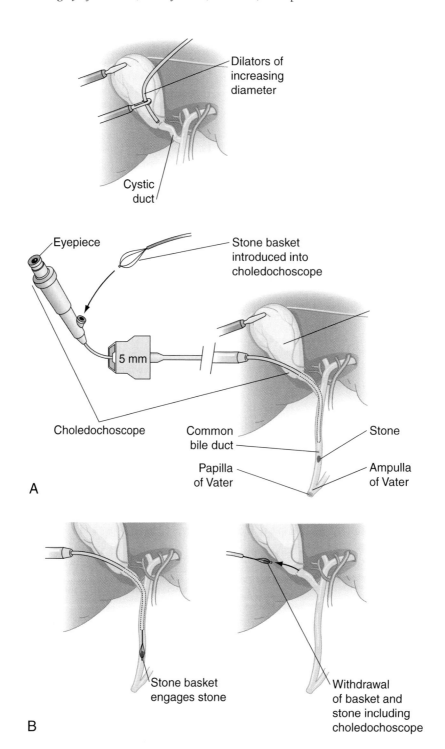

FIGURE 3-21 A, Laparoscopic common bile duct exploration. After dilation of the cystic duct, the flexible choledochoscope is inserted into the abdomen through the small trocar and maneuvered into the distal common bile duct. **B,** A stone basket is passed through the working channel of the choledochoscope and is used to snare a common duct stone. The stone basket and choledochoscope are then withdrawn together.

- Sterile IV tubing
- Pressure bag
- Light source for the choledochoscope

Distending the common duct is necessary for better visualization and is accomplished by irrigating the duct with copious amounts of sterile saline. A pressure bag is placed around an IV bag of 0.9% saline, and pressure to 300 mm Hg is applied. Sterile tubing is then passed from the sterile field and attached to the saline bag. The scrub person attaches the distal end of the sterile IV tubing directly to the irrigating stopcock on the scope.

Operative Procedure

1. The abdomen is opened through a subcostal incision or midline incision.
2. If the gallbladder has not been previously removed, it is exposed and removed or retracted by means of laparotomy packs and retractors.
3. The common duct may be identified by means of an aspirating syringe and fine-gauge needle to make certain that the suspected duct is not a blood vessel. Culture specimens may be obtained.
4. The common duct region is isolated with moistened laparotomy packs and narrow-blade retractors. A discard basin for contaminated instruments is placed at the lower end of the operative field and suction is prepared for immediate use.
5. Two fine traction sutures are placed in the wall of the duct, below the entrance of the cystic duct. A longitudinal incision is made in the common duct, between the traction sutures, with a long #3 knife handle and #15 or #11 blade, and enlarged with Potts angled or Metzenbaum scissors.
6. Visible stones are removed with gallstone forceps, after which exploration of the duct is begun with small, malleable scoops, proximal and then distal to the opening. Isotonic solution in an Asepto syringe and a soft, small-lumen catheter or a balloon-tipped catheter are used to facilitate the removal of small stones and debris as well as to demonstrate patency of the common bile duct in its entirety to the duodenum.
7. The choledochoscope may be used to identify additional stones. The scope is inserted into the common duct, which is then flushed with saline. After visualizing the duct to ensure that no stones remain, a T-tube is placed in the common bile duct and the choledochotomy is closed around the tube. A completion cholangiogram is performed to be certain all stones have been removed. The wound is closed, the T-tube anchored to the skin, and dressings applied. Sterile tubing is used to connect the T-tube to a small drainage container or bag.

Cholecystoduodenostomy and Cholecystojejunostomy

Cholecystoduodenostomy and cholecystojejunostomy create an anastomosis between the gallbladder and duodenum or the gallbladder and jejunum, respectively, to relieve an obstruction in the distal end of the common duct. An obstruction in the biliary system may be caused by a tumor of the ducts involving the head of the pancreas or the ampulla of Vater, an inflammatory lesion, a stricture of the common duct, or the presence of stones.

Procedural Considerations. Instrumentation includes a basic laparotomy set; gallbladder instruments with two curved Doyen intestinal forceps with guards, or similar atraumatic holding forceps; and a self-retaining retractor system. Fluoroscopy should be anticipated and radiation-protection devices for patient and surgical team should be available. The patient is positioned supine after administration of a general anesthetic. The anesthesia provider inserts an NG tube after intubation. An indwelling urinary catheter is inserted before abdominal skin preparation.

Operative Procedure

1. The abdomen is opened, the gallbladder exposed, the contents aspirated, and the pathologic condition confirmed.
2. The anastomosis site is prepared, posterior serosal silk sutures placed, and open anastomosis performed.
3. Anastomosis of the gallbladder to the duodenum or loop of the jejunum is usually performed as a two-layer anastomosis.
4. The serosa of the duodenum or loop of the jejunum is sutured to the full thickness of the fundus of the gallbladder.
5. A 1-cm to 1.5-cm opening is made into the small bowel and gallbladder in corresponding positions. GI technique (also referred to as bowel technique; see Chapter 2) is instituted.
6. Interrupted fine monofilament (5-0 or 4-0) sutures are then placed around the entire circumference.
7. Contaminated instruments are placed in the discard basin and the operative field is prepared for closure.
8. A drain may be inserted, the wound closed, and dressings applied.

Choledochoduodenostomy and Choledochojejunostomy

Choledochoduodenostomy is anastomosis between the common duct and the duodenum, and choledochojejunostomy is anastomosis between the duct and the jejunum. These procedures (referred to as choledochal drainage procedures) may be necessary in postcholecystectomy patients to circumvent an obstructive lesion and reestablish the flow of bile into the intestinal tract.

Procedural Considerations. Surgical approaches are similar to those for choledochostomy and cholecystojejunostomy. The patient is positioned supine after administration of a general anesthetic. The anesthesia provider inserts an NG tube after intubation. An indwelling urinary catheter is inserted before abdominal skin preparation.

Instrumentation and supplies necessary for this procedure include a basic laparotomy set with the addition of gallbladder instruments, a self-retaining retractor system, linear stapling devices, and T-tubes in varying sizes; a Silastic biliary stent should be available as should magnifying loupes. Fluoroscopy should be anticipated; radiation-protection devices will then be required for the patient and surgical team.

Operative Procedure
CHOLEDOCHODUODENOSTOMY
1. The abdomen is opened with a midline incision.
2. The common duct and duodenum are exposed.
3. The common duct is identified and dissected free, using forceps and Metzenbaum scissors.
4. The common duct and duodenum are approximated, side-to-side or with the end of the common duct to the side of the duodenum, and an anastomosis is established.
5. An intraluminal catheter is inserted.
6. The wound is closed and dressings applied.
CHOLEDOCHOJEJUNOSTOMY
1. The abdomen is opened with a midline incision.
2. The jejunum is mobilized, the common duct identified and opened, and the jejunum transected (Figure 3-22, *A*).
3. Anastomosis is established between the common duct and the transected jejunum.

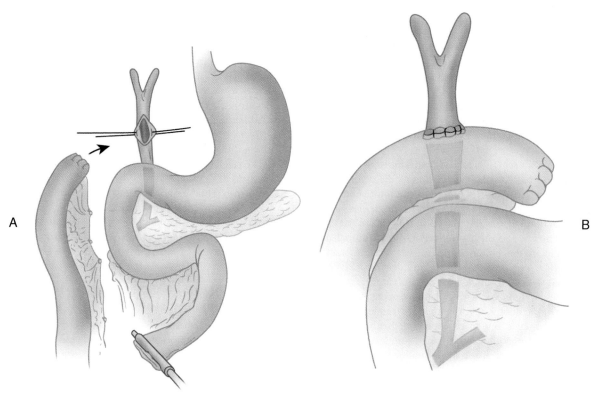

FIGURE 3-22 Choledochojejunostomy. **A,** The divided end of the jejunum is closed, and an end-to-side choledochojejunostomy is made in two layers to the jejunum. **B,** A jejunojejunostomy completes the operative procedure.

4. A catheter is introduced, as described previously for cholecystoduodenostomy.
5. Jejunal continuity is reestablished by jejunojejunostomy (Figure 3-22, *B*).
6. As an alternative, anastomosis may be fashioned from the end of the severed duct to the side of a loop of jejunum, with a side-to-side jejunal anastomosis.
7. Contaminated instruments are removed from the operative field.
8. A drain may be inserted, the wound closed, and dressings applied.

Transduodenal Sphincteroplasty

Transduodenal sphincteroplasty achieves a choledochoduodenostomy between the distal end of the common duct and the side of the duodenum. The sphincters normally affecting the distal common and pancreatic ducts are rendered functionless because the stoma is noncontractile and therefore remains permanently open. An indication for transduodenal sphincteroplasty is sphincter of Oddi dysfunction—a poorly defined clinical syndrome that is characterized by pain characteristic of biliary colic and recurrent acute pancreatitis. There may be a structural or functional abnormality of the sphincter, with or without fibrosis and elevated sphincter pressures. Both endoscopic sphincterotomy and transduodenal sphincteroplasty with transampullary septectomy have been used with similar results. The procedure described has the advantage of including division of the transampullary septum, which promotes pancreatic duct drainage.

Procedural Considerations. Instrumentation is as described for choledochotomy, with the addition of a GI set, since the duodenum is entered. The patient is positioned supine after administration of a general anesthetic. The anesthesia provider inserts an NG tube after intubation. An indwelling urinary catheter is inserted before abdominal skin preparation. The abdomen is prepped from nipple line to pubis. Supplies for an operative cholangiogram are necessary as are radiation-protection devices for the patient and surgical team.

Operative Procedure
1. A right subcostal or midline incision is made and the biliary tract exposed.
2. All structures are inspected and the normal configuration established before any structure is tied, clamped, or divided during biliary tract dissection.
3. Operative cholangiography is then performed by placing a cholangiocath through a small incision made with a #11 blade into the cystic duct.
4. If the gallbladder is present, cholecystectomy is performed.
5. The duodenum is mobilized by dividing the peritoneal reflection that covers the lateral portion of the second part of the duodenum and holds it in place.
6. The common duct is incised longitudinally between two stay sutures and explored.
7. Any residual stones are removed. Duodenotomy is performed with a longitudinal incision and the papilla of Vater located (Figure 3-23, *A*).

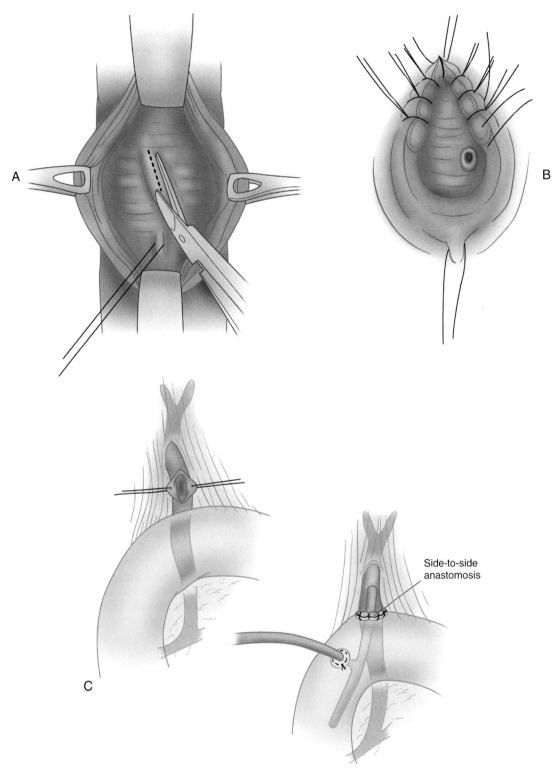

FIGURE 3-23 Transduodenal sphincteroplasty. **A,** The duodenum is opened longitudinally. **B,** The sphincter of Oddi is divided at 11 o'clock with angled Potts scissors, and the ductal mucosa is then sutured to the duodenal mucosa with 4-0 absorbable suture. The duodenum is then closed longitudinally in two layers. **C,** Choledochoduodenostomy. The common bile duct is joined to the apex of the mobilized duodenum in a two-layer anastomosis. A T-tube is placed to stent the anastomosis, with the external stem of the tube passed through the bile duct or through the wall of the duodenum.

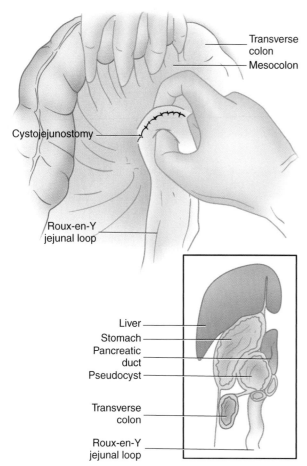

FIGURE 3-24 Internal drainage of a pancreatic pseudocyst by Roux-en-Y cystojejunostomy through the base of the transverse mesocolon.

8. The sphincter of Oddi is divided at the 11 o'clock position with angled Potts scissors, and the ductal mucosa is sutured to the duodenal mucosa with a fine monofilament synthetic absorbable suture on a small needle (Figure 3-23, *B*).
9. The duodenum is then closed in two layers.
10. The common bile duct is joined to the apex of the mobilized duodenum in a two-layer anastomosis.
11. A T-tube may be inserted to splint the anastomosis (Figure 3-23, *C*).
12. The abdominal cavity is closed.

SURGERY OF THE PANCREAS

Drainage or Excision of Pancreatic Cysts (Open Method)

Pancreatic pseudocysts are localized collections of pancreatic secretions in a cystic structure. The preferred operative therapy in patients with uncomplicated pseudocysts is internal drainage by one of three options: cystojejunostomy (use of a defunctionalized Roux-en-Y jejunal limb) (Figure 3-24); cystogastrostomy (drainage into the stomach); or cystoduodenostomy (drainage into the duodenum) (Steer, 2008). Cystogastrostomy is a faster and technically simpler procedure used

when the cyst adheres to the posterior wall of the stomach. Cystojejunostomy is the most versatile drainage procedure. Cystoduodenostomy is used in selected procedures, depending on cyst location, but has limited utility.

Procedural Considerations. The patient is positioned supine after administration of a general anesthetic. The anesthesia provider inserts an NG tube after intubation. An indwelling urinary catheter is inserted before abdominal skin preparation. Instrumentation and supplies necessary for this procedure include a basic laparotomy set, gallbladder instruments, a GI set, and a self-retaining retractor system.

Operative Procedure
1. A midline incision is made into the abdomen.
2. A self-retaining retractor system is used to expose the pancreatic area.
3. The pancreatic cyst is examined and the area isolated with moist packs.
4. Internal drainage may be accomplished by an incision into the anterior wall of the stomach, directly opposite the cyst if it adheres to the posterior wall, thereby providing drainage through the GI tract.
5. A fistula is established between the anterior wall of the cyst and the posterior wall of the stomach. Many surgeons prefer an anastomosis between the cyst and a Roux-en-Y loop of jejunum (see Figure 3-24) or into the duodenum directly, depending on the location of the cyst.
6. The anterior gastrostomy is closed, and wound closure completed.

Laparoscopic Pancreatic Cyst–Gastrostomy

Laparoscopic techniques may be used for internal drainage procedures for pancreatic pseudocysts. CT imaging is used to diagnose the pancreatic pseudocyst. An EUS may also provide additional information. The location, size, and thickness of the wall of the pseudocyst are all assessed to determine the most appropriate procedure for drainage, either a laparoscopic pancreatic cyst–gastrostomy or a Roux-en-Y pancreatic cystojejunostomy. Endoscopic drainage of pseudocysts may also be done in surgical centers where endoscopists are experienced in percutaneous drainage techniques (Steer, 2008).

Procedural Considerations. General anesthesia is induced and an NG tube inserted. The patient is positioned supine. Equipment and instrumentation are a 30-degree telescope (10 mm or 5 mm); a video camera; two high-density video monitors; a high-flow insufflator with CO_2 tank; an electrosurgical unit; two 12.5-mm trocar ports; two 5-mm trocar ports; an endodissecting instrument (5 mm) or atraumatic grasping forceps (5 mm); endoshears/scissors (5 mm) with electrocoagulation connection; an endo-Babcock instrument; a mechanical stapling device; a 10-mm endoclip applier; a 10-mm endosuturing instrument (optional); 2-0 suture material, 7-inch length (optional); an electrocoagulation hook; a long 5-mm laparoscopic needle; and an endoretractor.

Operative Procedure
1. Pneumoperitoneum is created and the trocars inserted by way of port sites as illustrated in Figure 3-25.

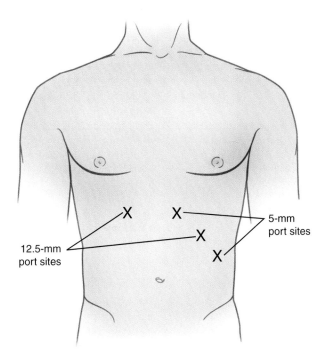

FIGURE 3-25 Port sites for trocar placement in laparoscopic pancreatic cyst–gastrostomy.

2. The pancreatic pseudocyst is located by entering the lesser sac by way of the greater curvature. Hemostasis is achieved by using the endoclip applier. An endostapling device (GIA type) with vascular cartridges is used to dissect the greater curvature.

3. The surgeon assesses the site for entry into the stomach. An endoretractor may be used to retract the left hepatic lobe.

4. Using electrodissection an incision centered between the lesser and greater curvatures is made on the anterior wall of the stomach and then extended.

5. A long laparoscopic aspiration needle is inserted into the intraabdominal and gastric cavity. The camera is advanced to visualize the posterior wall of the stomach.

6. The needle is inserted into the cyst and its presence is confirmed by aspiration.

7. A small incision is made into the cyst and the pancreatic fluid aspirated.

8. The endostapling device is inserted into the gastric cavity. The smaller jaw of this instrument is inserted into the pseudocyst. The stapling device is closed. It is important that the anastomosis not be under tension. The stapling device is fired and the anastomosis checked for integrity. An endosuturing instrument is used to close any defects in the anastomotic line.

9. An NG tube is directed into the pseudocyst.

10. The two edges of the anterior wall gastrostomy are approximated using endograsping forceps (atraumatic) or an endodissecting instrument. The gastrostomy is then closed using an endostapling device (thoracic-abdominal [TA] type).

11. A drain is placed, the abdomen deflated, trocar ports removed, and trocar sites closed and dressed.

Robotic-Assisted Laparoscopic Pancreatic Procedures

Procedural Considerations. Pancreatic lesions can be resected with robotic-assisted laparoscopy. Pancreaticojejunostomy may be performed following an open pancreaticoduodenectomy (Hanley and Talamini, 2004). Computer-assisted robotic surgery may be used to resect, drain, and reconstruct the pancreatic duct. Precise tissue manipulation and three-dimensional imaging allow better surgical approaches for reconstruction of the pancreatic or common bile ducts than open techniques (Melvin, 2003).

Pancreaticoduodenectomy (Whipple Procedure)

Pancreatic cancer is treated using a multidisciplinary approach that may include surgeons, gastroenterologists, oncologists, radiologists, nurses, and nutritionists (Hines and Reber, 2006). Tumors arise from the exocrine glands (95%) and endocrine glands (5%) in the pancreas. Ductal adenocarcinoma constitutes 80% of all pancreatic tumors. Most tumors begin in the head of the exocrine gland,

bile duct, and extend to the duodenum, intes-
... d spine. Metastasis occurs to regional lymph nodes,
... common metastatic sites include the liver and lungs. As
symptoms most often occur late in the disease, the prognosis
is usually poor (Research Highlight). Pancreaticoduodenectomy (Whipple procedure) is the removal of the head of the
pancreas, the entire duodenum, a portion of the jejunum, the
distal third of the stomach, and the lower half of the common
bile duct, with reestablishment of continuity of the biliary,
pancreatic, and GI tract systems.

Procedural Considerations. A basic laparotomy set, a GI
instrument set, a self-retaining retractor system (e.g., Bookwalter), linear stapling devices, and appropriate drains and
catheters are required. The perioperative nurse should ensure
that ordered blood and blood products are available. Pancreaticoduodenectomy may take 5 to 6 hours and require the
transfusion of many units of blood or blood products. The
patient is positioned supine after administration of a general
anesthetic. Attention is paid to padding positional pressure
points with gel pads or using a pressure-reducing OR bed
mattress. SCDs are applied as well as a forced-air warming
device and other active warming measures to prevent hypothermia. The anesthesia provider inserts an NG tube after
intubation. An indwelling urinary catheter is inserted before
abdominal preparation. The abdomen is prepped from nipple
line to midthigh.

Operative Procedure

1. The abdomen is entered through either an upper transverse, a bilateral subcostal, or a long paramedian incision. Resectability is assessed, exploring for hepatic
metastases, serosal implants of tumor, and lymph node
metastases. If these are outside the zone of resection, the
disease is unresectable.
2. Laparotomy packs and retractors are used to expose the
operative site and protect vital structures.
3. The duodenum is mobilized using the Kocher maneuver
(incision of peritoneal reflection lateral to the second portion of the duodenum) with Metzenbaum scissors and subsequent blunt dissection of loose areolar tissue.
4. Mobilization of the duodenum continues and bleeding vessels are ligated with silk.
5. The gastrocolic ligament and the gastrohepatic omentum
are divided between curved forceps and are ligated or
transfixed.
6. The gastroduodenal and right gastric arteries are clamped,
divided, and ligated.
7. The prepyloric area of the stomach is mobilized.
8. The operative field is prepared for open anastomosis by isolating the area with laparotomy sponges.
9. By placing two long Allen or Payr clamps near the midportion of the stomach, the transection is completed.
10. The duodenum is reflected, the common duct is divided, and
the hepatic end is marked or tagged for later anastomosis.
11. The jejunum is clamped with two Allen forceps and the
duodenojejunal flexure divided.
12. The pancreas is divided and the duct carefully identified.
13. Further mobilization of the duodenum and division of the
inferior pancreaticoduodenal artery are done to permit
complete removal of the specimen.

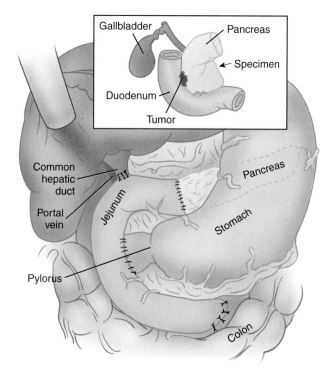

FIGURE 3-26 Illustration of a pylorus-preserving pancreaticoduodenectomy and the subsequent reconstruction. The inset at the top
depicts the resected specimen. The jejunal limb is passed through and
sutured to the transverse mesocolon.

14. The most common reconstructive technique anastomoses
the pancreas to the jejunum first, followed by the bile duct
and the duodenum (Figure 3-26).
15. Drains may be placed, the abdomen closed, and an abdominal dressing applied.

Pancreatic Transplantation

Pancreatic transplantation is the implantation of a pancreas
from a donor into a recipient for patients with type 1 (formerly
known as juvenile-onset) diabetes. Options for pancreatic
transplant include a pancreas transplant alone (PTA), an option
chosen for patients with functioning kidneys; a simultaneous
pancreas-kidney transplant (SPK), because severe diabetes is
often associated with chronic renal failure; or a pancreas transplant after a kidney transplant (PAK), in which the pancreas is
transplanted sometime after the kidney transplant. Pancreatic
transplantation differs from other organ transplants in that it
does not have immediate life-saving results. It is done in the
hope of preventing debilitating side effects of diabetes, such as
cardiovascular, retinal, and renal disease. For patients, a significant benefit is freedom from dependence on insulin. However,
pancreatic transplant in patients with brittle diabetes remains
a rare procedure because the trade-off of insulin dependence
is lifelong immunosuppression (Gruessner et al, 2008). Transplant is most effective in persons with few or no secondary diabetic complications and it can reverse or stop the progression
of these complications.

Procedural Considerations. The majority of pancreas transplants performed in the United States are SPK procedures
(Figure 3-27). Instrumentation includes a transplant set as

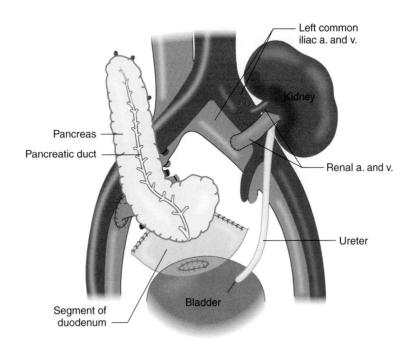

FIGURE 3-27 Transplantation of the pancreas with drainage of the bladder through a pancreatico-duodenocystostomy. A renal transplant is also shown with the common iliac vessels used for vascular anastomoses.

described for kidney transplantation in Chapter 6. In addition to the transplant set, vascular instruments and instruments for resection of the duodenal segment and management of the pancreatic duct are required. A linear stapling device may be used.

The patient is positioned supine after administration of a general anesthetic. The anesthesia provider inserts an NG tube after intubation. An indwelling urinary catheter is inserted before the abdominal skin prep and is attached to a urometer. Like other transplant procedures, these procedures are lengthy, lasting 5 to 7 hours. Positional pressure sites must be padded and a pressure-reducing mattress placed on the OR bed. Given the patient's diabetes, maintaining skin and tissue integrity is paramount. SCDs will likely be used. Careful monitoring of blood glucose level will occur throughout the procedure by the anesthesia provider. Blood and blood products will be ordered and their availability must be verified. Blood-warming devices, a forced-air warming device, warmed irrigating solution (<40.5° C [105° F]), and other measures are used to maintain normothermia. Communication among team members is essential in all transplant surgery. The patient is transferred to the SICU on completion of the procedure. Measures to address and reduce patient and family anxiety are usually part of all transplant programs. At-home rehabilitation is a gradual process and social services and other resources are part of the transplant team. The patient must take immunosuppressive drugs indefinitely. The verification process for organ transplant, established by the United Network for Organ Sharing (UNOS), must be followed to ensure that the organs of the donor and the recipient are compatible (Patient Safety).

Operative Procedure

1. The whole-organ pancreatic transplantation procedure is performed through an oblique incision opposite the side of the renal transplant in the lower abdominal quadrant. A midline incision may also be used for pancreatic transplant.

2. The external iliac artery and vein are skeletonized and lymphatics are tied off with 4-0 nonabsorbable ligatures.

3. The external iliac vein is clamped with noncrushing vascular clamps and a #11 blade used to make a venotomy.

4. The venotomy incision is extended with Potts scissors.

5. An end-to-side anastomosis of the donor portal vein to the recipient's external iliac vein is performed with four double-armed 5-0 polypropylene sutures.

6. The external iliac artery is then clamped and an aortic punch used to make an arteriotomy.

7. An end-to-side anastomosis of the recipient's external iliac artery with the donor aortic patch containing the origin of the superior mesenteric artery and the celiac axis is performed with four double-armed 6-0 polypropylene sutures.

8. Management of the pancreatic duct is then performed, according to the type of en bloc procedure performed.

9. Various enteric procedures for drainage of pancreatic duct secretions have been performed with whole-organ transplants en bloc with a segment of duodenum and the spleen. They include cutaneous jejunostomy, drainage into an ileal loop, and duodenojejunostomy with end-to-end or side-to-side anastomosis. Direct grafting of the pancreatic duct into the enteric or urinary system is also performed for management of exocrine secretions. Surgical procedures include pancreatico-jejunostomy with an established Roux-en-Y loop of jejunum (Figure 3-28), pancreaticoductoureterostomy, and pancreaticocystostomy. The whole-organ pancreas transplant may also be performed as a pancreaticoduodenal transplantation or a pancreaticoduodenal-splenic transplantation.

PATIENT SAFETY

Transplant of Donor Organs/Tissues: Example of Procedure for Establishing Identity and Matching Donor with Recipient

Before the transplant surgical procedure, a process of nine checkpoints is implemented to ensure identity and matching between the organs/tissues of the donor and the recipient.

Before the patient enters the OR the following must occur:

1. Once a transplant has been posted, Preliminary Transplant Crossmatch Reports are faxed from the human leukocyte antigen (HLA) lab to the OR where the transplant is to occur. The blood bank will fax ABO reports.
2. The OR charge nurse verifies the posted recipient's Preliminary Transplant Crossmatch Report and the ABO report.
3. The organ arrives at the OR.
4. The perioperative nurse applies an addressograph label to the box with the organ.
5. The perioperative nurse and another registered nurse together do the following:
   a. Verify the tag on the organ with the Preliminary Transplant Crossmatch Report to ensure the following match:
      i. Recorded ABO type of the recipient is the same or is compatible with the recorded ABO type of the donor.
      ii. The UNOS (United Network for Organ Sharing) number on the organ is the same as the UNOS number on the Preliminary Transplant Crossmatch Report.

   b. Identify the patient using the usual hospital policy.
   c. Sign the Transplant Verification form.
   In the OR the following must occur:
6. Preliminary anatomic checks are done by the surgeon. The transplant surgeon verifies that the UNOS number on the Preliminary Transplant Crossmatch Report is the same as the UNOS number on either the organ container or the paperwork provided and verifies the compatibility of the organ and the patient by ABO blood type. The transplant surgeon signs the Transplant Verification form.
7. Once the patient is taken into the OR, a time-out is taken with the OR team according to OR policy and procedure.
8. The Transplant Verification form and Preliminary Transplant Crossmatch Report are a permanent part of the patient's medical record.
9. The Transplant Verification form (deceased donor) is attached to the record.

Modified from *UNOS Policy 3.1.4.1: ABO verification prior to transplant,* 2005, available at www.unos.org/SharedContentDocuments/ABO_Verification_Processes_1_04.pdf. Accessed November 28, 2008.

SURGERY OF THE LIVER

Drainage of Abscess

Abscesses of the liver occur primarily by spread of bacteria or other organisms through the portal system (a direct route after trauma), the biliary tract, or the hepatic artery (in generalized

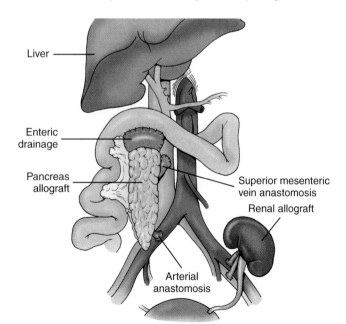

FIGURE 3-28 Pancreas and kidney transplants (PAK or SKP) with the donor pancreas vascularized to facilitate enteric exocrine drainage to a proximal portion of the jejunum (enteric drainage [ED] technique). The donor kidney is implanted in the left iliac fossa anastomosed to the femoral vessels and a ureteroneocystostomy is performed.

septicemia); in addition, direct extension from a subdiaphragmatic or subhepatic abscess can lead to a liver abscess. In most instances, percutaneous drainage is effective and safe in the drainage of hepatic abscesses. However, open procedures may be required, often by way of the transperitoneal route. This approach permits inspection of the abdominal cavity for the underlying source of the abscess.

Procedural Considerations. A basic laparotomy set is used. Biliary instrumentation, drainage materials, and aerobic and anaerobic culture tubes are needed. Safe practices for handling specimens such as cultures are initiated. The patient is positioned supine after administration of a general anesthetic. The anesthesia provider inserts an NG tube after intubation. An indwelling urinary catheter may be inserted before the abdominal skin prep.

Operative Procedure

1. The incision preferred by many surgeons is the transperitoneal route; the surgical approach may be modified, however, according to the location of the abscess (e.g., in a high posterior abscess, the transpleural approach may be selected).
2. The abdomen is opened as described for laparotomy and abdominal inspection carried out.
3. The abscess is mobilized and evacuated, and cultures obtained.
4. Surgical drains are placed and the wound closed.

Hepatic Resection

Anatomically, the liver is divided into left and right lobes with the caudate lobe lying in the dorsal segment. Resection of the liver is undertaken for primary tumors, benign conditions (e.g.,

RAPID RESPONSE TEAM

Treatment of nontraumatic shock can be delayed because of inadequate knowledge and/or skills of some clinicians. Some hospitals do not have system-wide resources to handle emergencies such as hypovolemic episodes, and the death rate can be high. Rapid response teams empower clinicians to identify and treat patients in shock using a multidisciplinary team approach. The team may consist of ICU nurses, respiratory therapists, emergency physicians, laboratory personnel, ECG and radiology technicians, pharmacists, and intensivists. These groups use evidence-based practice to promptly evaluate and treat deteriorating patients, which can lead to decreased inpatient cardiac arrests and postoperative morbidity and mortality.

Hypovolemia and sepsis are two typical reasons for team response. Early hemodynamic optimization improves survival in high-risk surgical patients and those with sepsis. Attitudes and behaviors of medical staff must be positive for this program to work effectively. Signs are posted that not only educate staff but also remind healthcare providers to use the team. Perioperative nurses are encouraged to call the team whenever something "doesn't feel right" about a patient or the patient is deteriorating rapidly.

In the case of hepatic, biliary, pancreatic, and splenic surgery, potential for bleeding exists postoperatively because of the high vascularity of these areas. When postoperative hypovolemia occurs and it becomes necessary to call the rapid response team, the surgical team members need to provide a short, but comprehensive, report on the type of surgery performed. For liver transplant patients, it is paramount that early intervention occurs in patients with hypovolemia or hypotension as renal dysfunction can worsen and renal failure can result.

Modified from Sebat FS et al: Effect of a rapid response system for patients in shock on time to treatment and mortality during 5 years, *Crit Care Med* 35(11):2568-2575, 2007; Biancofiore G, Davis C: Renal dysfunction in the perioperative liver transplant period, *Curr Opin Organ Transplant* 13(3):291-297, 2008.

hepatolithiasis), and metastatic tumors. Hepatic resection is usually approached in one of three ways. The *anatomic* approach is based on the premise that malignant cells distribute along the portal venous segmental supply. In the *enucleation* approach, specific benign lesions with limited chance of local invasion are removed. The third approach, the *nonanatomic*, includes resections appropriate for a pathologic process in which a limited margin is acceptable, such as in tumor debulking.

Procedural Considerations. Instruments used are a laparotomy set, biliary instruments, vascular instruments, noncrushing liver clamps, a self-retaining retractor, and a surgical stapler. Supplies and equipment should be available for thermoregulation, electrosurgery, measurement of portal pressure, and replacement of blood loss. For major liver procedures, intraoperative ultrasound (to guide vessel isolation and minimize vascular occlusion), the argon beam coagulator, and the CUSA are used. Special blunt needles for suturing liver tissue are also necessary.

The patient is placed in supine position. Mild Trendelenburg's position may be requested by the surgeon. The anesthesia provider inserts an NG tube after induction of general anesthesia and intubation. An indwelling urinary catheter is inserted before abdominal skin preparation. The abdomen is prepped from nipple line to midthigh. Surgeons often use a right subcostal incision, with the ability to extend with a left subcostal if necessary. In some instances, a median sternotomy or right thoracotomy incision is required, and chest instruments are then necessary. Liver sutures, absorbable or nonabsorbable according to surgeon's preference, vessel loops, and umbilical tapes should be available on the sterile field.

Hemostatic material, such as Gelfoam, Surgicel, or Avitene, and absorbable collagen sheets should be readily available when the resection begins. The potential for bleeding exists both intraoperatively and postoperatively because of the high vascularity of the liver. If postoperative bleeding and subsequent hypovolemia occur, it may become necessary to call the Rapid Response Team (Rapid Response Team box).

Surgeons use various methods to remove liver tissue. A CUSA allows the surgeon to dissect tissue using ultrasonic waves incorporated with fluid and suction. The ultrasonic waves cut through liver tissue, emulsifying it and diluting the tissue with fluid so that it can be suctioned. The electrosurgical pencil uses electrical current to cut through and desiccate liver tissue. Finger-fracture of the liver tissue is performed by digital pressure against the parenchyma to fracture the tissue.

Operative Procedure
1. Through a right subcostal incision, the abdominal cavity is opened and examined.
2. Pathologic condition is determined and resectability evaluated.
3. Moist laparotomy packs are inserted and a self-retaining retractor placed.
4. Intraoperative ultrasonography (US) is performed to assess all segments of the liver (Figure 3-29). Ultrasound-guided, digital intraparenchymal isolation of vessels is used during resection.
5. Lymph nodes in the porta hepatis and along the gastrohepatic ligament are then assessed by palpation to determine extrahepatic metastasis.
6. The intended resection line is scored with the blade tip of the electrosurgical pencil, and coagulation is set at the surgeon's selected setting (Figure 3-30).
7. The liver parenchyma is then delicately resected using the CUSA handpiece (Figure 3-31).
8. Once the portion of the liver is resected, the remaining liver resection margins are assessed for bleeding and bile leakage.
9. A laparotomy sponge may be placed against the transected surface for several minutes. The laparotomy sponge is gently rolled from the surface, which is then examined for bile leakage.
10. Areas may then be oversewn with 2-0 or 3-0 absorbable suture or an intended layer of eschar is applied using electrocoagulation or the argon beam coagulator.
11. Abdominal drains may be placed along the liver bed and exteriorized through the abdominal wall through separate stab wounds.
12. The abdominal wound is then closed and dressings applied.

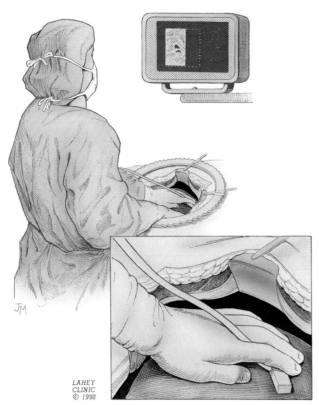

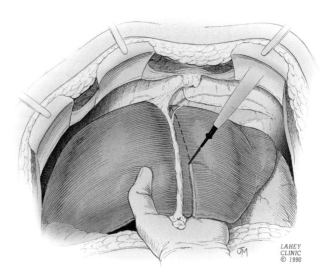

FIGURE 3-30 Use of electrosurgical pencil with blade tip to score the line of resection on the surface of the liver.

FIGURE 3-29 Use of intraoperative ultrasound using a 7-MHz T-probe to permit assessment of the liver.

Laparoscopic and Robotic-Assisted Laparoscopic Hepatic Surgery

Procedural Considerations. Laparoscopy for liver resection is a highly specialized field. It can present severe technical difficulties such as control of bleeding and risk of gas embolism (Belli et al, 2006; Borzellino et al, 2006). Other limitations relate to inadequate retraction, the inability to assess safe margins of resection with the loss of tactile sense, difficulty with safe parenchymal transection, and the potential for injury of adjacent structures (Poultsides et al, 2007). The use of stapling devices has made the procedure faster and safer. Results for laparoscopic resections have been similar to those of open surgical technique in carefully selected procedures (Borzellino et al, 2006). The benefits associated with robotic technology include less blood loss, faster recovery, less scarring, and reduced postoperative pain. The robot extends the surgeon's skills by providing a 360-degree range of motion not possible with traditional laparoscopic instruments. It also allows access to all the fine structures of the liver and better visualization of delicate blood vessels (First Robotic, 2005). Laparoscopic ultrasound navigation is often an important element in laparoscopic hepatic surgery as well (Kleemann et al, 2006). It enables determination of tumor location and the relationship to adjacent vascular and biliary structures (Santambrogio et al, 2007).

Radioimmunoguided Surgery

Radioimmunoguided surgery (RIGS) is a technique used intraoperatively to detect cancer that may not be readily

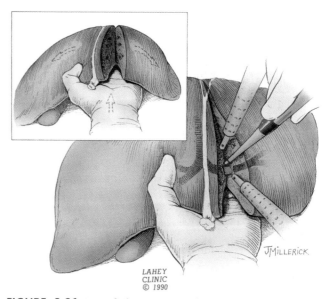

FIGURE 3-31 Use of the Cavitron ultrasonic surgical aspirator (CUSA) handpiece to dissect through the hepatic parenchyma.

detected by inspection or palpation. RIGS technique has been useful to determine safe margins of resection for metastatic colon cancer, as well as for extrahepatic disease and occult tumors in patients with rising serum carcinoembryonic antigen (CEA) levels.

About 2 to 3 weeks before surgery, patients receive an IV injection of radiolabeled monoclonal antibody, which binds reactive antigen on or near the surface of tumor cells. The antigen-antibody bond keeps minute amounts of radioactivity, or gamma emissions, localized in tumor tissue. An intraoperatively used, handheld gamma ray–detecting probe connected to a microcomputer emits an audible signal when the radioactive waves hit the crystal in the distal end of the probe. The Neoprobe instrument gives a digital reading as well as an audible pitch that rises or falls when placed on the gamma ray–emitting tissue. This advance in the intraoperative detection of adenocarcinoma and metastases can greatly assist in decision-making and resection of diseased tissue.

Procedural Considerations. Instrumentation includes a basic laparotomy set, biliary instruments, vascular instruments, and additional items such as a sterile marking pen, long clamps and a self-retaining retractor system (e.g., the Bookwalter retractor). Minimal suture (2-0 and 3-0 silk ties, 2-0 suture ligature) is added to the sterile field until the abdomen is explored and the extent of disease is assessed. The patient is positioned supine. The anesthesia provider inserts an NG tube after induction of general anesthesia and intubation. An indwelling urinary catheter is inserted before the abdominal prep. The abdomen is prepped from nipple line to midthigh. A midline abdominal incision provides access to the liver. Vertical abdominal incisions are sometimes used because they can be made and closed more rapidly and permit better exposure of all abdominal organs.

Operative Procedure

1. A midline abdominal incision is made from the xiphoid process to the pubis.
2. Intraoperative scanning of the liver and abdominal viscera is performed using the probe.
3. The digital readings as well as the anatomic structures being scanned are recorded.
4. Great care is taken to scan mesenteric, pelvic, and periaortic lymph nodes individually.
5. The liver is scanned and areas emitting strong-pitched tones are marked with a sterile marking pen. A very distinct change in pitch may be noted on liver tissue within a 2-cm to 3-cm radius of the tumor site.
6. Intraoperative ultrasonography and review of CT and MRI scans of the patient's liver are used to further confirm the liver lesions.
7. Margins for resection are drawn using an ESU tip on blend mode.
8. Resection of the lesion may be segmental, circumferential, or lobar.
9. After each resection, the margins of healthy liver tissue adjacent to the resection site are scanned and readings are recorded. This procedure continues until all tissue emitting high gamma ray waves has been resected.
10. Specimens are sent to the pathology laboratory for further pathologic and histologic analysis. The surgical team supports accurate correlation of pathologic diagnosis with intraoperative RIGS findings by using safe specimen practices. Tissue specimens are verified, and specifically and meticulously identified.
11. The surgeon determines the best plan of treatment for the patient based on the information obtained from intraoperative assessment of the extent of the patient's disease. Resection of RIGS-positive tissue may result in an extensive retroperitoneal lymphadenectomy, liver resection, gastrohepatic ligament lymphadenectomy, or the resection of colon, uterus, or bladder.

Liver Transplantation

Liver transplantation is the implantation of a liver from a donor into a recipient. The total procedure involves retrieving or procuring the liver from a donor, transporting the donor liver to the recipient's hospital, performing a hepatectomy on the recipient, and then implanting the donor liver. Reanastomoses are then undertaken of the suprahepatic vena cava, infrahepatic vena cava, portal vein, and hepatic artery; biliary reconstruction with end-to-end anastomosis of donor and recipient common bile ducts; or Roux-en-Y anastomosis if the recipient's bile duct is absent as a result of biliary atresia.

Liver transplantation is indicated for patients with chronic hepatocellular disease, chronic cholestatic disease, metabolic liver disease, primary hepatic cancer, acute fulminant liver disease, and inborn errors of metabolism. When malignancies are the cause of end-stage liver disease, the right upper quadrant may be radiated intraoperatively—after hepatectomy and before transplantation. The patient undergoes extensive physiologic and psychologic assessment and evaluation by physicians and transplant coordinators before being placed on a national-network waiting list. The potential for postoperative complications (Table 3-2) requires ongoing evaluation.

Procedural Considerations. Successful transplantation requires the cooperative efforts of the organ-procurement agency and the staffs of the donor and recipient hospitals. Usually two members of the surgical team from the recipient's hospital travel to the donor's hospital to procure the donated liver. Often, multiple transplant teams may arrive at the donor hospital to procure various organs for transplantation. UNOS policies dictate a detailed system for checking and rechecking organs for transplantation to ensure that organs of the donor and recipient are compatible (see Patient Safety box, p. 104). These policies must be strictly followed before any transplant can take place. Safe practice further requires that hospital policies are consistent with applicable law and organ donation regulations and should address patient and family preferences for organ donation, as well as specify the roles and desired outcomes for every stage of the donation process (NQF, 2009).

PREPARING THE OR FOR THE DONOR. The donor OR is set up for a major laparotomy procedure. Basic instrumentation and equipment include a basic laparotomy set, cardiovascular instruments, power sternal saw, and nephrectomy instruments. A sterile, draped, medium-size instrument table is needed for preparation of the liver away from the main sterile field and instrument tables. The procurement team provides special Collins solution for flushing the organs, sterile plastic containers and ice chests for organs, and in situ flush tubing. The liver is generally placed in two Lahey bags immediately after procurement.

PREPARING THE OR FOR THE RECIPIENT. Each transplant surgeon has preferred instruments, supplies, and sutures. In general, the following are needed in the recipient's OR: a basic laparotomy set, a cardiovascular instrument set, an assortment of T-tubes, a slush unit or means of providing iced lactated Ringer's solution, two ESUs, a forced-air warming device, a temperature probe, IV volumetric pumps on stands, two blood warmers or water baths, an indwelling urinary catheter, an insertion tray, and a urometer. An argon beam coagulator may be used and should be available. A defi-

TABLE 3-2

Assessment and Prevention of Common Postoperative Complications Associated with Liver Transplants

Assessment	Prevention
ACUTE GRAFT REJECTION	
Occurs from fourth to tenth postoperative day.	Use prophylaxis with immunosuppressant agents, such as cyclosporine, FK-506, CellCept, Prograf, Imuran, sirolimus, and prednisone.
Manifested by tachycardia, fever, right upper quadrant (RUQ) or flank pain, diminished bile drainage or change in bile color, or increased jaundice.	Diagnose early to treat with more potent antirejection drugs, such as muromonab-CD3 (Orthoclone OKT3).
Laboratory changes include increased levels of serum bilirubin, transaminases, and alkaline phosphatase and prolonged prothrombin time.	Use antibiotic prophylaxis.
INFECTION	
Can occur at any time during recovery.	Diagnose early and treat with organism-specific antiinfective agents.
Manifested by fever or excessive, foul-smelling drainage (urine, wound, or bile); other indicators depend on location and type of infection.	Perform frequent cultures of tubes, lines, and drainage. Remove invasive line as early as possible. Use good hand hygiene.
HEPATIC COMPLICATIONS (BILE LEAKAGE, ABSCESS FORMATION, HEPATIC THROMBOSIS)	
Manifested by decreased bile drainage, increased RUQ abdominal pain with distention and guarding, nausea or vomiting, increased jaundice, and clay-colored stools.	Keep T-tube in dependent position and secure to patient; empty frequently, recording quality and quantity of drainage.
Laboratory changes include increased levels of serum bilirubin and transaminases.	Report manifestations to physician immediately. May necessitate surgical intervention.
ACUTE RENAL FAILURE	
Caused by hypotension, antibiotics, cyclosporine, acute liver failure, or hypothermia.	Monitor all drug levels with nephrotoxic side effects. Prevent hypotension.
Indicators of hypothermia include shivering, hyperventilation, increased cardiac output, vasoconstriction, and alkalemia.	Observe for early signs of renal failure and report them immediately to physician.
Early indicators of renal failure include changes in urinary output, increased blood urea nitrogen (BUN) and creatinine levels, and electrolyte imbalance.	

Modified from Ignatavicius DD, Workman ML: *Medical-surgical nursing: patient-centered collaborative care,* ed 6, Philadelphia, 2010, Saunders.

brillator is always located in the room with sterile external paddles available.

Large-bore cannulae for IV monitoring and fluid or blood replacement lines are placed in addition to an arterial line and a central venous line.

Two surgeon headlights and light sources will be necessary to augment visualization of the abdominal site. A venovenous bypass system may be used to support peripheral blood flow. Extra drape sheets, table covers, gowns, towels, gloves, sponges, and laparotomy pads; cold IV Ringer's solution; sterile IV administration set for flushing the new liver; umbilical tape; booties; and vessel loops should be available to support the many steps of the transplantation procedure.

A cart containing sutures and the numerous other small items should be arranged and placed in the room for each procedure. This eliminates the need for the perioperative nurse to leave the patient and surgical team to obtain extra supplies.

The procedure for liver transplantation is a three-part process: retrieval of the donor organ, hepatectomy, and implantation of the donor liver. It is a lengthy procedure that takes many hours. The following aspects of implementing a plan of care deserve special attention.

Patient Positioning. The patient is placed supine with knees slightly flexed and padded. An indwelling urinary catheter is inserted after induction of anesthesia. Accurate body alignment is essential. A gel pad that is the length of the OR bed or a pressure-reducing OR bed mattress should be used, with attention to all potential pressure areas. Heel protectors are applied and SCDs are placed on the patient's legs. The safety strap is placed over the lower part of the thighs and secured. A forced-air warming device is applied over the upper body, neck, and head to assist in maintaining the patient's temperature. Fluid warmers are used to warm blood products and IV solutions.

Skin Preparation. The patient is prepped from the neck to midthigh, bedline to bedline. Prep solution should not pool at the bedline or wet the sheets on the OR bed. Fire safety precautions for prep solutions must be followed.

Blood Loss and Replacement. Blood loss may be extensive and replacement must be timely. The surgical team should confirm that blood products are available at the beginning of the procedure. These include 10 units each of packed red blood cells (RBCs) and fresh frozen plasma (FFP) and 1 unit of pooled donor platelets. The perioperative nurse should be available to assist the anesthesia provider during the insertion of peripheral and arterial lines. An autologous cell-saver device may be used to assist in blood replacement by way of autotransfusion.

Intraoperative Laboratory Testing. It is possible that as many as 50 blood specimens will be drawn for analysis during the procedure. Safe specimen collection practices are implemented. These specimens must be recorded on the blood-loss record and calculated into replacement needs. Specimens are delivered to the laboratory immediately. A telephone in the OR is useful for receiving and reading back critical test results/reports directly from the laboratory. Safe practices for reporting of critical test results require the perioperative nurse to verify the test result by "reading-back" the result (NQF, 2009). Standard precautions in collection of specimens must be observed.

Length of Procedure. Procedures may last from 6 to 20 hours. Special attention must be paid to maintaining the integrity of the sterile environment, given the length of surgery and number of people entering and exiting the OR.

Communication with Family. Frequent reports to the family are important. Family members often are knowledgeable about liver function tests and laboratory values and want this information in addition to reports on the condition of their loved one. One person should be assigned in advance to make regular contacts with family and support persons. The UNOS team often works closely in communicating with the donor's and recipient's families.

Communication Among Teams. Coordination among the procurement team, anesthesia team, and surgical teams is essential for a successful transplantation procedure. Perioperative nursing responsibilities also include monitoring and communicating blood-loss volume in suction canisters and on sponges, the availability of blood and blood products, laboratory results, time of organ arrival, ischemic time, and other events as they unfold in preparation for and during the transplant procedure.

Operative Procedure

1. Bilateral subcostal incisions are made with a midline incision extended toward the umbilicus. If necessary, the xiphoid is removed. The right side of the chest is entered if additional exposure is needed.
2. Initial dissection of the underlying tissues is achieved with electrosurgery and suture ligatures.
3. Isolation of all hilar structures and dissection to mobilize the lobes of the native liver are performed.
4. The retrohepatic vena cava is skeletonized, as are the hepatic artery, portal vein, common bile duct, and inferior vena cava.
5. The donor liver is examined.
6. Preparations may be made at this time for venovenous bypass using an extracorporeal assist device if the patient is unstable.
7. The infrahepatic vena cava and the suprahepatic vena cava are clamped, as are the portal vein, the hepatic artery, and the common bile duct.

8. Native hepatectomy is then performed.
9. The donor liver is placed in the right upper abdomen, and revascularization of the donor organ begins with end-to-end anastomoses in the vena cava and portal vein, with double-armed fine vascular suture.
10. At this point, the clamps on the portal vein, suprahepatic vena cava, and infrahepatic vena cava are released slowly, and blood flow through the vena cava and portal vein is restored.
11. The anastomosis sites are then checked for leaks.
12. If it was used, venovenous bypass is discontinued, and the cannulation sites are closed.
13. The postrevascularization phase focuses on achieving hemostasis. Complete hemostasis may require extensive time at this point. Bleeding may be exacerbated by a fibrinolytic episode associated with the reperfusion of the donor organ. The liver is monitored for a change in color from dusky to pink. An intraoperative Doppler may be used to confirm patency of the blood supply.
14. The anastomosis of the hepatic artery is then commenced, followed by bile duct reconstruction. This varies with the status of the recipient's biliary tract. If biliary atresia is the cause of the patient's end-stage liver disease, choledochoenterostomy into a Roux-en-Y loop of jejunum is performed (Figure 3-32).
15. The anastomoses are then checked for leaks.
16. Drains are placed behind and in front of the liver and exteriorized. The abdomen is then closed.

Donor Hepatectomy

Donor hepatectomy is performed for procurement of a healthy liver for transplant into a patient who has end-stage liver failure. This procedure occurs only after the donor patient has been determined to be brain dead and family consent for organ donation has been obtained. Donor hepatectomy can be performed at any hospital. Organ procurement agencies arrange contact with transplant centers when a viable organ donor has been identified.

Procedural Considerations. Once the liver transplant candidate has been identified, the procurement team from that transplant center travels to the institution where the organ donor is hospitalized. If multiple organs are being donated, surgeons from several transplant centers may arrive to procure the organs they will be transplanting to their respective centers.

The procedure for procurement of multiple organs will differ according to the transplant centers represented. Most commonly, the systemic cooling of the donor's body temperature is started before the procurement of the heart. Cannulation sites also vary according to which organs are procured.

The donor hospital supplies a basic laparotomy setup with instrumentation to open the sternum. Basic vascular clamps are also required to clamp the major vascular structures. Cold lactated Ringer's solution for parenteral infusion and cold Ringer's solution for irrigation are usually used in large amounts.

Operative Procedure

1. The donor patient is positioned supine on the OR bed. The skin area from neck to midthigh is prepped and draped.
2. A midline incision is made from the suprasternal notch to the pubis.

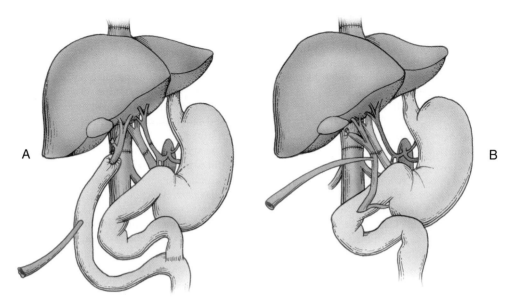

FIGURE 3-32 Completed orthotopic liver transplant with Roux-en-Y biliary reconstruction (**A**) and end-to-end anastomosis of the donor-to-recipient common bile ducts (**B**).

3. A subcostal incision is performed bilaterally on the abdomen for better exposure of the abdominal viscera.

4. Retractors are placed to provide optimal exposure of the organs that will be procured.

5. The aorta and vena cava, superior and inferior to the liver and kidneys, are skeletonized by dissection and ligation of the lymphatics and smaller vasculatures.

6. The porta hepatis is dissected; the superior mesenteric artery and celiac trunk are then dissected and delicately exposed as close to the aorta as is convenient.

7. The superior mesenteric vein is dissected and prepared for cannulation. The donor is heparinized and systemically cooled.

8. If the heart is to be procured, removal takes place at this time.

9. Further cooling and flushing of the pancreas, liver, and kidneys are achieved by cannulation and infusion of cold lactated Ringer's solution through the inferior vena cava just superior to the bifurcation.

10. The liver, pancreas, spleen, and a segment of the duodenum harboring the pancreatic duct are procured en bloc by placing clamps on the suprahepatic and infrahepatic venae cavae.

11. The suprahepatic vena cava is transected with a surrounding cuff of diaphragm intact.

12. The infrahepatic vena cava is transected above the level of the renal veins.

13. The celiac axis is detached from the aorta as an aortic patch or taken with a full aortic circumference.

14. The duodenal segment is procured, using a linear stapling device at opposite ends of the segment.

15. The en bloc organs are taken to a back table for further dissection and ligation to separate the liver from the en bloc pancreas, spleen, and duodenal segment graft. Meanwhile, other members of the procurement team continue working to free the kidneys and ureters if they are to be taken.

16. The liver is placed in a basin of cold Ringer's solution, double-bagged in sterile Lahey bags, and placed in an ice chest for transport to the recipient's hospital.

17. The kidneys are placed in sterile cassettes and mechanically perfused.

18. The pancreatic en bloc graft is also placed in a basin of cold Ringer's solution, bagged, and transported in a thermal chest of ice.

19. The abdomen is closed with a single layer of size 1 or 0 nonabsorbable suture.

20. Drapes are removed, and the donor patient is cleaned and washed. Tubes and infusion lines are tied off or clamped. Sometimes family members of the donor patient request to view the body after organ donation. This factor may be important in helping them face their loss. Before family viewing, the donor's body is covered with a warm blanket. The surgical team assists the family in their grieving process by providing a quiet and private environment in which to say good-bye to their family member.

21. The donor patient is then transported by stretcher to the morgue.

Living-Related Liver Transplantation

Just as kidney transplantation has evolved into living-related donor possibilities, so too has liver transplantation. The capacity of the liver to regenerate provided the scientific basis for development of the living-related donor transplantation procedure. Reduced-size and split-liver transplants have been performed successfully. Reduced-size liver transplantation has been performed for infants, children, or very small adults with results comparable to those obtained with whole-organ transplantation. Prospective living donors are thoroughly evaluated with a protocol that includes blood group compatibility, a comprehensive history and physical examination, laboratory studies, psychosocial evaluation, independent advocate opinion, anatomic compatibility, review of candidacy with the donor, and presentation to a selection committee (Patt and Thuluvath, 2003). As cloning, biogenetic engineering, and other technologic advances increase the possibilities for organ transplants, society will need to address ongoing debates of ethical dilemmas surrounding transplantation.

SURGERY OF THE SPLEEN

Splenectomy (Open Approach)

Splenectomy is removal of the spleen. It is performed for multiple reasons: trauma to the spleen; specific malignant conditions (Hodgkin's disease and non-Hodgkin's lymphomas; hairy cell, chronic lymphocytic, and chronic myelogenous leukemias); hemolytic jaundice or splenic anemia; idiopathic thrombocytopenia purpura (ITP); tumors, cysts, or splenomegaly; or accidental injury during vagotomy or other procedures involving mobilization of the splenic flexure of the colon. If accessory spleens are present, they are also removed because they are capable of perpetuating hypersplenic function. In most instances, patients evaluated for elective splenectomy are considered candidates for laparoscopic splenectomy. Contraindications to laparoscopic splenectomy include severe portal hypertension, uncorrectable coagulopathy, severe ascites, extreme splenomegaly, extensive adhesions, and most traumatic injuries to the spleen. For these patients, an open approach is indicated.

Procedural Considerations. Instrumentation is as described for a basic laparotomy, plus two large, right-angled pedicle clamps, long instruments, and hemostatic materials and devices. Abdominal suction apparatus is available and a cell-saver may be requested. The patient is positioned supine. After induction of general anesthesia and intubation, the anesthesia provider inserts an NG tube. An indwelling urinary catheter is inserted before the abdominal prep. The abdomen is prepped from nipple line to midthigh. The OR bed is moved to reverse Trendelenburg's position with a slight tilt to the right. A midline abdominal incision provides access to the spleen and allows maximal exposure of all abdominal organs. Occasionally, a subcostal approach is used for a patient without traumatic injury. Rarely, a thoracoabdominal approach is used.

Operative Procedure

1. The abdomen is opened through the selected incision.
2. Retractors are placed over moistened laparotomy packs and exploration is carried out.
3. The costal margin is retracted upward.
4. The splenorenal, splenocolic, and gastrosplenic ligaments are clamped and divided with long dressing forceps, long hemostats, sponges on holders, and long Metzenbaum or Nelson scissors.
5. Adhesions posterior to the spleen are freed.
6. The spleen is delivered into the wound.
7. The short gastric vessels are now easily identified, clamped, divided, and ligated.
8. The cavity formerly occupied by the spleen is packed with moist laparotomy pads, if necessary.
9. The splenic artery and vein are dissected free with fine dissecting scissors and forceps.
10. The artery is clamped and doubly ligated. The artery is ligated first to permit disengorgement of blood from the spleen and facilitate return of venous blood to the circulatory system.
11. The splenic vein is then clamped, divided, and ligated.
12. The specimen is removed, bleeding vessels controlled, and the wound closed in layers, as described for laparotomy. Dressings are applied.
13. Drainage is usually required only if extensive adhesions to the diaphragm were divided or if significant clotting abnormalities exist.

Laparoscopic Splenectomy

Laparoscopic splenectomy is standard procedure for surgical treatment of benign hematologic disorders (Beauchamp et al, 2008). Indications are the same as with open procedures, with the exception of the contraindications noted previously. Robotic assistance has improved visibility and motion control (Bodner et al, 2005b).

Procedural Considerations. After induction of general anesthesia, an NG tube and indwelling urinary catheter are inserted, and SCDs applied to the lower extremities. The patient is positioned in right lateral position, with the OR bed flexed and kidney rest raised to increase the distance between the lower rib and iliac crest. The anterior abdomen is brought close to the edge of the OR bed. A beanbag device may be used. Safety restraints must be placed, especially in anticipation of a possible slight backward patient tilt. Alternatively, supine or modified lithotomy position may be used. The surgeon stands on the patient's right side, as does the scrub person, and assistants stand to the left.

Instrumentation and equipment include a 30-degree telescope (10-mm or 5-mm); a camera (triple-chip or single-chip); a high-flow insufflator with CO_2 tank; a high-resolution monitor (second monitor optional for assistant); a printer (optional); a Surgineedle or Veress needle; four 12-mm trocars (trocar size depends on surgeon preference—some surgeons substitute one or two of the 12-mm trocars with 5-mm trocars or even 3-mm trocars); endoshears/scissors; ultrasonic endoshears; an endodissecting forceps or endograsper (atraumatic); an endoretractor; an endoclip applier; a linear stapling device (GIA type) with vascular cartridges; an endoretrieval pouch; and a suction-irrigation system. As with other laparoscopic procedures, instruments and supplies are available if it becomes necessary to convert to an open approach.

Operative Procedure

1. Pneumoperitoneum is created and the first trocar placed under direct visualization. Three to five 2- to 12-mm operating ports are used, with the camera port at the umbilicus.
2. The laparoscope is inserted through the port and the camera placed.
3. The stomach is retracted to expose the spleen and a search made for any accessory spleens.
4. Initial dissection is begun by mobilizing the splenic flexure of the colon.

5. The splenocolic ligament is divided using sharp dissection, mobilizing the inferior pole of the spleen. The spleen is now retracted cephalad, taking care not to rupture the splenic capsule during retraction.

6. The lateral peritoneal attachments of the spleen are then incised using either sharp dissection or ultrasonic endoshears.

7. The lesser sac is entered along the medial border of the spleen.

8. With the spleen elevated, the short gastric vessels and main vascular pedicle are visualized. The tail of the pancreas is also visualized and avoided.

9. The short gastric vessels are divided by means of an ultrasonic dissector, endoclips, or an endovascular stapling device.

10. After the short gastric vessels have been divided, the splenic pedicle is carefully dissected from both the medial and lateral aspects.

11. After the artery and vein are dissected, the vessels are divided by application of the endovascular stapler. Multiple vascular branches may be encountered and each is taken individually.

12. The spleen is now devascularized and ready for removal.

13. An Endo-Bag is introduced through one of the trocar sites, usually the left lateral site.

14. The bag is opened and the spleen placed into it. The drawstring is grasped and the bag closed, leaving only the superior pole attachments, which are now divided.

15. The open end of the bag is exteriorized from the abdomen through the supraumbilical port or epigastric trocar site. The spleen is then morcellated and removed in fragments.

16. The laparoscope is reinserted and the splenic bed is assessed for hemostasis.

17. If necessary, a drain is placed in the intraabdominal cavity, the abdomen deflated, and the trocars removed.

18. The trocar sites are then closed.

SURGERY OF THE LIVER, BILIARY TRACT, PANCREAS, AND SPLEEN SUMMARY

The expertise of a surgical technologist is highly valued in hepatobiliary surgery. As the field expands into uncharted territory with minimally invasive and robotic-assisted procedures, surgical technologists must stay current in their practice. Whether one of the 750,000 gallbladder surgeries or the highly technical liver transplant, the knowledge and skill of the surgical technologist can be appreciated from every vantage point of the operating suite. Knowledge of anatomy, physiology, instrumentation, surgeon's preferences, and aseptic technique combine to create a safe surgical environment for every patient. A passion for surgery, a willingness to learn, and openness to change make the surgical technologist a valued member of the surgical team.

GERIATRIC CONSIDERATIONS

The Elderly Patient—Surgery of the Liver, Biliary Tract, Pancreas, and Spleen

Populations in the Western world continue to age rapidly. Morbidity and mortality increase, primarily due to decreased reserves, increases in co-morbid and preexisting conditions, and sometimes a reluctance to perform surgery on an elderly population. For the most part, geriatric surgical patients can be managed well, and there is a strong emphasis on predicting risks and preventing them (Ergina and Meakins, 1993).

With aging, the pancreas secretes fewer bicarbonate and enzymes (exocrine functions) and the organ itself shrinks in size and becomes more fatty. There is an increased incidence of pancreatic adenocarcinoma, which has a very low survival rate (Fillit et al, 2010). Gallstones in the elderly can lead to acute pancreatitis. When pancreatic ducts distend and dilate, as they do with aging, lipase levels decrease, leading to decreased fat absorption and digestion. This results in steatorrhea (excess fat in the feces) (Ignatavicius and Workman, 2010).

The mass of functional hepatocytes and hepatic blood flow decrease with age. Although there are no specific liver diseases associated with advancing age, age does have an effect on metabolism of drugs and alcohol. Depressed drug metabolism can lead to an accumulation of drugs, perhaps to toxic levels. Both hepatitis C and alcoholic liver disease are becoming more prevalent in the elderly population. Liver biopsy is done to confirm the presence of and cause of liver disease. Age alone is not a contradiction to treating liver disease, and some healthy elderly patients are demonstrating improved outcomes following liver transplantation.

Diseases affecting the gallbladder and biliary tract are not uncommon in elderly patients. Cholecystitis more commonly has associated bile duct stones in the elderly than in younger populations. If there is biliary obstruction, ERCP and endoscopic techniques to remove the stones are safer than surgery in elderly patients. However, laparoscopic cholecystectomy remains the treatment of choice for patients with cholecystitis. In patients aged 65 to 69, mortality rates are similar to the general population. Those rates rise when the patient is older than 70. Some surgeons may opt for small incision cholecystectomy rather than a laparoscopic approach.

Risk-benefit ratios of the intended surgical procedure are thoughtfully analyzed in elderly patients, and careful planning by the surgical team is essential. Anticipating likely problems and subsequent early intervention are key to improving outcomes.

Modified from Ergina PL, Meakins JL: Perioperative care of the elderly patient. World Journal of Surgery, 17:192-198, 1993, available at www.springerlink.com/content/q4370r2874074982/fulltext.pdf. Accessed September 7, 2010; Fillit HM et al: *Textbook of geriatric medicine and gerontology*, ed 7, Philadelphia; 2010, Saunders; Hartford Institute for Geriatric Nursing: Geriatric nursing resources for care of older adults, available at consultgerirn.org/topics/normal_aging_changes/want_to_know_more#item_7. Accessed September 5, 2010; Ignatavicius DD, Workman ML: Medical-surgical nursing: patient-centered collaborative care, ed 6, Philadelphia, 2010, Saunders.

REVIEW QUESTIONS

1. Pancreatic transplant patients may remain on immunosuppression drugs postoperatively for:
   a. one week
   b. one month
   c. one year
   d. indefinitely

2. A patient with end-stage liver disease caused by biliary atresia will require what procedure in conjunction with their liver transplant?
   a. cholecystectomy
   b. gastrectomy
   c. choledochoenterostomy
   d. choledochoduodenectomy

3. The pancreas lies directly on top of what two blood vessels?
   a. inferior iliac vein and artery
   b. superior and inferior vena cava
   c. short gastric artery and phrenic artery
   d. superior mesenteric artery and vein

4. List three contraindications for laparoscopic splenectomy.

5. What is the most common nonemergent abdominal surgery performed today?

6. Explain why a cholangiogram setup must be free of bubbles.

7. List the four structures involved in a Whipple procedure.

8. Explain the difference between a clean-contaminated wound and a contaminated wound.

9. Define and briefly describe the following surgical procedures:
   Laparoscopic cholecystectomy
   Pancreatic transplantation
   Splenectomy (open and laparoscopic)

Critical Thinking Question

Patient John Smith is scheduled for a diagnostic laparoscopy with possible Whipple procedure. Mr. Smith is a 78-year-old male weighing 160 kilograms. The diagnostic laparoscopy is performed to rule out any malignancies. If it is determined laparoscopically that the mass cannot be resected, the procedure could be over in a few minutes; however if resectability is determined, the procedure could last several hours. During the procedure, it is determined that a Whipple procedure is indicated and the procedure converts to open. During the open procedure, the surgeon discovers the mass is connected to the portal vein and determines a reconstruction of the portal vein will be necessary. Explain what steps the surgical technologist should have taken preoperatively to facilitate a smooth transition from laparoscopy to open surgery. Also, explain what additional items, if any, will be needed for the portal vein reconstruction.

REFERENCES

Afdhal NH, Vollmer CM: Complications of laparoscopic cholecystectomy, available at www.uptodate.com/patients/content/topic.do?topicKey=~JduJa7QAGmGYd., 2008. Accessed Nov. 27, 2008.

Association of periOperative Registered Nurses (AORN): Recommended practices for a safe environment of care. In *Perioperative standards and recommended practices*, Denver, 2009, The Association.

Beauchamp RD et al: The spleen. In Townsend CM et al, editors: *Sabiston textbook of surgery*, ed 18, Philadelphia, 2008, Saunders.

Belli G et al: Laparoscopic left lateral hepatic lobectomy: a safer and faster technique, *J Hepatobiliary Pancreat Surg* 13(2):149–154, 2006.

Belli G et al: Laparoscopic versus open liver resection for hepatocellular carcinoma in patients with histologically proven cirrhosis: Short- and middle-term results, *Surg Endosc* 21(11):2004–2011, 2007.

Bodner J et al: Long-term follow-up after robotic cholecystectomy, *Am Surg* 71(4):281-288, 2005a.

Bodner J et al: A critical comparison of robotic versus conventional laparoscopic splenectomies, *World J Surg* 29(8):982-985, 2005b.

Borzellino G et al: Laparoscopic hepatic resection, *Surg Endosc* 20(5):787–790, 2006.

Chari RS, Shah SA: Biliary system, In Townsend CM et al: editors: *Sabiston textbook of surgery*, ed 18, Philadelphia, 2008, Saunders.

Denholm B: Tucking patient's arms and general positioning, *AORN J* 89(4):755–757, 2009.

First Robotic Complex Liver Surgery, available at www.medicalnewstoday.com/articles/22589.php.2005. Accessed March 30, 2009.

Gruessner RW et al: Over 500 solitary pancreas transplants in nonuremic patients with brittle diabetes mellitus, *Transplantation* 85(1):42–47, 2008.

Hanley EJ, Talamini MA: Robotic abdominal surgery, *Am J Surg* 188(4A, Suppl):19S–26S, 2004.

Hines OJ, Reber HA: Pancreatic surgery, *Curr Opin Gastroenterol* 22(5):520–526, 2006.

Insler SR, Sessler DI: Perioperative thermoregulation and temperature monitoring, *Anesthesiol Clin* 24(4):823–837, 2006.

Jacobsen G et al: Robotic surgery update, *Surg Endosc* 18(8):1186–1191, 2004.

Kleemann M et al: Laparoscopic ultrasound navigation in liver surgery: technical aspects and accuracy, *Surg Endosc* 20(5):726–729, 2006.

McPhee JT et al: Perioperative mortality for pancreatectomy: a national perspective, *Ann Surg* 246(2):246–253, 2007.

Meakins JL, Masterson BF: ACS Surgery: principles & practice, In Souba WW, editor: *American College of Surgeons*, ed. 6, New York, 2007, WebMD Professional Pub, p. 20.

Melvin WS: Minimally invasive pancreatic surgery, *Am J Surg* 186(3):274–278, 2003.

National Quality Forum (NQF): *Safe Practices for Better Healthcare, 2009 Update: A Consensus Report*, Washington, DC, 2009, NQF.

Nguyen NT et al: Application of robotics in general surgery: initial experience, *Am Surg* 70(10):914–917, 2004.

Patt CH, Thuluvath PJ: Adult living donor transplantation. Medscape Gastroenterology, 2003, available at www.medscape.com/viewarticle/458740?src=search. Accessed October 8, 2008.

Phillips NF: *Berry & Kohn's operating room technique*, 11th ed, St Louis, 2007, Mosby.

Poultsides G et al: Hand-assisted laparoscopic management of liver tumors, *Surg Endosc* 21(8):1275–1279, 2007.

Ramos AC et al: NOTES transvaginal video-assisted cholecystectomy: First series, *Endoscopy* 40:572–575, 2008.

Santambrogio R et al: Impact of intraoperative ultrasonography in laparoscopic liver surgery, *Surg Endosc* 21(2):181–188, 2007.

Steer ML: Exocrine pancreas, In Townsend CM, editor: *Sabiston textbook of surgery*, ed 18, Philadelphia, 2008, Saunders.

Universal Protocol for Preventing Wrong Site, Wrong Procedure and Wrong Person Surgery. The Joint Commission (TJC), available at www.jointcommission.org/PatientSafety/UniversalProtocol/. Accessed March 30, 2009.

Repair of Hernias

Overview

A hernia is an abnormal protrusion of a peritoneum-lined sac through the musculoaponeurotic covering of the abdomen. The word *hernia* is a Latin term that means "rupture" of a portion of a structure. Descriptions of hernia reduction date back to Hammurabi of Babylon and the Egyptian papyrus (History box). Weakness of the abdominal wall, congenital or acquired, results in the inability to contain the visceral contents of the abdominal cavity within their normal confines. This defect occurs frequently; hernia repair is the most common operation in general surgery (Menon, 2008). More than 700,000 surgical procedures are performed each year to repair congenital hernia defects; nearly 75% of all acquired hernias occur in the inguinal region. Of these, about 50% of hernias are indirect inguinal hernias and 24% are direct inguinal hernias. Incisional and ventral hernias account for approximately 10% of all hernias; as the frequency and magnitude of abdominal

surgeries have increased in recent years, so has the incidence of incisional hernia. Femoral hernias account for 3%, and unusual hernias account for the remaining 5% to 10%.

Hernias occur most often in males. The most common hernia in both males and females is the indirect inguinal hernia. Femoral hernias occur much more frequently in females, and only 2% of females will develop inguinal hernias in their lifetime. Also, hernias occur more commonly on the right side than on the left. Herniorrhaphy is one of the most common operative procedures performed and is the preferred treatment when a defect is detected.

Hernias have a tremendous economic significance in the United States. The number of workdays lost is substantial. The trend toward ambulatory surgery for hernia repair is one of many attempts to provide cost-effective healthcare that also leads to patient satisfaction.

A hernia can occur in several places in the abdominal wall, with protrusion of a portion of the parietal peritoneum and often a part of the intestine. The weak places or intervals in the abdominal aponeurosis are (1) the inguinal canals, (2) the femoral rings, and (3) the umbilicus. Any number of conditions causing increased pressure within the abdomen can contribute to the formation of a hernia. Contributing factors to hernia formation include age, gender, previous surgery, obesity,

This chapter was originally written by Maya N. Clark, ACNP-BC, and Jane C. Rothrock, PhD, RN, CNOR, FAAN, for the 14th edition of Alexander's Care of the Patient in Surgery *and has been revised by Crit Fisher, BS, CST, FAST, for this text.*

HISTORY

History of Hernia Repairs

Groin hernias were originally documented 3500 years ago, with surgical intervention starting approximately 1500 years after that. Before the intervention of surgical repair of the hernia, external supports called *trusses* were used to contain hernias that protruded from the body. A brief chronology of some of the events that laid the foundation for modern hernia repair is presented below.

Time Period	Breakthrough
2800 BC	Herodotus reported that physicians specialized in treating hernia.
1700 BC	Hammurabi described hernia reduction.
400 BC	Hippocrates described hernia as a tear in the abdomen.
200 BC	Galen described anatomy of the abdominal wall.
AD 100	Celsus described clinical signs to differentiate a hernia from a hydrocele.
1559	Maupassius performed the first surgical intervention to correct a strangulated hernia.
1724	Heister described direct hernias.
1804	Astley Cooper defines a hernia as a protrusion of any viscus from its proper cavity.
1814	Scarpa described sliding hernias.
1881	Lucas-Championniere laid the basis for the most important inguinal hernia repair procedure—reinforcing the posterior wall of the inguinal canal and narrowing the internal inguinal ring.
1887	Bassini introduced his repair technique that involved suturing the conjoined tendon to the inguinal ligament up to the inguinal ring; he is considered the father of modern-day hernia surgery.
1898	Lotheissen modified the Bassini repair, recommending the oblique internus and transversus abdominis muscles be attached to the Cooper ligament. (Cooper was the first to describe the superior pubic ligament, although he never used it to surgically repair a groin hernia.)
1918	Nursing textbook listed instruments for femoral, inguinal, umbilical, and ventral herniorrhaphy.
1940	Shouldice introduced multilayer closure; founded Shouldice Hospital near Toronto. Local anesthetic was used; patients walked to and from the OR.
1942	McVay again described Lotheissen repair; it became known as the *McVay/Cooper repair.*
1958	Usher introduced use of "Marlex" mesh for repair of both primary and recurrent hernias, describing it as "tension-eliminating."
1971	Nursing textbook described the Gallie method, in which fascia lata is removed from the thigh and stitched around the hernial orifice.
1982	Ger performed the first laparoscopic herniorrhaphy.

RESEARCH HIGHLIGHT

Prioritizing General Surgery Procedures for Quality Improvement Efforts

Despite growing reliance on quality improvement measures, there is no established protocol for determining which general surgical procedures should be the focus of these efforts. In this study, researchers sought to prioritize procedures for quality improvement efforts in general surgery in terms of morbidity, mortality, and excess length of stay. Using data from the American College of Surgeons' National Surgery Quality Improvement Program, they identified 129,233 patients who underwent general surgery between 2005 and 2006.

Patients were placed in 36 procedure groups. Of these, 10 groups accounted for 62% of complications and 54% of excess length of stay. Patients undergoing ventral hernia repair accounted for only 5% of complications. In contrast, the colectomy group accounted for the highest number of adverse events (24%), followed by small intestine resection (8%), inpatient cholecystectomy (6%), and pancreatic resection (4%).

In looking at ambulatory surgery, outpatient inguinal hernia repair, cholecystectomy, breast procedures, thyroidectomy, and parathyroidectomy accounted for 34% of procedures but only 6% of complications and less than 1% of excess hospital days.

Based on their analysis, researchers concluded that a relatively small number of general surgery procedures account for a disproportionate share of the morbidity, mortality, and excess hospital days. Therefore focusing quality improvement efforts on those procedures may be an effective strategy for improving care and reducing cost.

Adapted from Schilling PL et al: Prioritizing quality improvement in general surgery, *J Am Coll Surg* 207:698-704, 2008.

nutritional status, and pulmonary and cardiac disease. Loss of tissue turgor occurs with aging and in chronic debilitating diseases. Current evidence suggests that adult male inguinal hernias are likely associated with impaired collagen metabolism and weakening of the fibroconnective tissue of the groin (Gilbert et al, 2009). Smoking has also been noted as a contributing factor to hernia formation (Read, 2004). A successful herniorrhaphy is measured by the percentage of recurrence, the number of complications, the total costs, and the ability to return to normal activities of daily living (Research Highlight).

Surgical Anatomy

A hernia is a sac lined by peritoneum that protrudes through a defect in the layers of the abdominal wall. Generally, a hernia mass is composed of covering tissues, a peritoneal sac, and any contained viscera. Hernias may be acquired or congenital.

Depending on their location, hernias are classified as direct inguinal, indirect inguinal, femoral, umbilical, incisional, or epigastric (Figure 4-1). Hernias in any of these groups are either

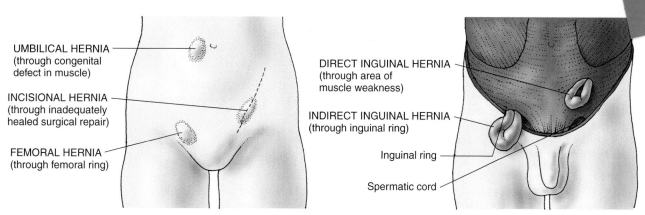

FIGURE 4-1 Types of abdominal hernias.

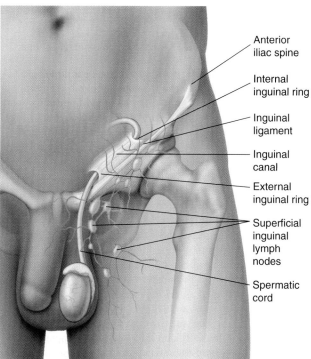

FIGURE 4-2 Structures of the inguinal area.

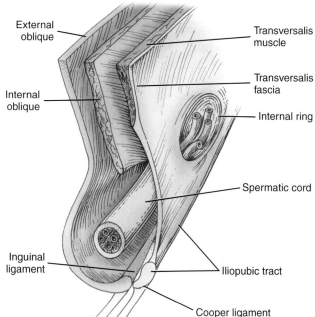

FIGURE 4-3 Right inguinal region, parasagittal section. Roof of inguinal canal is formed by external oblique aponeurosis, and floor is formed by transversalis aponeurosis and fascia.

reducible or nonreducible; that is, the contents of the hernia sac either can be returned to the normal intraabdominal position or are trapped in the extraabdominal sac (incarcerated). The conditions preventing the return of the hernia contents to the abdomen can result from (1) adhesions between the contents of the sac and the inner lining of the sac, (2) adhesions among the contents of the sac, or (3) narrowing of the neck of the sac. Patients with incarcerated hernias may have signs of intestinal obstruction, such as vomiting, abdominal pain, and distention. The greatest danger of an incarcerated hernia is that it may become strangulated. In a strangulated hernia, the blood supply of the trapped sac contents becomes compromised and eventually the sac contents necrose. When bowel is strangulated in such a hernia, resection of necrotic bowel, in addition to the repair of the hernia defect, becomes necessary. This is a surgical emergency.

Inguinal Hernias

The anterolateral abdominal wall consists of an arrangement of muscles, fascial layers, and muscular aponeuroses lined interiorly by peritoneum and exteriorly by skin (Figure 4-2). The abdominal wall in the groin area is composed of two groups of these structures: a superficial group (Scarpa's fascia, external and internal oblique muscles, and their aponeuroses) and a deep group (internal oblique muscle, transversalis fascia, and peritoneum).

Essential to an understanding of inguinal hernia repair is an appreciation of the central role of the transversalis fascia as the major supporting structure of the posterior inguinal floor. The inguinal canal, which contains the spermatic cord and associated structures in males and the round ligament in females, is approximately 4 cm long and takes an oblique course parallel to the groin crease. The inguinal canal is covered by the aponeurosis of the external abdominal oblique muscle, which

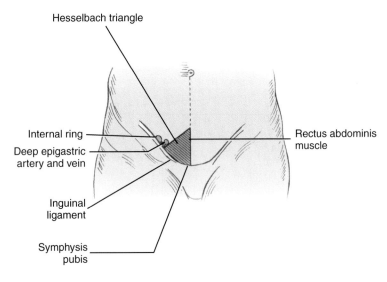

FIGURE 4-4 Schema of the Hesselbach triangle. Boundaries of the Hesselbach triangle are deep epigastric vessels laterally, inguinal ligament inferiorly, and rectus abdominis muscle medially.

forms a roof (Figure 4-3). A thickened lower border of the external oblique aponeurosis forms the inguinal (Poupart's) ligament, which runs from the anterior superior iliac spine to the pubic tubercle. Structures that traverse the inguinal canal enter it from the abdomen by the internal ring, a natural opening in the transversalis fascia, and exit by the external ring, an opening in the external oblique aponeurosis, to go to either the testis or the labium. If the external oblique aponeurosis is opened and the cord or round ligament is mobilized, the floor of the inguinal canal is exposed. The posterior inguinal floor is the structure that becomes defective and is susceptible to indirect, direct, or femoral hernias.

The key component of the important posterior inguinal floor is the transversalis muscle of the abdomen and its associated aponeurosis and fascia. The posterior inguinal floor can be divided into two areas. The superior lateral area represents the internal ring, whereas the inferior medial area represents the attachment of the transversalis aponeurosis and fascia to the Cooper ligament (iliopectineal line). The Cooper ligament is the site of the insertion of the transversalis aponeurosis along the superior ramus from the symphysis pubis laterally to the femoral sheath. The inguinal portion of the transversalis fascia arises from the iliopsoas fascia and not from the inguinal ligament.

Medially and superiorly the transversalis muscle becomes aponeurotic and fuses with the aponeurosis of the internal oblique muscle to form anterior and posterior rectus sheaths. As the symphysis pubis is approached, the contributions from the internal oblique muscle become fewer and fewer. At the pubic tubercle and behind the spermatic cord or round ligament, the internal oblique muscle makes no contribution and the posterior inguinal wall (floor of the inguinal canal) is composed solely of aponeurosis and fascia of the transversalis muscle.

None of the three groin hernias (direct and indirect inguinal hernias and femoral hernia) develops in the presence of a strong transversus abdominis layer and in the absence of persistent stress on the connective tissue layers. When a weakening or a tear in the aponeurosis of the transversus abdominis and the transversalis fascia occurs, the potential for development of a direct inguinal hernia is established.

Femoral Hernias

When the transversus abdominis aponeurosis and its fascia are only narrowly attached to the Cooper ligament, a femoral hernia may develop. This results in an enlarged femoral ring and canal, which allows for the prominence of the iliofemoral vessels, resulting in femoral herniation (Lawrence, 2006).

The walls of the femoral sheath are formed anteriorly and medially from the transversalis fascia, posteriorly from the pectineus and psoas fascia, and laterally from the iliaca fascia. The pelvis ostium consists of a relatively fixed rim of bone and connective tissue: anteriorly and medially the iliopubic tract, posteriorly the superior ramus, and laterally the iliopectineal arch.

The femoral sheath is subdivided into three compartments. The lateral compartment contains the femoral artery, and the intermediate compartment contains the femoral vein. The medial compartment is the smallest and constitutes the femoral canal, which is formed anteriorly and medially by the iliopubic tract. This opening is bound laterally by the iliofemoral vessels and posteriorly by the superior pubic ramus and pectineus fascia. Superiorly, laterally, and inferiorly the fossa is formed by the falciform margin of the fascia lata.

Abdominal Hernias

The anterior abdominal wall is composed of external abdominal oblique muscles attached to a thick sheath of connective tissue called the *rectus sheath*. The linea alba extends superiorly and inferiorly from above the xiphoid process to the pubis. Beneath the rectus sheath lies the rectus abdominis muscles, laterally to the right and left of the linea alba. Lateral to the rectus abdominis is the linea semilunaris. The transversus abdominis muscles originate from the seventh to the twelfth costal cartilages, lumbar fascia, iliac crest, and the inguinal ligament, and insert on the xiphoid process, the linea alba, and the pubic tubercle. The third layer of abdominal wall includes the internal abdominal oblique muscles originating from the iliac crest, inguinal ligament, and lumbar fascia, and inserting on the tenth to twelfth ribs and rectus sheath.

Direct and Indirect Inguinal Hernias

The deep epigastric vessels (inferior epigastric) arise from the external iliac vessels and enter the inguinal canal just proximal to the internal ring. The triangle formed by the deep epigastric

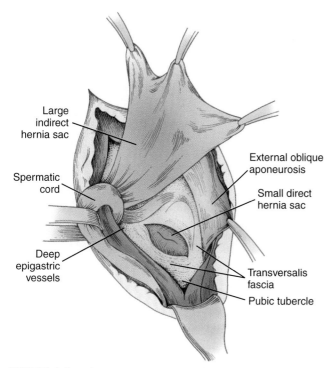

FIGURE 4-5 Defect in transversalis fascia, medial to deep epigastric vessels, results in direct hernia. Defect lateral to deep epigastric vessels results in indirect hernia.

Labels: Large indirect hernia sac; Spermatic cord; Deep epigastric vessels; External oblique aponeurosis; Small direct hernia sac; Transversalis fascia; Pubic tubercle

vessels laterally, the inguinal ligament inferiorly, and the rectus abdominis muscles medially is referred to as the *Hesselbach triangle* (Figure 4-4). Hernias that occur within the Hesselbach triangle are called *direct inguinal hernias*. Indirect inguinal hernias occur laterally to the deep epigastric vessels. Both direct and indirect hernias represent attenuations or tears in the transversalis fascia (Figure 4-5).

Direct hernias protrude into the inguinal canal but not into the cord and therefore rarely into the scrotum. Direct inguinal hernias usually result from heavy lifting or other strenuous activities. Indirect hernias leave the abdominal cavity at the internal inguinal ring and pass with the cord structures down the inguinal canal. Consequently, the indirect hernia sac may be found in the scrotum. Indirect hernias may be either congenital, representing a persistence of the processus vaginalis, or acquired. In a congenital hernia, the hernia sac has a small neck, is thin-walled, and is closely bound to the cord structures. In an acquired indirect hernia, the neck is wide and the sac is both short and thick-walled. When both direct and indirect hernias are present, the defect is called a *pantaloon hernia* after the French word for "pants," which this situation suggests.

Surgical Technologist Considerations

Assessment

Assessment of the patient should include the history of previous surgeries related to the herniated area as well as information relating to familial history. The patient's nutritional status, the duration of symptoms, and a history of obesity, increased intraabdominal pressure, chronic cough, constipation, benign prostatic hypertrophy, intestinal obstruction, colon malignancy, and, for women, pregnancy should all be taken into account. A list of the patient's current medications should be collected, as well as a history of chronic illness and allergies, including latex allergies (because a Penrose drain may be used during the procedure). The patient's occupation and physical activities should also be determined.

The diagnosis of hernias should be accompanied by clinical physical examination. Palpation of the herniated area reveals the contents of the hernia sac. Fingertip palpation allows the examiner to feel the edges of the external ring or abdominal wall. Having the patient stand and cough or prolonged strain during the examination also assists in the evaluation of the herniated area. If a definitive diagnosis is not confirmed, ultrasonic scanning and imaging techniques (e.g., computerized tomography [CT], herniography, standard radiography) may be employed.

In some patients, a hernia may cause no symptoms; its only sign may be a swelling or protrusion in a restricted area of the abdominal wall. If the hernia is unilateral, the patient notes the lack of a protrusion on the other side in comparison. The area may be visible when the patient stands or coughs and may disappear on reclining. Femoral hernias can be difficult to diagnose and may resemble an enlarged lymph node.

Preoperative testing includes a complete blood count. Patients older than 40 years may need an electrocardiogram (ECG) and chest radiograph. Patients with a history of more complex medical problems must be fully evaluated with appropriate laboratory tests. Preoperative assessment may also involve consultation with a pulmonologist or a cardiologist to ascertain whether surgical intervention is medically safe (this is referred to as *clearance* in patients with potential pulmonary or cardiac problems).

Planning

In planning for the surgeries on the hernia one must pay close attention to the operative approach and intended repair of the hernia, instrumentation, draping, and positioning of the patient depend on the type and approach—for example, open versus laparoscopic. With a laparoscopic approach, special video and recording equipment are needed. Also in most cases surgical mesh is used to repair the defect. The surgical technologist should be aware of the inventory levels of the styles and types of mesh and that there are enough resources available.

Instrumentation and Supplies

Instrumentation needed for an open hernia repair is a minor general surgery set. Depending on the location of the defect, a variety of supplies are needed. Mesh patches of synthetic material (Gore-Tex, Teflon, Dacron, Marlex, or Prolene) are now being widely used to repair hernias (hernioplasty). This is especially true for hernias that recur and for large hernias. Patches are sewn over the weakened area in the abdominal wall after the hernia is pushed back into place. The patch decreases the tension on the weakened abdominal wall, reducing the risk that a hernia will recur.

How Mesh Works. There are many types of mesh products available, but surgeons typically use a sterile, woven material made from a synthetic plasticlike material, such as polypropylene. The mesh can be in the form of a patch that goes under or over the weakness, or it can be in the form of a plug that goes inside the hole. Mesh is very sturdy and strong, yet extremely thin. It is also soft and flexible, to allow it to easily conform to body's movement, position, and size. Mesh is generally available in various measurements and can often be cut to size. Depending on the repair technique used, the mesh is placed either under or over the defect in the abdominal wall and held in place by a few sutures. Mesh acts as "scaffolding" for new growth of a patient's own tissue, which eventually incorporates the mesh into the surrounding area. Figure 4-6 shows an example of mesh.

Surgical Setup: Open Hernia

The mayo setup for the open hernia is similar to a minor general surgery setup. A #10 blade or #15 blade on a #3 handle is the instrument used on the skin. Typically the #15 blade will be used on the fascia. An Army/Navy or a small Richardson retractor will be used to gain exposure to the surgical site. A Weitlaner self-retaining retractor may be used as well. Metzenbaum scissors will be the instrument of choice for the soft tissue dissection. Once the defect is exposed the surgeon will use at least four Criles or small Kelly hemostats to clamp the outer rim of the defect, allowing the contents of the hernia sac to be reduced into the abdomen or groin. A standard needle driver and straight mayo scissors complete the setup.

Surgical Setup: Laparoscopic Hernia

The mayo setup and instrumentation for the laparoscopic hernia repair mimics the setup for a laparoscopic cholecystectomy. A #15 blade on a #3 handle is the instrument used on the skin to prep for the trocars. Three trocars are used for access to the abdomen. The surgeon may use a 0-degree or 30-degree laparoscope. Laparoscopic scissors, dissector, and atramatic graspers are the instrumentation used to complete the procedure. The final piece to the laparoscopic repair of a hernia is the stapler/tacker used to secure the mesh to the abdominal wall.

Other Considerations

The patient undergoing hernia repair may receive a general anesthetic, an inguinal nerve block, a field block, a spinal or

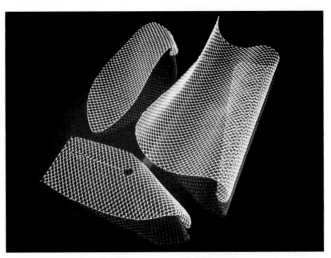

FIGURE 4-6 Mesh used in hernia repair procedures.

epidural block, a regional anesthetic with sedation, or a local anesthetic with sedation. Routine monitoring equipment, such as a three-lead or five-lead electrocardiogram (ECG), oxygen-saturation monitor, and blood pressure cuff, is used for a hernia repair. An intravenous (IV) line is inserted for fluid replacement and medication administration. The surgical site is marked as part of the preoperative verification process and rechecked during the time-out. In 2008 the World Health Organization (WHO) issued a surgical safety checklist as part of its "Safe Surgery Saves Lives" initiative. As part of the time-out, it recommends that all members of the surgical team identify themselves and their roles and ask simple questions such as, "Does everyone agree that this is Patient X, undergoing a right inguinal hernia repair?" The initiative also recommends an active role for the perioperative nursing team, who should review critical information such as confirming sterility of the instruments and supplies (including indicator results); discussing any equipment issues or concerns; noting whether antibiotic prophylaxis has been given within the last 60 minutes,

---

EVIDENCE FOR PRACTICE

Effectiveness of Preoperative Showers in Reducing Risk of Surgical Site Infections

First recommended by the CDC in 1999, preoperative showers have long been considered an important strategy for reducing the risk of surgical site infections. AORN's recommended practice for preoperative patient skin antisepsis states that patients undergoing open class I ("clean") surgical procedures below the level of the chin, such as inguinal hernia repair, have two preoperative showers with chlorhexidine gluconate (CHG) (AORN, 2009). This study from the Medical College of Wisconsin, Milwaukee, was conducted to validate effective skin surface concentrations of CHG using a standardized, timed protocol. It compared skin surface concentrations of CHG measured after showering with a 4% CHG liquid soap, as recommended by AORN, to those measured after cleansing the skin surface with a 2% CHG-impregnated polyester cloth. Researchers found that a timed, standardized preoperative shower was effective in achieving high skin surface levels of CHG that exceeded the concentration required to inhibit the growth of *Staphylococcus aureus,* the most common organism causing surgical site infections, and *Staphylococcus epidermidis.* Compared to use of 4% CHG soap, use of 2% CHG-impregnated polyester cloths resulted in considerably higher skin concentrations with no gaps in antiseptic coverage. CHG provides excellent activity against gram-positive organisms, and good antimicrobial activity with gram-negative bacteria and viruses, providing excellent residual activity. The researchers concluded that preoperative antiseptic showers are valuable in reducing surface skin colonization, which can play an important role in reducing the risk of surgical site infections.

Adapted from Association of periOperative Registered Nurses: Recommended practices for patient skin antisepsis. In *Perioperative standards and recommended practices,* Denver, 2009, The Association; Edmiston CE et al: Preoperative shower revisited: can high topical antiseptic levels be achieved on the skin surface before surgical admission? *J Am Coll Surg* 207:233-239, 2008.

SURGICAL TECHNOLOGY PREFERENCE CARD

HERNIORRHAPHY ADULT (OPEN)

The weight and age of your patient will direct you in setting up for the procedure. Discuss the equipment position with the perioperative team, taking into consideration additional equipment that may be needed for pediatric surgery. Understanding the room layout before setting up for the procedure allows the traffic pattern in the room to be maximized. This step can help insure sterility of the field and facilitate effective communication of additional supplies from the circulator to the scrub, as well as provide efficient space for other healthcare providers involved in the procedure.

Room Prep: Basic operating room equipment

Prep Solution: Males: betadine scrub and paint from nipples to mid thighs, including scrotum, side to side; females, chloraprep

Catheter: Foley catheter for ambulatory procedure only; removed after the procedure

PROCEDURE CHECKLIST

Instruments
- Basic appendix set/minor lap set
- Dull Weitlaner × 2

Suture
- Prolene 2-0, Vicryl 3-0, 4-0, and Proxi-Strips

Mesh
- Have three sizes of the Prolene Hernia Systems or the Bard PerFix Plugs in the room

Additional Supplies: both sterile and nonsterile
- If the physician is requesting supplies, instruments, or equipment not normally used, check to be sure all have arrived to the room before opening any other supplies
- Sponges
- Drapes
- Gowns and gloves for team members
- "Have ready" or "hold" supplies
- Penrose drain (males only)

Medications and Irrigation Solutions
- .25% Marcaine 50 cc for incision

Drains and Dressings
- Covaderm dressing for size of the incision

Specimen Care
- Proper container for each specimen
- Labels for each specimen
- Proper solution for specimen type

Before opening for the procedure, the surgical technologist should:
- Arrange furniture
- Gather positioning devices
- Damp dust lights, furniture, and surfaces
- Verify functionality of equipment
- Place items to be opened in their appropriate places

When opening sterile supplies:
- Verify exposure to sterilization
- Use sterile technique
- Open bundles in appropriate locations
- Open additional supplies onto sterile field
- Open all sterile supplies and equipment as close to the surgical start time as possible

if applicable; and verifying whether essential imaging is displayed, if applicable (WHO, 2008). Before the time-out, surgical team members may share any concerns about the planned procedure during a preoperative briefing (Research Highlight).

The patient is usually positioned supine with basic prepping and draping procedures followed. As with any surgical procedure, the prep solution must dry before the start of the surgical procedure as part of fire safety measures. To maintain the patient's dignity and modesty, expose only the part of the patient's body necessary for antimicrobial skin preparation (Beyea, 2007). Instruments used for herniorrhaphies are those found in standard laparotomy sets, laparoscopy sets, or minor sets.

A self-retaining retractor, such as a Weitlaner, facilitates the separation of tissue layers. A moistened Penrose drain is often used to retract the spermatic cord structures for better exposure. Because the peritoneal cavity may be entered in this procedure, sponge, sharp, and instrument counts are recommended.

With a sliding hernia or an incarcerated hernia, the possibility of having to enter the peritoneal cavity must be considered. If the hernia is strangulated, necrotic bowel must be resected and instruments for performing a bowel anastomosis must be available. For this procedure, antibiotics may be added to the irrigation to prevent an infection. Safe medication practices must be followed. All medications and solutions on and off the sterile field must be labeled. When the antibiotic solution is

SURGICAL TECHNOLOGY PREFERENCE CARD

LAPAROSCOPIC HERNIORRHAPHY ADULT

Room Prep: Basic operating room equipment, scope warmer, video cart and secondary monitor at the foot of the bed; patient is to be supine with arms on armboards

Prep Solution: Chloraprep nipples to midthighs, side to side; if male, prep genitalia with betadine scrub and paint

Catheter: Foley catheter for ambulatory procedure only; removed after the procedure

PROCEDURE CHECKLIST

Instruments
- Basic laparoscopy set
- 5-mm laparoscope, 0-30 degrees
- Camera and light cord
- Move major set into the room but DO NOT OPEN

Trocars
- 5-mm Trocar × 3

Suture
- Vicryl 0, 4-0, Mastisol, and Proxi-Strips

Mesh
- Have the desired mesh in the room per surgeon preference

Additional Supplies, both sterile and nonsterile
- If the physician is requesting supplies, instruments, or equipment not normally used, check to be sure all have arrived to the room before opening any other supplies
- Insufflation tubing
- Sponges
- Drapes
- Gowns and gloves for team members
- "Have ready" or "hold" supplies

Medications and irrigation solutions
- .25% Marcaine 50cc for incision
- If using mesh, antibiotic of surgeon's preference

Drains and Dressings
- Bandages for trocar site

Specimen Care
- Proper container for each specimen
- Labels for each specimen
- Proper solution for specimen type

Before opening for the procedure, the surgical technologist should:
- Arrange furniture
- Gather positioning devices
- Damp dust lights, furniture, and surfaces
- Verify functionality of equipment
- Place items to be opened in their appropriate places

When opening sterile supplies:
- Verify exposure to sterilization
- Use sterile technique
- Open bundles in appropriate locations
- Open additional supplies onto sterile field
- Open all sterile supplies and equipment as close to the surgical start time as possible

passed to the surgeon, the surgical technologist or other scrub person should announce the name and strength of the antibiotic solution to be used for irrigation.

Repair of an inguinal hernia includes approximation of the transversalis fascia with a heavy nonabsorbable type of suture; mesh may also be used. With some indirect hernias, only two or three sutures may be necessary. In other cases, however, up to 10 sutures in succession may be needed. Scarpa's fascia is approximated with absorbable sutures, and the skin is closed by one of several methods. Several types of prosthetic mesh are available and often used to support hernia repair.

A laparoscopic hernia repair is technically similar to an open laparotomy, but the instrumentation includes laparoscopic equipment. There is always a possibility that a laparoscopy may become a laparotomy, and instrumentation for this change in procedure must always be available.

Surgical Interventions

SURGERY FOR REPAIR OF GROIN HERNIAS

Repair of Inguinal Hernias

Several operative procedures for repair of inguinal hernias are currently used. Approaches that reestablish the integrity

RESEARCH HIGHLIGHT

Effect of Preoperative Briefings on OR Delays

In one study (Nundy et al, 2008), researchers at The Johns Hopkins University School of Medicine, Baltimore, sought an answer to the following question: "Do preoperative briefings reduce unexpected OR delays through improved teamwork and communication?" They implemented a preoperative briefing program in which the attending surgeon led OR personnel in a 2-minute discussion using a standardized format designed to familiarize team members with each other and with the operative plan. The researchers evaluated unexpected delays before and after the initiation of the OR briefings using an assessment tool that was distributed to OR personnel at the end of each surgical procedure. The tool was completed by 422 respondents. The use of preoperative OR briefings was associated with a 31% reduction in unexpected delays. A total of 36% of OR personnel reported delays before implementation of the briefings, and 25% reported delays after implementation. Among surgeons alone, an 82% reduction in unexpected delays was observed. Significantly, a 19% reduction in communication breakdowns leading to delays was associated with the briefings.

In another study (Lingard et al, 2008), Canadian researchers assessed whether structured team briefings that incorporated a preoperative checklist would improve communication in the OR. Over a 13-month period, surgeons, nurses, and anesthesia providers at a Canadian academic medical center completed a short team briefing guided by a checklist before 302 general surgery procedures. They found the mean number of communication failures per procedure declined from 3.95 to 1.31. A total of 34% of the briefings demonstrated utility, meaning they identified a problem, filled a critical knowledge gap, provoked a change in plan, or promoted follow-up actions.

Research shows that poor communication is the single most frequent cause of adverse events in healthcare. As in other research, these studies concluded that preoperative briefings reduce unexpected delays and decrease the frequency of communication breakdowns. Preoperative briefings have the potential to increase OR efficiency, improve quality of care, and reduce costs.

Adapted from Lingard L et al: Evaluation of a preoperative checklist and team briefing among surgeons, nurses, and anesthesiologists to reduce failures in communication, *Arch Surg* 143:12-17, 2008; Nundy S et al: Impact of preoperative briefings on operating room delays, *Arch Surg* 143:1068-1072, 2008.

▶▶ RISK REDUCTION STRATEGIES

Teamwork and Communication on Surgical Teams

Despite almost universal endorsement and knowledge of The Joint Commission's *Universal Protocol for Preventing Wrong-Site, Wrong-Procedure, Wrong-Person Surgery,* avoidable surgical errors continue to occur in U.S. healthcare facilities. Research has focused on communications' failures as the underlying cause of many errors. The Medical Team Training Questionnaire was developed as part of a national program in the Department of Veterans Affairs (VA) to improve communication. It assesses organizational culture, communication, teamwork, and awareness of human factors engineering principles. The questionnaire was pilot-tested with 300 healthcare clinicians. The final version of the questionnaire was then administered to an interdisciplinary group of 384 surgical staff in 6 facilities. Analysis of questionnaire results determined that nurses and anesthesia providers tend to perceive their environment similarly, and both differ significantly from surgeons' perceptions. Surgeons perceive their environment more positively, believing there is a stronger organizational culture for patient safety—

that all team members are comfortable intervening in a procedure if they have concerns about what is occurring. Surgeons also perceive better communication—that during surgical and diagnostic procedures, everyone on the team is aware of what is happening. Consistent with their positive beliefs, surgeons similarly perceive that there is good teamwork—that morale on their team is high and everyone on the team is comfortable giving feedback to other team members. Nurses and anesthesia providers did not agree with the positive perceptions of the surgeons.

According to the researchers, such disparities between team members pose a problem. If team members have disparate perceptions about how well they communicate or collaborate with each other, they do not collaborate optimally during care of their patients. Thus use of this or a similar questionnaire may prove helpful in identifying hidden problems with communication and may be useful in focusing efforts, such as team training, for improvement.

Adapted from Mills P et al: Teamwork and communication in surgical teams: implications for patient safety, *J Am Coll Surg* 206:107-112, 2008.

of the transversalis fascia and simultaneously reestablish and strengthen the posterior inguinal floor are favored. A surgical repair in which transversalis fascia is sewn to the Poupart ligament accomplishes this goal.

Procedural Considerations. The patient is in the supine position for abdominal wall and inguinal or femoral hernia repairs. Arms are placed on padded armboards with the palms up and fingers extended. Armboards are maintained at less than a 90-degree angle to prevent brachial plexus stretch. If there are surgical reasons to tuck the arms at the side, as may occur in laparoscopic hernia repair, the elbows are padded to protect the ulnar nerve, the palms face inward,

and the wrist is maintained in a neutral position (Denholm, 2009). A drape secures the arms. It should be tucked snugly under the patient, not under the mattress. This prevents the arm from shifting downward intraoperatively and resting against the OR bed rail.

The patient's skin surface area from above the umbilicus to midthigh is exposed, prepped with antimicrobial solution, and draped with sterile drapes. A sterile drape should be placed under the scrotum if it becomes necessary to enter the scrotum. Safe practices when using devices that generate surgical smoke, such as the electrosurgical unit (ESU), require the use of a smoke evacuation system and accessories in both open and laparoscopic procedures (AORN, 2009a).

Operative Procedures

McVAY, OR COOPER, LIGAMENT REPAIR. A McVay, or Cooper, ligament repair approximates transversalis fascia superior to the inferior insertion of the transversalis fascia along the Cooper ligament. It is accompanied by a relaxing incision to reduce tension on the suture line.

1. A transverse suprainguinal skinfold incision is made; some surgeons prefer an oblique incision, made parallel to the inguinal ligament, ending two fingerbreadths lateral to the pubic tubercle (Figure 4-7).
2. The incision is carried through the superficial and deep (Scarpa) fascia to the external oblique aponeurosis. Hemostasis is maintained with fine ties or electrocoagulation.
3. The external oblique aponeurosis is opened by way of a small incision over the inguinal canal, lateral to the inguinal ring and in the direction of its fibers, to the external ring. The aponeurotic flaps are reflected back along the iliohypogastric and ilioinguinal nerves, which are identified and preserved from injury (see Figure 4-7). The ilioinguinal nerve is a sensory nerve that innervates the medial thigh and the scrotum.
4. The cremaster muscles that form an envelope around the spermatic cord and represent the continuation of the internal oblique muscles are opened, and the cord is exposed. The medial fibrous portion of the internal oblique is called the *conjoined tendon.*
5. The cord and surrounding structures are dissected and freed circumferentially from the canal, and a moistened Penrose drain is often used to gently retract the vessels and vas deferens. The cord is then examined for an indirect her-

---

AMBULATORY SURGERY CONSIDERATIONS

Safe Use of Post-Op Pain Pumps for Surgical Analgesia

Elastomeric pumps, such as the ON-Q PainBuster, deliver local anesthetic intended to reduce pain after surgery to the tissue around the surgical site. The popular ON-Q PainBuster **Post-Op Pain Relief System** provides continuous infusion of a local anesthetic directly into the patient's surgical site for effective, non-narcotic postoperative pain relief for up to 5 days. Four pump models are available with this pain-relief system: one with a fixed flow rate that cannot be changed; one that delivers a basal infusion and also allows delivery of on-demand boluses; one that allows the user to adjust the flow rate within a predetermined range; and one with an adjustable rate controller and bolus device. Various sizes and types of catheters are available to deliver the medication. Pumps such as ON-Q pumps are used in many general surgical procedures. The following safe practice recommendations should be implemented to improve safety when using elastomeric pumps such as ON-Q pumps.

BEFORE USING THE PUMPS
- Establish protocols for use of ON-Q pumps, including indications; models and tubing to be used for each indication; steps for prescribing, preparing, and dispensing the pump of all associated medications; required testing of knowledge and skills; hand-off communication between providers; patient/family education; and patient monitoring.
- Have a committee, such as the Pharmacy and Therapeutics Committee, approve the drugs that can be administered through the ON-Q pump, taking into consideration the accuracy of the infusion rate (±15% to 20% of desired rate) and conditions that could influence the rate (e.g., heat and cold).
- Ensure clinical staff education before use. Include the signs of bupivacaine, ropivacaine, and lidocaine cardiotoxicity and risks associated with pump use (Surgical Pharmacology box).

PRESCRIBING THE PUMPS
- Establish standard order sets for prescribing the pumps and specific medications. Specify any concomitant analgesics that are acceptable or should be avoided. Require activation of the appropriate order set before the patient is transferred from the OR.

PLACING THE CATHETERS AND SETTING UP THE PUMPS
- Ensure proper insertion of the catheter(s) in the tissue and/or adjacent nerves surrounding a wound. Do not insert the catheter directly into a joint.
- Label the pump with the name of the drug, its concentration, infusion rate (in milliliters per hour and dose per hour), and start date.
- Ensure that the adjustable rate controller (available on some models) is clicked into place under the specified rate of infusion.
- Apply an occlusive dressing over the catheter insertion site.
- Tape the flow restrictor to the patient's skin. Do not tape over the filter.

DISPENSING PUMPS AND MEDICATION
- Establish standard concentrations for the local anesthetics (and other drugs, if appropriate) used in the pumps. Also establish pharmacy compounding procedures for preparing any mixtures of drugs.
- Establish order sets in the pharmacy computer that will facilitate automated screening of the drug(s) being used for appropriate dose, drug interactions, allergies, and duplicate therapy.
- Require pharmacy preparation of the medication reservoir balls following a protocol that specifies the exact amount of solution to instill based on the duration of therapy and expected rate of infusion.

PERIOPERATIVE NURSING CONSIDERATIONS FOR PATIENTS WITH PUMPS
- Ensure that all medications administered via the pump are listed on the intraoperative nursing record.
- Ensure the occlusive dressing over the catheter site is intact.
- Check that the flow restrictor is taped to patient's skin for accurate flow rates.
- Include information about the pump in the hand-off report to PACU or other discharge unit.

EDUCATING PATIENTS ABOUT PUMPS
- Educate patients and caregivers about how the pump works and items to periodically check (e.g., flow restrictor is taped to the skin, medication ball appears to be getting smaller each day, pain is under control).
- Educate patients about the signs of cardiotoxicity, when to call the physician, and how to clamp the tubing to prevent further drug administration, if necessary (Surgical Pharmacology).
- Send the Patient Guidelines provided by the manufacturer home with patients.

Modified from Institute for Safe Medication Practices (ISMP) Safety Alert: *Process for handling elastomeric pain relief balls (ON-Q PainBuster and others) requires safety improvements,* July 16, 2009, Newsletter, available at www.ismp.org/Newsletters/acutecare/articles/20090716.asp. Accessed August 1, 2009.

nia, the sac of which is located adjacent to the cord; the sac originates from the internal ring lateral to the inferior epigastric vessels and is initially adherent to the cord.

6. If an indirect sac is identified, it is carefully dissected away from the cord until the neck of the hernia is clearly delineated (Figure 4-8).

7. The sac is opened, and any abdominal contents are returned to the peritoneal cavity.

8. A suture ligature or purse-string suture is placed high in the neck of the sac, and the excess peritoneum of the hernia is excised. The ligated stump quickly retracts into the peritoneal cavity. (If the sac is long, the distal segment may be splayed open and left in place.) The inguinal floor is then inspected for evidence of a direct hernia. If only a direct sac is present, usually no resection of the hernia is done because the sac easily returns to the abdominal cavity.

9. If transversalis fascia is present on both sides of the hernia defect, it is sutured together or a piece of mesh is interposed (Figure 4-9). Suturing begins at the pubic tubercle and continues laterally to the internal ring. If the inferior transversalis fascia is weak or not present, the superior portion is sutured to the Cooper ligament, the site of insertion of the transversalis fascia. In this case, suturing again begins at the pubic tubercle and is continued laterally along the Cooper ligament to the medial border of the femoral sheath, where a transition stitch is placed. The repair is then car-

ried laterally, approximating transversalis fascia to inguinal ligament (Figure 4-10).

10. When the transversalis fascia is pulled down to the Cooper ligament, a relaxing incision in the rectus sheath is sometimes necessary to relieve excess tension. Essentially this incision is 5 to 7 cm long in the anterior rectus sheath. The incision begins immediately above the pubic crest, approximately 1 cm from the midline, and extends cephalad, following the line of fusion of the external oblique aponeurosis with the rectus sheath. The posterior rectus sheath and the rectus muscle itself guard against later herniation at the point where the relaxing incision is made. If too much tension makes direct approximation undesirable, a synthetic surgical mesh may be sutured in place as the new inguinal floor ("tension-free" mesh repair). The caudad edge of the mesh is sutured to the shelving edge of the inguinal ligament, the cephalad edge sutured to the conjoined tendon, and the lateral edge of the mesh split to accommodate the spermatic cord.

11. After the integrity of the posterior inguinal floor has been reestablished, the cremaster muscles are reapproximated around the cord. Repair is completed with the approximation of the external oblique aponeurosis, the Scarpa fascia, and the skin.

BASSINI REPAIR. The Bassini repair was introduced in 1887 and was formerly the standard of repair. In this procedure the

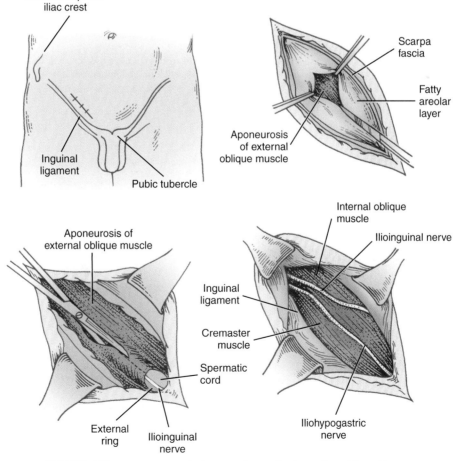

FIGURE 4-7 Skin incision with division of superficial muscle and fascial layers.

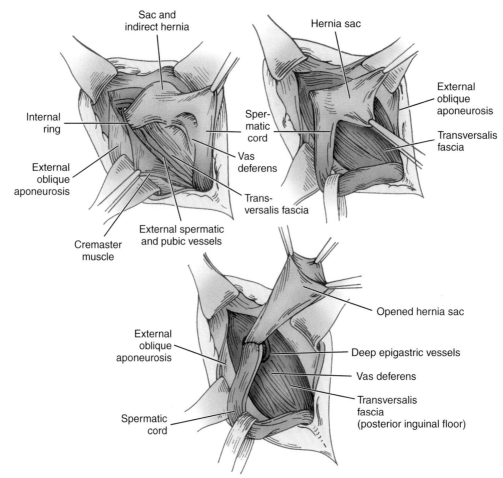

FIGURE 4-8 Indirect hernia sac is identified along with cord structures and dissected away from cord. Neck of hernia sac is clearly delineated, and sac is opened to check for abdominal contents.

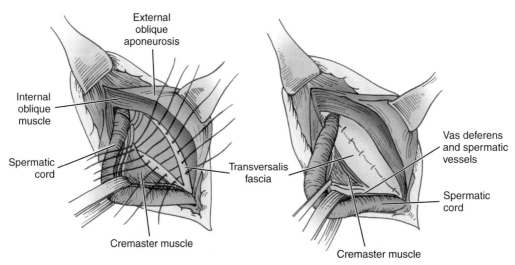

FIGURE 4-9 Transversalis fascia on either side of large hernia defect is approximated.

conjoined tendon and the shelving edge of the inguinal ligament are sutured together up to the internal ring (Bascom, 2004). The major difference with this repair is that the superior transversalis fascia is sutured to the inguinal ligament with no attempt made to approximate it to the inferior portion of the transversalis fas-cia or the Cooper ligament (pectineal ligament). Critics of this procedure claim that it is not anatomic because layers that origi-nally are not integrated (transversalis fascia and inguinal liga-ment) now are approximated. Nonetheless, this repair has been used successfully by many surgeons.

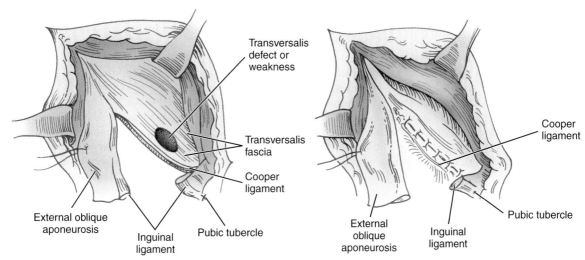

FIGURE 4-10 Defect in transversalis fascia repaired by approximation of fascia to the Cooper ligament.

SURGICAL PHARMACOLOGY

Bupivacaine, Ropivacaine, and Lidocaine Cardiotoxicity

Lidocaine (Xylocaine), bupivacaine (Marcaine), and ropivacaine (Naropin) all have similar actions. They produce analgesic effects via nerve conduction blockage. They are contraindicated in patients with hypersensitivity to amide local anesthetics. Compared to other local anesthetics, bupivacaine is markedly cardiotoxic. However, adverse drug reactions (ADRs) are rare when it is administered correctly. Most ADRs relate to systemic exposure, such as with pain pump failure.

Systemic exposure to excessive quantities of bupivacaine mainly result in central nervous system (CNS) and cardiovascular effects. CNS effects may include CNS excitation (nervousness, tingling around the mouth, tinnitus, tremor, dizziness, blurred vision, or seizures) followed by depression (drowsiness, loss of consciousness, respiratory depression, and apnea). Bupivacaine and ropivacaine are look-alike/sound-alike drugs.

Ropivacaine is found to have less cardiotoxicity than bupivacaine in animal models. Compared to bupivacaine, ropivacaine has similar CNS and cardiovascular effects.

Perioperative nurses providing discharge instructions to patients with pain pumps filled with one of these local anesthetics should be sure the medication is part of discharge medication reconciliation. An information sheet should be printed for the patient and their caregiver, and they should have one to take to their primary care physician. Be specific and direct in providing information about cardiotoxicity. Use descriptions of signs and symptoms that the patient can understand. For instance, you might tell the patient:

"The following symptoms may represent a serious medical condition. Immediately close the clamp on the pump tubing and call your doctor or 911 if you have any of the following:

◆ Difficulty breathing
◆ Dizziness, light-headedness
◆ Blurred vision
◆ Ringing, buzzing in your ears
◆ Metal taste in your mouth
◆ Numbness and/or tingling around your mouth, fingers, or toes
◆ Drowsiness
◆ Confusion"

SHOULDICE REPAIR. More than 250,000 hernias have been repaired at the Shouldice Hospital in Ontario, Canada, with a recurrence rate of less than 1%. In the Shouldice repair a double layer of transversalis fascia is sutured to the inguinal ligament. It is reinforced by a layer of internal oblique muscle and conjoined tendon approximated to the undersurface of the fascia of the external oblique.

MESH-PLUG REPAIR. The mesh-plug technique has been recommended for the treatment of primary and recurrent direct and indirect inguinal hernias. The various hernia types as classified by Gilbert have a corresponding relationship to the use of mesh plugs (Gilbert et al, 2009). Types I, II, and III are indirect hernias. Type I is characterized by a tight internal ring through which any size peritoneal sac can pass. The sac, when surgically reduced, is held within the abdominal cavity by the intact internal ring. Type II hernias have a moderately enlarged internal ring, 4 cm or smaller. Type III hernias have a patulous internal ring larger than 4 cm. In this type, the sac can have a sliding component that impinges on the direct space. Type IV and type V hernias are direct hernias. In type IV hernias, the defect involves virtually the entire floor of the inguinal canal. Type V is a diverticular defect of the floor and is generally in a suprapubic position, resembling a punched-out recurrent hernia. Type VI includes components of both indirect and direct hernias. Femoral hernias are classified as type VII.

Regardless of the hernia type, the mesh-plug technique is performed on an ambulatory basis, through a small incision, often laparoscopically. Repair of inguinal hernias with the mesh-plug technique has provided significant advantages when compared with conventional suture technique. A plug repair requires less overall dissection, has a decreased chance of nerve injury, and ensures a tension-free hernioplasty. These factors increase patient comfort, speed rehabilitation, and contribute to a very low recurrence rate.

Surgical Technique Using the PerFix Plug

1. An oblique incision, 6 cm in length, is made, and the external oblique fascia is opened through the external ring. Exposure is obtained by use of a self-retaining retractor (e.g., a Beckman); a handheld retractor such as a Gouley may also be required. Hemostasis is usually achieved with the use of electrocoagulation.

2. The spermatic cord is mobilized, as previously described in the McVay repair. The ilioinguinal and genital femoral nerves are identified and preserved. The medial external oblique fascia is separated from the underlying transversus abdominis aponeurosis with a sweeping motion of the index finger.

3. An indirect sac and any lipoma of the cord are dissected free (Figure 4-11, *A*). The sac and lipoma are allowed to drop back through the internal ring and into the abdominal cavity. Rarely is the sac opened except for incarcerated hernias.

4. Using the Gilbert classification, the internal ring is sized and the tapered end of the mesh plug is inserted through the internal ring and positioned just beneath the crura. The plug is designed such that its fluted outer layer, combined with its inside configuration of eight mesh petals, maintains its overall contour while allowing it to conform tension-free to the configuration of the internal ring (Figure 4-11, *B*).

5. *Repair of indirect hernias.* Type I indirect hernias require one or two synthetic absorbable sutures; in type II and type III hernias, more sutures are required because of the increased size of the internal ring.

6. *Repair of direct hernias.* In direct hernias, the fusiform or saccular defect is circumscribed near its base with an electrosurgical device and the hernia is reduced, providing a surrounding margin of intact tissue for securing the plug. The plug is then inserted through the floor of the defect (Figure 4-11, *C*). With type IV and type V (direct) hernias, the mesh plug is routinely secured with up to 10 interrupted synthetic absorbable sutures. Where there are both indirect and direct hernias (type VI), two mesh plugs may be needed. Type VII defects are treated similarly with mesh plugs.

7. *Repair of femoral hernias.* In femoral hernias, a small or medium-size plug is secured in position after the sac has been reduced.

8. In most types of mesh-plug hernia repairs, a second piece of flat mesh is used for reinforcement. The piece is cut to match the shape of the inguinal canal and then placed without sutures on the anterior surface of the posterior wall of the inguinal canal. The proximal portion is split to provide an opening for the spermatic cord, and the mesh tails are united with sutures to form a new internal ring (Figure 4-11, *D*).

9. With the spermatic cord structures placed on top of this flat mesh, the external oblique fascia is reapproximated over the structures with a running synthetic nonabsorbable suture.

10. An interrupted suture of a similar size is used to integrate the subcutaneous tissue, and the skin is closed with a subcuticular stitch.

LAPAROSCOPIC HERNIA REPAIRS. Ger was the first surgeon to perform a laparoscopic herniorrhaphy. In 1982 he described a laparoscopic transabdominal hernia approach. Variations in techniques for laparoscopic hernia repair continue to develop as surgeons gain experience with these procedures.

Techniques used today for laparoscopic herniorrhaphy include the transabdominal preperitoneal patch (TAPP) repair, the totally extraperitoneal patch (TEP) repair, and the intraperitoneal onlay mesh (IPOM) repair. The difference between TAPP and TEP is the manner in which access is gained to the preperitoneal space. The TAPP uses intraperitoneal trocars and the creation of a peritoneal flap over the posterior inguinal region. TEP provides access to the preperitoneal space without entering the peritoneal cavity (Research Highlight).

Studies indicating long-term postoperative hernia recurrence and complication rates with these approaches vary. The average recurrence rate for TAPP ranges from 2% to 7%; for TEP it approximates 1.8%. A laparoscopic hernia repair allegedly has the advantages of a quicker return to normal activity and some reduction of postoperative adhesions related to the minimal dissection required. Analysis of postoperative pain and paresthesia associated with laparoscopic hernia repair suggests that most patients experience minimal immediate postoperative pain and, after postoperative day 1, have minimal need for analgesics. In general, the procedure requires the placement of operative cameras and ports, identification of the inguinal floor, removal of an indirect hernia sac, insertion of mesh to fit around the spermatic cord and form a new inguinal floor, and closure of ports (Lawrence, 2006).

In 2007 the FDA granted 510(k) clearance for a hernia repair device (Rebound HRD, Minnesota Medical Development, Inc.) for the repair and/or reinforcement of hernia or other soft tissue defects where weakness exists and where the support of a nonabsorbable material is preferred. The device is a self-expanding framed/surgical mesh made of Nitinol, a family of intermetallic materials containing a nearly equal mixture of nickel and titanium that offers both superelasticity and shape memory. The device can be folded and inserted laparoscopically, after which it "rebounds" to its original shape for quick and easy placement over the hernia defect. Although ideally suited for laparoscopic surgery, the device also may be used in an open incisional approach (Taylor, 2007).

Procedural Considerations. After induction of general anesthesia the patient is placed in supine position with the arms tucked at the sides and padded. The anesthesia screen is moved as far to the head of the bed as possible to improve surgeon ability to maneuver the laparoscope. The skin is prepped and draped to include the lower abdomen, genital area (manipulation of the scrotal sac may be necessary), and upper thighs. Following introduction of the laparoscope, the patient is placed in deep Trendelenburg's position so that viscera fall away from the inguinal area (Feldman et al, 2007). Appropriately sized trocars and scopes, depending on the type of repair planned, ESU and appropriate smoke evacuation system, mesh, and the primary monitor and video cart

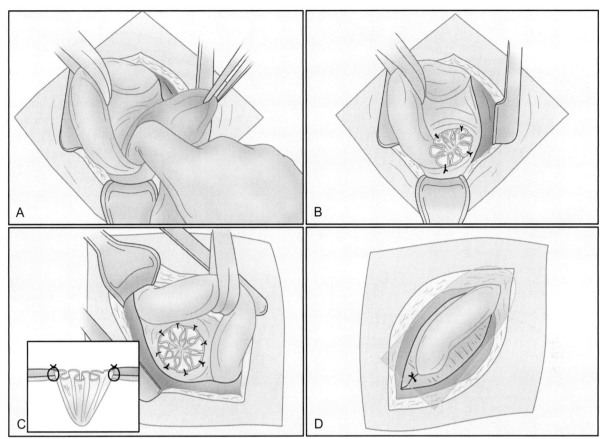

FIGURE 4-11 Mesh-plug repair using the PerFix Plug. **A,** The hernia sac is dissected free of the cord structure to the level of the internal ring. **B,** Typically, a large plug is used. Some of the internal petals may be removed if the plug is too bulky. **C,** Large or extra-large PerFix Plug is inserted. The plug should not be stretched to fill the defect. Typically, 8 to 10 sutures are used. **D,** Sutureless onlay patch. The tails of the onlay patch are taken around the cord and sutured together. The onlay patch is not sutured to the floor of the inguinal canal.

are required. If the patient has voided preoperatively, urinary catheterization can be avoided.

Operative Procedure—Totally Extraperitoneal Patch (TEP) Approach (Figure 4-12)

1. An infraumbilical incision is made. The anterior rectus sheath is incised and the ipsilateral rectus abdominis muscle is retracted laterally.
2. With blunt dissection, a space is created beneath the rectus.
3. A dissecting balloon (preperitoneal distention balloon, PDB) is inserted deep to the posterior rectus sheath, tunneled and advanced to the pubic symphysis, and inflated under direct laparoscopic vision.
4. The space is opened and the PDB removed and replaced with a blunt-tip trocar. The preperitoneal space is insufflated under low pressure and additional trocars are placed.
5. Using a 30-degree telescope, the inferior epigastric vessels and lower portion of the rectus sheath are identified and retracted anteriorly.
6. The Cooper ligament is cleared from the pubic symphysis medially to the level of the external iliac vein.
7. The iliopubic tract is identified. Care is taken to avoid injury to the femoral branch of the genitofemoral nerve and the lateral femoral cutaneous nerve.

RESEARCH HIGHLIGHT

Comparison of Different Types of Hernia Repair

This study was done to determine whether laparoscopic methods are more effective and cost-effective than open mesh methods of inguinal hernia repair. A secondary analysis was an exploration of whether laparoscopic transabdominal preperitoneal patch (TAPP) repair was more effective and cost-effective than laparoscopic totally extraperitoneal patch (TEP) repair. Laparoscopic repair was associated with a faster return to usual activities and less persisting pain and numbness. There also appeared to be fewer cases of wound or superficial infection and hematoma. However, operation times were longer, and there appears to be a higher rate of serious complications (e.g., bowel, bladder, and vascular injuries) with laparoscopic methods. Mesh infection is very uncommon, with similar rates noted among the surgical approaches. There is no apparent difference in the rate of hernia recurrence. The increased adoption of laparoscopic techniques may allow patients to return to usual activities faster. Economic savings in the form of fewer days of work missed and reduced workers' compensation have been reported.

Modified from McCormack K et al: Laparoscopic surgery for inguinal hernia repair: systematic review of effectiveness and economic evaluation, *Health Technol Assess* 9(1):218, 2005.

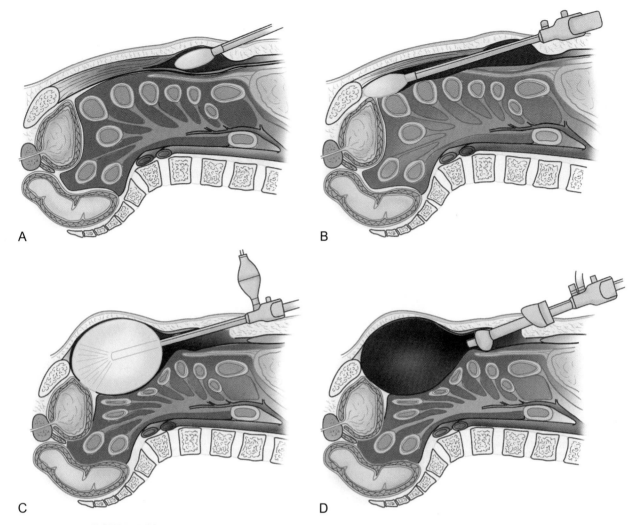

A

B

C

D

FIGURE 4-12 Totally extraperitoneal patch (TEP) laparoscopic hernia repair. **A,** The TEP approach for laparoscopic hernia repair is demonstrated. Access to the posterior rectus sheath is gained in the periumbilical region. A balloon dissector is placed on the anterior surface of the posterior rectus sheath. **B,** The balloon dissector is advanced to the posterior surface of the pubis in the preperitoneal space. **C,** The balloon is inflated, thereby creating an optical cavity. **D,** The optical cavity is insufflated by carbon dioxide, and the posterior surface of the inguinal floor is dissected.

8. Lateral dissection is carried out to the anterior superior iliac.
9. The spermatic cord is skeletonized.
10. A *direct hernia sac* is gently reduced by retraction if it has not already been reduced by balloon expansion of the peritoneal space. A *small indirect sac* is mobilized from the spermatic cord and reduced into the peritoneal cavity. A *large sac* may be divided with electrocoagulation near the internal ring. The proximal peritoneal sac is closed with a loop ligature to prevent pneumoperitoneum from occurring. A piece of polypropylene mesh is inserted; unfolded to cover the direct, indirect, and femoral spaces and rest over the cord structures; and carefully secured with a tacking stapler.

REPAIR OF INGUINAL HERNIAS IN FEMALES. Regardless of the specific technique used, the initial approach to the repair of a hernia in the female is the same as that used in the male.

After the cremaster muscles are opened to expose the round ligament, variations that may be encountered include the following: (1) with the sac exposed and cleared from the round ligament, the round ligament and accompanying vessels are dissected free from the inguinal floor to the labium; (2) at the labium the round ligament is clamped, ligated, and divided; (3) the sac at the internal ring is opened, checked to be sure that no abdominal contents are present, and ligated at its neck, together with the round ligament and associated vessels; or (4) the sac distal to the ligature is removed with the distal round ligament, while the ligated stump retracts promptly into the abdomen. The remainder of the repair is the same as that previously described.

REPAIR OF FEMORAL HERNIAS. A femoral hernia protrudes from the groin below the inguinal ligament into the thigh (Figure 4-13). In its most obvious form, a femoral hernia is an inflamed, tender mass below the inguinal ligament. Unfortunately, the presentation is frequently more subtle and the diagno-

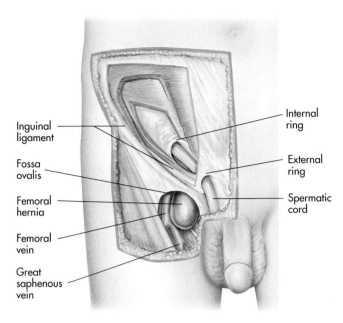

Inguinal
ligament

Fossa
ovalis

Femoral
hernia

Femoral
vein

Great
saphenous
vein

Internal
ring

External
ring

Spermatic
cord

FIGURE 4-13 Bulge from femoral hernia occurring below inguinal ligament.

sis is completely missed or confused with enlarged inguinal lymph nodes, a psoas muscle abscess, a saphenous varix, a lipoma, or an indirect or direct inguinal hernia. The defect is usually small and frequently nonreducible. Femoral hernias are highly likely to become incarcerated and strangulated; elective repair is clearly indicated unless serious contraindications to surgery exist.

Operative Procedure. The general approach is surgical treatment to free the tightly bound hernia, closely examine the contents of the hernia for ischemic change, and repair the hernia defect. The principles for repair of this type of hernia are the same as those described for inguinal herniorrhaphies. Ultimately, the defect must be obliterated. Repair of a femoral hernia requires approximating the aponeurotic margins of the femoral canal. The sutures are placed through the iliopubic tract superiorly and through the Cooper ligament and pectineus fascia inferiorly. Care is taken to not compromise the femoral artery and vein.

PREPERITONEAL (PROPERITONEAL) REPAIR—OPEN APPROACH. Preperitoneal (properitoneal) repair also is based on the essential role of the transversalis fascia in the cause and subsequent correction of a hernia. This repair is suitable for direct, indirect, and femoral hernias. It is particularly applicable in dealing with recurrent hernias and bilateral hernias, because exposure is obtained by operating through virgin surgical fields rather than through previous scars.

Operative Procedure
1. A transverse incision is made 2 cm above the symphysis pubis, through the rectus abdominis muscle on the affected side (Figure 4-14, *A*).
2. The wound is deepened by cutting the external oblique, internal oblique, and transversalis muscles.
3. The transversalis fascia is then cut, and the preperitoneal space is entered. This is the proper plane of dissection for the remainder of the operation.

4. Retraction on the lower side of the incision reveals the posterior inguinal wall and the hernia defect.

Variations in the procedure are performed for different types of hernias.
1. If the hernia is direct, it can be reduced easily and the superior edge of the hernia defect (the transversalis fascia) is sutured to the iliopubic tract (origin of the transversalis fascia) (Figure 4-14, *B*).
2. In an indirect hernia, the sac is gently retracted from the inguinal canal. A purse-string suture is placed around the peritoneal defect as the sac is excised (Figure 4-14, *C*). The lateral aspect of the internal abdominal ring is closed, and the posterior wall is reinforced as with the direct hernia.
3. In repair of a femoral hernia, the sac is again reduced by traction. After the sac is inspected for contents, a high ligation is performed. As it approaches the Cooper ligament, the defect in the posterior inguinal floor is clearly identified and is repaired by direct approximation (Figure 4-14, *D*).

After repair of any of the aforementioned hernias, the preperitoneal space is irrigated with saline solution and the appropriate layers are approximated.

REPAIR OF SLIDING HERNIAS. Direct or indirect hernias may occur as sliding hernias. A sliding inguinal hernia occurs when the wall of a viscus forms a portion of the wall of the hernia. The most common sliding hernias involve the bladder in direct hernias, the sigmoid colon in left indirect hernias, and the cecum in right indirect inguinal hernias (Figure 4-15). This hernia must be recognized early in the repair because attempts at surgical removal of the entire sac will injure the sliding viscus.

Operative Procedure. All operations designed to repair sliding hernias adhere to the basic principle of repairing the defect in the transversalis fascia. To free the bowel from the sac, the following steps must be taken:
1. The sac is opened in an area where no bowel is present and is excised medially and laterally to a point at which the bowel can be mobilized (Figure 4-16).
2. The lateral and medial peritoneal margins are approximated.
3. The bowel is reduced to the peritoneal cavity, and high ligation of the sac is performed.
4. Repair of the transversalis fascia is done by one of the methods previously described.

LITTRE, MAYDL, AND RICHTER HERNIAS. An inguinal hernia containing a Meckel's diverticulum is called a *Littre hernia,* and one containing two loops of bowel is called a *Maydl hernia.* A special type of strangulated hernia is a *Richter hernia* (Figure 4-17). In this hernia, only a part of the circumference of the bowel is incarcerated or strangulated in the hernia. Frequently it is described as a knuckle of bowel that becomes trapped and ischemic. Because initially a very small area is necrotic, diagnosis may be delayed. A Richter hernia most frequently occurs in femoral hernias because of the small size and sharp, relatively inflexible nature of the fascial ring in this area. A strangulated Richter hernia may be reduced spontaneously, and the gangrenous piece of intestine may be overlooked at the time of operation. Most commonly, the distal ileum is involved in a Richter hernia; however, omentum is frequently encountered in the sac. The favored approach for repair is through the preperitoneal space.

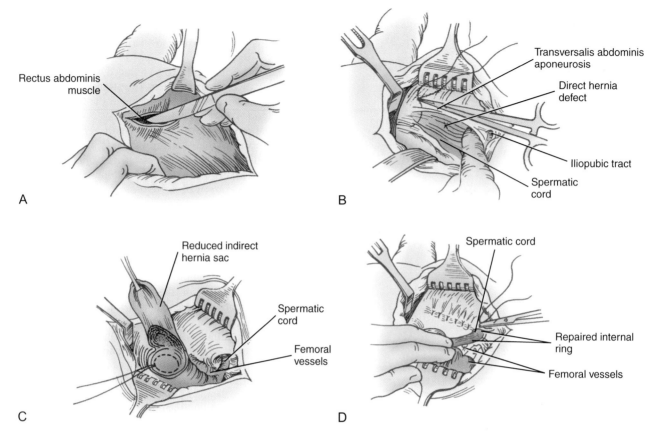

A

B

Transversalis abdominis
aponeurosis

Direct hernia
defect

Iliopubic tract

Spermatic
cord

Rectus abdominis
muscle

Reduced indirect
hernia sac

Spermatic
cord

Femoral
vessels

C

Spermatic cord

Repaired internal
ring

Femoral vessels

D

FIGURE 4-14 Preperitoneal repair. **A,** Skin incision starts 2 cm above symphysis pubis and is extended through external oblique, internal oblique, and transversalis muscles. **B,** With finger in direct hernia defect, the surgeon sutures the transversalis abdominis aponeurosis to the iliopubic tract. **C,** In case of indirect defect, the sac is reduced and then excised, with high ligation being achieved by use of a purse-string suture. **D,** Internal ring is tightened after transversus abdominis aponeurosis has been approximated to iliopubic tract.

SURGERY FOR REPAIR OF HERNIAS OF THE ANTERIOR ABDOMINAL WALL

Ventral or Incisional Hernias

Ventral hernias can appear either spontaneously or after previous operations. Spontaneously occurring ventral hernias include epigastric and umbilical hernias. Postoperative ventral hernias, called *incisional hernias,* appear more frequently when the original incision was T shaped or a vertical midline. Operations that involve a potential for contamination, such as that for acute perforated ulcer or other perforated abdominal viscera, or wounds that become infected, are more prone to developing subsequent ventral hernias. Patients taking steroids or diagnosed with chronic obstructive pulmonary disease (COPD), as well as patients with a poor nutritional state and resulting hypoproteinemia, are predisposed to ventral hernia formation. Finally, faulty surgical technique, such as the choice of inappropriate suture materials, may result in the ultimate appearance of a ventral hernia.

Several methods have been developed for repairing ventral hernias (Research Highlight). If all layers of the abdominal wall are easily identified, anatomic layer-by-layer repair may be done. Frequently a type of overlap method for repair is employed. Vertical and transverse overlap procedures are referred to as *vest-over-pants repair.* For large defects, in which approximation of tissue would result in closure with excessive tension or

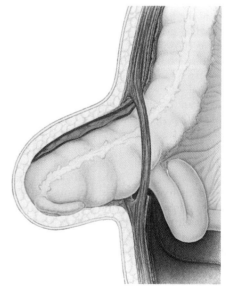

FIGURE 4-15 Sliding hernia.

would cause either circulatory or respiratory compromise, synthetic materials such as surgical mesh or patches are employed.

When a very large fascial defect is present, a technique that extrapolates on the principles of tissue expansion may be used. A Tenckhoff catheter is placed percutaneously into

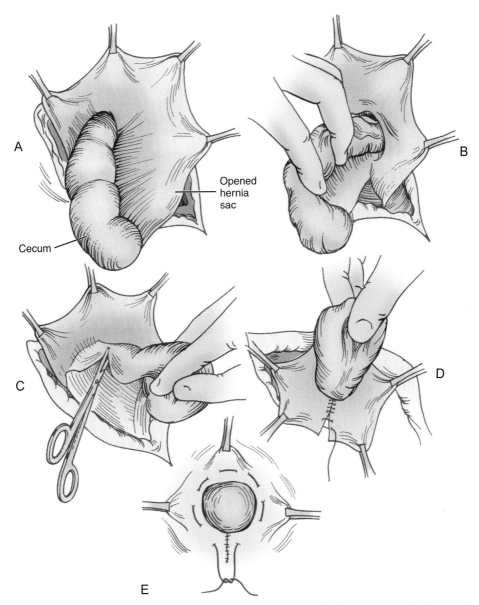

FIGURE 4-16 Right sliding hernia. **A,** Cecum forms posterior wall of hernia sac. **B,** Peritoneum is excised medially (**C**) and laterally (**D**) to allow mobilization of cecum for subsequent reduction to peritoneal cavity. Lateral and medial margins are approximated. **E,** After reduction, high ligation is accomplished using a purse-string suture.

the peritoneal cavity. Gradual expansion of the abdominal fascia is accomplished by insufflation of the abdomen with 1 to 2 liters of nitrous oxide gas, similar to the procedure for laparoscopy. The patient's vital signs are monitored during and after the insufflation procedure, which may be performed on a nursing unit or possibly in an outpatient clinical setting. The graduated expansion of the tissues sometimes allows for primary closure of the defect without the use of synthetic mesh or a patch.

Umbilical Hernias

Umbilical hernias are extraperitoneal and occur as small fascial defects under the umbilicus. They are common in children and frequently disappear spontaneously by 2 years of age. If the defect persists, a simple approximation of the overlying fascia is all that is necessary for repair (see Chapter 17 for a description of hernia repair in children). In adults, umbilical hernias represent a defect in the linea alba just above the umbilicus. These hernias tend to occur more frequently in obese people, making diagnosis more difficult. Umbilical hernias are potentially dangerous because they have small necks and frequently become incarcerated. Surgical repair is indicated for all adults with both symptomatic and asymptomatic umbilical hernias.

Epigastric Hernias

Epigastric hernias are protrusions of fat through defects in the abdominal wall between the xiphoid process and the umbilicus. Patients with epigastric hernias can have nausea, vague abdominal pain, or epigastric pain similar to that observed

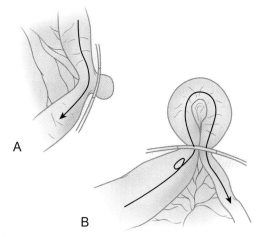

FIGURE 4-17 **A,** Richter hernia. Only a portion of bowel passes through hernial ring; arrow indicates that bowel need not be obstructed mechanically even with strangulation. **B,** Incarcerated hernia. Distended bowel in hernia cannot return to abdomen through narrow fascial defect.

RESEARCH HIGHLIGHT

Comparison of Laparoscopic versus Open Incisional Hernia Repair

In the United States, approximately 4 to 5 million laparotomies are performed annually, leading to at least 400,000 to 500,000 incisional hernias. Approximately 200,000 of these incisional hernias require surgical repair. This study focused on the United Kingdom (UK), where more than 124,000 laparotomies and 7000 subsequent incisional hernia repairs were performed from 2005 to 2006 using both open and laparoscopic techniques. UK researchers undertook a meta-analysis to compare the outcomes of laparoscopic versus open incisional hernia repair, examining surgical time, duration of hospital stay, perioperative complications, postoperative surgical site pain, and recurrence rates.

The analysis included 5 randomized controlled trials that involved 366 patients—183 in the open group and 183 in the laparoscopic group. Open repair was associated with significantly higher complication rates and longer hospital stays, as well as longer surgical times than laparoscopic repair. There was no statistical difference in surgical site pain or recurrence rates. The researchers concluded that laparoscopic repair of incisional hernias is a safe, feasible, and effective alternative to open repair techniques.

Adapted from Sajid MS et al: Laparoscopic versus open repair of incisional/ventral hernia: a meta-analysis, *Am J Surg* 197:64-72, 2009.

with cholecystitis or duodenal ulcers. Surgical repair of epigastric hernias is simple and very successful.

Spigelian Hernias

The linea semilunaris, often referred to as the *Spigelius line,* marks the transition from muscle to aponeurosis in the transversus abdominis muscle. The area of aponeurosis that lies between the linea semilunaris and the lateral edge of the rectus muscle is referred to as the *spigelian zone.* Protrusion of a peritoneal sac, preperitoneal fat, or other abdominal viscera through a congenital or acquired defect in this area is called a *spigelian hernia* (Menon, 2008). It is usually located between the different muscle layers of the abdominal wall. For this reason a spigelian hernia may be referred to as an *interstitial* or *intramuscular hernia.*

Spigelian hernias are uncommon and are generally difficult to diagnose. Ultrasonic scanning has improved the diagnosis of such hernias. When ultrasonic scanning is not conclusive, CT can better visualize the hernia orifice.

Interparietal Hernias

An interparietal hernia lies between the layers of the abdominal wall. These hernias may be classified by dividing them into those that present with ventral swelling and those without ventral swelling. Diagnosis is often made during an exploratory laparotomy for symptoms of intestinal obstruction.

Repair follows the same procedure as that done for a strangulated hernia. The sac contents are closely examined for ischemia, the sac is resected, and the defect is repaired.

Synthetic Mesh and Patch Repairs

An ideal prosthetic mesh should not be physically modified by tissue fluids; be chemically inert, noncarcinogenic, and nonallergenic; resist mechanical strain; be permeable, allowing tissue ingrowth; and be pliable. Synthetic meshes, such as Mersilene, Marlex, Prolene, and Dacron, have been particularly helpful in repairing recurrent or large ventral hernias. Closure of the

defect is obtained with minimal or no tension on the suture line. These synthetic materials are strong and durable, promoting fibrovascular growth within their pores, which lends extra strength to the repair. Single-dose antibiotic prophylaxis may be used to reduce wound infection rates with prosthetic hernia repair. Although there are studies that indicate that routine use of prophylactic antibiotics is not recommended for open non-implant herniorrhaphy, there is little direct clinical evidence on which to base recommendations when implantable mesh is used.

Another synthetic material, the Gore-Tex patch, has become popular for the reconstruction of abdominal wall defects and repair of soft tissue. Gore-Tex soft tissue patches are available in both 1-cm and 2-cm thicknesses. Impregnation of Gore-Tex patches with an antimicrobial agent has been associated with reduced incidence of infection. Gore-Tex is, however, very expensive, and surgical services departments should evaluate products such as surgical mesh with consideration to its performance, cost, effect on quality patient care, and value analysis (AORN, 2009b).

Essential to the use of mesh or patch in a hernia repair are the identification and cleaning of tissue planes to which the mesh or patch will be attached (Figure 4-18, *A*). In a ventral hernia, the peritoneum is dissected from the undersurface of the rectus abdominis muscle and the mesh or patch is placed between the peritoneum and the rectus (Figure 4-18, *B*). After the mesh or patch is positioned, it is sutured in place on one side, using the synthetic suture material compatible with the type of mesh or patch employed (Figure 4-18, *C*).

At this point the peritoneum can be closed, if possible. If the peritoneum cannot be closed, the mesh or patch can be placed directly over the omentum. The mesh or patch is then

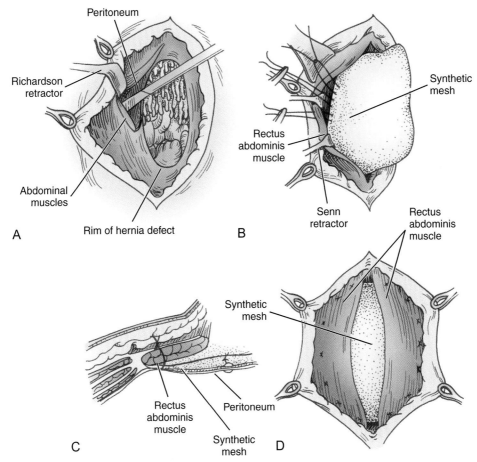

FIGURE 4-18 Use of mesh in hernia repair. After layers of abdominal wall surrounding ventral hernia are identified (**A**), mesh is inserted between rectus and peritoneum (**B**). **C**, Mesh is sutured into place on one side. **D**, With moderate tension, mesh is inserted between appropriate layers on opposite side and is sutured into place.

placed and sutured to the other side of the defect, with moderate tension maintained (Figure 4-18, *D*). If possible, the mesh or patch is then covered with a fascial or muscular layer before the subcutaneous fat and skin are closed. Closed-wound drainage catheters may be placed in the wound, and antibiotics are frequently used prophylactically. Using mesh or a patch to repair inguinal hernias is based on the same principles used for closing ventral hernias. With inguinal hernias, the mesh or patch is sutured to transversalis fascia on both sides of the defect.

GERIATRIC CONSIDERATIONS

The Elderly Patient—Hernia Surgery

A multidisciplinary team approach to surgical procedures on elderly patients is significant in providing effective care. Research by Hardin et al (2009) demonstrated that active co-morbid illnesses and emergency surgeries were indicators of successful surgical outcomes. Risk factors for surgery in elders include:

Surgical Risks

- ◆ Emergency surgery
- ◆ Site of surgery
- ◆ Vascular
- ◆ Aortic
- ◆ Intrathoracic
- ◆ Intraperitoneal
- ◆ Duration of procedure (more than 3.5 hours)

Continued

GERIATRIC CONSIDERATIONS—cont'd

Anesthetic Risks

◆ American Society of Anesthesiologists (ASA) classifications III to V
◆ Age older than 75 years
◆ Preexisting medical disease (hypertension; diabetes mellitus; cardiac, renal, liver, or respiratory disease)

Disease-Related Risks

◆ Cardiovascular
◆ Angina
◆ Previous myocardial infarction
◆ Congestive heart failure
◆ Pulmonary
◆ Bronchitis
◆ Pneumonia
◆ Cigarette smoking
◆ Digestive
◆ Poor nutritional status or malnutrition
◆ Protein deficiency
◆ Cirrhosis
◆ Active peptic ulcer
◆ Endocrine
◆ Adrenal insufficiency
◆ Hypothyroidism

Cognitive Impairment

◆ Dementia
◆ Acute confusional state (delirium)
◆ Alzheimer's disease

Other Factors

◆ Dehydration
◆ Anemia
◆ Recent stroke
◆ Malignancy
◆ Low albumin level
◆ Impaired mobility
◆ Patient living in institutional care

The estimated incidence of abdominal wall hernia in persons older than 65 years is 13 per 1000, with a fourfold to eightfold increase in the incidence in men. About 50% of all hernias are indirect inguinal, 20% are direct inguinal, 10% are ventral, 6% are femoral, 3% are umbilical, and 1% are esophageal hiatal (Berger et al, 2008). The elective repair of inguinal and femoral hernias is strongly advised because of the risk of incarceration with subsequent emergency surgery. Many hernia repairs in elderly patients are emergency procedures because of incarcerations and small bowel obstruction. When elective, the operation may be performed as an ambulatory procedure; IV sedation and local anesthesia provide a very satisfactory alternative to general or spinal anesthesia.

Laparoscopic techniques for hernia repair have gained popularity because of associated shorter hospital stay, minimal pain postoperatively, and early recovery. However, the necessity for general anesthesia makes this approach one that may not be advisable in elders. Decisions for local versus spinal or general anesthesia are made based on the patient's overall physiologic status and surgical risk.

In elderly men the co-existence of inguinal hernia and prostatism is fairly common. Depending on the size of the prostate, the hernia repair should be postponed until after the prostate surgery. Not unusual in elders are large, neglected scrotal hernias. The repair of these hernias is not routine in that the abdominal wall defect may be so large that primary repair cannot take place without tension. Synthetic abdominal wall replacements are helpful in the management of such large hernias. The repair of huge scrotal hernias can have a tremendous benefit on the personality of the geriatric patient, who is much relieved after removal of what can be considered an accessory appendage that is offensive, difficult to clean, and often an impedance to daily activities.

Modified from Berger DH et al: Surgery in the elderly. In Townsend CM et al: *Sabiston textbook of surgery,* ed 18, Philadelphia, 2008, Saunders; Hardin RE et al: Experience with dedicated geriatric surgical consult services: meeting the need for surgery in the frail elderly. *Clinical Interventions in Aging* 4:73–80, 2009, available at www.ncbi.nlm.nih.gov/pmc/articles/PMC2685228/. Accessed September 20, 2010; Kim SS, Zenilman ME: The elderly surgical patient. In Souba W et al, editors: *ACS surgery principles and practices,* ed 6, Ontario, Canada, 2007, BC Decker.

REPAIR OF HERNIAS SUMMARY

Hernias are common conditions that affect people of all ages. If left untreated they usually can cause severe pain and potentially serious complications. Surgery is usually the recommended treatment. Hernia surgery is very safe and effective and the risks and complications are rare. As a surgical technologist your role in the planning and implementation is essential to the success of the surgical procedure.

REVIEW QUESTIONS

1. All of the following are areas in the abdominal wall that a hernia can occur except:
   a. the inguinal canal
   b. the umbilicus
   c. the acromial process
   d. the femoral rings

2. All of the following are types of abdominal hernias except:
   a. umbilical
   b. incisional
   c. synovial
   d. inguinal

3. Which of the following anatomy is not part of the inguinal canal?
   a. deep epigastric vein
   b. spermatic cord
   c. Cooper's ligament
   d. internal ring

4. Which of the following are indications that a patient may have a hernia?
   a. swelling in the neck
   b. chronic cough
   c. fever
   d. pain in the abdomen

5. Which of the following is a treatment for an inguinal hernia?
   a. cholecystectomy
   b. Burch procedure
   c. simple mastectomy
   d. Bassini repair

6. All of the following are the compartments of the femoral sheath except:
   a. medial
   b. carotid
   c. lateral
   d. intermediate

7. When performing a laparoscopic repair of the hernia, which of the following is not an important procedural consideration?
   a. appropriate-sized trocars
   b. position of the patient
   c. prepped genital area
   d. correct catheter placement

8. Which of the following hernias deals with only a portion of the bowel passing through the hernia ring?
   a. Richter
   b. Shouldice
   c. Cooper
   d. McVay

9. All of the following are types of synthetic mesh except:
   a. Prolene
   b. Mersilene
   c. Dacron
   d. Ethibond

10. All of the following are causes for recurrent hernia except:
    a. chronic cough
    b. strong muscle tone
    c. infection of the surgical wound
    d. tension of the suture line

11. Define and briefly describe the following surgical procedures:
    McVay (Cooper's ligament) hernia repair
    Repair of sliding hernias
    Mesh-plug hernia repair

Critical Thinking Questions

1. Is there any benefit to having a hernia repaired laparoscopically versus open?

2. What are some of the ways that society today can reduce the need for hernia repairs?

REFERENCES

Association of periOperative Registered Nurses (AORN): Recommended practices for a safe environment of care. In *Perioperative standards and recommended practices*, Denver, 2009a, The Association.

Association of periOperative Registered Nurses (AORN): Recommended practices for product selection in perioperative practice settings. In *Perioperative standards and recommended practices*, Denver, 2009b, The Association.

Barclay L, Murata P: Evaluation of acute abdominal pain reviewed. From Medscape Medical News, April 18, 2008, available at http://cme.medscape.com/viewarticle/573206. Accessed August 1, 2009.

Bascom J: Inguinal hernia. In Harken AH, Moore EE, editors: *Abernathy's surgical secrets*, ed 5, Philadelphia, 2004, Hanley & Belfus.

Beyea SC: *Perioperative nursing data set, revised*, Denver, 2007, Association of Perioperative Registered Nurses (AORN).

Denholm B: Tucking patient's arms and general positioning, *AORN J* 89(4):755–757, 2009.

Feldman LS et al: Laparoscopic hernia repair. In Souba WW et al., *ACS surgery principles & practice,* ed 6, New York, NY, 2007.

Gilbert AI et al: Inguinal hernia: anatomy and management, available at www.surgery.medscape.com/ viewarticle/357. Accessed July 30, 2009.

Lawrence PF: *Essentials of general surgery*, ed 4, Philadelphia, 2006, Lippincott Williams & Wilkins.

Menon AS: Hernia reduction. eMedicine specialties, April 8, 2008, available at www.emedicinehealth.com/hernia/article_em.htm. Accessed August 1, 2009.

Read RC: Inguinal herniation in the adult, defect or disease: a surgeon's odyssey, Pioneers in Hernia Surgery, *Pioneer* 8:296–299, 2004.

Taylor J: FDA device clearances: hernia repair device, cryoablation system, automated perimetry device, available at www.medscape.com/viewarticle/562089. Accessed July 31, 2009.

World Health Organization. Implementation Manual WHO Surgical Safety Checklist (First edition), 2008, available at www.who.int/patientsafety. Accessed August 1, 2009.

CHAPTER 5

Gynecologic and Obstetric Surgery

After studying this chapter the reader will be able to:
- Identify the female reproductive anatomy and related structures
- Correlate physiology to conditions requiring surgical intervention
- Identify tissue layers involved in opening and closing sequences of gynecologic and obstetric surgery
- Identify the disorders and diseases associated with the female anatomy
- Compare diagnostic methods for determination of surgical interventions
- Contrast minimally invasive to open surgical procedures in gynecologic and obstetric surgery
- Identify specialized instrumentation, equipment, and supplies utilized in gynecologic and obstetric surgery
- List the pharmacologic/hemostatic agents in gynecologic and obstetric surgery
- Discuss the patient considerations of both the mother and the baby in Cesarean section
- Review specific procedural steps as a guide for clinical procedure consideration

CHAPTER OUTLINE

Overview

Whereas changes in science and technology have impacted every area in medicine over the past century, changes in the specialty of women's health have had enormous influence over the way women live. At some point in their lives, many women face the prospect of surgery. Surgical procedures on the structures of the female reproductive system are performed for diagnostic, therapeutic, or cosmetic purposes; for conditions such as abnor-

mal bleeding from the reproductive organs; for suspected malignant or benign neoplasms; and for infertility. Procedures are also performed to remove or repair weakened anatomic structures. Recent statistics show the majority of surgical procedures performed in the United States were performed on females (Healthcare Cost and Utilization Project [HCUPnet], 2007). A holistic approach with sensitivity to the special needs of this population is an essential component of perioperative care.

This chapter was originally written by Donna R. McEwen, RN, BSN, CNOR, for the 14th edition of Alexander's Care of the Patient in Surgery *and has been revised by Dana M. Fields, CST, for this text.*

Surgical Anatomy

The female reproductive organs and their relationships are shown in Figures 5-1 and 5-2. The adult female structures associated with the process of reproduction are the external organs (vulva), the associated ligaments and muscles, the soft tissues and contents of the pelvic cavity, and the bony pelvis.

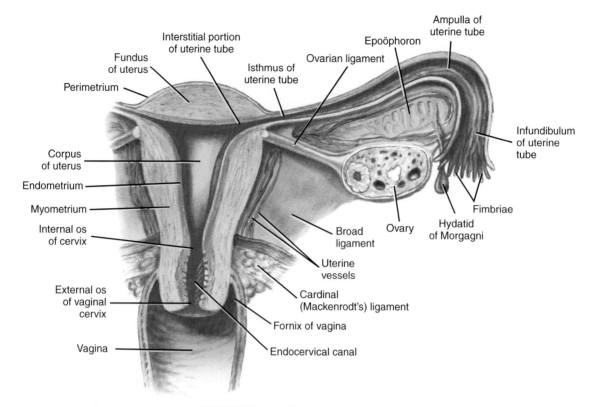

FIGURE 5-1 Female reproductive organs.

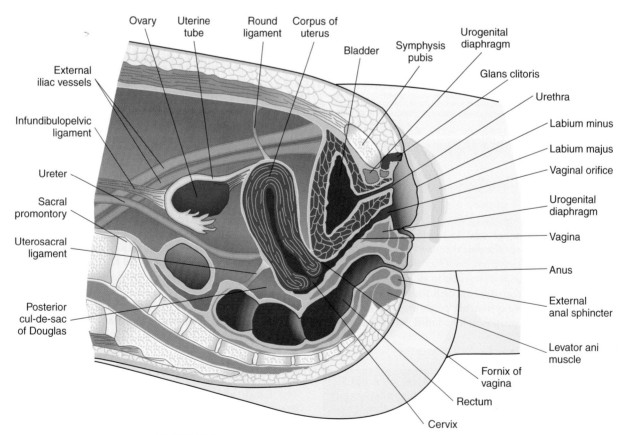

FIGURE 5-2 Female pelvic organs as viewed in midsagittal section.

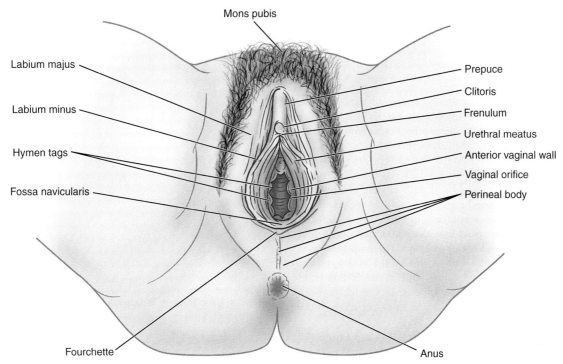

FIGURE 5-3 The structures of the external genitalia that are collectively called the *vulva.*

FEMALE EXTERNAL GENITAL ORGANS (VULVA)

The external organs, referred to collectively as the *vulva,* include the mons pubis, the labia majora and labia minora, the clitoris, the vestibular glands, the vaginal vestibule, the vaginal opening, and the urethral opening (Figure 5-3).

The mons pubis is a mound of adipose tissue covered by skin and, after puberty, by hair. It is situated over the anterior surface of the symphysis pubis.

The labia majora are two folds of adipose tissue covered with skin that extend downward and backward from the mons pubis. Varying in appearance according to the amount of adipose tissue, they unite below and behind the mons pubis to form the posterior commissure and in front of the mons pubis to form the anterior commissure. The labia minora are the two hairless, flat, delicate folds of skin that lie within the labia majora. Each labium splits into lateral and medial parts. The lateral part forms the prepuce of the clitoris, and the medial part forms the frenulum. The posterior folds of the labia are united by a delicate fold extending between them. This forms the fossa navicularis.

The clitoris is the homologue of the penis in the male. It hangs freely and terminates in a rounded glans (small, sensitive vascular body). Unlike the penis, the clitoris does not contain the urethra. The vaginal vestibule is a smooth area surrounded by the labia minora, with the clitoris at its apex and the fossa navicularis at its base. It contains openings for the urethra and the vagina.

The urethra, which is about 4 cm long in the premenopausal woman, is close to the anterior vaginal wall and connects the bladder with the urethral meatus. Two small paraurethral ducts, which are commonly known as *Skene's ducts,* lie on either side of the urethral meatus and drain *Skene's glands.*

The vaginal opening lies below the urethral meatus. The hymen surrounds the vaginal opening and may be circular, crescentic, or fimbriated.

Bartholin's glands and ducts are located on each side of the lower end of the vagina. These narrow ducts open into the vaginal orifice on the inner aspects of the labia minora. The glands secrete mucus and can become infected or inflamed.

PELVIC CAVITY

Uterus

The uterus is a pear-shaped organ situated in the pelvic cavity between the bladder and the rectum. It gains much of its support from its direct attachment to the vagina and from indirect attachments to nearby structures, such as the rectum and pelvic diaphragm. The uterus is supported on each side by the broad, round, cardinal, and uterosacral ligaments and levator ani muscles. The upper lateral points, the uterine cornua, receive the fallopian tubes. The fundus of the uterus is the upper, rounded portion positioned above the level of the tubal openings and just below the pelvic brim. Below, the body, or corpus, of the uterus joins the cervix. The corpus is separated from the cervix by a slight constriction (canal) called the *isthmus.* The cervix lies at the level of the ischial spines. The body of the uterus communicates with the cervical canal at the internal orifice, called the *internal os.* The constriction (canal) ends at the vaginal portion of the cervix at the external orifice, called the *external os.* The external os varies in appearance and may be oval, round, slitlike, or everted.

The uterine body has three layers: (1) the outer peritoneal, or serous, layer, which is a reflection of the pelvic peritoneum;

(2) the myometrium, or muscular layer, which houses involuntary muscles, nerves, blood vessels, and lymphatics; and (3) the endometrium, or mucosal layer, which lines the cavity of the uterus.

Fallopian Tubes (Oviducts)

The Greek word *salpinx,* meaning "trumpet" or "tube," is used to refer to the fallopian tubes (Figure 5-4). The tubes are paired and consist of a musculomembranous channel about 10 to 13 cm long, forming the canals through which the ova are conveyed to the uterus from the ovaries. The outer surfaces of the tubes are covered by peritoneum. The inner layers are composed of muscular tissue lined with ciliated epithelium. Each tube receives its blood supply from the branches of the uterine and ovarian arteries and has four parts. The infundibulum is trumpet-shaped, opens into the abdominal cavity, and has fingerlike projections called *fimbriae.* The ampulla forms more than half of the tube and is thin-walled and tortuous. The isthmus is cylindric and forms approximately one third of the tube. The remainder of the tube is the uterine portion. Measuring approximately 1 cm in length, it passes through the wall of the uterus.

It has been theorized that the transfer of the ova from the ruptured follicles into the uterus is accomplished through vascular changes that occur with contraction of the smooth muscle fibers of the tube. The peristaltic action of the muscular layer and the ciliary movement propel the ova toward the uterus.

The right tube and ovary are in close relationship to the cecum and appendix; the left tube and ovary are situated near the sigmoid flexure. The fallopian tubes are also in proximity to the ureters.

Ovaries

The ovaries are located on each side of the uterus. The ovaries and tubes are collectively known as the *adnexa.* Each ovary lies within a depression (ovarian fossa) on the lateral wall of the pelvic cavity and above the broad ligament (see Figure 5-1). The anterior border of each ovary is attached to the posterior layer of the broad ligament by a peritoneal fold (mesovarium) and is suspended by the ovarian ligament.

The ovaries are small, almond-shaped organs composed of an outer layer, known as the *cortex,* and an inner vascular layer, known as the *medulla.* The medulla consists of connective tissue containing nerves, blood vessels, and lymph vessels. The ovary is covered by epithelium, not peritoneum. The cortex contains ovarian (graafian) follicles in different stages of maturity. After ovulation, the corpus luteum arises from the graafian follicle that expelled the ovum.

The ovaries are homologous with the testes of the male. They produce ova after puberty and also function as endocrine glands, producing hormones such as estrogen, secreted by the ovarian follicles. Estrogen controls the development of the secondary sexual characteristics and initiates growth of the lining of the uterus during the menstrual cycle. Progesterone, which is secreted by the corpus luteum, is essential for the implantation of the fertilized ovum and for the development of the embryo.

Ligaments of the Uterus

The uterine ligaments are the broad, round, cardinal, and uterosacral ligaments (Figure 5-5).

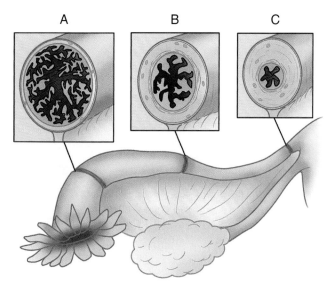

FIGURE 5-4 The longitudinal folds of the fallopian tube seen in cross section. **A,** Infundibulum. **B,** Ampulla. **C,** Isthmus

The pelvic peritoneum extends laterally, downward, and posteriorly from each side of the uterus. A double fold of pelvic peritoneum forms the layers of the broad ligament, enclosing the uterus. These layers separate to cover the floor and sides of the pelvis. The fallopian tube is situated within the free border of the broad ligament. The free margin of the upper division of the broad ligament, lying immediately below the fallopian tube, is termed the *mesosalpinx.* The ovary lies behind the broad ligament.

Round ligaments are fibromuscular bands attached to the uterus. Each round ligament passes forward and laterally between the layers of the broad ligament to enter the deep inguinal ring.

Cardinal ligaments are composed of connective tissue with smooth muscle fibers and provide strong support for the uterus.

Uterosacral ligaments are a posterior continuation of the peritoneal tissue. The ligaments pass posteriorly to the sacrum on either side of the rectum.

Vagina

The vagina is a rugated musculomembranous tube. It carries the menstrual blood from the uterus, serves as the organ for sexual intercourse, and is the terminal portion of the birth canal. The anterior wall measures 6 to 8 cm in length and the posterior wall 7 to 10 cm (see Figures 5-1 and 5-2). The anterior wall of the vagina is in proximity to the bladder and urethra. The lower posterior wall is anteriorly adjacent to the rectum. The upper portion of the vagina lies above the pelvic floor and is surrounded by visceral pelvic fascia. The lower half is surrounded by the levator ani muscles.

Cervix

The cervix consists of a supravaginal portion, which is closely associated with the bladder and the ureters, and a vaginal portion, which projects downward and backward into the vaginal vault. The projection of the cervix into the vaginal vault divides

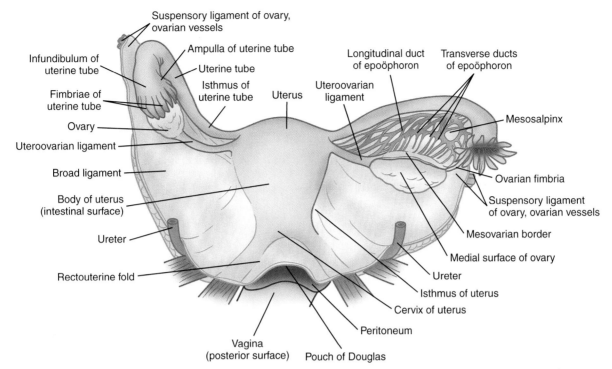

FIGURE 5-5 Schema of the broad ligament, posterior view. Note the many structures contained within the broad ligament. Note the posterior aspect of the rectouterine fold, called the *cul-de-sac*, or *pouch, of Douglas*.

the vault into four regions, called *fornices*: anterior, posterior, right lateral, and left lateral.

The posterior fornix is in contact with the peritoneum of the pouch, or cul-de-sac, of Douglas. The rectovaginal septum lies between the vagina and rectum. The dense connective tissue separating the anterior wall of the vagina from the distal urethra is termed the *urethrovaginal septum*.

BONY PELVIS

The pelvis is that portion of the trunk below and behind the abdomen. The bony pelvis is composed of the ilium, symphysis pubis, ischium, sacrum, and coccyx. The so-called *pelvic brim* divides the abdominal false portion, located above the arcuate line, from the true portion of the pelvis, located below this line. The bony pelvis accommodates the growing fetus during pregnancy and the birth process.

The true pelvis may be considered to have three parts: inlet, cavity, and outlet. The muscles lining the pelvis facilitate movement of the thighs, give form to the pelvic cavity, and provide a firm elastic lining to the bony pelvic framework. All organs located in the pelvis are covered by pelvic fascia, which is extremely important in the maintenance of normal strength in the pelvic floor.

The fascia covering the muscles is usually dense and firm, whereas that covering organs is often thin and elastic. The nerves, blood vessels, and ureters coursing through the anatomic structures are closely associated with muscular and fascial structures.

PELVIC FLOOR

The pelvic floor acts as a supportive sling for the pelvic contents. The pelvic fascia may be divided into three general groups: parietal, diaphragmatic, and visceral. The parietal pelvic fascia covers the muscles of the true pelvic wall and perineum. The diaphragmatic fascia covers both sides of the pelvic diaphragm, which is made up of the levator ani and coccygeal muscles. The visceral fascia is thin and flexible and covers the pelvic organs. The floor of the pelvis, known as the *pelvic diaphragm*, gives support to the abdominal pelvic viscera in this region. It consists of the levator ani and coccygeal muscles with their respective fascial coverings; it separates the pelvic cavity from the perineum.

The levator ani muscles, varying in thickness and strength, may be divided into three parts: the iliococcygeal, the pubococcygeal, and the puborectal muscles. The fibers of the levator ani muscles blend with the muscle fibers of the rectum and vagina. The pubovaginal fibers of the pubococcygeal portion of the levator ani muscles, lying directly below the urinary bladder, are involved in the control of micturition. The pubococcygeal fibers of the levator ani muscles control and pull the coccyx forward and assist in the closure of the pelvic outlet. The fibers pull the rectum, vagina, and bladder neck upward toward the symphysis pubis in an effort to close the pelvic outlet and are responsible for the flexure at the anorectal junction. Relaxation of the fibers during defecation permits a straightening at this junction. During parturition, the action of the levator ani muscles directs the fetal head into the lower part of the passageway.

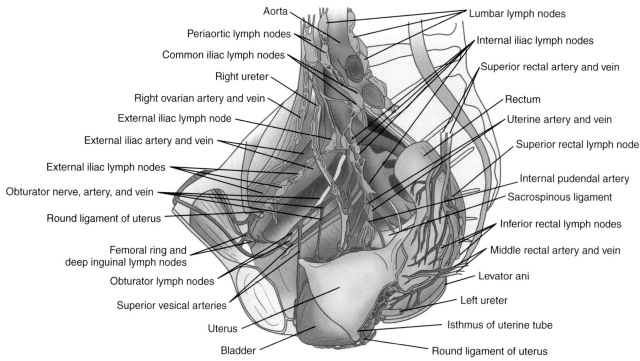

FIGURE 5-6 A lateral view of the female pelvis demonstrating the extensive lymphatic network. Note that most of the lymphatic channels follow the courses of the major vessels.

Vascular, Nerve, and Lymphatic Supply of the Reproductive System

The blood supply of the female pelvis is derived from the internal iliac branches of the common iliac artery and is supplemented by the ovarian, superior rectal, and median sacral arteries—branches of the aorta.

The nerve supply of the female pelvis comes from the autonomic nerves, which enter the pelvis in the superior hypogastric plexus (presacral nerve). The lymphatics of the female pelvis either follow the course of the vessels to the iliac and preaortic nodes or empty into the inguinal glands (Figure 5-6).

Surgical Technologist Considerations

As a part of the surgical team, the surgical technologist should check the chart and consult with the perioperative nurse and/or surgeon about the specifics of the procedure. For the surgical technologist to be adequately prepared for the procedure, the surgical technologist must have a clear understanding of the procedure and why the procedure is necessary (e.g., disorder, disease, infection). Ensuring patient safety is the number one goal of the surgical technologist. Understanding the dynamics of the procedure and the patient will prevent mistakes in the operating room. In addition to the patient allergies, it is necessary to be aware of the patient's medical history as noted by the perioperative nurse and surgeon. The medical history includes a chronological listing of each pregnancy with length of gestation, type of delivery, complications during pregnancy, duration of labor, and fetal weight. In addition to the medical history, the assessment also taken by the perioperative nurse and surgeon will add valid insight. This may include the patient's social history, sexual history, and any relevant cultural and/or religious preferences. Reviewing laboratory findings and other test results may also reveal vital information pertinent to the operative procedure preparation (Table 5-1).

Another important factor the surgical technologist should consider is the challenges of different approaches to OB/GYN procedures (sterile, clean, dirty, or a combination). As a rule, procedures utilizing an abdominal approach are sterile and those with a vaginal approach are clean/dirty. Please note: In procedures that utilize both abdominal and vaginal approaches (e.g., laparoscopic surgical interventions), the sterile field must be kept separate from the nonsterile field. Gloves should be changed when changing from the vaginal aspect of the procedure (clean) and moving to the abdominal aspect (sterile).

Also, the surgical technologist should consider the setup of tables for different OB/GYN interventions. Procedures using the vaginal approach (e.g., vaginal delivery, cerclage, and D&C) will not generally have a mayo stand. Back tables will be used and positioned at the patient's feet. It is not uncommon for the physicians to stand on one side of the back table and the surgical technologist on the other.

TABLE 5-1

Common Laboratory Studies Used in the Reproductive Assessment

Test	Normal Range for Adults	Significance of Abnormal Findings
Follicle-stimulating hormone (FSH) (follitropin)	Follicular phase, 1.37-9.9 milliinternational units/ml Midcycle, 6.17-17.2 milliinternational units/ml Luteal phase, 1.09-9.2 milliinternational units/ml Postmenopause, 19.3-100.6 milliinternational units/ml	Decreased levels indicate possible infertility, anorexia nervosa, neoplasm. Elevations indicate possible Turner's syndrome.
Luteinizing hormone (LH)	Follicular phase, 1.68-15 milliinternational units/ml Midcycle, 21.9-56.6 milliinternational units/ml Luteal phase, 0.61-16.3 milliinternational units/ml Postmenopause, 14.2-52.3 milliinternational units/ml	Decreased levels indicate possible infertility, anovulation. Increased levels indicate possible ovarian failure, Turner's syndrome.
Prolactin	0-20 ng/ml; 20-400 ng/ml in pregnancy	Increased levels indicate possible galactorrhea, pituitary tumor, disease of hypothalamus or pituitary gland, hypothyroidism.
Estradiol	Follicular phase, 20-350 pg/ml Midcycle, 150-750 pg/ml Luteal phase, 30-450 pg/ml Postmenopause, ≤20 pg/ml	Increased levels indicate normal pregnancy, precocious puberty, ovarian tumor. Decreased levels indicate failing pregnancy, Turner's syndrome, menopause, anorexia nervosa.
Progesterone	Follicular phase, <50 ng/dl Luteal phase, 300-2500 ng/dl Postmenopause, <40 ng/dl	Increased levels indicate possible ovarian luteal cysts. Decreased levels indicate possible inadequate luteal phase, amenorrhea.
Testosterone	<1 ng/dl	Increased levels indicate possible adrenal neoplasm, polycystic ovaries, ovarian tumors, trophoblastic tumors, idiopathic hirsutism.

Modified from Lowdermilk DL: Assessment of the reproductive system. In Ignatavicius DD, Workman ML, editors: *Medical-surgical nursing: patient-centered collaborative care*, ed 6, Philadelphia, 2010, Saunders.

▼ PATIENT SAFETY

Assessment Techniques for Intimate Partner Violence (IPV)

IPV can be defined as the actual or threatened physical, sexual, psychologic, or emotional abuse by a spouse, ex-spouse, boyfriend, girlfriend, ex-boyfriend, ex-girlfriend, date, or cohabitating partner. IPV may also include rape and stalking. Abuse or violence crosses all ages and segments of society; it is not limited to certain economic groups or educational level.

Healthcare providers may represent the first and only contact that an isolated woman will seek outside of the abusive relationship and are a primary source of relief; therefore screening for IPV should be an integral part of the perioperative assessment. A variety of screening tools are available and are summarized in the CDC publication, *Intimate Partner Violence and Sexual Violence Victimization Assessment Instruments for Use in Healthcare Settings.* Characteristics common to the tools include trying to normalize the conversation with neutral opening statements, such as "The staff at our facility are concerned about your safety. We know that many things can happen in our lives that affect our mental and physical health." In addition, healthcare providers should use direct questions when violence is suspected, such as "Are you with a partner who threatens or physically harms you?"

Cues to abuse include delay in seeking medical assistance (hours or days), vague explanations of injuries, nonspecific complaints, a partner who seems reluctant to leave the woman alone with the healthcare provider, and substance abuse. Physical signs include new and old injuries to the face, breasts, abdomen, and buttocks; fractures that have a suspicious etiology; injuries at various stages of healing; and patterns that indicate injuries made by biting or fist/hand patterns. Pregnant women have an increased risk for IPV and therefore should be thoroughly assessed.

If IPV is suspected, most states mandate the abuse be reported. Domestic violence is considered a crime in all states, but the category (e.g., misdemeanor or felony) varies by state definition. Healthcare providers must be aware of the reporting requirements for the state in which they reside. In addition to reporting the abuse or suspected abuse, healthcare providers must document the findings in the medical record. If appropriate to the situation, photographs can be taken and included in the record.

Healthcare providers must assess the patient's safety before she is discharged and provide her with written information about her legal options, shelters, crisis intervention services, and counseling. The National Domestic Violence Hotline (1-800-799-SAFE) is available 24 hours a day/7 days a week. Healthcare providers can also facilitate patient safety by providing education to women and empowering them to understand that abuse is a violation of their basic human rights; promoting assertiveness; and recommending resources that will enhance independence.

Modified from Centers for Disease Control and Prevention: *Intimate partner violence and sexual violence victimization assessment instruments for use in healthcare settings,* available at www.cdc.gov/ncipc/dvp/ipv/ipvandsv-screening.pdf. Accessed July 2, 2009; Rhynerson B: Violence against women. In Lowdermilk DL, Perry SE, editors: *Maternity and women's health care,* ed 9, St Louis, 2007, Mosby; World Health Organization (WHO): *Violence against women fact sheet,* 2008, available at www.who.int/mediacentre/factsheets/fs239/en/. Accessed July 2, 2009.

SURGICAL TECHNOLOGY PREFERENCE CARD

In OB/GYN, there are several factors to consider when preparing for a surgical intervention. Positioning and prepping will be determined by several factors including abdominal approaches, vaginal approaches, and even pregnant patients and their gestational age.

In many instances, hospitals have a dedicated unit or floor for women's health services. These services may encompass all health-related issues in addition to pregnancy. Therefore, the surgical technologist needs to evaluate each procedure and adjust the needs according to the specific patient and procedure. For example, when performing a D&C for a patient who has miscarried, the infant warmer and all visible supplies related to neonates should be removed from the OR.

Room Prep: Basic operating room furniture in place, sequential compression devices, thermoregulatory devices, extra blankets, padding, positioning supplies to achieve optimal patient safety and any additional equipment related to childbirth (as listed below)

Prep Solution: In room and warmed according to manufacturer's instructions
- Chlorhexidine gluconate
- Iodine and iodophors
- Duraprep
- Technicare
- Ivory soap
- Baby shampoo

Catheter: In room and correct size
- Catheter set and tray
  - Latex/rubber
  - PVC
  - Silicone
- Sizing
  - French
- Nonretaining
  - Red rubber (Robinson)
- Retaining
  - Foley
    - 2-way
    - 3-way
- Other urine collection devices

PROCEDURE CHECKLIST

Instruments
- Basic hysterectomy set
- Basic Cesarean section set
- Open instruments if needed to convert from laparoscopic to open
- Anticipated additional instruments

Specialty Suture
- As per surgeon's preference

Hemostatic Agents
- Mechanical
  - Staplers
  - Clip appliers and clips
  - Pressure
  - Ligatures
- Chemical
  - Absorbable gelatin
  - Collagen
  - Oxidized cellulose
  - Silvar nitrate
  - Epinephrine
  - Thrombin
- Thermal
  - Electrosurgical unit
  - Harmonic scalpel
  - Argon beam coagulator
  - Laser
  - Smoke evacuator

Additional Supplies: both sterile and nonsterile
- If the physician is requesting supplies, instruments, or equipment not normally used, check to be sure all have arrived to the room before opening
- Sponges
- Drapes
- Gowns and gloves for team members

SURGICAL TECHNOLOGY PREFERENCE CARD—cont'd

- ◆ "Have ready" or "hold" supplies
- ◆ Infant bulb suction and cord clamps, if appropriate

Medications and Irrigation Solutions
- ◆ Do these need to be warmed?
- ◆ Appropriate-sized syringes and hypodermic needles
- ◆ Sterile markers and labels for all medications on the sterile field

Drains and Dressings
- ◆ Correct size and type for planned surgery
  - • Open—not attached to a drainage system
    - • Penrose
    - • Cigarette
  - • Closed—attached to a closed reservoir for fluid collection
    - • Hemovac
    - • Jackson-Pratt
    - • Autologous blood retrieval drainage system

Specimen Care
- ◆ Proper container for each specimen
- ◆ Labels for each specimen
- ◆ Proper solution for specimen type

Supplies Needed for Delivery of Neonate
- ◆ Infant warmer
- ◆ Scale
- ◆ DeLee suction catheter
- ◆ Ambu bag
- ◆ Thermometer
- ◆ Tape measure
- ◆ Cord clamps
- ◆ Intubation box/cart
- ◆ Infant blankets and hats

Before opening for the procedure, the surgical technologist should:
- ◆ Arrange furniture
- ◆ Gather positioning devices
- ◆ Damp dust lights, furniture, and surfaces
- ◆ Verify functionality of equipment
- ◆ Place items to be opened in their appropriate places

When opening sterile supplies:
- ◆ Verify exposure to sterilization
- ◆ Use sterile technique
- ◆ Open bundles in appropriate locations
- ◆ Open additional supplies onto sterile field
- ◆ Open all sterile supplies and equipment as close to the surgical start time as possible

---

The gynecologic patient may undergo numerous diagnostic studies. The studies performed depend on the gynecologic problem or disorder. A laparoscopy may be performed for diagnostic or therapeutic reasons, such as infertility, pelvic pain, pelvic inflammatory disease, ova retrieval for in vitro fertilization (IVF), lysis of adhesions, evaluation of pelvic mass, removal of ectopic pregnancy, or sterilization.

Pelvic ultrasonography helps diagnose ectopic pregnancy and adnexal and uterine disease. Uterine fibroids and blood or fluid in the pelvis may be identified by means of ultrasonography. Computerized tomography (CT) scanning and magnetic resonance imaging (MRI) may be used in evaluation of the patient with suspected malignancy in the retroperitoneal lymph nodes or bone.

The gynecologic patient may have a hysterosalpingogram preoperatively to identify abnormalities in the uterine cavity and occlusions in the tubal folds. This diagnostic tool is useful in detecting potential reasons for infertility.

A colposcopy, with colpomicroscopy, is often performed in the physician's office. This examination is indicated for the patient with an abnormal Papanicolaou (Pap) smear suggestive of dysplasia. It identifies cellular abnormalities that may involve the vulva, vagina, or cervix and helps identify areas of dysplasia and carcinoma in situ. Endocervical curette samples may be obtained during the colposcopic procedure to rule out invasive carcinoma or to detect early adenocarcinoma.

Gynecologic Carcinoma. Gynecologic cancers commonly occur in the endometrium, the cervix, the ovaries, or the vagina. Less common sites are the vulva and fallopian tubes. Risk factors associated with the development of these cancers are noted in Table 5-2.

Endometrial cancer (Figure 5-7) is the most common gynecologic cancer and is responsible for approximately 42,160 new cases of cancer each year in the United States. Patients with this type of cancer may be asymptomatic, or they may experience

TABLE 5-2

Risk Factors for Cancers of the Reproductive System

Risk Factor	Endometrial Cancer	Cervical Cancer	Ovarian Cancer	Vulvar Cancer	Vaginal Cancer	Fallopian Tube Cancer
Age	50-65 yr	CIS: 30-40 yr Invasive: 40-60 yr	Infrequent before 35 yr; range usually is 40-65 yr	After 40 yr; peak is 60-70 yr	Most after 50 yr; adenocarcinoma: 14-30 yr	Most after 50 yr; range is 18-80 yr
Family history	Increased risk	—	Increased risk	—	DES exposure in utero	—
Personal history	Diabetes, hypertension	—	Breast, bowel, or endometrial cancer	Cervical cancer, diabetes, vulvar disease	Vulvar or cervical cancer	Ovarian or uterine cancer, infertility
Race	Caucasian	African American, Native American	Caucasian	—	—	—
Mother's age at delivery	—	<18 yr	>30 yr	—	—	—
Body size	Obese	—	—	Possibly obese	—	—
Parity	Nulliparity	Multiparity	Nulliparity	—	Multiparity	Nulliparity
Estrogen use	Prolonged use >3 yr after menopause	Possibly long-term birth control pill use	—	—	—	—
Smoking	Possibly increased risk	Possibly double the risk	—	—	—	—
Infection (STI)	—	Possibly STI (herpes simplex virus type 2 or papillomavirus infection)	—	Possibly STI (papillomavirus infection)	STI (herpes simplex virus type 2 or papillomavirus infection)	PID, chronic salpingitis

CIS, Carcinoma in situ; *DES,* diethylstilbestrol; *PID,* pelvic inflammatory disease; *STI,* sexually transmitted infection.
Modified from Gingrich PM: Interventions for clients with gynecologic problems. In Ignatavicius DD, Workman ML, editors: *Medical-surgical nursing: patient-centered collaborative care,* ed 6, Philadelphia, 2010, Saunders.

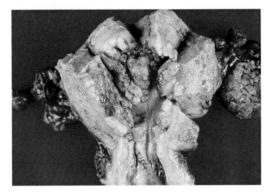

FIGURE 5-7 Endometrial cancer on posterior wall of uterus.

postmenopausal bleeding as their primary symptom (American Cancer Society [ACS], 2009).

Cervical cancer is the third most common cause of death related to gynecologic cancers. In its early, preinvasive stage, cervical cancer may be asymptomatic or associated with painless vaginal spotting or bleeding. During the early preinvasive stage, the disease may be described as dysplasia. From dysplasia, the disease progresses to carcinoma in situ (CIS). Preinvasive cancers may also be designated as cervical intraepithelial neoplasia (CIN) and classed according to severity (ACS, 2009; Lowdermilk, 2007a):

CIN 1: Mild
CIN 2: Moderate
CIN 3: Severe, to carcinoma in situ (Figure 5-8)

Ovarian cancer is often accompanied by symptoms attributable to other disease processes. It is the leading cause of death from gynecologic malignancies. These tumors are generally epithelial in nature and are associated with a poor prognosis (Figure 5-9). They spread directly to other organs in the pelvic space and distally to the lymphatics, or they seed into the peritoneum (ACS, 2009).

Vulvar cancer (Figure 5-10) represents the fourth most common gynecologic cancer and is typically slow-growing. It appears most often in women in their middle 60s to 70s. In younger women, the incidence is often linked to genital warts (condylomata acuminata) caused by human papillomavirus (HPV). Symptoms include irritation and pruritus in the perineal area or nonhealing lesions (ACS, 2009; Lowdermilk, 2007a).

Vaginal cancer ranks fifth of gynecologic cancers, causing fewer than 1000 deaths per year (ACS, 2009). This form of cancer is rare as a primary diagnosis and is usually an extension of cervical, endometrial, or vulvar cancers. It is generally

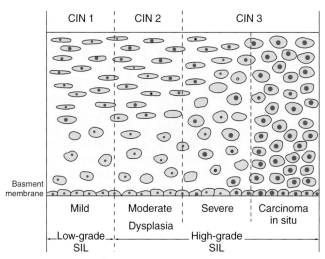

FIGURE 5-8 Diagram of cervical epithelium showing progressive changes and various terms used. *SIL,* Squamous intraepithelial lesion.

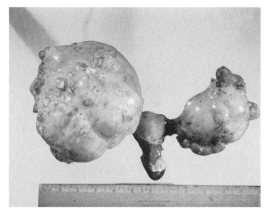

FIGURE 5-9 Bilateral ovarian carcinoma.

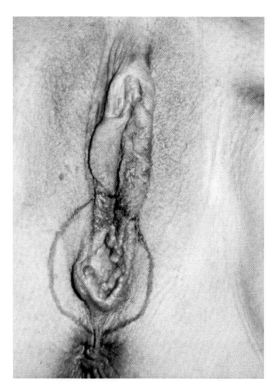

FIGURE 5-10 Vulvar/perineal carcinoma.

asymptomatic in the early stages and may be accompanied by pain, foul-smelling discharge, painless bleeding, pruritus, and urinary symptoms in the later stages (Lowdermilk, 2007a).

Fallopian tube cancer is very rare, with an incidence of less than 1%. It is seen primarily as a metastasis from ovarian and endometrial cancers (Lowdermilk, 2007a).

Other Considerations

Implementation includes gathering the appropriate instruments and patient care supplies, positioning the patient on the OR bed, performing antimicrobial skin preparation, inserting urinary catheters, draping the patient, creating and maintaining a sterile field, initiating safety measures, and monitoring the patient.

Instrumentation. A basic vaginal instrument set is required for vaginal and vulvar surgery. A basic abdominal gynecologic instrument set is required for abdominal gynecologic surgery. Laparoscopic, hysteroscopic, and robotic specific instrumentation may also be used. Surgeons' instrument preferences may vary, and the instrumentation described in this chapter is not meant to be all-inclusive.

For most abdominal gynecologic procedures, a dilation and curettage (D&C) set should be available.

Common instruments used in gynecologic and obstetric surgery are shown in Figures 5-11 through 5-19.

Positioning. Stirrups for the lithotomy position may support only the patient's feet (canvas, fabric, or gel-pad ankle straps) or may cradle and support the thighs, popliteal spaces, and lower legs. Padded cradle stirrups promote maintenance of skin integrity and assist in preventing nerve injury. The surgical team may anticipate that patient positions may be modified based on the surgical procedure and surgeon's preference. The patient is placed in the lithotomy position for most vaginal and vulvar surgery. Careful attention must be focused on placing the patient in the lithotomy position to prevent injury and vascular changes. Seek assistance during positioning the patient in lithotomy to ensure the legs are raised and lowered simultaneously. For abdominal gynecologic surgery, Trendelenburg's position may be used. Some surgeons use the low lithotomy position with the Trendelenburg position for abdominal oncology procedures to facilitate access to pelvic and para-aortic nodes. Patients placed in Trendelenburg's position for prolonged gynecologic procedures are at increased cardiovascular risk because of decreased pulmonary compliance and functional residual capacity (FRC) (Faust et al, 2005). Whenever possible position the patient's arms on padded armboards with the palms up and fingers extended. Armboards are maintained at less than a 90-degree angle to prevent stretching of the brachial plexus. If there are surgical reasons to tuck the arms at the side, the team members pad the patient's elbows to protect the ulnar nerve, face the palms inward, and maintain the wrists in a neutral posi-

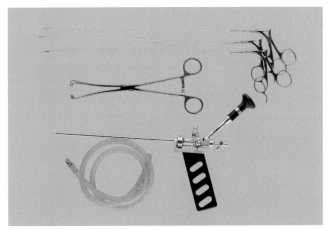

FIGURE 5-11 *Top to bottom:* Multitoothed semirigid grasping forceps, 5 Fr; semirigid Metzenbaum scissors, 5 Fr; semirigid cup biopsy forceps, 5 Fr; Gimpelson tenaculum; 20 degrees angled hysteroscope (adapter, on scope); and cable with adapter.

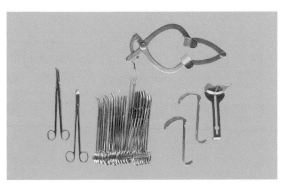

FIGURE 5-13 *Top, right:* 1 O'Sullivan-O'Connor retractor body. *Bottom, left to right:* Mayo dissecting scissors, curved, 9 inch; 1 Jorgenson dissecting scissors, curved, 9 inch; 4 Ochsner hemostatic forceps, 8 inch; 2 Heaney hysterectomy forceps, single tooth; 2 Heaney-Ballantine hysterectomy forceps, single tooth; 4 Ochsner hemostatic forceps, 8 inch; 1 Schroeder uterine tenaculum forceps, single tooth; 1 Schroeder uterine vulsellum forceps, double tooth; 2 Jarit hysterectomy forceps, straight 8½ inch; 2 Jarit hysterectomy forceps, curved 8½ inch; 2 Heaney needle holders; 2 medium blades for O'Sullivan-O'Connor retractor, side view; 1 large blade, front view.

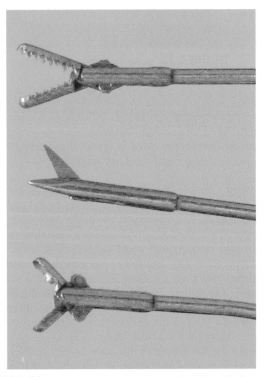

FIGURE 5-12 *Top to bottom:* Enlarged tips of multitoothed semirigid grasping forceps, 5 Fr; semirigid Metzenbaum scissors; and semirigid cup biopsy forceps.

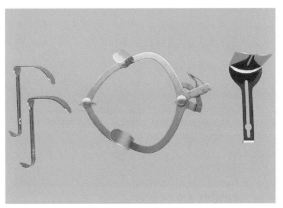

FIGURE 5-14 O'Sullivan-O'Connor retractor with 3 blades.

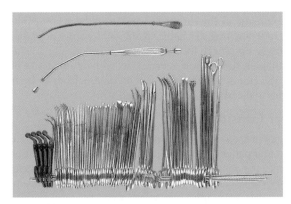

FIGURE 5-15 *Top to bottom:* 1 uterine sound; 1 Yankauer suction tube with tip. *Bottom, left to right:* 4 paper drape clips; 2 Backhaus towel clips; 8 Crile hemostatic forceps, 6½ inch; 4 Halsted hemostatic forceps; 12 Allis tissue forceps; 6 Allis-Adair tissue forceps; 4 tonsil hemostatic forceps; 2 Heanley needle holders; 2 Crile-Wood needle holders, 8 inch; 2 Heaney hysterectomy forceps, single tooth, curved; 2 Heaney-Ballantine hysterectomy forceps, single tooth, curved; 2 Ochsner hemostatic forceps, 8 inch; 2 Allis tissue forceps, long; 2 Babcock tissue forceps, medium; 2 Schroeder uterine tenaculum forceps, single tooth; 1 Schroeder uterine vulsellum forceps, double tooth, straight; 2 Foerster sponge forceps.

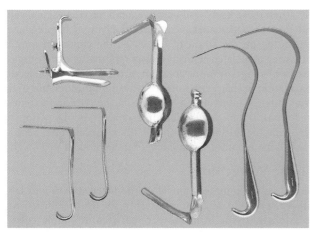

FIGURE 5-16 *Top, left to right:* 1 Graves vaginal speculum; 1 Auvard weighted vaginal speculum, medium lip. *Bottom, left to right:* 2 Heaney retractors; 1 Auvard weighted vaginal speculum, long tip; 2 Deaver retractors, narrow.

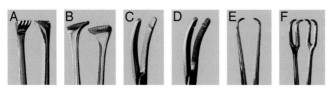

FIGURE 5-17 *Left to right:* Tips: **A,** Allis tissue forceps; **B,** Allis-Adair tissue forceps; **C,** Heaney hysterectomy forceps, single tooth, curved; **D,** Heaney-Ballantine hysterectomy forceps, single tooth, curved; **E,** Schroeder uterine tenaculum forceps, single tooth; **F,** Schroeder uterine vulsellum forceps, double tooth, straight.

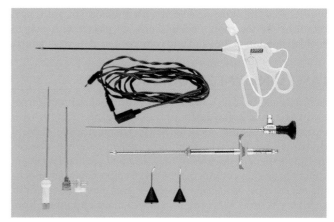

FIGURE 5-18 *Left to right, bottom:* Verres needle stylet with adapter. *Top to bottom:* bipolar forceps; bipolar cord; telescope; Cohen cannula; and two black tips.

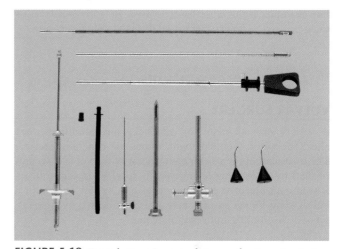

FIGURE 5-19 *Top to bottom:* 1 manipulation probe; 1 suction/irrigation cannula; 1 fallopian ring applicator. *Bottom, left to right:* 1 Cohen cannula, black nipple; 1 reducer cannula, 5 mm; 1 Verres needle stylet, medium; 1 trocar; trumpet-valve cannula; and 2 black Cohen nipples.

tion (Denholm, 2009). A drape secures the arms. It should be tucked snuggly under the patient, not under the mattress. This prevents the arm from shifting downward intraoperatively and resting against the OR bed rail. Care should be taken to protect all patients from integumentary, musculoskeletal, and nerve injury while ensuring adequate circulatory, renal, and respiratory functions.

Because pelvic and vaginal procedures involve manipulation of the ureters, bladder, and urethra, indwelling urinary drainage is frequently established before or during surgery with an indwelling urethral catheter or a suprapubic cystostomy catheter, depending on the type of procedure. The size of sutures, needles, and drains also varies, depending on the surgical procedure, surgeon preference, and patient needs.

Prepping. Care must be taken not to cross-contaminate when prepping multiple areas, such as for an abdominal hysterectomy. Always prep the abdomen before beginning the vaginal prep. Two separate prep trays should be used and the prep setups should be kept separate because the vaginal area is considered a "dirty" area and the abdominal area is considered a "clean" area. Special care must be taken when performing vaginal preps on patients who have been experiencing vaginal bleeding and may have clots in the vaginal vault. The clots and any gross blood on the thighs or vulva should be removed before beginning the prep to allow full contact of the prepping solution.

Examination Under Anesthesia (EUA). Many physicians will perform a pelvic examination after the patient is anesthetized and positioned. Surgical staff should anticipate this exam-

ination and ensure that nonsterile gloves and an appropriate lubricant are available. Culture specimens (e.g., gonococcal, chlamydial, trichomonal) and a Pap smear may be obtained during the examination. Verify with the surgeon that the prep agent and lubricant used are compatible with cytologic evaluation.

Dressings, Drains, and Packing. Various dressings are used in gynecologic surgery and may range from simple (e.g., wound closure tapes) to complex (e.g., multilayer gauze, ostomy appliances, binders). Perineal pads are used after vaginal surgery.

Closed and open drains are used. The surgeon may insert a Penrose drain through the vaginal cuff after a hysterectomy. Indwelling and suprapubic catheters are also commonly employed in gynecologic surgery. All drains and catheters should be secured for patient comfort and to avoid dislodgment. Verify that the patient has no latex allergy, as many of these drains contain latex.

Packing may be used in fistulas or other created cavities or to support and stent the vagina, absorb postoperative drainage, or aid in hemostasis. Products used for vaginal packing can include narrow fine-mesh gauze in various yardage, iodoform packing, and large-mesh gauze. Vaginal packing is usually moistened with saline or coated with antibiotic or antifungal cream before insertion. Packing must be placed with care to avoid distention of the vault and compression of its vasculature.

LASERS IN GYNECOLOGIC SURGERY

Carbon dioxide (CO_2), neodymium:yttrium-aluminum-garnet (Nd:YAG), and argon lasers are used in gynecology to treat extrauterine disease such as pelvic endometriosis, cervical dysplasia, condylomata acuminata, pelvic adhesive disease, and premalignant diseases of the vulva and vagina. Lasers are generally used in conjunction with the colposcope and operating microscope, or the laparoscope. A laser plume evacuator or suction system is necessary to remove smoke and fumes from the operative field (AORN, 2009). All accessories and instrumentation used should be laser-safe and secure, and tested or examined for working order before use. Safety precautions must be implemented by the OR team when the laser is used. For example, if the argon laser is used, pressure-relief valves must be used to prevent increased intraabdominal pressure.

Surgical Interventions

VULVAR SURGERY

A variety of malignant and nonmalignant conditions may affect the vulva. Nonmalignant lesions are generally excised. The treatment of early malignant disease of the vulva is accomplished by a skinning technique, by local wide excision, or, for more multicentric or extensive lesions, by simple or radical vulvectomy. Vulvar surgery may also be indicated in the treatment of vestibulitis and vestibulodynia.

Excision of Condylomata Acuminata

Vulvar/perineal condylomata are caused by the human papillomavirus (HPV) (Figure 5-20) and may be transmitted sexu-

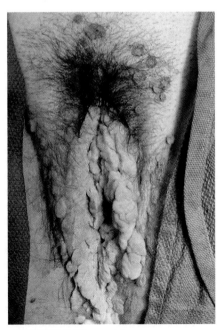

FIGURE 5-20 Condylomata acuminata.

ally. Often these warty lesions will extend into the vaginal vault and may be aggravated by hormonal changes in pregnancy. Depending on the strain of the virus, the condition may be benign or associated with dysplasia and malignancy. Surgical treatment ranges from desiccation of the lesions with electrocoagulation to sharp excision or eradication through use of the laser. Surgical intervention is based on the type and extent of the lesions. If removed by ESU or laser ablation, the perioperative team should take any and all laser precautions, because laser plume is considered a mode of transmission.

Simple Vulvectomy

Simple vulvectomy is removal of the labia majora and labia minora, possibly but not preferably the glans clitoris, and occasionally tissue from the perianal area. A simple vulvectomy is usually done to treat carcinoma in situ of the vulva when it is multicentric. Occasionally a vulvectomy is necessary for the treatment of either leukoplakia or intractable pruritus, especially when a skinning procedure is impractical or has failed.

Procedural Considerations. The basic vaginal instrument set is required, plus an electrosurgical unit (ESU), if desired. The surgical technologist may assist with placing the patient in the lithotomy position and perform a vaginal prep.

Operative Procedure

1. The surgeon incises the affected skin, usually starting anteriorly above the clitoris. The incision is continued laterally to the labia majora, to the midline of the perineum, and around the anus, if it is involved. A knife, hemostats, gauze sponges on sponge-holding forceps, tissue forceps, and Allis forceps are needed. Bleeding vessels are clamped and electrocoagulated or ligated.
2. Periurethral and perivaginal incisions are made. Bleeding of this vascular area can be controlled by means of Kelly or Crile hemostats and the ESU. Ligation of blood vessels should be minimal. Allis-Adair forceps are used for holding diseased tissues.
3. Using curved dissecting scissors, tissue forceps, Allis forceps, and sponges on holding forceps, the surgeon undermines and mobilizes the skin and subcutaneous tissues.
4. The wound is closed, usually by simple bilateral Z-plasty. In some cases, the surgeon excises the skin around the anus to accomplish a sliding skin flap.
5. Closed-wound drainage catheters may be placed in the dependent areas, an indwelling urinary catheter is inserted, and vaginal gauze packing may be placed in the vagina. Dressings are applied.

Skinning Vulvectomy

Skinning vulvectomy is the simple removal of the external skin from the affected area, which has been previously identified with a stain such as toluidine blue. The purpose of this procedure is to preserve the underlying structures of the external genitalia. A skinning procedure may be done to treat leukoplakia, intractable pruritus, or other types of skin lesions, such as kraurosis, vitiligo, and chronic venereal granulomas.

Procedural Considerations. The instrumentation required and patient position are as described for simple vulvectomy.

Operative Procedure. The external skin is simply excised from the affected area (Figure 5-21, *A*).

Radical Vulvectomy and Groin Lymphadenectomy

Radical vulvectomy and groin lymphadenectomy are the en bloc dissection of the following structures: a large segment of skin from the abdomen and groin, the labia majora, the labia minora, the clitoris, the mons veneris, and terminal portions of the urethra, vagina, and other vulvar organs, as well as the superficial and deep inguinal nodes, portions of the round ligaments, portions of the saphenous veins, and the lesion itself. It also involves reconstruction of the vaginal walls and pelvic floor and closure of the abdominal wounds. Full-thickness pinch or split-thickness grafts may be placed if the denuded area of the vulva appears too large for normal granulation. A plastic surgeon may immediately complete skin grafts or rotation flaps to cover defects (see Chapter 13).

Radical vulvectomy and groin lymphadenectomy involve abdominoperineal dissection and groin dissection, which may be performed as a one- or two-stage operation. When performed as a one-stage operation, it is optimally done by a four-person team. The skin prep is extensive, including the abdomen and thighs; if a skin graft will be done, the donor site will also need to be prepped.

Procedural Considerations. The patient lies supine and may be placed in the Trendelenburg's and low lithotomy positions, as required for the various stages. The skin prep includes the abdomen, vulva, and thighs. An indwelling urinary catheter is often inserted to act as a urethral marker and to prevent postoperative urethral trauma. As in other radical surgery, the surgical team should be prepared to measure blood loss and anticipate procedures to combat hypovolemia.

For radical vulvectomy, the basic vaginal instrument set is required, with the addition of assorted sizes of Richardson retractors, Richardson appendectomy retractors, Volkmann rake retractors, skin hooks, and closed-wound drainage systems.

For groin lymphadenectomy, the basic abdominal gynecologic instrument set is required, with the addition of Schnidt tonsil forceps, Kantrowitz thoracic clamps, ligating clips and appliers, and closed-wound drainage systems.

Operative Procedure
RADICAL VULVECTOMY

1. The skin incisions of the abdomen and thigh join with those for vulvectomy. The incisions in the vulva encircle the urethra.
2. In the vulvar dissection, the surgeon removes the terminal portions of the urethra and vagina, the mons veneris, the clitoris, the frenulum, the prepuce of the clitoris, Bartholin's and Skene's glands, and fascial coverings of the vulva with the specimen (Figure 5-21, *B*).
3. Reconstruction of the vaginal walls and the pelvic floor is completed.
4. An indwelling urinary catheter is inserted, closed-wound drainage catheters are placed in the denuded area, and pressure dressings are applied.

GROIN LYMPHADENECTOMY

1. The surgeon makes the first skin incision on the side opposite the primary lesion. The end of the incised skin is

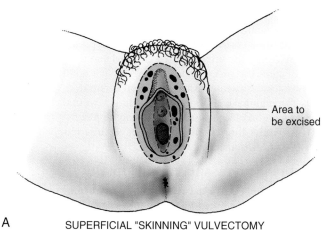

A   SUPERFICIAL "SKINNING" VULVECTOMY

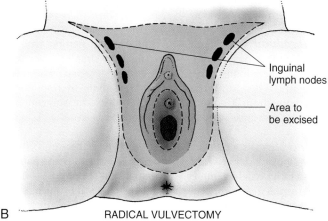

B   RADICAL VULVECTOMY

FIGURE 5-21 Outline of incisions used for (**A**) superficial skinning vulvectomy and (**B**) radical vulvectomy.

grasped with Allis forceps. The incision is extended to the aponeuroses of the external oblique muscle.
2. The fascia over the inguinal ligament and the fascia lata of the upper thigh are exposed, separated, and freed with retractors, knife, scissors, hemostats, and sponges.
3. Bleeding vessels, including the superficial iliac artery and vein, the epigastric artery and vein, and the superficial external pudendal artery and vein, are clamped and ligated. Smaller bleeding vessels are controlled with the ESU.
4. Using Metzenbaum scissors, tissue forceps without teeth, and long-bladed retractors the surgeon resects the fibers of the inguinal, hypogastric, and femoral nerves.
5. The lymphatic node beds may be identified with silk sutures or metal clips. Fine, long, sharp tissue dissection scissors are needed.
6. The large tissue surfaces are exposed for complete dissection by means of retractors and are protected by warm, moist laparotomy packs. High saphenous vein ligation is performed with scissors, forceps, and hemostats and then is doubly tied.
7. The surgeon cleans the femoral canal of its lymphatics; the round ligament is clamped, cut, and ligated.
8. The peritoneum is freed from the muscles; the fascia is dissected free; deep lymphatic nodes and areolar tissue are removed; and vessels and their attachments are clamped,

cut, and ligated, using long curved scissors, long tissue forceps, hemostats, and ligatures.

9. The surgeon removes the lesion. In deep pelvic lymphadenectomy, the ureter may be exposed and the area drained. In some instances, ureteral stents are placed; if that is necessary, cystoscopy instrumentation is required.

10. The inguinal canal is reconstructed, the wound closed with nonabsorbable suture, and dressings applied.

11. An indwelling urethral catheter is inserted before the patient is transferred to the PACU.

Vestibulectomy and Vestibuloplasty

Vestibulodynia is defined as severe pain or burning on vestibular touch or attempted vaginal entry or tenderness localized within the vulvar vestibule. It is often associated with erythema of varying degrees (vestibulitis) (Katz, 2007). Surgical intervention is often successful in relieving the symptoms associated with the condition.

Procedural Considerations. The instrumentation required and patient position are as described for simple vulvectomy. Before the administration of the anesthetic agent, the patient identifies the painful areas of the vestibule in response to pressure from a cotton-tipped applicator. The surgeon may mark these areas with a sterile skin marker.

Operative Procedure. For vestibulectomy, the surgeon uses a #15 blade to excise the vulvar area identified by the patient, carefully avoiding injury to the urethra. The mucosa of the hymen is removed, and the surgeon closes the mucosa and subcutaneous tissue with interrupted absorbable suture. For vestibuloplasty, the procedure is the same but closure is accomplished by advancing a vaginal flap and suturing it to the excision line.

GYNECOLOGIC SURGERY USING VAGINAL APPROACH

Plastic Reconstructive Repair of the Vagina (Anterior and Posterior Repair; Colporrhaphy)

A vaginal repair is done to correct a cystocele or a rectocele and to reestablish the support of the anterior and posterior vaginal walls, restoring the bladder and rectum to their normal positions.

A cystocele is a herniation of the bladder that causes the anterior vaginal wall to bulge downward (Figure 5-22). A defect in the anterior vaginal wall is usually caused by obstetric or surgical trauma, advanced age, or an inherent weakness. A large protrusion may cause a sensation of pressure in the vagina or present a mass at or through the introitus; it may also cause voiding difficulties.

A rectocele occurs when the anterior rectal wall (posterior vaginal wall) protrudes into the vagina. In general, the anterior rectal wall forms a bulging mass beneath the posterior vaginal mucosa (Figure 5-23). As the mass pushes downward into the lower vaginal canal, the rectum may be torn from the fascial and muscular attachments of the urogenital diaphragm and the pelvic wall. The levator ani muscles become stretched or torn. The patient may present with a mass protruding into the vagina, difficulty in evacuating the lower bowel, hemorrhoids, and a feeling of pressure.

An enterocele is a herniation of the pouch and almost always contains loops of the small intestine. An enterocele herniates into a weakened area between the anterior and posterior vaginal walls.

Procedural Considerations. The procedure is done with the patient in the lithotomy position. The basic vaginal instrument set is required. A D&C may be done in conjunction with the repair. Vaginal retractors are used for exposure. The

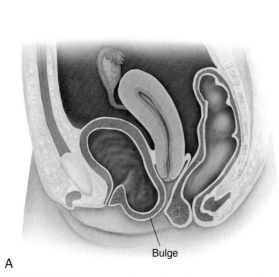

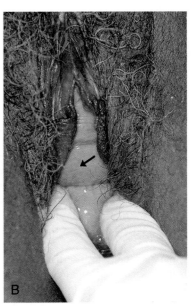

FIGURE 5-22 A, Cystocele resulting from unrepaired tears of muscles of pelvic floor and those under bladder, usually resulting from childbirth, surgical trauma, advanced age, or inherent weakness. **B,** Cystocele (*arrow*).

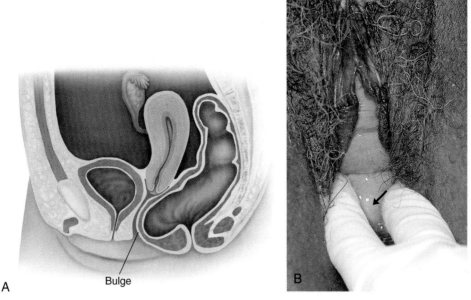

A

Bulge

B

FIGURE 5-23 **A**, Rectocele resulting from unrepaired tears of muscles of pelvic floor and those under bladder, usually resulting from childbirth, surgical trauma, advanced age, or inherent weakness. **B**, Rectocele (*arrow*).

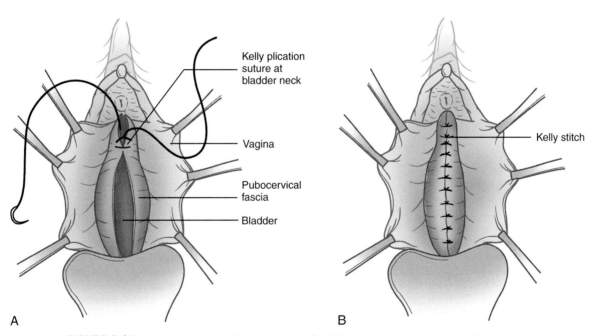

Kelly plication suture at bladder neck

Vagina

Pubocervical fascia

Bladder

Kelly stitch

A

B

FIGURE 5-24 Cystocele repair. **A**, The placement of a Kelly stitch in the pubocervical fascia at the junction of the urethra with the bladder neck. **B**, The repair of the cystocele as the pubocervical fascia is sutured. Thus the cystocele is plicated.

labia may be sutured to the mons pubis if the exposure is inadequate.

Operative Procedure
CYSTOCELE REPAIR

1. The bladder may be drained, or an indwelling urinary catheter or suprapubic cystostomy catheter may be inserted (surgeon's preference). Areolar tissue between the bladder and vagina at the bladder reflection is exposed. The full thickness of the vaginal wall is separated up to the bladder neck by a knife, curved scissors, tissue forceps, Allis-Adair or Allis forceps, and gauze sponges. Bleeding vessels are clamped and tied with ligatures or electrocoagulated.

2. The surgeon mobilizes the urethra and bladder neck with a knife, gauze sponges, and curved scissors.

3. Sutures are placed adjacent to the urethra and bladder neck in such a manner that, after they have been tied, the bladder neck and the posterior urethrovesical angle are narrowed (Figure 5-24, *A*).

4. The surgeon sutures the connective tissue on the lateral aspects of the cervix into the cervix to shorten the cardinal ligaments.
5. Allis-Adair forceps are applied to the edges of the incision, and the left flap of the vaginal wall is drawn across the midline. Edges are trimmed according to the size of the cystocele. The surgeon repeats the process on the right flap of the vaginal incision.
6. The anterior vaginal wall is closed in a manner resulting in reconstruction of an anterior vaginal fornix (Figure 5-24, *B*). Cystoscopy instrumentation may be required to evaluate the integrity of the urethra and ureteral orifices.

RECTOCELE REPAIR

1. The surgeon places Allis forceps posteriorly at the mucocutaneous junction on each side, at the hymenal ring, and just above the anus (Figure 5-25, *A*).
2. Skin and mucosa are incised and dissected from the muscles beneath with a knife, tissue forceps, curved scissors, and gauze sponges.
3. Allis-Adair forceps are placed on the posterior vaginal wall, scar tissue (from obstetric trauma) is removed, and the surgeon continues the dissection to the posterior vaginal fornix and laterally, depending on the size of the rectocele (Figure 5-25, *A* and *B*).
4. The perineum is denuded by sharp dissection, and the trimming of the posterior vaginal wall is carried out with Allis forceps and curved scissors (Figure 5-25, *C*).
5. The rectal wall proximal to the puborectal muscle is strengthened by placement of sutures.
6. Bleeding is controlled, and the surgeon closes the vaginal wall from above, downward to the anterior edge of the puborectal muscle. The rectocele is repaired from the posterior fornix to the perineal body. Remains of the transverse perineal and bulbocavernosus muscles are used to augment the perineum. The anterior edge of the levator ani muscle may be approximated (Figure 5-25, *D*).
7. The mucosa and skin are trimmed, and the remaining closure is performed with interrupted sutures.
8. The vagina may be packed with 2-inch vaginal gauze packing to which antibiotic or antifungal cream may be added. An indwelling urinary catheter or suprapubic cystostomy catheter is inserted, according to the surgeon's preference.

The surgeon will require an additional pair of sterile gloves if a rectal digital exam is performed during the procedure.

ENTEROCELE REPAIR. The procedure is illustrated in Figure 5-26. The peritoneal sac must be carefully dissected from the underlying rectum, the overlying bladder, or both, so that the peritoneal tissues are completely freed from the surrounding structures. The sac is opened to establish true identification and is then closed as high as possible by permanent purse-string sutures. The portion of peritoneal tissue distal to the purse-string ties is then excised, and the area is reinforced locally by transverse suture closures using any available supportive tissues. This technique is used to prevent recurrence.

PERINEAL REPAIR. The procedure is illustrated in Figure 5-27.

VESICOVAGINAL FISTULA REPAIR. A vesicovaginal fistula (a communication between the urinary bladder and the vagina) is repaired by free dissection of the mucosal tissue of the anterior vaginal wall, closing of the fistula tract, and repair of the fascial attachments between the bladder and vagina, with establishment of urinary drainage. Fistulas vary in size from a small opening that permits only slight leakage of urine into the vagina to a large opening that permits all urine to pass into the vagina (Figure 5-28). They may result from radiation therapy, radical surgery for the management of pelvic cancer, chronic ulceration of the vaginal structures, penetrating wounds, or obstetric trauma.

Vesicovaginal Fistula Repair (Transperitoneal Approach)
Procedural Considerations. In the presence of a high vesicovaginal fistula, a suprapubic incision is used. The opening from the bladder into the vagina is closed, and the fascial attachments are repaired.

The patient is supine with a slight Trendelenburg's angle. Ureteral catheters may be inserted just before surgery. An abdominal gynecologic instrument set is required. The vagina is cleansed and may be packed with moist gauze saturated with an antibiotic or antimicrobial solution before the abdominal site is prepped.

Operative Procedure
1. The surgeon makes a midline abdominal incision, as described for laparotomy.
2. The fistulous tract is identified; the vaginal vault and the adjacent adherent bladder are separated using scissors, forceps, and sponges.
3. The vesicovaginal septum is dissected down to healthy tissue beyond the site of the fistula.
4. The fistulous tract is mobilized. The bladder site of the fistula is inverted into the interior of the bladder with two rows of inverting sutures. The muscularis and mucosa layers of the vagina are inverted into the vaginal vault by means of two rows of sutures.
5. Flaps of peritoneum are mobilized, both from the bladder and from the adjacent vaginal vault, and closed to form a new vesicovaginal reflection of peritoneum below the site of the old fistulous tract.
6. The surgeon closes the wound in layers, as for laparotomy. Abdominal dressings are applied.

URETHROVAGINAL FISTULA REPAIR (VAGINAL APPROACH). A urethrovaginal fistula (a communication between the urethra and the vagina) usually causes constant incontinence or difficulty in retaining urine. This condition occurs after damage to the anterior wall and bladder, radiation therapy, or parturition.

Procedural Considerations. The basic vaginal instrument set is required, with the addition of Kelly fistula scissors, dressing forceps, probes, skin hooks, Frazier suction tips, urethral catheters, and sterile water for irrigation. The patient is in the lithotomy position; the team members seek assistance during positioning to safely raise and lower the patient's legs simultaneously to prevent injury.

Operative Procedure
1. After traction sutures are placed around the fistulous tract, the surgeon grasps the tissues with Allis-Adair forceps and plain tissue forceps.
2. The surgeon excises scar tissue around the fistula, locates the cleavage between the bladder and vagina, and mobilizes the flaps using scissors, forceps, and gauze sponges.
3. The bladder mucosa is inverted toward the interior of the bladder with interrupted sutures. The sutures are passed through the muscularis of the bladder down to the mucosa.

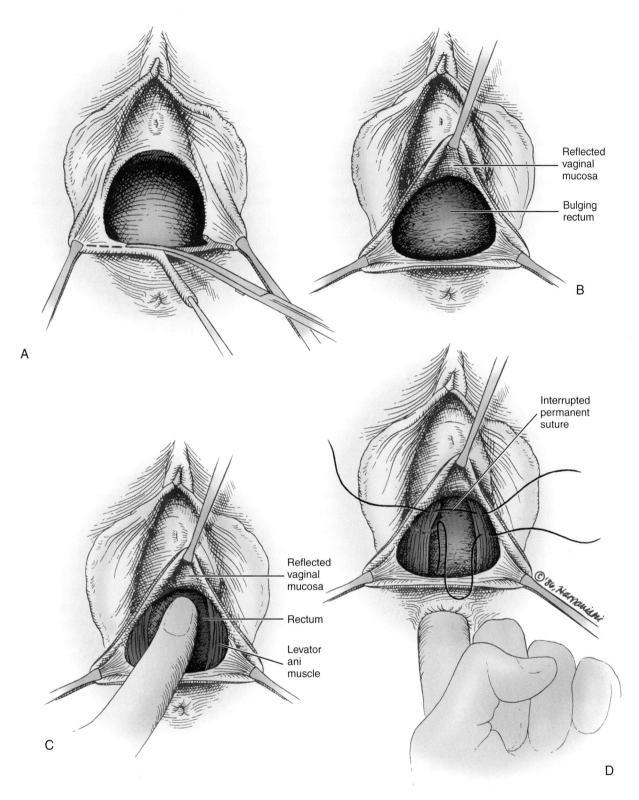

FIGURE 5-25 Rectocele repair. **A,** Placement of Allis clamps at margins of perineal incision; perineal incision is being made. **B,** Reflected vaginal mucosa with rectum bulging. **C,** Depression of rectum identifying margins of levator ani muscle. **D,** Placement of sutures in perirectal tissue and levator ani bundles.

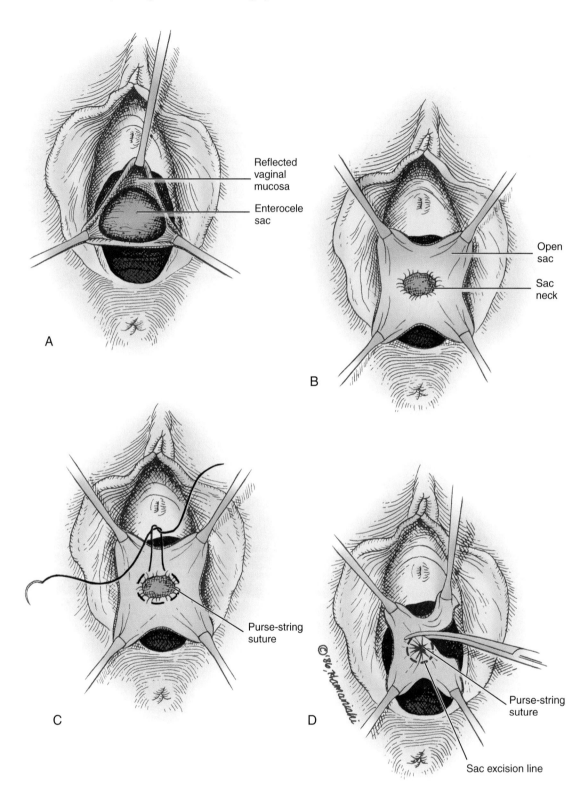

FIGURE 5-26 Enterocele repair. **A**, Appearance of enterocele sac with vaginal wall reflected. **B**, Appearance of open enterocele sac with sac neck identified. **C**, Placement of purse-string suture at neck of enterocele sac. **D**, Excision of enterocele sac.

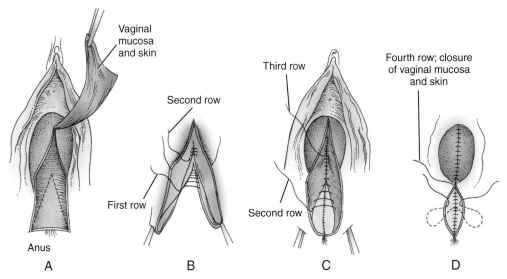

FIGURE 5-27 Repair of complete lacerations of the perineum. **A,** Lower margins of incision. **B,** Placement of first and second rows of sutures. **C,** Second and third rows of sutures. **D,** Fourth row of sutures.

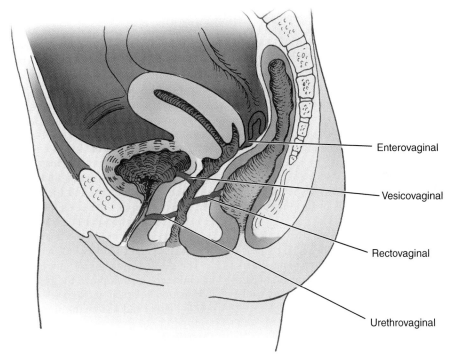

FIGURE 5-28 Genital fistulas may present as communications between the urethra, bladder, one of the ureters, or the bowel and some part of the genital tract. Two of the most common types are urethrovaginal and vesicovaginal, both of which empty into the vaginal canal.

4. A second layer of inverting sutures is placed in the bladder and tied, thereby completely inverting the bladder mucosa toward the interior.
5. The surgeon closes the vaginal wall with interrupted sutures in a direction opposite the closure of the bladder wall.
6. The bladder is distended with sterile saline to determine any leaks. An indwelling urinary catheter is inserted.
   URETEROVAGINAL FISTULA. A ureterovaginal fistula (a communication between the distal ureter and the vagina) develops as a result of injury to the ureter. In some cases, reim-

plantation of the ureter in the bladder or ureterostomy may be done.
   RECTOVAGINAL FISTULA REPAIR (VAGINAL APPROACH). Rectovaginal fistula repair by the vaginal approach includes repair of the perineum, fascia, and muscle-supporting structures between the rectum and vagina, thereby closing the fistula formed between the rectum and the vagina (Figure 5-29). In the presence of a large rectovaginal fistula, as in patients who have incurable cancer, a colostomy may be performed (see Chapter 2). The surgeon will require an addi-

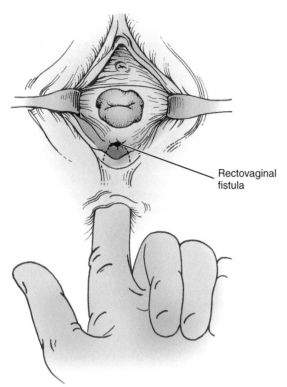

FIGURE 5-29 Rectovaginal fistula. Examiner's finger puts tension on rectovaginal septum.

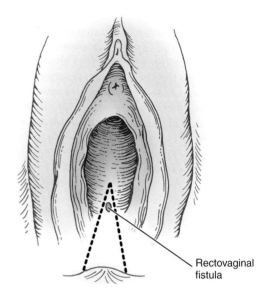

FIGURE 5-30 Repair of rectovaginal fistulas of all types is essentially the same as shown here. Portion of scar tissue to be excised is included within dotted lines; repair is as described for complete lacerations of perineum (see Figure 5-27).

tional pair of sterile gloves if a rectal digital exam is performed during the procedure.

Procedural Considerations. The basic vaginal instrument set is required for a rectovaginal fistula repair. The patient is placed in the lithotomy position.

Operative Procedure

1. The surgeon excises the scar tissue and tract between the rectum and vagina (Figure 5-30); edges of fresh tissue are approximated with absorbable sutures.
2. The rectum and vaginal walls are mobilized; the rectum is closed with inversion of the mucosa into the rectal canal.
3. The vagina is closed transversely or in a sagittal plane different from that of the rectal canal. The vaginal mucosal layer is inverted into the vaginal wall; an indwelling urinary catheter is inserted.

Operations for Urinary Stress Incontinence

Urinary incontinence describes the involuntary loss of urine. The three main types of incontinence include stress urinary incontinence (SUI), urge urinary incontinence (UUI), and mixed incontinence (MI), which describes the presence of both types of urinary incontinence simultaneously. Normal micturition depends on a finely coordinated group of voluntary and involuntary movements. As a result of volitional impulses, voiding may be inhibited or stopped by the intrinsic muscles of the bladder neck and proximal urethra and the puborectalis division of the levator ani muscle.

Previous pelvic procedures may have resulted in scarring and distortion, with displacement of the bladder neck. Conditions such as uterine prolapse, cystocele, urethrocele, cystourethrocele, or urogenital fistulas after radiation therapy may be associated with stress incontinence.

The type of operation selected depends on the severity of stress incontinence, the extent of the condition causing it, the patient's ability to use the anatomic mechanism for voluntary inhibition of urination, and any procedures that have previously been performed. States of stress incontinence are classified in relation to frequency and degree of incontinence, the presence of other diseases, and the function of the pubococcygeal muscle (levator ani). Surgery for urinary stress incontinence entails repair of the fascial supports and the pubococcygeal muscle surrounding the urethra and the bladder neck. This repair is performed through either a vaginal or an abdominal approach. In recent years, retropubic and transobturator suburethral tape has become important in the treatment of stress incontinence (Aschkenazi and Goldberg, 2009).

The desired outcome of any operation for urinary stress incontinence is to improve the performance of a dislodged or dysfunctional vesical neck, to restore normal urethral length, and to tighten and restore the anterior urethral vesical angle.

Operative Procedure

VAGINAL APPROACH

1. An indwelling urinary catheter or suprapubic cystostomy catheter is inserted, according to the surgeon's preference. The posterior vaginal wall is retracted, and the surgeon makes an incision through the anterior vaginal wall down to the urethra and bladder.
2. The vaginal wall is dissected from the bladder and urethra; the neck of the bladder is sutured together. The wound is closed as described for anterior vaginal wall repair.

VESICOURETHRAL SUSPENSION. The Marshall-Marchetti-Krantz procedure is fully described in Chapter 6. Basic steps of the procedure follow:

1. The surgeon enters the space of Retzius through a suprapubic abdominal incision, and frees the bladder and urethra from the underlying structures.

2. Mattress sutures are inserted through the perivaginal fascia on either side of the vesicourethral angle area and preferably at a right angle to the long axis of the urethra and bladder. These are then passed through the central portion of the undersurface of the symphysis pubis under direct vision. The application of the sutures to the perivaginal connective tissue is done with the surgeon's hand in the vagina to ensure that the suture material is not passed through the vaginal mucosa.
3. The wound is closed and may be drained if the vascularity of the area warrants. An abdominal dressing is applied.

Construction of a Vagina

Two basic approaches are used for repairing or overcoming a congenital or surgical defect of the vagina: obtaining a skin graft, which is applied to a mold and placed in the area of vaginal reconstruction; or making a simple opening in the area of vaginal reconstruction and placing a mold to permit spontaneous epithelialization of the area.

Procedural Considerations. For a skin graft, the plastic surgery instrument set (see Chapter 13) is required, with the addition of a dermatome, marking pen, and nonadherent gauze dressing. For vaginal construction, the basic vaginal instrument set is required, with the addition of iris scissors, skin hooks, a vaginal mold, Halsted mosquito hemostats, and a ruler.

Operative Procedure
1. The skin graft is taken from the abdomen or anterior area of the thigh. The donor site is dressed in the routine manner with nonadherent gauze and a pressure dressing.
2. The skin graft is kept in a moist gauze sponge until it is ready to be used.
3. The surgeon uses sharp dissection to create a vaginal orifice, taking care to prevent damage to the rectum and bladder. A mold is used to apply the donor skin or simply to hold the dissected area open to permit spontaneous epithelialization (Figure 5-31).

Trachelorrhaphy

Trachelorrhaphy is removal of torn surfaces of the anterior and posterior cervical lips and reconstruction of the cervical canal. It is performed to treat deep lacerations of a cervix that is relatively free from infection.

Procedural Considerations. The basic vaginal instrument set is required, plus the ESU and a conization loop electrode, if desired. An indwelling urinary catheter may be inserted into the bladder, depending on the surgeon's preference. The patient is in the lithotomy position.

Operative Procedure
1. The labia may be retracted with Allis-Adair tissue forceps or sutures. The surgeon grasps the cervix with a tenaculum.
2. The tissue of the exocervix is denuded with a knife. Using sharp dissection, the surgeon undermines the flaps. Bleeding vessels are clamped and ligated. The mucosa is dissected from the cervix.
3. A small distal portion of the cervical canal is coned with a knife or a loop electrode to remove tissue. Bleeding vessels are clamped and ligated.

4. The denuded and coned areas are covered by transversely suturing the mucosal flaps of the exocervix, using interrupted sutures. Tissue forceps, hemostats, and gauze sponges are needed. The sutures are placed in such a manner that the fibromuscular tissue of the cervix is included, thereby eliminating dead space where a hematoma may form, and providing a complete reconstructed cervical canal.
5. A vaginal pack may be inserted. A perineal pad is applied.

Dilation of the Cervix and Curettage (D&C)

D&C is done either for diagnostic purposes or as a form of therapy for a variety of pelvic conditions, such as abnormal uterine bleeding, or primary dysmenorrhea. D&C may also be performed when carcinoma of the endometrium is suspected, in the study of infertility, before amputation of the cervix, or before surgery for a prolapsed uterus. A common indication for D&C is incomplete abortion (e.g., miscarriage), or therapeutic abortion. The surgical team should be especially sensitive to the emotional needs of a patient experiencing a miscarriage (Box 5-1).

Procedural Considerations. In D&C, instruments are introduced through the vagina for the purpose of dilating the cervix. Dilation of the cervix can also take place by inserting laminaria tents into the cervical os before surgery; these tents are removed immediately before the procedure. The patient is in the lithotomy position for this procedure; the perioperative nurse ensures assistance is available for positioning.

Operative Procedure
1. The surgeon places a Jackson or Auvard weighted speculum in the vagina. A Sims or Deaver retractor is placed anteriorly to expose the cervix. The anterior lip of the cervix is grasped with a tenaculum (Figure 5-32).
2. The direction of the cervical canal and the depth of the uterine cavity are determined by means of a blunt probe or graduated uterine sound.
3. The surgeon dilates the cervix using graduated Hegar or Hank dilators and/or a Goodell uterine dilator.
4. Exploration for pedunculated polyps or myomas may be done with a polyp forceps.
5. Using a sharp curette the surgeon scrapes the interior of the cervical canal and uterine cavity to obtain either a fractional or a routine specimen. For specific identification of the site of specimens, the endocervix is scraped with the curette first, and the specimen is separated from the curetted matter of the uterine endometrium. In a routine curettage, all curetted matter is sent together for identification of tissue cells.
6. Fragments of endometrium or other dislodged tissues may be removed with warm, moist gauze sponges on sponge-holding forceps or with a teaspoon.
7. The surgeon may take multiple punch biopsies of the cervical circumference (at the 3, 6, 9, and 12 o'clock positions) with a Gaylor biopsy forceps to supplement the diagnostic studies.
8. Retractors are withdrawn; iodoform or plain gauze packing may be inserted into the uterus, using dressing forceps. The tenaculum is removed from the cervix. A vaginal pack may be inserted. A perineal pad is applied.

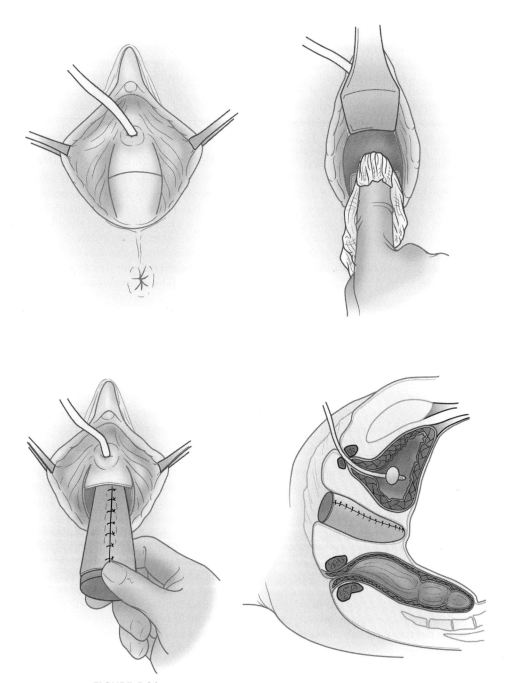

FIGURE 5-31 Vaginal reconstruction using split-thickness skin graft.

Suction Curettage

Suction curettage is vacuum aspiration of the uterine contents. Aspiration has proved to be a safe and effective method for early termination of pregnancy and for use in missed and incomplete spontaneous abortions. Advantages are smaller dilation of the cervix, less damage to the uterus, less blood loss, less chance of uterine perforation, and reduced danger of infection. Laminaria tents may be inserted approximately 4 to 24 hours before suction curettage to dilate the cervix; they are removed before the surgical prep begins. Suction curettage is the treatment of choice for benign gestational trophoblastic neoplasia, more commonly known as hydatidiform mole. Hydatidiform mole is a condition that arises from fertilization by the sperm in a defective egg that has no nucleus or fertilization of the egg by two sperm. This results in the synthesis of material that is termed a mole and consists of multiple fluid-filled vesicles resembling a cluster of grapes (Figure 5-33).

Procedural Considerations. The instrumentation required includes the D&C set, with the addition of one set of Pratt,

BOX 5-1

Supporting Patients through Miscarriage or Stillbirth

A diagnosis of pregnancy is often a joyous occasion; however, many women can experience perinatal loss, which is defined as ectopic pregnancy, miscarriage, or fetal death. Miscarriage occurs in approximately 15% of all pregnancies, and approximately 5 of every 1000 births result in stillbirth or fetal death (e.g., those occurring after 20 weeks of gestation). The primary cause of miscarriage and infant death is birth defects (127.6 per 100,000 births). Perinatal loss may occur with little or no advance warning for the mother, and unfamiliar and invasive procedures at this time can increase the woman's sense of vulnerability. The OB/surgical staff can play a sensitive and supportive role when providing care for patients who present to the OR with miscarriage or cesarean section for stillbirth.

By definition, a miscarriage is a pregnancy loss that occurs before 20 weeks of gestation. In the United States, state laws often stipulate that, in addition, the weight of the fetus is less than 350 g and signs of life are absent. Abortion is the medical term used for both spontaneous and elective pregnancy termination occurring before 20 weeks of gestation. Terms used to identify the diagnosis should also be carefully chosen. Many women find the term abortion harsh and unkind when referring to spontaneous events. Some may feel insulted or misunderstood, believing that abortion refers only to an elective procedure. The term miscarriage is more neutral and should be used consistently for early loss. Products of conception are better referred to as tissue and the embryo or fetus as baby. For infant death, use the words "dead and died" rather than "lost." Also, avoid the use of clinical terminology as this may convey a lack of sincere feeling on the part of the caregiver.

If discussing perinatal loss with a woman, the OB/surgical staff may want to initiate the conversation by referring to the pregnancy and listening for the patient's use of either the terms pregnancy or baby when referring to the loss. The staff's neutrality encourages the woman to express her feelings without being encumbered by what she "should" do and what she "should" feel and eliminates the perceived expectations negatively influencing the woman. Additional tips for communicating with parents include the use of phrases and open-ended questions such as follows:

- "I am sad for you."
- "How are you coping with all of this?"
- "I am sorry for your loss."
- "I am here, and I want to listen."
- "What can I do for you?"
  The following phrases should be avoided:
- "Be thankful you have another child."
- "I know how you feel."
- "You have to keep going."
- "You're young and you can have others."
- "Better for this to happen now, before you knew the baby."
- "There was something wrong with the baby anyway."

Compiled from Gilbert ES: *Manual of high risk pregnancy and delivery*, ed 4, St Louis, 2007, Mosby; Miles MS: Grieving the loss of a newborn. In Lowdermilk DL, Perry SE, editors: *Maternity and women's health care*, ed 9, St Louis, 2007, Mosby; March of Dimes: *Perinatal statistics*, available at www.marchofdimes.com/peristats/. Accessed June 28, 2009.

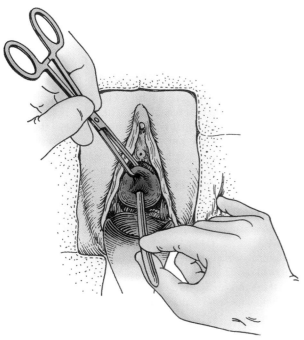

FIGURE 5-32 Dilation of cervix and curettage. Vaginal wall retracted; cervix held by tenaculum; cervix dilated with dilator. Uterine cavity curetted with sharp curettes.

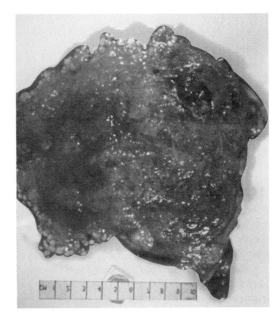

FIGURE 5-33 Hydatidiform mole. Note vesicles have appearance of grapes.

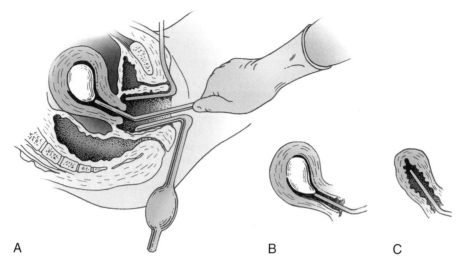

FIGURE 5-34 Suction curettage. **A**, Insertion of cannula. **B**, Gentle suction motion to aspirate contents. **C**, Uterine contents evacuated.

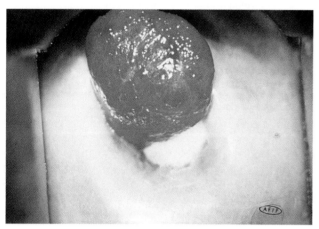

FIGURE 5-35 Cervical polyp. A large polyp protrudes from the external cervical os.

Hawkin, or Hank uterine dilators, placenta forceps, urethral catheter, sterile cannulae, aspirator tubing, a vacuum aspirator unit, and oxytocic drugs. The patient will be in the lithotomy position.

Operative Procedure

1. The surgeon exposes the cervix with an Auvard weighted speculum and an anterior retractor, grasps it with a sharp tenaculum, and draws it toward the introitus.
2. The cervix is dilated, allowing 1 mm of cannula diameter for each week of pregnancy.
3. The appropriate-size cannula is inserted into the uterus until the sac is encountered. The suction is turned on with immediate disruption and aspiration of the contents. Continued gentle motion of the cannula removes the uterine contents (Figure 5-34). Use of uterine curettes may supplement suction in removing the entire uterine contents.
4. Retractors and tenaculum are removed.
5. A perineal pad is applied.

Removal of Pedunculated Cervical Myomas (Cervical Polyps)

Cervical polyps (small pedunculated lesions) stem from the endocervical canal and consist almost entirely of columnar epithelium with or without squamous metaplasia (Figure 5-35). They may vary in size and are soft, red, and friable. Bleeding may result from the slightest trauma. Pedunculated lesions may be removed by the snare method or by dissection from the cervical canal with a knife, cold-knife conization, or resectoscope. Usually the surgeon performs an endometrial and endocervical curettage, and a cytologic smear is taken.

Procedural Considerations. A D&C set, a tonsil snare with medium-size snare wire, glass slides, the ESU, and a blade electrode or resectoscope are required. The patient is in the lithotomy position.

Operative Procedure

1. The surgeon grasps the anterior lip of the cervix with a Jacobs vulsellum or a tenaculum. The canal is sounded and dilated either to visualize or to palpate the base of the pedicle.
2. If the pedicle of the polyp is thin, the surgeon may place a tonsil snare over the body of the tumor, permitting the snare to crush the base of the tumor and to control bleeding. If the polyp is large, its base is dissected out with a knife. Bleeding may be controlled by the use of warm, moist gauze sponges with or without electrocoagulation. A resectoscope with the use of electrosurgery may be used to dissect the tumor.
3. Iodoform or plain gauze packing may be introduced into the cervical os. The tenaculum is removed from the cervix, and the retractors are withdrawn. A vaginal pack may be inserted for hemostasis. A perineal pad is applied.

Conization and Biopsy of the Cervix

Conization and biopsy of the cervix are generally performed for the diagnosis or treatment of cervical dysplasia. The procedure may be initiated with colposcopy and punch biopsy, followed by electrocoagulation, cryosurgery, cold-knife cone

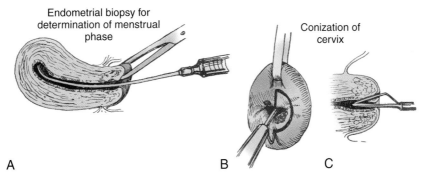

FIGURE 5-36 **A**, Endometrial biopsy technique. **B** and **C**, Conization loop used to treat cervical conditions or obtaining specimens for diagnostic tests.

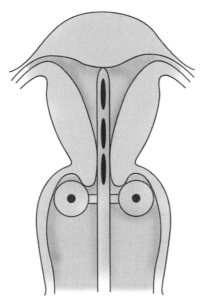

FIGURE 5-37 Intracavitary implant. Applicator in place in uterus.

biopsy, loop electrosurgical excision cone (LEEC), or laser excisional cone.

Procedural Considerations. The instruments required include a D&C set along with an ESU or laser, conization electrical loop, and ball-tipped electrode, depending on the procedure. The patient is in the lithotomy position.

Operative Procedure

1. The surgeon retracts the posterior vaginal wall with a speculum and the anterior vaginal wall with lateral retractors. The outer portions of the cervix are grasped with a tenaculum, and the cervix is drawn toward the introitus. Cystic areas of the cervix may be treated with a needle electrode or laser. Endometrial biopsy may be done (Figure 5-36, *A*). Bleeding points are coagulated or lased.
2. The electrode is passed into the cervical canal, and the diseased tissue is treated. Ferric subsulfate (Monsel's solution) may be used for hemostasis.
3. The surgeon uses the electrical loop (Figure 5-36, *B* and *C*) or the laser to remove the diseased tissue and obtain a histologic specimen for pathologic diagnosis.

4. If a wide conization is performed, the cervix may be sutured and vaginal packing may be used. An indwelling urinary catheter may be inserted. A perineal pad is applied.

Cesium Applicator Insertion for Cervical and Endometrial Malignancy

Cesium has generally replaced radium insertions for treatment of malignancy of the cervix and endometrium.

Procedural Considerations. The patient is in the lithotomy position. The bladder is drained with an indwelling urinary catheter. The catheter balloon is inflated with a radiopaque medium for radiographic visualization after insertion of the cesium. An indwelling rectal marker is also placed by the surgeon for radiographic visualization. Various types of cesium applicators may be used according to the surgeon's preference and the area of malignancy (Figure 5-37). The cesium is loaded into the applicators later in the radiation department or in the patient's room under controlled conditions, in which all personnel are monitored by use of a dosimeter.

Interstitial Therapy. Cesium needles are available in various lengths with small diameters for insertion into the tissue surrounding the cervix (Figure 5-38). They are inserted vaginally with a needle applicator and are used as a supplement to intravaginal or intrauterine sources. To facilitate removal, the needles have wires or threads attached to their distal ends.

Marsupialization of Bartholin Duct Cyst or Abscess

A cyst in a Bartholin gland usually follows acute infection and is treated by marsupialization. Such cysts result from retention of glandular secretions caused by blockage in the duct system (Figure 5-39). Marsupialization of a Bartholin duct cyst or abscess entails removal or incision of the cyst through the vaginal outlet and drainage of the area. In true marsupialization the cyst is surgically exteriorized by resecting the anterior wall and suturing the cut edges of the remaining cyst to the adjacent edges of the skin.

Procedural Considerations. The basic vaginal instrument set is required, with the addition of a 15-gauge needle, syringe, culture tubes (aerobic and anaerobic), iodoform or plain gauze packing, and a drain, if desired by the surgeon.

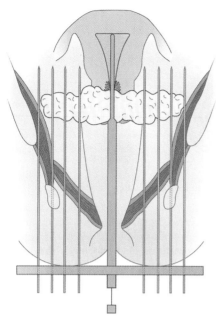

FIGURE 5-38 Interstitial intracavitary implant.

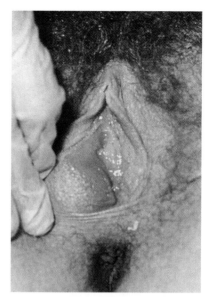

FIGURE 5-39 Bartholin abscess.

Operative Procedure

1. The labia minora may be sutured to the perineal skin on each side to expose the vaginal introitus.
2. A stellate incision is then made into the mucosa, which is distended over the cyst.
3. The surgeon dissects the cyst wall and, if indicated, removes the gland with blunt-pointed scissors. The tissue may be everted with sutures and left open. A drain or packing may be inserted, and a perineal pad is applied.

Vaginal Hysterectomy

Vaginal hysterectomy is removal of the uterus through an incision made in the vaginal wall and the pelvic cavity (History box). Contraindications to a vaginal approach are (1) a large uterine tumor, (2) a pelvic malignancy, and (3) the possibility of overlooked metastatic disease that might be present if malignancy is suspected.

Procedural Considerations. The instrumentation includes the basic vaginal instrument set with the addition of two 22-gauge needles and two 10-ml syringes. An abdominal gynecologic instrument set should be available in case laparotomy is indicated. To facilitate dissection and decrease bleeding, the vaginal walls may be infiltrated with normal saline or a local anesthetic (vasoconstrictors are optional). The patient is in the lithotomy position.

Operative Procedure

1. The labia may be retracted with sutures. The surgeon places a weighted vaginal retractor to retract the vaginal wall.
2. A Jacobs vulsellum, tenaculum, or suture ligature is placed through the cervical lips to permit traction on the cervix.
3. The surgeon incises the anterior vaginal wall with a knife through the full thickness of the wall (Figure 5-40, *A*). A circumferential saline with epinephrine injection of the

submucosa may be done at this point in the procedure. The bladder is then freed from the anterior surface of the cervix by sharp and blunt dissection. The bladder is then elevated to expose the peritoneum of the anterior cul-de-sac, which is entered by sharp dissection (Figure 5-40, *B*).

4. The peritoneum of the posterior cul-de-sac is identified and incised.
5. The surgeon clamps, cuts, and ligates the uterosacral ligaments (Figure 5-40, *C* and *D*). The ends of the ligatures are left long and are tagged with a clamp.
6. The uterus is drawn downward, and the bladder is held aside with retractors and moist, small laparotomy packs.
7. The surgeon clamps, cuts, and ligates the cardinal ligaments on each side. The uterine arteries are doubly clamped, cut, and ligated.
8. The fundus is delivered with the aid of a uterine tenaculum.
9. When the ovaries are not removed, the surgeon clamps and cuts the round ligament, the utero-ovarian ligament, and the fallopian tube on each side (Figure 5-40, *E*) and removes the uterus. These pedicles are then ligated.
10. The surgeon reapproximates the peritoneum between the rectum and vagina with a continuous suture. The retroperitoneal obliteration of the cul-de-sac is accomplished by passing sutures from the vaginal wall through the infundibulopelvic ligament and round ligament, through the cardinal ligament, and out the vaginal wall. The sutures are tied on the vaginal aspect of the new vault (Figure 5-40, *F* and *G*). The round, cardinal, and uterosacral ligaments may be individually approximated for additional support.
11. Any existing cystocele and rectocele and the perineum are repaired. In the presence of prolapse, reconstruction of the pelvic floor may be required.
12. An indwelling urethral or suprapubic catheter is usually inserted. The vagina may be packed, and a drain may be inserted. A perineal pad is applied.

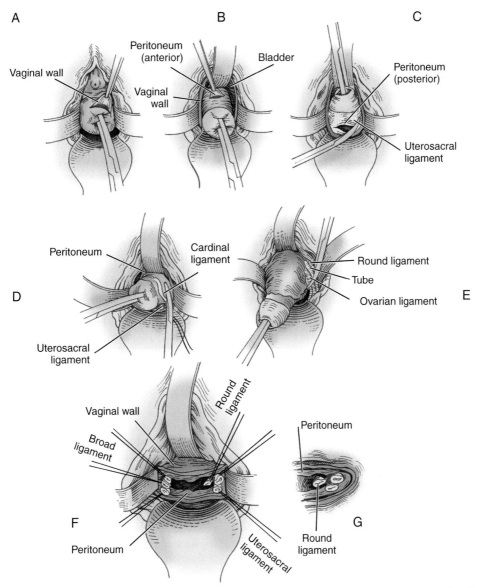

FIGURE 5-40 Vaginal hysterectomy. **A,** Incision of vaginal wall around cervix. Anterior vaginal wall slightly elevated. **B,** Deaver retractor on each side; one Deaver retractor under bladder. Peritoneum opened. **C,** Posterior cul-de-sac opened. Heaney clamp applied to left uterosacral ligament. **D,** Left uterosacral ligament cut and tied. Clamp applied to left cardinal ligament. **E,** Clamp applied to ovarian ligament, round ligament, and fallopian tube. **F,** Uterosacral ligament, broad ligament, and round ligament shown in their respective normal positions. **G,** Peritoneum closed and cardinal ligament, broad ligament, and uterosacral ligament reattached to angle of vagina. Left uterosacral and broad ligaments anchored.

GYNECOLOGIC SURGERY USING MINIMALLY INVASIVE TECHNIQUES

Hysteroscopy

Hysteroscopy is the endoscopic visualization of the uterine cavity and tubal orifices. The common indications for hysteroscopy include evaluation of abnormal uterine bleeding (with possible endometrial ablation), location and removal of "lost" intrauterine devices (IUDs), evaluation of infertility, diagnosis and surgical treatment of intrauterine adhesions, verification of submucous leiomyomas or endometrial polyps, resection of uterine septa or submucous leiomyomas, and tubal sterilization.

Laparoscopy may be done in association with hysteroscopy to assess the external contour of the uterus. Contraindications to either diagnostic or operative hysteroscopy include pelvic infection, cervical malignancy, and, in some instances, heavy bleeding.

A significant potential complication related to hysteroscopy is the intravasation of the fluid used to distend the uterine cavity. Intravasation can lead to hyponatremia. Signs and symptoms of hyponatremia may include bradycardia, hypertension followed by hypotension, nausea, vomiting, headache, visual disturbances, agitation, confusion, and lethargy. The surgical staff is responsible for accurately monitoring fluid intake and output

HISTORY

A Historical Look at Vaginal Hysterectomy

Women undergoing vaginal hysterectomy in the 1900s did so without the benefit of technology available today. The woman was admitted to the hospital several days in advance of the planned surgical procedure. Vigorous bowel preparation and thrice-daily douches with caustic solutions were a routine preoperative preparation, as was the removal of all hair from the abdomen and genitalia.

On the day of surgery, a douche was administered before transporting the patient into the OR. After positioning the patient for the procedure, green soap was used to cleanse the vulva and vaginal canal, followed by a rinse of saline and a douche of 10% creolin. The creolin was followed by an additional douche of corrosive sublimate in a 1:2000 concentration in sterile water. A glass catheter was placed to ensure the patient's bladder was empty before the start of the procedure.

During the vaginal hysterectomy, the surgeon controlled the patient's bleeding with clamps or ligatures. After the uterus was removed, as many as six clamps, which were equipped with detachable handles, were left in place for hemostasis. The clamps were surrounded with a roll of iodoform gauze extending up into the vagina. A retention catheter was placed in the bladder at the end of the procedure. The catheter would be used in the postoperative period for bladder irrigations.

Before the patient returned to consciousness, the patient's legs were tied with a broad towel to prevent strain on the clamps and any ligatures that had been placed. The towel was not removed until the patient regained consciousness and was able to cooperate.

The patient was transported back to her room, with the clamps in place, experiencing considerable pain. Two days after the procedure, the surgeon removed the clamps. The previously placed gauze packing was removed. The surgeon reattached the handles to the clamps and began removal, using a rocking motion, starting with the uppermost clamp. As the clamps were released, pieces of tissue would adhere, causing great discomfort for the patient. The healthcare personnel assisted the surgeon with repacking the patient's vagina with gauze and then returned the clamps, which were coated with rust, tissue, and secretions, to the instrument room.

The patient was allowed to sit up in bed 2 days after the clamps were removed; she was lifted to a chair on the fourth day, and began to ambulate on the fifth or sixth day.

Modified from Fowler R: *The operating room and the patient,* ed 3, St Louis, 1913, Mosby; Haubold HA: *Preparatory and after treatment in operative cases,* New York, 1910, D Appleton & Co.

---

during hysteroscopy. Monitoring may be manual (i.e., calculating the difference between inflow and outflow) or may be automatically calculated on commercially available hysteroscopy pumps, which decrease the chance of human error. Discrepancies of 500 ml or more must be communicated to the surgeon and the anesthesia provider (Cheong and Ledger, 2007).

Procedural Considerations. The instrumentation required includes a D&C set, with the addition of a hysteroscopy set, 50-ml syringes, polyethylene tubing, fiberoptic light source, the ESU or laser, hysteroscopic insufflator, pressure-infusion pump, and a video camera and monitor. The patient will be in the lithotomy position.

Operative Procedure

1. The surgeon places an Auvard weighted speculum and an anterior retractor to expose the cervix; the anterior lip of the cervix is grasped with a tenaculum and is drawn toward the introitus.
2. The direction of the cervical canal and the depth of the uterine cavity are determined by means of a graduated uterine sound.
3. The surgeon dilates the endocervical canal with graduated Hegar or Hank uterine dilators to 6, 7, or 8 mm, depending on the size of the hysteroscope.
4. A self-retaining vacuum cannula with obturator may be placed into contact with the cervix. The cannula is firmly applied to the cervix by vacuum created with a negative pressure.
5. The surgeon withdraws the obturator and introduces the hysteroscope to the level of the internal cervical os.
6. To achieve satisfactory visualization and sustained intrauterine pressure, the uterine cavity must be distended with one of the following media: 32% dextran 70 in dextrose (Hyskon), dextrose 5% in water (D_5W), sorbitol, mannitol, saline (normal saline solution [NSS]), sterile water, or by CO_2 gas insufflation. Because air or gas used for uterine insufflation may result in air or gas embolism, CO_2 pressures must be monitored closely. Injection of liquid media may be under continuous pressure from a 50-ml syringe or delivered by means of a pressure-controlled fluid-infusion (hysteroscopic) pump into the irrigating channel of the hysteroscope. When the syringe is used, care must be taken to prevent air bubbles, which distort the view or could lead to air embolism. Uterine distention with D_5W may be achieved by inserting a 500-ml plastic bag containing the medium into an intravenous pressure infusor or the infusion pump. The fluid runs freely within polyethylene tubing through the channel of the hysteroscope.
7. Exploration of the uterine cavity is begun. A video camera monitor may be used to enhance visibility for the OR team, and the procedure may be videotaped for record keeping and reevaluation.
8. The surgeon may introduce ancillary instruments, such as rigid and flexible biopsy forceps, scissors, grasping forceps, insulated coagulation electrodes, resectoscope with "rollerball" electrode, laser fiber tips, and tubal occlusive devices, for intrauterine manipulation or surgical intervention through the operating channel of the hysteroscope.
9. On completion of the procedure, the hysteroscope is withdrawn and the self-retaining vacuum cannula is removed.

If Hyskon is used for uterine distention, the instruments must be rinsed immediately and cleaned in hot water, because dextran has a tendency to harden and is difficult to remove if permitted to dry.

Endometrial Ablation

Endometrial ablation is performed to treat abnormal uterine bleeding. The overall goal of endometrial ablation is to create amenorrhea or to reduce menstrual bleeding to a normal, tolerable flow for the patient. It may be an alternative to hysterectomy in some patients with chronic menorrhagia. The procedure is performed through the hysteroscope with the use of either the laser, ESU, or microwave energy.

The Nd:YAG laser destroys the endometrium and results in scarring of the uterine lining. It is often the laser of choice for this procedure because of its ability to penetrate deep into the tissue, resulting in greater tissue destruction. The Nd:YAG, argon, and potassium titanyl phosphate (KTP) 532 lasers may be used hysteroscopically.

The two endometrial ablation techniques used with the Nd:YAG laser are *blanching* and *dragging*. In the blanching technique, the tip of the laser fiber is held away from tissue. In the dragging technique, the laser fiber tip is in direct contact with the endometrium. The endometrial lining is treated from the fundus to approximately 4 cm above the external cervical os. Air or gas is not used in cooling the laser fiber because of the risk of air or gas embolism. Because of the systemic effects of fluid absorption through open capillaries, Hyskon is not generally used as an irrigant for endometrial laser ablation.

A specially designed diode laser may also be used for endometrial ablation. The diode laser utilizes a disposable handset that emits laser beams through three separate parallel panels. The handset conforms to the shape of the uterus and delivers energy in all directions to destroy the tissue in the fundus and cornua, away from the cervical opening. A hysteroscopy may be performed at the conclusion of the therapy to evaluate the results.

Electrical energy delivered through an adapted urologic resectoscope, using continuous-flow irrigation, either coagulates or resects the endometrium. Endometrial ablation with the use of a resectoscope, with a rollerball electrode attached, is not an option for a patient who desires to remain fertile. When using the resectoscope, often Hyskon is chosen as the distending medium because it is electrolyte-free and compatible with electrosurgery.

Reported complications associated with endometrial ablation using the Nd:YAG laser and electrosurgery include hemorrhage, fluid overload, uterine perforation, recurrent bleeding, injury to bowel and bladder, cervical lacerations, and rupture of a fallopian tube.

A general anesthetic is usually administered, although endometrial ablation can be performed using a local anesthetic. If the Nd:YAG laser is to be used, ensure all laser safety precautions for the patient and the OR team are followed. The length of the procedure is typically less than that for a hysterectomy. Therefore the patient requires less anesthetic and may be discharged the same day, provided that her condition remains stable.

Balloon Endometrial Ablation. Endometrial ablation may also be accomplished using balloon therapy. The action of balloon therapy is thermal. The uterine balloon catheter conforms to the internal uterine contour and contains a heating element. The surgeon performs suction curettage before the therapy to provide maximal balloon contact with the uterine lining. The cervix is dilated to 5 mm, and the balloon catheter is inserted in the uterus until the tip touches the fundus. The surgeon inflates the balloon with sterile D_5W to a pressure of 160 to 180 mm Hg. The solution is heated to a temperature of 86.6° C (188° F) and maintained for 8 to 10 minutes. The procedure may be performed as an ambulatory surgical procedure and does not require hysteroscopy (Practice Committee, 2008).

Laparoscopy

Laparoscopy is the endoscopic visualization of the peritoneal cavity through the anterior abdominal wall after the establishment of a pneumoperitoneum. It is used to investigate and diagnose the causes of abdominal and pelvic pain and infertility and to evaluate pelvic masses. Ancillary procedures such as adhesiolysis, fulguration of endometriotic implants (Figure 5-41), aspiration of cysts, biopsy of tissue, aspiration of peritoneal fluid for cytologic study, ovarian biopsy, ovarian cystectomy, oophorectomy, removal of ectopic pregnancy, tuboplasty, and tubal sterilization may be performed. Laparoscopy also can be used for oocyte retrieval for IVF procedures. Lasers and electrosurgery may be used with the laparoscope.

Procedural Considerations. Although laparoscopy can be performed with a local anesthetic, more often the anesthesia provider administers a general anesthetic. Place the patient in the lithotomy position. The abdomen, perineum, and vagina are prepped. The abdomen and perineum are then draped for a combined procedure. Specially designed drapes with openings for the umbilical and perineal areas may be used. The bladder should be emptied with an in-and-out catheterization or through insertion of a Foley catheter.

The surgeon may perform a D&C in conjunction with laparoscopic procedures when indicated. After the cervix is exposed and the position and depth of the uterus are confirmed, the surgeon will introduce a uterine manipulator or dilator into the cervix to manipulate the uterus during the laparoscopy for better visibility. If chromotubation (e.g., injection of a dilute solution of methylene blue through the cervix to determine fallopian tube patency) will be performed during the laparoscopy, the surgeon places an intrauterine cannula in the cervical canal at the time of D&C.

The usual instrumentation for the vaginal portion of the procedure includes a D&C set, with the addition of a uterine manipulator, intrauterine cannula, diluted methylene blue or indigo carmine solution, and a syringe.

An abdominal gynecologic instrument set should be readily available in the event that a laparotomy is indicated.

Operative Procedure
1. The surgeon makes a small incision (0.7 to 1.2 cm) at the inferior margin of the umbilicus.
2. Elevating the skin with a towel clamp on either side of the umbilicus or grasping below the umbilicus with a gauze sponge for traction, the surgeon inserts a Veress needle through the layers of the abdominal wall into the peritoneal cavity.
3. Once the Veress needle is inserted into the peritoneal cavity, a 10-ml syringe partially filled with sterile saline is attached to the needle for aspiration. If the needle has entered a blood vessel, blood is aspirated. If a loop of intestine or the stomach has been entered, bowel contents or malodorous

gas is aspirated. If the needle is free in the peritoneal cavity, nothing is aspirated.

4. The surgeon attaches a plastic or Silastic tubing to the Veress needle and the gas insufflator. Approximately 2 to 3 liters of CO_2 or nitrous oxide gas is then delivered into the peritoneal cavity to achieve pneumoperitoneum. CO_2 is commonly used as the insufflation medium because it is nontoxic, highly soluble in blood, and rapidly absorbed from the peritoneal cavity. The intraabdominal pressure must be closely monitored to prevent overdistention of the abdomen and to ensure free passage of gas into the peritoneal cavity.

5. After insufflation is completed, the Veress needle is withdrawn.

6. The surgeon inserts the trocar, covered by the trocar sleeve, through the abdominal wall and into the peritoneal cavity. The angle taken by the trocar is approximately 45 degrees toward the concavity of the pelvis. The plastic or Silastic tubing is attached to the trocar sleeve, and insufflation is resumed. Some surgeons prefer a direct trocar insertion technique or the open laparoscopy technique of Hasson to establish the pneumoperitoneum through the valve of the trocar sleeve rather than through a Veress needle (see Chapter 2).

7. With the trocar sleeve in place, the surgeon withdraws the trocar and introduces the laparoscope.

8. Visualization of the pelvis and lower abdomen and the visceral contents is begun. If the lens of the laparoscope becomes foggy, application of a commercially available defogger solution may control the problem. Alternatively, the surgeon may touch the lens to a loop of intestine to clear it. Before use, warming the tip of the scope in warm saline or towels may prevent fogging of the distal lens.

9. The anesthesia provider places the patient in the Trendelenburg's position.

10. The video camera is attached to the scope to aid in the OR team's visualization, and the procedure may be recorded for future reference. If an ancillary instrument such as biopsy forceps or bipolar forceps is needed, the surgeon inserts a second trocar with sleeve under direct laparoscopic visualization through a suprapubic incision.

11. To test for tubal patency, the surgeon injects diluted methylene blue or indigo carmine solution through the intrauterine cannula into the cervical canal (i.e., chromotubation). If the fallopian tubes are patent, dye can be seen at the fimbriated ends.

12. On completion of the intraabdominal procedure, the surgeon withdraws the laparoscope and the insufflated gas is allowed to escape from the trocar sleeve or by suction. The trocar sleeve is removed and trocar sites closed.

13. Application of staples or subcuticular closure of the primary skin incision is followed by placement of a small bandage or wound closure strip.

14. The surgeon removes the uterine manipulator and checks the cervix for bleeding. If bleeding is present, pressure may

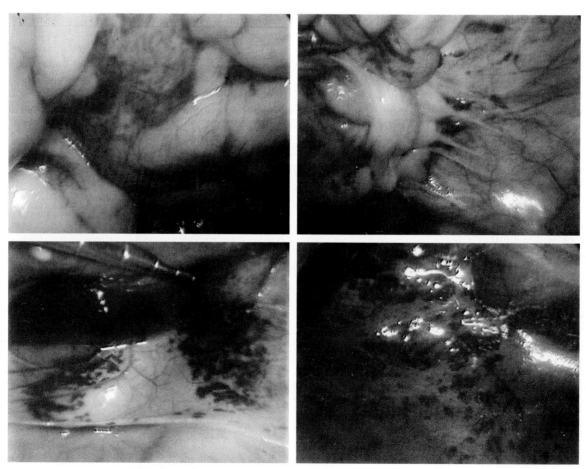

FIGURE 5-41 Laparoscopic view of endometriosis in the cul-de-sac.

be applied with a sponge stick or a suture ligature may be passed through the bleeding portion.

15. A perineal pad is applied.

Salpingostomy for Ectopic Tubal Pregnancy

Ectopic pregnancy is defined as any gestation developing outside of the endometrial cavity. Risk factors for developing an ectopic pregnancy include use of intrauterine devices (IUDs) for contraception, pelvic inflammatory disease, tubal ligation, tubal dysfunction (as with endometriosis), in vitro fertilization, and previous ectopic pregnancy. Although the fallopian tube is the most common site for ectopic pregnancies (occurring in up to 95% of all cases), they can develop in the cervix or broad ligament; in a previous cesarean section scar (myotomy), they can develop in the ovary and the peritoneal cavity (Genovese, 2007). Women who experience ectopic pregnancy generally present with abdominal pain, abnormal vaginal bleeding, and a palpable adnexal mass. Diagnosis is confirmed through measurement of human chorionic gonadotropin (hCG) levels and use of ultrasound to determine the absence of a gestational sac. A serious complication of ectopic pregnancy is tubal rupture and hemorrhage (Figure 5-42). The ultrasound is also useful in identifying free fluid in the peritoneal cavity. Ruptured ectopic pregnancy is considered a surgical emergency and is associated with severe abdominal pain, tachycardia, and hypotension. The woman with a ruptured ectopic pregnancy may also experience shoulder pain because of irritation of the phrenic nerve from the hemoperitoneum. Ectopic pregnancy may be treated medically with methotrexate or surgically through salpingostomy, segmental resection, fimbrial expression, and salpingectomy (Figure 5-43). Methotrexate destroys rapidly dividing cells and is often administered in conjunction with the surgical procedure to destroy any residual trophoblastic cells that might remain (Research Highlight) (Genovese, 2007). Laparoscopic and/or ultrasound-guided application of methotrexate to the extrauterine gestational sac may also be used as an alternative therapy (Lobo, 2007).

Procedural Considerations. Procedural considerations for laparoscopic salpingostomy are identical to those for any laparoscopic procedure with the addition of methotrexate.

Operative Procedure

1. The surgeon establishes a pneumoperitoneum, inserts the telescope, and mobilizes the distal end of the fallopian tube to perform an adhesiolysis. Grasping forceps are placed on either side of the fallopian tube, and gentle traction is applied.

2. Before making an incision, coagulation of the serial vessels on both sides of the anticipated incision may be performed. A dilute solution of vasopressin may also be injected into the mesenteric margin to avoid excessive bleeding (Figure 5-44).

3. A single incision is made with scissors from the mesenteric to the antimesenteric side of the fallopian tube, where the products of conception are exposed.

4. The tissue is removed gently with forceps while constant irrigation is maintained with an isotonic solution (Figure 5-45). Vigorous evacuation is avoided so that the highly vascular underlying interstitial layer is not disturbed.

5. Small bleeding vessels can be ligated with a fine, nonreactive suture. Simple traumatic compression of bleeding margins will also promote hemostasis. Mesosalpingeal vessel ligation may be performed.

6. The tubal incision may be allowed to close by secondary intention or, as in the instance of salpingotomy, the incision may be closed in one or two layers, with 6-0 interrupted sutures. On completion, the endoscope and instrumentation are removed. The insufflated gas is permitted to escape from

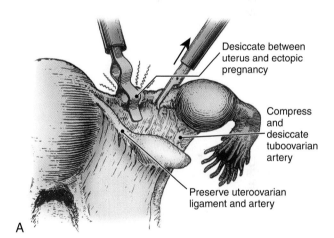

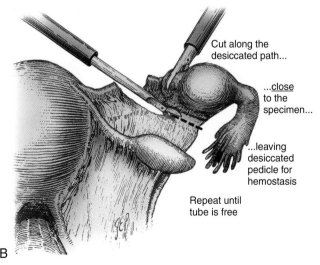

FIGURE 5-43 A, Electrodesiccation of the proximal fallopian tube during salpingectomy. **B,** Excision of the fallopian tube.

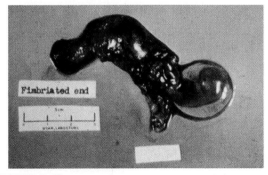

FIGURE 5-42 Ruptured ectopic pregnancy with fetus in sac.

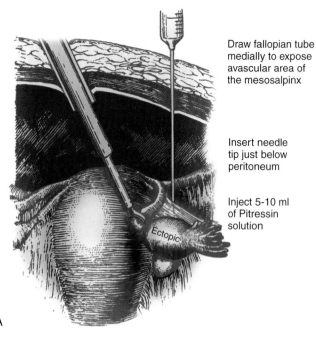

Draw fallopian tube medially to expose avascular area of the mesosalpinx

Insert needle tip just below peritoneum

Inject 5-10 ml of Pitressin solution

A

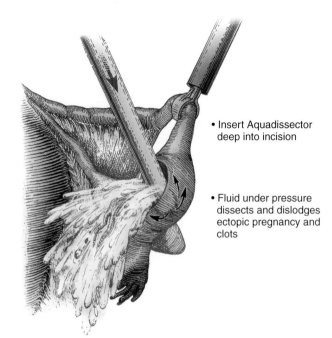

• Insert Aquadissector deep into incision

• Fluid under pressure dissects and dislodges ectopic pregnancy and clots

FIGURE 5-45 Hydrodissection used to separate ectopic pregnancy from fallopian tube during salpingostomy.

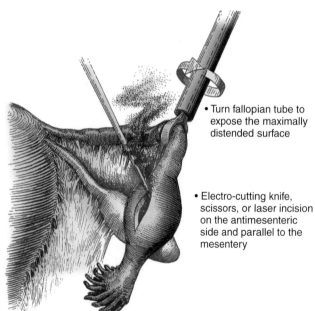

• Turn fallopian tube to expose the maximally distended surface

• Electro-cutting knife, scissors, or laser incision on the antimesenteric side and parallel to the mesentery

B

FIGURE 5-44 Salpingostomy. **A,** Injection of vasopressin into mesosalpinx. **B,** Incision made into fallopian tube.

the trocar sleeves. Trocar sleeves are then removed. Subcuticular closure of the primary skin incisions is followed by placement of wound closure strips or small dressings.

Ovarian Cystectomy

Ovarian cystectomy is frequently performed via the laparoscopic approach.

Operative Procedure

1. After successful laparoscopic entry, adhesiolysis is achieved.
2. On entry, peritoneal washings for cell block are obtained, if indicated.

3. The ovarian cyst is mobilized, and the cortex is grasped with a biopsy instrument.
4. The surgeon incises the cortex with scissors or the laser, exposing the cyst wall.
5. The incision is then enlarged with scissors, and pressurized hydrodissection is used to separate the cyst from the ovarian stroma.
6. The cyst is dissected and may be removed intact by a culdotomy incision, or the cyst may be opened, evacuated, thoroughly cleaned by lavage with the hydrodissector, and then removed.
7. If the cyst is opened intraperitoneally, the patient should be placed in the supine, not Trendelenburg's, position while the fluid is removed and the pelvis is cleaned by lavage.
8. Arterial bleeders are identified and desiccated.
9. The ovary usually does not require suturing; however, if the edges gape widely, the surgeon may loosely approximate the edges with interrupted 4-0 synthetic absorbable suture.
10. On completion, the endoscope and accessory instrumentation are removed. The insufflated gas is permitted to escape from the trocar sleeves. Trocar sleeves are then removed.
11. Closure of the primary skin incisions (fascia, if necessary, followed by a subcuticular stitch) is followed by placement of wound closure strips or small dressings.

Laparoscopic-Assisted Vaginal Hysterectomy

Laparoscopic-assisted vaginal hysterectomy (LAVH) offers an alternative to total abdominal hysterectomy (TAH) and vaginal hysterectomy (VH). The patient does not have the large abdominal incision, extended hospital stay, and long recovery period that occur with a TAH. LAVH may be associated with less pain than VH or TAH. Patients who are not candidates for traditional VH may be candidates for LAVH. Although not

RESEARCH HIGHLIGHT

Medical Management of Ectopic Pregnancy

Ectopic pregnancy is a devastating complication that affects up to 2% of all pregnancies. Although members of the surgical team are most familiar with the surgical treatment of ectopic pregnancy, the more cost-effective medical treatment for ectopic pregnancy is considered a front-line therapy in many major medical centers.

In this prospective study, researchers evaluated 100 women diagnosed with ectopic pregnancy who elected to have medical therapy for acceptability of the treatment and resolution of the pregnancy without surgical intervention. Participants received an intramuscular injection of methotrexate on days 0 and 4 and received additional doses on days 7 and/or 11 if their hCG levels did not decrease by 15% in the follow-up period. A total of 88 women were treated successfully with the methotrexate protocol; the others required surgery. Over half of the women (53%) treated with the protocol reported adverse effects related to the treatment, most commonly gastrointestinal complaints.

To assess satisfaction with the medical protocol, researchers mailed a questionnaire with a 5-point scale to collect data on the side effects of the treatment, missed work/school days, and the feasibility of choosing the medical protocol over surgery in the future, if necessary. A total of 64 women returned the questionnaire; 58 reported they were "satisfied" or "very satisfied" with their treatment and would also undergo the same treatment if they experienced another ectopic pregnancy in the future.

Modified from Barnhart K et al: Use of "2-dose" regimen of methotrexate to treat ectopic pregnancy, *Fertil Steril* 87(2):250-256, 2007.

described here, in laparoscopic-assisted supracervical hysterectomy (LASH), the body of the uterus is removed and the cervix is left intact (Goeser and Hasiak 2008).

The surgeon uses laparoscopy to visualize the pelvis and thereby determine whether disease is present. This is not possible with traditional vaginal hysterectomy. Conditions leading to LAVH include postmenopausal bleeding, pelvic pain, uterine leiomyomas, and adnexal masses. Indications for LAVH may be absence of genital prolapse, required adnexectomy, history of abdominopelvic surgery, salpingitis or endometriosis, lymphadenectomy, and endometrial cancer.

Procedural Considerations. Procedural considerations and accessory instrumentation and approach are similar to those used in other laparoscopic surgical procedures. The patient is placed in the low lithotomy position with attention to positioning interventions to protect the patient from injury.

Operative Procedure. The operative procedure may include the following:

1. Hydrodissection of the broad ligament
2. Desiccation of the round and infundibulopelvic ligaments with bipolar coagulation
3. Dissection of the broad ligaments
4. Freeing of the urinary bladder from the lower uterine segment
5. Opening of the vaginal vault with endoscopic scissors or monopolar electrode and removal of the uterus vaginally

Robotically Assisted Procedures

Robotic-assisted surgery represents the newest available technology for minimally invasive gynecologic procedures. The robotic system has the following three components: (1) a surgeon console with a stereoscopic viewer, hand manipulators, and foot controls; (2) the vision system that provides a three-dimensional image through an endoscope equipped with stereoscopic cameras and dual optics; and (3) an ancillary cart with telerobotic arms (Reynolds, 2006). Robotic technology has been used for myomectomies, sacrocolpopexies, hysterectomies, oophorectomies, and lymphadenectomies (Fanning et al, 2008) (Research Highlight). Advantages to robotic procedures include smaller incisions (often 1 to 2 cm in length), reduced blood loss, shorter hospital stays, and greater patient satisfaction.

Procedural Considerations. General anesthesia is used for robotic procedures. Procedural considerations applicable to laparoscopic surgery are appropriate for robotic surgery including prepping and draping practices. The surgical technologist must be familiar with the specialized equipment used for robotic surgery to minimize operative time and facilitate a smooth experience for the patient and surgical team. Instrumentation to convert the robotic procedure to an open procedure should be available.

Operative Procedure—Robotic-Assisted Hysterectomy

1. The surgeon places a uterine manipulator into the cervix and a vaginal balloon occluder into the vagina.
2. A Veress needle is placed and the surgeon establishes an adequate pneumoperitoneum. Alternately, the open Hasson technique (see Chapter 11) may be used.
3. The surgeon incises the skin at the umbilicus and places the endoscope port. Additional incisions are created and supplementary ports are inserted for instrumentation and suction.
4. The anesthesia provider positions the patient in steep Trendelenburg's position, and the circulator positions the surgical cart with the robotic arms between the patient's legs while observing the integrity of the sterile field.
5. Following the manufacturer's directions, the surgical technologist and surgical assistant dock the robotic system.
6. The surgeon moves to the console for the remainder of the procedure.
7. Using the hand and foot controls of the console, the surgeon surveys the operative field and opens the peritoneum using the ESU.
8. The surgeon skeletonizes and ligates the uterine artery pedicles and infundibulopelvic ligament with polyglactin suture or free ties.
9. Additional dissection is performed to divide the cardinal and uterosacral ligament complex on both sides.
10. The surgical assistant provides traction on the uterus while the surgeon performs an anterior and posterior colpotomy.
11. The uterus and cervix are detached and delivered into the patient's vagina; they remain in the vagina while the surgeon closes the vaginal cuff using interrupted polyglactin suture. When the cuff is closed and hemostasis is achieved, the specimen is removed from the vagina.

12. The surgical assistant disengages the robotic arms and removes the trocars.
13. Using polyglactin suture the surgeon or surgical assistant closes the fascia. Wound closure strips are used to close the skin incisions, and small dressings and a perineal pad are applied.

Uterine Artery Embolization

Uterine artery embolization (UAE, also referred to as "uterine fibroid embolization [UFE]") is an alternate treatment for fibroids that blocks the blood vessels supplying nutrients and oxygen to the tumors. The blockage causes the fibroid muscle cells to degenerate and form scar tissue, which causes the fibroids to shrink. The greatest period of shrinkage occurs in the first 6 months following the procedure with an additional 42% to 82% shrinkage over the next 6 months (Andrews et al, 2009). This procedure appeals to many women because of its minimally invasive nature and ability to be performed in the outpatient setting. The main complication associated with the procedure is postembolization syndrome, occurring in 2% to 10% of patients. Postembolization syndrome is characterized by pelvic pain, low-grade fever, vomiting, loss of appetite, and malaise in the first 48 hours after UAE (Parker, 2007). Occasionally, the procedure is complicated by inadvertent occlusion of the ovarian blood supply. Pregnancy is not recommended following UAE.

Procedural Considerations. A hysteroscope, light source, camera, and viewing tower are required along with uterine distention system, appropriate distention fluids, and energy sources (Dooley, 2007). The patient is placed in lithotomy position with appropriate positioning safety measures. An EUA is usually performed before the start of the procedure. A perineal pad will be used at the procedure conclusion.

Operative Procedure. The procedure is performed under fluoroscopic guidance using spinal anesthesia or local anesthesia supplemented with moderate sedation. A femoral artery sheath is inserted, and arteriography of the pelvic vasculature is performed by injecting radiologic contrast through a 5-French catheter as it passes through the femoral artery to the iliac artery to the uterine artery. An embolic agent is injected through the catheter until no more proximal arterial flow or reflux of contrast material is noted. Commonly used embolic agents are gelatin sponges, nonspheric polyvinyl alcohol (PVA) particles, and trisacryl gelatin microspheres. Gelfoam pledgets are cut into strips, rolled, and loaded into a nozzle of a syringe for injection. Nonspheric PVA particles are mixed with equal parts of saline and contrast and injected through the catheter until the vessel is occluded. The PVA particle size ranges from 350 to 700 micrometers, which is comparable in size to a grain of sand. Trisacryl microspheres range in size from 700 to 900 micrometers (Scheurig et al, 2008). Collateral circulation maintains the blood supply to the myometrium. The particles remain inert in the vessel.

GYNECOLOGIC SURGERY USING ABDOMINAL APPROACH

Total Abdominal Hysterectomy (TAH)

TAH is removal of the entire uterus, including the corpus and the cervix. When TAH is combined with bilateral salpingo-oophorectomy, the procedure is commonly termed *panhysterectomy* or *complete hysterectomy*. TAH may be performed for

---

RESEARCH HIGHLIGHT

Robotic Hysterectomy for Benign and Malignant Disease

Minimally invasive approaches to gynecologic surgery have recently expanded to include robotic-assisted procedures. Robotic-assisted surgery offers several advantages over standard laparoscopy including decreased tissue trauma, enhanced precision, and stereoscopic visualization.

To evaluate the use of robotic surgery in a minimally invasive approach to hysterectomy for benign uterine disease, a group of researchers performed a retrospective chart review to examine the operative and perioperative characteristics and trends for 200 patients before and after implementation of a robotic program in a community hospital. The researchers reviewed 100 charts of patients who underwent laparoscopic hysterectomy before the implementation of the robotic program to the charts of the first 100 patients to undergo robotic hysterectomy. Indications for surgery included myomas, endometriosis, ovarian cysts, dysmenorrhea, and dyspareunia. Both groups were similar in demographics and body mass index. Their review concluded that a twofold decrease in blood loss was realized in robotic hysterectomies compared to laparoscopic hysterectomies (e.g., 61 ml in the robotic group, 113 ml in the laparoscopic group), and hospital stays were decreased in the robotic group. They also reported that the rate of conversion to an open procedure was zero for the robotic group, but 11% in the laparoscopic group.

Robotic surgery may also have a place in the treatment of malignant gynecologic conditions. Researchers in Boston sought to determine if robotic hysterectomy would improve short-term outcomes in women being treated with open radical hysterectomy for cervical cancer. Using a retrospective chart review they compared 48 radical hysterectomies. Of the 48 cases reviewed, 16 were robotic radical hysterectomies and 32 were open radical hysterectomies. All patients were similar in body mass, age, and stage of cancer. They determined that operative time for the robotic hysterectomy was significantly longer than that for the open procedures; however, mean blood loss was significantly less in robotic hysterectomy patients (e.g., 81.9 ml for the robotic group vs 665 ml for the open group). Postoperative complications were less in the robotic group, and the mean length of stay was 1.7 days in the robotic group compared to 4.9 days in the open group.

As techniques for this relatively new technology evolve, research is needed to quantify the benefits and to determine future applications in the treatment of both benign and malignant uterine conditions.

Modified from Payne TN, Dauterive FR: A comparison of total laparoscopic hysterectomy to robotically assisted hysterectomy: surgical outcomes in a community practice, *J Minim Invasive Gynecol* 15(3):286-291, 2008; Ko EM et al: Robotic versus open radical hysterectomy: a comparative study at a single institution, *Gynecol Oncol* 111:425-430, 2008.

symptomatic pelvic relaxation or prolapse, pain associated with pelvic congestion, pelvic inflammatory disease, endometriosis, recurrent ovarian cysts, fibroids (myomas), bleeding with no apparent cause in postmenopausal women, adenomyosis, or dysfunctional uterine bleeding (Evidence for Practice). TAH, usually with bilateral salpingo-oophorectomy, is also indicated in malignancy, premalignant states, and conditions of high risk for development or recurrence of malignancy. The procedure can also be used to accomplish sterilization. Approximately 516,025 hysterectomies are performed each year in the United States (HCUPnet, 2007).

Procedural Considerations. Before the abdominal skin prep, perform an internal vaginal prep using a separate prep tray, ensuring contact of the prep solution with the cervix. An indwelling urinary drainage catheter is inserted to provide constant bladder drainage during the operation. The supine position, modified during the procedure with the Trendelenburg's position, is used. Instrumentation includes the abdominal gynecologic set. Provisions are made to remove those instruments used in separating the cervix from the vagina from the surgical field, thereby avoiding vaginal contamination of the pelvis.

Operative Procedure

1. In an obese patient or for exploration of the upper abdominal cavity, a left rectus or midline incision may be made. For simple hysterectomy, a Pfannenstiel incision may be used. The surgeon opens the abdominal layers and the peritoneum as described for laparotomy (see Chapter 10).
2. As the peritoneal cavity is opened, the anesthesia provider usually places the patient in the Trendelenburg's position to provide better visualization of the pelvic organs.
3. Vasopressin may be injected into the uterus. The round ligament is grasped with forceps, clamped, and ligated with sutures on long needle holders. The surgeon cuts the pedicles with a knife or Metzenbaum scissors; sutures are tagged with a hemostat to be used as traction later. This procedure is done on both sides (Figure 5-46, *A*).
4. Using blunt dissection the surgeon separates the layer of the broad ligament close to the uterus on each side. Bleeding vessels are clamped and ligated, and a moist laparotomy pack is inserted behind the flap. The fallopian tube and the utero-ovarian ligaments are doubly clamped together, incised, and doubly tied with suture ligatures (Figure 5-46, *B*).
5. The surgeon pulls the uterus forward to expose the posterior sheath of the broad ligament, and incises the ligament with a knife or Metzenbaum scissors. Ureters are identified. The uterine vessels and uterosacral ligaments are doubly clamped, divided by sharp dissection at the level of the internal os, and ligated with suture ligatures (Figure 5-46, *C*).
6. The severed uterine vessels are bluntly dissected away from the cervix on each side with the aid of sponges on sponge-holding forceps, scissors, and tissue forceps.
7. The bladder is separated from the cervix and upper vagina with sharp and blunt dissection assisted by sponges on sponge-holding forceps. The bladder may be retracted with a moist laparotomy pack and a retractor with an angular blade. The vaginal vault is incised close to the cervix with a knife or scissors (Figure 5-46, *D*).
8. The surgeon grasps the anterior lip of the cervix with an Allis, Kocher, or tenaculum forceps. Using scissors,

the surgeon dissects the cervix and amputates it from the vagina. The uterus is removed. The surgical technologist places any potentially contaminated instruments used on the cervix and vagina into a discard basin and passes them from the field (including sponge-holding forceps and suction). Bleeding is controlled with hemostats and sutures.

9. The vaginal vault is reconstructed with interrupted sutures. Angle sutures anchor all three connective tissue ligaments to the vaginal vault. The pedicles, fallopian tubes, and ovarian ligaments are left free of the vault.
10. The vaginal mucosa is approximated with a continuous suture on a long needle holder. The muscular coat of the vagina may be closed with figure-of-eight sutures to make the vault of the vagina firm and provide resistance against prolapse. A drain may be placed in the vagina.
11. The surgeon closes the peritoneum over the bladder, vaginal vault, and rectum (Figure 5-46, *E*). The laparotomy packs are removed, and the omentum is drawn over the bowel.
12. The abdominal wound is closed as described for laparotomy closure (see Chapter 2).
13. Abdominal dressings and a perineal pad are applied.

Abdominal Myomectomy

Uterine fibroids are benign tumors that arise from the muscular wall of the uterus (Figure 5-47). They may also be located in the submucosal area or the subserosal surface of the uterus. On occasion, they may become pedunculated and extend into the cervical canal. Rarely, a subserosal fibroid may pedunculate and migrate to become a parasitic fibroid attached to the omentum or mesentery. Another term for uterine fibroids is *uterine leiomyomas*. Abdominal myomectomy is removal of fibromyomas, or fibroid tumors, by carefully separating each fibroid from the uterine wall and its blood supply. Myomectomy is usually done in young women who have symptoms that indicate the presence of tumors and who wish to preserve their potential fertility. Uterine fibroids may cause pelvic pain and pressure or dysfunctional uterine bleeding, and they are a leading cause of infertility. Fibroids are more common in African-American women and become more common during the later reproductive years (Katz, 2007). Myomectomy may be performed as a prophylactic measure with other abdominopelvic surgery. Preoperative preparation may include injections of Lupron, a synthetic version of the naturally occurring gonadotropin-releasing hormone (GnRH), to reduce blood supply to the fibroid. This intervention mimics the postmenopausal state for women who receive it, as it reduces the amount of estrogen that the body synthesizes.

Procedural Considerations. The basic abdominal gynecologic instrument set and ESU are required. A laser may also be used. The patient is prepped as described for abdominal hysterectomy.

Operative Procedure

1. A midline or Pfannenstiel incision is used, and the uterus is exposed.
2. To contract the musculature of the uterine wall, a suitable drug may be injected into the fundus.
3. The surgeon grasps the fibroid tumor with a tenaculum. The broad ligament may be opened with curved hemostats and Metzenbaum scissors to determine the course of the ureter or to free the bladder.

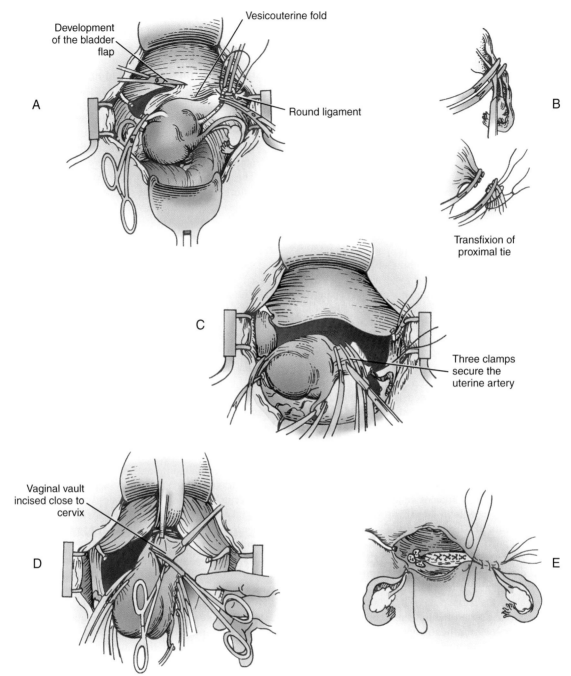

FIGURE 5-46 Abdominal hysterectomy for single fibroid uterus. **A,** Peritoneum retracted with self-retaining retractors, and organs protected with laparotomy packs saturated in warm normal saline solution. Transverse incision made through uterine peritoneum and extended to each side of uterine attachments of round ligaments. Bleeding vessels clamped and ligated. Round ligament grasped, ligated, and cut. **B,** Tube and ovarian ligaments clamped, cut, and sutured. **C,** Uterus pulled forward, posterior sheath of broad ligaments divided, and uterine artery and veins secured by three heavy curved clamps. Pedicle divided, leaving two hemostats on proximal pedicle. **D,** Bladder separated from cervix and upper vagina. Vaginal vault opened and grasped with Allis forceps. Allis forceps placed on anterior lip of cervix, and dissection of cervix carried out to complete its amputation from vagina. **E,** Three connective tissue thickenings anchored to vaginal vault, vaginal mucosa approximated, and vault closed. As shown, peritoneum closed with continuous suture.

EVIDENCE FOR PRACTICE

Alternatives to Hysterectomy

Hysterectomy is the most common non–pregnancy-related major surgery performed on women in the United States. It is widely accepted as appropriate treatment for cancer and various noncancerous conditions, such as pain, discomfort, uterine bleeding, emotional distress, and related symptoms. Although hysterectomy can alleviate uterine problems, less-invasive treatments are available. Alternatives to hysterectomy recommended by the Agency for Healthcare Research and Quality (AHRQ) are noted in the following table.

Condition	Conservative Surgery	Pharmacologic Therapies Hormonal	Nonhormonal	Other Strategies
Fibroids	Myomectomy	GnRH agonists with add-back therapy	NSAIDs	Watchful waiting
	Endometrial ablation	Oral contraceptives RU-486 (experimental) Gestrinone (experimental)		
Endometriosis	Adhesiolysis	GnRH agonists with add-back therapy	NSAIDs	Watchful waiting
	Excision or endometrial ablation	Danazol	Analgesics	Biofeedback
	Resection or cul-de-sac obliteration	Progestins	Anxiolytics	Hypnosis
	Nerve blocks	Oral contraceptives		Acupuncture
	Uterosacral nerve ablation	Tamoxifen (experimental) RU-486 (experimental)		Lifestyle modifications (nutrition/exercise)
Prolapse	Colporrhaphy	Estrogen		Watchful waiting
	Laparoscopic or vaginal suspension techniques			Kegel exercises Pessaries Electrical stimulation Urethral beads Periurethral injections (e.g., of fat, silicone)
Dysfunctional bleeding	Dilation and curettage	Progestins		Watchful waiting
	Endometrial ablation	Estrogens Oral contraceptives Danazol Prostaglandin inhibitors GnRH agonists Antifibrinolytic agents Luteinizing hormone agonists		Antidepressants
Chronic pelvic pain	Adhesiolysis	Danazol	NSAIDs	Watchful waiting
	Nerve blocks	GnRh agonists with add-back therapy	Analgesics	Counseling
	Denervation procedure		Nerve blocks	Biofeedback
	Uterosacral nerve ablation	Oral contraceptives Medroxyprogesterone acetate	Narcotics	Relaxation techniques Trigger-point injections Acupuncture Psychotropics Antidepressants Physical therapy

GnRH, Gonadotropin-releasing hormone; *NSAID,* nonsteroidal antiinflammatory drug.
Modified from *Common uterine conditions: options for treatment,* AHCPR Pub No. 98-0003, Rockville, Md, Dec 1997, Agency for Health Care Policy and Research, available at www.ahrq.gov/consumer/uterine1.htm. Accessed June 26, 2009.

4. Each tumor is shelled out of its bed, using blunt and sharp instruments, or the laser. Bleeding vessels are clamped and ligated or electrocoagulated.
5. The uterus is reconstructed with interrupted or continuous sutures.
6. The perimetrium is closed over the operative site, and the abdominal wound is closed.

Radical Hysterectomy (Wertheim)

Radical hysterectomy is en bloc dissection and wide removal of the uterus, tubes, ovaries, supporting ligaments, and upper vagina, together with careful removal of all recognizable lymph nodes in the pelvis (Figure 5-48). Extensive dissection of the ureters and of the bladder is also involved.

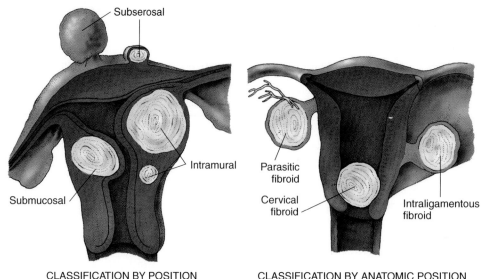

CLASSIFICATION BY POSITION
WITHIN UTERINE LAYERS

CLASSIFICATION BY ANATOMIC POSITION

FIGURE 5-47 Classification of uterine leiomyomas.

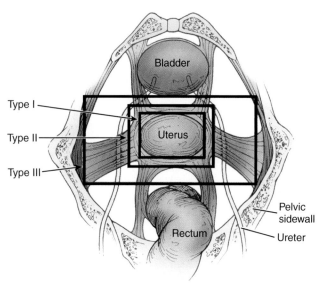

FIGURE 5-48 Different types of hysterectomy: type I—simple hysterectomy; type II—modified radical hysterectomy; type III—radical hysterectomy.

Radical hysterectomy is performed for gynecologic malignancy. Abdominal exploration determines lymph node involvement. With no lymph node involvement, a wide-cuff hysterectomy is performed. The uterus, tubes, and ovaries, together with most of the parametrial tissues and the upper portion of the vagina, are dissected en bloc. Dissection of the ureters from the paracervical structures takes place so that the ligaments supporting the uterus and vagina can be removed.

Procedural Considerations. Careful estimation of blood loss and calculation of urinary output are needed throughout the operative procedure. The patient is prepped as described for TAH. An indwelling urinary catheter is inserted. The basic abdominal gynecologic instrument set is required, with the addition of long and deep instruments and a self-retaining retractor.

Operative Procedure
1. The skin is incised, and the abdominal layers are opened, as described for laparotomy.
2. The surgeon cuts the peritoneum at its reflection on the anterior surface of the uterus between the round ligaments (Figure 5-49, *A*). Using blunt dissection, the surgeon frees the bladder surface from the cervix and vagina.
3. The right round and infundibulopelvic ligaments are clamped, cut with a knife or Metzenbaum scissors, and ligated with sutures to expose the external iliac artery. The ureter is identified and retracted with a vein retractor (Figure 5-49, *B*).
4. The lymph and areolar tissues are dissected from the iliac artery, obturator fossa, and ureter with Lahey forceps, Kitner sponges, and Metzenbaum scissors. A complete lymph gland dissection removes the tissue from the Cloquet node to the bifurcation of the iliac arteries bilaterally. The uterine artery and vein are clamped, cut, and doubly ligated.
5. The surgeon elevates the uterus and opens the cul-de-sac (Figure 5-49, *C*); the uterosacral and cardinal ligaments are clamped, cut with scissors, and doubly ligated with suture ligatures. The pararectal and paravesical areolar tissues are dissected free to skeletonize the upper vagina, and the paraurethral tissues are removed as near to the pelvic walls as possible.
6. The upper third of the vagina is cross-clamped with Heaney forceps (Figure 5-49, *D*) and divided using a long knife handle and #20 blade. The uterus and surrounding tissues are removed. Electrocoagulation is used to minimize venous oozing from small venules and capillaries. Lowering the head of the OR bed 15 degrees is also helpful in reducing the oozing of blood and serum.
7. The surgeon sutures the vagina with a running locked stitch, and inserts closed wound drains from above (Figure 5-49, *E*). The pelvis is peritonealized with a continuous suture.

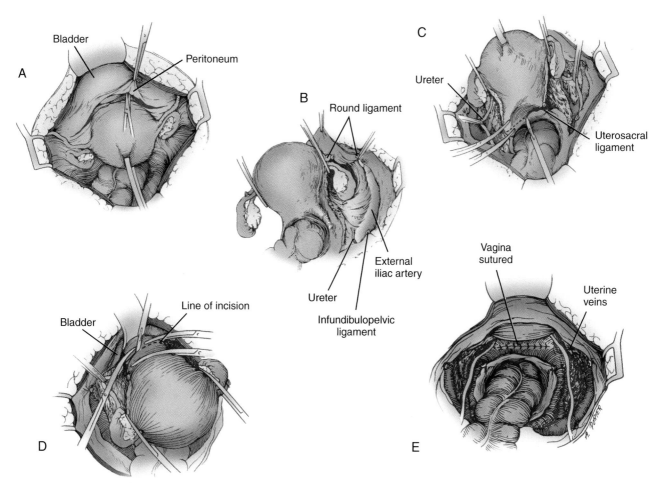

FIGURE 5-49 Wertheim radical hysterectomy. **A,** With upward traction applied on uterus, peritoneum is incised from round ligament to round ligament. **B,** Right round and infundibulopelvic ligaments are ligated and cut, thus exposing right external iliac artery. **C,** Uterus is held upward and forward, exposing cul-de-sac, which is incised as shown by dotted line. **D,** After dissection is completed, vagina is doubly clamped preparatory to transection, after which entire specimen is lifted out en bloc. **E,** Vagina is closed. Peritoneum remains to be reperitonealized.

8. The abdominal wound is closed (retention sutures may be used) and dressed in the usual manner. Vaginal packing and drains may be used. A suprapubic indwelling catheter may be placed to assist in preventing postoperative bladder spasm and for bladder drainage if the patient is unable to void after removal of the urethral catheter.
9. A perineal pad is applied.

Pelvic Exenteration

Pelvic exenteration is the en bloc removal of the rectum, the distal sigmoid colon, the urinary bladder and the distal ureters, the internal iliac vessels and their lateral branches, all pelvic reproductive organs and lymph nodes, and the entire pelvic floor with the accompanying pelvic peritoneum, levator muscles, and perineum. A partial exenteration, either anterior or posterior, may be performed, depending on the origin of the carcinoma and the extent of local tissue invasion (Figure 5-50).

Pelvic exenteration is the preferred treatment for recurrent or persistent carcinoma of the cervix after radiation therapy.

Advanced or recurrent vaginal, vulvar, or occasionally endometrial and rectal carcinomas are often amenable to exenteration (Jhingran and Levenback, 2007). Exenteration is considered only after a thorough investigation of the patient and disease status to determine if there is a reasonable chance of cure and of return to a productive life.

The need to create urinary and bowel diversions must also be considered, together with the patient's ability to cope with these diversions postoperatively. Plastic surgery may be required for creation of a neovagina. Psychologic preparation and support of the patient and family by the surgical team and physician are prime requisites.

Procedural Considerations. Utmost care must be taken in positioning the patient because of the duration of surgery. Pay strict attention to the patient's knees, hips, and lower back to prevent vascular and nerve damage. The patient is in the supine position with legs abducted in the ski position (i.e., lower extremities resting on a well-padded plantar surface rather than on the heel or popliteal area) or elevated in a modi-

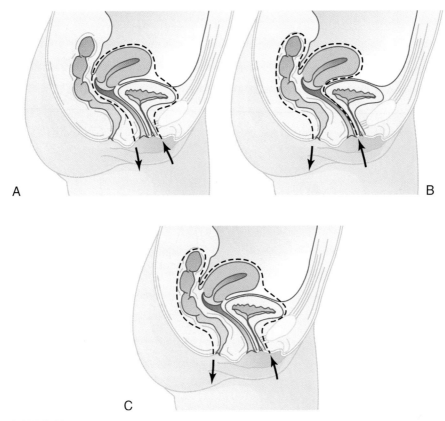

FIGURE 5-50 Organs removed in pelvic exenteration. **A,** Anterior exenteration. **B,** Posterior exenteration. **C,** Total pelvic exenteration.

fied lithotomy position to allow access to the perineum without disruptive position changes. Skin prepping includes the abdomen, thighs, perineum, and internal vaginal vault.

The circulator and surgical technologist must be alert to fluid and blood loss. Irrigation solutions must be accurately measured, laparotomy packs must be weighed to assess blood volume loss, and the anesthesia provider and surgical team must be apprised of the measurements.

When the colon is transected or ureteral drainage is diverted into a segment of the ileum the gastrointestinal technique (i.e., bowel technique) as described in Chapter 2 should be followed.

Separate instrument setups are required for the abdominal and perineal approaches. Extra drapes, gowns, and gloves should be available.

For the abdominal approach, the basic abdominal gynecologic instrument set and instrumentation for abdominoperineal resection (see Chapter 2) are required.

For the perineal approach, the basic vaginal instrument set is required. To prevent contamination, the anus may be closed with a purse-string suture.

Operative Procedure

1. A long midline incision from the symphysis pubis to the umbilicus is made, and the abdomen is opened in the usual manner. A second incision within the perineum encircling the vestibule and anus is also made.
2. The surgeon explores the peritoneal cavity for metastasis to the liver, the nodes of the celiac axis, the superior mesenteric artery, and the para-aortic tissues.
3. The pelvis is explored, and the peritoneum along the brim of the pelvis is examined for lymph node involvement. Frozen sections may be indicated. The obturator fossa and the region of the uterosacral ligaments are explored. When findings at exploration are negative, retractors are placed and the small bowel is isolated with moist laparotomy packs (Figure 5-51).
4. The surgeon frees the sigmoid mesocolon and sections it by means of intestinal clamps and a scalpel or a stapling device. The proximal end is exteriorized through an opening in the left side of the abdomen; an intestinal clamp is left across the lumen until later, when the permanent colostomy will be secured to the skin.
5. The remaining sigmoid mesentery is clamped with Rochester-Péan forceps, cut, and ligated down to and including the superior hemorrhoidal vessels. Long instruments and sutures are used to reach the deep pelvic structures.
6. The distal sigmoid colon is closed with an inverting suture. The sigmoid colon and rectum are freed from the sacrococcygeal area by blunt and sharp dissection.
7. The lateral pelvic peritoneum is cut along the iliac vessels; the ovarian vessels and round ligaments on each side are clamped with Rochester-Péan forceps, cut, and doubly ligated.
8. The surgeon incises the peritoneum over the dome of the bladder with a long knife and Metzenbaum scissors, and separates the bladder from the symphysis pubis down to the urethra.

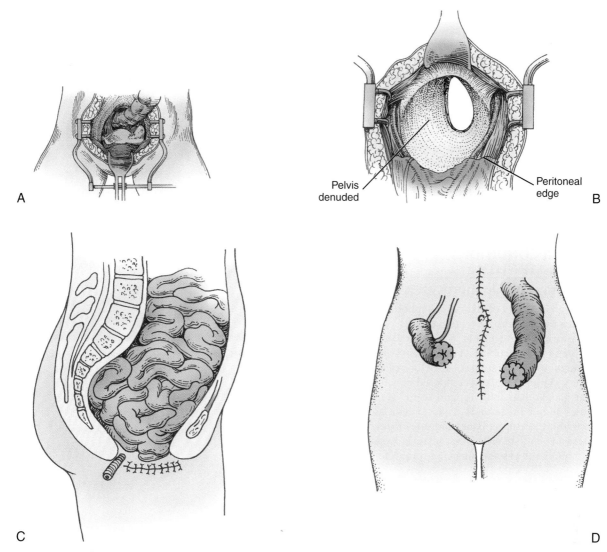

FIGURE 5-51 Pelvic exenteration. **A,** Pelvic viscera in situ as viewed from operating surgeon's vantage point after retractors are placed and small bowel is isolated with moist laparotomy packs. **B,** Empty pelvis after dissection of paravesical and paravaginal tissues and removal of specimen en bloc. **C,** Sagittal view of small bowel above pelvic defect. Perineal packing or drain may be used. **D,** After closure of abdominal wall, colostomy and ileostomy stomas are sutured to skin edges.

9. The ureters are identified and divided 2 to 3 cm below the brim of the pelvis. The proximal end is left open to allow urinary drainage, whereas the distal end is ligated.

10. The hypogastric artery, the internal iliac vein, and the superior and inferior gluteal vessels are exposed, clamped with hemostats, doubly ligated, and cut. The external iliac vein is retracted to allow evacuation of the contents of the obturator fossa, leaving the obturator nerve intact. Care must be taken in dissection not to damage the sacral plexus and sciatic nerve.

11. The surgeon isolates the internal pudendal vessels, ligates them with transfixion sutures, and cuts them. The remaining soft-tissue attachments of the pelvis are clamped and cut. Steps 10 and 11 are then performed on the opposite side.

12. The perineum is incised by an elliptic incision that includes the clitoris and anus. The ischiorectal fat is incised up to the area of the levator muscle.

13. The coccygeal attachment of the rectum is severed. The levator muscles are severed at their lateral attachments by using a long knife handle with #20 blade; hemostasis is maintained by pressure and traction.

14. The paravesical and paravaginal tissues are resected from the periosteum of the symphysis pubis and superior pubic rami by means of a knife. The specimen is completely freed and removed from the pelvis (Figure 5-52).

15. After residual bleeding vessels are identified and controlled by transfixing ligatures, the surgeon closes the subcutaneous tissue with interrupted sutures. A drain is placed in the wound, and the skin is closed.

16. Further residual bleeding vessels are controlled in the abdomen. Packs may be left in the pelvis, to be removed through the perineum after 48 hours.

17. The ileal segment is then fashioned, and the ureters are anastomosed to it. The external stoma is placed on the right side of the abdomen.

18. A jejunostomy catheter is inserted into the proximal jejunum to aid in postoperative bowel decompression. It is

connected to the bowel with a purse-string suture and exteriorized to the skin, where it is sutured in place.

19. A gastrostomy tube is placed into the stomach in the same manner.
20. Hemostasis is checked. The small intestine is carefully repositioned into the pelvis. Packs and retractors are removed.
21. The peritoneum, rectus muscles, and fascial sheaths are closed with interrupted figure-of-eight sutures. The skin is closed with interrupted sutures.
22. The colostomy stoma is prepared by removing the intestinal clamp from the sigmoid colon, opening the colon, and suturing the stoma to the skin edges.

The abdominal wound and tube sites are dressed in the usual manner. Drainage devices are applied to the colostomy and ileostomy stomas.

SURGERY FOR CONDITIONS THAT AFFECT FERTILITY

Oophorectomy and Oophorocystectomy

Oophorectomy is removal of an ovary. Oophorocystectomy is removal of an ovarian cyst. Functional cysts constitute the majority of ovarian enlargements, with follicular cysts being the most common. Functional cysts develop in the corpus luteum. Benign cystic teratomas, also known as dermoid cysts, are very common and are composed of ectodermal tissues (sweat glands, hair follicles, and teeth) (Figure 5-53). Other tissues found in dermoid cysts include adult brain, bronchus, thyroid, cartilage, bone, and intestinal cells (Katz, 2007). Ovarian epithelial tumors, serous cystadenomas, and pseudomucinous cystadenomas are prone to malignant change.

The choice of operation depends on the patient's age and symptoms, findings during physical examination, and direct examination of the adnexa during exploration. If the ovarian tumor is recognized as benign, only the visibly diseased portions of the adnexa are removed. In the presence of dermoid, follicular, and corpus luteum cysts, the cyst is usually enucleated and most of the ovarian parenchyma is preserved. In tubal pregnancy, the ectopic pregnancy may be removed from the tube or the pregnant fallopian tube may be removed concomitant with, in some instances, the ovary.

Procedural Considerations. The basic abdominal gynecologic instrument set is required, with the addition of a trocar and cannula, suction tubing, 10-ml syringe, and 21-gauge needle.

Operative Procedure

1. The surgeon opens the abdominal cavity as described for laparotomy.
2. After the abdominal cavity is opened, the surgeon has several options.
   a. For removal of a large ovarian cyst, a purse-string suture may be placed into the cyst wall and a trocar introduced in its center; the suture is tightened around the trocar as the fluid is aspirated. The trocar is removed, and the purse-string suture is tied. All normal ovarian tissue is preserved.
   b. For removal of a smaller ovarian cyst, a clamp is placed at the base of the cyst and the cyst is excised. The wound in the ovary is closed with absorbable suture (Figure 5-54).

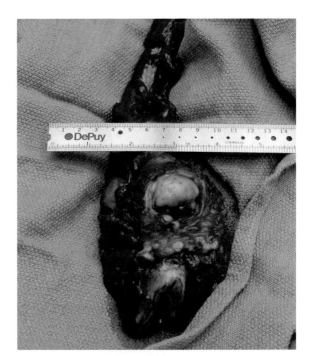

FIGURE 5-52 Pelvic exenteration specimen.

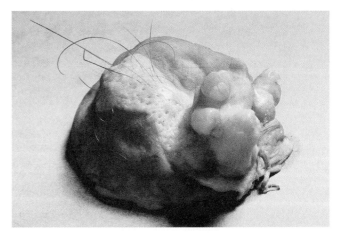

FIGURE 5-53 Dermoid cyst.

c. For removal of a dermoid cyst, the field is protected with laparotomy packs because the cystic contents produce irritation if they are spilled into the peritoneal cavity. An incision is made along the base of the cyst between the wall and normal ovarian tissue. The cystic wall is dissected away. The ovary is closed with interrupted or continuous sutures.
d. For decortication of the enlarged ovary and wedge resection, a large segment of the ovarian cortex opposite the hilum is removed. The cysts are punctured with a needle point and collapsed. A wedge of ovarian stroma, extending deep into the hilum, is resected with a small knife; the cortex of the ovary is closed with interrupted or continuous sutures.
3. To prevent prolapse of the tube into the cul-de-sac, the tube may be sutured to the posterior sheath of the broad ligament.

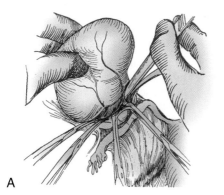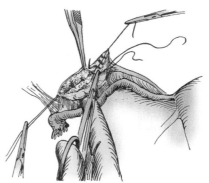

A   B

FIGURE 5-54 Resection of small cyst from ovary. **A,** Incision made around ovary near junction of cyst wall and normal ovarian tissue. Knife handle is convenient instrument for removal of cyst contents. **B,** Wound in ovary closed.

4. The abdominal wound is closed as described for laparotomy, and dressings are applied.

Salpingo-oophorectomy

Salpingo-oophorectomy is removal of a fallopian tube and all or part of the associated ovary. Unilateral salpingo-oophorectomy may be done to cure chronic salpingo-oophoritis, for ectopic tubal gestation, or for certain disease conditions of the adnexa or large adnexal cysts. If both tubes and ovaries are diseased, they are removed with total hysterectomy.

Procedural Considerations. The basic abdominal gynecologic instrument set is required.

Operative Procedure
1. The surgeon opens the abdominal cavity as described for laparotomy.
2. The affected tube is grasped with Allis or Babcock forceps. The infundibulopelvic ligament is clamped with hemostats, cut, and ligated.
3. The mesosalpinx is grasped with hemostats and divided with the suspensory ligament of the ovary.
4. The cornual attachment of the tube is excised with a knife or curved scissors. Bleeding vessels are clamped and ligated.
5. The edges of the broad ligament are peritonealized from the uterine horn to the infundibulopelvic ligament as described for total hysterectomy.
6. The wound is closed as described for laparotomy, and dressings are applied.

Microscopic Reconstructive Surgery of the Fallopian Tube

The obstructed portion of a fallopian tube may be removed and the tube reconstructed to create patency of the remaining portion of the tube, promoting the possibility of fertilization. Reconstructive surgery of the tube, broadly called *tuboplasty,* includes reanastomosis, salpingoneostomy, fimbrioplasty, and lysis of adhesions.

The development of microsurgical techniques has advanced surgical reconstruction of fallopian tubes. Microsurgical techniques may be used with mini-laparotomy or laparoscopy, or both. Microsurgical tubal anastomosis permits atraumatic, accurate alignment of fallopian tube segments. After surgery the fallopian tubes are shorter in length yet remain normal in other aspects. The laser may be adapted to the operating microscope, or the freehand approach may be used in tubal reconstructive surgery.

Procedural Considerations. The patient is in the supine position. The surgeon may place a Kahn, Calvin, Rubin, Hui, or Humi cannula or a pediatric Foley catheter into the uterine cavity for intraoperative chromotubation with diluted methylene blue or indigo carmine solution. Intraoperative chromotubation can also be achieved by applying a Buxton uterine clamp around the lower segment of the uterus and inserting an Angiocath catheter through the fundus into the cavity. A vaginal pack may be inserted to help elevate the uterus.

The basic abdominal gynecologic instrument set is required, with the addition of iris scissors (one curved and one straight), Adson forceps without teeth, Halsted mosquito hemostats, a set of Bowman lacrimal probes, Webster needle holders, Frazier suction tip, Kirschner retractor (if desired), and a Buxton uterine clamp (if desired).

Basic microsurgical instruments include microscissors (one curved and one straight), bayonet microscissors, jeweler's forceps, microforceps, fallopian tube forceps, petit-point mosquito hemostats, micro–needle holders (one curved and one straight), ball-tipped nerve hook, and glass or Teflon rods.

Accessory items include micro–needle electrodes, electrosurgical pencil, bipolar forceps with cord, irrigator, syringes and blunt needles for irrigation of the tissues, plastic or silastic tubing and connectors, diluted methylene blue or indigo carmine solution, diluted heparinized lactated Ringer's solution, microscope drape, microscope or operative loupes, ESU with monopolar and bipolar capabilities, and a video monitoring system (if desired).

Operative Procedure. Operative procedures for correction of postsurgical tubal occlusion are usually performed under the operating microscope. Other reconstructive procedures vary according to the nature of the pathologic condition of the tube and may be performed under the operating microscope or by use of operative loupes.

In microsurgery the surgeon must make sure that virtually no instruments are used in contact with the fallopian tube except those necessary to carry out the surgical technique. Microsurgery for infertility requires the use of specialized and delicate instruments. Each of these instruments is designed to permit gentle, atraumatic handling of tissues and prevent abrasions, lacerations, and vascular damage.

The tissues must be continually irrigated to prevent drying of the serosal surfaces. Lactated Ringer's solution alone or with heparin added may be used as the irrigating solution. Meticulous hemostasis is required in microsurgery. Irrigation is used to identify bleeding vessels or tissues. Hemostasis can be achieved by electrocoagulation with a micro–needle electrode or very fine bipolar forceps. When a CO_2 laser beam is used, the smoke from laser vaporization should be evacuated to prevent carbon deposits on the tissue.

Tubal Ligation

Tubal ligation is interruption of fallopian tube continuity, resulting in sterilization of the patient. In general, the indication for sterilization depends entirely on the desire of the patient. Certain medical indications and concern for the psychosocial needs of the patient are factors, and occasionally an obstetric indication exists, such as inherited fetal deformity. However, at least in the United States, sterilization is entirely a voluntary procedure. Depending on state law, a sterilization permit may have to be signed by the husband. Thorough presurgical counseling is needed for the patient and her husband or significant other because this procedure is not predictably reversible. Patients may elect to have the procedure performed on an ambulatory surgery basis at a time that is convenient for them.

Tubal ligation may be performed during or soon after delivery. This timing usually does not delay the normal discharge time for the patient. An objection to this practice is that the danger of hemorrhage still exists soon after delivery. With a vaginal delivery, tubal ligation is done on the first or second postpartum day. If a cesarean delivery is done, the tubes may be ligated at that time. Note that if performed postpartum, the incision may be at the umbilicus because the uterus is still large.

Operative Procedure. Many surgical methods and techniques are available for tubal ligation. The objective of each method is to achieve complete closure of the fallopian tube so that conception is prevented. When a segment of each fallopian tube is excised, it is preserved for pathologic examination. General surgical considerations are directed to excising a section of each fallopian tube, ligating the severed ends, achieving hemostasis, and incorporating the proximal stump within layers of the mesosalpinx. Another approach, involving insertion of an expandable spring coil into the fallopian tube to mechanically block it, is accomplished hysteroscopically via the transcervical route. The device is made from titanium, stainless steel, nickel, and Dacron fibers. Ultimately the device provides an inflammatory response and fibrosis of the intramural tubal lumen over a 3-month period (Hastings-Tolsma et al, 2006).

LAPAROSCOPIC TUBAL OCCLUSION

1. The operative approach is the same as that for laparoscopy.
2. An accessory suprapubic incision may be made for the occluding instrument.
3. Sterilization may take place by thermal coagulation or by placement of a spring clip or silastic band after the tube has been identified and isolated in the grasping forceps.

a. Bipolar coagulation occurs when electrical current passes only through the tube from prong to prong. At least 3 cm of the tube is destroyed, which therefore prevents spontaneous recanalization. It has been recommended that the tube be grasped at least 2 to 3 cm away from the uterocornual junction at the time of this procedure so that a stump of isthmus remains to absorb the intrauterine fluid under pressure and minimize fistula formation, which could result in an ectopic pregnancy for the patient in the future.

b. The *spring clip* occludes the isthmus of the tube by two plastic jaws (Figure 5-55, *A* and *B*). The tube is compressed by a stainless-steel spring that presses the jaws together. Spring clip application requires careful surgical technique to ensure that the clip is completely across the isthmus of the tube (Figure 5-55, *C*). Some surgeons apply two spring clips positioned close together on each tube when using this approach.

c. With a *silastic band,* the tube is drawn 1.5 cm into a 0.5-cm diameter metal cylinder, which destroys approximately 3 cm of the tube (Figure 5-56, *A*). A silastic ring stretched on the outside of the cylinder is released to form an occlusion (Figure 5-56, *B*). Over time, about 3 cm of the constricted tube undergoes necrosis and the tubes separate (Figure 5-56, *C*).

MINI-LAPAROTOMY APPROACH

1. The surgeon creates a 2-cm transverse incision above the pubic hairline.
2. A large bivalved speculum may be placed through the incision and into the peritoneal cavity. The large Graves bivalve speculum serves as a small abdominal retractor and permits easy access to the tubes.
3. Spring clips or silastic bands can be applied, or the original Pomeroy method of ligation can be carried out. The Pomeroy, modified Pomeroy, or Parkland techniques provide a tissue specimen of each tube. Suture material is tied around each tube, and a section of tube is removed. Over time, the tubes separate, destroying the passage between the ovary and the uterus.

TRANSCERVICAL APPROACH (ESSURE)

1. The operative approach is the same as that for hysteroscopy.
2. The uterus is distended, and the ostia are visualized.
3. The spring device (Figure 5-57) is placed on the tip of the plastic carrier provided in the kit and inserted through the hysteroscope's channel.
4. The device is guided to the tubal ostium, and the handle for the carrying device is stabilized.
5. The device is released from the plastic carrier, and the coil is deployed as the handle is retracted (Figure 5-58).
6. The surgeon counts the number of coils trailing into the uterine cavity. There should be three to eight visible coils (Figure 5-59).
7. The sequence is repeated for the remaining fallopian tube.

ASSISTED REPRODUCTIVE THERAPIES FOR INFERTILITY

Infertility is a condition that affects approximately 10% of reproductive-age couples. Infertility implies subfertility—a prolonged time to conceive—as opposed to sterility, which means inability to conceive (Lowdermilk, 2007b). Infertility is referred to as primary when it occurs without a prior preg-

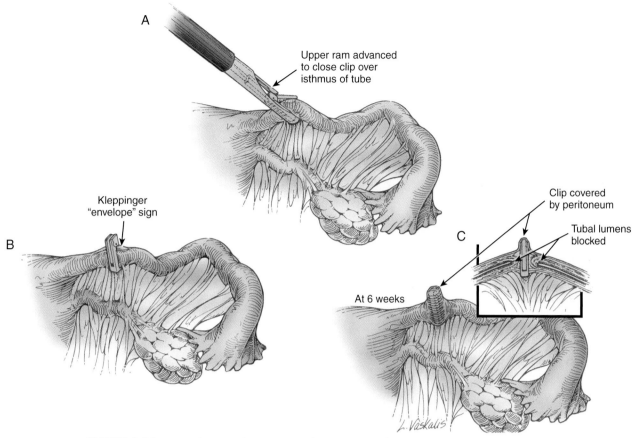

FIGURE 5-55 Spring clip. **A,** Isthmic portion (first 2 to 3 cm of tube) is maneuvered into the open jaws of the clip until it is snug against the hinge. **B,** Closing the clip will create the Kleppinger envelope sign—a fold of tubal peritoneum in the hinge of the clip. **C,** Failure to get the clip completely across the isthmus may result in pregnancy. Some surgeons routinely use two clips close together on each tube.

nancy and secondary if it occurs after a successful conception. Facing infertility is an emotionally stressful process for both partners. Treatment of infertility is multidimensional and may involve medical as well as surgical interventions. Often by the time a woman presents in the perioperative setting for a procedure related to infertility, she and her partner have undergone many months or years of testing and medical interventions. Individuals with infertility use various coping strategies, and the healthcare providers need to be aware of these in providing supportive care.

Eighty percent of couples that do not have fertility issues achieve conception within 1 year. A couple is considered infertile if they have not conceived after attempting for 1 year, although this landmark may be modified because of select clinical circumstances. Both partners undergo extensive testing to identify possible organic or functional causes for their infertility. Identifiable conditions contributing to infertility are attributed to the female partner in 50% of couples, the male partner in 18.5% of couples, and both partners in 18.4% of couples (Robins and Carson, 2008).

The term *assisted reproductive therapies (ARTs)* refers to the multiple options couples may select to assist them in the reproduction process. ARTs are described briefly in Table 5-3. Techniques for ART have evolved over time, with the majority of interventions conducted in the physician's office. The use of

ARTs has made it possible for women to successfully conceive and have children when they are older than 40.

OBSTETRIC SURGERY

Providing safe care for the perioperative patient is the goal of every healthcare provider. The interventions necessary to reach that goal intensify in the pregnant woman who presents for surgery. The team is now faced with the challenge of caring for at least two patients, the mother and her child (Risk Reduction Strategies).

Maternal changes in pregnancy increase as the gestation progresses and include hormonal fluctuations, mechanical changes to the viscera related to the enlarging uterus, increased metabolic and oxygen demands, and hemodynamic changes. The fetus also has unique metabolic and hemodynamic needs that must be considered. Hazards of performing surgery on the pregnant patient include fetal loss, fetal asphyxia, premature labor, premature rupture of the membranes, and thromboembolic events. Many medications used in the perioperative setting cross into the placental circulation on administration to the mother (Birnbach and Browne, 2005).

Special considerations for the obstetric surgical patient include continuous monitoring of the fetal heart rate, rapid induction for general gynesthesia, and preparation for the pos-

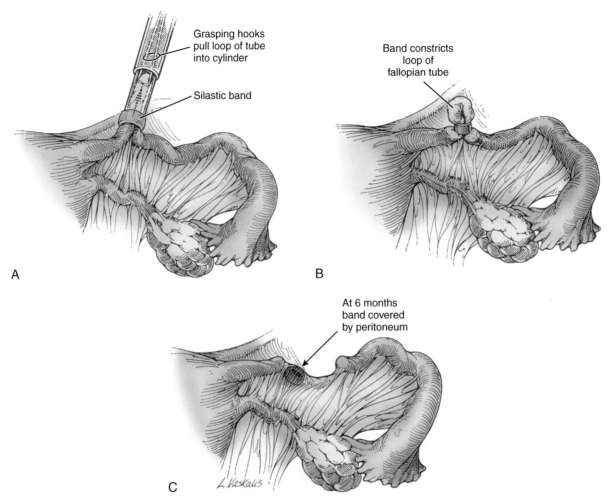

FIGURE 5-56 Silastic band. **A,** About 3 cm of tube is drawn into a 5-mm cylinder over which a silastic band has been stretched. **B,** Releasing the band constricts the knuckle of tube with eventual necrosis. **C,** As with the Pomeroy technique, 6 months later the stumps are about 3 cm apart.

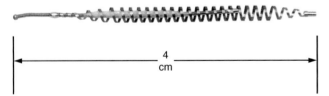

FIGURE 5-57 Essure implant.

sible use of tocolytics (e.g., medications to decrease uterine activity) to prevent labor (Surgical Pharmacology). Ready access to neonatal resuscitative drugs and equipment should be established when performing surgery on pregnant women in the second trimester and beyond. If permitted by the surgical approach, the pregnant woman should be positioned with a lateral tilt or with a wedge or pillow under her right hip to provide uterine displacement and relieve pressure on the maternal vena cava. This position promotes blood flow to the placenta.

Cervical Cerclage

Incompetence of the cervix is a condition characterized by habitual midtrimester spontaneous miscarriages. The condition is characterized by shortening of the length of the cer-

vix (observed on ultrasound) and occasional funneling of the cervix. Surgical intervention is designed to prevent cervical dilation that results in the release of uterine contents. Introduced by Shirodkar in 1951, the cervical cerclage provides a mechanical closure to the cervix. Cerclage is most commonly accomplished by way of the vaginal approach (Shirodkar and McDonald approaches) or, much less commonly, the abdominal or laparoscopic approach. The Shirodkar technique involves the *submucosal* placement of a purse-string type of ligature of Mersilene, Dacron tape, heavy nylon suture, or plastic-covered braided-steel suture at the level of the internal os to close it (Genovese, 2007). The McDonald cerclage uses a secured tie or tape placed horizontally and vertically across the cervix. The vaginal cerclage is generally removed in an office procedure when the woman reaches the thirty-seventh week of gestation, or the child may be delivered by cesarean.

Procedural Considerations—Vaginal Approach. Gentle vaginal preparation is carried out. The instrumentation includes the basic vaginal instrument set, with the addition of right and left Deschamps ligature carriers, trocar needles, sutures for the internal os, and the surgeon's preference for closure of the mucosal incisions.

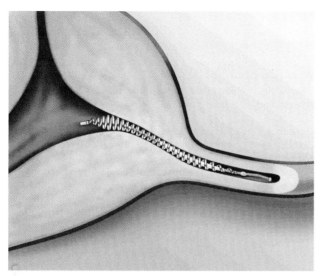

FIGURE 5-58 Essure device placed in fallopian tube.

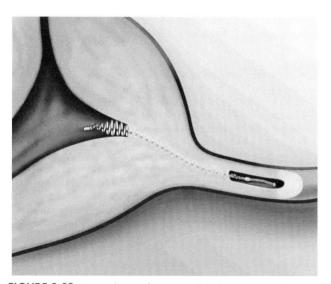

FIGURE 5-59 Essure device after carrier detached. Note coils in uterine cavity.

Operative Procedure—Shirodkar/McDonald

1. Anterior and posterior vaginal retractors are placed, and the cervix is pulled down with smooth ovum or sponge-holding forceps. With smooth tissue forceps and dissecting scissors, the mucosa over the anterior cervix is opened to permit the bladder to be pushed back (Figure 5-60).
2. The surgeon lifts the cervix and incises the posterior vaginal mucosa at the level of the peritoneal reflection. The corners of the anterior and posterior incisions are bilaterally approximated in the area of the lateral mucosa with curved tonsil or Allis forceps.
3. The prepared ligature is placed at the desired level by passage of the material through the approximated tissue and is drawn tight posteriorly to close the cervix. The suture material for the ligature is then tied. It is not necessary to suture the ligature to the underlying tissues. The suture material used for this ligation is 5-mm Dacron or Mersi-

lene tape. The anterior and posterior mucosal incisions are usually closed with 2-0 absorbable suture to complete the procedure.
4. The McDonald cerclage is performed in a similar manner, using the same instrumentation, supplies, and preparation. The suture is not buried in the submucosa in the McDonald technique (Figure 5-61).

►► RISK REDUCTION STRATEGIES

Preparation for Cardiac Arrest in the Pregnant Patient

Although rare, cardiopulmonary arrest does occur in the pregnant patient. The surgical team can reduce risk to the patient and her infant through familiarity with resuscitation techniques for pregnant patients. Guidelines for cardiac arrest during pregnancy include the following:

AIRWAY
◆ Determine unresponsiveness.
◆ Activate the code team and obtain the automated cardiac defibrillator.
◆ Position the woman supine on a firm surface with a roll or wedge placed under the right hip to displace the uterus laterally off the great vessels; or position her laterally.
◆ Open the airway with the head tilt-chin lift maneuver.

BREATHING
◆ Determine breathlessness (look, listen, and feel).
◆ If the woman is not breathing, give two breaths, 1 second apart.

CIRCULATION
◆ Determine pulselessness by checking the carotid pulse.
◆ If there is no pulse, begin chest compressions at a rate of 100 per minute. Chest compressions may be performed slightly higher on the sternum if the uterus is enlarged enough to displace the diaphragm into a higher position. Check the pulse after 2 minutes; if the pulse is not present, continue CPR.

DEFIBRILLATION
◆ If defibrillation is necessary, ensure the paddles are placed one rib space higher than usual because the heart is displaced slightly by the uterus.

If possible the fetus should be monitored during the cardiac arrest. If the fetus is delivered within 5 minutes of the arrest, intact neurologic survival (in fetuses of viable gestational age) is likely; beyond 15 minutes, impairment or death is likely.

Successful resuscitation may be associated with complications for the woman, including laceration of the liver, rupture of the spleen or uterus, hemothorax, hemoperitoneum, or fracture of the ribs or sternum. Fetal complications may include cardiac dysrhythmia or asystole associated with maternal defibrillation and medications, CNS depression related to antidysrhythmic medications and inadequate placental perfusion, possible hypoxemia, and acidosis.

If the resuscitation is successful, ongoing intensive monitoring, including fetal surveillance, is necessary as the woman is at increased risk for recurrent cardiac arrest and dysrhythmia. Fetal status and gestational age should be considered and used in decision-making regarding delivery or continuation of the pregnancy.

Modified from McAteer J: Medical-surgical problems in pregnancy. In Lowdermilk DL, Perry SE, editors: *Maternity and women's health care,* ed 9, St Louis, 2007, Mosby.

TABLE 5-3

Assisted Reproductive Therapies

Technology	Description	Use
Assisted hatching (AH)	The zona pellucida is micromanipulated chemically or mechanically to allow the embryo to hatch and attach to the uterine wall.	Recurrent miscarriage, failed IVF, advanced maternal age
In vitro fertilization embryo transfer (IVF-ET)	Follows in vitro fertilization. The fertilized ovum is implanted in the woman's uterus. Typically three embryos are transferred.	Tubal disease or blockage, endometriosis, unexplained infertility, cervical factors, immunity issues
Donor oocyte	Eggs are donated by an IVF procedure and the donated eggs are inseminated. Embryos are transferred into the recipient's uterus, which is hormonally prepared with estrogen/progesterone.	Early menopause, surgical removal of ovaries or congenitally absent ovaries, autosomal or sex-linked disorders, lack of fertilization in repeated IVF attempts because of subtle oocyte abnormalities or defects in oocyte-spermatozoa interaction
Donor embryo	A donated embryo is transferred to the uterus of an infertile woman.	Infertility not resolved by less aggressive forms of therapy; absence of ovaries; male partner azoospermic or severely compromised
Therapeutic donor insemination (TDI)	Donor sperm are used to inseminate the female partner.	Male partner azoospermic or has very low sperm count; couple has genetic defect; male partner has antisperm antibodies
Gamete intrafallopian transfer (GIFT)	Oocytes are retrieved from the ovary and mixed in a catheter with sperm. The solution is transferred into the fimbriated end of the tube for in situ fertilization.	Unexplained infertility with normal, patent fallopian tubes
Intracervical insemination (ICI)	Performed during a natural cycle or stimulated cycle. Sperm are placed inside the neck of the cervix by means of a catheter and syringe.	Immunity issues, desire or need to use donor sperm in otherwise fertile woman, male infertility, unexplained infertility
Intracytoplasmic sperm injection (ICSI)	Selection of single sperm injected directly into the egg to achieve fertilization.	Failed IVF, oligospermia, asthenospermia, obstructive azoospermia, immunity issues, failed vasectomy reversal
Intrauterine insemination (IUI)	Similar to ICI; performed during a natural cycle or stimulated cycle. Sperm are placed inside uterus by means of a catheter and syringe.	Immunity issues, desire or need to use donor sperm in otherwise fertile woman, male infertility, unexplained infertility; failure of ICI
In vitro fertilization (IVF)	Oocytes are retrieved from the ovary and fertilized with sperm in the laboratory and allowed to develop into embryos. Embryos are then transferred to the woman using a variety of techniques.	Tubal disease or blockage, severe male infertility, endometriosis, immunity issues, unexplained infertility, cervical factors
Zygote intrafallopian transfer (ZIFT)	In vitro fertilization is accomplished and embryo is placed in the fallopian tube during the zygote stage.	Unexplained infertility with normal, patent fallopian tubes

Modified from Lowdermilk DL: Infertility. In Lowdermilk DL, Perry SE, editors: *Maternity and women's health care*, ed 9, St Louis, 2007, Mosby.

Procedural Considerations—Abdominal Approach. The transabdominal cerclage is reserved for select women who have a cervix that is so short or damaged that the vaginal approach is not feasible. A vaginal and abdominal prep is performed. A Foley catheter may be placed to ensure the urinary bladder remains decompressed. A basic vaginal set and an abdominal set are needed for instrumentation. Sutures used for the transabdominal cerclage are identical to those used in the vaginal approach.

Operative Procedure—Abdominal Approach

1. The abdomen is opened and the viscera retracted. The Trendelenburg's position may be used to facilitate exposure.
2. The suture material or tape is placed around the uterine isthmus medial to the uterine vessels and fixed to the anterior isthmus, to Mackenrodt's ligaments, and to the insertions of the uterosacral ligaments.

3. The abdominal wound is closed as described for laparotomy closure (see Chapter 2).
4. Abdominal dressings and a perineal pad are applied.

Procedural Considerations—Laparoscopic Approach. The laparoscopic approach may be associated with decreased postoperative pain and morbidity compared with the laparotomy approach. Standard laparoscopic equipment commonly used in gynecologic procedures is required.

Operative Procedure—Laparoscopic Approach

1. The laparoscopic camera and ports are placed for a standard laparoscopic approach, and pneumoperitoneum is established.
2. The bladder peritoneum is opened at the level of the uterine isthmus.

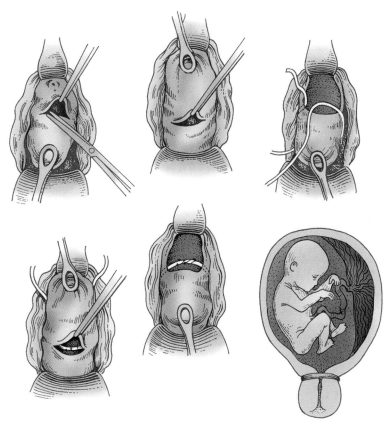

FIGURE 5-60 Principles of Shirodkar operation for treatment of incompetent internal cervical os during pregnancy.

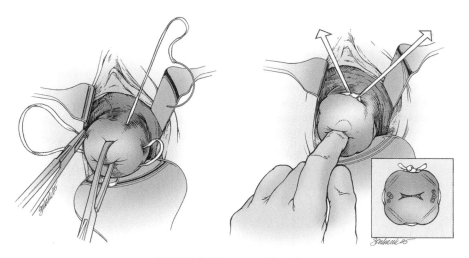

FIGURE 5-61 McDonald cerclage.

3. The surgeon creates a window through the broad ligament medially to the uterine vessels at the level of the internal os.
4. A strip of polypropylene mesh is placed retroperitoneally through the window circumferentially around the isthmus above the cardinal and sacrouterine ligaments.
5. The mesh is anchored with a nonabsorbable suture.
6. The laparoscopic instruments are removed, and the wounds are closed.

ABDOMINAL SURGERY DURING PREGNANCY

The incidence of the immediate need for abdominal surgery occurs as frequently among pregnant women as among nonpregnant women of childbearing ages. Diagnosis of the abdominal problems in the pregnant woman is challenging because of the enlarged uterus and displaced organs. Mild leukocytosis and increased levels of alkaline phosphatase and amylase

SURGICAL PHARMACOLOGY

Medications Used in Gynecology and Obstetrics

Part of safe perioperative patient care focuses on safe medication practices. Strategies for safe medication administration include standardizing medication labeling both on and off the surgical field, separating sound-alike and look-alike medications, and minimizing distractions.

In addition to practicing the "seven rights" (right patient, right drug, right time, right route, right dose, right documentation, and right technique) for the medications, the surgical staff must be familiar with medications administered to the patient by others (e.g., anesthesia providers, surgeons). Many of the medications used in gynecologic and obstetric surgery are unique to the specialty or have unique uses within the specialty.

OXYTOCICS

Medications that increase motor activity within the uterus by hormonal stimulation or direct stimulation on the smooth muscles, usually resulting in uterine contractions. Used intraoperatively and postoperatively.

Medication	Perioperative Uses	Actions	Dosage/Administration	Adverse Reactions
Oxytocin (Pitocin)	Postabortion bleeding, postpartum bleeding, improvement of uterine contractility after cesarean delivery	Acts on uterine myofibril activity	Given IV only, 10-40 units per liter of fluid	Hypertonicity with tearing of the uterus
Methylergonovine maleate (Methergine)	Postabortion bleeding, postpartum bleeding	Ergot alkaline that causes vasospasm of the coronary arteries and directly stimulates uterine muscle	May be given PO, IM, or IV; most frequent route in OR is IM; IM/IV dose is 0.2 mg; may be repeated q2-4hr for no more than a total of five doses	Nausea; cramping; vomiting; dizziness; diaphoresis; bradycardia; chest pain; tachycardia; pale, cool, and blotchy skin; facial swelling; increased uterine pain
Dinoprostone (Cervidil)	Postabortion bleeding, postpartum bleeding	Prostaglandin that directly acts on the myometrium, causing softening of the cervix; causes myometrial contractions in the gravid uterus	May be administered as an endocervical gel, vaginal insert, or vaginal suppository	Vomiting, nausea, bradycardia, chills/shivering, diarrhea

TOCOLYTICS

Medications that decrease uterine contractility. Most commonly used in the perioperative setting during fetal surgery or in surgical procedures on pregnant females. May also be used in the postanesthesia care unit.

Medication	Perioperative Uses	Actions	Dosage/Administration	Adverse Reactions
Ritodrine (Yutopar)	Prevention of preterm labor	β-Adrenergic that inhibits uterine activity by relaxing smooth uterine muscle tissue	May be given PO or IV; IV dose is 0.05-0.1 mg/min	Shortness of breath, tachypnea, tachycardia, palpitations, chest pain, fluid retention, hypotension, nausea, vomiting

are normal during pregnancy and may also indicate surgical intraperitoneal processes. Abnormally high or rising laboratory values should be noted. Radiographic evaluation is contraindicated in most instances during pregnancy (McAteer, 2007).

Laparotomy or laparoscopy may be required for conditions such as appendicitis and intestinal obstruction. Appendicitis is the most common nonobstetric surgical condition that complicates pregnancy and occurs with equal frequency in each of the trimesters and the postpartum period in approximately 1 in every 2000 pregnancies (McAteer, 2007).

Fetal Surgery

Developments in prenatal diagnosis have progressed to the point where clinicians may consider the fetus to be the patient. Serious congenital anomaly is diagnosable by ultrasonography, alpha-fetoprotein specimen, amniocentesis, chorionic villi sampling, or percutaneous umbilical blood sampling. When an anomaly is identified, a multidisciplinary team reviews the mother's complete medical history and prenatal ultrasonograms.

SURGICAL PHARMACOLOGY

Medications Used in Gynecology and Obstetrics—cont'd

Medication	Perioperative Uses	Actions	Dosage/Administration	Adverse Reactions
TOCOLYTICS—cont'd				
Terbutaline (Brethine)	Prevention of preterm labor	Adrenergic agonist that stimulates β-adrenergic receptors, resulting in relaxation of uterine smooth muscle	May be given PO, Sub-Q, or IV; usual IV dose is 2.5-10 mcg/min; may increase gradually q15-20 min up to 17.5-30 mcg/min; PO dose is 2.5-10 mg q4-6hr	Tremors, anxiety, nervousness, drowsiness, headache, nausea, heartburn, dizziness; flushing and weakness
Magnesium sulfate	Prevention of preterm labor, prevention/treatment of convulsions caused by pregnancy-induced hypertension (preeclampsia/eclampsia)	Relaxes smooth muscle of the uterus; blocks neuromuscular transmission to produce seizure control	Loading dose of 4-6 g diluted in 100 ml of IV fluid, given over 30-60 min; maintenance dose 2-4 g/hr	Reduced respiratory rate, decreased reflexes, decreased heart rate, hypotension, sedation
ANTIMETABOLITES				
Medications that interrupt cell division. May be given intraoperatively or postoperatively.				
Methotrexate	Used in ectopic pregnancy and hydatidiform mole surgery to eradicate any remaining trophoblastic cells	Inhibits RNA, DNA, and protein synthesis in rapidly dividing cells	PO, IM, IV Most commonly given IM in perioperative setting (15-30 mg)	Nausea, vomiting, stomatitis, dizziness, blurred vision, photophobia, hepatotoxicity, nephrotoxicity
MISCELLANEOUS AGENTS				
Misoprostol (Cytotec)	Used for cervical ripening; may be used instead of dilation and evacuation (D&E) for missed or incomplete abortion (off-label use)	Synthetic prostaglandin that acts directly on uterine muscle	Oral, rectal, or intravaginal; available in 100- and 200-mcg tablets; oral dose for missed abortion: 600 mcg; cervical ripening: intravaginal, 25 mcg (¼ of 100-mcg tablet) 2-3 hr before procedure	Diarrhea, abdominal pain; headache, nausea, uterine rupture
Estradiol cream (Estrace cream)	Lubricant for vaginal packing	Increased synthesis of RNA, DNA, protein in tissues; reduces release of gonadotropin hormone from the hypothalamus; reduces FSH and LH from the pituitary gland	Topical cream, 0.1 mg/g, intravaginally	Local irritation, vaginal discharge

Continued

Depending on the anomaly and the immediate danger posed to the fetus, the family will be counseled on their options. If no treatment is available and the condition is fatal, the family may elect to terminate the pregnancy if it is earlier than 24 weeks of gestation or may choose to carry the fetus to term. If postnatal correction is possible, the family may consider terminating the pregnancy or may continue the pregnancy with monitoring, hoping for successful correction after delivery. Lethal and nonlethal anomalies may be treated with prenatal surgery. If a family elects this option, both the mother and the fetus are evaluated to determine if they will be acceptable surgical candidates. Fetal surgery was previously confined to treatment of anomalies that would result in fetal death before term or during the immediate postnatal period, but it now includes treatment of nonlethal conditions in selected cases. Conditions treated by fetal surgery include congenital diaphragmatic hernia (Figure 5-62), congenital cystic adenomatoid malformation, bronchopulmonary sequestration, obstructive uropathy, sacrococcygeal teratomas (Figure 5-63), twin-to-twin transfusion syndrome, thoracic lesions, twin reversed arterial perfusion syndrome,

SURGICAL PHARMACOLOGY

Medications Used in Gynecology and Obstetrics—cont'd

Medication	Perioperative Uses	Actions	Dosage/Administration	Adverse Reactions
MISCELLANEOUS AGENTS—cont'd				
Miconazole nitrate cream (Monistat)	Lubricant for vaginal packing, treatment of vulvovaginal candidiasis	Inhibits synthesis of ergosterol (an important component of fungal cell formation)	2% topical cream intravaginally	Local irritation, vaginal discharge
Sulfathiazole/ sulfacetamide/ sulfabenzamide cream (Triple Sulfa)	Lubricant for vaginal packing, treatment of *Gardnerella* vaginitis	Exerts bacteriostatic action by competitive antagonism of PABA (a component of folic acid synthesis)	Topical cream used intravaginally; concentration: sulfathiazole 3.42%, sulfacetamide 2.86%, and sulfabenzamide 3.7%	Local irritation, vaginal discharge, Stevens-Johnson syndrome
Vasopressin (Pitressin)	Injected directly into uterus to decrease bleeding during hysterectomy	Causes vasoconstriction through direct stimulation of smooth muscle; pituitary hormone	20 units/ml to be diluted in injectable saline as directed by surgeon	Diaphoresis, circumoral pallor, wheezing, allergic reactions
Methylene blue	Indicator dye: intraoperative hysterosalpingogram; used to test patency of ureters	Converts ferrous iron to methemoglobin	0.1-0.2% ml/kg given IV push, slowly	Hypertension, dizziness, staining of skin, discoloration of urine or stool

ACOG, American College of Obstetricians and Gynecologists; *BP,* blood pressure; *DNA,* deoxyribonucleic acid; *FDA,* Food and Drug Administration; *FSH,* follicle-stimulating hormone; *hCG,* human chorionic gonadotropin; *I&O,* intake and output; *IM,* intramuscular; *IV,* intravascular; *LH,* luteinizing hormone; *PABA, para-*aminobenzoic acid; *PO,* by mouth; *RNA,* ribonucleic acid; *Sub-Q,* subcutaneous.

Modified from Hodgson BB, Kizior RJ: *Saunders nursing drug handbook 2010,* St Louis, 2010, Saunders; Skidmore-Roth L: *Mosby's drug guide for nurses with 2010 update,* ed 8, St Louis, 2010, Mosby; Wanzer LJ: Perioperative initiatives for medication safety, *AORN J* 82(4):663-666, 2005; Zhang J et al: A comparison of medical management with misoprostol and surgical management for early pregnancy failure, *N Engl J Med* 353:761-769, 2005.

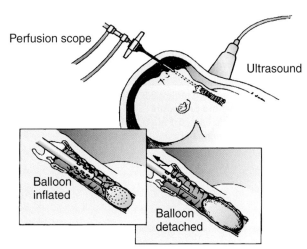

FIGURE 5-62 Fetal surgery for congenital diaphragmatic hernia. The trachea is isolated in preparation of hemoclip placement.

monochorionic twins, discordant twins, and myelomeningocele (Figure 5-64) (Jancelewicz and Harrison, 2009). Fetal surgery may be accomplished by way of laparotomy and hysterotomy or, in some instances, with endoscopic techniques.

Postoperatively, preterm labor is of great concern, and uterine contractions, fetal heart rate, and fetal electrocardiogram (ECG) are closely monitored. Tocolytic medications are titrated to control uterine contractions. The mother is educated in self-monitoring of uterine contractions, and tocolytic therapy is continued on an outpatient basis. Frequent fetal ultrasonic scans are performed postoperatively to monitor fetal growth, amniotic fluid volume, and the adequacy of the surgical repair. Fetal surgery may also place the mother at risk for uterine rupture in subsequent pregnancies.

Cesarean Birth

Cesarean birth, also referred to as *cesarean section* or *C-section*, is delivery of the fetus or fetuses through abdominal (laparotomy) and uterine (hysterotomy) incisions. In general, cesarean birth is employed whenever further delay in delivery may seriously compromise the fetus, the mother, or both, and vaginal delivery cannot be safely accomplished. In recent years the use of cesarean birth has increased as a result of fetal monitoring, fetal scalp blood sampling for pH determination, and the widespread emphasis on recognition of actual or suspected impairment of fetal well-being if delivery was delayed or vaginal delivery attempted. Reasons for cesarean birth include failure to progress, malposition and malpresentation, cephalopelvic disproportion, abruptio placentae, toxemia, fetal distress, uterine dysfunction, placenta previa, prolapsed cord, previous pelvic surgery, cervical dystocia, active herpes progenitalis, and diabetes. Multiple pregnancies may also be an indication for cesarean delivery. In certain situations, and after appropriate counseling, elective cesarean delivery may be a medically acceptable option. Thus

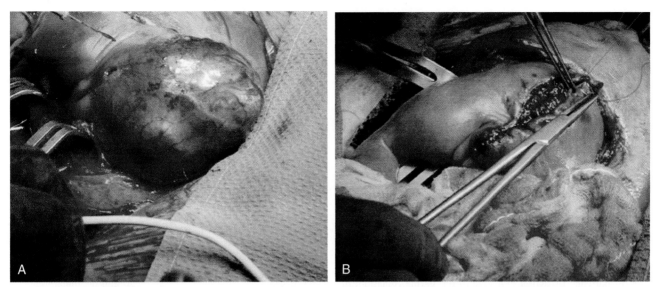

FIGURE 5-63 A, Start of fetal resection of a sacrococcygeal teratoma at 21 weeks of gestation. **B**, Closure of the defect.

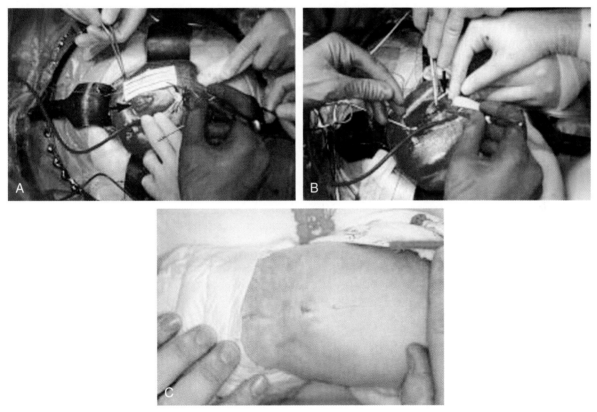

FIGURE 5-64 A, Myelomeningocele. **B**, Uterus is opened over defect. **C**, Myelomeningocele repair completed, appearance postdelivery.

cesarean births may be classified as primary (woman's first cesarean), repeat (indicates a previous cesarean birth), elective (a scheduled procedure in either of the previous categories or at maternal request), or emergency (there is an immediate need for intervention) (Roberts and Mangan, 2009).

Cesarean delivery is ranked as the second most frequently performed major surgical operation in the United States. Approximately 1,479,646 cesarean sections were performed in 2007 (HCUPnet, 2007). Rates have decreased slightly because of increased use of labor trials and vaginal birth after cesarean birth (VBAC) in selected patients.

Cesarean delivery may take place in the obstetric OR or main OR suite. Patients about to undergo cesarean birth need careful assessment and emotional support. Because cesarean

RAPID RESPONSE TEAM

Rapid response systems, endorsed by the American College of Obstetricians and Gynecologists, include case detection that triggers a crisis team response, and provision of a readily available response team. Within the OR setting, dedicated facility rapid response teams may or may not respond to perioperative emergencies, but in the case of obstetric emergencies, it may be necessary to summon a medical emergency team with experience in perinatal care. Surgical teams can positively impact outcomes by recognizing situations where early intervention is essential to prevent maternal morbidity. Amniotic fluid embolism (AFE) is an example of a situation that requires early recognition and swift action to save the mother and her child. Surgical teams summon an obstetric rapid response team for AFE if involved in cesarean section or assisting with a complicated vaginal delivery in the OR, or may be involved in assisting in the treatment of AFE in the labor and delivery department.

Although uncommon, AFE occurs when amniotic fluid containing particles of debris (e.g., hair, skin, vernix, meconium) enters the maternal circulation. The woman's pulmonary vessels become occluded and respiratory distress and circulatory collapse with coagulopathy may ensue. AFE can transpire at any point during labor and delivery and occurs in 7.7 per 100,000 births with a fatality rate between 21.6% and 37%.

The most common symptom of AFE is acute dyspnea followed by severe hypotension. Risk factors for AFE include multiparity, advanced maternal age, male fetus, cesarean section or operative vaginal delivery, abruptio placentae, placenta previa, and cervical laceration or uterine rupture. Emergency interventions by the rapid response team are summarized below:

♦ Administer oxygen by face mask (8-10 L/min) or Ambu bag with 100% oxygen.
♦ Prepare for mechanical intubation and ventilation.
♦ Initiate or assist with cardiopulmonary resuscitation. Tilt the pregnant woman 30 degrees to the left to displace the uterus.
♦ Administer IV fluids.
♦ Administer blood: packed cells, fresh frozen plasma.
♦ Insert indwelling catheter and monitor urine output.
♦ Correct coagulation failure.
♦ Monitor fetal and maternal status.

Newer treatment modalities for AFE that may be more easily accessed in the OR include the following:
♦ Cardiopulmonary bypass
♦ Cell salvage
♦ Extracorporeal membrane oxygenation
♦ Intra-aortic balloon counterpulsation
♦ Invasive cardiac and hemodynamic monitoring
♦ Nitric oxygen therapy
♦ Transesophageal echocardiography
♦ Ventricular assist device

Modified from Dobbenga-Rhodes YA: Responding to amniotic fluid embolism, *AORN J* 89(6):1079-1088, 2009; Gosman GG et al: Introduction of an obstetric-specific medical emergency team for obstetric crises: implementation and experience, *Am J Obstet Gynecol* 198:367e1-367e7, 2008; Piotrowski KA: Labor and birth complications. In Lowdermilk DL, Perry SE, editors: *Maternity and women's health care*, ed 9, St Louis, 2007, Mosby.

birth frequently involves emergency situations, the mother may express grave concern for the infant's well-being. If the mother has participated in childbirth classes, she may believe that she has failed in some way. All healthcare providers must be aware of the psychologic as well as physiologic needs of this patient population. Mothers may choose to remain awake after administration of a regional anesthetic; the mother's birthing partner may be permitted to accompany and support her in the OR and witness the birth (based on hospital policy). The birthing partner may need assistance in preparing for the delivery by washing hands and donning scrub attire or a protective gown. The surgical staff may need to reassure and encourage the birthing partner to coach and lend support to the mother during this intensely stressful time. The birthing partner can be included in the bonding process that is initiated at birth. The mother, if awake and stable, is shown and encouraged to hold the infant, thus promoting a positive family-oriented experience.

If the cesarean delivery is performed as an emergency, the family-oriented approach may not be feasible. In this emergency situation, the mother's support persons need to be directed to the surgical waiting area, where information will be communicated regarding the condition of the mother and infant. Support persons may then be able to accompany the infant as he or she is transferred to the nursery. In an emergency cesarean birth, certain perioperative procedures may be omitted, such as an initial surgical count. When this occurs, an abdominal x-ray is usually completed before the patient leaves the OR (Roberts and Mangan, 2009). The surgical team should follow the institution's protocol for documenting the x-ray and

its results, along with the reasons why the initial count was omitted.

A complication that may occur in conjunction with a cesarean delivery is amniotic fluid embolism. The surgical team must be familiar with this complication and recommended treatment to resolve it (Rapid Response Team box).

Procedural Considerations. The patient should be in a supine position with elevation of the right side to displace the uterus and prevent aortocaval compression. Bony prominences are padded, and the patient is positioned in good body alignment with a safety strap above the knees. Throughout this process, maternal vital signs and fetal heart tones are monitored and recorded per institutional protocol.

If a general anesthetic is to be employed, all preparations—including skin prep, bladder drainage, draping, suction connection, counts, and gowning and gloving of all scrubbed personnel—are done before induction. In many hospitals, healthcare providers qualified to deliver newborn care and resuscitation are in attendance for the delivery. A radiant warmer and resuscitative equipment for immediate postdelivery care of the infant are available in the OR because these infants are considered to be at risk until there is evidence of physiologic stability.

The skin is prepped as for abdominal surgery. The vagina is not prepped. An indwelling urinary catheter is inserted. Instrumentation includes the basic abdominal gynecologic set, with the addition of Lister bandage scissors, Foerster sponge-holding (ring) forceps, Pennington forceps, cord clamps, a DeLee

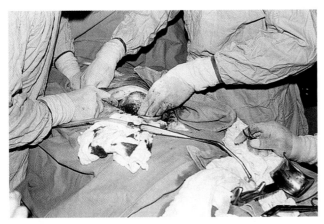

FIGURE 5-65 Fundal pressure applied. Infant's head emerging from hysterotomy.

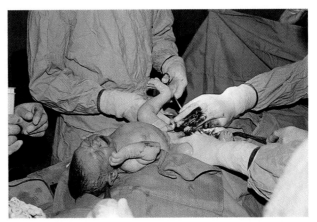

FIGURE 5-66 Cord clamped in preparation for passing infant off field.

retractor, delivery forceps, a head extractor (if desired), laboratory tubes for cord blood and blood gases, a drain (optional), and a bulb syringe.

Operative Procedure

1. The surgeon makes an infraumbilical vertical incision or lower transverse Pfannenstiel incision. The incision should be just long enough to allow the infant to be delivered without difficulty. Therefore the length of the incision varies with the estimated size of the fetus.

2. The abdominal wall is opened in layers. The rectus and pyramidalis muscles are separated in the midline by sharp and blunt dissection to expose the underlying transversalis fascia and peritoneum.

3. The peritoneum is elevated with two Crile hemostats about 2 cm apart. The peritoneum between the two clamps is palpated to rule out the inclusion of bowel, omentum, or bladder. The surgeon opens the peritoneum and enters the abdominal cavity.

4. Bleeding sites anywhere in the abdominal incision may be clamped but not ligated until later, unless the clamps obstruct exposure. When the patient has been administered a general anesthetic, speed is important to prevent an anesthetized infant. The ESU may be used for hemostasis, especially if the patient is awake and a regional anesthetic has been administered.

5. The surgeon quickly palpates the uterus to determine the size and presenting part of the fetus as well as the direction and degree of rotation of the uterus.

6. The reflection of the peritoneum (serosa) above the upper margin of the bladder and overlying the anterior lower uterine segment is gently separated by sharp and blunt dissection.

7. The developed bladder flap is held downward beneath the symphysis with a bladder retractor such as the DeLee.

8. The uterus is opened with a knife through the lower uterine segment about 2 cm above the bladder flap. Once the uterus is opened, the incision can be extended by cutting laterally with a large bandage scissors or by simply spreading the incision by means of lateral pressure applied with each index finger when the lower uterine segment is thin.

9. The presenting membranes are incised. Suction is imperative here, and many surgeons prefer no suction tip (only the large, open end of the suction tubing) during the expulsion and suctioning of amniotic fluid.

10. All retractors are removed. The fetal head is gently elevated, either manually or by use of obstetric forceps, through the incision, aided by transabdominal fundal pressure (Figure 5-65) to help expel the fetus.

11. As soon as the head is delivered, a bulb syringe or aspirator tip is used to aspirate the exposed nares and mouth to minimize aspiration of amniotic fluid and its contents.

12. Oxytocin (20 units per liter of fluid or as directed by the surgeon) may be administered intravenously by the anesthesia provider as soon as the shoulders are delivered (or after delivery of the infant), so that the uterus contracts. This use of oxytocin minimizes blood loss.

13. On delivery of the entire infant, the cord is clamped and cut (Figure 5-66), and the infant is given to the member of the team who is responsible for resuscitation efforts as needed. A sterile gown or sheet should be provided to the individual receiving the infant to avoid any break in aseptic technique and to maintain Standard Precautions during transfer of the infant.

14. The edges of the uterine incision are promptly clamped with Péan forceps, ring forceps, or Pennington clamps.

15. The placenta is delivered and placed in a large receptacle provided from the back table. Fundal massage or manual removal may be employed to hasten delivery of the placenta and reduce bleeding.

16. One or two separate layers of suture may be used to close the uterine incision. The circulator and surgical technologist conduct a count to verify no objects have been retained in the uterine cavity.

17. After determination that there is no further bleeding after closure of the uterine incision, the cut edges of the serosa overlying the uterus and bladder are approximated with a continuous suture.

18. Any blood, blood clots, vernix, and amniotic fluid in the pelvis and peritoneal cavity are removed. The fallopian tubes and ovaries are also inspected. Tubal ligation may be carried out at this point.

19. The peritoneum and each abdominal layer are closed.

20. After the wound is closed, the patient's fundus is massaged and any clots that are expressed from the vagina are cleared.

21. The abdominal dressing and a perineal pad are applied.

GERIATRIC CONSIDERATIONS

The Elderly Patient—Gynecologic Surgery

Gynecologic surgery often requires surgical positioning that can pull or shear the patient's skin. For that reason, it is important to consider the changes that occur in skin and the musculoskeletal system during aging.

The skin loses elasticity and subcutaneous fat and becomes more prone to shear force and pressure injury. Because of the thinness of the skin and small-vessel fragility, bruising and hemorrhaging are quite common. Dry skin develops because of decreased oil and sweat production from sebaceous and sweat glands, respectively. As a result, skin breakdown and pressure ulcers, as well as wound infections, develop more easily. The vascular system of the skin has nutritional and protective roles. It is necessary for body heat regulation, provides defenses against microbial and physical damage, provides nutrient supply to the avascular epidermis, and promotes wound healing. Having an intact vascular system to maintain these skin role characteristics is extremely important for a patient undergoing surgical intervention. However, papillary capillaries, responsible for epidermal nourishment and heat dissipation, degenerate with aging. What is left is only the horizontal arteriovenous plexus lying beneath the skin surface. This progressive impairment of vascular circulation and tissue nutrition and the loss of subcutaneous tissue predispose to a feeling of cold, especially in cool environments such as the OR. Therefore the ability to maintain thermoregulation is compromised in elders and must be controlled through external measures.

The following summarizes skin changes:

Physiologic Change	Results
Decreased vascularity of dermis	Increased pallor in white skin
Decreased amount of melanin	Decreased hair color (graying)
Decreased sebaceous and sweat gland function	Increased dry skin, decreased sweating
Decreased subcutaneous fat	Increased wrinkling
Decreased thickness of epidermis	Increased susceptibility to trauma
Increased localized pigmentation	Increased prevalence of brown spots (senile lentigo)
Increased capillary fragility	Increased purple patches (senile purpura)
Decreased density of hair growth	Decreased amount and thickness of hair on head and body
Decreased rate of nail growth	Increased brittleness of nails
Decreased peripheral circulation	Increased longitudinal ridges on nails, increased thickening and yellowing of nails
Increased androgen/estrogen ratio	Increased facial hair in women

The female reproductive system also undergoes changes. The cervix actually becomes flusher with the vaginal vault and the vagina itself thins. It is less elastic, which can lead to easier vaginal injury. There are decreased estrogen levels and increased vaginal alkalinity, reducing defenses against infection. The pelvic floor becomes weaker with age and uterovaginal prolapse often requires surgical correction. The female aging process, known to accelerate after menopause, is not a contraindication to either surgery or expressions of sexuality. Treatment for gynecologic carcinomas should be the same as offered to younger women, although management by a multidisciplinary team benefits the aging female.

Modified from Fillit HM et al: *Textbook of geriatric medicine and gerontology*, ed 7, Philadelphia, 2010, Saunders; Wold GH: *Basic geriatric nursing*, ed 4, St Louis, 2008, Mosby.

GYNECOLOGIC AND OBSTETRIC SURGERY SUMMARY

In addition to the gynecology anatomy, related diseases, procedures, and surgical interventions mentioned throughout this chapter, the surgical technologist specializing in the field of gynecology and obstetrics needs to be familiar with the typical OB/GYN unit. Many hospitals utilize the surgical technologist on the floor assisting the nursing personnel with patient care. The surgical technologist may also set up delivery tables for the vaginal deliveries as well as assist the obstetrician with the vaginal delivery (as per hospital policy). Others also may be involved in the bereavement system in the event of a miscarriage or fetal loss. This role is obviously outside the typical role of the surgical technologist and should be carefully considered when working on an OB unit.

REVIEW QUESTIONS

1. What procedure removes the warty lesions caused by HPV (human papilloma virus)?
   a. simple vulvectomy
   b. skinning vulvectomy
   c. suction and curettage
   d. excision of condylomata

2. Which of the following is NOT an indication of a hysteroscopy?
   a. evaluation of infertility
   b. diagnosis of urethral disorders
   c. location and removal of a lost IUD
   d. tubal sterilization

3. True or false: Pelvic exenteration involves the removal of the rectum?

4. A cervical cerclage is most commonly accomplished by way of what approach?
   a. abdominal
   b. vaginal
   c. laparoscopic
   d. fundal

5. True or false: Cesarean delivery is the fifth most commonly performed surgical procedure in the United States?

6. True or false: Ectopic pregnancies occur only in the fallopian tube?

7. In obstetrics, Methergine is given perioperatively to treat
   a. postpartum bleeding
   b. preterm labor
   c. convulsions caused by pregnancy
   d. ectopic pregnancies

8. Which of the following is NOT a contraindication to a vaginal approach of a hysterectomy?
   a. pelvic malignancy
   b. patient under age 40 who has never had children
   c. large uterine tumor
   d. possibility of overlooked metastatic disease

9. True or false: The vaginal prep should be completed before the abdominal prep for an abdominal hysterectomy.

10. The least common site for gynecologic cancers would include
    a. fallopian tubes
    b. vagina
    c. ovaries
    d. endometrium

11. Define and briefly describe the following surgical procedures:
    Vaginal hysterectomy
    Abdominal myomectomy
    Cesarean birth

Critical Thinking Question

Read the following scenario and utilizing the information in the chapter along with your critical thinking skills, determine the best plan of action as the role of the surgical technologist.

A patient presents to the OB unit for a scheduled induction of labor. After laboring for several hours, the physician determines the mother will not be able to deliver the infant vaginally because of fetal malposition. The physician con-sents the patient for cesarean section. After the cesarean birth, the mother postoperatively is hemorrhaging. The physician determines the patient needs to return to the OR for a D&C to remove retained placenta and/or blood clots. What special considerations, supplies, equipment, and instrumentation does the surgical technologist need to prepare to continue the care of the patient?

REFERENCES

American Cancer Society (ACS): *Cancer facts and figures 2009*, Atlanta, 2009, The Society.

Andrews RT et al: Patient care and uterine artery embolization for leiomyomata, *J Vasc Interv Radiol* 20:S307–S311, 2009.

Aschkenazi SO, Goldberg RP: Female sexual function and the pelvic floor, *Expert Rev of Obstet Gynecol* 4(2):165–178, 2009.

Association of periOperative Registered Nurses: *Perioperative standards and recommended practices*, Denver, 2009, The Association.

Birnbach DJ, Browne I: Anesthesia for obstetrics, In Miller RD, editor: *Miller's anesthesia*, ed 6, Philadelphia, 2005, Churchill Livingstone.

Cheong Y, Ledger WL: Hysteroscopy and hysteroscopic surgery, *Obstet Gynaecol Repro Med* 17(4):99–104, 2007.

Denholm B: Tucking patient's arms and general positioning, *AORN J* 89(4):755–757, 2009.

Dooley M: Innovative treatments for abnormal uterine bleeding, *OR Nurse* 6(1):18–21, 2007.

Fanning J et al: Robotic radical hysterectomy, *Am J Obstet Gynecol* 198:649. e1–649.e4, 2008.

Faust RJ et al: Patient positioning. In Miller RD, editor: *Miller's anesthesia*, ed 6, Philadelphia, 2005, Churchill Livingstone.

Genovese SK: Antepartal hemorrhagic disorders. In Lowdermilk DL, Perry SE, editors: *Maternity and women's health care*, ed 9, St Louis, 2007, Mosby.

Goeser AL, Hasiak MJ: An overview of hysterectomy: types of hysterectomy and methods of hysterectomy, *US Pharmacist* 33(9):HS11-HS20, 2008. available at www.medscape.com/viewarticle/582384_3. Accessed August 12, 2009.

Hastings-Tolsma M, et al: Essure: hysteroscopic sterilization, *J Midwifery Womens Health* 51:510–514, 2006.

Healthcare Cost and Utilization Project (HCUPnet): Statistics for U.S. community hospital stays, principle procedure based on clinical classifications software, 2007, available at www.hcup.ahrq.gov. Accessed June 26, 2009.

Jancelewicz T, Harrison MR: A history of fetal surgery, *Clin Perinatol* 36:227–236, 2009.

Jhingran A, Levenback C: Malignant diseases of the cervix: microinvasive and invasive carcinoma: diagnosis and management. In Katz VL et al: *Comprehensive gynecology*, ed 5, Philadelphia, 2007, Mosby.

Katz VL: Benign gynecologic lesions. In Katz VL, et al: *Comprehensive gynecology*, ed 5, Philadelphia, 2007, Mosby.

Lobo R: Ectopic pregnancy. In Katz VL et al: *Comprehensive gynecology*, ed 5, Philadelphia, 2007, Mosby.

Lowdermilk DL: Structural disorders and neoplasms of the reproductive system. In Lowdermilk DL, Perry SE: *Maternity and women's health care*, ed 9, St Louis, 2007a, Mosby.

Lowdermilk DL: Infertility. In Lowdermilk DL, Perry SE: *Maternity and women's health care*, ed 9, St Louis, 2007b, Mosby.

McAteer J: Medical-surgical problems in pregnancy. In Lowdermilk DL, Perry SE, editors: *Maternity and women's health care*, ed 9, St Louis, 2007, Mosby.

Parker WH: Uterine myomas: management, *Fertil Steril* 88(2):255–271, 2007.

Practice Committee of the American Society for Reproductive Medicine: Indications and options for endometrial ablation, *Fertil Steril* 90(5):S236–S240, 2008.

Reynolds RK, Advincula AP: Robot-assisted laparoscopic hysterectomy: technique and initial experience, *Am J Surg* 191:555–560, 2006.

Roberts C, Mangan S: Know the risks of cesarean delivery, *OR Nurse* 3(12):22–30, 2009.

Robins JC, Carson SA: Female fertility: what every urologist must understand, *Urol Clin N Am* 35:173–181, 2008.

Scheurig C, et al: Uterine artery embolization in patients with symptomatic diffuse leiomyomatosis of the uterus, *J Vasc Interv Radiol* 19:279–284, 2008.

Genitourinary Surgery

LEARNING OBJECTIVES

After studying this chapter the reader will be able to:
- Identify relevant anatomy of the male and female genitourinary systems
- Correlate physiology to conditions requiring surgical intervention
- Identify the etiology and pathology that leads to surgical intervention in the genitourinary system
- Identify relevant preoperative tests and procedures and assess resultant lab values
- Describe the names and uses of relevant instrumentation, equipment, supplies, and drugs used in genitourinary surgery
- Describe the role of the surgical technologist during genitourinary procedures
- Recognize the steps of genitourinary procedures
- Summarize the care of the genitourinary surgical patient

CHAPTER OUTLINE

Overview

Genitourinary surgery typically involves surgery of the kidney, adrenal gland, bladder, prostate, urethra, penis, and testicles, as well as the relevant accessory structures. Advances in genitourinary surgery, with the use of robotics, laparoscopy, cryotherapy, lasers, ultrasonography, lithotripters, innovative diagnostic measures, and minimally invasive surgical approaches, have expanded treatment options. As urologic surgery becomes more complex and far more precise, the surgical technologist is challenged to maintain up-to-date knowledge, documented competence, and new technical skills.

This chapter was originally written by Helene Korey Marley, RN, CNOR, CRNFA, for the 14th edition of Alexander's Care of the Patient in Surgery *and has been revised by Christopher Lee, CST, AAS, for this text.*

Surgical Anatomy

The normal genitourinary system includes one pair of kidneys, two ureters, the urinary bladder, the urethra, and the prostate gland in the male. Also considered essential to the genitourinary system are the adrenal glands, male reproductive organs, and the female urogynecologic system.

Urine is excreted by the kidneys and conveyed to the bladder through the ureters. Urine is stored in the bladder, which serves as a reservoir until its full capacity (350 to 700 ml) is reached, and is eliminated from the body by way of the urethra. Normal urinary output ranges from 0.5 to 1.0 ml/kg of body weight per hour for the average adult.

Kidneys

The kidneys are located in the retroperitoneal space along the lateral borders of the psoas muscle, one on each side of the vertebral column at the level of the twelfth thoracic to the third lumbar vertebrae. Usually the right kidney is several centimeters lower than the left because the liver rests superior and anterior to the right kidney (Figure 6-1).

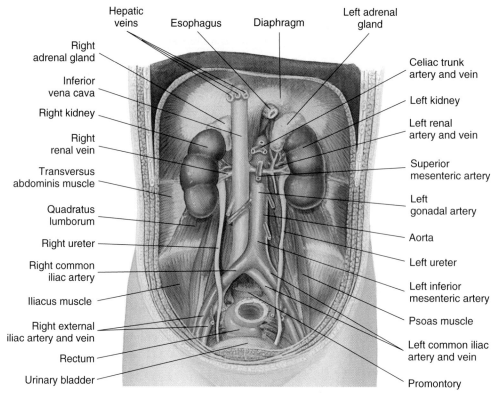

FIGURE 6-1 Location of urinary system organs.

Each kidney is surrounded by a mass of fatty and loose areolar tissue known as *pararenal fat.* A capsule enclosing the renal space is known as the *fascia renalis.* This is composed of *Gerota's fascia* (anterior renal fascia) and *Zuckerkandl fascia* (posterior renal fascia). These structures help keep the kidneys in their normal anatomic position. The anterior and posterior relationships of the kidneys are shown in Figure 6-2.

On the medial side of each kidney is a concave area known as the *hilum,* through which the renal artery and vein enter and exit. The renal pelvis, a funnel-shaped structure that lies within the kidney and posterior to the renal vascular pedicle, divides into several branches called *calyces* (Figure 6-3). When surgery is indicated in these structures, a posterior flank approach is preferred. When surgery for removal of a mass is anticipated, a transabdominal or thoracoabdominal incision may be chosen.

The kidneys are highly vascular organs that process approximately one fifth of the entire volume of blood at any one time. The blood supply to the kidney is conveyed through the renal artery (a large branch of the aorta) and leaves through the renal vein. On entering the kidney, the renal artery divides into anterior and posterior sections. These undergo further division into interlobular arteries from which smaller afferent branches pass to the glomeruli. Efferent arterioles in the glomeruli then pass to the tubules of the nephron.

The renal lymphatic supply originates beneath the capsule of the kidney and empties into the lumbar lymph nodes at the junction of the renal vascular pedicle and aorta. The nerves of the autonomic (involuntary) nervous system originate from the lumbar sympathetic trunk and from the vagus nerve. Removal of the nerve pathways does not impair renal function.

The renal artery and vein with their accompanying nerves and lymphatics are referred to as the *pedicle* of the kidney.

Adrenal Glands

The adrenal glands lie retroperitoneally beneath the diaphragm, capping the medial aspects of the superior pole of each kidney. On the right side, the gland is triangular and adjacent to the inferior vena cava; on the left side, it is a rounded, crescent-shaped gland posterior to the stomach and pancreas. Each adrenal gland has a medulla, which secretes epinephrine (adrenaline), and a cortex, which secretes steroids and hormones. Secretions from the adrenal cortex are influenced by the activity of the pituitary gland. The adrenal glands are liberally supplied with arterial branches from the inferior phrenic and renal arteries and from the aorta. Venous drainage is accomplished on the right side by the inferior vena cava and on the left by the left renal vein. The lymphatic system accompanies the suprarenal vein and drains into the lumbar lymph nodes.

Ureters

Each ureter is a continuation of the renal pelvis. The ureter extends in a smooth S curve from the renal pelvis to the base of the bladder (Figure 6-4). It is approximately 25 to 30 cm long and 4 to 5 mm in diameter in the adult. This fibromuscular cylindric tube is lined by transitional epithelium (urothelium) and lies on the psoas muscle, passing medially to the sacroiliac joints and laterally to the ischial spines. As urine accumulates in the renal pelvis, slight distention initiates a wave of muscular contractions. This peristaltic activity continues down the ureter, propelling urine into the bladder.

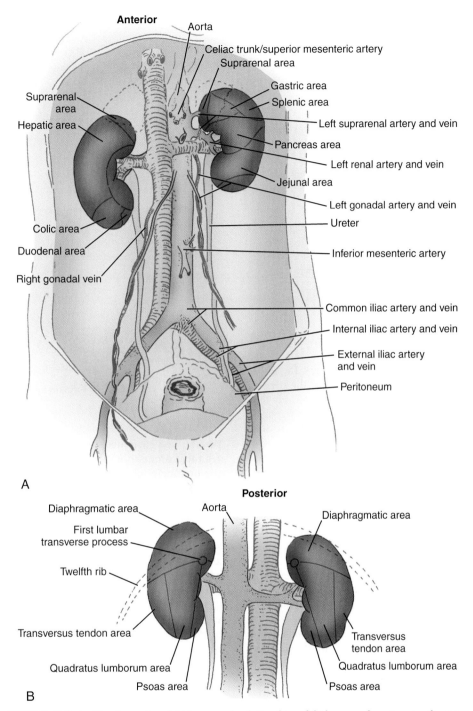

Anterior

Aorta
Celiac trunk/superior mesenteric artery
Suprarenal area
Gastric area
Splenic area
Left suprarenal artery and vein
Pancreas area
Left renal artery and vein
Jejunal area
Left gonadal artery and vein
Ureter
Inferior mesenteric artery
Common iliac artery and vein
Internal iliac artery and vein
External iliac artery and vein
Peritoneum

Suprarenal area
Hepatic area
Colic area
Duodenal area
Right gonadal vein

A

Posterior

Diaphragmatic area
Aorta
Diaphragmatic area
First lumbar transverse process
Twelfth rib
Transversus tendon area
Transversus tendon area
Quadratus lumborum area
Quadratus lumborum area
Psoas area
Psoas area

B

FIGURE 6-2 A, Blood supply of kidneys and relationship of kidneys and ureters to the main arteries and veins and the intraperitoneal organs. **B**, Relationship of the kidneys and ureters to the spinal column.

Urinary Bladder

The adult urinary bladder is a hollow, muscular viscus that acts as a reservoir for urine until micturition (voiding) occurs. It has an outer adventitial layer and inner urothelial layer. The trigone, a triangular area, forms the base of the bladder. The three corners of the trigone correspond to the orifices of the ureters and the bladder neck (opening of the urethra) (Figure 6-5). The ureteral orifices, on the prox-imal trigone at the interureteric ridge, are 2.5 cm apart. The bladder neck (internal sphincter) is formed from converging detrusor muscle fibers of the bladder wall that pass distally to form the smooth musculature of the urethra. Physiologically, the bladder fills with urine and expands into the abdominal cavity. The extraperitoneal location is advantageous because a suprapubic (above the pubic arch) incision may be performed without violating the peritoneum and potentially causing intraperitoneal complications.

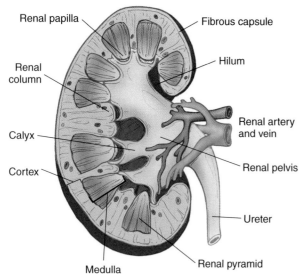

FIGURE 6-3 Normal kidney.

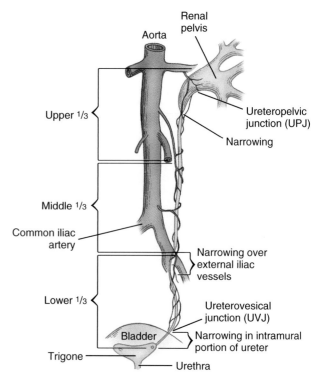

FIGURE 6-4 Anatomy of ureter.

The main arterial supply of the bladder comprises the superior, middle, and inferior vesical arteries. These vessels are derived from the internal iliac (hypogastric) artery, the obturator and inferior gluteal arteries, and in females the uterine and vaginal arteries. The bladder has a rich venous supply that drains into the internal iliac (hypogastric) vein. The lymphatic system is served by the vesical, external and internal iliac, and common iliac lymph nodes.

The bladder's size, position, and relation to the bowel, rectum, and reproductive organs vary according to the bladder's distention. In the female the vagina lies dorsal to the base of the bladder and parallel to the urethra (Figure 6-6). In the male the prostate gland is interposed between the bladder neck and the urethra (Figure 6-7). These anatomic relationships influence the symptoms that a patient experiences preoperatively and are important landmarks during pelvic surgery.

The process of bladder evacuation appears to be initiated by nerve cells from the sacral division of the autonomic nervous system. These sacral reflex centers are controlled by higher voluntary centers in the brain. Stimulation of the sacral centers results in contraction of the bladder muscles and relaxation of the bladder outlet sphincters. Muscles inside and adjacent to the urethral wall and from the pelvic floor maintain closure of the sphincters of the bladder, thus enabling continence.

Urethra

The male urethra, normally 20 to 25 cm long, extends from the bladder neck to the tip of the penis and varies in diameter from 7 to 10 mm. It is divided into two portions: the proximal (sphincteric) urethra and the distal (conduit or anterior) urethra, both of which undergo further subdivision. The proximal urethra is commonly referred to as the *posterior urethra,* where it is elevated by the verumontanum, extending from the bladder neck through the prostate and the membranous portion. Within the posterior urethra lie the prostatic and membranous portions (see Figure 6-5). As the urethra exits the prostate and crosses the pelvic (urogenital) diaphragm, it is called the *membranous urethra.* The distal urethra, commonly called the *anterior urethra,* is subdivided into the bulbar, pendulous

(penile), and glandular urethras. The bulbar urethra is the area most prone to urethral strictures in the male. The prostatic urethra is approximately 3 cm long and is the widest portion of the urethra. On the floor of the prostatic urethra is the verumontanum, which contains the openings of the ejaculatory ducts. The membranous urethra is the shortest portion, measuring approximately 2.5 cm and extending from the external sphincter to the apex of the prostate. The penile, or pendulous, urethra lies within the corpus spongiosum. The urothelium of the urethra is continuous with that of the bladder.

The female urethra is a narrow, membranous tube about 3 to 5 cm in length and 6 to 8 mm in diameter. Slightly curved, it lies behind and beneath the symphysis pubis, anterior to the vagina. It passes through the internal and external sphincters and the urogenital diaphragm. The periurethral glands of Skene open on the floor of the urethra just inside the meatus. Because the female urethra is so short and in proximity to the anal and vaginal areas, microorganisms find easy access to the bladder and can cause urinary tract infections (UTIs).

Prostate Gland

The prostate gland is a donut-shaped organ composed of fibromuscular and glandular components. It is located at the base of the bladder neck and completely surrounds the urethra. The gland is about 4 cm at the base, is about 2 cm in depth, and normally weighs 20 to 30 g (see Figures 6-5 and 6-7).

The four glandular regions within the prostate have two major zones (the peripheral zone and the central zone) and two minor zones (the transitional zone and the periurethral zone). Many clinicians still refer to prostate lobes as intraurethral lobes (right and left lateral) and extraurethral lobes (posterior

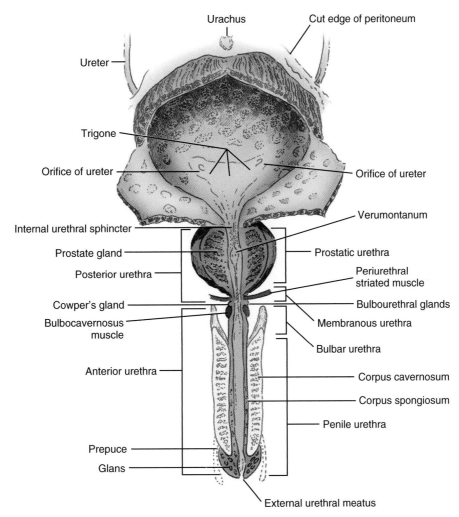

FIGURE 6-5 Anatomy of male urinary bladder, prostate gland, and urethra.

and median). The posterior lobe is readily palpable during rectal examination and prone to cancerous degeneration. Benign prostatic hyperplasia (BPH, often referred to as hypertrophy) generally occurs in the transitional zone (intraurethral lobe).

Behind the prostatic capsule is a fibrous sheath known as the *true prostatic capsule,* which separates the prostate gland and the seminal vesicles from the rectum. This fascia is an important landmark during perineal prostatectomy.

The lobes of the prostate gland secrete highly alkaline fluid that dilutes the testicular secretion as it is excreted from the ejaculatory ducts. These secretions are believed to be essential to the passage of spermatozoa and helpful in keeping them alive. The arterial supply to the prostate is derived from the pudendal, inferior vesical, and hemorrhoidal arteries.

Male Reproductive Organs

The male reproductive organs include several paired structures: the testes, epididymides, seminal ducts (vasa deferens), seminal vesicles, ejaculatory ducts, and bulbourethral glands. Other organs of the reproductive tract are the penis, prostate gland, and urethra.

The *scrotum* is located behind and below the base of the penis and in front of the anus. Within the scrotum are two

cavities, or sacs, that are lined with smooth, glistening tissue—the tunica vaginalis. Normally, a small amount of clear fluid is contained in the tunica vaginalis. Each loose sac contains and supports a testis, an epididymis, and some of the spermatic cord. The two sides of the scrotum are separated from each other by a median raphe (septum).

The *testes* manufacture the spermatozoa and also contain specialized Leydig's cells that produce the male hormone *testosterone.* Each testis consists of many tubules in which the sperm are formed, surrounded by dense capsules of connective tissue. The tubules coalesce and continue into the adjacent epididymis, where the sperm mature and are stored. At the upper pole of the testis is the appendix testis, a small body that may be pedunculated (stalked) or sessile (flat).

The *epididymis* is a long, convoluted duct located along the posterolateral surface of the testis. It is closely attached to the testicle by fibrous tissue and secretes seminal fluid, which gives the sperm a liquid medium in which to migrate. The vas deferens (ductus deferens, seminal duct) is a distal continuation of the epididymis as it enters the prostate gland and conveys the sperm to the seminal vesicle.

The *vas deferens* extends from the epididymis into the abdomen and lies within the spermatic cord in the inguinal region.

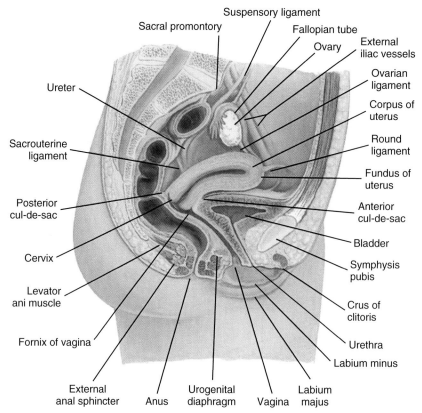

FIGURE 6-6 Female genitourinary and reproductive anatomy.

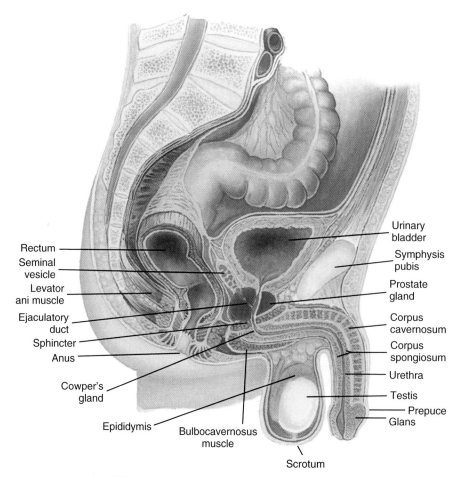

FIGURE 6-7 Male genitourinary and reproductive anatomy.

The spermatic cord also contains veins, arteries, lymphatics, nerves, and surrounding connective tissue (cremaster muscle), which give support to the testes. The terminal portion of each vas deferens is called the *ejaculatory duct;* it passes between the lobes of the prostate gland and opens into the posterior urethra.

The *accessory reproductive glands* include the seminal vesicles, prostate gland, and bulbourethral gland. The seminal vesicles unite with the vas deferens on either side, are situated behind the bladder, and produce protein and fructose for the nutrition of the sperm cell. Sperm and prostatic fluid are discharged at the time of ejaculation.

Cowper's glands (bulbourethral glands) are located on each side at the juncture of the membranous and bulbar urethras. Each gland, by way of its duct, empties mucous secretions into the urethra.

The *penis* is suspended from the pubic symphysis by the suspensory ligaments. The penis contains three distinct vascular, spongelike bodies surrounding the urethra: two outer bodies called the *right corpus cavernosum* and *left corpus cavernosum* and an inner body, the *corpus spongiosum urethrae*. These tissues contain a network of vascular channels that fill with blood during erection (see Figure 6-5). At the distal end of the penis, the skin is doubly folded to form the prepuce, or foreskin, which serves as a covering for the glans penis. The glans penis contains the urethral orifice.

Surgical Technologist Considerations

Assessment

Patients entering a hospital or ambulatory surgery unit for genitourinary surgery exhibit many emotions and reactions, including fear, embarrassment, helplessness, hostility, anger, and grief. To most, a successful surgical outcome is of prime importance. The urology patient population varies from infants with congenital anomalies to elderly people with physiologic impairments.

In addition to routine admission information, the patient's urologic and cardiac histories are obtained. This information includes but is not limited to vital signs, allergies (including latex), the patient's primary problem, history of the present illness, nature of symptoms, and limitations imposed by the disease condition. All data pertinent to the proposed operative procedure should be reviewed and shared with the entire surgical team.

The patient may undergo several studies preoperatively, including measurement of levels of serum and urine electrolytes, blood glucose, and blood urea nitrogen (BUN); urinalysis and urine cultures; cardiac enzymes; complete blood count (CBC); prothrombin time (PT) and partial thromboplastin time (PTT); blood chemistry profiles (Table 6-1); electrocardiogram (ECG); and chest x-ray examination. The nurse reviews the

TABLE 6-1

Common Preoperative Laboratory Analyses for Patients with Genitourinary Disorders

Laboratory Studies	Normal Range (Adult Values)	Laboratory Studies	Normal Range (Adult Values)
COAGULATION PROFILES		LDL (low-density lipids)	60-180 mg/dl
Bleeding time	<175 sec	VLDL (triglycerides)	7-32 mg/dl
Partial thromboplastin time (PTT)	60-70 sec	Creatinine	0.5-1.2 mg/dl
Platelet count	150,000-400,000/mm³	Glucose (blood sugar)	70-110 mg/dl
Prothrombin time (PT)	11-12.5 sec	Osmolality	285-295 mOsm/kg H_2O
		Potassium (K^+)	3.5-5 mEq/L
FERTILITY PROFILES (MALE)		Phosphorus (P)	3-4.5 mg/dl
Follicle-stimulating hormone (FSH)	1.42-15.4 milliinternational units/ml	Prostate-specific antigen (PSA)	<4 ng/dl
		Prostatic acid phosphatase (PAP)	0.013-0.63 unit/L
Luteinizing hormone (LH)	1.24-7.8 milliinternational units/ml	Protein	6.4-8.3 g/dl
		Sodium (Na^+)	136-145 mEq/L
Testosterone (total)	280-1080 ng/dl	Uric acid	2.7-8.5 mg/dl
Sperm count	≥20 million/nl; mobility ≥50% at 1 hr	**URINE PROFILES (VALUES NOT LISTED SHOULD BE NEGATIVE)**	
		Calcium (Ca^{++})	100-250 mg/day
HEMATOLOGY VALUES (LOW: FEMALE; HIGH: MALE)		Chloride (Cl^-)	110-250 mEq/L/day
Hematocrit (Hct)	37%-52%	Creatinine	88-137 ml/min
Hemoglobin (Hgb)	12-18 g/dl	Glucose (24 hr)	50-300 mg/day (<0.5 g/day)
Red blood cells (RBCs)	4.2-6.1 million/mm³	Osmolality (random)	50-1200 mOsm/kg H_2O
White blood cells (WBCs)	5000-10,000 million/mm³	Phosphorus	0.4-1.3 g/24 hr
		Potassium (K^+)	25-100 mEq/L/day
SERUM PROFILES (LOW: FEMALE; HIGH: MALE)		Protein	0-8 mg/dl
Bicarbonate	23-30 mEq/L (HCO_3^-)	Red blood cells (RBCs)	≤2 cells
Blood urea nitrogen (BUN)	10-20 mg/dl	Sodium (Na^+)	40-220 mEq/L/day
Calcium (Ca^{++})	9-10.5 mg/dl	Uric acid	250-750 mg/day
Chloride (Cl^-)	98-106 mEq/L	White blood cells (WBCs)	0-4 per lower field
Cholesterol	<200 mg/dl	pH	4.6-8 (average: 6)
HDL (high-density lipids)	Male: >45 mg/dl; Female: >55 mg/dl	Specific gravity	1.005-1.030

Data from Chernecky CC, Berger BJ: *Laboratory tests and diagnostic procedures,* ed 5, St Louis, 2008, Saunders; Pagana K, Pagana T: *Mosby's diagnostic and laboratory test reference,* ed 9, St Louis, 2009, Mosby.

patient's medical history, focusing on medication use (including the use of over-the-counter medications and herbal supplements), any infectious processes, or chronic diseases. Specific genitourinary studies can be found in the patient's medical record. They may encompass all or some of the following: computerized tomography (CT) scans, magnetic resonance imaging (MRI), bone and dual energy x-ray absorptiometry (DEXA) scans, positron emission tomography (PET), ProstaScint scans, intravenous (IV) pyelograms or urograms (IVPs or IVUs, respectively), genitourinary flat plate (KUB [kidney, ureter, bladder]), urinary flow studies, fluoroscopic examinations (angiography, cavernosography), prostate-specific antigen (PSA), and ultrasonography.

Planning

Frequently the urology patient presents a complex medical picture. Any alterations in the patient's physical, mental, or emotional status may greatly influence both the surgical and the postoperative course. A review of the patient's record; communication with the patient or family; recognition of specific psychosocial, cultural, ethnic, and spiritual needs of the patient and family; and knowledge gained from other members of the patient care team are all used to care for the intraoperative patient. The surgical technologist uses all preoperative information to plan for the surgical procedure and better anticipate the surgeon's needs.

Implementation

Patient Safety. Institutions have various protocols and processes in place to support patient safety. The rapid response team is one example of a protocol or process that focuses on safety (Rapid Response Team box). A critical safety protocol that the surgical team is responsible to follow is to ensure the correct patient, correct procedure, and correct site surgery. Such a protocol includes proper patient identification, proper operative site identification, proper procedure identification, and proper medication identification. All wrong site, wrong procedure, and wrong patient surgery occurrences are considered sentinel events by The Joint Commission.

To fulfill these requirements, preoperative verification, surgical site marking, and time-out processes must occur for every surgical procedure. What the patient expresses as the intended surgical procedure is compared with what is documented on the operative permit and other items, such as the OR schedule. Patient identification is achieved by also asking the patient to state his or her full name and birth date. This information is compared with the patient identification bracelet. Documentation of the processes implemented is completed on the designated institutional form or forms.

The surgical site is marked with a permanent nontoxic marking pen. A standard policy needs to be developed within the particular facility as to how marking will be accomplished for urologic, endoscopic, and abdominal procedures, particularly when they involve laterality. This mark should be clearly visible following prepping and draping.

"Time out" is a pause in the activity that occurs before the start or incision on all procedures. The entire team stops to verbally confirm the patient's identity, verify the patient's position, state and agree on the procedure and surgical site, and review that all implants and necessary equipment are available and ready (Patient Safety). The nurse documents this process according to hospital policy.

When medications are used intraoperatively the containers should always be marked with the medication and dose. The surgical technologist verifies the medication and dosage verbally when passing the drug in its administration device to the surgeon. Local anesthetics that contain epinephrine should be used with caution in urology. Many urologic interventions involve "end-organs," for example, the scrotum, testicles, and penis. The use of epinephrine in these areas can result in an ischemic situation and should be avoided.

Positioning. Thorough understanding of the urologic OR bed and its functions is essential for optimum patient positioning. The position in which the patient is placed for surgery is determined by the particular operation to be performed. For urologic operative procedures, the patient may be placed in the lateral, supine, prone, or lithotomy position. Any of these positions may be exaggerated to give optimum access to the organ involved, particularly in radical surgery of the prostate and bladder. When the patient is supine, his or her arms are placed on padded armboards with the palms up and fingers extended. Armboards are maintained at less than a 90-degree angle to prevent brachial

RAPID RESPONSE TEAM

A rapid response team (RRT) is used when patients display subtle warning signs of deterioration. These teams respond to the first sign of patient decline by bringing critical care assessment skills to the bedside of the patient in order to identify and treat issues before a patient codes. When activated, the RRT, which consists of a critical care nurse, respiratory therapist, med-surg nurse, ICU resident, admitting resident, and the surgical resident, assembles at the patient's bedside to assist with treatments and help determine if transfer to a higher level of care is necessary. The team is available 24/7.

In most cases, the RRT is not utilized in the perioperative setting. Exceptions occur when PACU is used as an overflow unit and ancillary staff is unavailable. At one particular institution, the RRT was only utilized twice in this respect. In both cases, the team was called to the scene because of apnea/shortness of breath and in neither case was CPR initiated.

Health professionals are not the only persons with access to the rapid response team. At this institution, a sign is placed in all public areas of the hospital to provide notice to patients, families, and visitors about the RRT. There is also an information sheet provided to all new admissions that details patient and visitor activation of the RRT. Each patient phone is equipped with a purple and white "glow in the dark" instruction to call the emergency operator and ask for the rapid response team in case of emergency. The operator will immediately alert healthcare professionals, who will soon arrive to assess the situation. Allowing family members and visitors to access rapid response ensures patients' medical, social, and spiritual needs will be met with compassion, skill, and respect.

Modified from University of Pennsylvania Health System: *Rapid response team, 2000,* available at Uphsxnet.Uphs.Upenn.Edu/Pahhome/Nursing/ Rapidresponse. Accessed April 10, 2009.

PATIENT SAFETY

Improving Teamwork to Reduce Errors

Publication of the 1999 Institute of Medicine report focused attention on medical errors and the critical importance of patient safety. Reducing errors (such as wrong person, wrong procedure, or wrong site surgery) requires, in part, human solutions, such as improving teamwork and communication in the OR team. Interdisciplinary teamwork is especially important in the so-called high-risk areas in hospitals, such as the OR. Perioperative nurses and surgical technologists have long believed that a team approach to patient care reduces errors. Effective teamwork in perioperative patient care consists of knowledge, attitudes, and skills. Developing sustainable efforts to improve teamwork requires thoughtful application. Interventions focused on changing the behavior of team members must first take into account their attitudes. Subsequently, skills and knowledge are assessed, and a training program can be designed to improve teamwork. The benefits of improved teamwork are well exemplified in the time-out process, which aims to enhance effectiveness, increase efficiency, and lower the possibility of error. Preoperative verification processes and the time-out result in fewer errors because these processes are planned by each institution and standardized through use of the Universal Protocol of The Joint Commission. Each member of the OR team knows his or her own responsibilities as well as those of teammates; members look out for each other and note errors before they happen; and members trust one another's judgments and concerns. Teamwork during preoperative verification and the time-out allows proper integration and execution of clinical activities, gives caregivers increased control over their work environment, and provides a safety net against error.

Modified from Kaissi A et al: Measuring teamwork and patient safety attitudes of high-risk areas, *Nurs Econ* 21(5):211-218, 2003; Rajnish P et al: Fires in the operating room and intensive care unit: awareness is the key to protection, *Anesth Analg* 102:172-174, 2006.

plexus stretch. If there are surgical reasons to tuck the arms at the side, the elbows are padded to protect the ulnar nerve, the palms face inward, and the wrist is maintained in a neutral position (Denholm, 2009). A drape secures the arms. It should be tucked snuggly under the patient, not under the mattress. This prevents the arm from shifting downward intraoperatively and resting against the OR bed rail. It is essential to avoid displacement of the joints and undue tension on neurovascular bundles or ligaments. A patient positioned laterally (flank position) for renal surgery has the spine extended for greater access to the retroperitoneal space. Padding and stabilized support with gel pads, pillows, sandbags, and straps should be available for precise anatomic positioning and safety. When an electrosurgical unit (ESU) is to be used, care must be taken that the patient does not contact metal parts of the OR bed.

In some procedures involving stones of the kidneys or ureters, intraoperative fluoroscopy may be required. When fluoroscopy (C-arm) is to be employed, the patient must be placed on an OR bed compatible with its use. Whenever possible, measures are taken to protect the patient from undue radiation exposure to the thyroid and chest areas by using small leaded shields. In urologic procedures it generally is not feasible to shield the reproductive organs.

Aseptic Techniques and Safety Measures. Prevention of infection is an important goal in the care of the genitourinary patient. It is, however, seldom possible to confirm freedom from infection intraoperatively or immediately postoperatively. Aseptic techniques must be carefully maintained and monitored. Skin preparation and draping procedures vary, depending on the surgery to be performed and institutional protocols. Special care must be taken when cleansing the perineal area to avoid contamination from the rectum to the urethra. Prepping solutions should be applied with downward strokes and the sponge discarded once it has contacted the inner vaginal or anal areas. Transurethral passage of instruments and catheters requires meticulous technique to prevent retrograde infections of the urinary tract, which account for 32% of all healthcare-associated infections (Scott, 2009).

Visualization of the bladder during transurethral procedures is often enhanced by darkening the room. Provision should be made for proper adjustments to lighting. ESUs and fiber-optic light systems are common adjuncts in urologic surgery. The nurse and surgical technologist must be familiar with the manufacturer's safety precautions and recommendations during their use.

Hemostasis. The organs and tissues of the genitourinary system are highly vascular. Therefore it is important to maintain hemostasis during these procedures. The potential for unexpected bleeding is increased during GU surgery, especially open procedures. The surgical technologist should be prepared with an adequate amount of lap sponges and vascular clamps during open procedures. In addition, hemostasic agents and coagulation devices such as the ESU and Argon Beam coagulator should also be available. Absorbable suture material such as chromic gut and polyglactin are preferred in GU surgery, and the surgical technologist should have a ready supply available.

Use of Irrigating Fluids. When the bladder is entered, sterile distilled irrigating fluid is administered to distend it for effective visualization. Commercially prepared sterile irrigation solutions with appropriate closed administration sets are highly recommended. Such closed systems prevent the inherent risks of cross-contamination. Large volumes of irrigating solutions are frequently used, particularly during more extensive endoscopic procedures. When these solutions are at the room temperature of the OR, they are cold compared with the patient's internal body temperature and can cause hypothermia. Solution-warming units are available commercially and are a useful tool to help decrease this risk. The drawback to these units may be that the warmth delays clotting, thus increasing the risk of blood loss.

Commercially prepared sterile irrigation solutions are available in collapsible bags and rigid plastic containers, both of which have the same advantages: neither depends on air, and each may be hung in series, thus providing continuous irrigation without interruption. Air bubbles, a problem that distorts visibility during the procedure, are eliminated with these systems.

For simple observation cystoscopy, retrograde pyelography, and simple bladder tumor fulgurations, sterile distilled water may be used without complication. However, during transurethral resection of the prostate (TURP), venous sinuses may be opened and varying amounts of irrigant are invariably absorbed

TURP Syndrome

Transurethral resection of the prostate (TURP) commonly is performed in older men. A variety of irrigants can be used to aid in visualization and electrosurgery during TURP. During TURP, venous sinuses within the gland may be opened and varying amounts of irrigant are invariably absorbed into the bloodstream. Depending on the type and amount of fluid used, several complications, collectively known as TURP syndrome, may occur. Patients may manifest signs and symptoms of hyponatremia and hypervolemia earlier when local and spinal anesthetics are used. Complications are more prevalent in the postoperative stage. A delay in recognizing the symptoms can be catastrophic. The perioperative nurse and surgical technologist play a critical role in reducing the risk of TURP syndrome and can have a positive impact through the following interventions:

♦ **Positioning and draping.** The surgical team assists with positioning the patient in the lithotomy position on the urologic table with the buttocks positioned slightly off the break in the table to provide a barrier to fluid escaping down the perineum and under the patient. The drapes should be applied in a manner that prevents pooling or loss of fluids so that losses can be monitored.

♦ **Maintenance of continuous irrigation.** Commercially prepared sterile irrigation solutions are available in collapsible bags and have the advantage of not depending on air, and each can be hung in series, providing continuous irrigation without interruption. The nurse retains the empty irrigation bags to assist with the fluid use calculation.

♦ **Volume monitoring.** The nurse monitors the amount of irrigation recovered and subtracts it from the amount of irrigation used. The total of the irrigation used minus the irrigation recovered is referred to as the volume deficit. If the cause for the deficit cannot be identified, it should be considered reabsorbed. Minimum amounts of fluids should be given and urine output carefully monitored. Irrigation fluid should be under as little pressure as possible and the bladder emptied before it reaches full capacity to prevent intravesical pressure.

♦ **Intraoperative observation.** Close observation during the intraoperative period is essential. Signs and symptoms such as sudden restlessness, apprehension, irritability, confusion, nausea, slow pulse rate, seizures, dysrhythmias, and rising blood pressure may be suggestive of TURP syndrome, a severe hyponatremia caused by systemic absorption of irrigating fluid used during surgery. IV diuretics such as furosemide (Lasix) may be required to prevent possible pulmonary edema associated with administration of hypertonic saline. If the patient's reaction is severe, surgery may have to be terminated.

♦ **Postoperative fluid management.** Immediate postoperative fluid management includes monitoring vital signs; confirming normal breath sounds in which no rales or wheezing are present; monitoring urinary output to ensure adequate volume (e.g., a minimum rate of 30 ml/hr); assessing skin color; observing blood count and electrolyte levels to confirm they are within normal limits; and maintaining IV therapy as needed.

Modified from Young E et al: Perioperative fluid management, *AORN J* 89:167-178, 2009.

into the bloodstream. Studies indicate that the use of distilled water during TURP may result in hemolysis of erythrocytes and possible renal failure. Other important complications include dilutional hyponatremia and cardiac decompensation (Risk Reduction Strategies).

Therefore a clear, nonelectrolytic, and iso-osmotic solution should be used. The most widely used urologic irrigating fluids are 3% sorbitol, an isomer of mannitol, and 1.5% glycine, an aminoacetic acid solution. In dilute solutions, sorbitol and glycine have many properties that make them particularly useful for irrigation during transurethral prostatectomy. At slightly hypotonic concentrations, they do not produce hemolysis. However, if too much intravasation occurs with glycine, an encephalitic state can result from the ammonia produced (Surgical Pharmacology). Because the solutions are nonelectrolytic, they do not cause dispersion of high-frequency current with consequent loss of electrosurgical cutting capacity, as occurs with normal saline.

During ureteropyeloscopy, sterile normal saline is the irrigant of choice unless electrosurgery is to be employed. This solution most closely approximates a physiologic solution—an important factor if perforation and extravasation of fluid into the retroperitoneum occur. If monopolar electrosurgery is required, as with a TURP, 3% sorbitol or 1.5% glycine should be used. If bipolar electrosurgery is required, as with a TURP, sterile normal saline should be used.

Thorough knowledge of the potential hazards encountered intraoperatively during transurethral surgery is extremely important. Although complications are more prevalent in the postoperative stage, close observation during the intraoperative period is essential. Signs and symptoms such as sudden restlessness, apprehension, irritability, confusion, nausea, slow pulse rate, seizures, dysrhythmias, and rising blood pressure may be suggestive of TURP syndrome, a severe hyponatremia caused by systemic absorption of irrigating fluid used during surgery (Han and Partin, 2007). Minimum amounts of fluids should be given and urine output carefully monitored. Irrigation fluid should be under as little pressure as possible and the bladder emptied before it reaches full capacity to prevent intravesical pressure. During ureteropyeloscopy it is frequently necessary to use a pressure bag to ensure adequate visualization of the upper urinary tract. Serum electrolyte values should be obtained, and if a low serum sodium value is reported, hypertonic sodium chloride is administered by means of a slow IV drip, often on a volumetric pump. IV diuretics such as furosemide (Lasix) may be required to prevent possible pulmonary edema associated with the administration of hypertonic saline. If the patient's reaction is severe, surgery may have to be terminated.

Endoscopic and Ancillary Equipment. Cystoscopic and ancillary equipment often varies from one institution to another. Therefore it is valuable to have a reference manual or standard setup cards that illustrate and describe in detail the required instrumentation for each specific procedure. Many common instruments used in genitourinary procedures are shown in Figures 6-8 through 6-16.

The basic cystoscopy tray should include instruments and accessory items that are routinely used for all cystoscopy procedures. If ureteral catheterization is planned, catheterizing telescopes or an Albarrán bridge, which can be packaged and

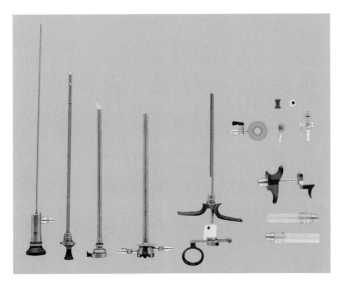

FIGURE 6-8 Resectoscopes: 30-degree telescope; obturator; inner sheath; outer sheath; working element. *Top to bottom:* 1 red port cap; 1 gray nipple; stopcock; 2 metal tubing connectors; bridge; and 2 peg clamps.

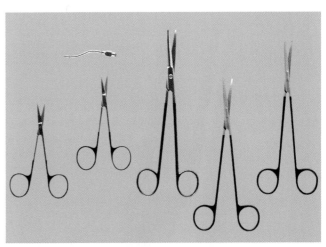

FIGURE 6-11 *Top:* Webster infusion cannula. *Bottom, left to right:* 2 iris scissors, straight, sharp, 4 inch; 1 facelift scissors, curved, 7¾ inch; 2 Metzenbaum scissors, curved, 7 inch.

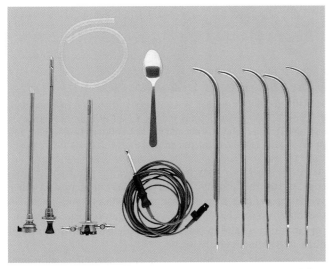

FIGURE 6-9 *Top, left to right:* plastic tubing; spoon. *Bottom, left to right:* inner sheath; obturator; outer sheath; light cord; van Buren urethral male sounds, 30F to 22F.

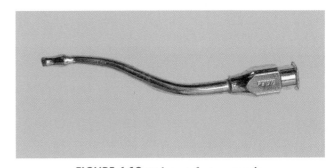

FIGURE 6-12 Webster infusion cannula.

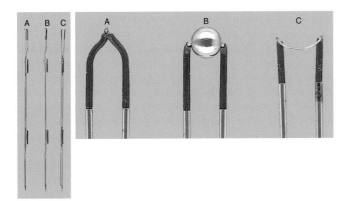

FIGURE 6-10 *Left to right:* **A**, cutting electrode with pointed end and tip; **B**, coagulating electrode with ball end and tip; **C**, cutting electrode with round wire and tip.

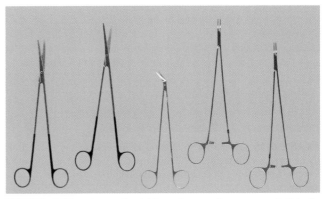

FIGURE 6-13 *Left to right:* 2 Metzenbaum scissors, curved, 9 inch; 1 Potts-Smith cardiovascular scissors; and 2 Ryder needle holders, 9 inch.

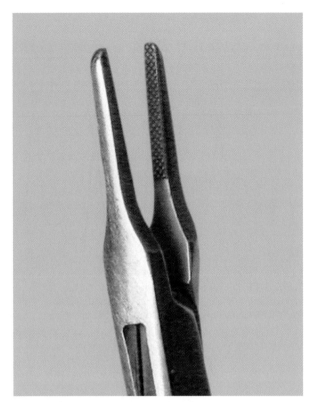

FIGURE 6-14 Tip of Ryder needle holder.

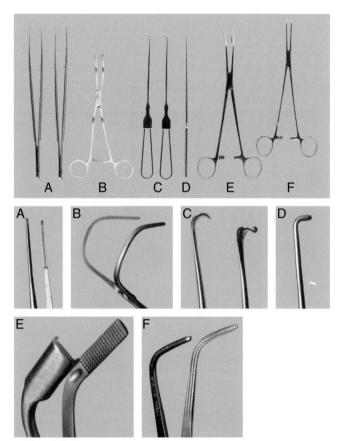

FIGURE 6-16 *Left to right:* **A,** 2 Autragrip tissue forceps, titanium, and tips; **B,** 1 Kay aortic clamp and tip; **C,** 2 Cushing vein retractors and tips; **D,** 1 nerve hook, dull, and tip; **E,** 1 bulldog clamp applier and tip; **F,** 1 Lahey gall duct forceps and tip.

sterilized separately, may be easily added to the basic cystoscopy setup. Instruments for transurethral surgery and other special procedures may be wrapped, sterilized, and placed on separate trays so that they are available on request. This concept minimizes handling of the delicate lensed instruments and ultimately reduces costly repairs.

Cystoscopic procedures frequently require additional instrumentation. Instruments of various types and sizes, such as a visual obturator, biopsy forceps, urethral sounds, Phillips filiforms and followers, and Ellik evacuators, are available as prepackaged, sterile, disposable items. The reusable products may also be packaged separately and sterilized.

Urethral and Ureteral Catheters. A variety of urethral and ureteral catheters are designed for specific procedures. Ureteral catheters are manufactured of polyurethane material and are graduated so that the urologist may determine the exact distance the catheter has been inserted into the ureter (Figure 6-17, *A*). Most manufacturers provide sterile disposable catheters wrapped in peel-open packages to allow aseptic handling during ureteral insertion. Some indications for the use of ureteral catheters are to (1) perform retrograde pyelography, (2) identify the ureters during pelvic or intestinal surgery, and (3) bypass partial or complete obstruction that may be present as a result of ureteral tumors, calculi, or strictures. Not uncommonly, it is necessary to insert a ureteral stent in a pregnant female because of hydronephrosis or obstructing calculi.

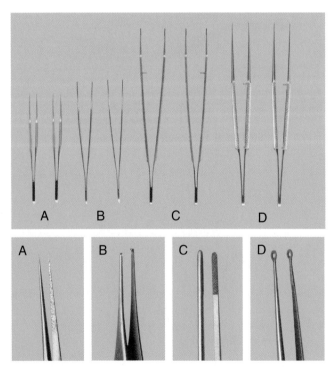

FIGURE 6-15 *Left to right:* **A,** 2 jeweler's forceps and tip; **B,** 2 Adson tissue forceps with teeth (1 × 2) and tip; **C,** 2 Gerald-DeBakey tissue forceps, 7 inch, and tip; **D,** 2 micro diamond dust ring forceps, 7 inch, and tip.

SURGICAL PHARMACOLOGY

Agents Used in Urologic Surgery

Category	Dose/Route	Purpose/Action	Adverse Reactions
BULKING AGENTS			
Contigen	Transurethral, periurethral	Correct UH, ISD, SUI	Swelling, urinary retention
Durasphere EXP	injection		Local tissue infarction/necrosis, vascular occlusion, embolus
IRRIGANTS			
Glycine (monocarboxylic amino acid)	1.5%, 3-5 L, intravesical	No hemolysis or dispersion of electrocurrent	Increased ammonia production Encephalitic reaction Biosynthesis of heme Blurred vision CNS disturbances TURP syndrome if absorbed
Sorbitol (nonelectrolytic, iso-osmotic, hypotonic aminoacetic acid)	3%, 3-5 L, intravesical	Isomer of mannitol, no hemolysis or dispersion of electrocurrent	TURP syndrome if absorbed
Water	Distilled, 3-5 L, intravesical	Irrigant, lyse cancer cells	Hyponatremia, hemolysis of erythrocytes
Normal saline	0.9%, 3-5 L, intravesical	Physiologic irrigant	Hypernatremia
IONIC RADIOPAQUE CONTRAST AGENTS (HIGH OSMOLAR)			
Conray 60 Hypaque 50 Renografin-60	30 ml half-strength; intraurethral, intraureteral, intravesical, intrarenal	Retrograde pyelography, renal arteriography, retrograde cystourethrography	Asthmatic response, rash, lactic acidosis, anaphylaxis
NONIONIC RADIOPAQUE CONTRAST AGENTS (LOW OSMOLAR)			
Omnipaque 300 Optiray 320	30 ml half-strength; intraurethral, intraureteral, intravesical, intrarenal	Retrograde pyelography, renal arteriography, retrograde cystourethrography	Back pain, dizziness, headache, diarrhea
INJECTABLES			
Indigo carmine	40 mg, IV or local	Colorize urine, vessels	Hypertension
Phenylephrine (Neo-Synephrine)	0.05% (5 mg), Sub-Q	Vasoconstriction for priapism	Hypertension, reflex bradycardia
Papaverine	30 mg/ml, 2 ml in solution, intercavernosal	Vasodilation, antispasmodic	Dizziness, dysrhythmia, hypotension, flushing, hypothermia
Vasopressin (Pitressin)	20 units/ml: 2 ml (40 units) in solution, local	Vasoconstriction	Water intoxication, dizziness, headache, pallor
TOPICAL			
Methylene blue	1 ml/100 ml NS, topical	Colorize tissues, vessels	Hypertension, dizziness, headache, anemia, diaphoresis
OTHER			
B&O suppository (belladonna/opium)	16.2 mg/30 mg, rectal	Prevent/decrease bladder/ureteral spasm	Constipation, decreased sweating

AV, Atrioventricular; *CNS,* central nervous system; *GI,* gastrointestinal; *ISD,* intrinsic sphincter dysfunction; *IV,* intravenous; *MAOIs,* monoamine oxidase inhibitors; *SubQ,* subcutaneous; *SUI,* stress urinary incontinence; *TURP,* transurethral prostatectomy; *UH,* urethral hypermobility.
Data compiled from Daily Med Current Medication Information, available at http://dailymed.nlm.nih.gov/dailymed/about.cfm. Accessed May 23, 2009; Hodgson BB, Kizior RJ: *Saunders nursing drug handbook 2009,* St Louis, 2009, Saunders; NCBI PubChem, available at http://pubchem.ncbi.nlm.nih.gov/. Accessed May 23, 2009.

The most commonly used catheters include the open-ended, whistle tip, cone tip, and olive tip. When a retrograde ureterogram is indicated, a cone-tipped ureteral catheter may be helpful in occluding the ureteral orifice to accomplish the x-ray study effectively. When a ureteral catheter is left indwelling, a special adapter (Figure 6-17, *B*) may be connected to the end of the ureteral catheter to facilitate connection to a closed urinary drainage system. A small slit may also be created in the Foley catheter, and the distal end of the ureteral catheter can be slipped into it and taped in place.

Indwelling double-pigtail or double-J stents are available and are passed cystoscopically to reside within the ureter (Figure 6-18). When the guidewire is removed from the core of the stent, a proximal and distal J or "pigtail" forms in the tubing

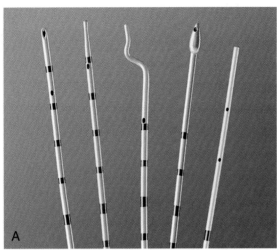
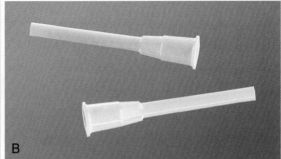

FIGURE 6-17 **A,** Ureteral catheters. **B,** Adapters.

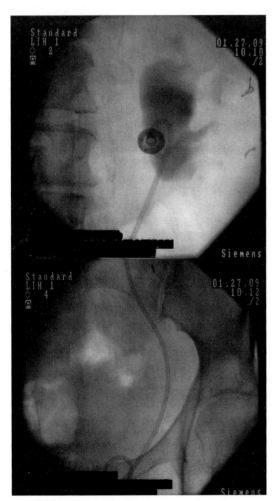

FIGURE 6-18 Double-pigtail stent set.

to retain the stents. Many of these stents have a nonabsorbable suture attached to the distal end, which extends through the urethral meatus. A suture may be easily tied to the distal end of those that do not. The surgeon can then remove the stent in

the office setting postoperatively without needing to perform a cystoscopy.

Urethral catheters have a multitude of functions as stents, as drainage tubes, and in diagnostic studies in the OR. They are generally divided into two categories—plain and indwelling (retention)—and range in different French (F) sizes, most commonly 10 through 30. The Foley catheter is the most frequently used retention catheter and is manufactured with a variety of balloon sizes, tip styles, lengths, and eye arrangements.

After transurethral prostatic surgery, a three-way Foley catheter with a 30-ml balloon capacity may be left indwelling. This type of catheter is preferred because it facilitates continuous bladder irrigation (CBI), and the large balloon aids in achieving hemostasis in the prostatic bed. The urologist may apply light traction on the Foley catheter with a leg strap, adhesive catheter anchor, tape, or a commercially available device such as the FoleyGoalie (Figure 6-19). This traction causes pressure against the bladder neck and aids in hemostasis (Figure 6-20). The FoleyGoalie is designed to prevent traumatic catheter removal in men. It is a cylindric device of helically arranged fibers that fits over the catheter and penis, secures with a Velcro strap to the base of the penis, and tapes to the catheter (Figure 6-21). If force is applied to pull out the catheter, the device tightens around the penis and catheter, holding it in position. When the force is released the FoleyGoalie loosens.

A hematuria catheter, a three-way Foley specifically for patients with excessive clot formation, is also available. This catheter is reinforced with a stretch spiral wire within the catheter lining that permits vigorous aspiration without fear of lumen collapse.

Diagnostic studies performed in the cystoscopy suite may require special catheters for specific studies. A Davis or Trattner triple-lumen double-balloon urethrographic catheter or any of a variety of urodynamic catheters may be used to diagnose lesions of the female urethra, such as urethral strictures, diverticula, and fistulas. To accomplish female urethrography, the catheter is inserted through the urethra into the bladder; the two balloons on the catheter are inflated, one in the bladder and one at the external urethral orifice, effectively isolating the urethra. Contrast medium is injected to visualize the entire urethra.

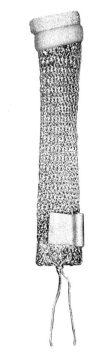

FIGURE 6-19 FoleyGoalie.

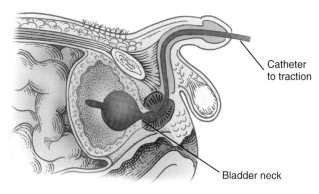

Catheter
to traction

Bladder neck

FIGURE 6-20 Balloon of Foley catheter inflated to size that prevents catheter from being pulled into prostatic fossa.

Another type of self-retaining catheter frequently used in the OR is Pezzer's catheter, also known as a *mushroom* catheter (Figure 6-22, *A*). It may be straight or angulated with a large single channel and a preformed tip in the shape of a mushroom. The flexible mushroom tip helps keep the catheter in place. This catheter is used primarily for suprapubic bladder drainage, often for poor-risk patients who have uremia, neurogenic bladder syndrome, or possibly long-standing urinary retention. The catheter is inserted into the bladder through a midline or small transverse abdominal wall incision and secured to the abdomen with suture or tape. The Malecot four-winged catheter, often used as a nephrostomy tube to provide temporary or permanent diversion of urine after kidney surgery and when renal tissue needs to be restored, may also be used for suprapubic drainage (Figure 6-22, *B*). A Foley catheter of preferred size is frequently chosen for either purpose. Nephrostomy tube replacement is accomplished by introducing the catheter into the surgical tract with a straight catheter guide and securing it in place with a suture or a nephrostomy retention disk that is

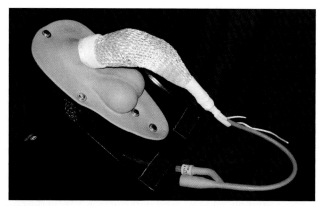

FIGURE 6-21 Attaching FoleyGoalie to catheter and penis; Velcro at base of penis, drawstring and Velcro at distal end of device to allow tightening in place.

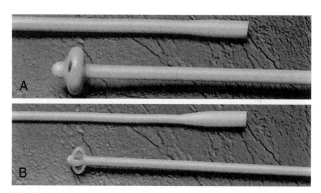

FIGURE 6-22 A, Pezzer (mushroom) catheter. **B,** Malecot (bat-winged) four-winged catheter.

one size smaller than the nephrostomy tube being used. The flanges of the disk are taped or sutured to the skin. The use of other variations of urethral catheters is described throughout the chapter.

Photography in Urology. The use of photographic and video imaging equipment in urologic surgery serves to document the patient's disease, the progress of a disease process, and long-term follow-up study. It is also an important teaching resource. Video equipment adapts to endoscopic instrumentation and has the capability of projecting an enhanced image on a television monitor, permitting members of the surgical team to observe and learn during the actual surgical procedure. Other visual aids, such as slides and photographs, are used in teaching, as visual references in publication, and as documentation in patient records.

When any form of photography or video imaging is used, the patient's privacy must be ensured and an informed consent should be obtained. Special release forms should also be signed preoperatively by the patient for any videotapes or photographs to be used in teaching or publications.

Evaluation

Before the patient is taken to the postanesthesia care unit (PACU) or observation unit, the patient's general condition is evaluated. The skin is assessed, and bony prominences, prepped and draped areas, and areas contacted by the attachment of ancillary equipment are observed for signs of pressure, irritation, or other changes from the preoperative status.

Many urology patients are discharged to the PACU with catheters and drains inserted, including urethral, ureteral, suprapubic, and wound drains. A local anesthetic may have been used for either primary analgesia or postoperative pain management (preemptive analgesia); preoperative or intraoperative infiltration of the surgical site blocks sensory input, resulting in postoperative analgesia. Documentation of medications administered from the sterile field should include time of administration, name of medication, dosage, site and route of administration, and the name of the person who performed the application or injection. Drains should be documented as to size and type, insertion site, time and date of insertion, type of collection device, name of the person who performed the insertion, and character of drainage. When several drains are in place, additional labeling on the collection devices is beneficial. Any postoperative observations before or during transport should be recorded.

Surgical Interventions

INTERVENTIONAL URORADIOLOGY

Many procedures that were once reserved for the OR are now being performed in the radiology department by specialists in uroradiology. As technology advances, procedures performed in the radiology department become a more common event. Those procedures include, but are not limited to, cystoscopy with stent placement, IV urogram, retrograde pyelogram, percutaneous antegrade stent placement and nephroscopic radiography, and ultrasound procedures with percutaneous access. The latter may be done to drain an abscess, to place a catheter or stent, or simply to introduce contrast material for direct fluoroscopic examination. Renal artery hypertension and stenosis may be treated successfully through new and advanced uroradiology methods, such as percutaneously placing stents in stenotic renal arteries (Novick and Fergany, 2007) (Figure 6-23).

DIAGNOSTIC AND ENDOSCOPIC PROCEDURES

Cystoscopy

Cystoscopy is an endoscopic examination of the lower urinary tract, including visual inspection of the interior of the urethra, the bladder, and the ureteral orifices. In a male patient, special attention is given to the examination of the verumontanum (which contains the ejaculatory duct), the bladder neck, and the median and lateral lobes of the prostate. In a female patient, the urethra, bladder neck, and bladder are examined.

Cystoscopy is an important diagnostic tool that provides the urologist with valuable information concerning the patient's urologic condition (History box). Indications for cystoscopy include hematuria, urinary retention, urinary tract infection, cystitis, tumors, fistulas, vesical calculus disease, and urinary incontinence. Urinary incontinence in postmenopausal women may be related to estrogen deprivation.

Procedural Considerations. Once in the preoperative area, all patients should be greeted by name and identified by their

HISTORY

How Cystoscopy Began

The blueprint for all other endoscopes is the cystoscope. In 1805 Philipp Bozzini of Germany lit the way with his *Lichtleiter,* a primitive prototype of what we now know as the cystoscope. In 1872 British scientist John Tyndall established the principle of internal light reflection inside glass rods. Then in 1877 Maximilian Nitze (the father of the cystoscope), in collaboration with Austrian manufacturer Joseph Leiter, turned Bozzini's prototype into the first direct-vision *kystoskop* for viewing the interior of the bladder, urethra, and larynx. This consisted of an incandescent platinum wire loop that fluoresced the bladder from the inside while magnifying the image externally through a system of lenses.

American physicians, in the meantime, worked with a German immigrant named Reinhold Wappler, who by the 1900s became known as a superior endoscope innovator. Endoscopic devices finally began to gain widespread popularity when Thomas A. Edison developed the incandescent lamp. Through miniaturization, a low-amperage mignon bulb was created from his lamp, allowing for simple, manageable, and low-cost cystoscopes to be produced.

Heinrich Lamm of Germany confirmed in 1930 that optical fibers could transmit images. But it was not until the mid-1950s that fiberoptics entered the scene, replacing these mignon bulbs with glass-fiber bundles. In 1954 fiberoptics became practical when British physicist Harold H. Hopkins produced the first usable system. A suggestion by a Dutch optics professor, Abraham van Heel, to coat the optic fibers with a transparent sheath led to unlocking the key to continuous illumination. This coating protected the fibers and prevented light from "leaking" out.

The contributions of Hopkins and van Heel became the inspirations behind the first fiberoptic gastroscope in 1957 and the first ureteroscope in 1960. Also in 1960, Hopkins introduced a refinement of his original technology, the "rod lens" rigid endoscope. This was created by combining air with long ground-up pieces of glass into an optical surface. In 1967 this method was applied to the cystoscope, thus replacing the previous prisms, mirrors, and lenses.

The 1980s brought the marriage of fibers and lenses into co-axial fiberoptic bundles through which one package of strands carried light and another returned images. These allowed increased flexibility and maneuverability without image distortion. Today endoscopy is so refined that visualization and treatment are achieved with flexible pencil-size tipped cystoscopes, ureteroscopes, and laparoscopes working through spearlike channeled sheaths and trocars.

Modified from Engel RM: Philipp Bozzini—the father of endoscopy, *J Endourol* 17(10):859-862, 2003; Wm. P. Didusch Center for Urologic History of the American Urological Association, Linthicum, Md, available at http://urologichistory.museum/content/milestones/cystoscopy/p1.cfm. Accessed May 16, 2009.

identification bracelet and number. The perioperative nurse should check the chart for operative consent and pertinent laboratory reports; IVPs and any other diagnostic x-ray studies ordered preoperatively should also be available for review. Customarily, the patient voids immediately before transport to the OR. The time of urination and the output volume should be documented for ruling out residual urine in the bladder.

SURGICAL TECHNOLOGY PREFERENCE CARD

In genitourinary surgery, patient positioning and temperature play a larger role in a successful outcome. As a significant majority of patients are middle aged to elderly, several factors need to be considered both preoperatively and intraoperatively. These patient populations have increased risk factors for vascular co-morbidities, and placing them in high or low lithotomy as well as lateral positions for extended periods of time can exacerbate these issues. Care should be taken to maintain proper body mechanics when placing them into position and sufficient padding should be placed at all pressure points to avoid creating a pressure ulcer. Thermoregulation is also an increased risk factor for these patients. Aging patients have decreased subcuticular fat stores and thinner skin, and coupled with cool irrigation fluids, can easily experience several degrees of core body temperature loss in a short period of time. As with all procedures, discuss the patient size, age, co-morbidities, position, estimated length of procedure, and other issues with the other members of the surgical team to ensure an optimal surgical outcome.

Room Prep: Basic operating room furniture in place, fluid warming devices, video equipment available for cysto/endoscopy, thermoregulatory devices, extra blankets, padding, positioning supplies to achieve optimal patient safety.

Prep Solution
- Iodine and iodophors
- Chlorhexidine gluconate
- Triclosan

Catheters: Have several sizes available. It is not unusual to insert a Foley catheter at the beginning of an open procedure and then change it out for another at the end.
- Catheter set and tray
  - Latex/rubber
  - PVC
  - Silicone
- Sizing
  - French
- Nonretaining
  - Red rubber (Robinson)—May be used to decompress the bladder or obtain a urine specimen preoperatively
- Retaining
  - Foley
    - 2-way
    - 3-way
    - 10 ml/30 ml balloon
  - Mushroom/Pezzer/Malecott
  - Ureteral catheters
    - Cone tip
    - Whistle tip
    - Olive tip
    - Open end
- Other urine collection devices

PROCEDURE CHECKLIST
Instruments
- Standard sets
- Various sizes of sheaths and obturators
- Rigid and flexible cystoscopes and ureteroscopes
- Have open instruments available if needed to convert from robotic/laparoscopic to open
- Anticipated additional/or surgeon-specific instruments

Specialty Suture
- As per surgeon's preference

Hemostatic Agents
- Mechanical
  - Clip appliers and clips
  - Staplers
  - Sutures/ligatures
  - Pressure
- Chemical
  - Collagen
  - Oxidized cellulose
  - Absorbable gelatin
  - Thrombin
- Thermal
  - Electrosurgical unit
  - Harmonic scalpel
  - Argon beam coagulator
  - Laser
  - Smoke evacuator

Continued

SURGICAL TECHNOLOGY PREFERENCE CARD—cont'd

Additional Supplies
- If the physician is requesting supplies, instruments, or equipment not normally used, check to be sure all have arrived before opening
- Gowns/gloves
- Drapes
- Sponges
- Guidewires
- Ureteral dilators
- Baskets/graspers
- Implants

Medications and Irrigation Solutions
- May need to be warmed for cystoscopic procedures, dependent on length of procedure
- Irrigation fluid determined by procedure/anatomy
  - Sterile water
  - Saline
  - Glycine
  - Sorbitol
- Viscous lidocaine for conscious sedation procedures
- Local anesthetics with epinephrine are contraindicated for use on the penis
- Appropriate-sized syringes, hypodermic needles, labels, and marking pen

Drains and Dressings
- Correct size and type for planned surgery
  - Open
    - Penrose
    - Cigarette
  - Closed
    - Jackson-Pratt
    - Hemovac

Specimen Care
- There may be many different types of specimens on certain procedures. Be sure to know the proper protocol for the handling and disposition of each type.
  - Frozen section
  - Permanent section
  - Cytology
  - Gram stain/fungal/acid fast
- Proper container for each specimen
- Labels for each specimen
- Proper solution for each specimen type
- Verify name and location of each specimen with both surgeon and circulator

Before opening for the procedure, the surgical technologist should:
- Arrange furniture
- Ensure proper equipment is in room and functioning
- Gather positioning devices
- Damp dust lights, furniture, and surfaces
- Check surgeon preference card to verify that all needed instruments, supplies, suture are picked and available for opening
- Place items to be opened in appropriate places

When opening sterile supplies:
- Check for holes in wrappers
- Verify exposure to sterilization
- Open bundles in appropriate locations
- Open additional supplies onto sterile field
- Use sterile technique
- Open all sterile supplies and equipment as close to the surgical start time as possible

After the patient is placed on the cystoscopy bed, correct positioning requires optimum relaxation of muscles of the legs and perineum. Proper positioning is a vital consideration for patient safety and comfort. Allen and Yellofin stirrups are boot-style stirrups that support the foot and calf. These have thick gel padding within the stirrup and provide optimum patient comfort and protection, relieving pressure on the popliteal space. They are especially beneficial for the patient who has limited hip mobility and altered peripheral circulatory status. The nurse should assess the patient's bilateral pedal pulses preoperatively and postoperatively when using any stirrups. Stirrups should be adjusted carefully to avoid undue pressure on the calf. If knee crutches are employed, the curve of the yoke suspension should flow outward from the perineum, in the same manner as the patient's legs. Padding the knee crutches reduces pressure on the popliteal areas. If sling stirrups that

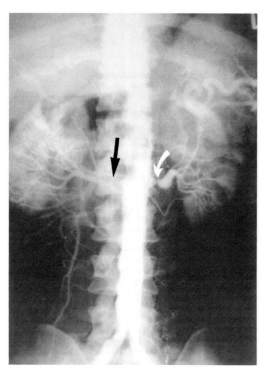

FIGURE 6-23 Bilateral renal artery stenosis. Severe stenosis of the right renal artery (*straight arrow*) is difficult to see because the artery overlies the vertebral body. The left renal artery stenosis is easier to identify (*curved arrow*).

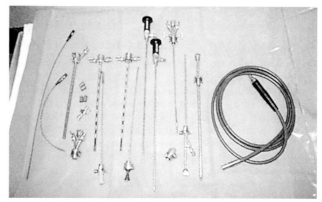

FIGURE 6-24 Basic instruments for cystoscopy, catheterization, electrosurgery, and retrograde ureteral pyelography (add ureteral catheter of choice). *Left to right,* Bugbee electrodes, single-horn Albarrán deflecting bridge, nipple adapters, stopcock, short double-horn bridge, 23F and 17F Foroblique cystourethroscopes and sheaths, 30-degree and 70-degree telescopes, double-horn Albarrán deflecting bridge, single-horn examining bridge, visual obturator, and fiberoptic cable.

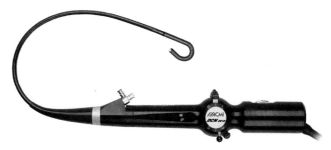

FIGURE 6-25 Flexible cystoscope.

support only the feet are employed, the post should be padded and positioned to prevent pressure on the peroneal nerve. Special pads are designed for use with both of these stirrups.

After the patient is properly positioned, the anesthesia provider may tilt the OR bed so that the patient's head is slightly higher than the buttocks to allow the prep solution to drain into the collecting pan. Pooling of solutions beneath the patient may cause skin reaction and chemical irritation, as well as the potential for burns if an ESU is used. If the cystoscopic procedure requires the use of an ESU, the nurse ensures that the dispersive pad is placed on the patient in direct contact with the skin as close to the operative site as is practical. When placing the ESU pad, the nurse avoids hairy areas, bony prominences, scar tissue, and proximity to prosthetic metal implants or pacemakers.

After properly positioning the patient, the nurse or urologist dons gloves and preps the entire pubic area, including the scrotum and perineum, with an antimicrobial solution. A disposable drape sheet with a sterile screen material incorporated into it is a standard part of the cystoscopy drape pack. The surgeon and surgical technologist drape the patient in a manner that ensures aseptic technique is maintained during the urologic procedure. If a general or spinal anesthetic is required, the anesthesia provider administers it before prepping and draping. If a local anesthetic is preferred, the surgeon instills it into the urethra of the male patient after prepping and draping but before instrumentation. For a female patient, the surgeon places a cotton applicator that has been dipped into the anesthetic solution in the urethral meatus. Usually, viscous lidocaine (Xylocaine), 1% or 2%, is used. If the patient is allergic to lidocaine, instillation of 50 to 60 ml of lubricant accompanied

by anesthesia-monitored sedation is often adequate to afford painless access to the urethra and bladder. The patient should be informed that a sensation of pressure is to be expected.

The basic cystoscopy setup requires a cystoscopy pack, a sterile gown or apron, sterile gloves, a fiberoptic light source, a prep cup and solution, gauze sponges, the cystourethroscope (Figure 6-24), a short bridge and fiberoptic light cord, lateral and Foroblique telescopes, a Luer-Lok stopcock, irrigation tubing and sterile water irrigant, and water-soluble lubricant. Additional items that should be sterile and available include a calibrated container to measure residual urine, test tubes with screw tops for urine specimens, an Albarrán bridge and rubber catheter nipples or adapters, a medicine glass for dye, anesthetic solution, disposable 10-ml and 20-ml syringes, medication labels and a marking pen, a penile clamp (to occlude male urethra after local anesthetic is instilled), contrast material, an ESU and dispersive pad, and a Bugbee electrode.

The flexible cystoscope (Figure 6-25) is used for patients with obstructive symptoms resulting from prostatic hyperplasia and rigid prostatic urethra. In addition, the flexible cystoscope can be used for patients who cannot assume a lithotomy position, such as those with spinal cord injuries or severe arthritis. Flexible cystoscopy may be accomplished with the use of a local anesthetic. It affords the patient a higher degree of comfort, is less traumatic to the urethra, and can be performed in the patient's bed on the nursing unit.

AMBULATORY SURGERY CONSIDERATIONS

Cystoscopy, Transrectal Guided Ultrasound of the Prostate

A commonly performed outpatient urologic procedure is a cystoscopy, transrectal ultrasound guided biopsy of the prostate (Cysto/TRUS). To minimize complications, patient selection is determined by the healthcare team. Patients classified as physical status 1 or 2, as per the American Society of Anesthesiologists, generally pose no great risk for procedures performed with general, intravenous moderate sedation (IV sedation), and local anesthetics. The majority of Cysto/TRUS patients have this procedure performed with IV sedation/local. To decrease pain during and immediately after the procedure, a viscous local anesthetic is injected into the rectum and also the urethra after IV sedation is initiated.

Preoperative and postoperative teaching of the patient and his family is most essential since the family will be the primary caregiver on discharge. Teaching begins in the surgeon's office. The office staff provides patients with a prescription for antibiotics with instructions to begin the medication 24 hours before the procedure and to continue oral antibiotics postoperatively until the prescription is completed. The office staff also advises the patient to take a cleansing enema 2 to 3 hours before the procedure. Both the antibiotics and the enema decrease the chances of postoperative infection.

Patient and family anxiety levels will be high pending the postoperative diagnosis. The patient may also be anxious because of the nature of the procedure and anesthetic used. The perioperative nurse plays a key role in supporting the patient and his family throughout the ambulatory surgical experience.

Discharge assessment following anesthesia includes the following:

- Airway patency, respiratory function, and oxygen saturation
- Stable vital signs
- Hypothermia resolved
- Level of consciousness and muscular strength
- Adequate pain control
- Mobility
- Skin color and condition
- Condition of the surgical site
- Intake and output
- Comfort
- Anxiety
- Significant other interaction
- Numeric score if used

Before discharge the nurse will instruct the patient to increase his clear liquid intake and monitor his urine output. Postoperative burning upon urination and blood in the urine as well as blood draining from the rectum are common. Patients are instructed to keep the perineum clean. The nurse ensures the patient has a prescription for pain medication, clarifies the instructions for dosage and frequency, and instructs the patient to call the surgeon for any temperature higher than 101° F. The nurse provides all instructions verbally and gives the patient and his family a written copy of the instructions. Patients call the physician as directed for results of the biopsy.

A postdischarge phone call to the patient is recommended. This phone call allows the nurse to review the patient's postoperative status, provide reassurance if necessary, and reinforce any teaching. The call also provides the patient and his family an opportunity to ask any additional questions.

Cleaning, sterilization, disinfection, and maintenance of endoscopic equipment are important procedures in the care of fiberoptic lensed instruments. Ultimately this process reduces costly repairs and ensures the availability of properly functioning instruments.

Endoscopy of the genitourinary tract is considered a class II (clean-contaminated) procedure and, according to the Centers for Disease Control and Prevention (CDC) and the Association for Professionals in Infection Control and Epidemiology (APIC) guidelines, presently requires disinfection rather than sterilization. High-level disinfection with an agent such as activated glutaraldehyde or dialdehyde that can destroy vegetative microorganisms, most fungal spores, tubercle bacilli, and small nonlipid viruses is recommended. In most situations, the routine of meticulous cleaning of endoscopic instruments and making sure that all channels are accessed, followed by appropriate high-level disinfection, provides reasonable assurance that the items are safe to use. The level of disinfection is based on the contact time, temperature, and concentration of the active ingredients of the disinfectant, as well as the nature of microbial contamination.

Many institutions are, however, treating endoscopic interventions as sterile procedures because the sterilization of instruments provides the greatest assurance that the risk of infections transmitted by contaminated instruments has been eliminated. Some options available include glutaraldehyde solution, hydrogen peroxide solution, an ETO (ethylene oxide, "gas") sterilizer, a hydrogen peroxide and plasma sterilizing unit, and high-vacuum or gravity steam autoclaving for those components that may be sterilized in this manner. The manufacturer's recommendations should always be followed. If soaking is chosen the lid should remain on the soaking container when not in use; masks should be worn when in direct contact with the fumes. It is also imperative that the instrumentation be thoroughly rinsed in sterile distilled water after removal from soaking solution and before use. Glutaraldehyde residue remaining in the channels or on the lens can result in chemical burns for the patient and the surgeon.

Stone removal, bladder biopsy, and bladder fulguration may be accomplished by using special cystoscopic accessories, such as the Hendrickson-Bigelow lithotrite, which crushes large bladder calculi. This procedure is called a *litholapaxy*. Lowsley forceps, Wappler rigid cup forceps, and flexible foreign body forceps may also be employed. Bladder fulguration requires the use of flexible-stem electrodes available in various French sizes and tip configurations such as the ball, cone, dome, and bayonet.

Operative Procedure

1. The surgeon lubricates the cystourethroscope and introduces it into the urethra, withdraws the obturator, and

drains the bladder. Residual urine may be measured at this time if the patient voided before the examination. The specimen may be saved for cultures or cytologic studies.

2. The surgeon connects the cystourethroscope to the irrigating system, and inserts and locks the telescope in place. If the patient is awake, telling the patient to try to urinate also helps facilitate passage of the scope. The surgeon controls the rate of flow and volume of fluid by adjusting the stopcock on the scope. If difficulty is encountered during insertion, the visual obturator may be used to introduce the scope under direct vision. This accessory is constructed to smooth the fenestrated edges of the cystourethroscope. It requires the use of the telescope for direct vision and permits irrigation during introduction.

3. For retrograde ureteral catheterization and pyelography, the surgeon passes ureteral catheters through the cystoscope sheath and then passes them through the ureteral orifice and into the ureter via the Albarrán bridge. A radiopaque substance (e.g., nonionic, low-osmolar agents Omnipaque 300 and Optiray 320; or ionic high-osmolar Renografin-60 and Hypaque 50) is injected (see Surgical Pharmacology, p. 211). Fluoroscopic imaging is used to outline the entire upper urinary collecting system.

Periurethral-Transurethral Injection of Bulking Agents

Collagen injection is an ambulatory surgery procedure achievable with the patient administered a local anesthetic with or without sedation. Collagen (Contigen) is a live bovine dermal natural protein and is prepackaged in a sterile syringe containing the collagen material. Injection needles available are an 8-inch, 23-gauge, noncoring needle for transurethral use or a 5-inch, 22-gauge needle for periurethral insertion. Female patients with intrinsic sphincter deficiency (ISD) demonstrated by urodynamic evaluation and male patients (usually after prostatectomy) with incontinence lasting more than 1 year may benefit from this procedure. Other indications for collagen injection include urethral hypermobility (UH), stress urinary incontinence (SUI) secondary to previous stricture treatment, trauma, or myelodysplasia (Appell and Winters, 2007).

Durasphere is a bulking product consisting of pyrolytic, carbon-coated beads within a water-based viscous medium. Needles for instillation include a 1.5-inch spinal-tip subcutaneous needle and a 15-inch spinal-tip transurethral needle. It is designed to treat women with SUI secondary to documented ISD. Durasphere is not absorbed as readily as collagen and may provide a more durable effect. Durasphere is currently approved by the U.S. Food and Drug Administration (FDA) for use in women only.

Procedural Considerations. Collagen must be kept refrigerated and the FDA guidelines for its use and documentation followed. Durasphere requires no refrigeration. Patients selected for collagen injection must be skin-tested with collagen 1 month before periurethral injection. The patient receiving Durasphere does not require skin testing. A urine culture and sensitivity will be done approximately 10 days preoperatively. It is optimal to use a video system for the procedure. A basic cystoscopy set is required. The patient will usually be in the lithotomy position.

Operative Procedure
1. The surgeon instills urethral anesthetic and may supplement the anesthesia with a perineal block of 1% or 2% lidocaine. Cystoscopic examination is performed before the bulking agent is injected to rule out any associated findings. It is recommended that the irrigation be instilled by use of a pressure bag to minimize extravasation of the material by increasing the intraurethral pressure.
2. The surgeon introduces the injection needle provided by the manufacturer through the cystoscope and places the tip transurethrally, below the urethral mucosa, just distal to the bladder neck. In the female the shorter needle may also be employed for periurethral introduction. Positioning of the needle tip is accomplished when the surgeon sees the indentation of the urethra by the tip while manipulating the needle.
3. The material is injected until the urothelium enlarges and meets in the midline, approximating the appearance of lateral lobe enlargement of the prostate.

Transurethral Ureteropyeloscopy

Transurethral ureteropyeloscopy is an endoscopic examination of the ureters and renal pelvis. The use of rigid or flexible ureteroscopes or ureteropyeloscopes provides the opportunity to diagnose filling defects in the ureter and renal pelvis, congenital anomalies (Figure 6-26), hematuria, ureteral obstruction, and damage from trauma. Manipulation, fragmentation, basketing of ureteral and renal calculi, and retrieval of foreign bodies are possible with transurethral ureteropyeloscopy. Extracorporeal shock-wave lithotripsy (ESWL), electrohydraulic lithotripsy (EHL), sonic lithotripsy, or laser lithotripsy may accompany the procedure. It may also be used to manage residual sludge after these treatments.

Ureteral strictures may be treated transurethrally, and biopsies of tumors of the ureter and renal pelvis are performed under direct visualization. Internal ureteral stents may also be inserted for ureteral patency. These range in size from 3F to 8.5F and are available in single-J, double-J, and pigtail configurations.

Procedural Considerations. The setup is similar to that for a cystoscopy with the addition of a rigid or flexible ureteroscope system (Figure 6-27). A critical factor in this procedure is allowing enough time for careful dilation of the ureter under C-arm fluoroscopy. The flexible ureteroscope has gained popularity because of its inherent tip mobility, which provides a more panoramic view of the entire circumference of the ureter. The perioperative nurse must be prepared to tilt the radiolucent operative bed at head and foot and laterally, as well as raise the bed.

In addition to the standard cystoscopy setup, the following items should be available: a rigid or flexible ureteroscope, ureteral dilators of graduated sizes and styles, size 3F to 5F ureteral stone baskets of various styles, a ureteral grasping forceps, biopsy forceps, snare, scissors, catheters of various styles and sizes, stents, guidewires, balloon dilators, and radiographic contrast material. Patient allergies should be checked before the use of radiographic contrast material.

Operative Procedure
1. The surgeon inserts the ureteropyeloscope and accesses the ureter with a guidewire under fluoroscopic control. The ureter is irrigated as the guidewire is advanced. The surgi-

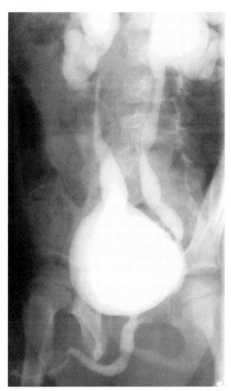

FIGURE 6-26 Grade 5 bilateral ureteral reflux.

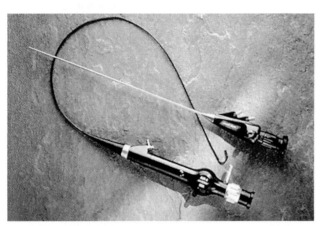

FIGURE 6-27 Flexible ureteropyeloscope and rigid ureteropyeloscope.

cal technologist assists by maintaining slight tension on the wire.

2. The ureter is dilated to 10F to 12F with a balloon dilator or co-axial dilators. If a balloon dilator is chosen, the balloon should be inflated with contrast material, using a pressure syringe to ensure that it does not exceed the maximum allowable atmospheric (ATM) pressure (burst pressure).

3. An additional working guidewire is placed by the surgeon to be used as a safety wire.

4. The surgeon passes the ureteroscope over the working guidewire, biopsies any suspicious lesions, and performs diagnostic pyeloscopy and ureteroscopy. The characteristics of calculi are observed to determine the best treat-

ment approach. Urine may be obtained for cytologic and microbiologic examination. If a calculus is small enough to be delivered through the ureter, the surgeon engages it in a retrieval basket and removes it under visual as well as fluoroscopic control. If, after ureteral dilation, the calculus does not appear to be small enough for delivery, lithotripsy (fragmentation) is performed through the ureteroscope, or ESWL may be performed later. Lithotripsy may be performed with ultrasonic (through a rigid ureteroscope) or electrohydraulic lithotripters or with the tunable pulse-dyed or holmium:yttrium-aluminum-garnet (Ho:YAG) lasers. Appropriate laser precautions must be enforced.

5. The surgeon assesses the ureter for integrity (perforation or laceration) with retrograde pyelography.

6. A ureteral stent is placed over the remaining safety guidewire, and the guidewire is removed.

SURGERY OF THE PENIS AND THE URETHRA

Laser Ablation of Condylomata and Penile Carcinoma

Laser ablation of condylomata or penile cancer is the eradication of diseased tissue by means of a laser beam. Laser therapy has been determined to be effective for condylomata and penile cancers that are refractory to other treatments. One of the major advantages of the laser is that heat is distributed evenly to the tissue underlying the lesion. When any laser is being used, precautions appropriate to that system must be initiated.

Procedural Considerations. Laser treatment may be performed successfully with local infiltration of an anesthetic. A U-shaped, craterlike lesion of predetermined depth with a 2-mm radius can be created. A power setting ranging from 2 to 20 watts on continuous or super-pulse mode is commonly used. With laser ablation, less edema and necrosis occur, fibrosis is minimized, and rapid healing is facilitated. The argon, CO_2, potassium-titanyl-phosphate (KTP), and neodymium (Nd):YAG lasers are all suitable for this therapeutic application.

Operative Procedure

1. The surgeon moves the beam transversely across the tissue and then in a crosshatch matrix, thereby treating all perimeters of the lesion. Throughout the procedure the surgeon wipes the area with a sponge moistened in acetic acid (5% vinegar), which results in greater visualization of the diseased tissue and allows therapy to deeper layers.

2. Postoperatively the affected areas may be coated with an antibiotic ointment. Wounds are generally left uncovered.

Circumcision

Circumcision is the excision of the foreskin (prepuce) of the glans penis. Circumcision in adult males is performed for the relief of phimosis, a condition in which the orifice of the prepuce is stenosed or too narrow to permit easy retraction behind the glans. Another condition that may require circumcision is balanoposthitis, an inflamed glans and mucous membrane with purulent discharge. Circumcision may also be done to prevent recurrent paraphimosis, a condition in which the prepuce cannot be reduced easily from a retracted position. (See Chapter 17 for pediatric considerations during circumcision.)

Procedural Considerations. The perioperative nurse assists in positioning the patient in the supine position. A plastic or minor instrument set and a local anesthetic with IV sedation are sufficient. The ESU should be available.

Operative Procedure

1. The surgeon clamps the prepuce in the dorsal midline and incises it toward the coronal margin (Figure 6-28, *A*), leaving about 5 cm of coronal mucosa intact. If the prepuce is adherent, a probe or hemostat may be used to break up adhesions.
2. A similar procedure is performed ventrally. The two incisions are then joined circumferentially. Alternatively, a superficial circumferential incision is made in the skin with a scalpel at the level of the coronal sulcus and the mucosa at the base of the glans.
3. The surgeon undermines redundant skin between the circumferential incisions and removes it as a complete cuff (Figure 6-28, *B*).
4. Bleeding vessels are coagulated or clamped with mosquito hemostats and ligated with fine absorbable ligatures.
5. The surgeon approximates the raw edges of the skin incision to a coronal cuff of mucosal prepuce, generally with 4-0 or 5-0 absorbable sutures on atraumatic, plastic cutting, or fine gastrointestinal (GI) needles (Figure 6-28, *C*).
6. The wound is dressed with petrolatum gauze.

Excision of Urethral Caruncle

A urethral caruncle is a benign lesion or inflammatory prolapse of the external urinary meatus in the female. Excision entails the removal of these papillary or sessile tumors from the urethra.

Procedural Considerations. The perioperative nurse assists with placing the patient in the lithotomy position. A minor or plastic set, an ESU, and a local anesthetic are used. A urethral catheter of an appropriate size may be required if the distal urethral prolapse is severe.

Operative Procedure

1. The surgeon uses a small, fine-tipped Metzenbaum or plastic scissors to expose the tumor and excise it within a wedge of ventral urethral tissue.
2. Figure-of-eight 4-0 absorbable sutures are placed at the edge of the incision to achieve hemostasis.

Urethral Meatotomy

Urethral meatotomy is an incisional enlargement of the external urethral meatus to relieve congenital or acquired stenosis or stricture at the external meatus.

Procedural Considerations. A male patient is placed in the supine position. Prepping and draping are as described for urethral catheterization. For a female patient, the lithotomy position is used. The surgeon administers local anesthesia. A plastic instrument set is required.

Operative Procedure

1. The surgeon places a straight hemostat on the ventral surface of the meatus.
2. An incision is made along the frenulum to enlarge the opening and overcome the stricture.

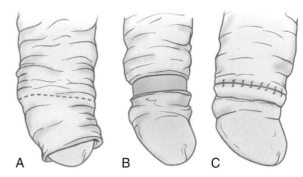

FIGURE 6-28 Circumcision.

3. Hemostasis is obtained by clamping the bleeding vessels and ligating them with fine absorbable sutures.
4. The surgeon sutures the mucosal layer to the skin with fine absorbable sutures.
5. A dressing of petrolatum gauze is applied.

Urethral Dilation and Internal Urethrotomy

Urethral dilation and internal urethrotomy entail the gradual dilation and lysis of a urethral stricture to provide relief of distal lower urinary tract obstruction. Urethral strictures or narrowing of the urethra may be caused by a congenital malformation that is usually found at the external urinary meatus. Infection or trauma may also contribute to stricture of the membranous and pendulous urethra. Urethral stricture disease may be treated by periodic dilation with Phillips filiforms and followers, Van Buren sounds, or balloon dilation catheters.

Procedural Considerations. The perioperative nurse assists with placing the male patient in the supine position for routine urethral dilation and in the lithotomy position for other procedures. The female patient is placed in the lithotomy position. Prepping and draping are conducted as appropriate to the patient's position and gender. The surgeon administers a local anesthetic either (1) by placing cotton-tipped applicators, which have been dipped into viscous 2% lidocaine (Xylocaine), into the urethral opening or (2) by using a urethral syringe to instill the lidocaine. Female urethral dilation is performed with short, straight metal dilators or with hollow McCarthy dilators. The latter allows a urine specimen to be obtained.

In addition to a cystoscopy setup, required instrumentation includes urethrotomes (Figure 6-29); the resectoscope working element with sheath, obturator, and cold knives; urethral dilators; Phillips filiforms and followers; Van Buren sounds; and a silicone Foley catheter. Before use, the filiforms and followers should be carefully inspected for damaged or weak points, particularly around the scored-threaded end.

Operative Procedure
GRADUAL DILATION

1. In a male patient, the surgeon lubricates and anesthetizes the urethra with a viscous anesthetic that is instilled into the urethra with a urethral or Uro-Jet syringe. A penile clamp occludes the penile urethra at the coronal sulcus and keeps the anesthetic within the urethra.
2. Phillips filiforms of various tips and sizes are introduced first in an attempt to pass an instrument beyond the urethral

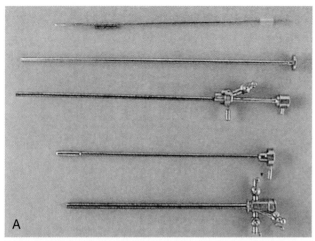

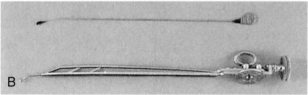

FIGURE 6-29 A, Optical internal urethrotome. B, Otis urethrotome.

stricture. Followers of increasing size are connected to the filiforms and passed through the strictured portion of the urethra, stretching the scarred area (Figure 6-30, A).

3. Slow dilation is also achieved with a small catheter or follower left in the urethra. It leads to softening of the stricture over the course of several days.

INTERNAL URETHROTOMY

1. The surgeon inserts the assembled visualizing urethrotome into the urethra using direct vision.
2. When necessary, the surgeon feeds a filiform or ureteral catheter into the catheterizing channel to help identify the patent portion of the urethra.
3. The surgeon advances the urethrotome to the desired position, and incises the urethral scar with the blade. The normal urethra is incised 1 cm proximally and distally beyond the stricture to achieve optimum results.
4. A silicone Foley catheter is usually left in place for 3 to 5 days after surgery.

Urethroplasty

Urethroplasty is reconstructive surgery of the urethra for strictures, urethral fractures, or narrowed segments of the urethral lumen that are congenital, inflammatory, or traumatic in origin. Urethral grafts are generally required and may include free skin grafts and mobilized vascular flaps. There are many combinations of these procedures, and in all of them some type of temporary urinary diversion may be used, depending on the location and severity of the condition.

Preoperatively, the patient usually complains of obstructive symptoms, frequently associated with a UTI. Techniques used to determine diagnosis include urodynamics (voiding pressures above and below the site of obstruction), urinary flow cytometry, IVU to rule out an upper tract lesion, cystoscopy, and urethrography. The length and density of the diseased urethra are determined to plan the appropriate reconstructive procedure. Any associated UTI must be treated and eradicated before surgical intervention. Definitive repair should not be done for 10 to 12 weeks after use of diagnostic instrumentation to allow the inflammatory reaction to subside.

Procedural Considerations. The patient is placed in the exaggerated lithotomy position by the perioperative nurse and one other person. Routine prepping and draping procedures are employed with precautions for isolating the anus (e.g., the use of an impervious plastic adherent drape). The setup includes a minor instrument set with fine plastic instruments for dissection and plastic repair. Strictures may be located deep, requiring fiberoptic lighting. An ESU may be required.

Operative Procedures

JOHANSON URETHROPLASTY. The Johanson urethroplasty is a two-stage procedure to repair and reconstruct the urethra for severe urethral stricture disease. Approximately 3 months after completion of the first stage, if the operative site is healing and the patient is voiding adequately, a second-stage procedure is performed. Vascularized flaps of preputial or penile skin may be mobilized to the ventrum by leaving them attached to the outer surface of the prepuce or as an island flap. One modification is the transverse preputial island flap neourethra with glans channel positioning for the meatus. Preputial skin is preferred because of its rich reliable blood supply and non–hair-bearing characteristics.

First Stage

1. The surgeon makes an inverted U incision in the perineum from the inner borders of the ischial tuberosities up to and including the base of the scrotum.
2. A Van Buren sound is passed into the urethra up to the stricture (Figure 6-30, B). The bulbocavernosus muscle is dissected and retracted laterally.
3. The surgeon makes an incision in the urethra over the strictured area and extends it in each direction at least 1 cm beyond the diseased area. The abnormal scar tissue is excised or simply incised, because scrotal skin ultimately increases the lumen.
4. A 28F sound is passed through both the proximal and the distal urethral lumens to rule out further stricture.
5. The surgeon sutures the remaining urethral mucosa to the scrotal skin with 4-0 absorbable sutures.
6. A cystotomy tube to divert the urinary stream may be left indwelling and removed in 5 to 7 days.

Second Stage (Mobilized Vascular Flap)

1. A red rubber catheter is temporarily inserted into the bladder through the proximal urethral stoma.
2. The surgeon incises the penoscrotal skin longitudinally, adjacent to the urethra.
3. A new urethra is constructed by developing the ventral preputial skin that is dissected free and fanned out. The rectangle of skin is rolled into the neourethra and measured.
4. A channel is sharply created on the ventral aspect of the glans, in a plane just above the corpora.
5. The surgeon removes the glans tissue, forming a groove approximately 14F in diameter.
6. Layers of subcutaneous tissue are dissected free from the dorsal penile skin to create an island flap that is spiraled to the ventrum. The surgeon brings the flaps together in the

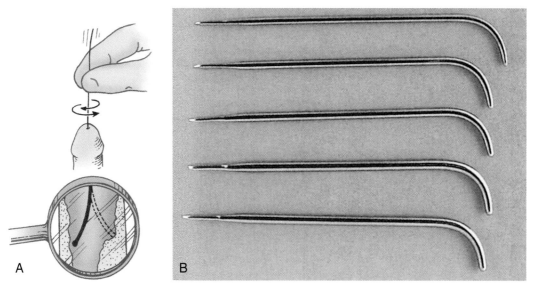

FIGURE 6-30 A, Method of using coudé-tipped bougie for passing stricture. B, Variety of urethral sounds (dilators).

midline and closes with a continuous or interrupted 4-0 absorbable suture.

7. The neourethra is anastomosed proximally to the urethra and carried to the tip of the glans.

8. The dorsal penile flaps are transposed laterally to the midline, and the surgeon excises the excess skin.

9. Closure is with 4-0 absorbable interrupted mattress sutures around the glans and down the penile shaft. A bulky pressure dressing is applied.

10. Suprapubic cystostomy drainage is an option, but a urethral catheter usually suffices.

HORTON-DEVINE URETHROPLASTY (URETHRAL PATCH GRAFT). Urethral patch graft is a one-stage operative procedure that incorporates a free skin graft to correct a urethral stricture. Free skin grafts should be at full thickness. Because the free graft must be revascularized, it is important that it have a perfect skin cover of well-vascularized dorsal, preputial, penile skin.

1. The surgeon passes a 17F panendoscope into the posterior urethra, and then passes a 20F urethral dilator into the posterior urethra.

2. A perineal vertical midline incision is made into the urethral lumen. The surgeon reinserts the panendoscope and examines the incision to determine if it crosses the stricture.

3. The defect is measured, and the surgeon makes a circumferential incision on the posterior penile shaft to harvest an oval piece of skin the size of the defect.

4. The epidermal side of the graft is defatted, and 4-0 absorbable sutures are placed at the apex and base.

5. The surgeon sutures the apex into position at the proximal and distal ends of the stricture with the epidermal side toward the urethral lumen.

6. The graft is anastomosed proximally to the urethra with the suture line of the graft next to the corpus. The middle glans dart is fixed to the corpus. The graft is formed into a neourethra over a Silastic stenting catheter.

7. The surgeon reinserts the panendoscope and irrigates the urethra to check for suture-line leaks.

8. A Foley or fenestrated catheter is inserted to serve as a stent.

9. The surgeon approximates and closes the corpus spongiosum over the patched area as a separate layer with interrupted 3-0 absorbable sutures. Subcutaneous 4-0 absorbable sutures are placed.

10. The skin and the graft site are closed with interrupted 4-0 sutures.

11. A suprapubic catheter is inserted to divert urine for healing. Petrolatum gauze is wrapped around the penis and covered with gauze sponges and fluffed dressings. A scrotal support is applied to provide support and pressure.

Penectomy

Penectomy is the partial or total removal of a cancerous penis. The procedure selected depends on the extent of involvement and disease stage. Invasive penile cancer not suited for irradiation because of its size, depth, or location is best dealt with by penectomy. Excision of a 2-cm gross tumor margin is adequate for local management. Partial penectomy may afford a sufficient length for directable and upright urination. At least 3 cm of viable proximal shaft is necessary for consideration of a partial penectomy. If the residual stump is inadequate in length, detachment and mobilization of the suspensory ligaments may be an option in selected patients. A total penectomy is generally required when tumor margins are beyond a 2-cm retrievable length from the penoscrotal junction.

Options are available to limit the extent of the disfiguring surgery previously indicated for penile cancer. Chemotherapy agents, often combined with irradiation, are proving effective in shrinking penile carcinomas that would have previously mandated radical penectomy.

Reconstruction is possible after penectomy. Evaluation must take into account sexual, urinary, and cosmetic factors. Extensive or proximally invasive lesions that include the scrotum, perineum, abdominal wall, and pubis necessitate emasculation as well as expanded resection of involved tissues.

Procedural Considerations. The setup necessary is similar to that for any inguinal surgery, with the addition of a medium Penrose drain for use as a tourniquet.

Operative Procedure
PARTIAL PENECTOMY
1. The lesion is excluded by a towel attached to the planned amputation line. The surgeon applies a penile tourniquet at the base of the penis (Figure 6-31, *A*).
2. After circumferential skin incision, the surgeon divides the cavernous bodies to the urethra with a 2-cm gross margin (Figure 6-31, *B*).
3. Dorsal vessels are ligated, margins of the tunica albuginea are approximated, and the urethra is dissected proximally and distally (spatulated) to obtain a 1-cm redundant flap (Figure 6-31, *C*).
4. Without sacrificing the tumor margin, the surgeon divides the urethra. Interrupted sutures are placed on the opposite margins of the tunica albuginea to secure the corpora. The tourniquet is removed, and hemostasis is achieved.
5. After the dorsal urethrotomy, a skin-to-urethra anastomosis is performed. The redundant skin flap is then dorsally approximated (Figure 6-31, *D*).
6. A small urinary catheter is inserted, and a nonadherent dressing is applied.

TOTAL PENECTOMY
1. A vertical elliptic incision is made around the penile base (Figure 6-32, *A*).
2. The distal urethra and its ventral traction are divided through an incision in Buck's fascia, mobilizing the urethra and aiding its dissection, which extends from the corpora to the bulbar region.
3. The surgeon separates and ligates the corpora (Figure 6-32, *B*). The suspensory ligaments and dorsal vessels are divided as corporal dissection is carried out.
4. The urethra is transected from the corpora (Figure 6-32, *C*).
5. An ellipse of skin approximately 1 cm in size is taken from the perineal area. A tunnel is fashioned in the perineal subcutaneous layer of tissue. A traction suture through the tunnel, at the penile base, aids dissection for transposition of the urethra to the perineum (Figure 6-32, *D*).
6. The surgeon grasps the urethra with forceps and transfers it to the perineum. The urethra is spatulated, and a skin-to-urethra anastomosis is performed through a buttonhole incision in the perineum (Figure 6-32, *E*).
7. The primary incision is closed horizontally, elevating the scrotum away from the urethral opening (Figure 6-32, *F*).
8. An indwelling urinary catheter is inserted, and the wound is covered with a nonadherent dressing.

Penile Implant

A penile prosthesis is implanted for treatment of organic sexual impotence. Sexual impotence may be caused by (1) diabetes mellitus, (2) priapism, (3) Peyronie's disease, (4) penile trauma, (5) pelvic surgery, (6) neurologic disease (in selected cases), (7) vascular disease, (8) hypertension, and (9) idiopathic impotence. The penile implant serves as a stent to enable vaginal penetration for sexual intercourse. Penile implants are

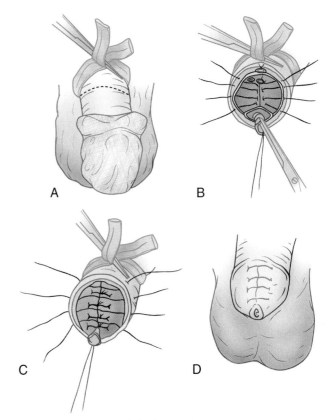

FIGURE 6-31 Partial penectomy.

available as malleable one-piece devices, self-contained inflatable devices, and two- and three-piece devices. The procedure described for the inflatable penile implant is for the three-piece device.

Procedural Considerations. The anesthesia provider administers either a spinal or a general anesthetic. The perioperative nurse assists with positioning the patient in either the supine or the lithotomy position, as directed by the surgeon. A 5- to 10-minute skin prep is usually performed before draping is carried out. To prevent urethral injury and potential urinary retention, the surgeon may insert a 14F or 16F Foley catheter to identify the urethra intraoperatively. The ESU may be required. The surgeon may inject a local anesthetic of 0.5% plain bupivacaine (Marcaine) or 1% etidocaine (Duranest) at the beginning of the procedure into the incisional sites. Often, a penile block, composed of 0.9% saline (150 ml), 1% plain lidocaine (50 ml), and 30 mg/ml papaverine (2 ml), is instilled intraoperatively before the incision into the corpus cavernosum. This enables the surgeon to evaluate erectile size and provides some postoperative pain management.

The surgical technologist sets up a separate sterile Mayo stand or small table covered with a plastic drape for the implants. It is recommended that the implants not be in contact with paper or cloth that may shed fiber particles.

The instrument setup includes a minor set with fine instruments, plus Hegar dilators, the penile prosthesis of choice (Figure 6-33), the Furlow inserter, the closing tool, the assembly tool for clamping connectors (Figure 6-34, *A*), and the connectors of choice (Figure 6-34, *B*). Medications needed in the operative field include 50 ml of 1% lidocaine, 150 ml of inject-

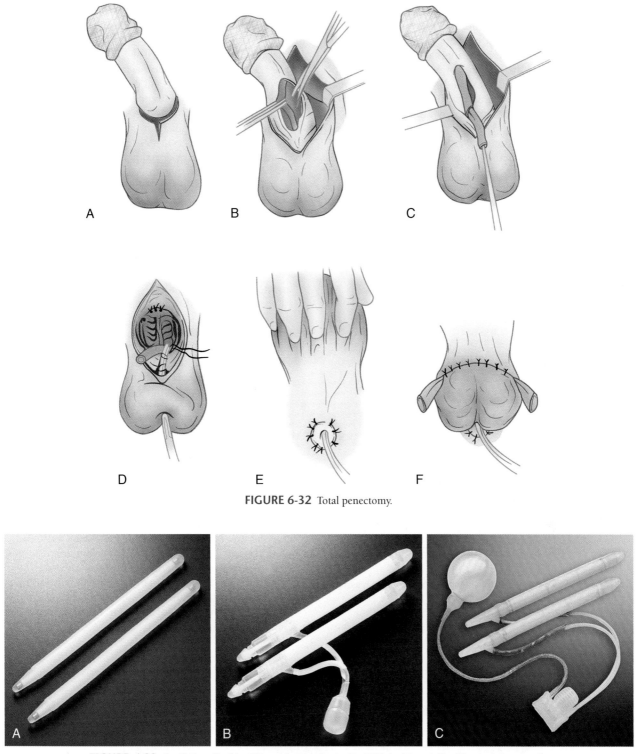

FIGURE 6-32 Total penectomy.

FIGURE 6-33 A, AMS malleable 650 penile prosthesis. **B**, AMS Ambicor inflatable two-piece penile prosthesis. **C**, AMS tactile inflatable penile prosthesis, three-piece with rifampin (Inhibizone).

able 0.9% normal saline, 1 ml of methylene blue (optional by surgeon preference), 2 ml of papaverine, 50 ml of 0.5% bupivacaine (Marcaine) or 1% etidocaine (Duranest), 50,000 units of bacitracin, and 80 mg of kanamycin. Medication safety practices must be implemented for all medications on the sterile field.

A serious risk with a penile implant is infection. Infection rates for first-time implantation are low at 1%, but the rate can rise to as high as 18% with reimplantation procedures. Because of the high risk of infection, models that have been irradiated and embedded with minocycline hydrochloride and rifampin (Inhibizone) are now available (American Medical Systems

[AMS], 2009). The sterile team should be double-gloved throughout the procedure. A 5-minute antimicrobial prep of the operative area is critical in reducing skin flora. The anus should be isolated in the perineal approach. Intraoperatively and before insertion of the implant components, a prophylactic antibiotic irrigant of bacitracin and kanamycin in normal saline is used on the implants without Inhibizone and in the insertion sites. Systemic antibiotics may also be required. As with any implant procedure, it is vital to maintain an environment conducive to infection prevention. The perioperative nurse ensures that traffic in and out of the OR is minimized.

It is recommended that the implants with Inhibizone not be soaked in any solution before implantation because this may cause the antibiotic component to disintegrate. The area to be implanted may be irrigated with antibiotic solution, and the implant itself may be dipped in a sterile solution of 0.9% normal saline to assist with insertion if desired. Prophylactic antibiotic protocols remain the same.

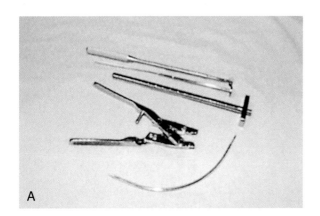

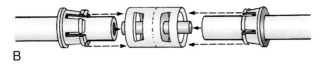

FIGURE 6-34 **A,** *Top to bottom,* Closing tool, Furlow inserter, assembly tool, tubing passer. **B,** Quik-connectors.

Operative Procedure

IMPLANTATION OF NONINFLATABLE (SEMIRIGID) PROSTHESIS

1. The surgeon inserts a 14F or 16F Foley catheter and attaches it to a drainage collection device to be maintained within the sterile field. The amount and color of urine are noted. The catheter is left in place intraoperatively to assist in identifying the urethra.
2. A midline incision is made from the base of the penis into the scrotum for approximately 3 cm. Some surgeons may choose a suprapubic or dorsal penile approach.
3. The surgeon incises the tunica albuginea over the most proximal portion of the corpora in a longitudinal manner, and places stay sutures.
4. The corpora are dilated proximally and distally with 7-mm to 14-mm Hegar dilators, depending on the diameter of the implant chosen. The corpora are dilated to 1 mm more than the implant size. Care is taken to not perforate the urethra.
5. The surgeon measures the corporal length with a Furlow inserter or sizing instrument.
6. After placement of the closure sutures, the surgeon inserts the prostheses into the corpora. Proper placement is evident immediately by a change in the configuration of the penis with no buckling of the glans.
7. The surgeon closes the tunica albuginea using the previously placed 2-0 absorbable continuous suture; 3-0 or 4-0 absorbable interrupted sutures are used for skin closure.
8. Petrolatum gauze or 2-inch Kling tube gauze may be used for the dressing.

IMPLANTATION OF INFLATABLE PROSTHESIS

1. The surgeon inserts a 14F or 16F Foley catheter and attaches it to a drainage collection device to be maintained within the sterile field. The amount and color of urine are noted. The catheter is left in place intraoperatively to assist in identifying the urethra.
2. A midline incision is made from the base of the penis into the scrotum for approximately 3 cm (Figure 6-35, *A*).
3. The surgeon incises the tunica albuginea of each corpus in the most proximal portion, and places stay sutures.
4. The corpora are dilated distally and proximally with 7-mm to 14-mm Hegar dilators. Dilation should be 1 mm more than the diameter of the chosen implant. The 700CX

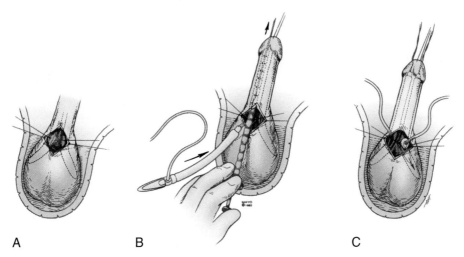

FIGURE 6-35 Penoscrotal approach for inflatable penile implant.

implant is 12 mm at its widest point. When this is used the dilation at the distal end should be 13 mm. The proximal end, however, should be 14 mm to accommodate the input tubing.

5. The surgeon measures the corporal length with the Furlow inserter.

6. Corporal sutures of 2-0 absorbable material are placed along the tunica incision and tagged. Some surgeons prefer to place these sutures last and employ the closing tool to prevent puncture of the cylinders.

7. The cylinders are packaged with attached traction sutures of 4-0 braided polyester at the distal end. The surgeon places the suture through the eye of a 2½-inch Keith needle, and slides the needle into the groove of the Furlow inserter.

8. The surgeon guides the Furlow inserter along the corporal tunnel, and pushes the plunger to release the Keith needle, which punctures the glans (Figure 6-35, *B*).

9. The Keith needle is grasped with a heavy hemostat and pulled through the glans, allowing the cylinders to slide to the channel opening. The surgeon removes the Furlow inserter, inserts the cylinder, and guides it to its proper position beneath the glans penis (Figure 6-35, *C*).

10. If necessary, rear tip extenders are added to the proximal end of the cylinder. The proximal end is positioned in the crus.

11. The procedure is repeated on the other side.

12. The surgeon palpates the external inguinal ring and uses blunt dissection to create a path. Dissecting scissors are used to separate the transversalis fascia on the inguinal floor. If the Ambicor implant with self-contained reservoir is being placed, steps 12 through 14 are eliminated.

13. The perivesical space is enlarged to allow palpation of the Cooper ligament. The reservoir is then positioned into the perivesical space.

14. The surgeon fills the reservoir with 65 or 100 ml of saline solution (dependent on the reservoir size selected) and pulls it against the floor of Hesselbach's triangle.

15. The pump is then placed into the most dependent portion of the scrotum. It is generally positioned on the patient's dominant side. The space is created by blunt dissection lateral to the testicle.

16. The rods and reservoir tubings are connected to the pump with the connectors of choice, using the assembly tool to clamp them in place, and tested for inflation and deflation.

17. The surgeon closes the tunica of the scrotum over the pump with a running stitch of 3-0 absorbable suture.

18. The prosthetic device is left in a partially inflated position to reduce bleeding and promote healing for 24 hours postoperatively (Figures 6-36 and 6-37). (Following this period the implants are deflated for the remainder of the "healing phase" so the reservoir pocket heals with the reservoir in "full position" to prevent autoinflation.)

19. The surgeon closes the incision with 4-0 absorbable suture in a running subcuticular stitch, and a dressing is applied.

20. The penis is positioned flush with the lower abdomen for patient comfort. Mesh pants are useful as a nonadherent support dressing. An ice pack may be applied to reduce swelling.

21. The Foley catheter is left in place during the immediate 24-hour postoperative period and then usually removed.

Deep Dorsal and Emissary Vein Ligation

Undertaken for vascular compromise–related impotence, this procedure entails the ligation or elimination of the penile deep dorsal vein and its tributaries. Care is taken to avoid damage to the arteries and nerves lying alongside the deep dorsal vein. A common cause of erectile dysfunction in patients with organic impotence is vascular compromise. Before surgical intervention is undertaken, a definitive diagnosis of a corporal leak is made through dynamic infusion cavernosometry and cavernosography. Diagnostic results may indicate failure-to-store or failure-to-fill impotence. Patients with vascular compromise in a given anatomic region tend to be compromised elsewhere as well. Many have diabetes or hypertension. Because of this, the surgical team must exercise great care in positioning the patient to prevent further damage to the patient's altered tissue perfusion. The cavernous and crural veins are suture-ligated. All circumflex and emissary branches are ligated or coagulated. The suspensory ligament is detached, and the entire deep and accessory dorsal vein is removed.

Revascularization of the Penile Arteries

The relationship of focal arterial occlusive disease to sexual dysfunction has prompted efforts to rectify the resulting impotence. Reconstructive surgery has been attempted in patients who demonstrate correctable vascular disease in the large arteries. The most widely attempted repairs are end-to-end and end-to-side microscopic anastomoses of the distal inferior epigastric artery to the proximal deep dorsal artery near the pubic level, below the rectus muscle and Buck's fascia. Paramedian and infrapubic incisions are made, and the arteries are freed and tunneled. This procedure requires both urologic and vascular surgeons.

SURGERY OF THE SCROTUM AND TESTICLES

Hydrocelectomy

A hydrocele is an abnormal accumulation of fluid within the scrotum. The fluid is contained within the tunica vaginalis. Excessive secretion or accumulation of hydrocele fluid may be the result of infection or trauma. A hydrocelectomy is the excision of the tunica vaginalis of the testis to remove the enlarged, fluid-filled sac.

Procedural Considerations. The patient is placed in the supine position. Prepping and draping of the patient include routine cleansing of the external genitalia and draping with a fenestrated sheet. A minor instrument set is required, plus a small drain, a 30-ml syringe with a 20-gauge, 2-inch aspirating needle, and a suspensory dressing.

Operative Procedure

1. The surgeon administers a local anesthetic into the cord at the base of the scrotum with 10 to 15 ml of plain lidocaine 1%.

2. An anterolateral incision is made in the stretched skin of the scrotum over the hydrocele mass with a #10 or #15 blade.

3. Bleeding is controlled with Crile hemostats, electrocoagulation, or vessel ligation with 3-0 absorbable ligatures. Stretching the skin of the scrotum compresses the scrotal vessels.

4. An incision is then made between the blood vessels. The fascial layers are incised to expose the tunica vaginalis.
5. The surgeon uses sharp and blunt dissection to free the hydrocele.
6. The sac is opened, and clamps are placed on each side incorporating the tissue adjacent to the tunica vaginalis and the skin.
7. Using Martius clamps, the surgeon everts the incised edges. The tension placed by the Martius clamp compresses the incised edge, controls bleeding, and prevents dissection between the tissue layers.
8. A pouch is created by dissecting between the tunica vaginalis and the dartos layer. Scrotal pressure is released. This pouch will hold the testis after the repair.
9. The surgeon opens the tunica vaginalis and evacuates the fluid contents.
10. The testis is lifted, and the sac is inverted so that it surrounds the testicular attachments and epididymis.
11. Excess tunica vaginalis may be excised. The surgeon sutures the tunica edges along the peritoneal surface with 3-0 absorbable suture in an interrupted fashion to the juncture of the testis. Six to eight sutures are placed around the circumference of the testis (Figure 6-38). Some surgeons elect to sew the sac behind the spermatic cord in an interrupted fashion, and others may choose a continuous radial stitch around the posterior testis and epididymis.
12. The testis is replaced into the scrotum.
13. A drain may be placed into the scrotum and exteriorized through a stab wound in its most dependent portion. The drain is loosely sutured to the external scrotal wall to prevent migration.
14. The surgeon closes the scrotal incision with 3-0 absorbable sutures in a full-thickness continuous manner or in layers with 3-0 and 4-0 continuous absorbable sutures.
15. A fluff compression dressing contained in a scrotal support or mesh underwear aids in reducing postoperative scrotal edema.

Vasectomy

A vasectomy is the excision of a section of the vas deferens. The operation is usually performed selectively as a permanent method of sterilization. Because of the serious implications of permanent sterilization, particular attention must be paid to acquiring informed consent. Although studies have raised the question of a correlation between prostate cancer and vasectomy, a definitive causal relationship has not been established.

The patient having elective sterilization for birth control is encouraged to return to the office setting for sperm-count analysis. Generally, two successive negative counts are sufficient to indicate that sterility has been achieved. Elective vasectomies are frequently performed in the office setting.

Procedural Considerations. The patient usually lies in the supine position. A local anesthetic is used. A minor instrument set and scrotal support are needed.

Operative Procedure
NO-SCALPEL APPROACH
The no-scalpel technique was devised in China and has five fundamental principles:

1. Fixation of the vas deferens without entering the scrotal skin
2. Performance under direct vision to prevent damage from blind sharp scrotal penetration
3. Simplified instrumentation
4. Decreased operative time by simplification of the procedure
5. Elimination of an incision or use of a scalpel

The procedure is as follows:

1. The right vas deferens is fixed under the scrotal skin with three fingers.
2. Using a syringe with 1% or 2% plain lidocaine and a small needle, the surgeon raises a small wheal in the median raphe of the scrotum. The needle is advanced along the vas toward the external inguinal ring. Additional lidocaine is injected into the perivasal region.
3. The procedure is repeated on the left side. Pressure is applied to the wheal site to minimize edema.
4. Once adequate anesthesia is accomplished, the right vas is again fixed with three fingers.
5. The surgeon applies a vas ring clamp over the scrotal skin, encircling the vas. Lifting the clamp upward, the skin over the vas is stretched as thin as possible, leaving minimal tissue between the vas and the clamp.
6. The ring clamp is locked in place, and the scrotal skin cephalad to the clamp is stretched with an index finger.
7. The surgeon punctures the skin directly into the vas deferens with the inner prong of the pointed dissecting hemostat. Both prongs of the dissecting hemostat are placed into the puncture site and spread directly on top of the vas.
8. When the surface of the vas is visualized, one prong is used to penetrate the vas itself. The vas is brought out of the wound by twisting the hemostat 180 degrees.
9. The ring clamp is moved to directly encircle the vasal tissue. The vas may then be divided and occluded by intraluminal electrocoagulation, clips, or suture ligation. Fascia should be placed between the severed ends of the vas.
10. The surgeon repeats the procedure on the left side. It is usually possible to place the ring clamp around the left vas through the initial entry site. Sutures are not necessary.
11. After ensuring that there is no bleeding, antibiotic ointment, pressure dressings, and a scrotal support are applied.

Vasovasostomy

Vasovasostomy is the surgical reanastomosis of the vas deferens, using the operative microscope. The number of vasal reanastomosis procedures has increased dramatically. Reanastomosis may often alleviate chronic testicular pain, a not infrequent complication after vasectomy. In addition, a significant number of men who underwent a vasectomy want to regain their fertility. A precise reconnection can be performed with the use of a microscope and a modified two-layer anastomosis. Success rates vary, but in general, patency can be demonstrated by the presence of sperm in the semen within 4 weeks after vasovasostomy (Lipshultz et al, 2007). When there are no longer two viable segments of vas deferens, a similar procedure, the epididymovasostomy, may be performed. This involves anastomosis of a vas deferens to a segment of the epididymis. Postoperative precautions include no lifting or ejaculation for a minimum of 2 weeks. The sperm count and viability of sperm are rechecked at 3- and 6-month intervals. If sperm are not present by 6 months, the operation is considered a failure (Lipshultz et al, 2007).

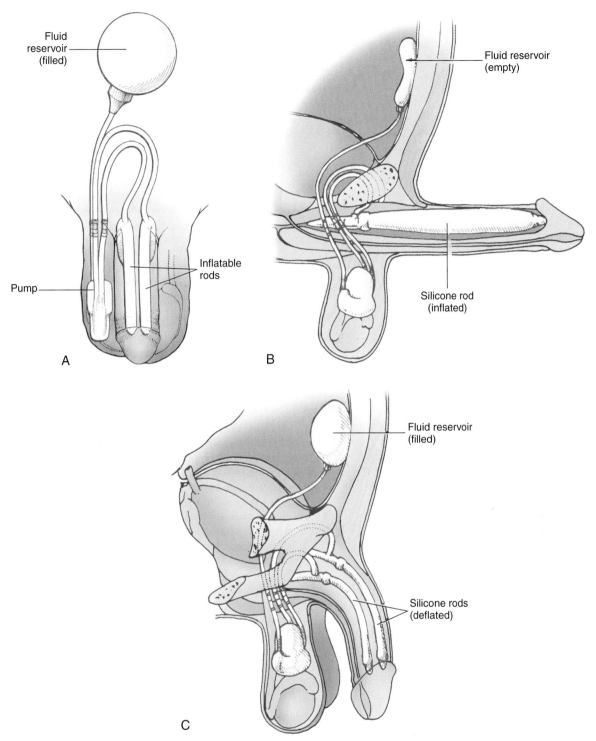

Fluid
reservoir
(filled)

Pump

Inflatable
rods

A

Fluid reservoir
(empty)

Silicone rod
(inflated)

B

Fluid reservoir
(filled)

Silicone rods
(deflated)

C

FIGURE 6-36 AMS inflatable 700CX penile prosthesis. **A,** Frontal view. **B,** Sagittal view—penis in erect position. **C,** Sagittal view—penis in flaccid position.

Procedural Considerations. A minor instrument set is required, with the addition of selected microsurgical instruments and sutures. The procedure is frequently done under monitored anesthesia care with local injection of 0.5% plain bupivacaine (Marcaine) and 1% lidocaine (Xylocaine) in a 50:50 ratio.

Operative Procedure
1. After the vas deferens has been located by external manipulation, the surgeon makes a vertical scrotal incision.
2. The testicle, epididymis, and vas are displaced from the scrotum. The vasectomy site is identified, and the scarred area is excised.

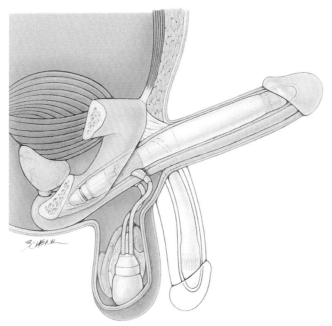

FIGURE 6-37 AMS Ambicor inflatable two-piece implant, sagittal view.

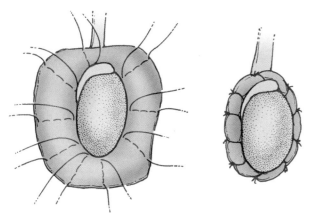

FIGURE 6-38 Hydrocelectomy.

3. The surgeon trims the proximal end of the vas deferens until fluid is expressed. Fluid is collected on a glass slide and examined for the presence of live sperm. Surgery continues even if results for sperm are negative unless an epididymal obstruction exists.
4. The distal end of the vas is resected until a normal lumen is visible.
5. The distal and proximal lumens are then dilated.
6. The surgeon places the two portions of the vas in an approximator clip and inserts a piece of background material underneath to provide contrast and improve visibility. Six stitches of 10-0 nonabsorbable microsuture are placed in the inner layer. The proximal end is sutured through the serosa to the mucosa, and the distal end is sutured through the mucosa to the serosa (Figure 6-39).
7. A second layer of 8 to 10 stitches of 9-0 nonabsorbable suture is placed without penetrating the lumen of the vas.
8. The surgeon closes the incision in two layers with interrupted 3-0 and 4-0 absorbable sutures.

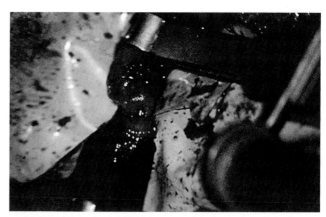

FIGURE 6-39 The two portions of the vas in approximator clip with background material as the proximal end is sutured through the serosa to the mucosa with 10-0 nylon.

9. Gauze sponges and a scrotal support are placed on the patient to provide a pressure dressing.

Microscopic Epididymal Sperm Aspiration

Microscopic epididymal sperm aspiration (MESA) requires the availability of an in vitro fertilization team so that the aspirated sperm may be immediately processed and used for the selected in vitro technique or frozen for later use. The procedure must be timed according to the partner's cycle of ovulation. Ova are aspirated as an office procedure just before MESA is performed.

MESA should be done using the micropipette technique. The surgeon inserts the tip of a 250- to 350-micrometer (μm) pipette into an epididymal tubule to retrieve sperm cells without contamination by red blood cells. After aspiration, the fluid is given to the in vitro fertilization team to process the sperm cells. Processing involves washing debris from the cells, retrieving the most active cells from the sample, and removing any red blood cells, if possible. This is critical because red blood cells significantly interfere with sperm cell function.

After the sperm cells are aspirated, the surgeon closes the epididymal tubule using microscopic technique. If adequate numbers of sperm cells can be obtained from one testis, the other side may be aspirated to add to the sperm bank if this is desirable. It may be necessary to aspirate sperm cells from the rete testis (tubules between the testicles and the epididymal head that carry cells to the head of the epididymis) if sperm cells are not found in tubules closer to the vas deferens.

The sperm cells retrieved may be used for intracytoplasmic injection into the partner's egg (ICSI), the most successful of the in vitro techniques available. This technique is not as dependent on the quality of the sperm as earlier techniques of in vitro fertilization.

Epididymectomy

An epididymectomy is the excision of the epididymis from the testis. Epididymectomy is rarely performed, usually only as a last-choice treatment for degenerative cystic disease, chronic infection, and intractable pain of the epididymis.

Procedural Considerations. The perioperative nurse assists with positioning the patient in the supine position with his legs slightly abducted. The anesthesia provider administers a general, spinal, or regional anesthetic. Setup is as described for hydrocelectomy, plus an ESU, if desired.

Operative Procedure

1. The surgeon makes an anterolateral incision over the testis in the scrotum to expose the tunica vaginalis. The tunica is incised to expose the testis and overlying epididymis.
2. An incision is made along the superior head of the epididymis, which is then sharply dissected from the testis. A portion of the vas deferens may also be excised.
3. Bleeding is controlled by electrocoagulation and absorbable ties.
4. The skin wound is closed with 4-0 absorbable sutures.
5. A small drain may be left intrascrotally for 24 to 48 hours.

Spermatocelectomy

Spermatocelectomy is removal of a spermatocele—a lobulated intrascrotal cystic mass attached to the superior head of the epididymis. Spermatocele is usually caused by an obstruction of the tubular system that conveys the sperm and may be a late complication after vasectomy.

Procedural Considerations. The setup for a spermatocelectomy is as described for a hydrocelectomy, plus a microscope and slides, if desired.

Operative Procedure

1. The mass is approached through a scrotal incision as described for hydrocelectomy.
2. The surgeon identifies the structures of the testis and spermatic cord and dissects the cystic structure free.
3. Bleeding is controlled with electrocoagulation.
4. The wound is closed and dressed as described for hydrocelectomy.

Varicocelectomy

A varicocelectomy is the high ligation of the gonadal veins of the testes. Varicocelectomy is done to reduce venous backflow of blood into the venous plexus around the testes and to improve spermatogenesis.

Varicoceles occur more frequently on the left side because the gonadal vein of the left testis unites retroperitoneally with the renal vein at a 90-degree angle and is consequently under greater backpressure. As a result of this unusual backpressure, the pampiniform plexus of the spermatic cord becomes tortuous and engorged, resembling a bag of worms.

Procedural Considerations. The setup for inguinal varicocelectomy is as described for an inguinal hernia repair (see Chapter 4). A microscope may be employed to better visualize the vessels involved.

Operative Procedure

The incision may be through a suprainguinal approach or an oblique inguinal approach over the external inguinal ring.

1. The surgeon identifies the structures of the spermatic cord and dissects the vessels free from the vas deferens.
2. The abnormal dilated veins in the inguinal canal are clamped and ligated. The redundant portions are excised. A drain may be placed.
3. The incision is closed in layers.

Testicular Biopsy

A biopsy of the testicle involves a wedge excision of suspicious tissue for diagnostic confirmation. Men experiencing infertility who are azoospermatic or oligospermatic with a normal or minimally elevated level of follicle-stimulating hormone may be evaluated through this means. Biopsy may also be performed to obtain sperm cells for in vitro fertilization techniques.

Procedural Considerations. The perioperative nurse assists with positioning the patient in the supine position and the anesthesia provider administers a general, regional, or spinal anesthetic. A minor instrument set is used. Special fixatives, such as Bouin's or Zenker's solution, must be available when pathologic confirmation is required. If retrieval of sperm cells is planned the perioperative nurse and surgical technologist ensure the biopsy specimen is placed in a small amount of saline, kept warm, and taken immediately to the fertility laboratory for aspiration of cells. Formalin destroys the germinal epithelium and should not be used.

Operative Procedure

1. The scrotum is held firmly on its posterior aspect. This causes the skin on the anterior aspect to stretch tightly over the incisional site, forcing the epididymis to remain posterior and allowing the scrotal skin to part without retraction.
2. The surgeon makes a 1-cm to 2-cm vertical incision taking care to avoid injury to the epididymis.
3. The incision is continued to the tunica vaginalis. As the tunica is incised, there should be a normal efflux of clear fluid.
4. Absorbable 4-0 stay sutures are placed in the tunica vaginalis. Two more are placed in the tunica albuginea.
5. Using the scalpel in a shaving action, no-touch technique, the surgeon resects a small ellipse of tunica with its tubules. The tissue is placed in the fixative or sent to the histology department as a fresh specimen.
6. The wound is closed in three layers with 3-0 and 4-0 absorbable suture.
7. Gauze sponges and fluffed dressings are placed over and around the scrotum. A scrotal support is applied to provide pressure and support.

Orchiectomy

An orchiectomy is the removal of the testis or testes. Removal of both testes is castration and renders the patient sterile and deficient in the hormone *testosterone,* which is responsible for development of secondary sexual characteristics and potency. This operation, like vasectomy, has legal implications that require attention to acquiring informed consent for surgery. Bilateral orchiectomy is usually performed to control symptomatic metastatic carcinoma of the prostate gland. A unilateral orchiectomy is indicated because of testicular cancer, trauma, or infection. Testicular implants are available for cosmetic purposes. These must be ordered preoperatively based on preoperative measurements for size. This procedure has recently been approached through endoscopic techniques, usually in conjunction with laparoscopic herniorrhaphy.

Procedural Considerations. The perioperative nurse assists with positioning the patient supine and the anesthesia provider administers a general, spinal, or regional anesthetic. A minor instrument setup is required.

Operative Procedure
SCROTAL APPROACH

1. For benign conditions the incision is made over the antero-lateral surface of the midportion of the scrotum.
2. The surgeon carries the skin incision through the subcutaneous and fascial layers through the tunica vaginalis, exposing the testicle.
3. Retractors are placed, and bleeding vessels are clamped and ligated.
4. The spermatic cord is divided into two or three vascular bundles. Each vascular bundle is doubly clamped, cut, and ligated, first with 0 absorbable suture ligature and then with a proximal free 0 absorbable tie.
5. The vas is separately ligated with a 0 absorbable tie. The testis is removed.
6. The procedure is repeated on the opposite side if bilateral excision is planned.

INGUINAL APPROACH

1. For malignant conditions the incision is begun just above the internal ring, extending downward and inward over the inguinal canal to the external inguinal ring.
2. The surgeon exposes the inguinal canal and dissects the spermatic cord free, cross-clamps it, and divides it into vascular bundles at the internal ring.
3. Gentle forward traction is applied to the cord, which is dissected from its bed.
4. The testis is everted into the wound from the scrotum and excised.
5. The procedure is repeated on the opposite side if bilateral excision is planned.
6. Bleeding is controlled with electrocoagulation. A small drain may be placed in the empty hemiscrotum if desired.
7. The surgeon reapproximates the external oblique fascia with 2-0 absorbable interrupted sutures.
8. Subcutaneous tissue, including Scarpa's fascia, is closed with 4-0 absorbable sutures.
9. The skin is reapproximated with surgical staples or 4-0 subcuticular sutures.

Radical Lymphadenectomy (Retroperitoneal Lymph Node Dissection)

Radical lymphadenectomy is a bilateral resection of retroperitoneal lymph nodes. Dissection usually includes lymph nodes, channels, and fat around both renal pedicles; the vena cava; and the aorta, including the bifurcation of the aorta. Lymph node dissection is performed for treatment of nonseminomatous testicular tumors or in conjunction with an open prostatectomy for prostate cancer.

Procedural Considerations. The perioperative nurse assists with placing the patient in the supine position. The anesthesia provider administers a general anesthetic. If the dissection is unilateral, the patient is supine with the operative side tilted upward. Long, fine dissection instruments along with basic laparotomy instruments are required.

Although this procedure may be performed laparoscopically, this approach has not yet become the standard of practice because of its technical difficulty.

Operative Procedure

1. The surgeon makes a midline abdominal incision from the xiphoid process to the symphysis pubis.
2. The abdominal contents are explored to determine the degree of gross nodal involvement. The colon is either packed within the abdominal cavity or mobilized and kept moist outside the abdomen.
3. The surgeon opens the posterior peritoneum between the aorta and the vena cava.
4. Using blunt and sharp dissection, the surgeon removes the lymphatic structures and fat en bloc from around both renal pedicles, the vena cava, and the aorta from above the renal hilum to beyond the bifurcation of the iliac vessels on the side of the original testicular neoplasm.
5. The spermatic vessels of the affected side are removed down to and including the stump of the previous orchiectomy.
6. The inferior mesenteric artery may be sacrificed if technically necessary, but the superior mesenteric artery is not disturbed.
7. The ureter on the affected side is skeletonized to remove any perilymphatic tissue.
8. If reperitonealization is desired, the posterior peritoneum is closed with a 2-0 absorbable continuous suture.
9. The surgeon repositions the viscera into the abdominal cavity, and closes the wound in layers, usually without placement of a drain.

SURGERY OF THE PROSTATE GLAND

Glandular hyperplasia of the prostatic urethra usually manifests itself after 50 years of age. Prostatic enlargement may be benign or malignant and may occur in one or more lobes of the prostate but most frequently occurs in the lateral or median lobes. Progressive growth of the hyperplastic gland compresses the remaining normal prostatic tissue, forming what is called a *surgical capsule.* The growth of adenomatous tissue slowly encroaches on the prostatic urethral lumen, causing obstruction of urinary outflow. The surgeon must consider several factors when determining the best route for removal of the prostatic obstruction: the age and medical condition of the patient, the size of the gland and location of the pathologic condition, and the presence of associated medical disease.

Prostate cancer is the most frequently diagnosed cancer in men and is the leading cause of cancer death in men (American Cancer Society, 2008). Because of the prevalence of prostate cancer and the similarity of symptoms to benign prostatic hyperplasia (BPH), the American Urological Association (AUA) recommends that starting at age 40 the prostate-specific antigen (PSA) test and digital rectal examination (DRE) be offered to men at average risk.

A blood sample is drawn to determine the PSA level, followed by a DRE. The blood is often drawn first, since manipulation of the gland has been known to alter the efficacy of the PSA test. The PSA test is considered a valuable tool for early detection of carcinoma of the prostate, but if used alone, it will miss 20% to 30% of all prostate cancers. If the test value is elevated, the patient is at risk for carcinoma of the prostate; a PSA value above 10 ng/ml is highly suggestive of prostatic carcinoma. Clinical evaluation and an elevated PSA usually indicate the need for a transrectal ultrasound needle biopsy to confirm the diagnosis. When the results of the biopsy are positive for malignancy, additional diagnostic studies are indicated including measurement of free and total serum PSA II levels, bone scans, and CT and MRI scans of the pelvis (Ignatavicius, 2010).

The most commonly used system to grade prostate cancer is the Gleason score. To calculate the Gleason score, the pathologist evaluates the prostatic tissue to determine which type of cell is the most common and which type is the second most common and gives each of the two cell types a score from 1 to 5. The two scores are combined to determine the total score. Higher numbers are an indication of more abnormal, aggressive cancer cells. Men with a Gleason score of 2 to 4 are generally cured by surgery; scores from 5 to 6 indicate mildly aggressive cancer cells; a score of 7 indicates the cancer is moderately aggressive. Scores between 8 and 10 indicate highly aggressive tumors and are associated with a poor prognosis after surgery (Epstein, 2007). Additional prostate cancer staging tools are the TNM (tumor, node, metastasis) system and the American Urological Association (AUA) system (Box 6-1).

If the prostate gland is cancerous, a radical retropubic or radical perineal prostatectomy, in conjunction with open or laparoscopic pelvic lymph node dissection, is usually performed. TURP may also be used in men who cannot have a radical prostatectomy, or to relieve symptoms caused by prostate cancer before other treatments begin. Select patients with well-differentiated or moderately differentiated lesions may be candidates for transperineal, ultrasonically guided implantation of radium seeds (brachytherapy) or cryoablation of the prostate (cryotherapy). Newer therapies for prostate cancer are being developed (Research Highlight). Many patients desire to retain sexual function. The surgeon may attempt to save the neurovascular bundles in what is termed a nerve-sparing approach. The site and size of the prostatic lesion, however, often determine if this can be achieved successfully and without undue risk to the patient.

Three open surgical approaches are possible in removing the benign hyperplastic obstructive prostate gland: retropubic prostatectomy, suprapubic prostatectomy, and perineal prostatectomy. Of these, the one most commonly employed is the suprapubic prostatectomy. All open prostatectomies hold the risk for loss of sexual potency.

TURP is the endoscopic (closed) surgical approach that has been traditionally used. Alternative modalities that have shown moderate to good success in the treatment of BPH are photoselective vaporization of the prostate (PVP), interstitial laser coagulation of the prostate (ILC), transurethral incision of the prostate (TUIP), transurethral laser incision of the prostate (TULIP), holmium laser enucleation of the prostate, and holmium laser ablation of the prostate (HoLAP). A visual laser ablation of the prostate (VLAP) was originally performed with the Nd:YAG laser but may now also be accomplished with the holmium laser (Fitzpatrick, 2007). Proper laser protocol must be followed for the type of laser being employed. The standard

---

RESEARCH HIGHLIGHT

High-Intensity Focused Ultrasound Prostate Cancer Treatment: A Safe Alternative to Surgery or Radiotherapy

High-intensity focused ultrasound (HIFU) is a noninvasive technique used in the treatment of prostate cancer. It is available in North America, but has not yet been approved by the FDA for use in the United States. Researchers in Europe are reporting impressive results with the technique; a multicenter trial studied 402 patients with localized cancer treated with HIFU. Although 28% of the patients required two treatment sessions, 87% of the treated patients had negative biopsy findings on follow-up; a median PSA level of 0.4 ng/ml was achieved at a minimal follow-up appointment of 6 months. These same investigators later reported a 5-year actuarial negative biopsy rate of 90%. Another group of researchers studied the long-term results in patients with low-risk disease (initial PSA level <10 ng/ml, Gleason score ≤6). In this study, 78% of the patients were considered free of disease (stable PSA level according to American Society for Therapeutic Radiology and Oncology criteria) and had negative biopsy results at 5 years. For those with intermediate-risk cancer, the disease-free rate was 53%; for those with high-risk cancer, the disease-free rate was 36%.

HIFU is highly focused into a small area, creating intense heat of 80° to 100° C, which is lethal to prostate cancer tissue. HIFU destroys tissue by heat, rather than by cavitation or mechanical shearing. Since ultrasound is nonionizing, there is no collateral tissue damage.

For the majority of patients, HIFU is indicated as a curative therapy. The best candidates are clinical/pathologic stages T1c to T3. Because of the limited focal length of HIFU, gland volume cannot be 40 ml or larger. If the gland is larger, then downsizing is required with total androgen ablation. Aside from primary therapy, HIFU can be utilized as salvage therapy, primarily after

radiation. HIFU can also be repeated without any increase in risk or complications. In addition, HIFU can be used to treat cryosurgical failures. If necessary, radical prostatectomy can be performed after HIFU.

HIFU is performed as an outpatient procedure, usually after induction of anesthesia with an epidural anesthetic. The HIFU unit consists of a control console, a power generator, a cooling system, and a probe that contains a standard imaging and high-intensity treatment ultrasound head. The HIFU probe is placed into the rectum and multiple gland images are taken. The surgeon selects the treatment zones. The procedure usually lasts 2 to 4 hours. The procedure is completed without blood loss or exposure to radiation.

There will be edema secondary to the thermal effects: therefore at the end of the procedure, a urethral Foley catheter is placed into the bladder. This catheter will remain in place for 2 to 4 weeks. There may be some bladder discomfort for several days, but full activities can be resumed the day following surgery. Once the catheter is removed, the urinary stream may take several months to improve, as the urethra needs to heal, and the gland will take up to 3 months to start shrinking. During this time, some prostate tissue may slough and pass in the urine. The rest of the gland forms scar tissue.

Although HIFU is a relatively new procedure for prostate cancer treatment, it represents what may become the next generation of minimally invasive therapy for prostate cancer. The control and precision that HIFU provides truly allows the surgeon to precisely ablate the prostate gland with pinpoint accuracy and thereby preserve the adjacent structures. Furthermore, because HIFU is nonionizing, there is no collateral tissue damage.

Modified from Chinn D: *Transrectal HIFU: the next generation?* Prostate Cancer Research Institute, available at www.prostate-cancer.org/education/novelthr/Chinn_TransrectalHIFU.html. Accessed May 27, 2009; Marberger M et al: New treatments for localized prostate cancer, *Urology* 72(suppl 6A):36-43, 2008.

STAGE A: CLINICALLY UNSUSPECTED DISEASE

A1   Focal carcinoma, well differentiated
A2   Diffuse carcinoma, usually poorly differentiated

STAGE B: TUMOR CONFINED TO PROSTATE GLAND

B1   Small, discrete nodule of one lobe of the gland
B2   Large or multiple nodules or areas of involvement

STAGE C: TUMOR LOCALIZED TO PERIPROSTATIC AREA

C1   Tumor outside prostate capsule, estimated weight ≤70 g, seminal vesicles uninvolved
C2   Tumor outside prostate capsule, estimated weight >70 g, seminal vesicles involved

STAGE D: METASTATIC PROSTATE CANCER

D1   Pelvic lymph node metastases or ureteral obstruction causing hydronephrosis, or both
D2   Bone, soft tissue, organ, or distant lymph node metastases

Modified from Nelson WG et al: Prostate cancer. In Abeloff MD et al, editors: *Abeloff's clinical oncology*, ed 4, Philadelphia, 2008, Churchill Livingstone.

TUIP procedure involves the use of electrosurgery only. Transurethral microwave therapy (TUMT) is another alternative that is performed as an office procedure.

Prostatic Core Needle Biopsy

Needle biopsy of the prostate is indicated for patients in whom prostatic cancer is clinically suspected. It may be accomplished transrectally with a needle designed for this purpose or transperineally.

Procedural Considerations. Needle biopsy of the prostate has the risk of both intraoperative and postoperative bleeding. A cystoscopic examination may accompany a needle biopsy. Most needle biopsies are performed in the urologist's office or ultrasound department.

The most significant potential complication of a biopsy is systemic infection. This risk can be decreased with antibiotic administration before and after the procedure and bowel cleansing before the examination. The patient is given antibiotic therapy 24 hours before the procedure and is advised to use a sodium phosphate enema 2 to 3 hours before the test is performed. Before the examination, an antiseptic solution mixed with a viscous local anesthetic often is instilled into the rectum and allowed to coat the tissues for 5 to 15 minutes. The surgeon may also inject local anesthetic into the prostate and seminal vesicles transrectally with a 22-gauge, 22-cm injection needle through the needle guide on the transducer.

Operative Procedure
TRANSRECTAL, ULTRASONICALLY GUIDED BIOPSY. Transrectal, ultrasonically guided biopsy is commonly performed in the urologist's office using a high-frequency transrectal ultrasound transducer to assess the prostate gland. The technique allows the urologist to assess the size, volume, and shape of the prostate and the likelihood of the presence of a malignancy. Biopsy specimens of suspicious areas or lesions may be obtained with a needle passed across the rectal wall, with the aid of ultrasound guidance. The needle penetrates the rectal mucosa with a core biopsy system. Color-flow imaging may also be used to help identify areas that are likely invaded with prostatic carcinoma or have acute and chronic inflammation. Highly vascular areas carry a greater probability of harboring a carcinoma. A full bladder helps delineate the base of the prostate.

The urologist visualizes the prostate in three dimensions, allowing more accurate localization of abnormalities and extent of disease. For the axial view, the transrectal transducer is placed deeply into the rectum, just proximal to the seminal vesicles, to about 10 cm above the anal verge. Here the vas deferens may be distinguished. The transducer is slowly withdrawn to the level of the base of the gland, enabling visualization of the inner gland. Seminal vesicles are seen in cross section. To evaluate the prostate in the sagittal planes, the urologist rotates the probe clockwise or counterclockwise (Figure 6-40). A series of 12 biopsy specimens is generally taken with a disposable "core biopsy" needle. These are taken from the right and left medial and lateral apices, the right and left midline, and the right and left medial and lateral bases. Lesions as small as 2 to 3 mm are visible with this procedure.

TRANSPERINEAL BIOPSY. The perioperative nurse assists with placing the patient in the lithotomy or lateral position. The procedure may be performed with the patient receiving a general, regional, or local anesthetic. The surgeon performs a rectal exam to identify the induration. The needle is inserted through the perineal skin and guided ahead until the tip is against the lesion. The biopsy specimen is taken in the same fashion as described for the transrectal approach. Some surgeons may incise the site with the #11 or #15 scalpel and place a 4-0 absorbable closing suture.

The surgeon may also use the transperineal approach to perform template biopsies with ultrasound guidance, utilizing the brachytherapy (seed implant) template. The perioperative nurse assists with placing the patient in the lithotomy position, and secures his scrotum toward the abdomen with a transparent adhesive dressing. The surgeon positions the brachytherapy grid, template fixation device, and probe with cradle adjacent to the patient's perineum. Using the ultrasonic transrectal transducer the surgeon measures the prostate and calculates its total volume. Biopsies are then obtained transperineally through the template grid.

Transurethral Resection of the Prostate Gland

In transurethral resection of the prostate gland (TURP), the surgeon passes a resectoscope into the bladder through the urethra and resects successive pieces of tissue from around the bladder neck and the lobes of the prostate gland, leaving the capsule intact. The resectoscope has a stabilized cutting loop that is used to resect tissue and coagulate blood vessels by means of electric current. The electric current that powers the electrode is supplied by a high-frequency ESU. The current settings are specified by the surgeon, who activates the cutting or coagulating current with a foot pedal during the course of the procedure.

TURP is one surgical method of treating benign obstructive enlargement of the prostate gland. Several factors influence the surgical approach: size of the gland and location of the pathologic condition, age and condition of the patient, and presence of associated diseases.

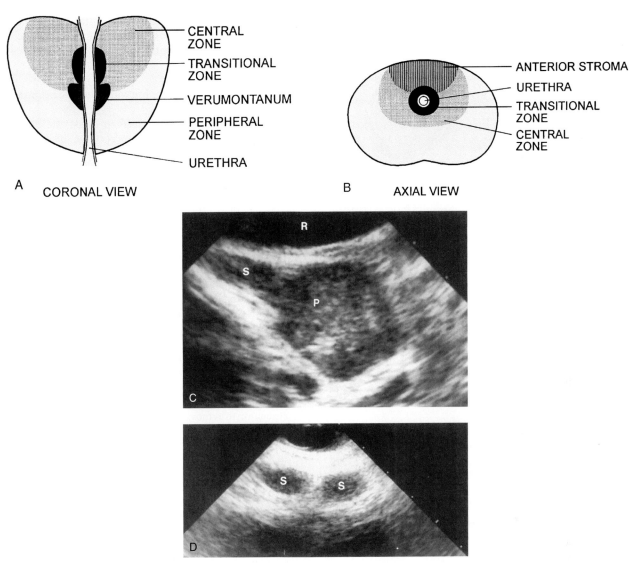

FIGURE 6-40 Schematic drawing of zonal anatomy of the prostate (*nonshaded area* is peripheral zone). **A,** Coronal view. **B,** Axial view and transrectal ultrasound views of prostate during biopsy. **C,** Sagittal image showing prostate *(P)*, seminal vesicles *(S)*, and rectum *(R)*. **D,** Transverse image of seminal vesicles *(S)*.

Procedural Considerations. The instrument setup for TURP is as described for cystoscopy with additional necessary instruments. The four principal types of resectoscopes are McCarthy, Nesbit, Iglesias, and Baumrucker. Adult resectoscopes range in size from 24F to 28F and have the following components: Foroblique telescope, operating element, cutting loops, and postresectoscope sheaths and obturators (Figure 6-41). A TURP requires a resectoscope (multiple working elements); a Foroblique telescope as well as a backup telescope; stabilized or unstabilized cutting loops; a postresectoscope sheath with its corresponding articulated obturator; a high-frequency cord; a short bridge; a Toomey syringe or the Ellik or Urovac evacuator; van Buren sounds; a 22F or 24F, 30-ml, three-way Foley catheter; a disposable urologic drape with rectal sheath; and a system for continuous bladder irrigation and urinary drainage. Supplementary instruments include a resectoscope adapter and a lateral telescope.

The continuous-flow resectoscope (CFR) (Figure 6-42) has unique components that include an outlet stopcock to which a suction tube is attached, an inflow tube on the inner sheath, and outflow holes on the outer sheath. These features enable the surgeon to resect tissue without interruption to empty the bladder, as must be done with the standard resectoscope. In addition to the CFR, which replaces the standard resectoscope, the setup includes thick-walled Silastic suction tubing and a continuous-flow pump. The continuous-flow technique decreases intravesical pressure on the bladder during the procedure, provides a clearer field of vision because of the constant inflow and outflow of irrigant, reduces the operating time because the resection process need not be interrupted to evacuate the bladder, and provides a "still" bladder for the resection of bladder tumors.

A continuous flow of isotonic and nonelectrolytic irrigating fluid is necessary to ensure transmission of electric current

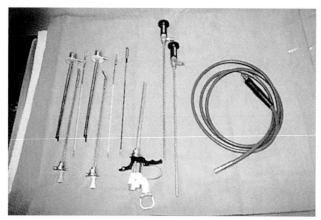

FIGURE 6-41 Resectoscope components: 24F and 26F Timberlake obturators and postresectoscope sheaths with fulgurating electrodes and Iglesias operating element, Foroblique 30-degree and 70-degree telescopes, and fiberoptic cable.

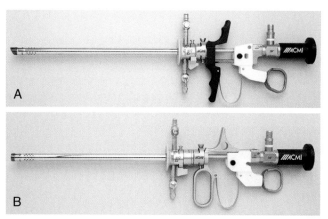

FIGURE 6-42 **A,** Continuous-flow resectoscope (CFR). **B,** Vista CFR bipolar resectoscope.

and clear visualization throughout surgery. Irrigating solution such as 3% sorbitol or 1.5% glycine, 3 to 5 liters, may be connected in tandem to provide a constant flow. Warming units, available for these solutions, help to eliminate the hypothermia often experienced when large amounts of cold irrigants are employed. On the other hand, when solutions are warm, the patient may show a tendency to bleed more. The surgical team must remain alert as to the status of the irrigation solution and replace it as required.

During transurethral prostatic surgery, the return of irrigation fluid must be monitored because intravasation and absorption of fluid into open prostatic venous sinuses or bladder perforation may occur. The perioperative nurse should be aware of the early signs and symptoms and measures employed to remedy these complications (Young et al, 2009). The patient usually experiences significant respiratory changes and abdominal discomfort. Continued extravasation and absorption can lead to hypovolemia and hyponatremia. Other important observations are rigidity and swelling of the lower abdomen, coupled with changes in sensorium. If extravasation of irrigating fluid is evident, the surgical procedure is discontinued and a cystogram is obtained immediately to determine if bladder perforation has occurred. Insertion of a Foley catheter is gen-

erally all that is necessary to control the situation. In the rare instance of a major perforation, surgical closure may be accomplished through a cystotomy incision.

Operative Procedure

1. The surgeon dilates the urethra with sounds sized from 20F to 30F.
2. Cystourethroscopy is performed to assess the degree of prostatic obstruction and to inspect the bladder. Some surgeons perform this diagnostic procedure several days before surgery, whereas others perform the examination in the OR immediately before surgery.
3. The surgeon passes a well-lubricated postresectoscope sheath with its fitted Timberlake obturator into the urethra.
4. The Timberlake obturator is removed, and the working element (resectoscope), assembled with the Foroblique telescope and cutting loop, is inserted through the sheath.
5. The irrigation tubing, light cord, and high-frequency cord are appropriately connected, and the surgeon opens the stopcock to allow the irrigation fluid to fill the bladder.
6. With the bladder distended, the surgeon inspects the prostatic urethra and bladder trigone.
7. After determining the location of the ureteral orifice, the surgeon begins electrodissection, alternating cutting and coagulating currents as required (Figure 6-43).
8. The bladder is drained, washing out prostatic tissue and small blood clots. At times the surgeon may use the Ellik evacuator to remove resected prostatic tissue. The Ellik is used by removing the working element of the resectoscope, fitting the nozzle of the evacuator onto the resectoscope sheath, and removing the bladder contents by manual pulsatile pressure. The surgical technologist ensures an Ellik or Urovac evacuator or a Toomey syringe is readily available for manual irrigation. Fluid may be drawn from the irrigant directly into the resectoscope sheath through the already attached tubing.
9. When the resection is completed, the surgeon inspects the prostatic fossa to ensure that all bleeding points have been coagulated.
10. The resectoscope is then removed, and a Foley catheter (22F or 24F, two-way or three-way, 30-ml balloon) is inserted into the bladder for urinary drainage. The balloon is inflated (Figure 6-44, *A*), pulled gently in traction against the bladder neck, and secured, to help control venous bleeding (Figure 6-44, *B*). The Foley balloon must not be inflated within the prostatic fossa (Figure 6-44, *C*), where it may cause excessive bleeding from the resected prostatic capsule. If desired, continuous irrigation with gravity drainage is initiated, with normal saline as the bladder irrigant instead of sorbitol or glycine. A 3-liter to 4-liter urinary drainage system is suggested to avoid frequent emptying of the drainage bag.
11. When VLAP, TUIP, or TULIP is performed, the surgeon may choose to place a standard 18F Foley with a 5-ml or 30-ml balloon connected to straight drainage. If irrigation is required postoperatively, it is then performed manually with sterile solution and a Toomey syringe.

Transurethral Incision of the Prostate (TUIP)

TUIP is a procedure in which the prostate is incised at the 5 and 7 o'clock positions to provide relief of obstruction, with results

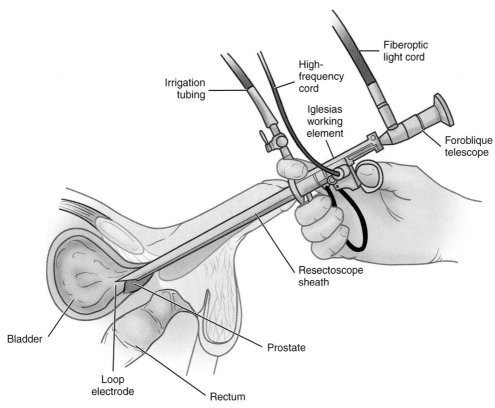

Fiberoptic
light cord

High-
frequency
cord

Irrigation
tubing

Iglesias
working
element

Foroblique
telescope

Resectoscope
sheath

Bladder

Prostate

Loop
electrode

Rectum

FIGURE 6-43 Sectional view illustrating removal of portion of hypertrophied middle lobe of prostate
gland with Iglesias resectoscope.

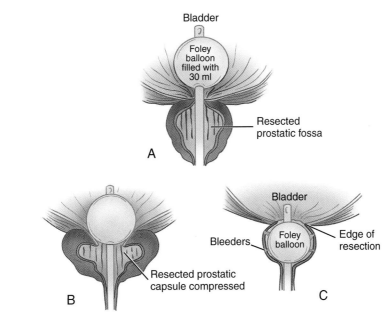

Bladder

Foley
balloon
filled with
30 ml

Resected
prostatic fossa

A

Resected prostatic
capsule compressed

B

Bladder

Bleeders

Foley
balloon

Edge of
resection

C

FIGURE 6-44 A and **B,** Proper position for Foley catheter with inflated balloon beyond prostatic
capsule. **C,** Improper position.

similar to those provided by a complete transurethral resection
but with a lower incidence of bladder neck contracture and retrograde ejaculation. The shorter operative time inherent with
the procedure minimizes fluid absorption and may decrease
postoperative pulmonary and cardiovascular complications.
The procedure may be performed with cold or hot knives

as well as the standard resectoscope, or laser fiber (TULIP).
This procedure is appropriate for sexually active patients with
moderate to small obstructive prostates without a significant
middle-lobe component. One major disadvantage is the potential for missing occult prostatic cancer. Despite this, some clinicians view this as an underused, feasible form of treatment.

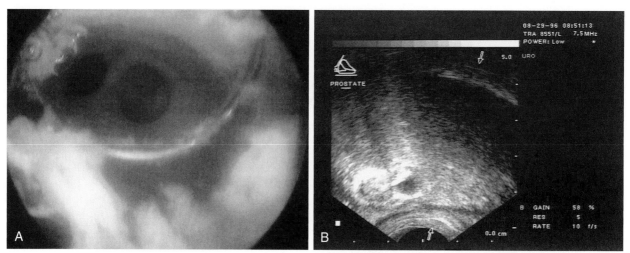

FIGURE 6-45 A, Dilated seminal vesicle (ejaculatory duct) with resectoscope loop approaching. B, Resectoscope loop entering dilated seminal vesicle (ejaculatory duct).

Transurethral Incision of the Ejaculatory Ducts

Transurethral incision of the ejaculatory ducts is performed for the relief of obstructed ejaculatory ducts, a common condition in men with chronic prostatitis and prostatic calculi. Symptoms closely mimic prostatodynia and include aching in the perineal and genital areas with no lasting or significant improvement from conservative therapy (antibiotics and analgesics). The resectoscope loop is guided with transrectal ultrasound imaging to the dilated ejaculatory ducts, and the obstructed ducts are resected (Figure 6-45). Calculi may be fragmented if necessary and removed. A catheter generally is not needed.

Photoselective Vaporization of the Prostate

The KTP laser is now being used to treat BPH or prostatic enlargement. *Green-light PVP* is photoselective vaporization of the prostate and a new minimally invasive approach performed on an outpatient basis. The approach is the same as with other endoscopic techniques. A noncontact laser fiber is used to heat the prostate tissue and rapidly vaporize it to a penetration depth of 0.8 mm with minimal to no blood loss. Vaporization occurs from within the tissues where the collagen matrix eventually bursts as a result of the vapor buildup. The laser is operated in a continuous wave mode and induces a coagulation zone of only 1 to 2 mm in thickness. This prevents the excessive sloughing of necrotic tissue. The patient may not always need a Foley catheter following the procedure.

Interstitial Laser Coagulation of the Prostate

Interstitial laser coagulation (ILC) with the Indigo laser is a minimally invasive procedure for treatment of urinary outflow obstruction secondary to BPH. It is indicated for men older than 50 years with a median or lateral prostatic lobe volume of 20 to 85 ml. Designed for those men who wish to minimize the risk for incontinence and impotence found with conventional TURP, this procedure is now performed in the office setting about 80% of the time.

The procedure is contraindicated for the treatment of prostate cancer and for those patients who had previous brachy-therapy with radioactive seeds. However, some physicians may elect to perform ILC before brachytherapy (or cryotherapy) in the hopes of minimizing, if not relieving, the postoperative voiding symptoms associated with these more definitive treatments.

Procedural Considerations. The patient is placed in the lithotomy position and prepped as for cystoscopy. An optional local anesthetic with oral or monitored IV sedation is generally adequate. Oral sedation is used more commonly with the office-based procedure; if the surgery takes place in the hospital or ambulatory center, monitored IV sedation may be used. An ultrasound machine with transrectal capability is often used to measure the size of the prostate gland and determine the appropriate number of laser applications (sticks). Some surgeons choose to measure by cystoscopy alone.

The setup includes a 17F or 23F panendoscope and 30-degree fiberoptic lens, ultrasound and transrectal transducer, and the Indigo laser machine with laser fiber (Figure 6-46). The fiber has graduated black depth markings used to guide placement into the prostate gland. The laser machine automatically times each "stick" for 2 minutes, 30 seconds. The surgical team ensures that all laser safety precautions are observed.

Operative Procedure
1. The surgeon inserts the transrectal transducer and measures the prostatic volume. (This may have been performed as an office procedure preoperatively.) Local anesthetic may be injected through the transducer guide pin with an 8-inch spinal needle or with the 8-inch collagen injection needle if ultrasound is not employed.
2. Cystoscopy is performed, and the prostatic urethra is evaluated.
3. The surgeon introduces the laser fiber through the panendoscope and passes it into the lateral lobe of the prostate gland through the urethral wall to the desired depth.
4. This is repeated one to three times on each side, depending on the measured prostatic volume.
5. A TUIP may be performed utilizing the bare-tip fiber (Figure 6-47).

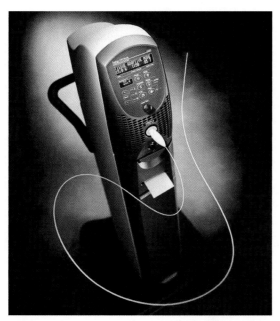

FIGURE 6-46 Indigo Optima Laser unit with diffuser-tip fiber.

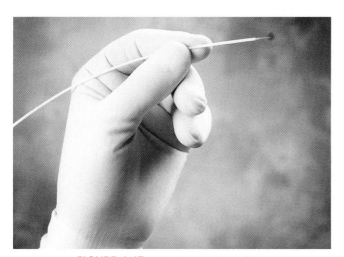

FIGURE 6-47 Indigo bare-tip laser fiber.

6. A 16F or 18F urethral catheter is inserted and connected to straight drainage. A 16F suprapubic Foley catheter may also be employed and attached to irrigation or drainage.

Transurethral Microwave Therapy (TUMT)/Transurethral Needle Ablation (TUNA)

TUMT is a minimally invasive method of applying heat to the prostate gland for the relief of the symptoms associated with BPH and bladder-outlet obstruction. TUMT maintains temperatures in the urethra, sphincter, and rectum at a level that is physiologically safe while heating the tissue deep within the transitional zone of the prostate. A water-cooled catheter is combined with microwave radiation to the lobes of the prostate. This treatment is an office-based procedure.

Transurethral needle ablation (TUNA) is also a minimally invasive office procedure for the treatment of BPH of the median and lateral lobes. This technique delivers radiofre-

quency (RF) energy through two electrodes that are embedded in a special urethral catheter. Specific target areas of the prostate are thermally ablated by the RF energy and combined inductive heating of water molecules, leaving the urethra and the remainder of the prostate intact.

Simple Retropubic Prostatectomy

Simple retropubic prostatectomy is the enucleation of hypertrophic prostatic tissue through an incision in the anterior prostatic capsule by an extravesical approach. The retropubic approach offers excellent exposure of the prostate bed and vesical neck and readily controllable intraoperative and postoperative bleeding.

A preoperative bowel prep and antibiotic therapy are the standard of care for all open prostatectomies.

Procedural Considerations. The perioperative nurse assists with positioning the patient in a slight Trendelenburg position with the pelvis elevated and the legs slightly abducted. Although the draping procedure must conform to individual OR policies, the following procedure is suggested for draping the patient:

1. The first towel, with a cuff, is placed under the scrotum.
2. The next three towels are placed around the lower abdominal incision site, followed by a sterile laparotomy sheet.
3. A fifth towel, folded in half, is placed over the penis and scrotum below the retropubic incision site and secured with two nonperforating towel clamps.

The instrument setup includes a basic laparotomy set and bladder and prostatic instruments (Figures 6-48 and 6-49). The following supplies should be readily available: Jackson-Pratt drains; water-soluble lubricant; Toomey and Asepto syringes; urinary drainage system; 20F, 5-ml Foley catheter; 22F or 24F, 30-ml Foley catheter; 10-ml and 30-ml syringes; and a self-retaining retractor such as the adjustable Omni-Tract Surgical UO400 Urology Retractor System (Figure 6-50).

Operative Procedure

1. The surgeon inserts a 20F or 22F Foley catheter with 30-ml balloon into the urethra and through the bladder neck and inflates it. This is clamped and maintained within the sterile field. Frequently, a three-way catheter is used for continuous bladder irrigation.
2. Through a Pfannenstiel or low vertical midline incision, the surgeon incises the anterior rectus sheath along with portions of the internal and external oblique muscles.
3. The rectus abdominis muscles are retracted laterally to expose the space of Retzius.
4. After placement of traction sutures, the anterior portion of the prostatic capsule is incised transversely (Figure 6-51, *A*).
5. The prostatic adenoma may be dissected or finger-enucleated from the surgical capsule (Figure 6-51, *B*).
6. The surgeon places hemostatic sutures at the 5 and 7 o'clock positions, encompassing the vesical neck and prostatic capsule, to ligate the primary blood supply to the prostate. Other bleeding points within the capsule may be suture-ligated with 2-0 absorbable sutures.
7. The prostatic capsule incision is closed with either a continuous or an interrupted 0 absorbable suture (Figure 6-51, *C*).
8. A drain is placed in the space of Retzius and exteriorized through the fascia and skin via a separate stab incision.

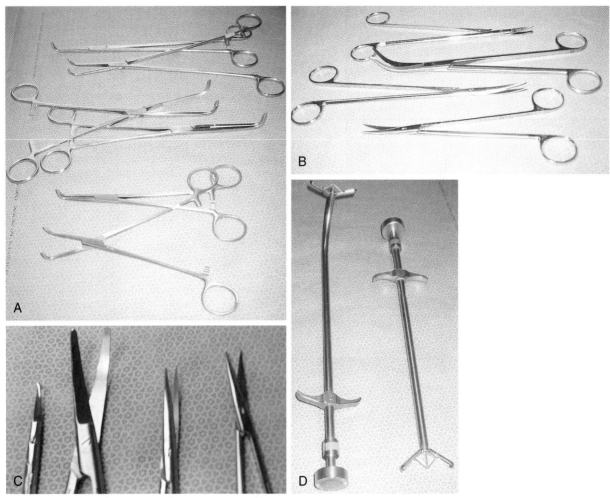

FIGURE 6-48 **A**, Right-angle (Mixter) clamps in various tip lengths. **B**, Scissors (*top to bottom*): Strully, curved Jorgenson, long sharp-tip Metzenbaum, standard sharp-tip Metzenbaum. **C**, Same scissor tips, *left to right*. **D**, Curved and straight Lowsley tractors in open position.

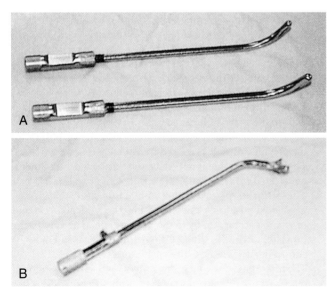

FIGURE 6-49 **A**, Urethral suture guides. **B**, Roth grip-tip urethral suture guide.

9. The abdominal incision is then closed in layers, and the wound is dressed.
10. If continuous bladder irrigation is to be used, normal saline solution irrigation is initiated through a 3-liter closed irrigation system.

Suprapubic Prostatectomy

Suprapubic prostatectomy is the removal, through a transvesical approach, of benign periurethral glandular tissue obstructing the outlet of the urinary tract. A low midline, or Pfannenstiel, incision may be used. One advantage of the suprapubic approach is that it allows access for surgical correction of any existing bladder condition such as vesical calculi or vesical diverticula. Control of bleeding is a major consideration in any prostatectomy and is one disadvantage of the suprapubic approach. Because the prostate is located beneath the symphysis pubis, ligation of bleeding capsular vessels is difficult. However, control of hemorrhage and replacement of blood loss, coupled with skilled perioperative nursing care and early mobilization of the patient, have greatly minimized complications.

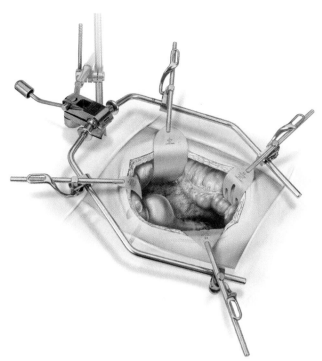

FIGURE 6-50 Adjustable Omni-Tract Surgical UO400 Urology Retractor System.

Procedural Considerations. Spinal, epidural, or general anesthesia may be selected for patients having a suprapubic prostatectomy, depending on their medical condition. The patient is placed in a slight Trendelenburg's position with the umbilicus elevated and the legs slightly abducted. Draping and instrumentation are as described for retropubic prostatectomy.

Operative Procedure

1. The surgeon inserts a 20F or 22F Foley catheter with 30-ml balloon into the urethra and through the bladder neck and inflates it. This is clamped and maintained within the sterile field. This maneuver facilitates identification of the bladder.
2. A transverse or midline lower abdominal incision is made through the skin and the two layers of superficial fascia (Figure 6-52, *A*).
3. The external and internal oblique muscles are cut along the lines of the original incision.
4. Bleeding vessels are clamped, electrocoagulated, or ligated with fine absorbable ties.
5. The rectus muscles are separated in the midline and retracted laterally.
6. After the placement of traction sutures, the surgeon opens the bladder at the dome with a scalpel. Liquid contents are aspirated, and the bladder incision is enlarged.
7. The bladder is visually and manually explored for calculi, a tumor, or diverticula.
8. The surgeon manually enucleates the adenomatous tissue using the tip of the index finger inserted through the vesical neck into the prostatic urethra (Figure 6-52, *B*). If difficulty is experienced with the enucleation, the surgical assistant may place a finger into the rectum to elevate the prostate gland. Aseptic technique is maintained during enucleation with the use of a sterile second glove on the hand used in the rectum.

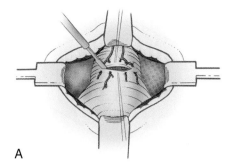

A

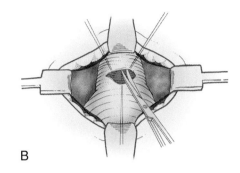

B

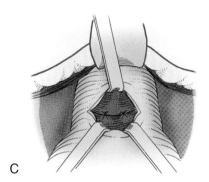

C

FIGURE 6-51 Retropubic prostatectomy.

9. After enucleation is completed, attention is directed to maintaining good hemostasis by suture ligation of the vesical neck at the 5 and 7 o'clock positions. Other significant bleeding points may also be ligated.
10. A suprapubic catheter is placed into the bladder lumen through a small stab incision.
11. A 22F or 24F, two-way or three-way Foley catheter with a 30-ml balloon is inserted into the urethra in place of the original one, and the balloon is inflated to a size that prevents the catheter from falling or being pulled into the prostatic fossa (Figure 6-52, *C*).
12. The surgeon closes the cystotomy incision with interrupted 2-0 absorbable sutures.
13. A drain is left along the cystotomy incision, exteriorized through a separate stab wound, and secured to the skin with a silk suture.
14. The muscles, fascia, and subcutaneous tissues are closed in layers, and a dressing is applied.
15. To reduce clot formation and maintain catheter patency, normal saline irrigation solution may be connected to the Foley catheter to provide continuous irrigation to the bladder. Continuous irrigation may be initiated during closure.

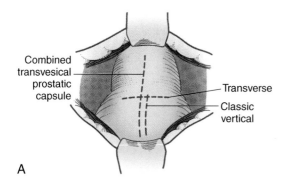

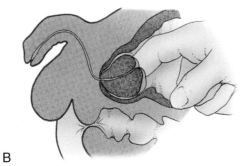

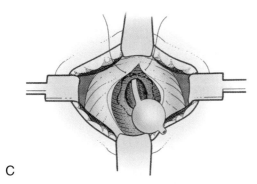

FIGURE 6-52 Suprapubic prostatectomy.

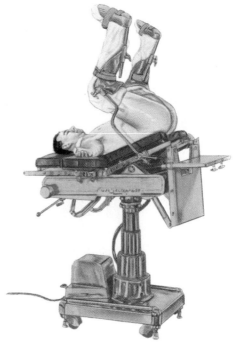

FIGURE 6-53 Exaggerated lithotomy position for perineal prostatectomy.

Simple Perineal Prostatectomy

Simple perineal prostatectomy is the removal of a prostatic adenoma through a perineal approach. A perineal approach to the prostate gland is most suitable when open prostatic biopsy is desired and, after receipt of pathologic confirmation, radical excision is to follow. Other advantages include preservation of the bladder neck, improved urethrovesical anastomosis, and easier control of bleeding. Some surgical disadvantages are (1) inability to perform biopsy of the iliac and obturator nodes for determining extension of disease and (2) possible formation of urethrorectal fistulas.

Procedural Considerations. The patient is placed in an exaggerated lithotomy position with the legs above the level of the pelvis (Figure 6-53). The perioperative nurse places a bolster beneath the sacrum to allow the perineum to be as parallel to the OR bed as possible, with the buttocks extending several inches over the bed edge. Stirrups should be well padded to protect the popliteal fossa. Sequential compression stockings are recommended to assist peripheral vascular flow.

The patient is often placed in a steep Trendelenburg's position. Well-padded shoulder braces, placed over the acromial processes in a manner to prevent stretch or pressure injury, may be required to prevent the patient from sliding upward on the bed. Routine skin preparation is carried out and includes an interior rectal prep. Special draping is as follows:

1. A towel folded in half is placed over the pubic area.
2. Two towels with a cuff are placed on either side of the perineum.
3. Two leggings, with points down, are placed over the legs.
4. One impervious drape is placed over the anus.
5. A large sheet fully opened with a large cuff is placed across from one stirrup to the other and secured by towel clamps.
6. A laparotomy sheet follows, with the short end to the floor.

The instrument setup is as described for suprapubic prostatectomy, omitting abdominal self-retaining retractors and adding straight and curved Lowsley tractors (Figure 6-54), Roux retractors, Jackson retractors with short and long blades, Doyen vaginal retractors, Young retractor, perineal prostatic retractors (Figure 6-55), Sauerbruch retractors, and a narrow and wide self-retaining perineal retractor, such as the Thompson retractor or the Omni-Tract Surgical UO100 Pelvic Retractor System (Figure 6-56).

Operative Procedure

1. A curved Lowsley tractor is placed through the urethra into the bladder and held back by the surgical assistant, causing the prostate to be pushed down toward the perineum.
2. An inverted U-shaped incision is made from one ischial tuberosity to another, curving just anteriorly to the anus (Figure 6-57, *A*).
3. Three Martius or Allis clamps are secured to the posterior edge of the incision and retracted downward, over the anal drape.

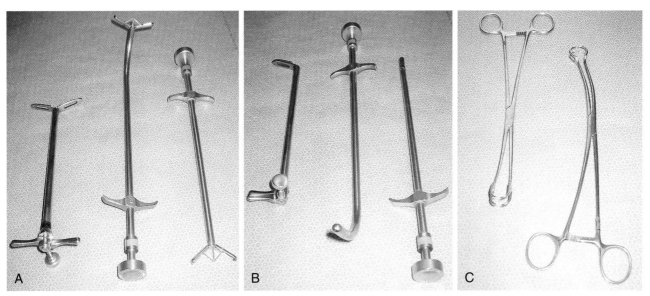

FIGURE 6-54 Young, curved Lowsley, and straight Lowsley tractors in open (A) and closed (B) positions. C, Curved double-prong prostate clamps.

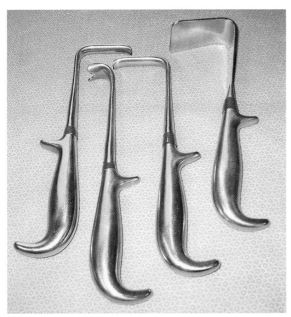

FIGURE 6-55 Lateral, bulb, and anterior perineal prostatectomy retractors.

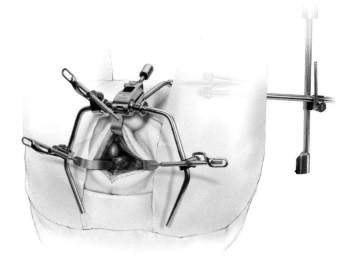

FIGURE 6-56 Adjustable Omni-Tract Surgical UO100 Pelvic Retractor System.

4. The surgeon clamps any subcutaneous bleeders with straight mosquito hemostats and electrocoagulates or ties them with 3-0 absorbable ligatures.
5. The central tendon is isolated, clamped, and cut distally to the external anal sphincter (Figure 6-57, *B*).
6. The rectourethral muscle is incised and pushed downward from the central tendon.
7. The levator ani muscle is exposed and retracted laterally (Figure 6-57, *C*).
8. The prostate gland is exposed. The surgeon may send biopsies of the prostate for pathologic confirmation. If the results are negative, the prostatic adenoma is removed. If the frozen section reveals malignancy, a radical prostatectomy may be done at this time.

9. If simple enucleation is to be performed, the prostatic capsule is incised and the Lowsley tractor is removed (Figure 6-57, *D*).
10. The urethra is divided, and the Young prostatic retractor is inserted.
11. The blades are opened, drawing the prostate down, and the adenoma is manually enucleated from the surgical capsule.
12. A 22F Foley catheter with a 30-ml balloon is inserted through the urethra into the bladder.
13. Bleeding is controlled at the 5 and 7 o'clock positions.
14. The capsulotomy incision is repaired with a continuous 2-0 absorbable suture (Figure 6-57, *E*).
15. A drain is left in place at the level of the capsulotomy incision.
16. The surgeon reapproximates the subcutaneous tissue with 3-0 absorbable suture.
17. The skin incision is reapproximated with 4-0 absorbable subcutaneous sutures.

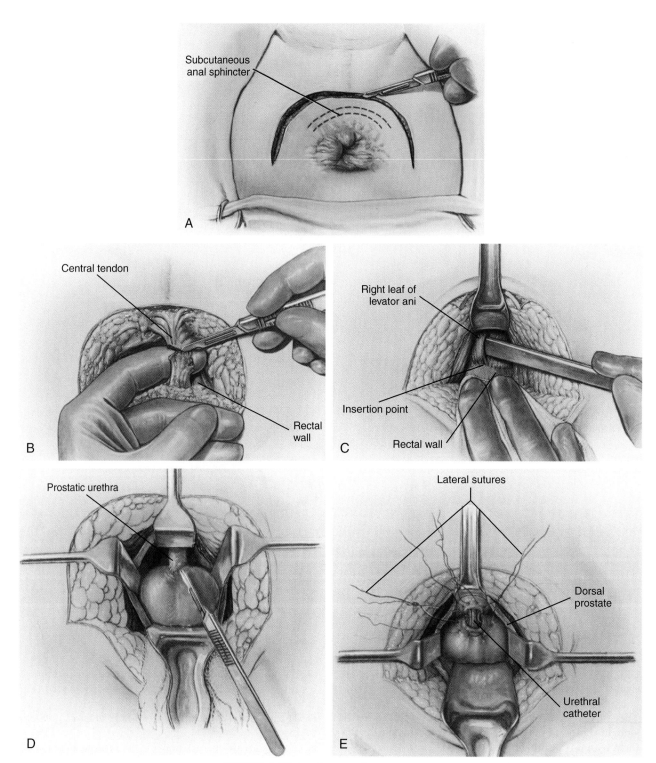

FIGURE 6-57 Simple perineal prostatectomy.

18. The wound is dressed according to the surgeon's preference and taped or held with a supportive device, such as mesh pants.

Transrectal Seed Implantation (Interstitial Radiotherapy with Brachytherapy)

Brachytherapy of the prostate gland is a procedure that requires a collaborative, multidisciplinary approach to patient care. The radiation oncologist and medical physicist, in addition to the surgeon, are vital to an optimum outcome from the initial planning stage throughout the postoperative surveillance. Preplanning is required to determine the size of the prostate, dose of each seed, the spacing necessary between each seed, and the number of seeds required. A template plan is developed preoperatively by using the ultrasound and the probe-anchoring equipment to measure and map the appropriate seed sites within the prostate. This may be accomplished in the surgeon's office, radiology department, or oncology clinic. The implant plan is finalized at the time of surgery.

The facility that offers this treatment must be licensed for "Group 6" with the radioactive materials licensing department of their respective state. If seed implantation is indicated as an adjunct to radiation therapy, it should be performed 3 to 4 weeks after the radiation treatment.

During percutaneous implantation of iodine-125 or palladium-103 seeds, the patient is positioned in the lithotomy position. The surgeon visualizes the prostate with transrectal ultrasonic imaging, and locates the midportion of the prostate on a transverse image. This location becomes an index for positioning the axial ultrasound plane at the base of the prostate. Approximately 2 to 3 hours should be allowed from start to completion. The procedure is amenable to outpatient management using a regional or general anesthetic.

Iodine seeds are commercially available in titanium-encased rods called magazines that absorb the electrons. The magazines can be sterilized in the OR at the beginning of the procedure. These seeds may also be obtained embedded in an absorbable suture that allows them to remain positioned appropriately in relation to themselves and their location within the prostate and minimizes the risk of seed migration. Palladium seeds, not presently available prethreaded, are plated onto a graphite pellet. The pellets are loaded into titanium tubes with a lead marker. The half-life of iodine-125 (60 days) is longer than that of palladium-103 (17 days) and allows the therapy to be delivered over the duration of tumor cell replication, altering the ability of the tumor cells to multiply. Compared to iodine-125, palladium-103 affords a larger dose of radiation in a shorter time interval to more rapidly growing tumors.

Procedural Considerations. Percutaneous implantation of radioactive seeds allows the delivery of significantly higher doses of radiotherapy to the prostate than provided by external beam therapy. The radius of penetration around each seed is only 5 mm, thus sparing adjacent organs. The typical radiation dose that can be delivered by external beam may be 6500 centigrays (cGy), whereas the dose that can be delivered with implantation of seeds alone is in the range of 12,000 to 16,000 cGy. Some patients may receive hormone therapy, to shrink the prostate gland, for 3 months before implantation, and some will undergo radiation therapy before implantation. Patients with stage A or stage B prostate cancer are appropriate candidates, and selection is not influenced by a rise in the PSA level, biopsy specimens indicative of further involvement, or age. Ideal patients for brachytherapy treatment as monotherapy are those with low-risk parameters (PSA ≤10, Gleason score 6 or less, low-volume disease on biopsy).

Possible complications include the risk of intraoperative seed displacement into the bladder; implantation too close to the urethra, resulting in postoperative urethral stricture or prolonged dysuria; and implantation into the perineum if the needles are withdrawn too quickly. There is also the chance of migration of seeds, placed just outside the periphery of the gland and in the periprostatic plexus, to the lung. The nurse instructs the patient to avoid extended contact with children and pregnant females and to keep a 6-foot distance from this population group for 6 to 8 weeks. The patient must strain his urine, and any seeds expelled should be retrieved and returned to the oncologist. Body wastes are not considered hazardous, however.

Bleeding from the percutaneous sites is minimal, but postoperative ecchymosis of the perineum is to be expected. Other postoperative complications that may occur in the first 12 months include acute cystitis, prostatitis, and urinary retention. Late complications may include chronic prostatitis with cystitis, urethral stricture with contracture, stress with urge or total incontinence, proctitis, and impotence. Some patients have required posttreatment TURP, bladder-neck incision, suprapubic catheter insertion, or urethral dilation to alleviate the aforementioned conditions. Much less commonly, rectovesical or rectoprostatic fistula can occur, requiring interventions such as laparotomy, colostomy, and urinary diversion. Patients are generally able to void 24 to 48 hours after implantation. The patient is positioned in the lithotomy position with assistance. The scrotum must be secured cephalad to allow a clear operating field. The surgeon places a traction stitch through the lateral edges of the scrotum and anchors it to the groin region.

With an experienced team, seeding is done with real-time ultrasound imaging. Throughout the procedure, random room checks with the Geiger counter will be performed to determine radiation levels. All personnel, surgical equipment, and trash (including disposable drapes) are scanned before leaving the room at the end of the procedure.

Operative Procedure

Before seeding is begun, the surgeon positions the ultrasound transducer so that the posterior margin of the prostate is parallel to the axis of the ultrasound transducer. The direction of seed insertion and the transverse images of the prostate must have a similar appearance to those on the preoperative volume study. The volume study and implant worksheet are used for continual verification of coordinates. The surgeon attaches a stabilizer bar to the OR bed. This secures the "stepping unit," which allows a 5-mm incremental forward-and-backward motion of the probe. The sled that holds the transducer is attached to the stepping unit. The probe must be securely anchored so that the position of the prostate relative to the needles used to implant the seeds remains unaltered throughout the procedure. For the needles to be positioned appropriately, the template with labeled grid is attached to the transrectal transducer so that the needles placed through the probe grid match the grid locations on the plan. The grid is labeled alphabetically *Aa, Bb, Cc,* and so on, with the center of the prostate corresponding to D on the grid. The plan is designed to avoid the urethra, bladder neck, and rectum to prevent urethrorectal fistula formation, irradiation of the bladder, and scarring at the bladder neck level.

1. At the beginning of the procedure the surgeon inserts a urethral catheter, drains the bladder, and then refills it with 150 ml of sterile water. The bladder then provides an "acoustic void" to better visualize the prostate. If fluoroscopy is used, contrast medium can be instilled into the bladder to delineate the position of the bladder neck.

2. The surgeon removes the urethral catheter during implantation of seeds to avoid placement of seeds close to the urethra. The catheter causes the tissue surrounding the urethra to be compressed, and if attempts are made to implant seeds into this compressed tissue, penetration of the catheter and urethra may occur. The catheter also causes an acoustic shadow that prevents visualization of the anterior prostate gland.

3. The surgical technologist covers the ultrasound probe with a sterile probe cover filled with 15 ml of sterile water to remove the artifact. Alternatively, a gel-filled probe cover can be placed on the end of the ultrasound probe. Filling with too much fluid will change the configuration of the prostate and alter the anatomic presentation. The transducer will be aimed with the tip upward at a 10- to 20-degree angle (Figure 6-58). The posterior wall of the prostate must be far enough away from the probe so that the posterior row of seeds is placed just inside the posterior capsule. Seeds are implanted by means of loaded needles placed into the prostate according to the template plan, with the midline seeds placed slightly off center to avoid the urethra. Alternatively, individual seeds can be placed through the hollow needles using a mick applicator that utilizes a long plunger.

4. Stabilization of the prostate may be achieved with stabilization needles placed laterally to the center into the right and left lobes and then removed once the anterior seeds are in place. Another method is to use a Foley catheter as a retractor for implantation of the periphery and until implantation near the urethra occurs. The best method may be to overcompensate for the rotation of the prostate by angling or turning the needle slightly opposite to the direction desired.

5. The most anterior seeds are placed first so that imaging of the anterior portion of the gland is not obscured by the ultrasonic shadows created by seeds placed posteriorly. If strands are used, Anusol-HC (hydrocortisone) is used to seal the bevel before implantation. Strands should be cut cleanly with electrosurgery to seal the ends and avoid frayed ends, which may be split further when the stylet is inserted into the needle, adversely affecting seed placement.

6. Contrary to normal needle insertion with the bevel up, these needles are placed into the prostate with the solid, or back, side up. Every effort is extended to avoid implanting seeds into the bladder or too close to the urethra, which causes significant postoperative irritative symptoms.

7. When placing the anterior needles, passage of the needle may be prevented by the inferior arch of the pubic bone. The needle tip is visualized as a bright echo, and the angle may be altered to compensate for the bone. Alternatively, the placement of the anterior seeds may be postponed until the end when the template may be dropped down, the probe positioned parallel to the pubic arch, and the needles inserted past the anterior portion into the prostate. Rarely, the template may need to be removed from the ultrasound probe at the conclusion of the procedure to allow "freehand" placement of anterior needles.

8. The needle is inserted beyond the desired site and then retracted. The first seed will then determine where the balance will lie because the seeds will fall into a plane that follows the first seed in a specific needle. The target volume is greater than the actual volume of the prostate so the capsular edge of the prostate and just beyond are also subjected to seed penetration (Figure 6-59). These peripherally placed seeds have a higher energy and may also have a greater tendency for migration if the tissue is not dense enough to hold the seed in place.

9. The distribution of seeds is generally 80% peripheral and 20% central.

10. The surgeon performs a cystoscopy at the end of the treatment so that seeds protruding into the urethra or left in the bladder may be removed.

11. A Foley catheter is placed and left for 24 to 48 hours.

Transrectal Cryosurgical Ablation of the Prostate Gland

Cryoablation of the prostate is a feasible, minimally invasive option for patients with localized or locally advanced prostate cancer. This method of treating the prostate gland can be used either as primary therapy or as a salvage procedure for local recurrence of prostate adenocarcinoma after previous external radiation therapy, brachytherapy, or even previous cryoablation. Cryoablation causes cell death through crystallization within the intercellular and extracellular spaces that exert mechanical shear forces on the cell membranes, osmotic changes, and cellular hypoxia. Complications related to the procedure include urinary incontinence, urethral slough, rectourethral fistula, UTI, and post-cryoablation erectile dysfunction (Langenhuijsen et al, 2009).

Procedural Considerations. The perioperative nurse assists with positioning the patient in a dorsal lithotomy position with the legs raised high enough to allow placement of a stabilizer bar that is affixed directly to the operating table. The ultrasound probe can then be placed on a sled with the use of brachytherapy. Because of the positioning required for the pro-

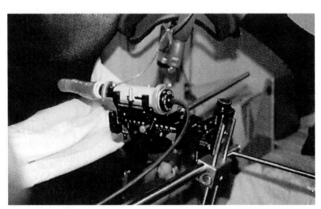

FIGURE 6-58 Transducer on stepping unit and slide, angled upward to "get under" the pubic bone.

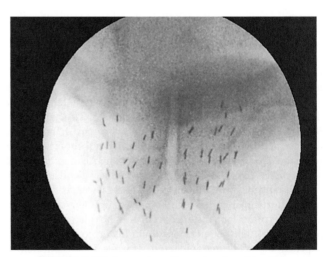

FIGURE 6-59 C-arm view of completed seed implant.

cedure and the length of the procedure (e.g., average 2 hours), the patient is at increased risk for developing deep vein thrombosis (DVT). The surgical team initiates DVT precautions (e.g., elastic stockings, sequential compression device sleeves) as part of the plan of care. Patients treated with cryosurgery are generally admitted to the hospital after the procedure and discharged the following morning, unless bleeding, fever, or anesthetic complications prevent their discharge.

Operative Procedure

1. The surgeon performs a cystoscopy to assess the external sphincter, prostatic urethra, bladder neck, and location of the ureteric orifices on the bladder trigone.
2. At the conclusion of the cystoscopy the surgeon fills the bladder with sterile irrigant to facilitate percutaneous insertion of a suprapubic cystotomy tube.
3. A guidewire is then introduced into the bladder upon removal of the cystoscope, to facilitate later passage of the urethral warming device.
4. The surgeon tacks the scrotum away from the perineum with suture.
5. The transrectal ultrasound probe is then affixed to the table and inserted for visualization of the prostate gland. Volume and length measurements of the prostate are made at this time.
6. The perioperative nurse attaches the needles to the cryosurgery machine to allow circulation of the argon and helium gases through the device tubing. Before insertion of the needles into the perineum, the perioperative nurse and surgical technologist test the needles in the saline to ensure production of an ice ball.
7. Once all needles are in place, the surgeon advances the urethral warming device over the guidewire previously placed in the urethra. This warming catheter remains for the duration of the procedure, and is often left in place for up to 1 hour following the cryoablation treatment. The use of the urethral warming catheter is crucial to the safety of this procedure, and cryoablation of the prostate should not be done without its use.
8. Using ultrasound guidance in the transverse and longitudinal planes, the surgeon inserts the cryosurgery treatment needles and thermocouple needles for temperature monitoring. The needles are positioned according to a template that allows for uniform freezing of the prostate gland. Alternatively, needle placement can be tailored by the surgeon to allow for focal cryoablation as clinically indicated. The needle probes are placed at least 1 cm from the location of the urethra, to minimize risk of damage to this structure and to the urinary sphincter.
9. Freezing is initiated in the anterior portion of the prostate (upper needles), and progress of the ice ball is monitored with ultrasound as the ice front progresses to the posterior aspect and apex of the prostate gland.
10. After all tissue has been frozen using a double-freeze technique, the surgeon removes the cryoprobes. Active warming of the prostate can be achieved with circulation of helium through the hollow needles, and this also facilitates removal of the needles at the conclusion of the procedure.
11. If the urethral warming catheter is to remain in place, the patient is transferred to the recovery room with the urethral warmer and circulating machine, which can be transported on an IV pole. One hour following the procedure, the warming catheter is removed and replaced with a Foley catheter, which is usually removed the morning after surgery.
12. The suprapubic catheter allows for urinary drainage for the first 1 to 2 weeks. The tube can then be clamped for a voiding trial after prostate swelling has subsided enough to allow micturition to occur.

Nerve-Sparing Radical Retropubic Prostatectomy with Pelvic Lymphadenectomy

Radical prostatectomy is the treatment preferred for patients with organ-confined carcinoma of the prostate. This procedure involves removal of the entire gland, its capsule, and the seminal vesicles. Important anatomic structures that impact erectile function are within the surgical field. Whenever possible, the surgeon attempts to spare the posterolateral neurovascular bundles, supplying the corpora cavernosa, to preserve potency. Those with tumors confined in the prostatic capsule are the best candidates for nerve-sparing procedures. In the presence of more advanced tumor extension, the surgeon attempts to spare one of the bundles, allowing the chance for potency.

Procedural Considerations. Patient preparation and basic surgical instrumentation are as for the simple retropubic approach. Additional supplies include long-tipped, right-angled clamps; urethral suture guides; a Bookwalter or Wishbone (UO400) self-retaining retractor; long Martius clamps; straight and right-angled clip appliers and clips; and right-angled scissors.

Operative Procedure

1. The surgeon creates a vertical midline lower abdominal extraperitoneal incision.
2. A bilateral pelvic lymphadenectomy is performed, removing the external iliac, obturator, and hypogastric nodes en bloc. Lymphadenectomy is done primarily for tumor staging.
3. The surgeon exposes the puboprostatic ligaments, and incises the endopelvic fascia on each side of the gland to the puboprostatic ligaments (Figure 6-60, *A*). Right-angled scissors are employed to divide the puboprostatic ligaments. The dorsal vein complex is easily subject to injury, and excessive venous bleeding may occur during this phase of the procedure. The surgical technologist and the perioperative nurse need to be alert to this potential complication.
4. A plane is developed between the lateral prostatic border and the levator ani muscles with sharp and blunt dissection. Once visualized, the muscle is dissected laterally to the urogenital diaphragm.
5. The surgeon ligates and divides the collateral veins originating from the levator ani muscle and running laterally to the puboprostatic ligaments to free the apex of the prostate.
6. The dorsal venous complex, supplying the penis, is carefully retracted medially. Once a plane is developed, the venous complex is separated from the urethra with a long-tipped, right-angled clamp. The venous complex is ligated with 0 or 2-0 absorbable ligatures. Some surgeons opt to use a stapler designed for this purpose. The complex is then transected with a #15 scalpel. Backbleeding, from the vessels onto the anterior surface of the prostate, is suture-ligated.

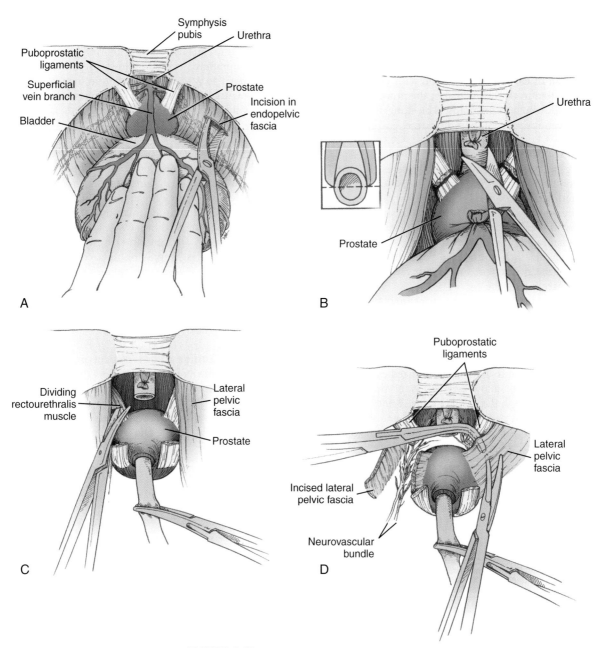

FIGURE 6-60 Radical retropubic prostatectomy.

7. The surgeon uses a right-angled clamp to mobilize the urethra from the rectourethralis muscle between the two neurovascular bundles, avoiding damage to them.

8. A Penrose drain or vessel loop is passed around the urethra. The surgeon elevates and divides the urethra with a long-handled scissors or scalpel (Figure 6-60, *B*). The catheter is clamped proximally and pulled upward through the urethral incision, where it is cut and held cephalad.

9. The posterior urethra is transected (Figure 6-60, *B*).

10. The surgeon dissects the rectourethralis fibers free from and medial to the neurovascular bundles (Figure 6-60, *C* and *D*).

11. Next, the surgeon enucleates the prostate, divides the bladder neck, and clip-ligates the seminal vesicles (Figure 6-60, *E* and *F*).

12. Once bleeding is controlled, the urethral suture guide is inserted in place of the Foley and six 2-0 absorbable sutures on a ⅝-inch curved needle are placed inside to outside on the distal urethral segment. These are tagged and left uncut to be anastomosed to the bladder neck (Figure 6-60, *G*).

13. The surgeon trims and everts the bladder neck and creates a rosebud stoma. The sutures are placed from the urethra to a corresponding position on the bladder neck. When all are placed, they are brought together in single fashion and tied.

14. Closure is as for simple retropubic prostatectomy. Continuous postoperative irrigation is rarely used. A 22F, 30-ml Foley catheter is inserted and placed to gentle traction, and dressings are applied.

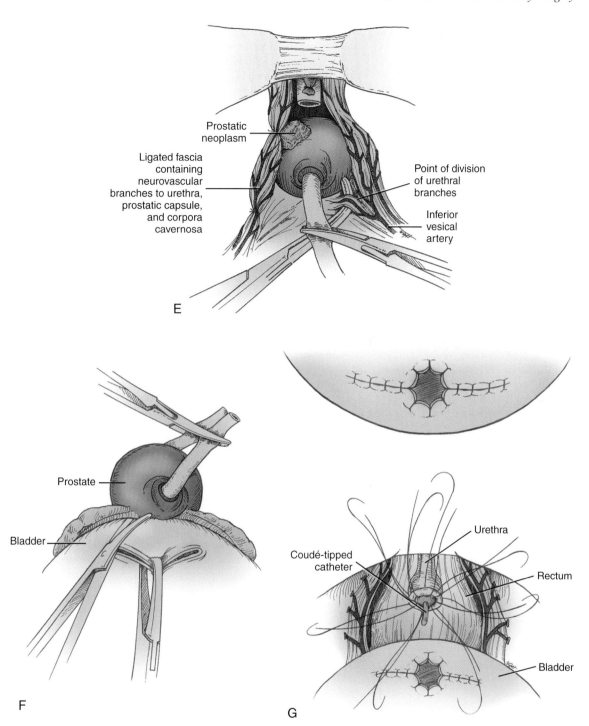

FIGURE 6-60, cont'd. Radical retropubic prostatectomy.

Radical (Total) Perineal Prostatectomy

Patient preparation and instrumentation are the same as for simple perineal prostatectomy. The radical approach is accompanied by laparoscopic or low abdominal lymph node dissection, if not previously performed as a separate procedure. Currently, laparoscopy is performed more frequently than the standard incisional approach. Supplies needed for laparoscopy include standard laparoscopic instrumentation, three 10-mm trocars, one 5-mm trocar, an insufflation needle, a video camera unit, and CO_2 insufflation supplies.

Procedural Considerations. Two operative setups are necessary. Most commonly, laparoscopy precedes prostatectomy. The patient is in the supine position for the laparoscopy, with the area of the umbilicus slightly elevated. Sequential compressive stockings and preoperative Foley catheterization are necessary. Instruments should be available in the OR to convert to an open procedure if necessary. Lymph nodes may be sent for frozen section, primarily for tumor staging.

Operative Procedure
LAPAROSCOPIC LYMPH NODE DISSECTION

1. The surgeon inserts the Veress needle and insufflates the abdomen.
2. Trocars are placed as follows: 10-mm trocars at the 12 o'clock (umbilicus), 3 o'clock, and 9 o'clock positions; a 5-mm trocar at the 6 o'clock position.
3. The surgeon grasps the peritoneum over the vas deferens, and incises it with scissors. The vas is identified, clipped or electrocoagulated, and divided.
4. The peritoneal dissection is continued laterally and cephalad to the sigmoid colon on the left and the ascending colon on the right.
5. After identification of the spermatic cord structures, iliac vessels, ureters, and psoas muscle, the surgeon extends the incision to the pubic ramus.
6. The Cloquet node is identified and freed from under the external iliac vein.
7. Dissection continues until the obturator nerve is isolated.
8. At the level of the bifurcation of the common iliac vein, the large lymph channel is located and removed. Endoclips or scissor-coagulation may be employed. Clips offer a lower risk of postoperative lymphocele.
9. In a similar fashion, the tissue overlying the external iliac artery is removed.
10. The procedure is repeated on the opposite side.
11. Hemostasis is achieved and the trocars are removed. Each trocar is removed under direct observation with the laparoscope, to allow for identification of inner abdominal wall bleeding sites.
12. After evacuation of the gas from the abdomen, the fascia layers are closed at the 12, 3, and 9 o'clock positions.
13. The surgeon closes the skin with 4-0 absorbable subcuticular sutures and dresses the wound.

14. The patient is then repositioned and prepared for radical perineal prostatectomy.

RADICAL PERINEAL PROSTATECTOMY. Surgical approach is as for simple perineal prostatectomy (Figure 6-61).

1. The surgeon incises a layer of subcutaneous fascia and uses blunt dissection to create a space within the ischial rectal fossa (Figure 6-62, *A*).
2. The central tendon is incised, permitting dissection to be carried out beneath the triangle formed by the superficial external anal sphincter (Figure 6-62, *B*).
3. The assistant retracts the sphincter to provide visualization of the rectourethralis (Figure 6-62, *C*).
4. The true prostatic capsule is exposed by incision of the overlying fascia (Figure 6-62, *D*).
5. After dissection of the periprostatic fascia unilaterally, the surgeon passes a right-angled clamp around the membranous urethra and incises it (Figure 6-62, *E*).
6. Using a knife, the surgeon severs the posterior bladder neck and retracts the bladder superiorly (Figure 6-62, *F*).
7. Blunt dissection is used to develop a plane between the anterior bladder and the posterior prostate and seminal vesicles (Figure 6-62, *G*).
8. The surgeon identifies the vascular pedicles at the 5 and 7 o'clock positions, and incises and divides them (Figure 6-62, *H*).
9. Before closure of the bladder neck, the surgeon may place vest sutures of 0 or 2-0 absorbable material in a mattress fashion in the open bladder neck at the 2 and 10 o'clock positions and left long for later lateral perineal placement (Figure 6-62, *I*).
10. Once the reanastomosis is accomplished, the vest sutures are crossed, passed through the perineal body laterally and parallel to the urethra (anterior to the incision), and secured either just beneath the skin or to the skin with suture buttons.
11. After placement of the Foley catheter, the surgeon reanastomoses the urethra to the bladder neck with four to six

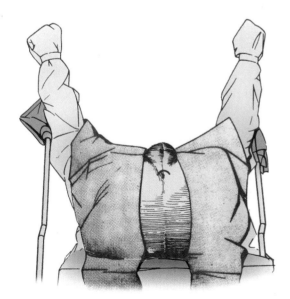
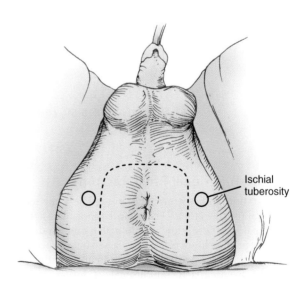

Ischial tuberosity

FIGURE 6-61 Radical perineal prostatectomy, draping and incision.

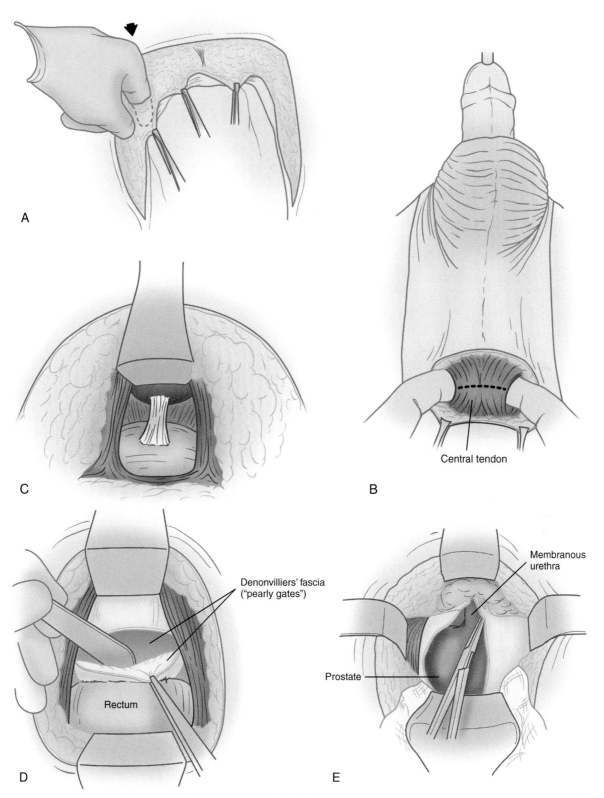

A

B

Central tendon

C

D

Denonvilliers' fascia
("pearly gates")

Rectum

E

Membranous
urethra

Prostate

FIGURE 6-62 Radical perineal prostatectomy.

Continued

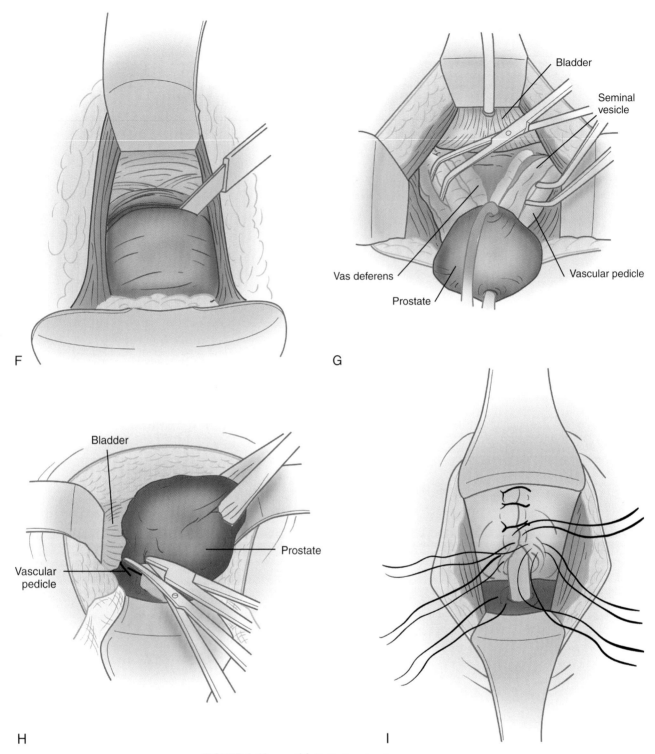

F

G

Bladder

Seminal vesicle

Vas deferens

Prostate

Vascular pedicle

H

Bladder

Vascular pedicle

Prostate

I

FIGURE 6-62, cont'd Radical perineal prostatectomy.

2-0 absorbable sutures placed at the 2, 4, 8, and 10 o'clock positions. Some surgeons opt to place sutures at the 6 and 12 o'clock positions as well.

12. A drain is placed anteriorly to the rectal surface and exteriorized through the incision line or through a separate stab wound.

13. The wound is closed as described in the simple procedure.

Laparoscopic Radical Prostatectomy

Laparoscopic radical prostatectomy (LRP) is a minimally invasive approach that may be offered to some patients in centers where practitioners are skilled in the technique. Patient selection is the same as that for radical retropubic or perineal prostatectomy. Those patients who have undergone androgen deprivation, radiation, or perineal surgery may not be good candidates for the procedure, however. Advantages to an LRP over an open procedure are decreased intraoperative blood loss (attributable to the tamponade effect of the pneumoperitoneum on the venous sinuses, and improved access to and visualization of vascular structures), shorter hospital stays, and decreased postoperative pain. The return to continence and sexual potency is reported to be comparable with other approaches. Some practitioners suggest that retaining sexual potency is more likely because the neurovascular bundles may be visualized under magnification and therefore are more readily preserved (Gonzalgo, 2008). Because of the high cost of the numerous disposable items needed, many institutions may opt to not offer this approach to their patients.

Procedural Considerations. Generally no bowel prep is performed preoperatively. Intravenous administration of a third-generation cephalosporin and 2500 units of low–molecular weight subcutaneous heparin on the morning of surgery is standard treatment.

With the assistance of at least one additional person, the patient is positioned in low lithotomy position with his arms at the sides. The abdomen, entire perineal area, and the upper and inner thigh region are prepped. This entire area is draped open, and separate leggings are employed. The anesthesia provider places the patient in the Trendelenburg position. The perioperative nurse positions the video monitor between the patient's legs. A Foley catheter is inserted into the urethra and attached to drainage. After the procedure, heparin is given once daily for 2 weeks postoperatively. The drain and Foley catheter are generally removed on the third postoperative day, and the patient is discharged.

Operative Procedure
1. The surgeon inserts the Veress needle and insufflates the abdomen. Once an internal pressure of 15 mm Hg of CO_2 is achieved the needle is removed and replaced with a 10-mm trocar.
2. The laparoscope is used to inspect the interior of the abdominal wall. A second incision is then created at McBurney point, a 10-mm trocar is inserted, and the CO_2 line is moved and reattached to this port to prevent fogging of the lens.
3. Three small incisions are made for 5-mm trocar placement: one inferolateral to McBurney point, one in the left iliac fossa, and the third midline between the umbilicus and pubis.
4. If a lymph node dissection is to be performed, this is accomplished first as described in laparoscopic lymph node dissection.
5. The surgeon incises the peritoneal reflection to expose the vas deferens and seminal vesicles. The vasal artery is coagulated, and the vas is transected bilaterally. The seminal vesicles are transected bilaterally and well mobilized.
6. Denonvilliers' fascia is incised longitudinally close to the ampulla of the vas and seminal vesicles and placed on mild traction. Once the prerectal fat is visible, the surgeon begins inferior blunt dissection to the posterior surface of the prostate. Dissection is carried to the rectourethralis muscle.
7. The bladder is filled through the Foley catheter with approximately 120 ml of sterile saline to pull it posteriorly and help identify the bladder contours.
8. An incision is made medial to the medial umbilical ligament for the initiation of bladder dissection. This is carried to the vas and up the abdominal wall anteriorly and caudally until contact is made with the pubic ramus.
9. The urachus is divided in the midline and dissected to the level of the symphysis pubis, across the space of Retzius. A bipolar or monopolar dissector is often employed for this purpose.
10. After the bladder is freed anteriorly and laterally, the surgeon manually empties it with a suction or syringe device.
11. The surgeon coagulates and incises the dorsal vein. The fascia of Zuckerkandl (fat) covering the prostate is resected or pushed laterally cephalad. The periprostatic space is entered, and the endopelvic fascia is incised on its line of reflection.
12. The puboprostatic ligaments are incised to allow dissection of the dorsal venous complex. This is accomplished with a curved monopolar or bipolar scissors. The vessels surrounding the dorsal venous complex are electrocoagulated with bipolar forceps and then ligated with 2-0 absorbable ligature passed from one side to the other.
13. Using sharp and blunt dissection, the surgeon develops a plane between the bladder neck and prostate. The anterior wall of the urethra is incised, and the Foley catheter is deflated and pulled into the operative field. The lateral and posterior urethral walls are then incised.
14. The posterior bladder neck is finally incised and the retrovesical space entered. The prostatic pedicles are bilaterally electrocoagulated with bipolar forceps.
15. A lateral incision is made to expose and preserve the neurovascular bundles on each side. They are dissected free of the prostatic base to the entrance of the pelvic floor and posterolateral to the urethra.
16. The surgeon transects the dorsal vein complex and retracts it anteriorly to expose the anterior urethral wall. A knife is used to cut across the anterior urethra, and a urethral suture guide is pushed through the urethrotomy into the pelvis. The posterior wall is then transected.
17. The prostate is retracted superiorly and the remaining attachments freed.
18. The surgeon creates the urethrovesical anastomosis with interrupted 3-0 absorbable sutures using two needle holders. Once all sutures are placed and tied, the Foley is reinserted and the bladder filled to check the patency of the anastomosis.
19. A specimen collection bag is passed through the second port at McBurney point and opened. The prostate is placed in the sac, the sac is closed, and the string is cut. The port is removed and the string to the sac is placed on the abdomen outside the port, a mosquito clamp is attached to the end, and the port is reinserted.
20. Abdominal pressure is lowered to 5 mm Hg, and peritoneal incisions are left open. A drain is placed in the pelvis through the lower left port and sutured to the skin. The abdominal muscles are split, and the specimen is extracted after removal of the trocar. All trocars are then removed and the incisions closed in a routine manner.

Robotic-Assisted Laparoscopic Radical Prostatectomy

Robotic-assisted surgery uses robotic equipment to imitate the surgeon's movements, allowing for operative access through five small portal incisions rather than large incisions, which results in shorter recovery times. The robotic system enhances the surgeon's range of motion and precision and allows surgeons to preserve nerves crucial to urinary continence and erectile function. Benefits of robotic-assisted prostatectomy are similar to benefits of laparoscopic surgery. Patients have only five to six small incisions, a shorter hospital stay, decreased blood loss, and a shorter time period before the catheter is removed. Men who have undergone the procedure also have decreased incidence of postoperative urinary incontinence and improved sexual function compared to patients who undergo open prostatectomy (Gonzalgo, 2008).

The robotic surgical system consists of a surgeon console, a cart with interactive robotic arms, jointed instruments that mimic the dexterity of the human hand and wrist, and a high-resolution three-dimensional endoscope and image processing equipment. The system provides a three-dimensional stereoscopic display as the surgeon uses the master arms to make surgical movements that are translated into real-time movements of the instrument tips (Figure 6-63). The surgeon's movements are transferred to the robot 13,000 times per second (Rigdon, 2006).

The role of the surgical technologist during robotic laparoscopic radical prostatectomy procedures begins with competency in the OR. Because use of this technology requires special skills, surgical technologists should become familiar and proficient with all aspects of the procedure.

Procedural Considerations. Before the patient's arrival to the OR the perioperative nurse and surgical technologist collaborate to ensure all the necessary instrumentation and equipment is available for the procedure. Depending on the robotic system used, a standard laparoscopic setup is utilized with the addition of the robotic instrumentation and equipment, including the control station, the surgeon's console that provides the interface to the robot, and the robotic arms.

Patients undergoing robotic prostatectomy receive a general anesthetic. The perioperative nurse assists with positioning the patient in the supine position with his legs in Allen stirrups. Once the procedure begins, the anesthesia provider will place the patient in the Trendelenburg position to displace the viscera from the pelvis into the upper abdomen to improve visualization. Surgeons may use a transperitoneal or extraperitoneal approach to the prostatectomy. The transperitoneal approach is described in the next section.

Operative Procedure

1. The surgeon inserts a 22F Foley catheter and maintains it within the sterile field.
2. Pneumoperitoneum is established using either a Veress needle placed at the base of the umbilicus or an open trocar placement with a Hasson technique, depending on the surgeon's preference.
3. The surgeon inserts the 0-degree endoscope through the 12-mm cannula and places the remaining ports as described under direct vision: Two ports are inserted on each side of

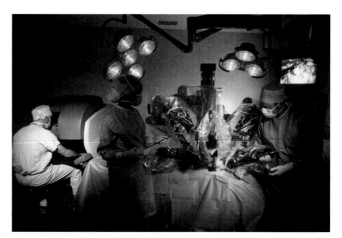

FIGURE 6-63 Minimally invasive robotic surgery system.

the pararectus and two additional ports are placed two to three fingerbreadths medial to the patient's right and left anterior superior iliac spine.

4. The sterile team docks the robot and the perioperative nurse transfers the cart with the robotic arms to the field and assists the surgical technologist with draping. The surgical technologist assists with connecting the robotic manipulators and other system components.
5. The surgeon moves to the console and the assistant remains in the sterile field to operate the clip applicator and suction devices.
6. From the remote location at the console, the surgeon incises the peritoneum over the vas deferens and divides them.
7. The seminal vesicles are dissected and the surgeon incises Denonvilliers' fascia.
8. Using blunt dissection, the surgeon develops a plane between Denonvilliers' fascia and the rectum. The surgeon identifies the endopelvic fascia, dissects it, and makes a bilateral incision.
9. The Foley catheter is removed and the assistant replaces it with a metal sound. Using a figure-of-eight 2-0 polyglactin suture, the surgeon suture-ligates the deep dorsal venous complex. The sound ensures that the urethra is not incorporated into the ligature (Figure 6-64).
10. Using ultrasonic shears or the monopolar ESU, the surgeon incises the anterior and posterior bladder neck. EndoClips are placed along the lateral pedicles as necessary for hemostasis.
11. Dissection continues along the lateral surface of the prostate and the neurovascular bundles are identified.
12. The surgeon divides the dorsal vein and divides the urethra distal to the apex of the prostate.
13. The gland is freed and placed in an entrapment bag.
14. Using a running or interrupted 2-0 polyglactin suture, the surgeon performs the urethrovesical anastomosis (Figure 6-65). The assistant fills the bladder with 100 to 150 ml of irrigant to test the anastomosis. Any visible leaks are repaired with additional suture.
15. A closed-suction drain is placed in the prevesical space.
16. The assistant extends the incision at the umbilical port site and removes the specimen.
17. The surgeon closes the port incisions.

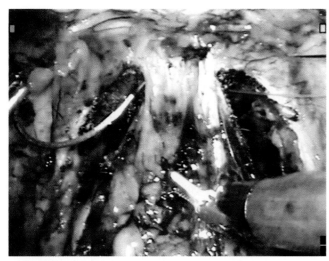

FIGURE 6-64 Intraoperative view demonstrating passage of a suture incorporating the deep dorsal vein complex during robotic-assisted laparoscopic radical prostatectomy.

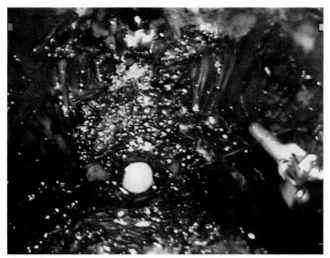

FIGURE 6-65 Intraoperative view demonstrating the use of a running continuous suture for the vesicourethral anastomosis.

SURGERY OF THE BLADDER

Operations on the urinary bladder may be performed through an open abdominal incision or a transurethral route. Diagnostic procedures are often undertaken via the transurethral route. Bladder tumors, diverticula, congenital defects, or trauma may necessitate an open abdominal approach. A thorough diagnostic workup and endoscopic examination help to determine the appropriate surgical approach to be employed. Radical procedures, such as total cystectomy, are performed for the treatment of invasive carcinoma of the bladder and require permanent urinary diversion.

For most open-bladder surgery the patient is placed in the supine position with a bolster under the pelvis. The Trendelenburg position may be desired because this position tilts the head down and allows the viscera to fall cephalad. This allows excellent exposure of the pelvic organs, including the bladder. The patient is draped as described for routine suprapubic prostatectomy, using a disposable impermeable

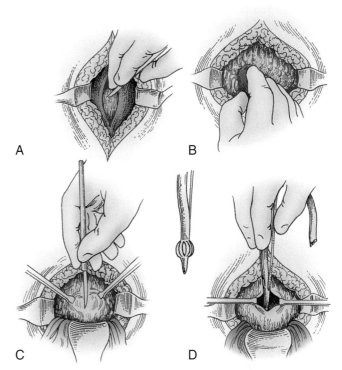

FIGURE 6-66 Suprapubic cystostomy.

drape that is placed immediately below the bladder incision. A catheter may be inserted into the urethra and the bladder distended with sterile saline at the start of surgery for easy identification. The ESU is required. The instrument setup for open-bladder operations requires a basic laparotomy set, plus Mason-Judd bladder retractors, long and short thyroid traction forceps, retropubic needle holders (or other long needle holders), one trocar, vessel loops, a catheter stylet, a closed-wound suction system, and assorted Foley, Pezzer, and Malecot catheters.

Suprapubic Cystostomy

Cystotomy is an opening made into the urinary bladder through a low abdominal incision. When a drainage tube is inserted into the bladder through an abdominal incision, the procedure is a cystostomy.

Procedural Considerations. The patient is in the supine position. Anesthesia may be general, spinal, or local with sedation. A basic laparotomy set is generally sufficient for the procedure. Foley catheters ranging from 22F to 30F should be available, as well as Malecot suprapubic catheters and a drainage bag. Frequently, a flexible cystoscopy is incorporated as part of the procedure.

Operative Procedure
1. After making a vertical or Pfannenstiel incision the surgeon divides the rectus fascia along the midline (Figure 6-66, *A*).
2. The bladder is distended with saline solution that is instilled with an Asepto syringe through a catheter.
3. The surgeon uses sharp and blunt dissection to dissect free the dome of the bladder (Figure 6-66, *B*).

4. Using a pair of Martius forceps, the surgeon grasps the walls of the bladder on either side of the midline (Figure 6-66, *C*).

5. Two traction sutures may be placed through the bladder wall and held with straight hemostats.

6. The surgeon incises the bladder downward with a scalpel. Bleeding vessels in the bladder wall are clamped and ligated.

7. The bladder contents are aspirated with a suction device.

8. The bladder opening may be extended if the bladder is to be explored for diverticula or calculi.

9. The surgeon inserts a large-size Malecot or Pezzer catheter into the bladder (Figure 6-66, *D*).

10. The incision is closed snugly about the catheter with absorbable sutures to render the closure watertight around the cystostomy tube.

11. The muscle, fascia, and subcutaneous tissue are closed with absorbable suture.

12. The surgeon closes the skin with staples or suture.

13. The cystostomy tube is secured to the skin with a 0 or 2-0 nonabsorbable suture to prevent it from being inadvertently dislodged from the bladder. A drain such as a Jackson-Pratt may be left in the prevesical space.

14. The wound is dressed, and the cystostomy tube is connected to a straight urinary drainage system.

Transurethral Resection of Bladder Tumors

Bladder lesions may be removed using a standard resectoscope, working element, loop, and a Foroblique telescope, which is passed through the urethra into the bladder. A 24F cystoscope sheath with a catheterizing bridge and biopsy forceps may be used to remove bladder tumors located at the very top or dome of the bladder (Figure 6-67). Transitional cell carcinoma of the bladder is one of the most difficult lesions to track because it can occur wherever there is transitional cell lining of the urinary tract. Bladder cancer has a tendency to recur in other areas of the bladder, even after complete resection of the original lesion.

Usually the surgeon removes not only the bladder lesion but also a portion of the bladder muscle underlying the lesion so that the pathologist can determine if any tumor has invaded the muscle. Random biopsy specimens of the normal bladder lining are also taken to ascertain if microscopic transitional cell carcinoma in situ is present. Lesions that deeply invade the muscle must be treated with an open surgical procedure, such as a partial cystectomy or total cystectomy.

The resection technique, setup, and preparation of the patient are virtually the same as those for TURP. The anesthesia provider administers a general, spinal, or regional anesthetic. A retrograde pyelogram may be done to check for lesions existing in the upper urinary tract.

Sterile water is recommended as an irrigating solution in transurethral resection of bladder tumors. Because few vessels are uncovered during this short resection procedure, water absorption with hemolysis and systemic complications such as hyponatremia do not occur. In addition, cancer cells released during the procedure tend to absorb water, causing them to rupture and lyse rather than remain viable and capable of implanting themselves into the raw surface of the bladder created by the surgery. When the procedure is completed, the surgeon passes a large catheter, usually a 24F, into the bladder and connects it to drainage.

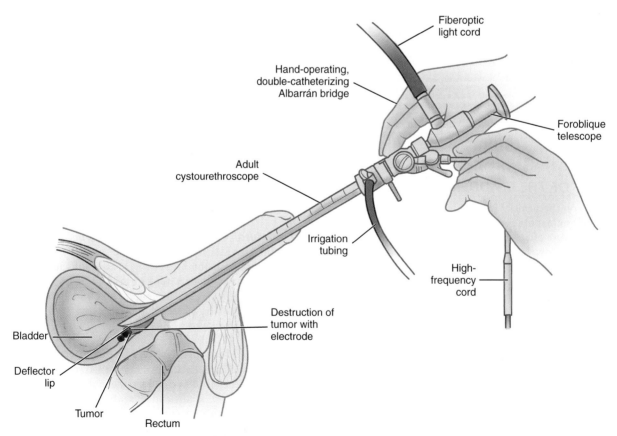

FIGURE 6-67 Fulguration of a bladder tumor.

Transurethral Laser Ablation of Bladder Tumors

The neodymium (Nd):YAG or holmium (Ho):YAG laser may be used to destroy small recurrent bladder tumors and to coagulate the tumor bed of larger bladder tumors resected with an electrosurgical loop. A powerful, highly focused beam of light in the near-infrared range is transmitted to the tumor site through a flexible glass fiber. This laser fiber is passed through the catheter channel of a cystoscope, and the fiber is directed by a deflecting laser bridge (Figure 6-68). The advantages of a laser in the eradication of bladder tumors are as follows: (1) bleeding is minimized, (2) only sedation is required, (3) the operating time is shortened, (4) there is minimal damage to healthy tissue, and (5) postoperative drainage of the bladder by a urethral catheter is not needed.

Alternatives to Surgery for Superficial Bladder Cancer

Patients with various types of cancer may be treated in the urology office setting with various therapeutic modalities including the instillation of chemotherapeutic solutions. These measures may be initiated instead of surgery or as an adjunct to surgery. Instillations are aimed at eradicating existing disease, reducing tumor recurrence and progression, and improving overall patient survival (Lamm et al, 2005).

Patients with bladder cancer that has been staged as Ta, carcinoma in situ (CIS), and T1 may be treated with intravesical, antineoplastic chemotherapy agents such as *thiotepa* (Thioplax), *mitomycin C* (Mutamycin), *doxorubicin* (Adriamycin), and *etoglucid* (Epodyl). Chemotherapy has become the treatment of choice for low-risk patients.

Immunotherapy with TheraCys or Tice *bacille Calmette-Guérin (BCG)* is used to treat patients considered to have high-risk tumors. BCG, through an unknown mechanism, strengthens the body's immune reaction to cancer and is considered the most effective therapy for recurrent and residual bladder cancer.

Combination chemotherapy and immunotherapy have become standard treatment for patients with metastatic transitional cell carcinoma. BCG has been combined with *mitomycin C* and with *interferon alfa-2b*. The latter combination has been highly effective, rescuing approximately 60% of those who failed with BCG alone (Lamm et al, 2005).

Trocar Cystostomy

Trocar cystostomy consists of draining the bladder by puncture with a needle or trocar and inserting a catheter.

Procedural Considerations. A minor instrument set along with a metal probe and grooved director, an Anthony suction tube and tubing, and trocar catheters or a prepackaged cystostomy kit is required. A local anesthetic may be used.

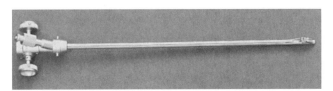

FIGURE 6-68 Rectoscope with bridge.

Operative Procedure
1. The surgeon nicks the skin at the site of the puncture with a scalpel and inserts the trocar into the bladder.
2. The trocar obturator is withdrawn, the bladder is drained through the trocar by suction, and a catheter is passed through the trocar cannula into the bladder.
3. The surgeon removes the cannula and sutures the catheter to the wound edges. The wound is dressed.

Suprapubic Cystolithotomy

Suprapubic cystolithotomy is the removal of calculi from the bladder. Obstructions, such as prostatic enlargement or foreign bodies, are common causes of bladder calculi and may be corrected at the time of surgery. In the past, special transurethral instruments such as the lithotrite were commonly used to crush vesical calculi manually. Bladder stones are often eradicated via the electrohydraulic lithotripter, which fragments the stone within the bladder by using an electric current to initiate shock waves (Figure 6-69, *A*), or by ultrasonic lithotripsy.

During ultrasonic lithotripsy ultrasound waves are transmitted through a hollow metal probe, which creates vibration at the tip. When applied to the surface of a calculus, the vibrating tip drills and fragments the calculus. This mechanical disintegration is continued until the stone is reduced to small fragments that are evacuated by suction through the hollow center of the probe (Figure 6-69, *B*). The holmium:YAG laser (Ho:YAG) may also be used for fragmentation of bladder calculi (Figure 6-70).

Procedural Considerations. Instruments for open-bladder operations along with Millin T-shaped stone forceps, Millin capsule forceps, and Lewkowitz lithotomy forceps are required.

Operative Procedure. The surgical approach is similar to that described for suprapubic cystotomy. When the bladder is opened, calculi are identified and extracted. If indicated, bladder outlet obstruction is repaired.

Repair of Vesical Fistulas

Vesical fistulas occurring between the bladder and the intestines or vagina may be repaired surgically. *Vesicointestinal fistulas* may be caused by ulcerative colitis, diverticulitis, or neoplasms of the colon or rectum. *Vesicovaginal fistulas* may be a complication of radiotherapy for cervical cancer, endoscopic procedures involving surgery of the trigone or vesical neck, obstetric injuries, and hysterectomies.

Procedural Considerations. The instrument setup is as described for open-bladder operations. Intestinal instruments are necessary for vesicointestinal fistulas. For vesicovaginal fistulas, vaginal preparation and a colporrhaphy set with colostomy or ileostomy instruments are used.

Vesicointestinal fistulas are more common than vesicovaginal fistulas. Of the intestinal fistulas, the sigmoid colon is most often involved (Figure 6-71). A colostomy proximal to the fistula may be performed to protect the repaired segment of bowel. The communicating area of bladder and bowel is totally resected. Generally, an end-to-end bowel resection is performed after excision of the involved intestinal segment. The bladder is then repaired in three layers.

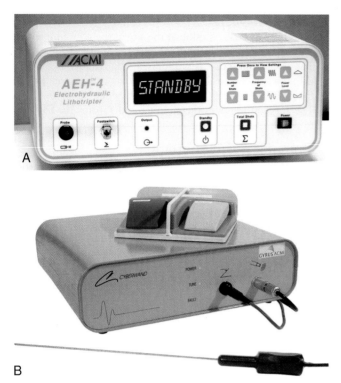

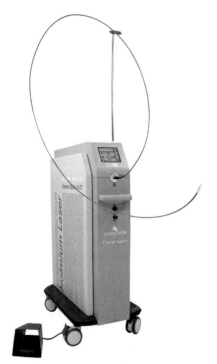

B

FIGURE 6-69 A, Electrohydraulic lithotripter. **B**, Ultrasonic lithotripter.

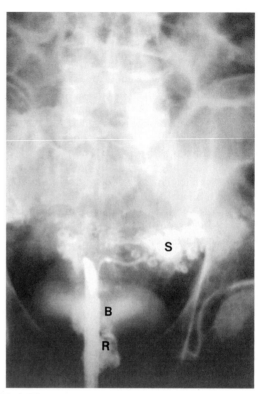

FIGURE 6-71 Vesicoenteric fistulogram (cystogram) showing contrast material in bladder (*B*), sigmoid colon (*S*), and rectum (*R*).

FIGURE 6-70 Holmium laser unit.

If the fistula is at the dome of the bladder, the approach will be transperitoneal, transvesical, or a combination of the two. If the fistula is in the trigone of the bladder, a vaginal approach may be employed. A suprapubic tube is usually left in the bladder.

Operative Procedure
VESICOVAGINAL FISTULA REPAIR—VAGINAL APPROACH
1. Before placing the patient in the hyperflexed lithotomy or Kraske position (jackknife), the surgeon inserts a suprapubic catheter, clamps it, and connects it to closed drainage. If the intended position is Kraske, separate draping material and instrumentation are set up for the suprapubic catheter insertion with the patient supine. The catheter is secured, and the patient is turned for the procedure.
2. The area is draped with a lithotomy or laparotomy sheet as indicated per the patient's position.
3. The surgeon sutures the labia to the outer groin or inner thigh for retraction and visualization.
4. A weighted vaginal retractor is placed posteriorly, and the defect is examined. A relaxing vaginal incision may be necessary at the 5 or 7 o'clock position.
5. The surgeon inserts a 4F ureteral catheter through the fistula, and dilates the tract to admit an 8F balloon catheter. The balloon is inflated, and the catheter is used as a retractor.
6. The area is infiltrated with vasopressin (Pitressin) solution.
7. The surgeon incises the vaginal mucosa and perivesical fascia around the defect outside of the scarred tissue.
8. Two planes are developed—one between the mucosa and fascia and one between the fascia and the bladder wall—with fine scissors, forceps, and gauze (Kittner) dissectors.
9. The bladder wall is freed from the vaginal wall.
10. The vesical defect is grasped with Martius clamps, the scarred edges are everted, and the defect is closed vertically with interrupted 3-0 absorbable sutures after removal of the catheter previously placed. In some instances,

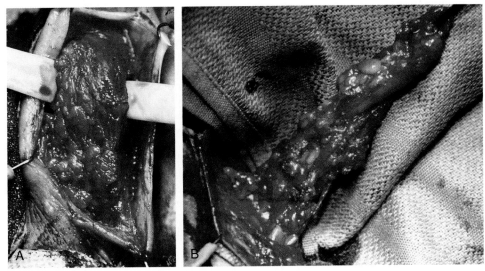

FIGURE 6-72 Creation of Martius flap.

a labial pedicle or full-thickness flap (Martius flap) may be placed between the vesical closure and the vaginal closure (Figure 6-72). This prevents suture-line stress and overlay and removes the need for a relaxing incision. Larger fistulas that do not adequately reapproximate may necessitate a vascularized muscle flap to reinforce closure.

11. The surgeon approximates the perivesical fascia and vaginal mucosa separately with transverse interrupted 3-0 absorbable sutures. A one-sided ellipse of vaginal mucosa may be excised to offset the closure.
12. Alternatively, an inverted-U incision may provide more exposure than other incisions and result in a posterior flap that completely covers the site of the defect.
13. The surgeon unclamps the suprapubic catheter, removes the labial stitches, and loosely packs the vagina.

VESICOVAGINAL FISTULA—TRANSPERITONEAL (TRANSVESICAL) APPROACH

1. The patient is placed in the low lithotomy and moderate Trendelenburg's position. Both the perineum and the abdomen are prepped and draped appropriately. A laparoscopy pack works well for this approach.
2. The surgeon inserts ureteral catheters and places a 16F Foley catheter in the bladder and clamps it.
3. A tight gauze pack or vaginal ball is placed into the vagina.
4. The surgeon makes a vertical midline or Pfannenstiel incision.
5. The peritoneum is incised and bluntly dissected from the dome of the bladder.
6. The small bowel is packed cephalad.
7. Stay sutures of 2-0 absorbable material are placed in the bladder dome, and the bladder is opened.
8. The surgeon divides the bladder wall and overlying peritoneum down to the fistula. Stay sutures are placed periodically to serve as retractors for bladder elevation.
9. The peritoneum is incised transversely at the level of the fistula, forming a pedicle flap.
10. The vagina and bladder are separated widely on each side of the fistula. An assistant places upward pressure on the vaginal ball or pack to facilitate dissection.
11. As the fistula is exposed, the surgeon excises it until it is completely removed. A probe may be used to localize it, if

small, or an 8F balloon catheter may be inserted and used for traction during dissection.
12. The bladder and vagina are freed from each other until there is enough mobility for separate closures.
13. The surgeon closes the vagina, without tension, with inverting 2-0 or 3-0 interrupted sutures in two layers.
14. The peritoneal flap is swung into the defect and sutured in place for reperitonealization. A long, attached peritoneal or free peritoneal pedicle flap may be needed for reperitonealization. Alternatively, the omentum may be manipulated from behind the right side of the colon for an omental graft. A vascularized muscle flap may be placed for fistulas resulting from radiation necrosis.
15. A 22F Malecot catheter and a wound drain are inserted and pulled through separate stab wounds in the abdomen.
16. The ureteral catheters are removed, and the bladder mucosa and submucosa are closed in separate layers with 2-0 or 3-0 absorbable suture in a running fashion.
17. The muscularis and adventitia are externally approximated with interrupted 3-0 sutures.
18. The wound is closed in layers.
19. Dressings are applied, the Foley is unclamped, the vaginal ball or gauze pack is removed, and the vagina is loosely repacked.

VESICOSIGMOID FISTULA REPAIR—ABDOMINAL APPROACH

1. With the patient in the Trendelenburg position, a 20F or 22F, 5-ml Foley catheter is inserted and the bladder filled with 100 ml of sterile water. Once the patient is prepped and draped as described for laparotomy, a midline, or paramedian, and transperitoneal incisions are made.
2. The surgeon explores the abdomen.
3. The descending colon and sigmoid colon are mobilized by incising along the fascia fusion line of Toldt.
4. The involved loop of colon is identified. If a walled-off inflammatory mass is found, a transverse colostomy may be performed and a two-stage intervention considered.
5. Using blunt dissection, the surgeon separates the fistulous tract.
6. A probe is inserted to determine the extent of involvement.

7. The defects in the bladder and bowel are debrided to obtain healthy tissue. Large inflammatory masses require a colon resection.

8. The surgeon closes the bladder in two layers with a 3-0 absorbable submucosal running stitch and a 2-0 absorbable interrupted muscularis and adventitial stitch.

9. The edges of the bowel defect are trimmed to reach normal tissue, and stay sutures are placed on each side.

10. The cavity is pulled transversely, and the mucosa and submucosa are closed in one pass with a Connell stitch of 3-0 chromic catgut.

11. The surgeon approximates and closes the muscularis and serosa in one pass with 4-0 silk Lembert sutures.

12. The abdomen is irrigated with 2000 ml of sterile saline with an attempt to reach all areas.

13. A sump-style drain is placed intraperitoneally, and a Penrose or small Jackson-Pratt drain is placed suprapubically, exiting through separate stab wounds.

14. The surgeon closes the abdomen in layers in the conventional manner. If a colostomy was performed, it is opened for fecal diversion and the appropriate appliance applied.

15. Gauze and bulky absorbable dressings are applied and secured; Montgomery straps may be used.

Vesicourethral (Marshall-Marchetti-Krantz) Suspension

A Marshall-Marchetti-Krantz suspension is performed for the correction of stress incontinence caused by an abnormal urethrovesical angle. The intent of the Marshall-Marchetti-Krantz operation is to bring the bladder and urethra into the pelvis by suturing paraurethral vaginal tissue to the back of the symphysis pubis. A modification of this technique is the Burch procedure. The approach mimics the Marshall-Marchetti-Krantz until placement of the buttressing sutures. Instead of attempting difficult periosteal sutures, the surgeon places nonabsorbable size 0 sutures into the Cooper ligament from each side of the bladder neck. The Burch procedure is technically easier, and long-term results are fairly equivalent.

A large percentage of patients with stress incontinence are obese and have diabetes. It is important to evaluate for these conditions and prepare for proper patient management (i.e., positioning concerns relating to peripheral vascular circulation and pressure points, skin breakdown, risk for infection, wound healing).

Procedural Considerations. The patient is usually placed in a moderate Trendelenburg's position, frog-legged, with supports under each knee to allow for intraoperative vaginal manipulation. Abdominal and vaginal preps are required. A Foley catheter is inserted at the beginning of surgery. Both the surgeon and assistant double-glove for vaginal manipulation. Basic laparotomy and abdominal hysterectomy instruments, if needed, are used. Postoperatively, the patient commonly has a vaginal pack, a urethral catheter with or without a suprapubic catheter, and possibly a wound drain.

Operative Procedure

1. The surgeon makes a suprapubic transverse incision and exposes the prevesical space of Retzius.

2. The bladder retractor is positioned with small, moist laparotomy packs in place.

3. Using blunt dissection, the surgeon frees the bladder and urethra from the posterior surface of the rectus muscle and symphysis pubis.

4. The assistant places two fingers into the vagina, lifting the urethra upward against the symphysis pubis to facilitate ease of repair of the periurethral musculofascial structures.

5. A heavy, nonabsorbable atraumatic suture on a Heaney needle holder is placed through the supporting fascia of the vaginal wall on each side of the urethra. The suture is passed through the symphysis pubis, providing support to the urethra and bladder neck. Generally, a row of three heavy, nonabsorbable sutures is placed on each side of the urethra, the most proximal being located just at the vesical neck.

6. The surgeon closes the wound in layers.

7. The vagina may be packed with 2-inch packing, which is removed after 24 to 36 hours.

TVT Sling (Tension-Free Vaginal Tape)

A TVT sling is indicated for women diagnosed with urethral hypermobility, intrinsic sphincter deficiency, and pure stress incontinence caused by pelvic floor relaxation. It will not correct urge incontinence, although it may be used in women with combination stress and urge incontinence. This patient will need to have her urge incontinence controlled in another manner. It appears to be a viable option for the overweight and older female and for women who have had previous corrective measures that failed. It is not recommended for younger women who are pregnant or intend to become pregnant. Other contraindications include patients with intrinsic bleeding problems or who are receiving anticoagulant therapy. Risks include bladder perforation, perforation of pelvic viscera adherent to the pubis, retropubic hemorrhage and hematoma formation, infection, and urinary retention.

The tape is composed of polypropylene mesh (Figure 6-73) encased in a plastic sleeve that has a center slit and is secured to a large, curved trocar needle at each end. A T-shaped introducer is attached to these needles for passage of the sling material. The mesh is passed through the pelvic tissue and positioned under the urethra, creating a supportive sling. Unlike other corrective procedures for incontinence, no screws, anchors, or internal sutures are required.

Procedural Considerations. The procedure may be performed using a local anesthetic with monitored sedation. After the sedation is administered, the perioperative nurse places the patient in the lithotomy position.

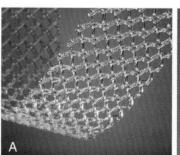
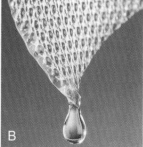

FIGURE 6-73 A, Uretex self-anchoring urethral support system.

Operative Procedure

1. A 16F or 18F Foley catheter is inserted to drain the bladder.
2. The surgeon injects local anesthetic through the skin and into the muscle and fascia lateral to the midline and just above the symphysis pubis, bilaterally. Vasopressin (Pitressin) is commonly added to the anesthetic to help control bleeding.
3. Additional local anesthetic is injected suburethrally into the anterior vaginal mucosa to the retropubic space, bilaterally.
4. The surgeon performs a cystoscopy to confirm integrity of the bladder wall, urethral patency and length, and location of the ureters.
5. Two incisions, 0.5 to 1 cm in length, are made in the abdominal skin over each injection site.
6. The surgeon places a weighted speculum in the vagina, and grasps the anterior vaginal mucosa with two Allis clamps.
7. Using a #10 or #15 scalpel the surgeon makes a 1.5-cm incision into the anterior vaginal mucosa, 1 cm to the right of the external meatus.
8. Blunt Metzenbaum scissors are used to dissect suburethrally and periurethrally to the level of the endopelvic fascia.
9. The surgeon inserts a rigid stylet into the Foley catheter, and inserts the catheter into the bladder.
10. The bladder neck and urethra are deflected away to allow passage of the first needle by holding the Foley with its stylet against the inner ipsilateral thigh. An Allis clamp or hemostat may be placed in the center of the sling material to prevent twisting of the mesh or its sleeve.
11. After attaching the introducer, the first needle is passed 1 cm lateral to the urethra with the curve of the needle in the palm of the surgeon's hand. The needle penetrates the urogenital diaphragm behind the symphysis pubis.
12. Two fingers of the other hand are placed over the skin incision, the needle is pushed through the retropubic space, and the introducer is removed. The needle is guided up to partially protrude through the abdominal wall.
13. Before the trocar needle is extracted and removed, the surgeon removes the Foley and performs a cystoscopy. When bladder integrity has been confirmed, the first needle may be brought out through the abdominal wall and cut from the sling material, and a hemostat is attached to the mesh and sleeve.
14. The procedure is then repeated on the other side with the Foley directed toward the ipsilateral inner thigh during insertion and passage of the needle.
15. Once the tape is in place, the surgeon positions an 8F Hegar dilator between the tape and the urethra for tension testing. The patient is asked to cough, and the tape is adjusted until there is no leak or only a few drops of fluid are lost during coughing. The plastic sleeves are then removed by pulling them up through the abdominal incisions. The excess mesh that protrudes is cut at the skin surface.
16. The surgeon closes the vaginal mucosa with a running stitch of 2-0 chromic suture. Wound closure strips or skin sutures are used to close the abdominal incisions.
17. A perineal pad may be placed to absorb any vaginal bleeding. Abdominal dressings are applied at the surgeon's discretion. Vaginal packing and a postoperative Foley catheter are usually not necessary.

Transvaginal Sling with Bone Anchor

Indications and contraindications for this procedure are the same as those for the TVT sling procedure. In addition, the patient with severe osteoporosis may not be a good candidate for this technique because the bone anchors may not integrate into the pubic bone properly.

Risks with this technique include bladder perforation, inadequate fixation of the bone anchor (this generally requires abandoning the method and using a different type of sling approach), urinary retention, pain, osteitis pubis or osteomyelitis of the pubic bone, and recurrent incontinence.

Procedural Considerations. The procedure may be performed using a local anesthetic with monitored sedation. After the sedation is administered, the perioperative nurse places the patient in the lithotomy position. A formal incision may not be necessary for this procedure.

Operative Procedure

1. Before the procedure the surgical technologist loads a bone screw with preloaded #1 polypropylene suture onto the bone drill. A plastic cover fits over the screw, protecting the patient during insertion.
2. A Foley catheter is inserted, the bladder drained, and the catheter clamped.
3. The surgeon places Allis clamps on the mucosa and pulls gently upward to expose the anterior vaginal wall.
4. Tension is put on the polypropylene stitch that protrudes through the handle of the bone drill. The surgeon inserts the drill into the vagina in a line parallel to the plane of the symphysis pubis, and holds the drill head against the pubic bone (Figure 6-74).
5. Insertion is complete when the polypropylene stitch stops rotating. Fixation of the screw is tested with a gentle downward tug on the suture. The bone screws should lie lateral to the symphysis pubis in the posterior midthird of the pubic bone.
6. The Foley is opened and drained. If the urine is bloody a cystoscopy is performed. Some surgeons choose to routinely perform cystoscopy after each screw insertion to evaluate bladder patency.
7. A right-angle clamp is employed to follow the tunnel of the polypropylene suture upward. A small puncture is created in the urethropelvic ligament to allow passage of the sling material into the retropubic space. The sling material may be cadaveric fascia or polypropylene mesh.
8. The surgeon creates a 2-cm tunnel between the midurethra and bladder neck, behind the vaginal wall.
9. The sling material is perforated with a Keith needle, and the polypropylene suture is passed through the eye of the needle. The suture is then transferred to the sling material. This is done twice on each end of the material.
10. The material is passed through the tunnel (Figure 6-75).
11. Following cystoscopy, steps 4 through 6 are repeated on the contralateral vaginal wall. The polypropylene sutures are tied individually so that the material lies in close proximity to the pubic bone.

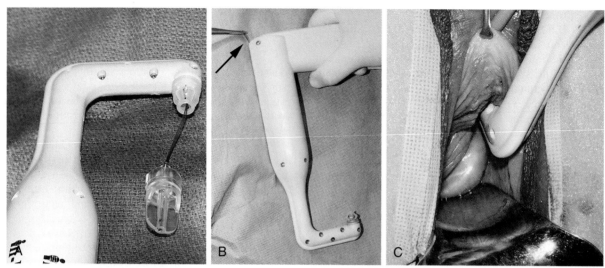

FIGURE 6-74 **A,** Bone anchor on bone drill with #1 polypropylene. **B,** Bone drill ready; polypropylene extends out handle. **C,** Bone drill in place.

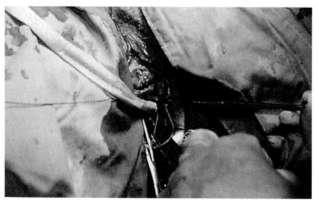

FIGURE 6-75 Fascia lata graft being placed for suburethral sling procedure.

12. The vagina is sutured on each side with a single stitch of absorbable 2-0 sutures.
13. A vaginal pack soaked in antibiotic or estrogen cream is inserted. The Foley catheter is drained and attached to a closed drainage system.

Implantation of InterStim Sacral Nerve Stimulator (Neuromodulator)

The InterStim System is indicated for the treatment of urinary urge incontinence, urinary retention, and significant urgency-frequency in patients who have failed or could not tolerate other measures (Sherman and Amundsen, 2007). The procedure is performed in two stages. During the first stage, a lead is implanted and connected to an external stimulator. The patient is discharged and undergoes a trial period that lasts from 2 to 4 weeks to determine if the device will be effective. During this trial period, the patient maintains a diary to track symptoms and post void residuals. If the trial is successful, the patient will return for the subcutaneous implantation of a pulse generator.

Some precautions must be taken by the patient who has had this device implanted. MRI studies are not recommended. Caution should be taken and the device turned off if electrocoagulation will be employed during any future surgery the patient might undergo. Female patients should be instructed to carry their purses on the opposite side of the implant.

Procedural Considerations. The perioperative nurse assists with positioning the patient in the prone position with a 30-degree flexion at the hips. Pillows may be placed under the patient's abdomen to support the lumbar area and decrease lordosis. Pillows are also placed under the ankles to elevate the feet and prevent pressure on the toes.

C-arm fluoroscopy is employed to visualize sacral landmarks and verify lead position intraoperatively. Although general anesthesia may be employed, monitored sedation with a local anesthetic is preferable so that the patient may verbally respond to nerve stimuli during the procedure. It is suggested that no IV muscle relaxants be administered, because this will affect the physiologic response to the stimulator. If electrocoagulation is needed, a bipolar system should be employed, because unipolar current could potentially travel into the sacral foramen. The patient is typically discharged from the hospital on the same day.

The nurse preps the patient's sacral area, buttocks, and perineum and applies the test stimulation ground pad to the patient's heel. An alternative to this placement is the calf or skin below the rib cage or iliac crest. The pad is approximately 5 to 8 cm in size. The pad will be attached by a test stimulation cable to the external stimulator. The patient is draped to expose the entire buttock area so that responses to nerve stimulation may be assessed. The feet and lower legs are also exposed to allow visualization of muscle response.

The surgeon locates and marks the sacral outline, S3 foramen, posterior iliac spine, coccygeal tip, and midline. To locate these landmarks, the surgeon palpates the upper border of the greater sciatic notch. The S3 sacral foramen is approximately one fingerbreadth from the midline whereas the S2 and S4 foramina are one fingerbreadth above and below S3. The sacral crest corresponds to S4, and the S3 foramen is 9 cm above the coccygeal tip and 2 cm from the midline.

Operative Procedure

1. The surgeon inserts the needle into the S3 foramen. The external stimulator is activated to confirm correct placement of the needle. A bellows response (flattening of the perineum) and flexion of the great toe indicate the needle is in the S3 foramen.
2. The guidewire is inserted into the foramen needle.
3. A 5-mm stab wound is created for the lead introducer.
4. The surgeon slides the lead introducer, consisting of dilator and sheath, over the guidewire and advances it into the foramen. The depth marker on the directional guide is aligned with the top of the dilator.
5. The dilator is then removed, and the sheath remains in place.
6. The surgeon inserts the tined lead, with its stylet (Figure 6-76), and passes it through the sheath until the second white marker is aligned with the back of the sheath. The four electrodes on the lead are now exposed and visible on fluoroscopy.
7. Nerve responses are again assessed at this time by connecting the mini-J hook on the patient cable to the uninsulated section of the foramen needle. The electrodes are numbered zero to three, and the connector contacts on the needle correspond to these numbers. Beginning at the distal tip of the needle, all four electrodes are tested. The lead is repositioned according to the verbalized and visualized responses of the patient. The foramen producing the best results is chosen.
8. Once the electrodes are in optimal position the lead body proximal to the sheath is held in place and the sheath is slowly backed out of the wound. This is often accomplished under live fluoroscopy.
9. As the sheath is withdrawn the tines on the lead open, anchoring it in place.
10. The surgeon creates a tunnel for the subcutaneous neurostimulator generator pocket by means of the same incision. Placement is in the upper buttock below the beltline.
11. A pocket is created with the bipolar ESU. The pocket depth should not be greater than 4 cm to avoid interference with programming and shifting of the neurostimulator. The ideal pocket is 3 to 5 cm below the superior iliac crest and lateral to the outer sacral edge.
12. The surgeon uses the tunneling tool with its metal tip and plastic tube to develop the tunnel from the lead to the intended pocket. Once tunneling is achieved the metal tip is removed and the tool is withdrawn, leaving the plastic tubing in place. The proximal lead end is then fed through the tubing to the pocket, and the tubing is removed. The protective boot is placed over the end of the lead. Leads may be placed bilaterally at the surgeon's discretion.
13. The percutaneous extension is then tunneled from the eventual generator site to the opposite posterior iliac side and exits the skin. This is then attached to the external device.
14. The incisions at all wound sites are closed. The wounds are dressed with small gauze and an occlusive dressing.

If the patient has a good response (50% or greater decrease in symptoms), then the area of generator site is extended in a second stage and the generator is connected to the lead (Figures 6-77 and 6-78). The percutaneous extension is pulled out through the other side and taken away from the field.

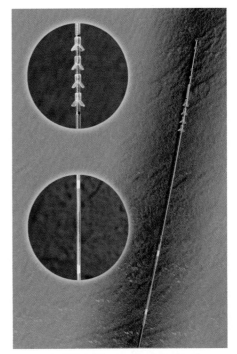

FIGURE 6-76 InterStim tined lead.

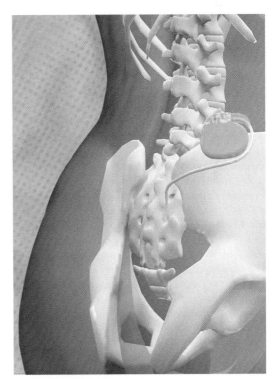

FIGURE 6-77 Graphic placement of InterStim.

Male Sling

The male perineal sling is designed to improve male incontinence by increasing outlet resistance. Using cadaveric dermis, fascia lata, or pericardium, the surgeon places a triangular sling under the bulbous urethra and anchors it with six screws that are placed into the inner portion of the descending ramus just below the symphysis pubis. Other treatments for incontinence,

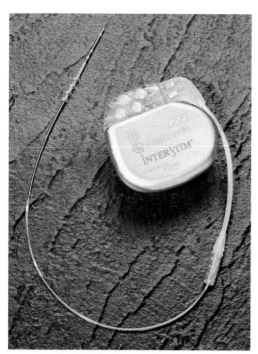

FIGURE 6-78 InterStim implant.

Botox Treatment for Urinary Incontinence

Researchers evaluated the use of Botox in the treatment of idiopathic overactive bladder in a two-stage, randomized, double-blinded study comparing Botox to a placebo. The toxin, which is more commonly used in cosmetic treatments, works by paralyzing one of the muscles that controls the bladder, preventing it from emptying involuntarily. Stage 1 of the study consisted of a 6-week randomized, placebo-controlled trial, and stage 2 was a 9-month randomized trial of two doses of Botox without a placebo control.

A total of 22 patients participated in stage 1 of this two-stage study. Criteria for the study were overactive bladder refractory to anticholinergic medications, multiple daily incontinence episodes, and a 24-hour incontinence pad weight of 100 g or greater. Researchers injected the detrusor muscle in 8 to 10 locations above the trigone.

In analyzing the study results, the researchers reported improvements in daily incontinence episodes, number of incontinence pads used per day, and quality-of-life questionnaires in the botulinum-A toxin group with no changes in the placebo group. Complications experienced during the study were minor, and included urinary tract infection in 13% of the botulinum-A toxin group and 28% in the placebo group. One participant required intermittent catheterization.

Modified from Flynn MK et al: Outcome of a randomized, double-blind, placebo controlled trial of botulinum A toxin for refractory overactive bladder, *J Urol* 181:2608-2615, 2009.

including the use of botulinum A toxin, are being investigated (Research Highlight).

Bladder Augmentation

Augmentation enterocystoplasty is a procedure performed to surgically enlarge the bladder capacity. A wide range of conditions that were previously treated with urinary diversion may now be successfully managed with this technique. Indications include reflex incontinence unresponsive to medical management, detrusor hyperactivity with compromised bladder function, chronically contracted bladder resulting from radiation or repeated infections, and neuropathic bladder combined with recurrent urinary tract infections or compromised renal function. A segment of bowel is used to augment the bladder. The bowel is re-formed into a semispheric shape to decrease peristaltic contractions and anastomosed to the opened bladder dome. The result is a low-pressure reservoir that provides improved bladder capacity and urinary compliance. Almost all segments of bowel as well as the stomach have been employed for bladder augmentation. Selection depends on anatomic factors, functional characteristics, and the surgeon's preference. In some cases, ureteral reimplantation or associated bladder-outlet procedures are incorporated in a one-stage procedure.

Postoperatively, intermittent catheterization and bladder irrigations may be necessary. The patient must be able and willing to learn and perform these procedures and must be accepting of this alteration in lifestyle.

Procedural Considerations. The nurse assists with positioning the patient in the supine position after the anesthesia provider administers a general or regional anesthetic. The female patient may be in a frog-leg or lithotomy position, particularly if access to the perineum is necessary. The entire abdomen and genitalia are prepped and draped. The surgeon inserts a Foley catheter after the patient has been prepped and draped so that the bladder can be filled to capacity for visualization during the procedure. Basic laparotomy and intestinal instruments are required.

Operative Procedure
1. The surgeon makes a supraumbilical to symphysis midline abdominal incision.
2. The peritoneal cavity is exposed using a Bookwalter or similar retractor.
3. The surgeon examines the intestines and stomach, and chooses the appropriate segment for reconstruction (Figure 6-79, *A*).
4. A sagittal bladder incision is made from 2 cm cephalad to the bladder neck anteriorly across the anterior bladder wall, the peritonealized dome surface, and the posterior bladder wall to 2 cm above the posterior interureteric ridge. This causes the bladder to be bivalved in a clam-shaped design.
5. The surgeon places bilateral traction sutures along the bladder incision.
6. The length of the incision is measured to correlate with the corresponding segment of bowel or stomach. Average length required is 25 cm.
7. The surgeon mobilizes the segment of bowel and closes the mesentery cephalad so that the segment is on the retroperitoneum. The segment is left attached to its mesentery to maintain blood supply (Figure 6-79, *B*).
8. The isolated segment is opened, trimmed, and detubularized. The surgeon then folds it double and sutures it to form a cup patch (Figure 6-79, *C*).
9. Anastomosis is accomplished with a running, intermittent locking, absorbable suture, beginning at the posterior apex and running up each side.

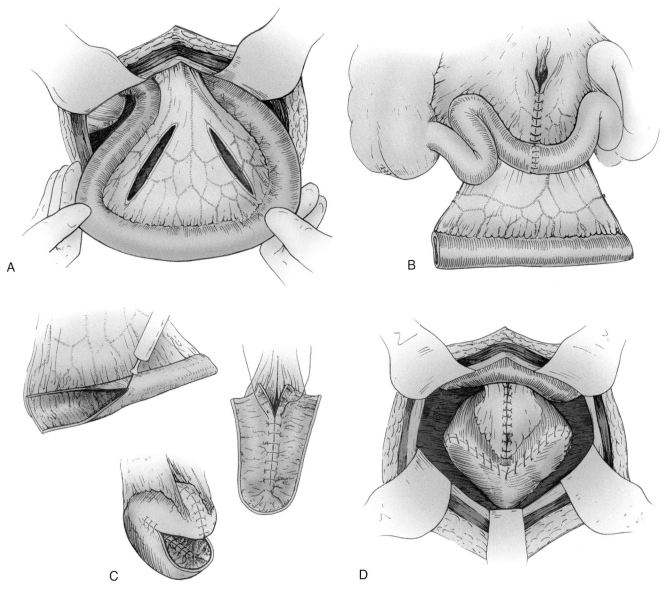

FIGURE 6-79 Ileocystoplasty for bladder augmentation.

10. With one third of the attachment complete, the surgeon places sutures at the anterior apex and runs them bilaterally to meet cephalad (Figure 6-79, *D*).
11. The surgeon fills the bladder to check the integrity of the anastomosis.
12. Abdominal closure is performed, and dressings are applied. The Foley catheter will remain for 7 to 14 days. Some surgeons may choose to place a suprapubic catheter instead of a Foley.

Implantation of Prosthetic Urethral Sphincter

Implantation of a prosthetic urethral sphincter is usually done as a last measure for patients with stress incontinence for which other modalities have failed. Problems with the device have included foreign-body reaction, persistent urethral pressure causing urethral erosion, and fluid hydraulic failure. The artificial sphincter unit has an abdominally placed, pressure-regulated reservoir that maintains a constant predetermined pressure on the periurethral cuff. Because of the connection between the reservoir and cuff, any increase in intraabdominal pressure transmits more fluid into the cuff. This connection allows for a compensatory increase in urethral resistance during coughing or straining.

The scrotal or labial pump shifts the fluid into the cuff to the reservoir to allow bladder emptying. The fluid reenters the cuff through a resistor in about 60 to 120 seconds. The locking button in the AMS Sphincter 800 artificial sphincter unit traps fluid in the reservoir to allow activation of the cuff. The sphincter is available in a single-cuff and double-cuff model.

Procedural Considerations. Standard laparotomy and lithotomy setups are required, as well as the sphincter components, contrast material diluted according to the manufacturer's recommendations, and an antibiotic solution. The patient is placed in a modified lithotomy position.

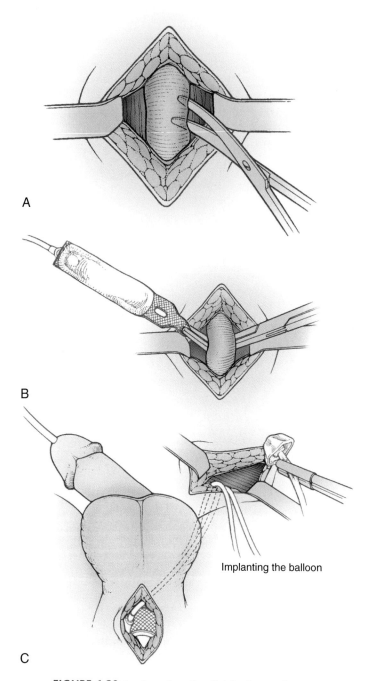

A

B

Implanting the balloon

C

FIGURE 6-80 Implantation of artificial urinary sphincter.

Stricture disease is more commonly found in the male population, and the most common cuff placement is around the bulbous urethra. Bladder neck placement of the cuff is generally reserved only for females.

Operative Procedure

BULBOUS URETHRAL CUFF

1. Perineal and transverse suprapubic incisions are made.
2. The surgeon mobilizes the bulbous urethra through a midline perineal incision (Figure 6-80, *A*).
3. A 2-cm space is created beneath the bulbocavernous muscle and around the bulbous urethra.

4. The surgeon places the cuff, tab end first, around the bulbous urethra (Figure 6-80, *B*).
5. The reservoir is placed beneath the rectus muscle through the suprapubic incision (Figure 6-80, *C*).
6. The surgeon attaches the pump to the tubing passer, introduces it through the suprapubic incision, and transfers it to the scrotum through a subcutaneous tunnel created between the two incisions. The reservoir, cuff, and pump are connected and filled with contrast material or injectable saline to the appropriate volume (Figure 6-81).
7. The wound is closed and dressed with gauze sponges. A urethral catheter is usually not inserted.

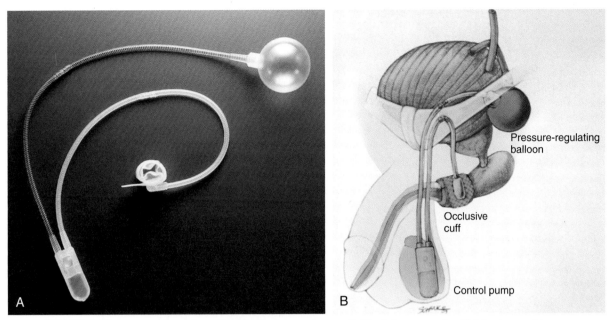

FIGURE 6-81 **A,** AMS 800 single-cuff artificial urinary sphincter. **B,** Final placement of artificial urinary sphincter.

Radical Cystectomy with Pelvic Lymphadenectomy

Cystectomy is the total excision of the urinary bladder and adjacent structures along with pelvic lymph nodes. Cystectomy is a surgical consideration when a vesical malignancy has invaded the muscular wall of the bladder or when frequent recurrences of widespread papillary tumors do not respond to endoscopic or chemotherapeutic management. The patient should be medically able to withstand surgery with the expectation of reasonable longevity. Total cystectomy necessitates permanent urinary diversion into an ileal or colonic conduit. In a male patient, the prostate gland, seminal vesicles, and distal ureters are removed with the bladder and its peritoneal surface. In a female patient, the bladder, urethra, distal ureters, uterus, cervix, and proximal third of the vagina are removed.

Procedural Considerations. The perioperative nurse places the patient in the supine position. Instruments are as described for major abdominal procedures. For a male patient, if the prostate and seminal vesicles are to be removed, prostatectomy instruments should be added. For a female patient, vaginal and abdominal hysterectomy as well as plastic surgery instruments should be added.

Operative Procedure. A midline incision from the epigastrium to the symphysis pubis, curving to the left of the umbilicus, is generally used.

1. The surgeon enters the peritoneal cavity above the umbilicus. The entire urachal remnant is clamped, divided, and ligated with heavy silk ligatures (Figure 6-82, *A*). It will be removed en bloc with the bladder.
2. The bladder dome is lifted at its peritoneal surface, and dissection proceeds laterally on either side with ligation of the major vesical arteries to the level of the vas deferens or round ligament (Figure 6-82, *B*).
3. The surgeon divides the vas deferens and cuts the urethra at the level of the pelvic diaphragm.

4. The ureters are identified and traced to the bladder. Care is taken to preserve the adventitial tissue (Figure 6-82, *C*).
5. Abdominal exploration and pelvic lymphadenectomy with frozen sections are performed to rule out metastatic disease.
6. In the male patient, the bladder is then retracted to expose the endopelvic fascia and puboprostatic ligaments. The prostate, dorsal venous complex, and seminal vesicles are dissected free, as described for a radical retropubic prostatectomy (Figure 6-82, *D*). These will be removed in continuity with the bladder.
7. In the female patient, the broad ligament is bilaterally incised posterior to the fallopian tube and ovary to the level of the posterior vagina to be removed en bloc with the bladder (Figure 6-82, *E*). The endopelvic fascia is incised at the bladder neck to expose the proximal urethra. The vagina is then incised along the lateral walls to the level of the proximal urethra and bladder neck. The anterior vaginal wall is incised in a U fashion to circumscribe the urethra (Figure 6-82, *F*). The vagina is reconstructed.
8. The surgical specimen consists of the bladder, distal ureters, prostate, seminal vesicles, and distal vas in the male and the uterus, fallopian tubes, and ovaries in the female and is removed en bloc.
9. The surgeon ligates the urethra with absorbable suture. If urethrectomy is indicated, this is done en bloc with the bladder.
10. Lap pads are placed in the denuded pelvis, and pressure is applied to reduce blood loss from oozing.
11. Urinary diversion is accomplished by means of an isolated ileal or colonic conduit, an orthotopic diversion, or a continent urinary diversion.

Bladder Substitution (Substitution Cystoplasty)

The ideal candidate for a bladder replacement after cystectomy for carcinoma is a patient with a normal urethra; a proximally located, well-differentiated bladder tumor; absence of carcinoma in situ; and proof, in the male patient, that the prostatic urethra is free of disease. High-dose radiation offers appreciable

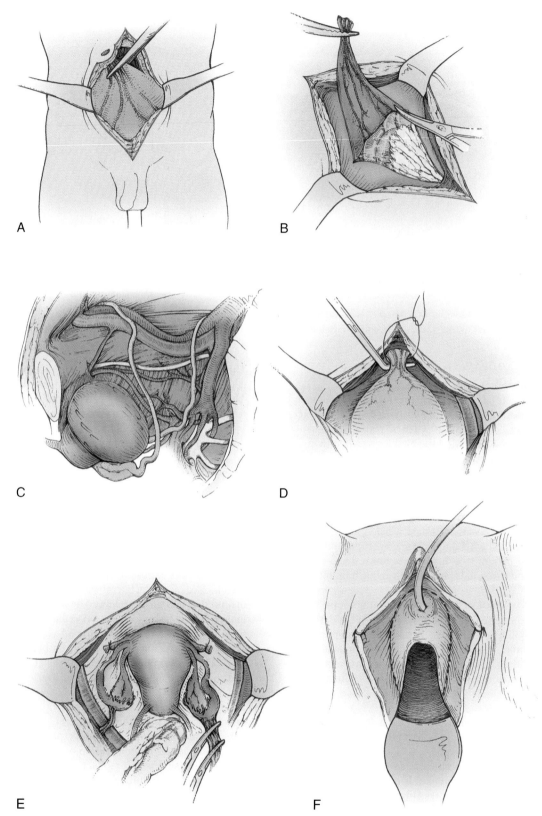

FIGURE 6-82 A, The urachal remnant is identified and divided just below the umbilicus. **B,** The peritoneum is divided laterally to the umbilical ligaments to the level of the vas deferens or round ligament. **C,** The ureter crossing the bifurcation of the iliac vessels is identified. **D,** Right-angled clamp is passed beneath the dorsal venous complex, anterior to the membranous urethra. **E,** In female patients the ovaries, fallopian tubes, and uterus are removed en bloc with the bladder and anterior vaginal wall. **F,** U-shaped incision is made on the anterior vagina to circumscribe the urethra.

risks for postoperative complications and is contraindicated with enterourethral anastomosis. A discussion of techniques to create a neobladder follows.

Right Colocystoplasty.

Depending on the extent of involvement, the right side of the colon may be used to replace the bladder, the bladder and prostatic urethra, or the bladder and prostate with a direct enteric-to-proximal bulbar urethral anastomosis. This procedure has become more functionally effective with the use of intermittent self-catheterization and selective implantation of a prosthetic urinary sphincter.

Ileocecal Bladder Substitution.

The ileum has been used as a reservoir to restore urinary continuity because it possesses a low intraluminal pressure. However, the short mesentery does not always permit the bowel to reach the urethra and results are not consistently successful. There have been significant incidences of recurrent carcinoma, renal damage, incontinence, postoperative strictures, fistula, hypokalemia, anemia, suture-line breakdown, and stone formation. Although most patients attain daytime urinary control, a small percentage still have problems with enuresis. Deterioration of the upper urinary tract as a result of infection and obstruction has historically been a significant risk with this procedure, and therefore ileocecal substitution is met with mixed reactions and recommendations.

Sigmoidocystoplasty.

Because of the sigmoid colon's ease of construction, bladder proximity, decreased obstruction from mucus, and large capacity, it has been more appealing to many surgeons in their attempt to create a new bladder. More efficient emptying with a larger reservoir capacity seems to occur with a sigmoid replacement. Results yield higher intraluminal pressures, more effective urinary flow rates, and less nocturnal incontinence than with ileal segments.

Ileoascending Bladder Substitution.

In an effort to improve the intestinal reservoir's capacity and antirefluxing effectiveness, the use of the ascending colon as a continent reservoir was introduced. This technique has several anatomic advantages over other methods of bladder replacement. The segment used can include the hepatic flexure and proximal transverse colon. A large-capacity reservoir is obtained, and colonic incision or tailoring is not required to achieve an appropriate shape. It easily reaches any site within the pelvis and can be anastomosed directly to the urethra without tension.

Orthotopic Ileocolic Neobladder.

The Le Bag continent diversion technique utilizes the right colon and ileum as an orthotopic bladder replacement. Bladder substitution relies on meticulous dissection of the prostatic apex with preservation of the urinary sphincter and neurovascular bundles, as well as a watertight urethral anastomosis. Most patients have achieved a high degree of daytime continence and a minimum of nocturnal enuresis. Short-term complications encountered include bleeding, infection, urinary extravasation, bladder perforation, urethral stricture, fistula formation, urinoma, and small-bowel obstruction. Long-term problems include chronic constipation or diarrhea, compromised enterohepatic circulation, vitamin B_{12} deficiency, and urinary incontinence in a small percentage of patients.

Considerations influencing patient selection include age, general health, and fitness for extensive, complicated surgery. Contraindications include previous radiation therapy, bowel disease (diverticulosis, Crohn's disease, colitis), and other major medical problems. Preoperative urethral biopsy specimens are frequently taken to rule out tumor or cellular atypia in the urethra, which would prevent this particular intervention.

PROCEDURAL CONSIDERATIONS. The patient is placed in the supine position. SCDs are applied before the induction of anesthesia. A cystectomy and prostatectomy or hysterectomy are performed. Major deep intestinal, bladder, and prostate or hysterectomy instruments, as well as a large self-retaining retractor, are needed.

OPERATIVE PROCEDURE

1. After cystoprostatectomy, the right side of the colon is reflected medially along the mesentery to the hepatic flexure. The distal ileum that is to be used in the neobladder is inspected.
2. The surgeon divides the small bowel, positions it in an S shape, and places stay sutures of 2-0 or 3-0 absorbable material.
3. The posterior walls are sewn from inside to outside with running 3-0 absorbable suture.
4. A seromuscular wedge of the dependent cecum is excised, and the mucosa is everted with 4-0 absorbable sutures to form a bladder neck.
5. The left ureter is brought retroperitoneally under the sigmoid mesentery, a submucosal tunnel is created, and the ureters are reimplanted through the colonic wall. Anastomosis is done from the interior of the pouch.
6. The surgeon places anchor sutures of 3-0 or 4-0 silk at the outer entry point. The wall of the colon is anchored to the psoas muscle with 3-0 or 4-0 silk to prevent migration of the neobladder.
7. Ureteral stents are placed and exteriorized through the colonic segment and a separate abdominal stab wound, along with a catheter, to serve as a suprapubic tube.
8. Sutures of 2-0 absorbable material are placed around the urethral stump and tagged.
9. The surgeon inserts a Foley catheter into the urethra in a retrograde manner, and the urethra is anastomosed to the neobladder at the point of the new bladder neck.
10. The neobladder is closed in an intestinal fashion or with a GI stapler in a side-to-side anastomosis. Wound drains are placed, the bladder filled to test for leaks, and the wound closed.

Cutaneous Urinary Diversions

Ileal Conduit.

The ileal conduit is the classic method by which the urine flow is diverted to an isolated loop of bowel. One end of the isolated loop is exteriorized through the skin so that the urine can be collected in a drainage bag, which is intermittently emptied. The surgeon consults with the enterostomal therapist preoperatively to determine the stoma site. The selected site, usually in the right lower quadrant of the abdomen, above the beltline, is marked with a fine needle dipped in methylene blue to prevent erasure during skin preparation. The goal is to create a round, protruding stoma without wrinkles in the skin, to prevent urine leakage under the collecting device. The candidate for ileal diversion must have a retrievable ureter at least 1 cm in diameter with a thick, well-vascularized wall. The patient must be able to care for the appliance. Conditions amenable to diversion include neurogenic bladder, interstitial cystitis, and bladder carcinoma. Cystectomy may be performed before or after this procedure, depending on the patient's diagnosis. In cases that do not involve bladder cancer, the surgeon may choose to leave the bladder in situ rather than subject a debilitated patient to further surgery. In certain cases of extensive bladder carcinoma, the surgeon may elect to treat the patient with radiation in an attempt to decrease the size of the tumor and neutralize the regional lymph nodes before performing cystectomy.

PROCEDURAL CONSIDERATIONS. The perioperative nurse assists with positioning the patient in the supine position. Abdominal and GI instruments are required. A cystectomy, prostatectomy, or hysterectomy may also be done at the time of the surgery. Endostapling devices, with absorbable staples, should be available.

OPERATIVE PROCEDURE

1. The bladder is decompressed with a catheter.
2. The surgeon enters the abdomen through a midline abdominal incision and places a self-retaining abdominal retractor to exclude the viscera from the region of dissection.
3. The ureters are identified and severed approximately 2.5 cm from the bladder.
4. The surgeon creates a retroperitoneal tunnel so that the left ureter lies close to the right ureter.
5. The distal ileum and mesentery are inspected to identify the bowel's blood supply.
6. A drain is passed through the mesentery, midway between the two main arterial arcades adjacent to the ileum at the proximal and distal ends of the selected segment. This segment usually makes up 15 to 20 cm of the terminal ileum, a few centimeters from the ileocecal valve. The ileocecal artery is preserved to maintain adequate circulation to the isolated ileal segment.
7. The surgeon incises the peritoneum over the proposed line of division of the mesentery.
8. Intestinal clamps are placed across the ileum, and the bowel is divided flush with the clamps.
9. Using GI technique (also referred to as bowel technique; see Chapter 2), the surgeon closes the proximal end of the isolated ileal segment first with a layer of absorbable sutures and then with a second layer of interrupted 2-0 nonabsorbable sutures.
10. The proximal and distal segments of ileum are reanastomosed end-to-end in two layers.
11. The surgeon closes the mesenteric incision with interrupted nonabsorbable sutures.
12. The closed proximal end of the conduit segment is fixed to the posterior peritoneum.
13. The ureters are implanted in the ileal segment, using fine instruments and 4-0 absorbable ureteral sutures on atraumatic needles.
14. The surgeon separates the peritoneum and muscle of the abdominal wall lateral to the original incision with blunt dissection.
15. The abdominal opening for the stoma is made, and the distal opening of the ileal conduit is then drawn through a fenestration in the muscle, fascia, and skin.
16. The ileum is fixed to the fascia with 2-0 sutures. A rosebud stoma is constructed as the ileum is sutured to the skin using subcuticular stitches (Figure 6-83).

17. Ureteral stents are usually left in the stoma, and a urinary collecting pouch is placed over the rosebud stoma to collect urine.
18. The surgeon inserts closed-suction wound drains and closes the abdominal incision. The skin is reapproximated.

Continent Urinary Diversions

The Kock pouch, the right colocystoplasty, and the Camey version of the ileocystoplasty have been modified for anastomosis to a urethral stump or the prostatic capsule, resulting in effective continent bladder replacement. All continent urinary diversions create an easily catheterized stoma and a nonrefluxing ureteral anastomosis. Different parts of the bowel and the stomach have been used as continent reservoirs. The choice of the antireflux mechanism depends on the implantation site. The stoma does not require an appliance; therefore the site may be placed below the beltline or bikini line, permitting it to be catheterized when the patient is sitting. It may be anastomosed to the proximal urethra, thus forming an orthotopic bladder.

Ileal Reservoir (Kock Pouch)

PROCEDURAL CONSIDERATIONS. A continent reservoir formed into a U configuration is constructed from a section of ileum proximal to the ileocecal valve. The legs of the U are sewn together at the antimesenteric border. The intestine is opened adjacent to the antimesenteric border, and the back wall of the pouch is reinforced with absorbable suture.

Continence is achieved by the valve mechanism with the nipple valve attached to the skin. Nipple valves are created proximally and distally by intussusception of the bowel into the reservoir cavity. Once the nipples are fixed to the sidewall of the reservoir with absorbable suture or polyglycolic staples, the anterior wall is closed. The ureters are anastomosed to the afferent limb of the pouch, preventing reflux. The efferent limb is drawn through the stoma site and anchored to the abdominal wall fascia.

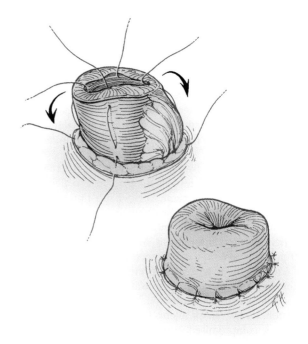

FIGURE 6-83 Rosebud suture technique for stoma.

OPERATIVE PROCEDURE

1. The mesentery is divided and suture-ligated or staple-ligated along the avascular plane between the superior mesenteric artery and the ileocolic artery.
2. The surgeon divides the bowel, and four segments are measured and marked with silk suture tags. These segments will serve as the efferent conduit, the pouch, and the afferent limb.
3. A portion of the proximal ileum is resected and discarded along with a wedge of mesentery. Suction is passed down the lumen to clear any fecal material or mucus.
4. The surgeon closes the proximal end of the bowel with suture or staples.
5. The segment to be employed is spread out in a U-shaped fashion. The sides are sewn together with 3-0 absorbable suture in a running stitch or connected using a GI endostapler.
6. The surgeon uses the ESU to incise the bowel laterally to the suture in the two loops. The medial edges are oversewn with 3-0 or 4-0 silk.
7. The mesentery is cleared on the limb segments, and the lumens are intussuscepted into the open pouch.
8. Synthetic mesh is used to serve as a strut to prevent peristomal herniation and to fix the base of the efferent nipple to the abdominal wall, facilitating catheterization. The TA or similar endostapler is used to form each nipple and to attach the nipples to the back wall of the pouch.
9. An 8F stenting catheter is placed inside the nipple of the efferent conduit to prevent the formation of a collar that is too tight.
10. The surgeon secures the limbs with 3-0 or 4-0 silk suture.
11. The pouch is closed with sutures or the endostapler.
12. The ureters are anastomosed, as described in the "Ileal Conduit" discussion, to the afferent limb.
13. A small stoma site is prepared, as described in the Ileal Conduit discussion. A catheter of choice is placed in the stoma for postoperative care. Stents may be placed in the ureters for the immediate postoperative period. This will necessitate initial placement of an ileostomy appliance until all systems are functioning.
14. A drain is placed, which exits through a separate stab wound.
15. The surgeon closes the wound. Retention sutures may be employed. Bulky absorbent dressings are applied; Montgomery straps may be used.

Indiana Pouch

PROCEDURAL CONSIDERATIONS. The Indiana pouch technique is a modification of the original ileocecal diversion. The surgeon constructs a continent reservoir from the right side of the colon, which may include the ileum and cecum, the ileocecal valve, and ascending colon. Surgery proceeds as for any diversionary procedure. The ileocecal valve is reinforced with nonabsorbable suture. Two rows of nonabsorbable suture are used to then imbricate the ileal segment, which serves as a limb that can be catheterized once it is exteriorized to the skin level as a stoma. The cecal segment is detubularized by incising along the taenia and anastomosing the distal edge horizontally to the proximal portion. Intussusception of the ileocecal valve into the cecum and narrowing of the ileal segment attached to the skin allow for continence.

OPERATIVE PROCEDURE

1. The large bowel is split down the antimesenteric border for approximately three fourths of its length.
2. The U-shaped defect is closed.
3. The surgeon sutures the terminal ileum along its length over a small Robinson catheter in an intestinal fashion.
4. The pouch is filled with 400 ml of saline, and a larger catheter is placed to determine ability to be catheterized.
5. The ureters are tunneled into the cecum through its taenia and then tacked to the outer bowel wall. The cecum is secured to the pelvic wall. Ureteral stents may be placed.
6. The pouch is secured to the abdominal wall.
7. The surgeon prepares the stomal site as described in the Ileal Conduit discussion.
8. A 22F Malecot drain is placed in the reservoir to drain the cecostomy, exiting through a separate stab wound.

SURGERY OF THE URETERS AND KIDNEYS

Stones, infections, and tumors are the most common causes of urinary tract obstruction, necessitating surgery to prevent renal obstruction and subsequent renal failure. Obstruction may also result from congenital malformations or previous operations on the urinary tract (Figure 6-84).

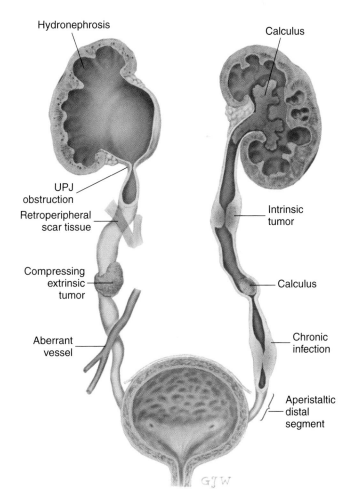

Hydronephrosis

Calculus

UPJ obstruction

Retroperipheral scar tissue

Intrinsic tumor

Compressing extrinsic tumor

Calculus

Aberrant vessel

Chronic infection

Aperistaltic distal segment

FIGURE 6-84 Some common causes of urinary tract obstruction. *UPJ,* ureteropelvic junction.

The ureter has three areas of narrowing where calculi may become lodged and pose a potential problem with pain and obstruction: (1) the ureteropelvic junction (UPJ), (2) the crossing of the ureter over the external iliac vessels, and (3) the ureterovesical junction (UVJ). Urine may sometimes cause calculi to be washed down the ureter to produce severe ureteral colic. The majority of renal calculi are spontaneously passed into the bladder. However, if they become lodged in the ureter, surgical intervention may be indicated.

Although the causes of many kidney stones are obscure, certain conditions, such as obstruction, stasis, and imbalance of metabolism, predispose to their formation. Stones consist of various elements: calcium oxalate, calcium phosphate, magnesium ammonium phosphate, uric acid, calcium carbonate, and cystine. An increase in the concentration of any of these compounds can cause tiny crystals to form; as these clump together, they begin to form a stone. Stones removed during surgery are subjected to chemical analysis and should be submitted in a dry jar. Fixative agents such as formalin should not be used.

Stones in the renal pelvis may fall into the ureteropelvic junction and obstruct the flow of urine. However, stones less than 3 cm in diameter may also pass down the ureter and lodge at a more distal location. A stone may remain in a renal calyx and continue to enlarge, eventually filling the entire renal collecting system (staghorn calculus). Diverticula may form and harbor stones that can be difficult to reach and treat. Hydroureteronephrosis, infection, and destruction of renal parenchyma frequently result from unrelieved obstruction.

Hypothermia may be used as an adjunct to renal stone surgery as a means of prolonging the safe period of renal ischemia. Several methods enable renal cooling: ice slush or cold saline solution, surface cooling coils, perfusion of cold solutions through the renal artery, or a variation of these basic techniques, such as perfusion of the renal pelvis with saline that has been cooled by a coil immersed in ice slush.

A refrigeration unit "slush machine" that produces sterile slush provides a cost-effective, time-saving alternative to the other methods of slush preparation. Commercially synthesized ultrafiltrate of sterile plasma in liter bottles is also available for use as the slush. Alternatively, a rigid plastic container of 1000 ml of normal saline or lactated Ringer's solution may be placed on its side in a freezer several hours before surgery. To prevent the solution from solidifying, the container should be rotated one-half turn every 20 to 30 minutes. Sterile slush may then be poured directly into a sterile basin as required.

The surgical approach in renal surgery depends on the patient's condition, the amount of exposure needed, and the surgical procedure to be performed. There are three principal surgical approaches to the kidney. The simple *flank,* or *transabdominal,* incision is most frequently used and may include removal of the eleventh or twelfth rib. The incision begins at the posterior axillary line and parallels the course of the twelfth rib. It extends forward and slightly downward between the iliac crest and the thorax. For the *lumbar* incision, the patient may be initially positioned supine and then rotated to lateral and slightly forward over protective bolsters with the operative side up. This effectively places the flank in an oblique position, causing the abdominal viscera to fall away from the operative incision, and affords an excellent approach to the renal pedicle. Alternatively, the patient may be placed prone with bolsters under the affected side to provide elevation. The *thoracoabdominal* exposure is employed primarily for large upper-pole renal neoplasms. The tenth and eleventh ribs are usually removed, and the chest cavity is opened, collapsing the lung. The leaves of the diaphragm are separated to expose the kidney.

Ureteral Surgery

Ureterostomy (ureterotomy) is opening the ureter for continued drainage from it into another body part. Cutaneous ureterostomy is diversion of the flow of urine from the kidney, through the ureter, away from the bladder, and onto the skin of the lower abdomen. A suitable urinary collecting device is then placed over the ureteral stoma.

Ureterectomy is complete removal of the ureter. This procedure is generally employed in collecting system tumors and includes nephrectomy and the excision of a cuff of bladder.

Ureteroureterostomy is segmental resection of a diseased portion of the ureter and reconstruction in continuity of the two normal segments.

Ureteroenterostomy is diversion of the ureter into a segment of the ileum (ureteroileostomy, or more commonly, ileal urinary conduit) or into the sigmoid colon (ureterosigmoidostomy). Ureteroneocystostomy (ureterovesical anastomosis) is division of the distal ureter from the bladder and reimplantation of the ureter into the bladder with a submucosal tunnel.

Reconstructive operations may be indicated because of a pathologic condition of the bladder or lower ureter that interferes with normal drainage. Conditions requiring urinary diversion or reconstruction of the urinary tract include malignancy, cystitis, stricture, trauma, and congenital ureterovesical reflux. Invasive vesical malignancy requiring surgical removal of the bladder necessitates urinary diversion.

Ureterocutaneous transplant, ureterosigmoid anastomosis, and ileal conduit are urinary diversionary procedures performed when the bladder is no longer functioning as a proper urine reservoir. Etiologic factors causing irreparable vesical dysfunction are chronic inflammation, interstitial cystitis, neurogenic bladder, exstrophy, trauma, tumor, and infiltrative disease (amyloidosis). Ureterolithotomy is incision into the ureter and removal of an obstructing calculus.

Procedural Considerations. The site of the incision and position of the patient depend on the nature of the proposed surgery. The patient may be placed in the supine position for abdominal surgery, in the modified Trendelenburg's position for low abdominal or pelvic surgery, or in the lateral position for high- or mid-ureteral obstructing calculi. The perioperative nurse ensures that the patient's arms are supinated when on armboards; in lateral position the upper arm is placed on an overbed armboard such as the Allen lateral arm support and the lower arm is supinated on a padded armboard. The kidney rest should lie just under the dependent iliac crest.

Instruments include the nephrectomy set, plus plastic instrumentation for pyeloplasty. Additional instruments may be required, depending on the type of operation and the surgical approach used.

Operative Procedure
URETERAL REIMPLANTATION
1. The surgeon exposes the ureter through an incision determined by the location of the pathologic condition. A ureteral catheter, passed retrograde, may be used to facilitate identification and isolation of the ureter.

2. The ureter is dissected free with long forceps and scissors, picked up with fine traction sutures, freed from the surrounding tissues, and severed at the desired level.

3. The surgeon ligates the distal end of the ureter and transfers the proximal stoma to the site of anastomosis. The anastomosis is accomplished with fine dissection instruments and fine atraumatic sutures.

4. A soft splinting stent is usually left in place until healing has taken place and free drainage is ensured. The wound is closed in layers and dressings applied.

URETEROCUTANEOUS TRANSPLANT (ANASTOMOSIS). The surgical approach is the same as that for a low ureterolithotomy.

1. The ureter is divided as far distally as possible.

2. The surgeon passes the severed ureter retroperitoneally through the lower abdominal wall and sutures it to the skin with an absorbable everting suture of 4-0 on an atraumatic needle to form a stoma. The ureter is handled gently with plastic instruments, fixation forceps, and iris scissors.

3. A small Silastic stenting catheter is passed up into the ureter and left in place for 48 to 72 hours, as ureteral edema subsides. The patient requires a urine-collecting device after surgery.

URETEROSIGMOID ANASTOMOSIS

1. The surgeon enters the peritoneal cavity through a lower left paramedian incision.

2. The major portion of the large bowel is protected with moist laparotomy packs.

3. Deep retractors are placed, and the surgeon uses long forceps and scissors to incise the posterior peritoneum.

4. The ureters are identified, divided close to the bladder, mobilized, and brought through the posterior peritoneal incision to lie near the sigmoid. Traction sutures and smooth tissue forceps are used to handle the ureters.

5. The sigmoid colon is mobilized to prevent tension on the ureteroenteric anastomosis.

6. Using 3-0 nonabsorbable suture material, the surgeon sutures the sigmoid colon to the pelvic peritoneum at a point where the ureter falls easily on the bowel.

7. Using a scalpel with a #15 blade, the surgeon makes an incision into the taenia of the sigmoid down to the mucosal layer. The edges of the taenia are undermined to create two parallel flaps.

8. The ureter is laid on the bowel mucosa, and a small slit is made through the mucosa into the lumen of the colon.

9. With fixation forceps and iris scissors, the surgeon bevels the ureter to lie flat in the tunica incision.

10. The distal ureter is anchored to the bowel mucosa with 4-0 absorbable ureteral sutures on atraumatic needles. The other ureter is anastomosed in the same manner in a position slightly above the first.

11. The tunicae are then loosely reapproximated over the ureter with 4-0 absorbable sutures, creating an antireflux anastomosis.

12. The surgeon closes the posterior peritoneum with absorbable sutures. Drains are exteriorized retroperitoneally. The incision is closed and dressings applied.

Ureterolithotomy

PROCEDURAL CONSIDERATIONS. A KUB x-ray examination should be done immediately before surgery to determine the exact location of the stone. The surgeon may also schedule a cystoscopic examination preoperatively and may attempt to remove the stone endoscopically. The location of the stone determines the surgical approach. A stone high in the ureter requires a flank incision with possible removal of the twelfth rib; a more distal ureteral stone requires a lower abdominal incision.

OPERATIVE PROCEDURE

1. After exposure of the ureter, the stone may be kept stationary with Babcock clamps or vessel loops applied above and below it.

2. With a #15 blade, the surgeon makes an incision in the ureter directly over the stone, which may be easily removed with Randall stone forceps.

3. A 10F catheter is passed proximally up and distally down the ureter while irrigating with saline to check for ureteral patency and to dislodge any remaining stone fragments.

4. The surgeon closes the ureter with 4-0 or 5-0 absorbable sutures. All stones should be placed in dry receptacles and sent to the chemistry laboratory for analysis.

Kidney Surgery

See Box 6-2 for terms pertaining to kidney surgery.

Procedural Considerations. Patient preparation and instrument setup are as described for ureteral surgery.

Operative Procedure
PYELOTOMY AND PYELOSTOMY

1. The surgeon incises the pelvis of the kidney with a small scalpel blade. Fine traction sutures may be placed at the edges of the incision for gentle retraction while the pelvis and calyces are explored.

2. In pyelostomy a small Malecot or Foley catheter is placed through the incision into the renal pelvis. Pyelotomy is used only for very short periods of renal drainage because tubes tend to be dislodged easily from the renal pelvis.

BOX 6-2

Terms Pertaining to Kidney Surgery

Term	Definition
Nephrostomy	Creation of an opening into the kidney to maintain temporary or permanent urinary drainage. A nephrostomy is used to correct an obstruction of the urinary tract and to conserve and permit physiologic functioning of renal tissue. It is also used to provide permanent urinary drainage when a ureter is obstructed or for temporary urinary drainage immediately after a plastic repair on the kidney.
Nephrotomy	Incision into the kidney, usually over a collecting system containing a calculus
Pyelolithotomy	Removal of a calculus through an opening in the renal pelvis
Pyelostomy	Making an opening in the renal pelvis for temporarily or permanently diverting the flow of urine
Pyelotomy	Incision into the renal pelvis used as an access to stones in the renal pelvis or collecting system

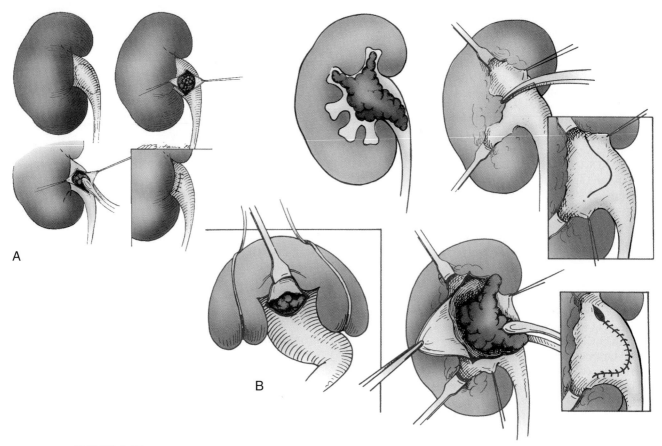

FIGURE 6-85 Pyelolithotomy. **A,** Technique of simple pyelolithotomy. **B,** Technique of extended pyelolithotomy.

NEPHROSTOMY

1. The surgeon passes a curved clamp or stone forceps through a pyelotomy incision into the renal pelvis and then out through the substance of the renal parenchyma through a lower pole minor calyx.
2. The tip of a Malecot, Foley, or Pezzer catheter is drawn into the renal pelvis, and the pyelotomy incision is sutured closed.
3. The distal end of the nephrostomy tube is exteriorized through a separate stab incision in the flank.
4. A drain is placed at the level of the pyelotomy incision, and the wound is closed.

PYELOLITHOTOMY AND NEPHROLITHOTOMY

1. The surgeon opens the renal pelvis (Figure 6-85, *A*), and removes the calculus.
2. The pelvis and collecting systems are thoroughly irrigated with saline using an Asepto syringe to dislodge and remove any small remaining stones from the kidney.
3. Nephrolithotomy or extended pyelolithotomy is employed when stones are locked in the calyceal system and cannot be removed through a pyelotomy incision. In such cases, the renal parenchyma above the stone is incised and the stone removed. In many instances, such a situation is associated with a calyceal diverticulum (Figure 6-85, *B*).
4. After the stone is removed, the collecting system is closed and the renal cortex reapproximated with deep hemostatic 2-0 absorbable sutures.
5. A nephroscope is sometimes used to localize and remove calyceal stones. The nephroscope is also useful with staghorn

calculi to remove residual fragments in the pelvic portion of the calculus.
6. An incision in the renal pelvis may be closed with 4-0 absorbable atraumatic sutures.
7. The renal fossa is drained and closed, as described for nephrectomy. Reinforced absorbent dressings are useful because some urinary leakage occurs for 3 to 4 days after surgery.

PERCUTANEOUS NEPHROLITHOTOMY. Percutaneous nephrolithotomy facilitates the removal or disintegration of renal stones using a rigid or flexible nephroscope (Figure 6-86) passed through a percutaneous nephrostomy tract. Accessory instrumentation, such as the ultrasound wand, electrohydraulic lithotripter probe, laser fiber, stone basket, and stone grasper, is passed through the lumen of the nephroscope.

Ideally, the patient is in good health and not obese and the calculus is 1 cm or less in diameter, free-floating, radiopaque, and solitary. However, advances in technology complemented by the experience gained by the uroradiology team have allowed patients with more complex problems to be managed in this manner. Patients who have undergone previous renal surgery, have stone recurrence, or have an established nephrostomy tract may also benefit from this procedure.

Creation of the nephrostomy tract and removal of the stone can be accomplished by three different methods. Proper placement of the nephrostomy wire can decrease the operating time significantly. In the *one-step procedure*, creation of the nephrostomy tract, tract dilation, and stone removal are completed in a

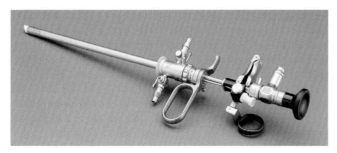

FIGURE 6-86 Kuntz laser working element.

single session. This method is generally preferred unless there are contraindications. In the *immediate two-step procedure,* the radiologist places the nephrostomy tube under radiographic guidance and the urologist removes the stone later the same day or the next morning. The second step is usually done in the OR with the patient administered a general anesthetic. In the *delayed two-step procedure,* the nephrostomy tract is established after the patient has been administered a local anesthetic. The patient is discharged the following day with a 22F or 24F nephrostomy tube connected to drainage. The patient is readmitted to the hospital 5 to 7 days later for the percutaneous removal of the stone after the patient has been administered a general anesthetic.

Of basic concern during the operative phase are the patient's position and body temperature, the potential for sudden and rapid blood loss, the type of anesthesia, medications required during surgery, and catheter management during and after the procedure. The patient's position, which may be prone or up to 30 degrees prone-oblique, and the draping procedure depend on whether the surgery is performed in the radiology department or the OR and the type of x-ray equipment that will be used.

Extracorporeal Shock-Wave Lithotripsy (ESWL). ESWL units use water-filled cushions adjacent to the kidney area. An x-ray image intensifier with two monitors is used to visualize the kidney stone at the focal point of the shock wave. After every 100 shocks, fluoroscopy is used to locate remaining stone particles. Adjustments are made, and the patient is repositioned before further treatments. ESWL is often used with percutaneous nephrolithotomy and transurethral ureteropyeloscopy if the patient does not pass the gravel.

Stones that are treated with ESWL are fragmented by the energy focused on the stone with the lithotripter. The shock waves are administered over a time that can vary from 30 minutes to 2 hours. Shock waves reverberate inside the stone, causing fragmentation with ultimate complete or partial destruction of the calculus. The amount of destruction depends on the number and energy of the shock waves delivered and the hardness of the stone. This technique is effective because shock waves can be transmitted and focused through tissue without loss of energy. A loud, reverberating, popping sound occurs each time a wave pulse is activated. It is advisable that earplugs be worn.

The requirement for anesthesia is determined by the power of the shock wave, the area of shock-wave entry at the skin level, and the size of the shock-wave focal point. The summation of shock waves used during the procedure can cause pain at the skin level. Typically, a general, spinal, or local anesthetic is used with the older lithotripters. Modern versions allow for lithotripsy with only IV sedation, oral sedation, or a transcutaneous electric nerve stimulator (TENS) unit.

The use of a stent before ESWL depends on the patient and the character of the stone or stones. The patient should have a negative urine culture before stent placement. Studies show that complication rates decrease if a stent is used with a stone larger than 1.5 cm. A stent placed before ESWL tends to decrease the need for ancillary interventions, reduces overall complications, and assists in proper positioning for ESWL by delineating the ureteral anatomy and the precise stone location. On the other hand, those patients who tend to readily form stones may demonstrate calcification of the ureteral stent in a relatively short time. Without a stent, the risk of silent renal obstruction resulting in loss of kidney function, obstruction of the ureter, nephritis, and sepsis is increased.

Complications related to ESWL are attributable to the cavitation effects of treatment and are proportional to the number of shocks. The ability of the kidney's tubular cells to survive shock waves is related to the number of shock waves to which the kidney is exposed and not to the energy level. Gross hematuria is seen almost universally, resolves in 12 to 48 hours, and is believed to be attributable to parenchymal edema that spontaneously heals within 1 week. Subcapsular or perirenal hematoma caused by perinephric fluid collections may occur and appears to be higher in the hypertensive patient. Subcapsular hematoma may resolve in 6 weeks or may take up to 6 months, whereas perirenal hematoma will be relieved usually in a matter of days. Impairment of renal function may be seen in patients with solitary kidneys. Iliac artery and vein thromboses have been reported with lithotripsy for ureteral stones. The majority of lithotripsy patients will demonstrate little or no long-term morbidity (Gayer, 2006).

Laser Lithotripsy. Laser lithotripsy has become an exciting alternative to ESWL and electrohydraulic lithotripsy (EHL). The Ho:YAG (holmium:yttrium-aluminum-garnet), tunable pulse-dyed (coumarin), Er:YAG (erbium:yttrium-aluminum-garnet), the tunable Alexandrite (a chromium-doped mineral), or the Q-switched Nd:YAG (neodymium:yttrium-aluminum-garnet) laser systems have the ability to disintegrate stones without damaging soft tissue. The technique may be used during a ureteropyeloscopy or nephroscopy or to manage ureteral stones instead of performing a ureterolithotomy. When the laser probe is discharged in direct contact with the calculus, plasma (ionized gas) coats the stone's surface. This plasma expands with repeated firings, creating a shock wave that fractures the stone. Normal saline is used for continuous irrigation throughout the procedure. It is not necessary to immobilize the calculus. All persons in the room wear laser goggles, and all laser precautions apply.

Dismembered Pyeloplasty. Pyeloplasty is revision or plastic reconstruction of the renal pelvis. Pyeloplasty is performed to create a better anatomic relationship between the renal pelvis and the proximal ureter and to allow proper urinary drainage from the kidney to the bladder. A temporary nephrostomy is often included to protect the plastic reconstruction of the ureteropelvic junction (UPJ). Tissue healing usually occurs in 10 to 12 days, and the nephrostomy tube is removed once ureteral patency is demonstrated. *Ureteroplasty* is reconstruction of the ureter distal to the UPJ. A *dismembered pyeloplasty* is the combined correction of the redundant renal pelvis and resection of a stenotic portion of the UPJ.

PROCEDURAL CONSIDERATIONS. The instrument setup is as described for nephrectomy, plus fine plastic and vascular instrumentation and Randall stone forceps. A ureteral stent and red rubber catheters will also be employed. The perioperative nurse assists with positioning the patient in the lateral position.

OPERATIVE PROCEDURE

Open Approach

1. The surgeon exposes the kidney and upper ureter through a supracostal flank incision.
2. Gerota's fascia is entered, and the renal pelvis and ureter are freed while the kidney is rotated medially.
3. The surgeon frees the ureter and stabilizes it with a vessel loop below the level of the UPJ.
4. A 4-0 stay suture is placed in the tip of the ureter, and the ureter is incised, trimmed, and shaped to the desired contour with fine forceps and scissors.
5. Anchoring sutures of 4-0 material are placed for traction during reconstruction of the renal pelvis. A diamond-shaped incision is made into the renal pelvis, and the tissue is removed. The Y-V-plasty technique may be followed. It converts a Y-shaped surgical incision of the renal pelvis into a V by drawing the apex of the arms of the Y to the foot of the Y with absorbable sutures.
6. Sutures are placed at each end of the refashioned renal pelvis, passed to the ureteral stoma, and tagged. The pelvis is irrigated free of clots. The sutures are run in a continuous manner, creating the anastomosis.
7. A Silastic tubing may be used to stent the repaired pelvis until adequate healing has occurred. A nephrostomy tube is also placed within the pelvis to divert urine safely while the edema in the area of the repair resolves.
8. The surgeon closes Gerota's fascia over the repair.
9. A drain is placed where the pelvis was reconstructed, and the surgical incision is closed in layers.

Laparoscopic Approach. UPJ obstruction has recently joined the rank of surgeries that may be treated laparoscopically. Generally, a standard transperitoneal approach is used. The patient may be placed supine with a lateral tilt or in lateral decubitus and the bed rotated to access the ports.

After placement of four trocars as in laparoscopic nephrectomy, the surgeon frees the proximal ureters and renal pelvis. The obstruction at the UPJ is excised, and a spatulated anastomosis is performed using running or interrupted sutures. A ureteral stent is usually left in place.

Decreased postoperative pain and shorter hospitalization make this approach appealing. A higher degree of skill is required for this technique, however, making it an option that has not become standard treatment as yet.

Nephroureterectomy—Open Approach. Nephroureterectomy is removal of a kidney and its entire ureter. This procedure is indicated for hydroureteronephrosis of such a degree that reconstructive repair is impossible. It is also employed for collecting system tumors of the kidney and ureter.

PROCEDURAL CONSIDERATIONS. Open nephroureterectomy requires an extension of the incision anteriorly with the patient positioned semilaterally and fully prepped and draped

for the surgeon to access the flank and lower abdomen. Only one instrument set is required, but a second skin-prep setup and set of sterile drapes may be necessary. An alternative to open nephroureterectomy is laparoscopic nephroureterectomy.

OPERATIVE PROCEDURE

1. The surgeon exposes the kidney and upper ureter and performs a nephrectomy as described in the following procedure. The kidney may be placed in a plastic bag to prevent possible spillage of tumor cells.
2. The ureter is mobilized as far distally as possible. The OR bed is adjusted so that surgery on the lower ureter may proceed. The lower ureter and bladder are identified and mobilized.
3. The ureter and a small cuff of the bladder are removed in continuity, and the bladder is repaired with a single layer of 2-0 absorbable interrupted sutures. The ureter and cuff of bladder are pulled superiorly, and the intact kidney and ureter are removed.
4. An 18F or 20F Foley catheter is left in the bladder, and a drain is placed behind the bladder. The incision is closed in layers.

Nephrectomy—Open Approach. Nephrectomy is the surgical removal of a kidney. It is performed as a means of definitive therapy for many renal problems, such as congenital UPJ obstruction with severe hydronephrosis, renal tumor, renal trauma, calculus disease with infection, cortical abscess, pyelonephrosis, and renovascular hypertension.

In routine renal surgery the patient is placed in the lateral position with the dependent iliac crest over the kidney rest. The operative flank is uppermost, with the patient's back brought to the edge of the OR bed. The upper arm is supported on an overhead arm support, and the lower arm is supinated on a padded armboard. It may be flexed slightly at the elbow and angled cephalad to promote better access to the flank. The patient's legs are positioned by placing a pillow between them and flexing the lower leg at the knee. The upper leg remains extended. The kidney rest is then raised, and when the desired bed flexion is achieved, 3-inch adhesive tape is used to stabilize the patient throughout surgery. Routine skin preparation and draping procedures are carried out.

PROCEDURAL CONSIDERATIONS. The nephrectomy setup includes a routine laparotomy setup; kidney instruments (Figure 6-87); a variety of red rubber, Malecot, or Pezzer catheters; a wound drainage system; and vessel loops. In certain nephrectomies the chest or the GI tract may be opened. If the chest is opened, appropriate instruments and postoperative chest drains are needed. Rib resection requires the addition of a Finochietto rib retractor, a large Matson costal periosteotome, an Alexander costal periosteotome, right and left Doyen rib raspatories, a Bethune rib cutter, a double-action duckbill rongeur, a Bailey rib approximator, and a Langenbeck periosteal elevator. When the GI tract is opened, GI technique is used for the anastomosis.

OPERATIVE PROCEDURE

1. The incision is carried through the skin, fat, and fascia. Bleeding vessels are clamped and ligated.
2. The surgeon exposes and incises the external oblique, internal oblique, and transversalis muscles in the direction of the initial skin incision.

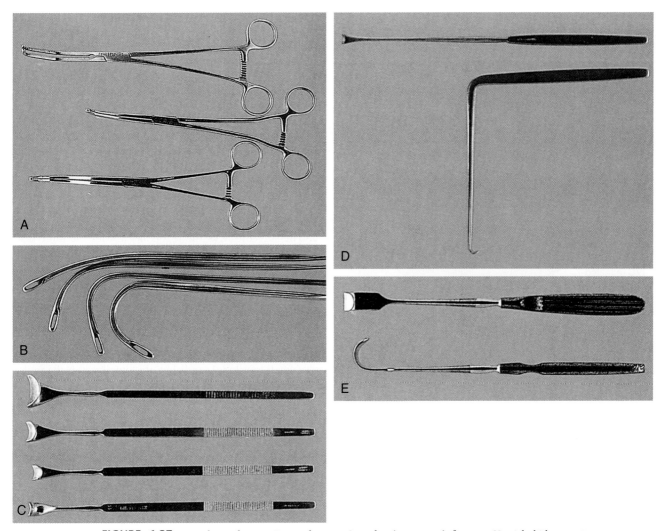

FIGURE 6-87 A, Kidney clamps. *Top to bottom,* Satinsky (vena cava) forceps; Herrick kidney forceps; Mayo-Guyon kidney forceps. **B**, Randall stone forcep tips. *Top to bottom,* ¼ curved, ½ curved, ¾ curved, full curved. **C**, Gil-Vernet retractors, front view. **D**, *Top to bottom,* Love nerve retractors: straight, front view; 90-degree angle, side view. **E**, *Top to bottom,* Little retractors, medium: front view, side view.

3. If necessary, a rib or ribs (eleventh and/or twelfth) may be resected to provide better access to the kidney. The surgeon strips the periosteum with an Alexander costal periosteotome and Doyen rib raspatory. A scalpel and heavy scissors are used to cut through the lumbocostal ligaments. The rib is grasped with an Ochsner clamp and cut with rib shears, removing the portion necessary to expose the kidney. Gerota's fascia is identified and incised with Metzenbaum scissors.

4. The surgeon extends the incision and uses blunt and sharp dissection to expose the kidney and perirenal fat. The surgical technologist should save all perirenal fat that is removed during surgery, placing it in a small basin of normal saline for possible use as a bolster to stop bleeding.

5. The ureter is identified, separated from its adjacent structures, doubly clamped, divided, and ligated with absorbable 0 suture.

6. The kidney pedicle containing the major blood vessels is isolated and doubly clamped; each vessel is triply ligated with heavy nonabsorbable ties. Each vessel is then severed, leaving two ligatures on the pedicle, and the kidney is removed (Figure 6-88).

7. The renal fossa is explored for bleeding, and necessary hemostasis is achieved. The fossa is then irrigated with normal saline, and the irrigant is removed by suction.

8. The surgeon closes the fascia and muscle in layers with interrupted absorbable sutures. Retention sutures may be used in obese or chronically ill patients in whom wound healing may be delayed.

9. The skin edges are approximated with sutures or skin staples, and the dressing is applied.

Laparoscopic Nephrectomy. The approach for laparoscopic nephrectomy may be transabdominal (transperitoneal), extraperitoneal (retroperitoneal), or intraperitoneal. Transabdominal is the most common approach. Indications for laparoscopy are generally for benign disease, although more radical surgeries have been accomplished in this manner. A full mechanical antibiotic bowel prep is prescribed. Although surgery time is

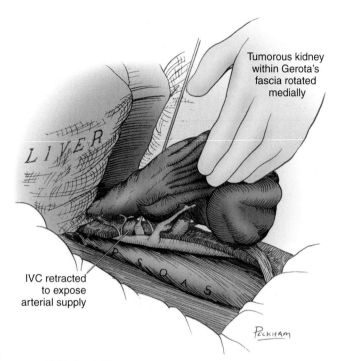

Tumorous kidney within Gerota's fascia rotated medially

LIVER

PSOAS

IVC retracted to expose arterial supply

PECKHAM

FIGURE 6-88 Nephrectomy. *IVC*, inferior vena cava.

longer (an average of 3½ to 5 hours), postoperative recovery time, analgesia requirements, and total hospital stay are lessened. The procedure always includes cystoscopy with placement of a renal balloon catheter, a ureteral catheter, and a Foley urethral catheter under C-arm fluoroscopy. Indigo carmine may be injected into the skin overlying the renal pelvis.

The patient is initially placed on a beanbag in the supine position. A standard laparoscopy instrument and equipment setup that includes three 5-mm trocars, an insufflation needle, and two 10-mm to 12-mm trocars is used. Cystoscopic and ureteroscopic supplies will be needed, as well as an 0.035-gauge Bentson guidewire, an occlusion balloon catheter, an 0.035-gauge Amplatz stiff guidewire, a 16F Foley catheter and drainage bag, indigo carmine, an irrigator-aspirator, a 1-liter bag of saline, a 1-liter pressure bag (to pressurize the irrigant to 250 mm Hg), a #12 or #11 knife blade, 10-mm clip appliers, the entrapment sack, and tissue morcellator. An open setup should always be available in the event laparoscopy is unsuccessful.

PROCEDURAL CONSIDERATIONS. The patient is prepped and draped as for laparotomy. Use of a draping pack with four large adherent drape sheets, instead of a standard laparotomy sheet, affords better access for the port sites.

The patient may be placed in lateral decubitus position on a deflated beanbag positioner at the outset or turned after endoscopic intervention. Ensuring that the patient is adequately secured to the OR bed is critical. Before prepping the patient, the bed is tilted laterally to afford a central abdominal access. The patient is prepped and draped, and access of the first three ports is achieved. Before the surgeon inserts the remaining trocars, the anesthesia provider returns the bed to its normal configuration so that the patient is again in lateral decubitus position. The kidney rest is then elevated, and the operation continues.

Some surgeons begin the procedure with the patient supine. The contralateral arm is padded with thick foam from the

shoulder to the fingertips. The patient is prepped and draped for thoracoabdominal surgery. Extra draping materials are used when the patient is repositioned.

OPERATIVE PROCEDURE

1. The surgeon accesses the peritoneal cavity through a 1-cm transverse, subumbilical, stab-wound incision. After elevation of the anterior abdominal wall with towel clips, the Veress needle is inserted with the stopcock valve control in the closed position.

2. Once the Veress needle is in place, sterile saline is dropped into the lumen of the needle and the valve of the needle is opened. If the saline enters freely (a successful test), the abdominal cavity is inflated with CO_2 until a pressure of 15 to 20 mm Hg is obtained. If saline does not enter freely, it indicates improper placement of the needle.

3. The surgeon nicks the rectus fascia with the knife blade, and replaces the Veress needle with the 10-mm trocar. Towel clips are again used on each side of the incision to stabilize the abdominal wall during insertion.

4. The 10-mm laparoscope is inserted.

5. A second incision is made immediately below the costal margin in the midclavicular line, and a 10-mm to 12-mm trocar is inserted.

6. The surgeon inserts the first of three 5-mm trocars through a small incision 2 cm below the umbilicus in the midclavicular line.

7. The last two 5-mm trocars are placed, one in the anterior axillary line level with the umbilicus and one subcostal in the anterior axillary line. All trocars are then withdrawn until 2 to 3 cm of each sheath protrudes into the abdomen. The surgeon may use polypropylene suture to secure the side arm ports to the patient's skin. Each trocar site is laparoscopically inspected after trocar insertion to identify any bleeding or perforation. On occasion, it may be necessary to extend the incision for trocar insertion.

8. The ascending or descending colon is completely mobilized with electrosurgical scissors and deflected medially. The retroperitoneum is opened.

9. Using gentle motion on the ureteral catheter, the surgeon identifies and dissects the ureter. A Babcock forceps is clamped around the dissected ureter for retraction.

10. The ureter is dissected until the lower pole of the kidney is visualized (Figure 6-89). Any veins encountered are clipped twice proximally and twice distally. The kidney is cleared of surrounding tissue and freed laterally and superiorly. Gerota's fascia is entered to free the adrenal gland and exclude it from the dissection.

11. The renal artery and vein are identified and cleared to create a 360-degree window around each vessel. The clip applier is inserted through the 10-mm to 12-mm port. Two clips are placed on the specimen side, and three clips are placed on the stump side of both the artery and the vein, which are then sharply incised.

12. Two pairs of clips are placed proximally and distally on the ureter, which is sharply incised. The specimen end is grasped, and the kidney is moved into the upper abdominal quadrant.

13. The surgeon introduces the entrapment sac through the 10-mm to 12-mm port. The bottom of the sac is pulled into the abdomen with graspers until the neck of the sac clears the end of the port and is then unfurled.

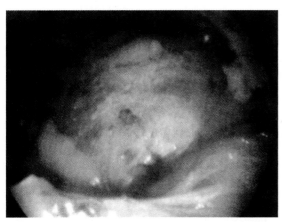

FIGURE 6-89 Interior view of exposing right kidney laparoscopically.

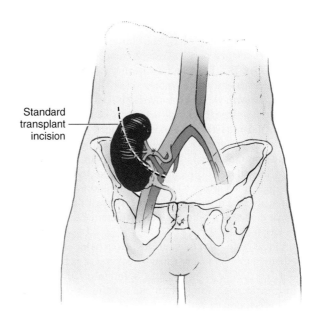

Standard transplant incision

FIGURE 6-90 Transplanted kidney in recipient's iliac fossa.

14. The sac is opened, and the ureteral stump with attached kidney is placed inside. The drawstrings are pulled tight, closing the mouth of the sac.
15. The anesthesia provider returns the patient to the supine position by tilting the OR bed, and the sac strings are extracted through the umbilical port. Under laparoscopic observation, the surgeon removes the port and the neck of the sac is brought to lie on the abdominal surface. The tissue morcellator is inserted into the sac, and the kidney is morcellated under suction in a clockwise fashion.
16. The abdominal cavity is exited with laparoscopic observation of each trocar site, during and after removal, to ensure that hemostasis has been achieved. Fascial layers at the 12-mm trocar sites are closed with 2-0 or 3-0 absorbable suture in a figure-of-eight pattern.
17. Using a 4-0 absorbable suture, the surgeon performs a subcuticular closure of all port sites.

Heminephrectomy. Heminephrectomy is removal of a portion of the kidney. It is usually indicated for conditions involving the lower or upper pole of the kidney, such as calculus disease, or trauma limited to one pole of a kidney. In rare instances in which a patient has only one kidney, such surgery may be used for renal neoplasms to avoid the need for dialysis and subsequent renal transplantation.
    PROCEDURAL CONSIDERATIONS. The setup is as described for nephrectomy with the addition of vascular and bulldog clamps.
OPERATIVE PROCEDURE
1. The kidney and its pedicle should be completely mobilized as described for nephrectomy. The main vessels may be temporarily occluded for only 20 to 30 minutes, after which progressive renal damage may occur. Local hypothermia may be indicated to prolong ischemic operating time.
2. The renal capsule is incised and stripped back.
3. A wedge of kidney tissue containing the diseased or damaged cortex is excised. The surgeon clamps the interlobar fat or arcuate and interlobular arteries with Hopkins clamps and suture-ligates them with 4-0 absorbable suture on urologic needles.
4. The surgeon reapproximates the open collecting system with a continuous 4-0 suture.

5. Perirenal fat is placed in the area in which tissue was excised, and the renal parenchyma is reapproximated with horizontal mattress sutures.
6. If possible, the renal capsule is reapproximated with a continuous 2-0 suture.

Radical Nephrectomy. Radical nephrectomy is excision of the kidney, perirenal fat, adrenal gland, Gerota's capsule (fascia), and contiguous periaortic lymph nodes. This procedure is performed for parenchymal renal neoplasms. In the open approach, a lumbar, transthoracic, or transabdominal approach to the kidney is used, depending on the size and location of the lesion. The transthoracic or transabdominal approach is preferred because the blood vessels of the kidney can be more easily reached and ligated before the tumor is mobilized, decreasing the possibility of tumor embolization into the bloodstream. For the laparoscopic approach a retroperitoneal or transperitoneal approach may be employed.
    PROCEDURAL CONSIDERATIONS. The setups are as described for open nephrectomy and laparoscopic nephrectomy.
    OPERATIVE PROCEDURE. In general, the procedure is as described for nephrectomy with two exceptions: (1) the renal pedicle is ligated before the kidney is mobilized, and (2) Gerota's capsule is not incised but is removed en bloc with the kidney. Involved lymph nodes surrounding the renal pedicle are excised. A chest tube is inserted if the transthoracic approach is used.

Kidney Transplant

Kidney transplant entails transplantation of a living-related or cadaveric donor kidney into the recipient's iliac fossa (Figure 6-90). It is performed in an effort to restore renal function and thus maintain life in a patient who has end-stage renal disease.

Transplant from a Living Donor. The kidney donor must be in good health. ABO (blood typing) and histocompatibility (human leukocyte antigen [HLA] tissue typing) along with a negative white cell (lymphocyte) crossmatch determine donor-recipient compatibility. It is not necessary to match the Rh factor. Once the donor has been chosen, a complete workup that includes history, physical examination, chest x-ray examination, ECG, CBC, BUN and creatinine values, blood chemistry profiles, coagulation studies, viral titers, and serologic testing is performed. Renal function is assessed by monitoring three creatinine clearances, urinalysis, and blood and urine cultures if hospitalized 72 hours or longer, followed by IVP and excretory urography. A flush aortogram assesses the vascular anatomy, and renal angiography pinpoints the kidney of choice while ruling out the presence of renal lesions. A kidney with a single renal artery is preferred, but kidneys with double and triple arteries may be used if necessary. If there is a family history of diabetes, a 5-hour glucose tolerance test is also performed (UNOS, 2009).

The ideal living donor is an identical twin, although any immediate family member (usually a sibling or parent) may be a donor. The donor is given an IV solution of 1000 ml of 5% dextrose in lactated Ringer's on the evening before nephrectomy. This is followed with 500 ml of 5% dextrose in water over the next 10 to 12 hours. The morning of surgery, about 45 minutes before transport to the OR, 12.5 g of mannitol is administered to ensure diuresis during the induction of anesthesia.

PROCEDURAL CONSIDERATIONS. Two adjacent ORs are prepared for the procedures; surgery on the donor and surgery on the recipient proceed simultaneously.

Usually the right kidney is chosen for removal because of its smaller size, leaving the donor patient with the left and larger kidney. Two IV lines are required. The patient is placed on a beanbag positioning device and moved into the left lateral decubitus position following endotracheal intubation. The lower arm is positioned extended outward on a well-padded armboard at a right angle to the torso; the upper arm is positioned on an elevated lateral armboard. The sternum and anterior superior iliac spine are brought near the edge of the OR bed. A pillow is placed between the patient's legs, and the ankles and feet are appropriately padded. The bed is flexed to 30 degrees, and the upper portion is angled downward to approximately 140 degrees. The skin is prepped from midchest to midthigh and draped to expose the flank area.

Required instruments and equipment are identical to those for a nephrectomy plus an IV pole and supplies for the sterile perfusion table. These include electrolyte solution (placed in an iced basin until needed), two IV extension tubes, a kidney basin with cold (4° C) IV saline solution, a three-way stopcock, an 18-gauge needle catheter, mosquito hemostats, vascular forceps, Metzenbaum scissors, suture scissors, and Kelly hemostats.

An electrolyte solution of Ringer's lactate that contains procaine and heparin may be used to perfuse the harvested kidney. A more common perfusion is CUW (Chelex-treated University of Wisconsin) solution. It contains hydroxyethyl starch, providing a better metabolic substrate for organ metabolism.

Collins or Sachs solution may be used to perfuse cadaveric kidneys after harvest but should never be used to perfuse a kidney from a living donor because of the potential effect of elevated potassium in the recipient from residual perfusate in the kidney.

OPERATIVE PROCEDURE

Open Approach

1. The donor nephrectomy procedure is as described for nephrectomy; however, the ureter and renal vein and artery require meticulous dissection.

2. Maximum length of the ureter is achieved by dividing it at or below the pelvic rim if possible. To preserve adequate ureteral vascularization, the surgeon is cautious not to skeletonize the ureter.

3. Particular care is taken to remove the maximum length of the renal vein and artery. Obtaining the maximum length of the right renal vein sometimes requires partial occlusion of the inferior vena cava with a Satinsky clamp and dissection of a portion of the inferior vena cava. This is done after the ureter has been freed.

4. Repair of the inferior vena cava is made with a continuous 4-0 or 5-0 vascular suture.

5. Five minutes before the surgeon clamps the renal vessels, 5000 units of heparin sodium and 12.5 g of mannitol are systemically administered to the patient to prevent intravascular clotting and maximize diuresis.

6. Immediately after the kidney is removed from the donor, the anesthesia provider administers 50 mg of protamine sulfate intravenously to reverse the heparinization.

7. Furosemide, mannitol, and IV fluids are administered to the donor to maintain adequate urinary output from the donor's remaining kidney.

8. Gentle handling of the kidney is essential. Team members must prevent undue traction on the vascular pedicle, which may induce vasospasm and reduce perfusion of the kidney.

9. To reduce warm ischemia time, the surgeon double-clamps the vein and the artery, excises the kidney, and immediately places it in cold saline solution on a sterile back table, where the kidney is flushed with the designated electrolyte solution. Warm ischemia time (from the clamping of renal vessels to a point at which the kidney is perfused with cold electrolyte solution) should be kept to a minimum to prevent acute tubular necrosis and to maintain maximum renal function after transplantation.

10. Mosquito clamps and fine vascular forceps are used to expose the renal artery to permit insertion of a needle catheter. The cold electrolyte solution passes through the IV tubing and the needle catheter, flushing any remaining donor's blood from the kidney. This also decreases the kidney's metabolic rate by lowering its temperature. Flushing time is usually 2 to 5 minutes.

11. After flushing, the surgeon may trim the vessels of adventitia to facilitate the vascular anastomosis to the recipient's iliac vessels.

12. The kidney, in cold saline solution, is covered with sterile drapes and taken by the surgeon to the room in which the recipient's iliac vessels have been exposed.

13. Wound closure for the donor is as described for nephrectomy.

Laparoscopic Approach. Five trocars are used (four trocars if the left kidney is chosen). Generally the operating trocar is 12 mm, the second and third trocars are 10 mm, and the last two trocars are 5 mm. Instruments required include the following: four 5-mm fenestrated graspers, 5-mm straight and curved dissecting scissors, a coagulating hook, a bipolar grasper, ultrasonic scissors, two 5-mm curved graspers and a 10-mm curved grasper, two needle holders, a clip applier, a vascular stapler, and an atraumatic retrieval bag without a system for opening and closing it and a minimal opening of 15 cm. In addition, the standard open setup needs to be ready with open vascular instrumentation, a smooth perfusion tip, sterile IV tubing, and sterile ice for ex vivo perfusion.

1. The first 12-mm trocar is introduced through an open technique at a level 2 to 5 cm cephalad to McBurney point to allow access to the superior pole and as far caudad as possible so the renal vein may be divided parallel to the vena cava.
2. The surgeon inserts the second 10-mm trocar in the periumbilical position about 3 cm lateral and cephalad to the umbilicus. This will be used for the laparoscope.
3. The third 10-mm trocar is placed 6 to 8 cm cephalad to the second trocar.
4. A 5-mm trocar is inserted into the flank at the convex border of the kidney.
5. The surgeon places the final 5-mm trocar below the xiphoid process to the left of the round ligament.
6. The OR bed is rotated vertically, and the small intestine and omentum are pushed into the inferior pelvic cavity.
7. Beginning at the foramen of Winslow, the subhepatic parietal peritoneum is incised and followed by division of the triangular ligament of the liver. Grasping forceps are placed posterior to the liver and used to retract the right lobe ventrally.
8. The surgeon incises the pericolic gutter beginning at the cecal base, extending to the hepatic flexure, and ending at the duodenum.
9. The duodenum is then freed of its attachments to the mesenteric root. The entire length of the subhepatic vena cava is exposed to the level of the iliac bifurcation.
10. The renal vein is identified and a vessel loop placed around it. Dissection of the right border of the subhepatic vena cava is carried out along the entire length. The right gonadal vein is clipped and divided at its caval origin.
11. A vessel loop is then passed around the right renal artery.
12. The ureter lies anterior to the iliac vessels. It is located, controlled with a vessel loop, and dissected caudad to cephalad, also removing areolar tissue. Once dissection reaches the inferior pole of the kidney, Gerota's fascia is incised and dissection continues to the renal parenchyma.
13. Pararenal fat is removed and a dissection plane is created against the renal capsule. When the anterior surface of the kidney has been freed the superior pole is separated from the adrenal gland.
14. Dissection is now directed to the inferior renal pole to free the kidney posteriorly from pararenal fat. Once free it is rotated ventrally to expose the vessels already marked with the vessel loops. The vessels are circumferentially dissected, and the kidney is freed.
15. The surgeon clips the distal end of the ureter and divides it at its bifurcation with the iliac vessels. Copious diuresis generally occurs at this point.
16. A 6-cm incision is made just above the pubic symphysis. The aponeurosis is transversely divided, and the rectus abdominis muscles are retracted.
17. The retrieval bag is introduced directly into the peritoneal cavity. It is placed around the kidney and held firmly without obstructing the vessels.
18. The grasper that has been placed in the suprapubic area is used to keep the retrieval bag closed and exert enough traction on the renal vessels to promote maximum length.
19. The renal side of the renal artery is left open while the surgeon applies one or two clips on the aortic side. This is divided in two steps to ensure occlusion.
20. The vein is divided with a vascular stapler, including a small cuff of the vena cava to add extra length.
21. The suprapubic peritoneal opening is widened manually, allowing the kidney to be extracted. It is immediately perfused on ice with 4° C CUW solution. Vessels are individually perfused. The volume corresponds to about 300 ml. This continues until the outflow from the vein becomes completely transparent.
22. The surgeon irrigates the peritoneum and achieves hemostasis. A drain may be inserted into the peritoneal space for a short time postoperatively.
23. The wounds are sutured and dressings applied.

Transplant from a Cadaveric Donor. The ideal cadaveric donor is young, free from infection and cancer, normotensive until a short time before death, and under hospital observation several hours before death. Permission to harvest the donor kidney must be obtained from the family and the medical examiner after brain death has been unequivocally established. Awareness of existing state legislation in this complex area is advisable.

The donor is completely evaluated. The medical history is reviewed for any possible contraindications, such as chronic disease, ongoing systemic infection, IV drug abuse, malignancy, heart or lung disease, trauma to the donor organ, and the presence of human immunodeficiency virus (HIV). Laboratory studies include blood typing, urinalysis, urine and blood cultures, BUN, serum creatinine, CBC, hepatitis B antigen evaluation, Venereal Disease Research Laboratories (VDRL) for the presence of venereal disease, and p24 antigen capture assay for the presence of HIV antigen. Evaluation of arterial blood gases, electrolyte values, and liver enzymes is also necessary. Because of improvements in medical therapy, the only absolute contraindications to organ donation are HIV and metastasis.

Preoperative management of the cadaver donor is vital to the success of the transplant. Organ perfusion, oxygenation, and hydration must be maintained. Arterial blood gas (ABG) evaluation determines ventilatory support, and dopamine may be administered if fluids alone are not able to maintain an adequate systolic blood pressure. Urine output is monitored, and antibiotics may be administered to combat and prevent infection.

PROCEDURAL CONSIDERATIONS. After brain death has been established, the donor is taken to the OR with respiratory and cardiac function maintained mechanically. The donor is placed in the supine position and is prepared for a laparotomy. Anticoagulant and α-adrenergic receptor blocking agents are administered systemically during the procedure. Adequate renal perfusion and function are maintained with IV fluids and diuretics.

Instruments and equipment are the same as those for nephrectomy, with the addition of Metzenbaum scissors, suture scissors, vascular forceps, DeBakey forceps, Dean hemostatic forceps, mosquito hemostats, DeBakey clamps, angled clip appliers with medium and large clips, bulldog clamps, vascular clamps, Deaver retractors, Harrington splanchnic retractors, vascular needle holders, a sternal saw or Lebsche knife and mallet, umbilical tapes, electrolyte solution (lactated Ringer's, Sachs, or Collins), cold packing in an iced basin until needed, an IV pole, IV extension tubes, a kidney basin with cold (4° C) IV saline solution, a three-way stopcock, an 18-gauge needle catheter, a centimeter ruler, the perfusion machine or kidney transplantation equipment, and ice.

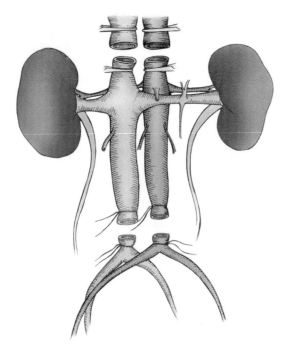

FIGURE 6-91 En bloc resection.

OPERATIVE PROCEDURE

1. The surgeon makes a midline incision from the xiphoid process to the symphysis pubis with bilateral supraumbilical transverse extensions through the skin, subcutaneous layer, fascia, and muscle.
2. Hemostasis is obtained with clamps, ties, suture ligatures, and electrocoagulation.
3. The kidney, renal vessels, and ureter are carefully dissected with Metzenbaum scissors, DeBakey forceps, and Dean hemostatic forceps.
4. The anesthesia provider administers 15,000 units of heparin sodium intravenously 5 to 10 minutes before the renal vessels are clamped.
5. The usual method of resection is en bloc resection (harvesting of donor kidneys) (Figure 6-91), which involves the removal of sections of the inferior vena cava and aorta with both kidneys in continuity.
6. The surgeon makes an incision along the route of the small bowel mesentery up to the esophageal hiatus.
7. The entire GI tract, spleen, and inferior portion of the pancreas are mobilized by dividing the celiac axis and the superior mesenteric artery, exposing the entire retroperitoneal region.
8. Using vascular clamps, the surgeon clamps and divides the inferior vena cava and aorta below the renal vessels.
9. Lumbar tributaries are secured with metal clips and are divided.
10. The kidneys and ureters are freed from their surrounding soft tissues.
11. The ureters are divided distally at the pelvic brim.
12. The surgeon clamps and divides the suprarenal aorta and inferior vena cava at the level of the diaphragm, close to the bifurcation.
13. The vessels and kidney are severed and the aorta and vena cava ligated.

14. After removal of the kidneys, immediate perfusion with cold (4° C) CUW or electrolyte solution is carried out. The kidneys are placed in a container of cold saline solution and surrounded by saline slush in an insulated carrier or placed on a hypothermic pulsatile perfusion machine for transport. While kidney perfusion is begun, the abdominal lymph nodes and spleen are removed for use in tissue typing.
15. The incision is closed with interrupted sutures, and artificial life-support systems are terminated. The perioperative nurse and surgical technologist care for the patient's body, preserving privacy, dignity, and humanity at the patient's death.

Transplant Recipient. Each potential recipient is judged individually in regard to kidney transplantation. Most persons younger than 55 years are acceptable; older patients are less tolerant of postoperative complications. Contraindications for renal transplantation include (1) systemic disease that precludes major surgery, (2) oxalosis (a metabolic disorder), (3) a positive HLA cytotoxic antibody screen, (4) untreatable cardiovascular disease, (5) active cancer, and (6) noncompliance (Ibrahim and Kasiske, 2008). If required, a patient may need to undergo bilateral nephrectomy before renal transplantation for uncontrollable hypertension, for kidney infections, or for reflux when there is a significant history of infections. Occasionally a large polycystic kidney may need to be removed to create a space for the new kidney. Splenectomy may be performed at this time to improve leukopenia and enhance the effects of myelosuppressive and immunosuppressive drugs.

The transplant recipient requires optimal nutritional support and adequate dialysis. All potential sources of infection must be treated. Most commonly these include teeth, bladder, nasal sinuses, and skin. The patient may need a short hemodialysis to control fluid overload or electrolyte imbalances. A repeat cytotoxic crossmatch with fresh serum specimens should follow hemodialysis. Preoperative antibiotics are commonly administered. Other important diagnostic tools for preoperative evaluation are chest x-ray examination, abdominal ultrasonography, voiding cystourethrography, liver function studies, hematologic assays, and serum values for screening hepatitis, HIV, and viral diseases.

PROCEDURAL CONSIDERATIONS. The patient is positioned in the supine position. A Foley catheter with an attached Silastic stenting catheter is inserted into the bladder by sterile technique. From 50 to 75 ml of antibiotic solution is instilled into the bladder through a sterile, catheter-tipped syringe, allowed to remain for 20 minutes, and drained. The patient is prepped from nipples to knees and draped.

OPERATIVE PROCEDURE

1. The surgeon makes a curved right lower quadrant incision through the skin, subcutaneous layer, fascia, and muscle.
2. Bleeding is controlled with clamps, ties, and electrocoagulation.
3. The inferior epigastric vessels are divided between suture ligatures.
4. Retroperitoneal dissection is performed by mobilizing the peritoneum superiorly and medially.
5. A Balfour self-retaining retractor is placed in the wound for exposure, and a wide Deaver retractor used to reflect the peritoneum superiorly and medially.

6. Using Metzenbaum scissors and DeBakey forceps, the surgeon dissects along the entire length of the hypogastric artery and the external and common iliac arteries to the bifurcation of the aorta, continuing down the internal iliac artery.

7. The internal iliac artery is ligated distally and divided, with proximal control maintained by a vascular clamp.

8. The iliac vein may be dissected free by ligating and dividing the internal iliac venous branches with 3-0 nonabsorbable sutures or ligating clips. More commonly, only the hypogastric artery and that portion of iliac vein to be anastomosed are dissected free.

9. The donor kidney is brought into the operative field and placed in cold (4° C) IV saline solution.

10. The surgeon uses mosquito hemostats, 4-inch DeBakey forceps, and curved and straight fine scissors to make the necessary alterations on the donor kidney vessels to facilitate the anastomoses.

11. The donor kidney is returned to the cold IV saline solution until the time of the anastomosis.

12. Two angled DeBakey vascular clamps are placed on the internal iliac vein.

13. A #11 blade is used to make a 1-cm incision in the iliac vein between the clamps.

14. The vessel is rinsed with heparin sodium solution (10 units/ml) in the Asepto syringe.

15. Angled Potts scissors are used to extend the incision to accommodate the donor renal vein.

16. The donor kidney is placed in a 3-inch by 10-inch, cold saline–soaked stockinette, with the renal vessels leaving from a hole in the side. Use of the stockinette prevents direct contact with the kidney and therefore trauma.

17. The surgeon performs the anastomosis of the donor kidney renal vein to the side of the recipient's iliac vein with 5-0 double-armed vascular sutures.

18. In like manner the renal artery is anastomosed end-to-end with the proximal portion of the internal iliac artery using 5-0 vascular sutures.

19. Before placing the final sutures, the vessels are irrigated proximally and distally with heparin sodium solution by using the 10-ml syringe attached to a catheter.

20. The stockinette is removed for adequate visualization of the entire kidney. The angled DeBakey clamps are removed from the venous vessels, and the anastomosis is checked for leakage.

21. The clamps on the internal iliac artery are then released, and the anastomosis is checked.

22. Meticulous inspection is made of the hilum and surface of the kidney for bleeding and infarction.

23. The anesthesia provider administers diuretics intravenously as needed.

24. Attention is then directed to the ureter and bladder.

25. Two long Martius forceps are used to grasp the anterior bladder wall.

26. Using a scalpel with a #10 knife blade, the surgeon makes a 4-cm anterior incision.

27. Two narrow Harrington retractors and one narrow Deaver retractor are inserted into the bladder for exposure.

28. The ureter is passed through the bladder wall and tunneled suburothelially for 2 to 2.5 cm.

29. The surgeon sutures the spatulated end of the ureter into the bladder urothelium with four to six 4-0 or 5-0 atraumatic absorbable sutures, creating a ureteroneocystostomy.

30. A 5F pediatric infant feeding tube is passed through the ureteroneocystostomy, up to the renal pelvis, and out through the urethra with the Foley catheter. This stenting catheter will remain in place for 36 to 48 hours to ensure ureteral patency during a period in which ureteral edema may occur.

31. Retractors are removed, and the bladder is closed in three layers.

32. Continuous 4-0 absorbable suture is used for urothelial closure and interrupted 2-0 absorbable suture for closure of bladder muscles.

33. An overlapping layer of 2-0 nonabsorbable material is used to bury the suture line.

34. The bladder is irrigated with an antibiotic solution to check for leaks.

35. The renal anastomoses are again checked for bleeding.

36. The surgeon places three metal clips on the superior, inferior, and lateral aspects of the kidney to radiographically measure renal size and determine postoperative swelling.

37. Retractors are removed from the incision.

38. Closed-wound suction drains are inserted into the wound, exteriorized through the skin laterally, and secured with 2-0 nonabsorbable suture on a cutting needle.

39. Muscle and fascial layers are closed with a single layer of 0 nonabsorbable sutures on a large atraumatic needle.

40. The subcutaneous layer is closed with 3-0 absorbable sutures on an atraumatic needle.

41. Skin closure is accomplished with skin staples, and dressings are applied.

42. The bladder is irrigated with 50 to 75 ml of antibiotic solution to prevent infection and free any blood clots.

Adrenalectomy

Adrenalectomy is partial or total excision of one or both adrenal glands. It may be performed for several reasons: hypersecretion of adrenal hormones; neoplasms of the adrenal gland; secondary treatment of neoplasms elsewhere in the body that depend on adrenal hormonal secretions, such as carcinoma of the prostate and breast; and pheochromocytoma.

Care of the patient with pheochromocytoma carries with it particular concerns for the surgical team. These patients are subject to extreme elevations in blood pressure, often accompanied by tachycardia, and hypovolemic states that can induce vascular collapse. If an adrenal tumor is being excised, early ligation of the adrenal vein is crucial in avoiding a sudden blood pressure elevation from the manipulation of the gland. After tumor removal there will be a rapid drop in blood pressure that can be minimized by maintenance of blood volume and administration of norepinephrine. With bilateral adrenalectomy, cortisone replacement will be instituted.

Procedural Considerations. Adrenalectomy may be approached as a laparoscopic or an open procedure. The laparoscopic approach is generally associated with less morbidity and shorter hospital stays. For unilateral adrenalectomy, the patient may be placed in the lateral or supine position, depending on the intended approach. If both glands are to be removed the supine or prone position is selected. The prone position is especially useful for a known disorder, such as aldosteronism, localized benign lesions, and solitary adenomas of Cushing's disease, and for debilitated patients with an advanced neoplasm.

The setup for a lateral approach is like that described for nephrectomy, including rib resection instruments, vascular instruments, and vessel clips and appliers. The setup for an abdominal approach is like that described for laparotomy, including vascular instruments, extralong scissors, tissue forceps, Rochester-Péan forceps, Mixter forceps, and needle holders. Penrose tubing is needed for retraction. Vessel clips and appliers also may be needed, as well as various sizes of nonabsorbable braided sutures.

The setup for the posterior approach is like that described for the lateral approach. The patient is placed prone in a 35-degree jackknife position with the kidney rest under the inferior margin of the anterior rib cage. Both arms should be carefully extended cephalad with adequate support under each shoulder.

Operative Procedure

LAPAROSCOPIC APPROACH

1. A 1.5-cm incision is made at the tip of the twelfth rib. The thoracolumbar fascia is entered by blunt dissection, and the 12-mm balloon dissector is placed behind Gerota's fascia and along the anterior axillary line. The balloon is inflated with 800 ml of saline, and the laparoscope is used to confirm balloon placement.
2. The operating balloon trocar is then placed in this position.
3. The surgeon inserts two 10-mm trocars on each side of the initial trocar, along the costal margin, in the anterior and posterior axillary line.
4. The fourth trocar is placed along the posterior costal margin.
5. Dissection begins near the renal hilum, incising into Gerota's fascia.
6. The surgeon identifies, clips, and divides the adrenal arteries.
7. The anterior, lateral aspect of the gland is freed from the upper pole of the kidney.
8. The adrenal vein is clipped and divided.
9. The surgeon mobilizes the posterior, superior, and anterior surfaces of the adrenal gland. A fan retractor is employed to retract the pancreas and spleen, or pancreas and liver, depending on which side the gland is being excised.
10. The adrenal branches of the inferior phrenic vessels and any accessory vessels are clipped and divided. The gland is removed through the original port using a retrieval sac. Hemostasis is achieved. The trocars are then sequentially removed, the incisions closed, and dressings applied.

LATERAL APPROACH—OPEN

1. A flank, thoracolumbar, or transthoracic incision is performed as described for nephrectomy.
2. The rib underlying the chosen approach is resected or deflected for optimum exposure of the upper pole of the kidney.
3. Entry is between the eleventh and twelfth ribs in a flank approach, the tenth and eleventh ribs in a thoracolumbar approach, and the ninth and tenth ribs in a transthoracic approach.
4. An opening is made with scissors through the transverse fascia.
5. The pleura and diaphragm are protected with moist laparotomy packs, and Gerota's fascia is incised to expose the kidney and adrenal gland.
6. The surgeon identifies the gland and dissects it free from the upper pole of the kidney with scissors and Babcock forceps.
7. The blood supply of the gland is identified, clamped or clipped, fescia and divided. Bleeding vessels are ligated.

8. To release the gland, the left adrenal vein, a branch of the left renal vein, is separated by clamping and cutting. The right adrenal vein, a tributary of the vena cava, is also divided. Fine vascular sutures may be required to repair inadvertent injury to the vena cava.
9. When hemostasis has been ensured, the wound is closed sequentially in layers: muscle, fascia, subcutaneous tissue, and skin. Dressings are then applied.

ABDOMINAL APPROACH

1. The abdominal wall is incised with an upper abdominal incision, and the peritoneal cavity is opened and explored.
2. Hemostasis is established.
3. The abdominal wound is retracted, and the surrounding organs are protected with moist laparotomy packs.
4. The surgeon opens the retroperitoneal area near the diaphragm on the left side, exposing the renal fascia.
5. The renal fascia is opened to reveal the left kidney and adrenal gland.
6. Using blunt and sharp dissection, the surgeon frees the adrenal gland from the kidney, clamps all bleeding vessels, and ligates them with 3-0 nonabsorbable sutures.
7. After all bleeding is controlled, the surgeon replaces the kidney in the renal fascia, and closes it with interrupted 0 absorbable sutures.
8. The peritoneum is closed over the left kidney and renal fascia.
9. The abdominal retractors are rearranged to provide access to the peritoneum over the right kidney and adrenal gland. Care must be taken to prevent trauma to the liver.
10. The surgeon repeats the procedure on the right side, taking care to clamp and ligate the short adrenal vein.
11. The abdomen is inspected for bleeding vessels, which are clamped and ligated.
12. The wound is closed and dressings applied.

POSTERIOR APPROACH

1. The surgeon makes an incision over the eleventh or twelfth rib.
2. The periosteum is elevated, avoiding the nerve and vessels on the inferior margin.
3. The diaphragm and pleura are displaced superiorly, and the appropriate rib is resected.
4. Hemostasis is achieved.
5. Gerota's fascia is incised, and through sharp and blunt dissection the surgeon exposes the posterior aspect of the upper pole of the kidney.
6. The upper pole is mobilized, and a padded retractor is placed to deflect the kidney downward for the approach to the adrenal gland.
7. The suprarenal fat is meticulously dissected.
8. Vessel clips are used for control of smaller vessels.
9. Dissection continues superiorly, laterally, and inferiorly while the integrity of the hilum of the adrenal gland is maintained.
10. With right-angled clamps, the adrenal vein and artery are freed, divided, and ligated with 0 or 2-0 braided nonabsorbable ties.
11. Babcock clamps are employed for manipulation and removal of the adrenal gland.
12. Bleeding is controlled, and the wound is inspected for injury to renal structures.
13. The surgeon closes Gerota's fascia with interrupted absorbable sutures.
14. The wound is closed and dressings applied.

GERIATRIC CONSIDERATIONS

The Elderly Patient—Genitourinary Surgery

The predominant reason for urologic surgery in elderly men is benign prostatic hypertrophy (BPH). BPH may be silent or have minimal symptoms in the presence of severe bladder decompensation. As part of history taking, symptoms such as dysuria, straining at micturition, and hematuria are noted. Prostate surgery, especially transurethral resection of the prostate (TURP), is relatively safe and generally well tolerated. The majority of BPH operations are performed to relieve symptoms, such as nocturia, slow stream, intermittency, and double voiding. TURP is indicated if the surgeon believes that total resection can be accomplished in 1 hour and that no bladder disease or impairment to urethral access is present.

A surgical alternative to TURP is transurethral incision of the prostate (TUIP). The complications associated with TUIP are significantly fewer than those occurring after TURP, especially bleeding, retrograde ejaculation, and impotence. It is a more desirable alternative to TURP for patients with prostates weighing less than 30 g. Other alternatives are laser prostatectomy, transurethral vaporization of the prostate, microwave hyperthermia, and transurethral needle ablation. These techniques are gaining acceptance because they can be done as outpatient procedures using local anesthetic. Genitourinary (GU) procedures may also be performed to correct incontinence. Incontinence in elderly men can result from nerve-damaging events such as radical prostatectomy and spinal cord injury. Surgical treatments can include artificial sphincter creation, formation of a bulbourethral sling, and a urinary diversion procedure (*Men's Guide to Urinary Incontinence,* 2008).

Prostate cancer is the second most common cancer in American men and accounts for approximately 28% of all cancers in men; the median age of diagnosis for cancer of the prostate is about 68 years of age (Meiner, 2011). Because treatment can have long-term implications, conversations with the older male and his partner should include consequences for sexual function. Perioperative personnel need to keep in mind that age alone does not dictate sexual interest or activity; some degree of sexual activity is reported in about 70% of those over 70 years of age. Thus, loss of sexual function can have a serious impact on the quality of life of the older man and should be part of treatment decisions.

Older women experience overactive bladder (OAB) or urinary incontinence more frequently than younger women. Sneezing, coughing, and laughing may cause urine to leak from the bladder. The decision to have surgery should always be based on appropriate diagnosis, evaluation of all treatment modalities, and realistic expectations from surgical intervention. Surgical choices can include urethral sling, retropubic suspension, and tension-free vaginal tape (TVT) surgery. This procedure may be performed under local anesthesia, carrying a low morbidity with a reported 2-year cure rate of 84% (Fillit et al, 2010). Factors that can impair a positive outcome include, but may not be limited to, obesity, radiation therapy, aging, chronic cough, poor nutrition, low estrogen level, postmenopausal, and strenuous physical activity (*Women's Guide to Urinary Incontinence in Females,* 2008).

Modified from Fillit HM, et al: *Textbook of geriatric medicine and gerontology,* ed 7, Philadelphia, 2010, Saunders; Meiner SE: *Gerontologic nursing,* ed 4, St. Louis, 2011, Elsevier; Men's guide to urinary incontinence, 2008, available at www.webmd.com/urinary-incontinence-oab/mens-guide/urinary-incontinence-in-men-surgery. Accessed April 13, 2009; Women's guide to urinary incontinence in females, 2008, available at www.webmd.com/urinary-incontinence-oab/womens-guide/urinary-incontinence-in-women-surgery. Accessed April 13, 2009.

GENITOURINARY SURGERY SUMMARY

The genitourinary system is comprised of the following organs: kidneys, adrenals, ureters, bladder, urethra, prostate gland, penis, testicles, and the female urogynecologic system. The kidneys excrete urine, which is then transported to the bladder by the ureters. The adrenal glands sit on the medial side of the superior pole of each kidney, and secrete epinephrine, steroids, and hormones. Both the kidneys and adrenal glands lie retroperitoneally beneath the diaphragm. The bladder is a hollow, muscular viscus that acts as a reservoir for the urine excreted by the kidneys until it reaches capacity when it then excretes the stored urine out of the body via the urethra. The male urethra, at 20 to 25 cm long, is 4 to 5 times the length of the 3- to 5-cm female urethra. It is surrounded at the base of the bladder by the prostate gland, which, in conjunction with the bulbourethral glands, secrete the seminal fluid that transports the sperm from the testicles out of the body via the urethra.

Surgery of the genitourinary system is accomplished primarily in one of three ways: open laparotomy, laparoscopically, or transurethrally. The majority of procedures are conducted in either supine, lateral, or lithotomy position. Because of the vascular nature of the genitourinary organs, hemostasis is a key concern. Various hemostatic devices, mechanical, chemical, and thermal, should all be available. There are a variety of irrigation fluids available for use during transurethral procedures. The type, temperature, and amount are determined by the organ undergoing the procedure and the patient's own physiological status. Open and laparoscopic genitourinary surgery is similar in many ways to both general and gynecologic surgery. With the increasing utilization of more advanced medical technology, such as robotics, lasers, and imaging techniques, patients are enjoying better outcomes with less trauma.

REVIEW QUESTIONS

1. The kidneys lie retroperitoneally along the lateral borders of the _____ muscle.

2. The anterior fascia covering the kidneys is known as _____.

3. The renal pelvis is divided into several branches called _____.

4. The renal vein and artery are collectively known as _____.

5. Each adrenal gland is comprised of a _____ and a _____.

6. Urine is transported down each ureter by _____.

7. The male urethra is divided into two portions. They are known as the _____ and _____.

8. Benign prostate hyperplasia (BPH) generally occurs in the _____ zone of the prostate gland.

9. An abnormal accumulation of fluid in the tunica vaginalis of the scrotum is known as _____.

10. The normal range for a prostate-specific antigen (PSA) test is _____.

11. The use of epinephrine in local anesthetics is typically avoided in urology because of the change of _____.

12. Which surgical positions are more frequently utilized in genitourinary surgery?

13. Which irrigating fluids are indicated for a patient undergoing a TURP?

14. What fixative solution should not be used for testicular biopsy?

15. Why is a three-way catheter used following a TURP?

16. Which patients are best candidates for nerve-sparing radical retropubic prostatectomy?

17. Which irrigating fluid is best for a patient undergoing a transurethral resection of bladder tumor?

18. The most common causes of urinary tract obstruction are _____, _____, and _____.

19. What surgical procedure is indicated when a vesical malignancy has invaded the muscular wall of the bladder?

20. Which kidney is typically removed from a living donor?

21. What are the only two absolute contraindications to organ donation?

22. Define and briefly describe the following surgical procedures:
    Transurethral ureteropyeloscopy
    Robotic-assisted laparoscopic radical prostatectomy
    Laparoscopic nephrectomy

Critical Thinking Question

Tom is undergoing surgery as a living kidney donor. What should the surgical technologist anticipate in the OR during this procedure? How should the ST prepare the room and ensure Tom is ready for the surgery?

REFERENCES

American Cancer Society: *Cancer facts and figures 2008*, Atlanta, 2008, American Cancer Society.

American Medical Systems (AMS): Erectile dysfunction, 2009, available at www.americanmedicalsystems.com/prof_erectile_restoration_product_objectname_prof_male_700_inflatable.html. Accessed May 17, 2009.

Appell RA, Winters JC: Injection therapy for urinary incontinence. In Wein AJ, editors: *Campbell-Walsh urology*, ed 9, Philadelphia, 2007, Saunders.

Association of periOperative Registered Nurses (AORN): Creating a patient safety culture guideline. In *Perioperative standards and recommended practices*, Denver, 2009, The Association.

Denholm B: Tucking patient's arms and general positioning, *AORN J* 89(4):755–757, 2009.

Epstein JL: Pathology of prostatic neoplasia. In Wein AJ et al, editors: *Campbell-Walsh urology*, ed 9, Philadelphia, 2007, Saunders.

Fitzpatrick JM: Minimally invasive and endoscopic management of benign prostatic hyperplasia. In Wein AJ et al, editors: *Campbell-Walsh urology*, ed 9, Philadelphia, 2007, Saunders.

Gayer G: Minimally invasive management of urolithiasis, *Semin Ultrasound CT MRI* 27:139–151, 2006.

Gonzalgo ML: Minimally invasive surgical approaches and management of prostate cancer, *Urol Clin N Am* 35:489–504, 2008.

Han M, Partin AW: Retropubic and suprapubic open prostatectomy. In Wein AJ et al, editors: *Campbell-Walsh urology*, ed 9, Philadelphia, 2007, Saunders.

Ibrahim HN, Kasiske BL: Donor and recipient issues. In Brenner BM, Levine SA, editors: *Brenner & Rector's the kidney*, ed 8, Philadelphia, 2008, Saunders.

Ignatavicius DD: Care of male patients with reproductive problems. In Ignatavicius DD, Workman ML, editors: *Medical-surgical nursing: patient-centered collaborative care*, ed 6, St Louis, 2010, Saunders.

Lamm DL et al: Bladder cancer: current optimal intravesical treatment, *Urol Nurs* 25(5):323–332, 2005.

Langenhuijsen JF et al: Cryosurgery for prostate cancer: an update on clinical results of modern cryotechnology, *Eur Urol* 55:76–86, 2009.

Lipshultz LI et al: Surgical management of male infertility. In Wein AJ et al: *Campbell-Walsh urology*, ed 9, Philadelphia, 2007, Saunders.

Novick AC, Fergany A: Renovascular hypertension and ischemic nephropathy. In Wein AJ et al: *Campbell-Walsh urology*, ed 9, Philadelphia, 2007, Saunders.

Rigdon JL: Robotic-assisted laparoscopic radical prostatectomy, *AORN J* 84(5):760–770, 2006.

Scott RD: The direct medical costs of healthcare-associated infections in U.S. hospitals and the benefits of prevention. March 2009, Centers for Disease Control and Prevention, available at www.cdc.gov/ncidod/dhqp/hai.html. Accessed May 17, 2009.

Sherman ND, Amundsen CL: Current and future techniques of neuromodulation for bladder dysfunction, *Curr Urol Rep* 8(6):448–454, 2007.

UNOS: Critical pathway for the organ donor 2009, available at www.unos.org/qa.asp. Accessed May 27, 2009.

Young E et al: Perioperative fluid management, *AORN J* 89:167–178, 2009.

Thyroid and Parathyroid Surgery

Overview

The first documented thyroid surgery occurred in the twelfth century (History box). Today surgeons continue to perform surgical procedures on the thyroid gland for various underlying causes. Surgery ranges from lobectomy and isthmectomy for papillary microcarcinomas (lesions smaller than 1 cm) to near-total and total thyroidectomies for symptomatic multinodular goiters. Technologic advances have added new approaches to thyroid and parathyroid surgery, such as minimally invasive surgery (MIS) techniques.

This chapter was originally written by Joanne C. Wentzell, RN, MSN, CNOR, CRNFA, for the 14th edition of Alexander's Care of the Patient in Surgery *and has been revised by Sherri M. Alexander, CST, for this text.*

Surgical Anatomy

Thyroid Gland

The thyroid gland (Figure 7-1) is a highly vascular organ that lies in the anterior portion of the neck, deep to the paired strap muscles, resting on the midline of the trachea. It is attached to the cricoid and trachea by the ligament of Berry. The inferior border of the thyroid varies and may be located above or below the sternal notch. It consists of right and left lobes united by a middle portion, the isthmus, and it weighs approximately 20 g. The isthmus is situated near the base of the neck, between the second and fourth tracheal rings, and the lobes lie beside the larynx, trachea, and esophagus. The pyramidal lobe, a long, thin projection of thyroid tissue protruding cephalad from the isthmus, is found in about 30% of patients at surgery; it is the vestige of the embryonic thyroglossal duct and migrates from the foramen cecum at the base of the tongue. If the migratory tract fails to degenerate, a fistula or cyst may be present (Loevner and Mukherji, 2008).

HISTORY

Formerly Hazardous, Thyroid Surgery Now Minimally Invasive and Focused

Since 2700 BC, long before the thyroid gland was identified, goiters (from Latin *gutter* for "throat") have been described. Europeans living 2000 years ago, especially those living in the Alps, noted a swelling in the neck and called it *bronchocele,* ancient Greek for "tracheal out-pouching." Thousands of years later, Hieronymus Fabricius ab Aquapendente in 1619 recognized that goiters arose from the thyroid gland.

With the Italian Renaissance came an expansion of inquiry into the human body. During this time, the thyroid gland was identified. Around 1500 Leonardo da Vinci depicted the gland and in 1543 Vesalius called the thyroid gland the "laryngeal glands." da Vinci's drawings portrayed the thyroid as two separate glands on either side of the larynx. Thomas Wharton, with his 1656 publication *Adenographia,* is credited for replacing the term "laryngeal gland" with the term "thyroid gland" (Greek *thyreoeides,* for "shield shaped").

In 1170 Roger Frugardi first described thyroid surgery. Thyroid surgery was hazardous, with death rates of more than 40%. High death rates continued until the 1800s when increased knowledge and advances in general anesthesia, antisepsis, and hemostasis became the norm.

In the late 1800s two notable thyroid surgeons—C.A. Theodor Billroth (1829 to 1894) and Emil Theodor Kocher (1841 to 1917)—revolutionized the treatment of thyroid diseases. Despite Billroth's earlier success with thyroidectomies, Kocher is regarded as the father of thyroid surgery. Kocher performed more than 2000 thyroid surgeries in the late 1800s, with only a 4.5% death rate, and he received the Nobel Prize in 1909 for his contributions to this field. In 1914 Kendall isolated the hormone *thyroxine (T_4).* Since 1941 thyroidectomy as treatment of thyroid mass (goiter) has become less frequent because of the use of radioactive iodine (RAI) and antithyroid drugs, which reduce the activity of the thyroid gland.

Over the last 10 years new technology and techniques have been introduced that have greatly improved thyroid and parathyroid surgeries. Minimally invasive and focused approaches have enhanced and refined treatment and surgery for thyroid and parathyroid disease.

Modified from Kaplan EL: Thyroid and parathyroid. In Schwartz SI et al, editors: *Principles of surgery,* ed 6, New York, 1994, McGraw-Hill; Sadler GP et al: Thyroid and parathyroid. In Schwartz SI et al, editors: *Principles of surgery,* ed 7, New York, 1999, McGraw-Hill; Sawin CT: The heritage of the thyroid. In Braverman LE, Utiger RD, editors: *Werner and Ingbar's the thyroid: a fundamental and clinical text,* ed 7, Philadelphia, 1996, Lippincott-Raven; Yousem DM, Scheff AM: Thyroid and parathyroid. In Som PM, Curtin AD, editors: *Head and neck imaging,* ed 3, St Louis, 1996, Mosby.

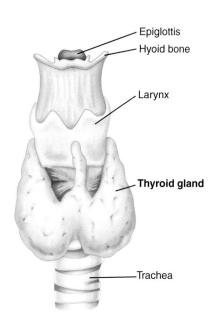

- Epiglottis
- Hyoid bone
- Larynx
- **Thyroid gland**
- Trachea

FIGURE 7-1 Thyroid gland.

Blood supply to the thyroid is from the superior thyroid artery, which originates from the external carotid artery, and from the inferior thyroid artery, which originates from the thyrocervical trunk of the subclavian artery. The points at which these two arteries enter the thyroid gland are referred to as "poles" of the thyroid and are important anatomic landmarks during surgery. The thyroid gland is drained by three pairs of veins (superior, middle, and inferior thyroid veins). Occasionally a single thyroid artery (thyroidea ima) may arise directly from the arch of the aorta or the innominate artery and rise in front of the trachea to enter the midline of the gland inferiorly.

The recurrent laryngeal nerve, a branch of the vagus nerve, innervates the intrinsic muscles of the larynx. The right recurrent laryngeal nerve loops under the subclavian artery and ascends in an oblique direction lateral to the tracheoesophageal groove. The recurrent laryngeal nerve contains both motor and sensory fibers. The motor component innervates the abductor muscles of the true vocal cords. The sensory component supplies sensation to the larynx below the vocal cords. During surgery, care is taken to identify and protect this nerve. Immediate hoarseness occurs if the nerve is divided on one side. If the recurrent nerve is injured bilaterally, acute paralysis of both vocal cords may obstruct the airway and require emergency tracheotomy. Injury to the external branch of the superior laryngeal nerve, which innervates the cricothyroid muscle, results in difficulty shouting or singing high notes.

The thyroid gland produces three hormones: thyroxine (T_4) and triiodothyronine (T_3) (together known as the *thyroid hormones [TH]*) and calcitonin. T_3 and T_4 cannot be synthesized without iodine. Calcitonin increases calcium storage in the bone and decreases blood calcium levels. The primary function of thyroid hormones is to regulate energy metabolism, but they also play an important role in growth and development. Thyroid-stimulating hormone (TSH) is synthesized by the anterior pituitary, and stimulates the production and release of thyroid hormones and the uptake of iodine.

Parathyroid Gland

The parathyroid glands usually consist of four small, mahogany-to-yellow, flat, ovoid masses (Figure 7-2) (Gauger and Doherty, 2004). Normal parathyroid glands are generally

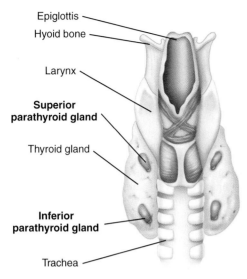

Epiglottis

Hyoid bone

Larynx

Superior parathyroid gland

Thyroid gland

Inferior parathyroid gland

Trachea

FIGURE 7-2 Parathyroid gland.

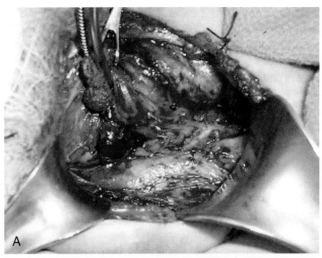

A

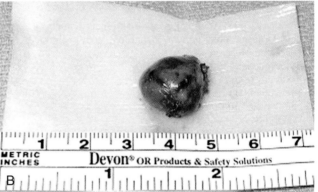

B

FIGURE 7-3 A, A right upper parathyroid adenoma in situ. The thyroid gland is retracted to the midline. The recurrent laryngeal nerve enters the operative field inferiorly and tracks superiorly in the tracheoesophageal groove. The carotid sheath lies lateral to the nerve. The adenoma is the lobular mahogany mass located at the superior pole of the thyroid. **B,** Parathyroid adenoma after removal.

small, lobular, and yellow in color, about the size of a lentil bean. It can be challenging to differentiate the gland from a lobule of fat, a thyroid nodule, or lymph node. Thyroid adenomas generally, although not always, tend to be larger, asymmetric, and more of a red-brown hue than normal parathyroids (Figure 7-3). The upper pair of glands lies in proximity to the posterior portion of the superior pole of the thyroid; the lower pair usually (about 60% of the time) lies near the posterior lateral aspect of the lower pole of the thyroid. Ectopic parathyroid glands, more common in the inferior parathyroid glands, may be found in the superior mediastinum, especially within the thymus and as low as the pericardium. Parathyroids may also be buried under the strap muscle, in the carotid sheath, or embedded in the thyroid beneath the capsule (Loevner and Mukherji, 2008). Each parathyroid gland measures approximately 3 mm × 3 mm × 3 mm and generally weighs less than 50 mg; the upper glands are generally smaller than the lower ones. Both the upper and lower parathyroid glands receive their blood supply from the inferior thyroid artery. As the blood supply to the superior parathyroid stems from that of the supply to the inferior parathyroid, disrupting supply to the inferior parathyroid necessarily compromises the supply to the upper parathyroid.

The parathyroid glands secrete parathyroid hormone (PTH), an antagonist to calcitonin. Both PTH and calcitonin work together to maintain calcium homeostasis by increasing calcium removal from storage in bone and increasing absorption of calcium by the intestines.

Surgical Technologist Considerations

Surgery on the neck is performed with the patient in supine position and the head on a specific headrest. Large thyroid nodules may cause a tracheal shift and present a challenge to the anesthesia provider for intubation and airway management. It may be prudent to have the "difficult airway" cart available.

Grossly enlarged thyroid gland may be more difficult to excise, and intraoperative bleeding is more common and pro-

fuse. Hemorrhage may cause tracheal compression and airway compromise. It is wise for the surgical technologist to have a tracheal tray in the operating room for this reason.

General surgery instruments are used for neck surgery, with the addition of special instruments from both vascular and otorhinolaryngology sets. The surgical technologist should also have vessel loops, suture boots, and a nerve stimulator for the procedure.

There may be several specimens on these procedures. When setting up, the scrub should have several containers to keep the specimens separated and labels to properly identify each specimen as it is handed off to the circulator.

Thyroid Assessment. In addition to palpation of the thyroid gland for size, contour, consistency, lymph nodes, fixation, tenderness, and bruits (Wilson and Giddens, 2009), scans are used to clarify thyroid anatomy. CT and MRI scans are used to assess a thyroid with suspected malignancy for encroachment of the tumor outside the thyroid capsule into the adjacent tissue of the neck. Scans are the most effective means to evaluate local invasion of surrounding tissue.

While palpable thyroid nodules are present in 3% to 5% of healthy adults, ultrasound and autopsy studies show rates of

Common Symptoms and Signs of Thyroid Dysfunction

HYPOTHYROIDISM

◆ Fatigue
◆ Weight gain
◆ Cold intolerance
◆ Hair dryness or loss
◆ Dry skin
◆ Depression
◆ Hoarse voice
◆ Poor concentration
◆ Muscle stiffness and pain
◆ Edema
◆ Bradycardia
◆ Constipation
◆ Menstrual irregularity (especially heavy menses; infertility)

HYPERTHYROIDISM

◆ Vision changes—myopathy, ophthalmopathy, such as extra-ocular muscle enlargement, visual loss with prolonged optic nerve compression
◆ Emotional lability, mood changes
◆ Irritability
◆ Exercise intolerance
◆ Fatigue
◆ Weight loss
◆ Heat intolerance and flushing
◆ Hyperactivity—especially children
◆ Increased sweating
◆ Insomnia
◆ Tremor
◆ Muscle weakness
◆ Dyspnea
◆ Frequent bowel movements
◆ Menstrual irregularity (oligomenorrhea; infertility)
◆ More common in elderly—tachycardia and atrial tachydys-rhythmias, palpitations, cardiomegaly

Modified from Roberts CG, Ladenson PW: Hypothyroidism, *Lancet* 363(9411):793-803, 2004; Surks MI et al: Subclinical thyroid disease: scientific review and guidelines for diagnosis and management, *JAMA* 291(2):228-238, 2004.

---

more than 50%. Although most nodules are benign, 7% to 29% will be cancerous. Consequently, the most common endocrine malignancy is thyroid cancer, estimated to be the thirteenth most common cause of any new malignant neoplasm in the United States for 2007, ranking seventh in women (25,480 cases; 3.8%), while causing just over 1% of new cases in men. Prevalence figures are likely to increase further, as the yearly incidence of thyroid cancer has been growing exponentially from 7800 cases in 1974 to 33,550 cases in 2007 (Tuttle, 2007). Thus thyroid cancer is poised to become one of the most common cancer diagnoses in living cancer patients (Grebe, 2009).

PREOPERATIVE TESTING

Thyroid Isotope Scan (Thyroid Scintigraphy). A thyroid nodule, the most common endocrine problem in the United States, is any abnormal growth of thyroid cells. Most nodules are discovered during routine physical examination, because they rarely are symptomatic. Imaging of the normal thyroid with radionuclide agents shows normal size, shape, position, and function of the thyroid, with no areas of decreased or increased

---

EVIDENCE FOR PRACTICE

Screening for Thyroid Dysfunction

A number of symptoms and signs are well-established manifestations of thyroid dysfunction. A thorough history and physical is indicated in screening for thyroid cancer. A history of being exposed to neck or whole-body radiation or being raised in iodine-poor areas should be assessed. A rapidly expanding neck mass, new onset of hoarseness, neck or ear pain, or cough are symptoms of concern. Patients with a fixed, immobile mass and/or hoarseness, dysphagia, or respiratory symptoms require CT or MRI imaging as part of evaluation. These symptoms may be indicative of metastasis (Loevner and Mukherji, 2008). Although calcifications were formerly considered a benign finding, some thyroid cancers demonstrate eggshell calcifications.

The American Association of Clinical Endocrinologists (AACE) practice guidelines for the diagnostic evaluation of hyperthyroidism and hypothyroidism recommend TSH assay as the single best screening test. Hyperthyroidism results in a lower-than-normal TSH level (suppressed TSH secretion). To diagnose hyperthyroidism accurately, TSH assay sensitivity, the lowest reliably measured TSH concentration, must be 0.02 milliinternational unit/liter or less.

Serum TSH level is the most sensitive test for detecting mild (subclinical) thyroid hormone excess or deficiency. An elevated serum TSH concentration is present in both overt and mild (subclinical) hypothyroidism. In the latter, the free thyroid hormone (fT_3 and fT_4) levels are, by definition, normal.

Hypothyroidism results from undersecretion of thyroid hormone. In the United States, hypothyroidism affects close to 11 million people each year. The most common cause of primary hypothyroidism is chronic autoimmune thyroiditis (Hashimoto's disease). The most valuable laboratory test is a sensitive measurement of TSH level. Clinical hypothyroidism is treated with levothyroxine replacement therapy. The AACE supports treating subclinical hypothyroidism if TSH levels are greater than 10 microunits/ml or if TSH levels are between 5 and 10 microunits/ml in conjunction with goiter or positive antibodies or both.

Serum TSH measurement is the single most reliable test to diagnose all common forms of hypothyroidism and hyperthyroidism, with high sensitivity (98%) and specificity (92%).

---

fT₃, Free triiodothyronine; *fT₄*, free thyroxine; *TSH*, thyroid-stimulating hormone.
Modified from American Association of Clinical Endocrinologists: Medical guidelines for clinical practice for the evaluation and treatment of hyperthyroidism and hypothyroidism, *Endocr Pract* 8(6):457-469, 2002; Loevner LA, Mukherji SK: *Thyroid and parathyroid glands: imaging, treatment, and beyond*, Philadelphia, 2008, Saunders; Mauk KL: Rooting out hypothyroidism in the elderly, *Nursing 2005* 35(12):65-66, 2005; Screening for thyroid disease: *Recommendation statement, U.S. Preventive Services Task Force* 140(2):125-127, 2004.

---

uptake. Nodules that are *hot* demonstrate increased uptake of radionuclide agent; this may indicate benign adenoma or localized toxic goiter. *Cold* nodules are hypofunctioning or nonfunctioning and may indicate cyst, nonfunctioning adenoma or goiter, lymphoma, localized area of thyroiditis, or carcinoma. Two commonly used agents in thyroid imaging are radioactive iodine and technetium 99m-pertechnetate ($^{99m}TcO_4^-$).

Ultrasonic Scan. Ultrasonic scans are the treatment of choice to evaluate thyroid nodules and are useful to determine the size and number of nodules within the thyroid as well as to monitor size progression during follow-up. Involvement

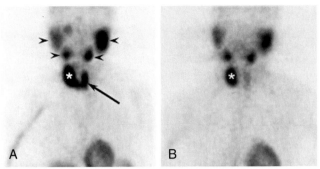

FIGURE 7-4 A, Early three-dimensional sestamibi image shows uptake in mass (*asterisk*), in salivary glands (*arrowheads*), and in thyroid gland (*arrow*). **B,** Late three-dimensional sestamibi image shows retention of radiotracer in the adenoma (*asterisk*), with absence of radiotracer in the thyroid gland. Salivary glands normally retain radiotracer on late images.

of the vessels in the neck or mediastinum, although rare, can occur. It is critical that the surgeon and operative team know this before surgery. Radiologic evaluation frequently dictates the extent of the surgery. Several new ultrasonic techniques have been applied to the thyroid. The three-dimensional (3D) ultrasound has proven to be more accurate. Tissue harmonic imaging (THI) uses the first harmonic of the transmitted frequency for image formation and results in images with less "noise." These new techniques improve image clarity but do not improve lesion characterization.

Ultrasonography also helps to facilitate accurate needle placement and sampling of the target nodule during fine needle aspiration (FNA). Ultrasound-guided FNA with cytologic evaluation remains the mainstay for palpable and incidentally found thyroid nodules (Loevner and Mukherji, 2008).

Fine Needle Aspiration. FNA is the most useful diagnostic tool currently available in the management of thyroid nodules. It is the accepted standard of care for all patients who have palpable nodules with normal functioning thyroids, has high accuracy and low risk, and is cost-effective (Lansford and Teknos, 2006). The procedure is usually performed under ultrasound guidance, but may be performed in the surgeon's office. Several samples are usually taken from various parts of the nodule. Pathologic examination of FNA specimens reveals a benign nodule in 70% of biopsies, a nondiagnostic or inadequate biopsy 15% of the time, a suspicious nodule in 10% of cases, and malignancy in 5% of biopsies (American Thyroid Association, 2005). A suspicious nodule usually implies a follicular neoplasm, which can be benign or malignant, and requires removal for histologic evaluation.

Patient preparation for FNA should include the following information:

- You will be lying down for the procedure and may expect coldness on your neck from the prepping solution.
- Local anesthesia may or may not be used.
- Once the prick of the needle is felt, no talking, swallowing, or moving is allowed.

FNA may be an emotionally stressful procedure for the patient. Vials of ammonia should be kept in the room in case the patient feels faint. Lowering the head (using Trendelenburg's position or sitting with the head down) is also important to treat vasovagal syncope. Postprocedure education should

include (1) the necessity of refraining from using aspirin or aspirin-containing medications or nonsteroidal antiinflammatory drugs (NSAIDs) for the next 24 hours, and (2) the expectation of seeing a half-dollar–size bruise at the FNA site. There are no restrictions on food or activity.

Parathyroid Assessment. Elevation of serum PTH level in association with hypercalcemia is diagnostic of hyperparathyroidism in most cases. PTH normal levels are between 10 and 65 pg/ml (values vary with specific laboratory); the concentration of serum ionized calcium (4.5 to 5.6 mg/dl) is usually measured at the same time (Pagana and Pagana, 2009). Causes of primary hyperparathyroidism are single adenoma (80% to 85%), four-gland hyperplasia (10% to 15%), and rarely parathyroid carcinoma (less than 1%). Preoperative localization studies with a parathyroid sestamibi scan (Figure 7-4) or high-resolution ultrasonography can identify parathyroid adenomas with high sensitivity (70% to 80%). Sensitivity decreases significantly for hyperplasia (less than 50%).

Hyperparathyroidism causes an increase in the level of serum calcium and a decrease in the level of serum phosphate. Nursing diagnoses and plans of care are based on these imbalances and the severity of associated symptoms. Some patients are asymptomatic while others have symptoms that manifest themselves as disturbances in the central nervous system or cardiovascular, renal, gastrointestinal, or musculoskeletal system (Box 7-1).

Assessment includes determining whether the patient is apathetic or emotionally irritable; whether there is muscle weakness and atrophy, back or joint pain, nausea, vomiting, constipation, peptic ulcer disease, or cardiac dysrhythmia; and whether there is renal damage, stones, or disease (Canobbio, 2006). If any of these are present, the plan of care is adjusted. Otherwise, perioperative patient education and nursing management of the patient undergoing parathyroidectomy are essentially the same as those for thyroidectomy. In the early postoperative period for both thyroidectomy and parathyroidectomy, the patient is closely observed for any signs of hypocalcemia. The serum calcium level reaches its lowest level in 48 to 72 hours after surgery and returns to normal within the following 2 to 3 days. Symptoms include numbness and tingling of extremities and around the lips. Hyperactive tendon reflexes and a positive Chvostek's sign (tapping on the facial nerve elicits contraction of facial muscles) can be demonstrated on physical examination. Tetany may develop and is exhibited by carpopedal spasms, tonic-clonic convulsions, and laryngeal stridor, which can be fatal.

Planning

The entire surgical team has mutual accountability for patient safety (Banschbach, 2008). The perioperative nurse and surgical technologist should know the OR team members who will participate in the procedure as well as the roles each team member will assume (Haynes et al, 2009). Careful planning, assessment, and tailoring the plan of care to the surgery and specific patient needs reduce inherent risks (Risk Reduction Strategies). The surgical team should consider a patient who is not at optimal weight at high risk for pressure ulcer development and plan on padding pressure areas to prevent skin and tissue damage. Intraoperatively, warm saline should be provided for irrigation and a forced-air warming device used.

BOX 7-1

Parathyroid Dysfunction

HYPERPARATHYROIDISM
Definition
Overactivity of one or more of the parathyroid glands; excessive secretion of parathyroid hormone causes an increase in the level of calcium (hypercalcemia)

Signs and Symptoms
◆ Polyuria, polydipsia, kidney stones
◆ Abdominal pain, constipation, nausea, anorexia
◆ Fractures of ribs, spine
◆ Joint or back pain
◆ Depression, paranoia, mood swings
◆ Muscle weakness and atrophy

Complications
◆ Cardiac dysrhythmias, cardiac failure
◆ Gastric ulcer
◆ Pathologic fractures
◆ Renal disorders: kidney stones, urinary tract infections, renal failure
◆ Pancreatitis
◆ Stupor/coma

HYPOPARATHYROIDISM
Definition
Deficiency of parathyroid hormone, necessary to maintain normal levels of serum calcium; may occur as a result of radiation therapy for head and neck cancer or as a postoperative complication from thyroid or parathyroid surgery; symptoms are related to reduced calcium levels (hypocalcemia)

Signs and Symptoms
◆ Personality disturbances: anxiety, depression, irritability
◆ Tetany: muscle cramps, spasms (hands, face, feet); paresthesias: numbness and tingling (around mouth, lips, and tongue)
◆ Dry, scaly skin; brittle nails; thin, patchy hair
◆ Weak tooth enamel/dental caries
◆ Cataracts

Complications
◆ Cardiac dysrhythmias
◆ Seizures
◆ Psychoses
◆ Cardiac arrest

Modified from Canobbio MM: *Mosby's handbook of patient teaching*, ed 3, St Louis, 2006, Mosby; Workman LM: Care of patients with problems of the thyroid and parathyroid glands. In Ignatavicius DD, Workman ML, editors: *Medical-surgical nursing: patient-centered collaborative care*, ed 6, Philadelphia, 2010, Saunders.

BOX 7-2

Thyroid Storm

MORTALITY/MORBIDITY
Thyroid storm is a fulminating state that is fatal if untreated, with death rates of 20% to 30%.

PHYSICAL SYMPTOMS
◆ Thyroid storm may be difficult to differentiate from signs of uncomplicated thyrotoxicosis. It is an accentuation of the same signs. Onset is heralded by high-grade fever, mental obtundation, and decompensation of one or more organ systems as a result of severe hypermetabolism.
◆ Only guidelines are presented in the following table that compares symptoms of uncomplicated thyrotoxicosis and thyroid storm.

Uncomplicated Thyrotoxicosis	Thyroid Storm
Heat intolerance, diaphoresis	Hyperpyrexia, temperature in excess of 106° C, dehydration
Sinus tachycardia, heart rate 100-140 beats/min	Heart rate faster than 140 beats/min, hypotension, atrial dysrhythmias, congestive heart failure
Diarrhea, increased appetite with weight loss	Nausea, vomiting, severe diarrhea, abdominal pain, hepatocellular dysfunction with jaundice
Anxiety, restlessness	Confusion, agitation, delirium, frank psychosis, seizures, stupor, or coma

CAUSES
Causes of rapid rise in thyroid hormone levels:
◆ Thyroid or parathyroid surgery
◆ Radioiodine therapy
◆ Withdrawal of antithyroid drug therapy
◆ Vigorous thyroid palpation
◆ Iodinated contrast dye
◆ Thyroid hormone medication
Other common precipitating factors:
◆ Infection
◆ Emotional stress
◆ Tooth extraction
◆ Diabetic ketoacidosis
◆ Hypoglycemia
◆ Trauma
◆ Bowel infarction
◆ Parturition
◆ Pregnancy toxemia
◆ Pulmonary embolism
◆ Cerebrovascular accident
◆ Gestational trophoblastic disease

Modified from Kuwajerwala NK et al: *Thyroid, thyrotoxic storm following thyroidectomy*, available at emedicine.medscape.com/article850924. Accessed January 24, 2009.

Patients with hypothyroidism are at increased risk of becoming hypothermic (Hegarty et al, 2009).

A rapidly progressive and potentially fatal complication for patients with hyperthyroidism is thyroid storm (thyrotoxic crisis) (Kuwajerwala et al, 2007). The perioperative staff must recognize and differentiate between uncomplicated thyrotoxicosis and thyroid storm (Box 7-2) and be prepared to act quickly. The use of a rapid response team (RRT) for patients in crisis impacts treatment and patient outcomes (Rapid Response Team box) (Steel and Reynolds, 2008). Thyroid storm can occur in patients who have been partially controlled or whose hyperthyroidism is untreated. Thyrotoxic crisis can be precipitated by a stressful event, such as surgery. By planning a quiet, calm atmosphere and helping the patient relax, the perioperative staff can reduce the risk of thyroid storm. Collaborating with the surgical and anesthesia team, the perioperative staff can plan for appropriate interventions to assist in reducing body temperature and heart rate, provide oxy-

➤➤ RISK REDUCTION STRATEGIES

Perioperative Care of Thyroid and Parathyroid Surgery Patients

Risk reduction springs from the adage that "an ounce of prevention is better than a pound of cure." It is much better to prevent a problem than to treat one. A strong base of knowledge coupled with skills, experience, clinical judgment, and caring helps ensure the best possible patient outcomes (Benner et al, 2009).

Risk reduction strategies for patients undergoing thyroid and/or parathyroid surgery include the following:

PREOPERATIVELY
- The appropriate scans and preadmission testing are done.
- Patients are thoroughly screened for inpatient versus ambulatory status (Patient Screening and Assessment in Ambulatory Surgical Facilities, 2009).
- A detailed history and physical is completed.

INTRAOPERATIVELY
- Appropriate body alignment and padding are used to prevent nerve injury and postoperative discomfort.
- The OR team recognizes and is prepared for patients who are at risk for difficult intubation.
- Attention to sterile technique is a core team value.
- Gentle tissue handling reduces the risk of damage to nerves, parathyroid glands, and surrounding structures.
- Achieving and maintaining hemostasis promotes visibility and reduces postoperative bleeding.
- Hypertension is treated and controlled.
- The scrub person keeps instruments sterile for those patients who are at risk for postoperative bleeding. This would include patients with large thyroids that necessitated finger dissection and those who were difficult to intubate.

POSTOPERATIVELY
- The patient is monitored closely for airway difficulty.
- Hypertension is treated and controlled.
- The incision site is observed for swelling and/or bleeding. Ice packs may be applied to reduce swelling.
- Coughing should be minimized and neck support during coughing demonstrated.
- Complications of hemorrhage, compromised airway, thyroid storm, and hypocalcemia are recognized and treated immediately.
- The patient's condition is carefully assessed to determine that criteria are met for discharge to home on the day of surgery.
- Discharge instructions are clear, concise, and thorough; reviewed verbally; and provided in written format. Patients "teach-back" the instructions in their own words (TJC, 2007). Questions are encouraged and time allotted for answering them.

RAPID RESPONSE TEAM

Rapid response teams (RRTs) handle many critical situations, all of which require skill, knowledge, quick thinking, and immediate action. RRTs are called to treat patients who show signs of developing rapidly deteriorating conditions. Early response and treatment by a specialized, proficient, and experienced team can prevent further deterioration and greatly enhance outcomes for many patients.

The team's assessment and diagnostic skills must complement their abilities to respond to and treat the particular crisis appropriately. The team members should have advanced certification in critical care, PALS and ACLS. They are called a team because they must be able to work together efficiently and smoothly.

Perioperative staff and other caregivers, and in some institutions members of the patient's family, should be encouraged to initiate the RRT early when there is a concern about a patient's condition or they believe that "something's not right." The earlier the treatment, the less likelihood there is of a problem escalating out of control.

There must be a rapid response cart with all the medications and equipment needed to deal with a crisis. Supplies should also include airway equipment, a defibrillator, IV supplies, and monitoring equipment.

In the instances of potential patient complications described in this chapter, the RRT would treat hypocalcemia, hemorrhage, or thyroid storm appropriately.

---

gen and intravenous solutions, and administer medications as prescribed in the event thyrotoxic crisis occurs (Surgical Pharmacology).

Implementation

Positioning. Proper patient positioning on the OR bed is crucial for optimal exposure of the thyroid gland. The patient is positioned supine. Some surgeons prefer a beach chair position or a wedge under the back. Hyperextension of the neck is required for maximal exposure. A headrest provides proper support, keeps the head straight, and prevents aggravation of prior neck problems. Alternatively, a shoulder roll may be used. The arms are tucked at the side, the elbows are padded to protect the ulnar nerve, the palms face inward, and the wrist is maintained in a neutral position (Denholm, 2009). A drape secures the arms. It should be tucked snuggly, but not tightly, under the patient, not under the mattress. This prevents the arm from shifting downward intraoperatively and resting against the OR bed rail. All pressure points should be padded, especially for patients not at optimal weight. Should

SURGICAL PHARMACOLOGY

Thyroid Storm

PREOPERATIVE PROPHYLACTIC CARE FOR THYROID STORM

Potassium iodide (KI) is used preoperatively in thyrotoxicosis to decrease thyroid blood flow.

EMERGENCY CARE DURING THYROID STORM

◆ Maintain a patent airway and adequate ventilation.

◆ Give antithyroid drugs as prescribed: propylthiouracil (PTU, Propyl-Thyracil), 300-900 mg/day; methimazole (MMI) (Tapazole), up to 60 mg/day.

◆ Administer sodium iodide solution, 2 g/day IV as prescribed.

◆ Give propranolol (Inderal, Detensol), 1-3 mg IV as prescribed. Administer slowly, over 3 minutes. The patient should be connected to a cardiac monitor and a central venous pressure line should be in place.

◆ Esmolol (Brevibloc), 500 mcg/kg IV followed by 50-200 mcg/kg, minimum maintenance dose, is useful in patients at risk for complications from beta-blockade.

◆ Guanethidine or reserpine is substituted for propranolol in patients with congestive cardiac failure, bronchospasm, or history of asthma, although they cannot be used for patients who are in cardiovascular shock or collapse.

◆ One hour after administration of PTU or MMI, hormone release can be inhibited by large doses of iodine, which reduce thyroidal iodine uptake. Lugol's solution, 30 gtt/day PO in 4 divided doses, or a saturated solution of potassium iodide, 5 gtt orally or via an NG tube q6hr, can be used.

◆ Ipodate sodium, 0.5-3 g/day PO, can be administered instead of iodine.

◆ Patients unable to take PTU or MMI also can be treated with lithium 300 mg PO q6hr in conjunction with iodine. The lithium dose is adjusted as necessary to maintain levels at about 1 mEq/L.

◆ Plasmapheresis, plasma exchange, peritoneal dialysis exchange transfusion, and charcoal plasma perfusion are other techniques used to remove excess circulating hormone for patients who do not respond to the initial line of management.

◆ Monitor continuously for cardiac dysrhythmias.

◆ Monitor vital signs every 30 minutes.

◆ Provide comfort measures, including a cooling blanket.

◆ Give nonsalicylate antipyretics such as acetaminophen (FeverAll, Panadol) as prescribed (normally 650 mg PO q4hr).

◆ Aggressive fluid and electrolyte therapy, 3-5 L/day, is needed for dehydration and hypotension. Therefore invasive monitoring is advisable in elderly patients and in those with congestive cardiac failure. Fluid therapy should include glucose.

◆ Multivitamins, especially vitamin B_1, are added to prevent Wernicke's encephalopathy.

◆ Glucocorticoids reduce iodine uptake and antibody titers of thyroid-stimulating antibodies with stabilization of the vascular bed. They must be used with caution, however, as they have significant adverse effects. Dexamethasone (Decadron, Dexone), 2 mg IV q6hr, or hydrocortisone (Cortef, Solu-Cortef), 100 mg IV q8hr, may be given.

◆ Hypertension must be controlled with agents such as guanethidine (Ismelin), 1-2 mg/kg/day PO, or reserpine, 2.5-5 mg IM q4-6hr.

◆ Treat heart failure if present.

IM, Intramuscularly; *IV,* intravenously.

Modified from Kuwajerwala NK et al: *Thyroid, thyrotoxic storm following thyroidectomy,* available at emedicine.medscape.com/article850924. Accessed January 24, 2009; Workman LM: Care of patients with problems of the thyroid and parathyroid glands. In Ignatavicius DD, Workman ML, editors: *Medical-surgical nursing: patient-centered collaborative care,* ed 6, Philadelphia, 2010, Saunders.

the patient be too large to tuck the arms safely at the sides, arm sleds or side extensions for the OR bed may be used to accommodate the arms. Reduction of venous congestion can be accomplished by a 30-degree reverse-Trendelenburg's tilt of the OR bed.

Skin Preparation. The operative area (chin and anterior neck region, lateral surfaces of the neck from the earlobes down to the outer aspects of the shoulder, and upper anterior chest region to the nipples) is prepped with an antimicrobial solution. Appropriate precautions must be taken to prevent pooling of solution under the neck or in the axillary area. Alcohol-based prep solutions around the head and neck area present a risk for surgical fire. They must be used with caution, allowing time for the prep to dry and the fumes to dissipate. Bed sheets that become soaked with a flammable prep solution should be removed from the OR. After the skin prep, the patient is draped

with sterile towels and a fenestrated sheet. A sterile towel, lap sponge, or self-adherent tape strips may be placed on each side of the neck to prevent pooling of blood under the neck during surgery. Self-adherent tape strips or drapes also promote maintenance of the integrity of the sterile field and reduce the risk of intraoperative fire hazard by sealing off the operative site from anesthetic vapors that may have leaked and become trapped under the drapes. If lap sponges are used, they should be noted on the count sheet to avoid confusion in accounting for all counted items. After draping is complete, the time-out is taken. The following must be verified: correct patient, correct site, and correct procedure to be performed; and supplies may also be included (Perioperative Grand Rounds, 2009). The time-out is documented. The surgeon then marks the incision site with a marking pen or the pressure of a full-length fine silk tie to help ensure a wound line that blends with the patient's neck creases and skin lines.

SURGICAL TECHNOLOGY PREFERENCE CARD

Understanding the possibility of the patient experiencing airway difficulties and hemostasis issues, the room personnel should prepare themselves appropriately. Having a difficult airway cart, sponges, suture, and vascular clamps will facilitate this. Anticipating the possibilities of multiple specimens, the surgical technologist and circulator should prepare themselves with the proper supplies for specimen care. The scrub should maintain sterility until after the patient leaves the room, because of the possibility of postoperative bleeding.

Room Prep: Basic operating room furniture, thermoregulatory devices, sequential compression devices, extra blankets, padding/positioning devices, and safety/restraining devices

Prep Solution: In room
- Iodine and iodophors
- Chlorhexidine gluconate (CHG)

Note: If using an alcohol-based product, please be aware of pooling of product because these can cause a fire.

PROCEDURE CHECKLIST

Instrument Sets
- Standard set
- Vascular set
- Otolaryngology set

Equipment
- Difficult airway cart
- Electrosurgical unit—monopolar/bipolar
- Nerve monitoring system
- Suction

Additional Supplies: both sterile and nonsterile
- Peanuts
- Specialty suture
- Hemoclips
- Suction
- Sponges
- Drapes
- Gown and gloves for team members

Medications and Irrigation Solutions
- Lidocaine with epinephrine
- Thrombin
- Absorbable gelatin
- Oxidized cellulose

Drains and Dressings
- Penrose
- Jackson-Pratt

Specimen Care
- Proper container for each specimen
- Labels for each specimen
- Proper solution for specimen type

Surgical Interventions

UNILATERAL THYROID LOBECTOMY, SUBTOTAL LOBECTOMY, BILATERAL SUBTOTAL LOBECTOMY, NEAR-TOTAL THYROIDECTOMY, AND TOTAL THYROIDECTOMY

Unilateral thyroid lobectomy or hemithyroidectomy is the removal of one thyroid lobe with excision of the isthmus. The isthmus is completely removed to prevent postoperative hypertrophy in response to the lobectomy with subsequent airway impingement. *Subtotal lobectomy* is a lobectomy that spares the posterior capsule and a portion of adjacent thyroid tissue. *Bilateral subtotal thyroidectomy* is removal of both lobes of the thyroid in the fashion stated for subtotal thyroidectomy. *Near-total thyroidectomy* is a total lobectomy with contralateral subtotal thyroidectomy. *Total thyroidectomy* is the removal of both lobes of the thyroid and all thyroid tissue present. For patients with cancer of the thyroid, total thyroidectomy is the desired surgical treatment (Sarkar, 2004; Tuttle, 2007), followed by iodine-131 remnant ablation. Preventing thyroid cancer recurrence does not depend on surgical approach, but on complete surgical excision of the tumor (Loevner and Mukherji, 2008). Following surgery, the thyroid cancer patient is prescribed thyroid hormone suppression therapy and monitored by physical examination, laboratory studies (serum thyroid function and thyroglobulin levels), and scans.

The purpose of the surgical intervention relates to the patient's medical diagnosis. *Goiter* refers to any enlargement of the thyroid gland and includes both benign and malignant nodules; the enlargement is visible over the anterior neck (Wilson and Giddens, 2009). *Benign adenomas* are encased in a fibrous capsule, distinct from surrounding thyroid tissue. *Malignancies* occur most commonly in patients under 20 or over 60 years of age. Excising the lymph nodes with suspected or known cancer of the thyroid remains a standard therapy. Radiologic studies

AMBULATORY SURGERY CONSIDERATIONS

Patient Teaching, Preparation, and Screening

If the patient will be discharged home on the same day as surgery, thorough patient teaching and preparation with written instructions is critical. It is paramount that nursing staff have strong critical thinking and assessment skills to screen patients for problems that may preclude same-day discharge. Safe and successful ambulatory surgery depends, in part, on recognizing which patients can be sent home and which patients should be admitted.

The nursing staff must verify that the patient has arranged for someone to drive him/her home and for a caregiver (family/friend) to assist during the first 24 hours at home. Surgery cannot be done on an ambulatory basis if these arrangements have not been made.

Patients must be thoroughly and carefully screened as to eligibility for ambulatory thyroidectomy or parathyroidectomy (Patient Screening and Assessment, 2009). Ambulatory surgery is contraindicated in patients with grossly enlarged thyroids or comorbid medical conditions, such as cardiac disease, uncontrolled hypertension, brittle diabetes, and sleep apnea. Intraoperatively, patients who had a difficult intubation or who bled excessively should be excluded from discharge on the same day as surgery.

The nursing staff should ascertain the patient's ability to understand and cooperate with discharge instructions.

The patient is sent home with prescriptions for pain management, calcium supplements, thyroid hormone (if indicated), and other medications specific to preexisting conditions. All medications should be reviewed (discharge reconciliation) and a list provided.

The patient must meet discharge criteria: the patient must be fully awake, alert, and oriented and be able to void, swallow, and drink fluids without nausea or vomiting.

The need for deep breathing, mobility, and hydration must be emphasized.

The patient should be cautioned not to drive or drink alcohol for at least 24 hours.

Patients and families are under physical and emotional stress and often will find the environment and information received overwhelming. Standardized printed discharge instructions from the surgeon, specific to the surgery performed, with space available to customize information for the patient, provide a valuable tool and reference resource for the patient and family/caregiver to use at home.

Perioperative staff must ascertain that the patient and caregiver understand the symptoms indicating a significant problem that needs immediate attention, as well as actions to take and persons to contact in case of an emergency. These include signs and symptoms of dyspnea, hemorrhage, thyroid storm, and hypocalcemia.

The patient should be instructed to call the physician's office for a follow-up visit if this has not been arranged.

▶▶ RISK REDUCTION STRATEGIES

Discharge Medication Reconciliation

Medication reconciliation is an ongoing National Patient Safety Goal (NPSG). Up to 75% of potential adverse drug events occur during discharge (Pippins et al, 2008) as patients and their caregivers review, as part of discharge preparation, new medications and must understand which medications to stop or change. Their ability to concentrate or ask questions may be compromised by other needs such as making follow-up appointments and planning for multiple, and sometimes complex, changes in routine activities. In one study, only 27.9% of discharged patients were able to identify their medications, 37.2% knew the purpose of all their medications, 14.0% were able to state the common side effect(s) of all their medications, and 41.9% were able to state their diagnosis or diagnoses (Makaryus and Friedman, 2005).

Discharge reconciliation has several specific aspects. Drug formulary and related changes that occurred at admission must be addressed. If, for example, the patient's home medication was one drug but the patient was switched to another in the drug formulary, this change must be reconciled. A resolution must be made and clearly communicated to prevent the patient from taking both, or neither, of these medications. Prescriptions must be provided. The full medication list must be communicated clearly to both the patient and the caregiver. A simple printed discharge summary that includes details of the medications, including dose, indication, and directions, can reduce post-discharge medication errors. This same form can be sent to the next provider of care (i.e., primary care provider or specialist).

Adapted from Makaryus AN, Friedman EA: Patients' understanding of their treatment plans and diagnosis at discharge, *Mayo Clin Proc* 80:991-994; 2005; Meisel S: *Falling through the cracks: medication reconciliation at admission and discharge,* Medscape CME, March 2009, available at cme.medscape.com/viewprogram/19223?src=cmemp. Accessed April 6, 2009; Pippins JR et al: Classifying and predicting errors of inpatient medication reconciliation, *J Gen Intern Med* 23:1414-1422, 2008; The Joint Commission, Accreditation Program for Hospitals: *National Patient Safety Goals,* Oakridge, Ill, 2009, Author.

aid in the understanding of nodal metastasis and determining which levels of the neck to dissect. Contralateral metastasis is generally associated with large tumors. Young patients tend to respond favorably to treatment and have a better prognosis than older patients (Loevner and Mukherji, 2008).

Graves' disease, the most common cause of hyperthyroidism, is associated with diffuse, bilateral enlargement of the thyroid gland. Surgery is not the first response for Graves' disease, but is reserved for those patients who fail medical therapy (antithyroid drugs and radioactive iodine) or have a contrain-dication to medical therapy. *Hashimoto's thyroiditis* is believed to be an autoimmune disease in which nontender enlargement of the gland occurs. Surgery is performed to relieve tracheal obstruction. *Nontoxic nodular goiter* involves production of insufficient hormones and is noninflammatory in character; in such cases thyroid tissue proliferates in an apparent attempt to produce the minimal hormonal requirement. Surgery may be indicated to relieve tracheal or esophageal obstruction or to rule out a malignant nodule of the thyroid. *Total thyroidectomy* may be done for malignant tumors (Box 7-3). An intraopera-

RESEARCH HIGHLIGHT

Transoral Access for Endoscopic Thyroid Resection

Advances in thyroid surgery have been facilitated by intraoperative neuromonitoring to prevent laryngeal nerve paralysis, early measurement of intraoperative parathyroid hormone (IoPTH) levels to avert symptomatic hypocalcemia, and improved devices for hemostasis and dissection to better control bleeding. The authors of this study suggest the sublingual transoral approach as a promising minimally invasive endoscopic access to the thyroid gland from outside the neck region.

Sublingual transoral access was first evaluated in two fresh human cadavers. An experimental investigation then was performed using a porcine model. A total of 10 endoscopic transoral thyroidectomies were performed using a modified axilloscope with an obturator, ultrasonic scissors, and a neuromonitoring system to identify the recurrent laryngeal nerve.

Complete transoral thyroid resection was achieved with both human cadavers and live pigs. Despite the complexity of the anatomic region, the transoral procedure was successfully and smoothly performed. The neuromonitoring system ensured normal function of the recurrent laryngeal nerves on both sides after removal of the thyroid gland. No complications occurred during the procedures or afterward.

Endoscopic transoral thyroid resection is possible. A follow-up study undertook preclinical investigation in human cadavers, again demonstrating adequacy of access and feasibility of the procedure. The next step will be its broad application in living pigs before it may be applied in humans. Finally, large prospective, randomized trials comparing the outcomes of different endoscopic procedures are needed to establish levels of evidence and grades of recommendation for transoral access.

Modified from Benhidjeb T et al: *Natural orifice surgery on thyroid gland: totally transoral video-assisted thyroidectomy (TOVAT): report of first experimental results of a new surgical method*, 2009, available at www.ncbi.nlm.nih.gov/pubmed/. Accessed April 4, 2009; Witzel K et al: Transoral access for endoscopic thyroid resection, *Surg Endosc* 22(8):1871-1875, 2007.

BOX 7-3

Malignant Thyroid Nodules

PAPILLARY CARCINOMA
◆ Most common form (>70%)
◆ Poorly encapsulated
◆ Calcifications present—uncommon in other carcinomas

FOLLICULAR CARCINOMA
◆ Second most common form (15%)
◆ Well-differentiated
◆ Associated with iodine deficiency

HÜRTHLE CELL TUMOR
◆ Derived from follicular epithelium
◆ Associated with regional nodal metastasis

MEDULLARY CARCINOMA
◆ Undifferentiated tumor
◆ Higher death rate than differentiated

ANAPLASTIC CARCINOMA
◆ More common in females and elderly
◆ Highly aggressive
◆ Rapidly fatal; death usually occurs within 1 year of diagnosis

UNCOMMON CARCINOMAS
◆ Primary lymphoma
◆ Primary squamous cell
◆ Metastatic thyroid tumors

Modified from Deitch M: Thyroid cancer, *Adv Nurses* 10(14):24, 2008.

tive frozen section may be indicated to confirm the diagnosis. If the diagnosis is not definitive on frozen section, a hemithyroidectomy may be the treatment of choice. If the permanent histologic report is benign, the patient has the unaffected thyroid lobe preserved and intact. If the pathology, however, proves to be carcinoma, a complete thyroidectomy is then performed as soon as possible.

Minimally invasive approaches to thyroid surgery arose in the late 1990s and early twenty-first century for treatment of small thyroid nodules. These include minimally invasive open thyroidectomy (MIT) and minimally invasive video-assisted thyroidectomy (MIVAT). Minimally invasive thyroid surgery is performed for both partial and total thyroidectomies (Dhingra, 2008). Researchers are conducting studies on natural orifice transendoscopic surgery (NOTES); in the future, skin incisions may become obsolete for some surgeries.

Minimally invasive thyroidectomies reduce postoperative pain, decrease hospital length of stays, and improve cosmetic results (Research Highlight, p. 580, bottom) and may be done using a local anesthetic. Minimizing dissection and resultant

dead space eliminates the need for external drains in most cases. Smaller incisions, minimal use of surgical drains, and prophylactic calcium supplementation have enabled thyroid surgery to be performed safely on an ambulatory basis (Dinghra, 2008).

MIVAT is generally reserved for thyroid nodules within specific size limits as well as for low-stage papillary thyroid carcinomas. As MIVAT has evolved and surgeons have become more proficient with the technique, the only absolute contraindications for its use are thyroid malignancies beyond low-stage papillary carcinoma and preoperative evidence of lymph node metastasis. Relative contraindications include prior conventional thyroidectomy, nodules larger than 35 mm and 30 ml, and a history of thyroiditis (Dinghra, 2008). Studies indicate that it is safe to perform MIVAT thyroidectomies as ambulatory procedures under certain conditions (Terris, 2006).

Procedural Considerations

The patient is positioned supine. A drape pack with fenestrated sheet is required along with a basic instrument set and the addition of thyroid instruments. An electrosurgical unit (ESU),

RESEARCH HIGHLIGHT

Cosmetic Surgery Techniques Can Enhance Thyroid Surgery Results

As noted in the plan of care for patients undergoing thyroid and parathyroid surgery, concern about appearance after surgery is not unusual. This prospective analysis included 248 patients (198 women and 50 men) who underwent varying approaches to thyroid surgery—from a standard (i.e., several inches long) neck incision for large thyroids, to minimally invasive techniques that cut the incision size in half, to endoscopic approaches that further reduced incision size. The following techniques were reported to improve aesthetic results:

♦ Having the patient sit or stand while incision sites were marked to ensure that they blend with the natural lines of the body
♦ Minimizing incision size
♦ Trimming skin edges at the incision sites. In minimal access techniques, skin edges sometimes become frayed as large nodules are removed from relatively small incisions. Rather than make a bigger incision, skin edges are excised to improve reapproximation.

♦ Using surgical glue instead of sutures. Surgical glue allows accurate skin edge apposition without the risk of "railroad-tracking" from skin sutures. It is also convenient for patients. Instead of returning for suture removal, they can peel the glue off.
♦ Minimizing trauma to surrounding skin. Instead of creating extensive flaps, as described in conventional approaches, a modified approach involves minimal flap creation, sparing extensive tissue dissection.
♦ Avoiding use of drains
♦ Using other techniques, such as the ultrasonic harmonic scalpel, to reduce overall surgical trauma

In this analysis, only 1 of the 248 patients required additional treatment for the surgical scar; that female patient required steroid injections for hypertrophic scarring. The application of well-known cosmetic surgery principles improved optimal outcomes relating to the appearance of postoperative incision sites.

Modified from Terris D: Cosmetic surgery techniques can enhance thyroid surgery results, *Medical College of Georgia, available at https://my.mcg.edu/portal/page/portal/News/archive/2007. Accessed January 24, 2009.*

an exhaust system for surgical smoke (AORN, 2008), gauze dissectors, and a small drain (optional) are commonly used. A headlight for the surgeon and assistant may be required. A nerve monitor may be used during surgery to protect the laryngeal nerve. The patient is prepped from the chin to the upper chest, using fire safety precautions. Surgeons may use the harmonic scalpel or LigaSure Precise. The heated blade of the harmonic scalpel retains its heat longer than an electrosurgical unit blade. Appropriate precautions must therefore be used to avoid inadvertent burning of adjacent tissue. Thyroidectomies are done through a small incision and visualization is critical for successful extraction. Bleeding can obscure the view and hinder the progress of the surgery. Therefore, surgeons may use hemostatic agents intraoperatively to maintain hemostasis (Research Highlight).

Open Thyroidectomy Operative Procedure

Figure 7-5 provides an overview of safe thyroidectomy principles.

1. A transverse incision (slightly curved and symmetric) is made parallel to the normal skin line crease of the neck, through the skin and first layers of the cervical fascia and platysma muscle, about 2 cm above the sternoclavicular junction.
2. An upper skin flap is undermined to the level of the thyroid notch of the thyroid cartilage; double skin hooks or Allis clamps are placed on the dermis and retracted anteriorly and superiorly to facilitate dissection. A lower flap is then undermined to the sternoclavicular joint. A knife, fine curved scissors, tissue forceps, and gauze sponges are used to undermine the flaps. Bleeding vessels are clamped with hemostats and ligated with fine nonabsorbable sutures. Lateral retraction with a vein retractor or Army-Navy retractor helps identify the plane for dissection.
3. Flaps are held away from the wound with stay sutures inserted through the cervical fascia and platysma muscle or by a self-retaining retractor.
4. The fascia in the midline is incised between the strap (sternohyoid and sternothyroid) muscles with a knife.

Care must be taken to preserve the anterior jugular veins. The fascia may be lifted on either side with forceps during the dissection to help define the plane of dissection and protect the jugular vessels. The sternocleidomastoid muscle may be retracted with a loop retractor. Ordinarily, it is not necessary to divide the strap muscles. However, if additional exposure is required, such as with a very large gland, they may be divided between clamps using Mastin muscle clamps, Kocher clamps, or hemostats and a knife. The divided muscles are retracted from the operative site to expose the target lobe.

5. The inferior and middle thyroid veins are ligated with fine nonabsorbable sutures or hemoclips, and divided with Metzenbaum scissors.
6. The lobe is first rotated medially, and loose areolar tissue is then divided posteriorly and medially toward the tracheoesophageal sulcus with hemostats and Metzenbaum scissors. Small sponges are used for blunt dissection. Bleeding is controlled with hemostats, hemoclips, and ligatures, as well as with the ESU; a bipolar ESU may be used. The recurrent laryngeal nerve, which enters the cricothyroid muscle at the level of the cricoid cartilage, is identified and carefully preserved. Electrocoagulation should not be used in the vicinity of the recurrent or superior laryngeal nerve because the spread of current could damage the nerve. Nerve integrity monitoring systems (NIMSs) are helpful in identifying the branches of the laryngeal nerve. NIMSs should supplement, not replace, good surgical technique and anatomic awareness (Loevner and Mukherji, 2008). Vigorous suction and dissection may cause injury to the nerve and parathyroid glands. The scrub person should prepare a radiopaque 4 × 8 inch sponge on the end of a forceps for the surgeon or assistant to use in gently blotting the area.
7. The thyroid lobe is pulled downward, a Lahey goiter or polar retractor inserted as necessary, and the avascular tissue between the trachea and upper pole of the thyroid dissected by means of Metzenbaum scissors.

Dissection and Hemostasis with Hydroxylated Polyvinyl Acetal Tampons in Open Thyroid Surgery

The objectives for thyroidectomy are avoidance of injury to the recurrent laryngeal nerves, conservation of the parathyroid glands, accurate hemostasis, and excellent cosmesis. To achieve these objectives major improvements and new technologies have been proposed and applied in thyroid surgery; among these are performing mini-invasive thyroidectomies, using a regional anesthetic, conducting intraoperative neuromonitoring, and implementing new devices for dissection and hemostasis. Minor bleeding from small vessels, however, can still present major complications in thyroid surgery. Bleeding obscures visualization and is the major cause of converting minimally invasive to open thyroidectomies.

Hydroxylated polyvinyl acetal (HPA) tampons are made with a synthetic, open cell foam structure able to absorb fluids up to 25 times their initial weight. Their surface is smooth and they do not stick to tissues. They have an initial, mildly hard, firmness that allows their use as blunt dissection devices. They are designed in different shapes, forms, and sizes. Specific tests demonstrated that HPA tampons are fully biocompatible and able to reduce bacterial growth.

Studies were performed to test the efficacy of HPA tampons for tissue dissection and minor bleeding control during several thyroid procedures. They were found to be exceptionally useful for absorbing blood from minor and diffuse loss, helping to control bleeding by a combined action of fluid absorption and local compression. The tampon's porous design allowed use of a suction device through the tampon itself. The initial mildly hard consistency of the HPA tampons allowed their use in blunt tissue dissection.

The authors concluded that the use of HPA tampons was efficient for controlling minor bleeding, removing fluids, and performing blunt tissue dissection during thyroid surgery.

Modified from Dionigi G et al: Dissection and hemostasis with hydroxylated polyvinyl acetyl tampons in open thyroid surgery, *Ann Surg Innov Res* 1:3, 2007, available at www.aornjournal.org/article/S0001-2092(07)00583-2/fulltext#further-reading. Accessed April 6, 2009.

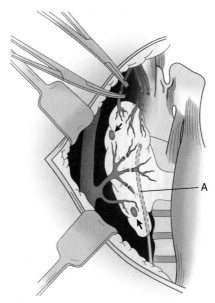

FIGURE 7-5 Safe thyroid principles emphasize the following: division of all branch vessels on the capsule of the thyroid with fine mosquito hemostats to prevent injury to the superior laryngeal nerve while detaching the superior thyroid artery and to prevent injury to the parathyroid glands while detaching the inferior thyroid artery; mobilization of parathyroid glands (*arrows*) by medial-to-lateral dissection to preserve their vascular pedicle; constant awareness of the location of the recurrent laryngeal nerve (*A*), especially near its penetration into the larynx.

8. The superior thyroid artery is defined by blunt dissection with a peanut sponge on a clamp; it is then isolated with a right-angle clamp. The artery is ligated with nonabsorbable suture or clamped with hemoclips, and divided. Care is taken here to avoid injury to the superior laryngeal nerve. The upper parathyroid gland is often identified at this time.

9. The inferior thyroid artery is identified and preserved. The inferior parathyroid is likewise identified. Only branches of the inferior thyroid artery that do not supply the parathyroid glands are ligated, using fine forceps, sutures, and scissors. The thyroid lobe is then dissected away from the recurrent laryngeal nerve with Metzenbaum scissors and hemostats. Bleeding vessels are clamped with hemostats or hemoclips, and ligated with fine nonabsorbable sutures.

10. The lobe is elevated with Babcock clamps and freed from the trachea with fine scissors, forceps, knife, and hemostats, or with cautious electrodissection. The fibrous bands attached to the trachea and cricoid cartilage are divided.

11. The isthmus of the gland is elevated with fine forceps and divided between hemostats with scissors, removing the lobe and isthmus. The cut edge of the remaining thyroid may be oversewn to maintain hemostasis. If a pyramidal lobe is present, it is removed, along with the lobe to which it is attached, to its termination in the neck, which may reach the hyoid bone. If it is necessary to transect the hyoid bone, a small bone cutter is used.

12. The cut surface of the opposite lobe requires careful hemostasis. Interrupted sutures may be used for this purpose as well as for reapproximation to the pretracheal fascia.

13. The excised thyroid is examined for inadvertent parathyroid inclusion. If a parathyroid is present, it is removed and reimplanted.

14. The strap muscles, if severed, are reapproximated with fine interrupted absorbable or nonabsorbable sutures. If necessary, a drain is inserted into the thyroid bed and exteriorized through the midline. Some surgeons prefer to drain the wound laterally through the sternocleidomastoid muscle and the lateral extremity of the incision, believing that this produces better healing and cosmetic results. A hemostatic agent may be placed in the lateral gutter to facilitate hemostasis.

15. The edges of the platysma muscle are reapproximated. The skin edges are then reapproximated with subcuticular fine absorbable sutures.

16. Wound closure tapes (e.g., Steri-Strips) are applied to the wound edges and gauze dressings, if required, are placed on the wound with minimal tape.

SUBSTERNAL OR INTRATHORACIC THYROIDECTOMY

Extensions of goiters enlarging into the substernal and intrathoracic regions may occur. If they cause tracheal and esophageal obstruction, they are usually excised surgically. Longer instruments are sometimes required. Splitting the sternum is rarely necessary because access to the substernal part of the gland is usually satisfactory through the standard thyroid incision.

MINIMALLY INVASIVE THYROIDECTOMY

Minimally Invasive Open Thyroidectomy

The length of the incision is the major difference between minimally invasive and traditional thyroidectomy. An incision of less than 6 cm is considered minimally invasive. Because of its smaller size, the site of the incision is critical for optimum access and visualization. After the incision is made, the remaining procedure is the same as that for conventional thyroidectomy (Dinghra, 2008).

Minimally Invasive Video-Assisted Thyroidectomy (MIVAT)

Procedural Considerations. The possibility of conversion to open thyroidectomy should be included on the operative consent form. Instruments and supplies for a possible open procedure are readied. Surgical skin preparation is done as in an open procedure in the event conversion is necessary. A set of long Miccoli instruments is added to the standard thyroid or neck dissection setup (Figure 7-6, *A*). A 30-degree endoscope and harmonic scalpel with scissors are used to ligate and divide vessels (Figure 7-6, *B*). Fire safety precautions are implemented for illuminated light cords, endoscopes, light sources, and cable connections.

Intraoperative Procedure
1. The patient is positioned and draped as for thyroidectomy. A horizontal incision of 3 cm or less is marked and then carefully made between the sternal notch and cricoid cartilage, usually less than 2 cm inferior to the cricoid (Figure 7-7).
2. Subcutaneous tissue is electrodissected and the raphe of strap muscle is then separated superiorly and inferiorly for about 3 cm. The anterior jugular veins are preserved.
3. Blunt dissection is used to separate the strap muscle from the thyroid.
4. The middle thyroid vein is clipped and divided.
5. Miccoli retractors are used to retract the strap muscles and soft tissue, exposing the superior lobe and vascular bundle.
6. The endoscope is introduced to visualize the upper pole. Three persons are needed: the surgeon, an assistant for retraction, and an endoscopist.
7. Miccoli spatula-shaped and aspirator dissectors are used to dissect the superior pole and vascular bundle (Figure 7-8). Care is taken to identify and preserve the external branch of the superior laryngeal nerve.
8. The thyroid lobe is then retracted medially and its lateral and posterior attachments are dissected. The recurrent laryngeal nerve and parathyroids are protected and preserved (Figure 7-9).
9. After sufficient mobilization of the lobe, the remainder of the procedure is accomplished under direct visualization. The isthmus is transected to complete the lobectomy.
10. The same procedure is repeated on the other side for complete thyroidectomy.

11. Hemostasis is achieved, the wound is irrigated, strap muscles are reapproximated, and the skin is closed (Figure 7-10).

Postoperatively, analgesics, antiemetics, and prophylactic antibiotics are administered in PACU. Preoperative thyroid hormone supplementation is continued. For inpatients, ionized calcium and albumin levels are checked in PACU and then every 6 to 8 hours. Hypocalcemia is a serum calcium level below 8.0 mg/dl. If patients are discharged the same day as surgery, prophylactic calcium supplements will be prescribed for several weeks. Ambulatory patients are provided with contact information and told to notify their surgeon immediately if they experience signs of hypocalcemia. Early signs include perioral numbness or paresthesia and a positive Chvostek's sign.

THYROGLOSSAL DUCT CYSTECTOMY

Thyroglossal duct cyst is the most common congenital cyst found in the neck. Although this cyst may be found in patients of any age, 50% usually are seen before 20 years of age and about 70% by 30 years of age. The thyroglossal duct is an embryonic structure arising from the descent of the thyroid gland into the anterior portion of the neck. When present in an adult, it exists as a pretracheal cystic pouch attached to the hyoid bone, with or without a sinus tract to the base of the tongue at the foramen cecum (Figure 7-11). Thyroglossal duct cystectomy requires complete excision of the cyst in continuity with its tract, the central portion of the hyoid bone, and the tissue above the hyoid bone extending to the base of the tongue to avoid recurrent cystic formation and to prevent infection (Warner, 2004).

Procedural Considerations

The perioperative nursing assessment should be appropriate to the patient's age because the patient is frequently a child or teenager. Reassurance and age-appropriate information about the procedure are given. The patient is positioned supine, with the neck supported in extension. Bone instruments are needed in addition to the basic instrument set.

Operative Procedure

1. After the head is extended and the chin elevated, a transverse incision is made between the hyoid bone and thyroid cartilage through the subcutaneous tissue.
2. The platysma muscle is incised and flaps raised as described for thyroidectomy.
3. The strap (sternohyoid and sternothyroid) muscles are separated in the midline.
4. Sharp and blunt dissection is used to mobilize the cyst and duct, up to the attachment to the hyoid bone. The hyoid bone is transected twice, removing the center section with bone-cutting forceps. The segment of bone and the cyst are freed from adjacent structures.
5. The duct is traced superiorly through or near the hyoid up to the musculature of the tongue and removed completely. Methylene blue dye injection is used occasionally to visualize the whole tract.
6. The cyst is removed and the strap muscles closed with interrupted fine nonabsorbable sutures. A drain may be placed. The skin is then closed with subcuticular fine absorbable sutures and dressings are applied.

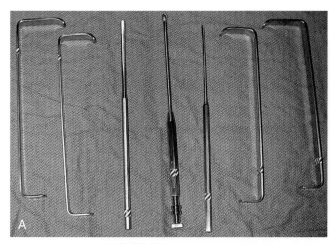

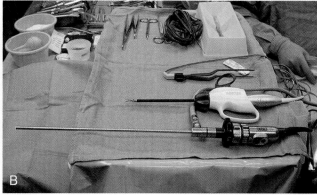

FIGURE 7-6 **A**, Miccoli instrument set designed for MIVAT. **B**, Endoscope and harmonic scalpel.

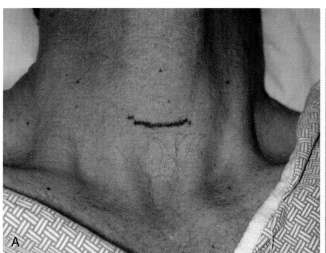

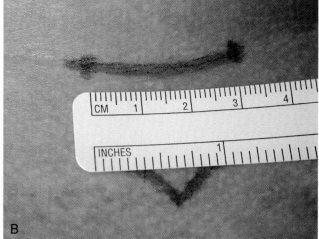

FIGURE 7-7 **A**, MIVAT incision location. **B**, MIVAT incision length.

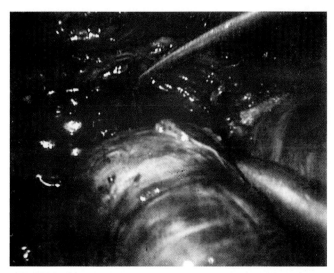

FIGURE 7-8 Video-assisted dissection of the right superior pole.

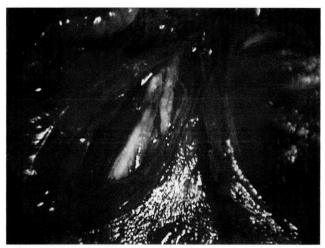

FIGURE 7-9 Identification of the recurrent laryngeal nerve during video-assisted right thyroid lobectomy. A parathyroid gland is also identified.

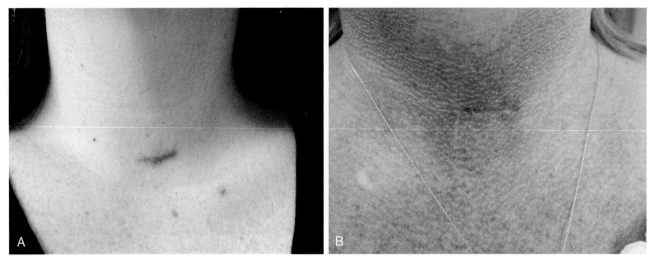

FIGURE 7-10 **A**, Surgical scar at 2 weeks. **B**, Surgical scar at 6 weeks.

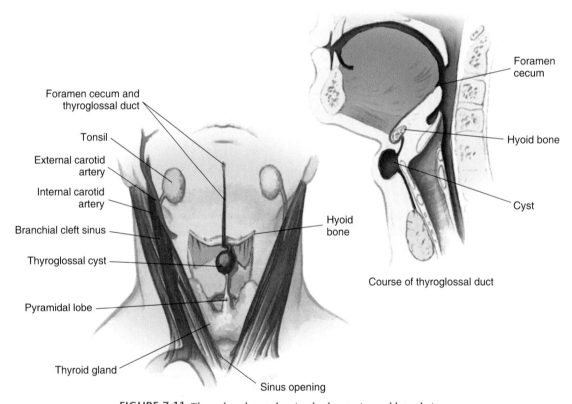

FIGURE 7-11 Thyroglossal cyst showing both anterior and lateral views.

NECK DISSECTION

Neck dissection for metastatic node disease remains controversial as there is a high correlation of recurrence of cancer with little impact on long-term survival despite neck dissection. Lateral neck dissection is reserved for patients who have clinically proven lateral neck disease or gross metastasis along the jugular vein. Central compartment dissection is reserved for those who have clinically apparent or suspicious nodes first noted during the primary surgery.

Patients are closely monitored postoperatively with ultrasound and thyroglobulin to screen for recurrence. Adjuvant radioactive iodine ablation is used for high-risk thyroid cancer patients, including those with residual disease in the thyroid bed, large tumors, multifocal disease, nodal metastasis, vascular and extrathyroidal invasion, and cancer with an aggressive history as well as younger patients with distant metastasis (Loevner and Mukherji, 2008). Surgery is the treatment of choice for resectable recurrent thyroid carcinoma. The overall 10-year survival rate is 90%.

Handling Multiple Specimens

The perioperative nurse and surgical technologist are accountable for specimen collection, identification, and handling. During parathyroidectomy, multiple specimens may be collected. To accurately identify and safely manage these specimens, they should do the following:

◆ Verify specimen collection and handling needs with the surgeon. This should occur before the procedure starts and may be part of the time-out or preoperative briefing (Paige et al, 2008).

◆ Have available an adequate number of specimen containers, labels, laboratory forms, and appropriate preservative.

◆ Take an additional time-out when the specimen is collected, in which the surgeon, scrub person, and nurse agree on the name of the specimen, its type, and source location.

◆ Label the specimen with a patient label naming the contents of the container. When multiple specimens are collected, they may be labeled A, B, C, etc. to indicate the order of harvesting.

◆ Communicate to the pathology department the nature of the procedure and anticipated specimens. Plan for direct communication about specimens between the surgeon and pathologist or perform a read-back or repeat-back of pathology findings.

◆ Use Standard Transmission–Based Precautions.

◆ Log (chain of custody) specimens according to institutional protocol.

◆ Arrange for timely transport of specimens to the pathology department.

◆ Document specimen collection in the intraoperative nursing record according to institutional protocol.

Modified from AORN recommended practices for the care and handling of specimens in the perioperative environment. In *Perioperative standards and recommended practices*, Denver, 2009, The Association.

PARATHYROIDECTOMY

Parathyroidectomy is excision of one or more parathyroid glands. Normal or atrophic glands are generally not removed. The presence of adenomas (hypersecreting neoplasms), hyperplasia, or carcinoma requires surgical excision. For carcinomas, resection of the ipsilateral thyroid lobe and lymph nodes is essential, although metastasis may still occur by way of the bloodstream. Any residual parathyroid cancer may secrete parathormone, causing hypercalcemia and its attendant problems.

Previously, the gold standard for parathyroidectomy was bilateral neck exploration with biopsy of all four glands to confirm the presence of adenoma or hyperplasia. New technologies, however, have offered less invasive surgical options that pinpoint the affected gland and obviate the need to biopsy, and potentially damage, healthy parathyroid glands. The four-gland exploration for single-gland involvement is being replaced by radio-guided, minimally invasive ambulatory procedures utilizing intraoperative PTH levels and/or the gamma probe. Patients with a negative sestamibi scan are excluded from minimally invasive parathyroidectomy protocols although intraoperative PTH levels are still helpful in identifying multiple adenomas (Loevner and Mukherji, 2008). Often, the diagnosis of an adenoma can be made by gross inspection of the glands

by the surgeon, but such diagnoses must be confirmed histologically by the pathologist.

Minimally invasive techniques cannot be used for hyperplasia. Hyperplasia requires removal of three and one-half glands through a bilateral neck exploration. A portion of a gland must remain to prevent hypocalcemia and its complications.

Procedural Considerations

During bilateral neck exploration multiple biopsies may be performed to determine the presence or absence of parathyroid tissue. Numerous specimen containers should be available (Patient Safety). Some surgeons perform parathyroidectomy using a minimally invasive approach with intraoperative parathyroid hormone assays to determine if the gland removed was the cause of hypersecretion. The perioperative nurse should ascertain that a pathologist is alerted and ready to analyze blood samples and tissue specimens. Preoperative localization studies, if done, should be conducted in the OR. If the surgeon is performing a focused parathyroidectomy (as described under Minimally Invasive, Focused Parathyroid Surgery), several blood tubes will be required to measure parathyroid levels intraoperatively. The circulating nurse will note excision time and collaborate with the anesthesia provider to anticipate and handle postexcision blood samples. Mediastinotomy instruments should be available. The patient is positioned, prepped, and draped as described for thyroidectomy. Hemoclips should be available.

Operative Procedure (Open Approach)

Although it is quickly being replaced with the focused approach to parathyroidectomy, in the classic open approach, with the thyroid gland visible, bilateral neck exploration of the "normal" locations of the four parathyroid glands is conducted. Meticulous hemostasis by means of mosquito hemostats and fine ligatures is a prerequisite to location and identification of these small glands.

The thyroid gland is gently rotated anteriorly to provide access to the posterior thyroid sulcus, where the parathyroid glands are almost always found. Identification of the parathyroid vascular pedicle, as it leaves either the superior thyroid artery or the inferior thyroid artery, is a means of locating both the inferior and superior glands. Metzenbaum scissors, mosquito hemostats, hemoclips, and gauze dissector (Kittner or peanut) sponges are used during dissection.

Attention then turns to the posterior lateral surface of the thyroid lobe or just beneath the lower thyroid pole, where the lower parathyroid glands are frequently found. Finding the vascular pedicle from the inferior thyroid artery may aid in identification. Occasionally, the lower pair is found in the thymic capsule or tissue, in which case a portion of the thymus is resected. A mediastinotomy is indicated for a small percentage of patients. Thoracoscopy is also a successful, minimally invasive technique that may be used to remove parathyroid tumors that are deep in the mediastinum.

If one of the parathyroid glands shows evidence of disease, an effort is made to find other glands on the same side to ensure that they are disease-free. When found, biopsy is performed, using a marker such as a hemoclip. The surgeon resects the diseased gland by clamping the vascular pedicle with mosquito hemostats, dividing with small scissors or a knife, and ligating with a fine nonabsorbable suture or hemoclip. The amount of parathyroid tissue that should be removed remains controversial and relates to whether single or multiple glands are involved. As previously noted, a portion of a gland must remain to prevent hypocalcemia and its complications.

A current alternative for multiple gland involvement is to excise all four glands and to transplant a portion of one in an accessible site, such as the neck or forearm, for later removal if hypercalcemia recurs. The amount of remaining parathyroid tissue can then be adjusted to regulate PTH to the desired level. This eliminates reexploration and potential injury to the recurrent laryngeal nerve. The parathyroid is morselized and divided into several segments. An incision is made in the forearm or neck and four separate grooves with purse-string sutures are made in the muscle. Some parathyroid tissue is placed and secured in each groove. The sites are then marked with one, two, three, and four hemoclips, respectively. If PTH levels remain high, the sites can be easily identified by the clips and more parathyroid tissue excised.

The neck region is then explored for aberrant parathyroid tissue, which is also resected. The remainder of the procedure is as described for the thyroid gland.

Minimally Invasive, Focused Parathyroid Surgery

A variety of minimally invasive techniques have evolved over the last decade. The most widely used is the focused minimally invasive open approach (focused parathyroidectomy, [FP]) where imaging has identified a single parathyroid lesion (Simpson et al, 2007). A localization study with sestamibi scan or ultrasound is used to identify the offending adenoma and to determine an optimum incision site. FP can be performed using a local anesthetic. Ambulatory surgery patients are provided specific education about postoperative oral calcium supplementation. In their study, Norman and Politz (2007) concluded that use of a specific calcium dosing protocol prevented postoperative development of symptomatic hypocalcemia in 93% of patients, identified patients at high risk of hypocalcemia, and allowed most patients who developed symptoms of hypocalcemia to self-medicate in a simple and predictable fashion.

PTH-Guided Parathyroidectomy. One relatively new approach is the intraoperative intact, rapid assessment PTH approach. Given that blood samples must be drawn before, during, and after the procedure to measure PTH levels, an arterial line is inserted and a baseline PTH measurement is taken preoperatively.

A small 2-cm incision is made in the neck based on the localization studies. Once the suspect parathyroid gland is exposed, a pre-excision blood sample is taken. As a result of manipulation, the pre-excision blood level may test higher than the baseline level. The pre-excision level becomes the marker for measuring the post-excision drop in PTH level.

The excised gland is placed in sterile saline and kept on the instrument table until the pathologist confirms a sufficient drop in PTH blood levels. A drop of 50% or more is considered verification that the parathyroid adenoma was excised. Blood levels are also drawn at 5, 10, and 20 minutes post-excision. When the adenoma is excised a dramatic drop in PTH level

GERIATRIC CONSIDERATIONS

The Elderly Patient—Thyroid Surgery

Surgical procedures that are common among the elderly population are governed more by pathologic condition than by anatomy and are directly related to the common diseases affecting older adults. In the elderly population, thyroid gland dysfunction is common and associated with significant morbidity because the symptoms are often subtle, absent, or confused with co-existing diseases. Hypothyroidism occurs in 10% to 15% of patients older than 60 years and is more frequent in females than males (Rehman et al, 2005). Both metabolic rate and production of thyroid hormone decrease with age. This is particularly true among patients older than 80. However, laboratory findings alone should not dictate thyroid hormone therapy in older patients, as lower levels of T_3 and T_4 may only signify "normal values" established for younger patients (Ignatavicius and Workman, 2010). In healthy aging patients, thyroid function may actually be preserved until about the 8th decade; advanced old age is associated with reduced thyroid activity and a decrease in TSH secretion (Fillit et al, 2010).

Typical symptoms of thyroid disorders may be absent or erroneously attributed to co-morbid conditions or normal aging. The polypharmacy used in the treatment of elderly patients can interfere with normal thyroid function. Drugs such as lithium or amiodarone may cause primary hyperthyroidism. For example, an elderly man taking medication for hypertension, congestive heart failure, and atrial fibrillation with complaints of fatigue, weakness, constipation, and weight gain may be considered to have these symptoms because of medication or medical conditions, whereas the symptoms could also be caused by hypothyroidism.

A rare complication of hypothyroidism, myxedema coma, affects patients older than 75 years. Confusion, disorientation, lethargy, thinning eyebrows and hair, hoarse voice, bradycardia, cardiomegaly, pericardial effusion, hypothermia, hyponatremia, and pseudomyotonic reflexes characterize this condition.

The great masquerader in the elderly population is hyperthyroidism and can easily be missed in patients older than 60 years. It can be severe and even life-threatening. Elderly patients may not have a goiter, exophthalmos, or other ophthalmopathy. Hyperthyroidism may also cause osteoporosis. Almost any condition that can make a person ill can cause euthyroid sick syndrome; so elders are more susceptible because of their co-morbid conditions. Medication to suppress hormone secretion by the gland, surgery to remove the hyperfunctioning tissue, and radioactive iodine (RAI) to destroy the gland are the three treatment options. Although surgery is a less attractive option, it must be employed when RAI is ineffective in the presence of a single nodule or multinodular toxic goiter or when the patient has dysphagia, tracheal compression, or suspected malignancy. Following surgery, the perioperative staff must keep in mind the possibility of a hyperthyroid storm that can be precipitated by the stress of the procedure, systemic infections, and anesthesia induction.

Modified from Fillit HM et al: *Textbook of geriatric medicine and gerontology,* ed 7, Philadelphia, 2010, Saunders; Ignatavicius DD, Workman ML: *Medical-surgical nursing: patient-centered care,* ed 6, Philadelphia, 2010, Saunders; Rehman SU et al: Thyroid disorders in elderly patients, *South Med J* 98(5):543-549, 2005.

is frequently achieved by the 10-minute post-excision PTH sample. If the 10-minute drop is significant, the surgeon may opt not to have the pathologist run a 20-minute post-excision blood sample. If the hormone level fails to drop sufficiently, the ipsilateral parathyroid is explored as the next most likely adenoma. False positives have been reported in patients who have slow metabolic rates, are renal insufficient, or have large adenomas, 3 g or greater (Loevner and Mukherji, 2008).

Any normal parathyroid that was excised and placed in saline is then morselized with a #15 blade to increase surface area and then reimplanted. After the fascia is reapproximated, a clamp or scissors is used to create a groove in the strap muscle. A purse-string stitch of fine nonabsorbable suture is placed around the groove. The morselized parathyroid tissue is placed inside the groove and the purse-string tightened and tied. Parathyroids respond well to reimplantation.

Sestamibi-Guided Parathyroidectomy. Another minimally invasive technique is the sestamibi-guided, or radio-guided, parathyroidectomy. Sestamibi is given preoperatively and a gamma probe used intraoperatively to pinpoint the adenoma. When this technique is used postoperative normocalcemia has been reported in 97% of patients (Loevner and Mukherji, 2008).

THYROID AND PARATHYROID SURGERY SUMMARY

To review, as with any surgical service, in thyroid and parathyroid surgery it is imperative to know the anatomy and physiology of the surgical area. The surgical technologist needs to be able to think several steps ahead in the procedure to have the items needed ready when the surgeon asks for them. Planning ahead will help greatly by having any items that may be needed ready and available either on the sterile field or in the room.

Understanding that neck surgery can present difficulty with the airway and intraoperative bleeding, the surgical technologist should be prepared with sponges, suture, vascular clamps, and specific retractors to gain the necessary exposure. A difficult airway cart in the operating room may prove to be helpful in this situation.

Because there may be several specimens, the surgical technologist should have the proper specimen, containers and supplies to store and label each specimen, avoiding specimen errors. Having the appropriate drains and dressing ready will facilitate an efficient and effective closure of the procedure.

REVIEW QUESTIONS

1. True/false: Thyroid surgery is performed with the patient in lateral position.

2. True/false: Vascular clamps may be needed in thyroid surgery.

3. True/false: During thyroid surgery, the patient's head will be secured on a headrest.

4. True/false: The thyroid gland lies in the anterior portion of the neck.

5. True/false: There are generally six parathyroid glands.

6. Blood supply to the thyroid is from the superior _____.

7. The parathyroid glands secrete _____.

8. With the patient in supine for a thyroidectomy, the neck should be _____.

9. Removal of one thyroid lobe with excision of the isthmus:
   a. Total thyroidectomy
   b. Subtotal lobectomy
   c. Hemithyroidectomy
   d. None of the above

10. A lobectomy that spares the posterior capsule and a portion of the adjacent thyroid:
    a. Total thyroidectomy
    b. Subtotal lobectomy
    c. Hemithyroidectomy
    d. None of the above

11. Removal of both lobes of the thyroid:
    a. Total thyroidectomy
    b. Subtotal lobectomy
    c. Bilateral subtotal thyroidectomy
    d. None of the above

12. Minimally invasive thyroidectomies (MIT):
    a. reduce postoperative pain
    b. decrease hospital stays
    c. improve cosmetic results
    d. all of the above

13. Define and briefly describe the following surgical procedures:
    Open thyroidectomy
    Neck dissection
    Minimally invasive video-assisted thyroidectomy

Critical Thinking Question

Because large nodules on the thyroid gland can cause a tracheal shift and prove to be more difficult to excise with more intraoperative bleeding, how should the surgical technologist be prepared for this situation?

REFERENCES

Association of PeriOperative Registered Nurses: AORN Position Statement on Surgical Smoke and Bio-Aerosols, 2008, available at www.aorn.org/PracticeResources/AORNPositionStatements/SurgicalSmokeAndBioAerosols. Accessed April 4, 2009.

Banschbach SK: Mutual accountability for the common goal of patient safety, *AORN J* 88(1):11–13, 2008.

Benner P et al: *Expertise in nursing practice: caring, clinical judgment, and ethics,* ed 2, New York, 2009, Springer.

Burman KD: Advances in thyroid cancer treatment, *Medscape Diabetes & Endocrinology* 7(1), 2005, available at www.medscape.com/viewarticle/496261. Accessed April 12, 2009.

Canobbio MM: *Mosby's handbook of patient teaching,* ed 3, St Louis, 2006, Mosby.

Denholm B: Tucking patient's arms and general positioning, *AORN J* 89(4):755–757, 2009.

Dhingra JK: Minimally invasive surgery of the thyroid. Emedicine from WebMD, 2008, available at www.WebMD.com. Accessed November 19, 2008.

Elberling TV et al: Impaired health-related quality of life in Graves' disease: a prospective study, *Eur J Endocrinol* 151:549–555, 2004.

Frost L et al: Hyperthyroidism and risk of atrial fibrillation or flutter: a population-based study, *Arch Int Med* 164:1675–1678, 2004.

Gauger PG, Doherty GM: Parathyroid gland. In Townsend CM et al, editors: *Sabiston textbook of surgery,* ed 17, Philadelphia, 2004, Saunders.

Grebe SKG: Diagnosis and management of thyroid carcinoma: a focus on serum thyroglobulin, *Expert Rev Endocrinol Metab* 4(1):25–43, 2009.

Haynes AB et al: A surgical safety checklist to reduce morbidity and mortality in a global population, *N Engl J Med* 360(5):491–499, 2009.

Hegarty J et al: Nurses' knowledge of inadvertent hypothermia, *AORN J* 89(4):710–713, 2009.

Kuwajerwala NK et al: Thyroid, thyrotoxic storm following thyroidectomy, 2007, available at emedicine.medscape.com/article850924. Accessed January 24, 2009.

Lansford CD, Teknos TN: Evaluation of the thyroid nodule, *Cancer Control* 13(2):89–98, 2006.

Loevner LA, Mukherji SK: *Thyroid and parathyroid glands: imaging, treatment, and beyond,* Philadelphia, 2008, Saunders.

Mirnezami R et al: Day-case and short-stay surgery: the future for thyroidectomy? *Int J Clin Pract* 61(7):1216–1222, 2007.

Norman JG, Politz DE: Safety of immediate discharge after parathyroidectomy: a prospective study of 3,000 consecutive patients, *Endocrinol Pract* 13(3):105–113, 2007.

Pagana KD, Pagana TJ: *Mosby's diagnostic and laboratory test reference,* ed 9, St Louis, 2009, Mosby.

Paige JT et al: Implementation of a preoperative briefing protocol improves accuracy of teamwork assessment in the operating room, *Am Surg* 74(9):817–823, 2008.

Patient Screening and Assessment in Ambulatory Surgical Facilities, *Pennsylvania Patient Safety Advisory* March 6(1):3–9, 2009, available at www.patientsafetyauthority.org. Accessed April 2, 2009.

Perioperative Grand Rounds: The inside of a time out, *AORN J* 89(4):808, 656, 2009.

Sarkar SD, Savitch I: Management of thyroid cancer, *Appl Radiol* 33(11):34–45, 2004.

Simpson H et al: Long term follow up following focused parathyroidectomy for primary hyperparathyroidism. Presented at Society for Endocrinology BES 2007, Birmingham, UK. Endocrine Abstracts 13 P85, 2007.

Steel AC, Reynolds SF: The growth of rapid response systems, *Jt Comm J Qual Patient Saf* 34(8):489–495, 2008.

Terris D: *Outpatient thyroid surgery safe for most patients, study shows,* Medical College of Georgia, 2006, available at https://my.mcg.edu. Accessed January 24, 2009.

The Joint Commission Public Policy Initiative: *"What Did the Doctor Say?" Improving Health Literacy to Protect Patient Safety,* TJC, Oak Bridge Terrace, IL, 2007.

Thyroid nodules, 2005, American Thyroid Association, available at www.thyroid.org. Accessed April 12, 2009.

Tuttle RM: NCCN Thyroid Carcinoma Guidelines Update, 2007. cme.medscape.com/viewarticle/555684. Accessed April 12, 2009.

Warner BW: Pediatric surgery. In Townsend CM et al, editors: *Sabiston textbook of surgery,* ed 17, Philadelphia, 2004, Saunders.

Wilson SF, Giddens JF: *Health assessment for nursing practice,* ed 4, St Louis, 2009, Elsevier.

Breast Surgery

Overview

Most surgical procedures on the breast are performed to establish a definitive diagnosis or to treat breast cancer. Changing hormone levels from puberty throughout the remainder of life affect breast tissue in its physical and microscopic characteristics. In association with these changes, numerous aberrations and tumors can occur.

The occurrence of breast changes, benign or malignant, are some of the most emotionally upsetting health problems

confronting women. Breast cancer is the most common cancer in women (Weaver, 2009); it accounts for nearly one of every three cancers diagnosed. The probability of developing breast cancer increases with age. Estimates are that one in eight women in the United States will develop breast cancer during her life. If the cancer is detected early, there is a 97% 5-year survival rate. Breast cancer risk increases if a woman's mother, sister, or daughter had breast cancer, especially if the cancer developed before menopause. Early menarche (before 12 years of age) and a late natural menopause (after 50 years of age) are associated with a slightly increased risk for developing breast cancer. Further, a woman who has cancer in one breast is at increased risk for cancer in the other breast (American Cancer Society, 2009). Heightened public awareness, an increased number of women practicing self-examination, and early detection of breast masses by mammography have started to slow the annual increase in breast cancer mortality.

This chapter was originally written by Elizabeth B. Pearsall, RN, BSN, CNOR, RNFA, for the 14th edition of Alexander's Care of the Patient in Surgery and has been revised by James S. Miazga, Jr., CST, BS-Psy, for this text.

Surgical Anatomy

The breasts are bilateral mammary glands that lie on the pectoralis major fascia of the anterior chest wall. They are surrounded by a layer of fat and are encased in an envelope of

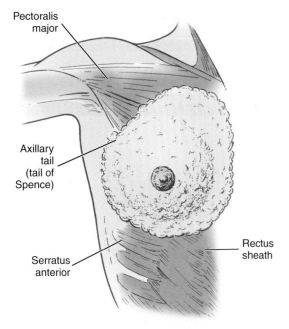

skin. The breasts extend from the second to the sixth rib and horizontally from the lateral edge of the sternum to the anterior axillary line. The largest part of the mammary gland rests on the connective tissue of the pectoralis major muscle and laterally on the serratus anterior (upper outer quadrant of the breast), with a normal globular contour occurring as a result of fascial support (Cooper's ligaments). An elongation of mammary tissue normally extends laterally on the pectoralis major toward the axilla and is known as the *tail of Spence* (Figure 8-1).

Each breast is made up of 12 to 20 glandular lobes separated by connective tissue. Each lobe drains by a single lactiferous duct that opens on the nipple. The nipple, located at about the fourth intercostal space, forms a conical projection into which the ducts open independently of each other on the surface. A pigmented circular area called the *areola* surrounds the nipple. Smooth muscle fibers of the areola contract to allow for nipple projection.

Three major arterial systems (Figure 8-2) supply the mammary glands with blood. The two main sources are branches of the internal mammary and lateral branches of the anterior aortic intercostal arteries, all of which form an extensive network of anastomoses over the breast. The third source is the pectoral branch, deriving from a branch of the axillary artery. The veins that mainly drain the breasts follow the course of the arteries. Superficial veins frequently dilate during pregnancy.

Lymph drainage generally follows the course of the vessels. Lymphatics drain into two main areas represented by the axillary nodes and the internal thoracic chain of nodes (Figure 8-3). The internal thoracic nodes are few, but are responsible for most lymph drainage from the inner half of the breast. Thus the lymph system can also be a channel for the spread of malignant

FIGURE 8-1 Normal distribution of mammary tissue of adult female breast.

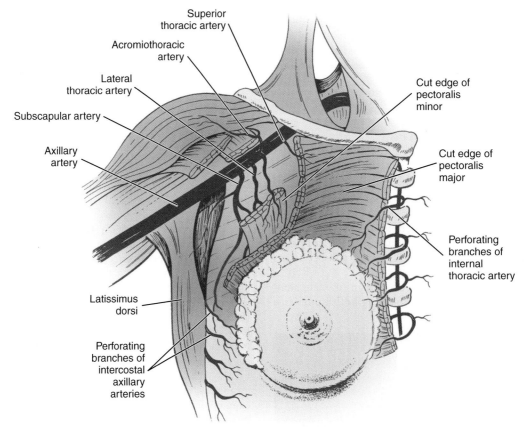

FIGURE 8-2 Normal arterial blood supply of the breast.

disease from the breast to associated areas of the chest wall or to the axilla.

The breast's sensory nerve supply is primarily threefold: the anterior cutaneous branches of the upper intercostal nerves, the third and fourth branches of the cervical plexus, and the lateral cutaneous branches of the intercostal nerves.

The mammary glands are affected by three types of physiologic changes: (1) those related to growth and development, (2) those related to the menstrual cycle, and (3) those related to pregnancy and lactation. The mammary glands are present at birth in both males and females. Hormonal stimulation, however, produces the development and function of these glands in females. Estrogen promotes growth of the ductal structures, whereas progesterone promotes lobular development. Occasionally, developmental errors of the breast occur. Additional nipples or extramammary tissue in the axilla or over the upper abdomen may be present. Absence of one or both nipples may also occur and may be associated with absence of the underlying pectoral muscle and chest wall.

BENIGN LESIONS OF THE BREAST

Fibrocystic change in the breast is an all-encompassing term used to describe many different breast changes. Examples of benign lesions that are generally considered when fibrocystic changes are discussed are multiple lesions of fibrous disease, intraductal papillomas, cysts, and solid masses, such as fibroadenomas (Table 8-1). These changes affect almost all women at some time in their lives. Frequently pain is present, which calls attention to the problem. Pain, fluctuations in size, and multiple lesions are common features that help differentiate these generally benign lesions from cancer.

Nipple discharge is more commonly associated with benign lesions than with cancer. A postmenopausal woman who has some duct ectasia or who has borne children can manually produce nipple discharge. Discharge is usually significant only if it is spontaneous and persistent. Chronic unilateral nipple discharge, especially if bloody, should prompt an investigation for occult carcinoma.

BREAST CANCER

Breast cancer affects primarily women, although it can occur in the mammary gland of men. Until it can be prevented, early

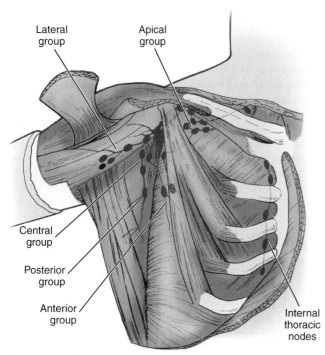

FIGURE 8-3 Distribution of axillary and thoracic lymph nodes.

Lateral group
Apical group
Central group
Posterior group
Anterior group
Internal thoracic nodes

HISTORY

Breast Surgery through the Ages

Over 3500 years ago, ancient Egyptians first noted breast cancer, describing it as "bulging tumors" with no cure. In 460 BC, Hippocrates described breast cancer as a "humoral" disease caused by an excess of black bile. Hippocrates believed the body consisted of four "humors" (blood, phlegm, yellow bile, and black bile) and any imbalance of the humors caused sickness or death. He claimed surgery was dangerous because he had noted that women who had the tumor excised died quickly and those who did not have surgery lived longer. Galen, in 200 AD, believed that some tumors were worse than others and surgery was not an option.

By the eighteenth century, the humoral theory of the origin of breast cancer was losing credibility. Some theories of the cause of breast cancer were that it was derived from curdled milk or a sedentary lifestyle, or that it occurred more frequently in childless women. People also thought the disease was localized. Dr. LeDran, a French physician, and Dr. LeCat were both of the opinion that surgery was the only way to cure the cancer.

By the mid-nineteenth century, most doctors agreed that surgery was the answer. Dr. William Halstead of New York dominated breast cancer surgery with radical mastectomy for most of the next century. He theorized that the cancer was a cellular disease. He urged women to have radical mastectomies before the tumor spread to the lymph nodes. Scottish physician Bealson discovered that a bilateral oophorectomy shrank his patients' breast tumors. Surgeons then began to perform radical mastectomy and bilateral oophorectomy, but the surgery was debilitating to the patient. Other radical surgeries to halt estrogen supply to the breast tumor were removal of the pituitary gland and adrenalectomy.

In 1955 Dr. George Crile argued cancer was not localized, but it spread throughout the body. Dr. Bernard Fisher theorized that cancer cells spread systemically by the circulatory and lymph system and that surgery could not cure cancer. Crile and Fisher both advocated a more systemic approach to breast cancer.

In the 1990s, after an initial increase in breast cancer rates, the number of breast cancer deaths reached a plateau in 1995 and then started to decline. By 1995 less than 10% of women inflicted with breast cancer had a mastectomy. Improvements in chemotherapy, radiation, hormone treatment, mammography, and surgery helped reposition breast cancer from an urgent disease to a chronic condition. Breast cancer theory has come full circle, from Hippocrates' theory of systems of imbalanced humors to the present view of breast cancer as a systemic condition.

Modified from *A history of breast cancer,* 2008, available at www.random history.com/1-50/029cancer.html. Accessed April 6, 2009.

detection is the best hope for cure. All women should practice monthly self-examination to detect palpable lesions, and they should immediately report any changes or masses to a physician. External physical changes, such as dimpling of the skin, can also indicate the presence of a benign or malignant pathologic process. The older the patient, the more likely it is that a mass is malignant. The most common form of breast cancer is infiltrating ductal carcinoma (Table 8-2).

The cause of breast cancer remains unknown. Many factors, including environmental, dietary (National Cancer Institute, 2007), and familial influences, have been suggested as contributors to its development (Table 8-3). The belief that breast cancer spreads by direct extension from its initial site in the breast to adjacent lymph nodes may not always be correct. Breast cancer may be a systemic condition at the time of diagnosis (History box). Distant metastases may have already occurred without adjacent lymph node involvement at the time of its palpable detection. This could explain why radical breast surgery of the past, which involved removal of the affected breast and all axillary and thoracic lymph nodes, did not greatly lower mortality. Survival from breast cancer is best when detected early, reducing axillary lymph node involvement and improving long-term survival. Tumor size can usually be correlated with involvement of lymph nodes. The larger a tumor is, the more likely it is that lymph nodes are involved.

Less radical surgery is the treatment of choice today. Surgical excision of the tumor, the use of radiation therapy alone, or a combination of surgery, chemotherapy, and radiation therapy are current treatment recommendations. The use of adjuvant chemotherapy is particularly recommended for premenopausal women with axillary-node metastasis. Studies show that similar therapy can benefit node-negative breast cancer patients. New studies and new therapeutic options are continually being developed and tested. Clinical use of accelerated partial breast irradiation (APBI) is the subject of ongoing clinical trials. In APBI the radiation is focused on the area of greatest risk for tumor recurrence, the lumpectomy site, instead of whole breast irradiation (WBI). Such focused radiation treatment therapies reduce the traditional 6-week radiation treatment plan to 1 week (Fearmonti et al, 2007).

Minimally invasive cryoablation technology to freeze and destroy core biopsy–proven fibroadenomas has been approved by the U.S. Food and Drug Administration (FDA) and is now performed safely in an office setting (Bland et al, 2009). Another breast surgery alternative is focused ultrasound (FUS) with magnetic resonance guidance (MRgFUS), which allows for imaging and tissue temperature monitoring while controlling the FUS beam direction during ablation of breast lesions (Bland et al, 2009).

SCREENING TECHNOLOGIES

Imaging methodologies, such as mammography and ultrasonography, have helped to detect breast masses too small for clinical detection (Hulvat et al, 2009). The American Cancer Society recommends clinical breast exams by a physician every 3 years for women ages 20 to 39 years and annual clinical breast exams and mammograms for women 40 and older (Table 8-4). The American College of Physicians recommends that women who are not at high risk for breast cancer should have regu-

TABLE 8-1

Typical Presentation of Benign Breast Disorders

Breast Disorder	Description	Incidence
Fibroadenoma	Most common benign lesion; solid mass of connective tissue that is unattached to surrounding tissue	Teenage years into 30s
Fibrocystic breast disease (FBD)	*First stage:* characterized by premenstrual bilateral fullness and tenderness *Second stage:* presence of bilateral, multicentric nodules *Third stage:* presence of microscopic and macroscopic cysts	Late teens and 20s
Ductal ectasia	Hard, irregular mass or masses with nipple discharge, enlarged axillary nodes, redness, and edema; difficult to distinguish from cancer	Women approaching menopause
Intraductal ectasia	Mass in duct that results in nipple discharge; mass is usually not palpable	Women 40-55 yr of age

Data from American Cancer Society: *Noncancerous breast conditions, 2009,* Atlanta, Author; Ignatavicius DD, Workman ML: *Medical-surgical nursing: patient-centered collaborative care,* ed 6, St Louis, 2010, Saunders.

lar mammograms starting at age 50. High-risk women, such as those who have a family history of breast cancer or who have detected a lump in the breast, should start annual mammograms at age 40 (Zuckerman, 2007).

The most common screening mechanism for asymptomatic women is x-ray (film-screen) mammography (Figure 8-4). In mammography, the entire breast is visualized as x-ray beams are directed in several planes through it. Mammograms detect abnormal-appearing densities, irregular or spiculated margins, microcalcifications, and clusters of calcium deposits that are clinically nonpalpable. These masses may be as small as 1 cm in diameter (Mulholland et al, 2006). Often, previous mammograms are used for comparison. Screening mammography has led to identification of more nonpalpable breast masses. The accuracy of mammography depends on careful x-ray technique and breast size, structure, and density. Radiation dosage varies with individuals and techniques. As a result of improved radiologic techniques, radiation exposure in a mammogram is very low. The benefits of this screening mechanism far outweigh the minute risks of radiation exposure. Advances in computer-assisted detection allow the computer to analyze the mammogram, placing asterisks and triangles on small potential problem areas, which a radiologist then reviews. If screening mammography reveals a suspicious area, the patient is asked to return for diagnostic mammography (explained in the following paragraphs).

TABLE 8-2

Types of Invasive Breast Cancer

Breast Cancer Type	Percent of Breast Cancers	Specific Features
Ductal carcinoma	≈80	Can appear as microcalcifications, can vary widely in appearance, can have features of other histologic subtypes of breast cancer
Lobular carcinoma	10-15	Begins in milk (lobules) glands of breast, high rate of bilaterality, grows as single file of malignant cells around ducts and lobules, poorly defined mass
Medullary carcinoma	1-5	Forms distinct boundary between tumor tissue and normal tissue, well circumscribed, frequent phenotype of *BRCA1* hereditary breast cancer
Tubular	2	Infrequently metastasizes to lymph nodes, slow growing, long-term survival approaches 100%
Inflammatory carcinoma	≈1	Rapidly growing, often with metastasis present at diagnosis, first manifestations are breast skin edema and redness and warmth with dimples or ridges

Data from Imaginis: *What is breast cancer? 2008,* available at www.imaginis.com/breasthealth/breast_cancer2.asp. Accessed June 1, 2009; Mulholland M et al: *Greenfield's surgery: scientific principles & practice,* ed 4, Philadelphia, 2006, Lippincott Williams & Wilkins; Brunicardi FC et al: *Schwartz's principles of surgery,* ed 8, New York, 2005, McGraw-Hill.

TABLE 8-3

Risk Factors for Breast Cancer

Factors	Comments
HIGH INCREASED RISK (RELATIVE RISK >4.0)	
Female gender	99% of all breast cancers occur in women.
Age >65 yr	Incidence increases with age and peaks in sixth decade.
Genetic factors	Inherited mutations of *BRCA1* and/or *BRCA2* increase risk.
Family history	Two or more first-degree relatives with breast cancer at an early age increases risk.
History of previous breast cancer	Risk for developing cancer in opposite breast is 5 times greater than average population at risk.
Breast density	Dense breasts contain more glandular and connective tissue.
MODERATE INCREASED RISK (RELATIVE RISK 2.1-4.0)	
Family history	One first-degree relative with breast cancer moderately increases risk.
Biopsy-confirmed atypical hyperplasia	Overactive growth of cells increases risk.
Ionizing radiation	Women who received frequent low-level radiation exposure to thorax have increased risk, especially if exposure occurred during periods of rapid breast formation.
High postmenopausal bone density	High estrogen levels over time both strengthen bone and increase breast cancer risk.
LOW INCREASED RISK (RELATIVE RISK 1.1-2.0)	
Reproductive history	Childless women have an increased risk, as do women who bear their first child near or at age 30.
Menstrual history	Risk for breast cancer rises as interval between menarche and menopause increases. Women who undergo bilateral oophorectomy before age 35 have only 40% of risk for breast cancer compared to women who undergo natural menopause.
Oral contraceptives	There is a slight increase in breast cancer risk in women taking oral contraceptives.
Hormone replacement therapy (HRT)	Recent and long-term use of hormone replacement therapy slightly increases risk.
Obesity	Postmenopausal obesity (especially increased abdominal fat), increased body mass, insulin resistance, and hyperglycemia have been reported to be associated with increased risk for breast cancer.
OTHER RISK FACTORS	
Alcohol	The equivalent of two drinks per day may increase risk by 21%.
High socioeconomic status	Breast cancer incidence is greater in women of higher education and socioeconomic background. This relationship is possibly related to lifestyle differences, such as age at first birth.
Jewish heritage	Women of Jewish Ashkenazic heritage have higher incidences of *BRCA1* and *BRCA2* genetic mutations.

Modified from American Cancer Society: *Breast cancer facts and figures 2007-2008,* Atlanta, 2009, Author; Ignatavicius DD, Workman ML: *Medical-surgical nursing: patient-centered collaborative care,* ed 6, St Louis, 2010, Saunders.

TABLE 8-4

American Cancer Society Breast Cancer Screening Guidelines for Asymptomatic Women*

Age	Screening Activity
20-39 yr	Breast self-examination (BSE) monthly
	Clinical breast examination (CBE) every 3 yr
40 yr and older	BSE monthly
	CBE annually
	Screening mammography (two views of each breast) annually

*Asymptomatic women who are identified to be at higher risk need to have an individualized screening plan that may differ from these guidelines. From American Cancer Society: *Breast cancer facts and figures 2007-2008*, Atlanta, 2009, Author.

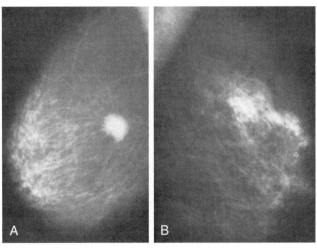

FIGURE 8-4 Mammographic features of malignancy. **A,** A stellate mass. The combination of a density, surrounding spicules, and distortion of the breast architecture strongly suggests a malignancy in this mammogram. **B,** Clustered microcalcifications. Fine, irregular, and branching forms suggest malignancy in this mammogram. Fine calcifications, less than 0.5 mm in size, are more often associated with cancer than are larger, coarse calcifications.

Digital mammography takes an electronic image of the breast and stores it directly in a computer. Digital mammography uses less radiation than film mammography and improves image storage and transmission, as images are stored and sent electronically. Radiologists also can use software to interpret digital mammograms. One obstacle to greater use of digital mammography is its cost, currently about 1.5 to 4 times more than film systems. Digital screening mammograms are more accurate than film screening mammograms, with a 70% detection rate compared with 55% for film screens. Women most likely to benefit from digital screening are those younger than 50 with dense breast tissue and who are premenopausal or perimenopausal (Hulvat et al, 2009).

When there is a palpable mass or other abnormality identified on screening mammography, a diagnostic imaging evaluation is done (Mikula, 2008). Additional diagnostic mammographic views are obtained, and the radiologist assigns

BOX 8-1

BI-RADS Assessment Scores

Category 0: The screening mammogram indicates additional screening is necessary. Prior mammograms, if available, are used for comparison. Additional imaging may include spot compression, magnification, special mammographic views, or ultrasound.
Category 1: The results are negative.
Category 2: The findings are benign.
Category 3: The findings are probably benign. Short-term follow-up is advised.
Category 4: The findings are suspicious. Biopsy is considered.
Category 5: The findings are highly suggestive of malignancy. Preliminary biopsy is needed; surgical treatment likely required.
Category 6: Known biopsy-proven malignancy. This category may be used for a second opinion before excisional biopsy, radiation therapy, chemotherapy, or mastectomy or for following tumor response during chemotherapy.

Modified from Mikula C: Mammography and biopsy, *Adv Nurs* 10(9):21-23, 2008.

a BI-RADS (Breast Imaging Reporting and Data System) score (Box 8-1). An ultrasound may then be ordered.

Ultrasonography differentiates between solid and cystic lesions. As a screening methodology, its sensitivity and specificity are less definitive than mammography. Ultrasonography can be useful with dense or dysplastic breasts and in pregnant or lactating women.

Magnetic resonance imaging (MRI) is another technique used as an adjunct to mammography in the detection of breast lesions. Breast MRI can image dense breast tissue, which shows poorly with conventional mammography. There is interest in the use of MRI to improve selection for breast-conserving therapy (BCT). In 2007 the American Cancer Society recommended that MRI be used for women at high risk. Such women include those who have known breast cancer–associated *BRCA1* or *BRCA2* gene mutations, have a first-degree relative with a *BRCA1* or *BRCA2* gene mutation, have a lifetime risk of breast cancer of 20% to 25% or greater according to risk assessment tools, had radiation therapy to the chest between 10 and 30 years of age, or have certain rare syndromes. The 2008 study by Martinez-Cecilia found that preoperative MRI improved tumor staging and changed the surgical approach for 13% of study patients; MRI discovered an additional malignant lesion in 8% of patients, and showed a tumor larger than originally believed in 16 patients, altering the planned surgery.

Molecular breast imaging (MBI) involves injection of a short-lived radiotracer, which is absorbed by breast tissue and preferentially so by breast tumors. MBI is especially useful in detecting breast cancer in women with dense breasts and who are at higher risk of developing the disease. This new technique has shown good promise as a helpful adjunct to screening mammography (U.S. Department of Health and Human Services, 2008).

Positron emission tomography (PET) scans with the glucose analog 2 are also being used for breast cancer detection. This scan is about 88% accurate for large breast tumors. For lesions less than 1 cm, the sensitivity of PET is 57% (Hulvat et al, 2009).

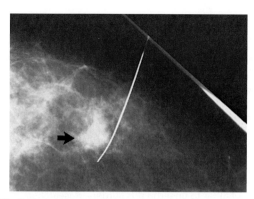

FIGURE 8-5 Mammogram section. Craniocaudal view of breast. Arrow indicates breast lesion localized by wire before surgical excision.

DNA-based genetic testing for *BRCA1* and *BRCA2* is not reommended for women without family histories that suggest risk for these gene mutations. A recent meta-analysis estimated that the lifetime risk for breast cancer was 47% to 66% in carriers of *BRCA1* and 40% to 57% in carriers of *BRCA2*. Other studies have shown even higher estimates. Managing breast cancer risk for women with these mutations includes frequent screening and prophylactic surgeries (Nelson, 2009).

In some instances, such as when a lesion previously detected by mammogram is too small to palpate, mammograms are repeated immediately before surgery. The lesion is localized by the insertion of a needle or a wire within a needle (the procedure is often referred to as "needle" or "wire" localization). The wire is placed within the suspect area, and the distal end is left on the outside of the skin. The needle may be left in place or removed after insertion of the wire (Figure 8-5). The needle or wire is then taped in place, and the patient sent to the OR for surgical biopsy. Wire localization and surgical biopsy occur on the same day. After biopsy, the specimen is sent to the radiology department for mammographic validation of correct surgical excision of the questionable breast tissue. The tissue is then sent for pathologic examination.

DIAGNOSTIC TECHNIQUES

Once a mass is identified, the physician has multiple techniques to establish a diagnosis. During a fine needle aspiration biopsy (FNAB), the physician anesthetizes a small area of the breast with lidocaine. A 22- or 25-gauge needle attached to a 20-ml syringe is inserted into the mass, and a small amount of the contents is aspirated. Cytologic examination of the aspirate can assist in microscopic evaluation of the mass. FNAB yields greater diagnostic accuracy if the physician has been thoroughly trained in the technique. In a review of 31,340 procedures, FNAB sensitivity ranged from 65% to 98%. False-positive rates were less than 1%. As diagnosis of malignancy by FNAB is extremely reliable, treatment options can then be discussed with the patient and definitive surgery performed without the need for a surgical biopsy (Mulholland et al, 2006).

Advances in instrumentation now allow for simultaneous biopsy and removal of mammographic densities that are up to 20 mm in size using digital stereotactic imaging and minimally invasive instruments to locate and remove tissue for diagnosis. The patient is assessed preoperatively for neck or back problems. In addition, the patient should not be receiving antico-

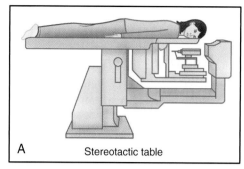

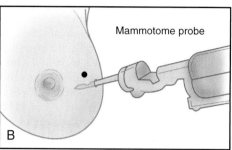

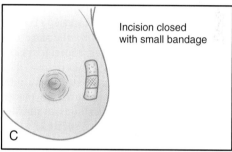

FIGURE 8-6 A, In stereotactic procedures, patients lie facedown on a special table. The woman's breast protrudes through a hole in the table's surface, where it is lightly compressed and immobilized while a computer produces detailed images of the abnormality. **B,** Once the biopsy area has been located and mapped, the Mammotome probe is inserted through a small ¼-inch incision in the breast, where it gently vacuums, cuts, and removes breast tissue samples. **C,** The incision is then closed with a small adhesive bandage.

agulant therapy. Masses located near the patient's areola, high in the axilla, or near the chest wall are not appropriate for this technique. The patient is placed on a specially designed table (Figure 8-6) in the prone position with the affected breast through the table's 10-inch aperture to the work area below. The patient's head is turned away from the physician. Padding is placed under bony prominences to improve comfort. When the suspicious area in the breast is located through stereotactic imaging, its coordinates are transferred to the table's automated instrument. After preparing the skin with an antiseptic solution while the patient is administered a local anesthetic, the physician makes a small incision in the breast. The physician positions the disposable device to remove the identified tissue. Additional biopsies can be made if indicated, and coagulation can be used if necessary. A titanium vessel clip can be placed at the base of the biopsy specimen as a point of reference for future evaluations. A postoperative dressing is then applied to the area. The benefits to the patient include small incisions for cosmetic results, decreased disfigurement, shortened time between detection and diagnosis, and elimination of the need for more involved surgical intervention (Stephan, 2009).

SURGICAL TREATMENT OPTIONS

Surgical treatment ranges from minimally invasive breast biopsy, lumpectomy, and wide excision of the tumor mass; to modified radical mastectomy involving the breast and axillary lymph nodes; to salpingo-oophorectomy (Research Highlight). The goal of surgery is removal of the cancerous mass with a margin of normal tissue and a good cosmetic result. When a specimen of breast tissue is sent to the laboratory, it is inked to mark the relationship between the tumor and the surgical margins of the excision. The pathologist evaluates these margins on all sides of the tumor for malignant cells. If a margin is positive, it indicates that malignant cells may remain in the breast. Additional surgery is usually required until the margins contain only normal tissue (Re-excision for Close Margins, 2008).

The choice of procedure depends on the size and site of the mass, the characteristics of the cells, the stage of the disease, and the patient's choice. A breast cancer diagnosis is usually staged to measure the extent of the disease and to classify patients for possible treatment modalities (Figure 8-7). The TNM (T = tumor; N = node; M = metastasis) classification has been adopted as a mechanism to clinically stage this disease. Staging results are used in designing a specific treatment plan. Radiation therapy, chemotherapy, or hormonal therapy may be used with surgery or as alternative treatment methods. An intravenous (IV) access port may be surgically placed for later infusion of chemotherapeutic drugs, fluids, or nutrition as well as to withdraw blood and laboratory specimens (Ambulatory Surgery Considerations).

RESEARCH HIGHLIGHT

Salpingo-Oophorectomy to Reduce Cancer Risk in Women with *BRCA* Mutations

According to a meta-analysis undertaken by Rebbeck and colleagues, prophylactic salpingo-oophorectomy reduces the risk for breast cancer by 50% and the risk for ovarian and fallopian tube cancer by 80% in women who carry mutations in the *BRCA1* or *BRCA2* gene. Their study quantified cancer risk reduction and is currently the most authoritative review. Salpingo-oophorectomy surgery reduces risk but is not 100% risk-eliminating. These new risk estimates should help women decide whether to undergo this surgery. Researchers and clinicians need to find ways to improve the efficacy of this surgical intervention by using optimal timing and type of surgery. Breast cancer reduction with prophylactic salpingo-oophorectomy was greater in *BRCA1/2* mutation carriers younger than 50 years than in women ages 50 and older. However, removal of both ovaries before age 45 increases risk for cardiovascular death 20 to 30 years later. Women with inherited mutations in *BRCA1* or *BRCA2* genes have a substantially elevated risk for breast and ovarian cancer, with a lifetime risk for breast cancer of 56% to 84%. This meta-analysis provides strong data about risk reduction estimates, which provide surgeons and patients with better information about risk-reducing salpingo-oophorectomy (RRSO). Discovering that RRSO is associated with a large reduction in *BRCA* mutation–related breast cancer risk, especially among women who are premenopausal at RRSO, makes this surgery much more acceptable to high-risk women.

Adapted from Greene MH, Mai PL: What have we learned from risk-reducing salpingo-oophorectomy? J Natl Cancer Inst 101(2):70-71, 2009; Rebbeck TR et al: Meta-analysis of risk reduction estimates associated with risk reducing salpingo-oophorectomy in BRCA1 or BRCA2 mutation carriers, J Natl Cancer Inst 101(2):80-87, 2008.

AMBULATORY SURGERY CONSIDERATIONS

Port Insertion

A breast cancer patient who needs further medical treatment may opt to have an implanted venous access port placed under the skin in either the chest, abdomen, or upper arm. This access port is used for repeated infusions of chemotherapeutic agents, solutions, other drugs, pain management medication, or blood products as well as for procurement of blood samples. Consequently, the patient's veins do not need to be repeatedly accessed. Port insertion is commonly done in an ambulatory surgery setting by a surgeon or in an interventional radiology department by a radiologist. The port has a soft, pliable plastic catheter that is threaded into the subclavian vein or right atrium by way of the subclavian or internal jugular vein under x-ray guidance. The catheter is then attached to a metal base with a rubber dome, which is placed under the skin by the interventionist. Preoperatively, the patient is instructed to refrain from consuming solid foods or full liquids for at least 6 hours before the procedure. Clear liquids may be ingested 2 hours before the procedure. Regular medications may be taken the morning of the insertion unless instructed otherwise. No aspirin, aspirin products, or antiinflammatory medications may be taken for 1 week before port insertion. Drug allergies are noted. The Universal Protocol is observed. After the procedure, the patient will be observed for approximately 1 hour before discharge. Discharge instructions are as follows:

- Give both the patient and the caregiver verbal and written instructions and the telephone numbers of the physician and nurse so that questions or concerns can be addressed.
- Review the purpose of the port insertion and discuss how long it will stay in place.
- Discuss protecting the skin over the port and keeping the incision clean and dry.
- If fever, chills, swelling, redness, bleeding, discharge, shortness of breath, or chest pain develops, seek prompt medical attention.
- No blood pressure measurement or blood draws are to be done from the arm containing an arm port.
- The port needs to be flushed monthly to keep it patent. Demonstrate this technique and have the patient repeat critical steps for port flushing.
- Explain that removal of the port will be an outpatient procedure when it is no longer needed medically.

Adapted from Canobbio MM: Mosby's handbook of patient teaching, ed 3, St Louis, 2009, Mosby; Department of Radiology, Abington Memorial Hospital Interventional Radiology: Patient information—implanted venous access device, available at www.abingtonir.com/images/uploaded/Abington/venousaccess_Info.pdf. Accessed May 12, 2009.

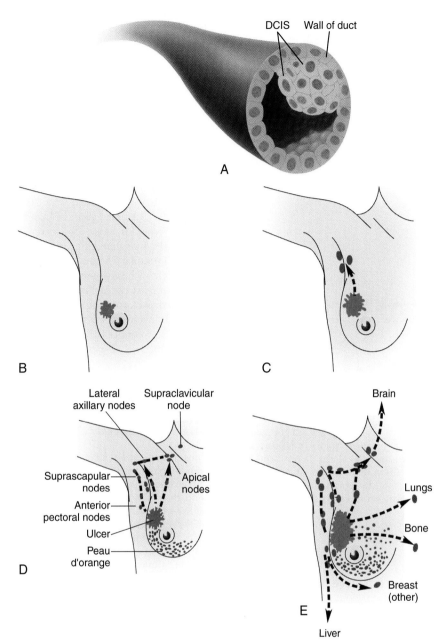

FIGURE 8-7 Staging of breast cancer. **A,** *Stage 0* is carcinoma in situ. Lobular carcinoma in situ (LCIS) is defined as abnormal cells that are in the lining of a lobule. LCIS seldom becomes invasive cancer. However, having LCIS in one breast increases the risk of cancer for both breasts. Ductal carcinoma in situ (DCIS) is defined as abnormal cells that are in the lining of a duct. DCIS is also called intraductal carcinoma. The abnormal cells have not spread outside the duct. They have not invaded the nearby breast tissue. DCIS sometimes becomes invasive cancer if not treated. **B,** *Stage I:* tumor <2 cm with no axillary lymph node involvement. **C,** *Stage IIa:* cancer cells found in axillary lymph nodes, or tumor ≤2 cm with metastasis to axillary lymph nodes, or tumor >2 cm but not >5 cm with no metastasis to axillary lymph nodes. *Stage IIb:* tumor >2 cm but not >5 cm with positive axillary lymph node involvement, or tumor >5 cm with negative axillary lymph node involvement. **D,** *Stage IIIa:* tumor ≤5 cm with metastasis to axillary lymph nodes that are attached to each other or to other structures, or has spread to lymph nodes behind breast bone; or tumor >5 cm and has spread to axillary lymph nodes that are alone or attached to each other or to other structures, or has spread to lymph nodes behind the breast bone. *Stage IIIb:* tumor of any size that has grown into the chest wall or skin of the breast, causing swelling of the breast or nodules in breast skin; may have spread to axillary lymph nodes that are attached to each other and to other structures and may have spread to lymph nodes behind the breast bone. Inflammatory breast cancer: breast is red, swollen (at least stage IIIb). *Stage IIIc:* tumor of any size that has spread either to the lymph nodes behind the breast bone and axillary lymph nodes or to the lymph nodes above or below the collarbone. **E,** *Stage IV:* distant metastatic cancer.

Excised tumors or core needle biopsies are evaluated for their estrogen-binding and progesterone-binding abilities. Techniques have been developed to assess the ability of breast cancer to bind with estrogen and progesterone. This positive binding capability identifies the patient with a hormone-dependent tumor (Figure 8-8). It is estimated that about two thirds of all breast cancers are positive for estrogen binding, and a majority of these tumors are also positive for progesterone binding. The presence of these receptor sites is conducive to hormone manipulation, with the goal of preventing breast cancer cells from receiving stimulation from estrogen. The use of anti-estrogen tamoxifen, in addition to surgery and chemotherapy, increases disease-free survival in premenopausal women with positive binding for estrogen.

Another therapy can be offered by aromatase inhibitors (AIs). These may be nonsteroidal, such as anastrozole and letrozole. Aromatase inhibitors are only effective in postmenopausal women. They appear to work better than tamoxifen on certain breast cancers, with fewer side effects. A large study found that anastrozole may prevent 70% to 80% of the most common breast cancer tumors that occur in postmenopausal women; this was compared with 50% for tamoxifen (Hulvat et al, 2009). A new class of parenteral hormone therapy, estrogen receptor (ER) down-regulators (e.g., fulvestrant [Faslodex]), is available for the treatment of metastatic breast cancer (Hormonal Therapy Changes, 2007).

Some of the most promising data reported in recent years for advanced breast cancer have involved HER-2 (human epidermal growth factor receptor 2), a cellular proto-oncogene coding for a transmembrane receptor. Agents such as trastuzumab (Herceptin) to target HER-2 were first approved for treatment of metastatic HER-2–positive breast cancer in 1998 (Surgical

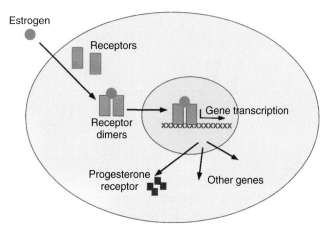

FIGURE 8-8 Physiology of estrogen and the estrogen receptor, shown schematically. Estrogen binds to estrogen receptors, translocates to the nucleus of the cell, and interacts with cellular deoxyribonucleic acid (DNA). This interaction results in the transcription of estrogen-responsive genes, such as the receptor for progesterone. In addition, other genes are induced by the estrogen receptors that influence cell growth and differentiation.

TABLE 8-5

Complementary and Integrative Therapies for Breast Cancer Patients

Symptom	Complementary and Integrative Therapies
PHYSICAL	
Pain	Acupuncture, chiropractic therapy, hypnosis, massage, music, reiki, shiatsu
Nausea/vomiting	Acupuncture, aromatherapy, ginger, hypnosis, progressive muscle relaxation, shiatsu
Fatigue	Acupuncture, massage, meditation, reiki, tai chi, yoga
Hot flashes	Acupuncture, black cohosh, flaxseed
Muscle tension	Aromatherapy, massage, shiatsu
EMOTIONAL	
Anxiety/stress/fear	Aromatherapy, guided imagery, hypnosis, journaling, massage, meditation, music therapy, progressive muscle relaxation, prayer, support groups, tai chi, yoga
Depression	Aromatherapy, yoga, journaling, progressive muscle relaxation

From Ignatavicius DD, Workman ML: *Medical-surgical nursing: patient-centered collaborative care*, ed 6, St Louis, 2010, Saunders.

SURGICAL PHARMACOLOGY

Herceptin

Trastuzumab (Herceptin) is a recombinant humanized immunoglobulin B (IgB) monoclonal antibody that targets the extracellular domain of HER-2. Trastuzumab interferes with the many steps in the tumor cell cycle and sensitizes HER-2–positive cancers to other cytotoxic therapies. HER-2–positive patients usually have more aggressive disease. Data from trials sponsored by the National Cancer Institute, which were terminated prematurely because of the superiority in the groups treated with trastuzumab, reported a 52% reduction in the risk of recurrence and a 33% reduction in the risk of death in the trastuzumab group compared with patients who received standard regimens. A major limitation to the use of trastuzumab in all studies is cardiotoxicity, especially when given concurrently with Adriamycin. Cardiotoxicity lowers considerably when given after Adriamycin therapy. Resistance to trastuzumab eventually occurs in most metastatic breast cancer patients who initially respond to the treatment. Additional research is being conducted on other members of the epidermal growth factor family. One agent is lapatinib, which targets epidermal growth factor and HER-2. Lapatinib in combination with trastuzumab in vitro shows a synergistic effect. Lapatinib also inhibits growth of HER-2–overexpressing breast cancer cells when long-term trastuzumab therapy becomes resistant. Observed side effects are tachycardia, congestive heart failure, nausea, vomiting, diarrhea, anemia, leukopenia, edema, arthralgia, bone pain, rash, acne, herpes simplex virus, anaphylaxis, and flulike symptoms of fever, headache, and chills. It is contraindicated in patients hypersensitive to Chinese hamster ovary cell protein. Teach patients to take acetaminophen for fever, avoid hazardous tasks, report signs of infection, and notify the physician if emotionally labile.

Modified from Hulvat MC: Multidisciplinary care for patients with breast cancer, *Surg Clin North Am* 87:133-164, 2007; Skidmore-Roth: *Mosby's nursing drug reference*, St Louis, 2010, Mosby.

Pharmacology). Research and understanding of the immune system, the development of methods to evaluate aspects of the immune response, and ongoing development of monoclonal antibodies are transforming the field of immunotherapy and breast cancer treatment.

A new drug class in experimental targeted therapy medicine called poly (ADP-ribose) polymerase enzyme (PARP) inhibitors is being studied for triple-negative breast cancer patients (O'Shaugnessy et al, 2009). The biopsy of patients with triple-negative breast cancer (TNBC) is estrogen and progesterone hormone receptor negative and HER-2/neu negative (Kassam et al, 2009). TNBC is found in younger women, women of African American or Hispanic descent, and women with lower socioeconomic status (Winkeljohn, 2008).

Breast cancer patients are increasingly seeking and using complementary and alternative medicine (CAM) and integrative therapies to enhance their surgical and medical treatment (Table 8-5). Besides using products such as green tea, vitamins E and C, and flaxseed, breast cancer patients are incorporating massage therapy and meditation and enlisting the help of dietitians and nutritionists (Boon et al., 2007) as they battle breast cancer.

Surgical Technologist Considerations

When preparing for surgery it is necessary to review the surgical preference cards and use these as a guide to pull the equipment, instrument sets, sterile supplies, and any other items listed in the preference card list. Be sure that any x-rays or other related studies are in the room with the patient. It is the responsibility of the surgical technologist to have the operating room suite ready for each procedure to ensure the best possible patient outcomes. The equipment needed in the room includes the electrosurgical unit (ESU), suction canisters, smoke evacuators, specialized equipment such as vacuum-assisted breast biopsy systems and sentinel node machine, and special positioning devices. Be sure to have the correct armboards for the OR bed.

Basic instruments will include a major surgery tray. In addition, the facility may have a special reconstructive or plastic surgery tray. Clip appliers and clip cartridges should be available. It is wise to have extra items such as hemostats and suction tips available. Have a Mayo stand and a large back table to work from. Be sure to have two complete sur-

SURGICAL TECHNOLOGY PREFERENCE CARD

Discuss the OR bed position with the perioperative team, taking into consideration additional equipment that may be needed for breast surgery. Understanding the room layout before setting up for the procedure allows the traffic pattern in the room to be maximized. This step can help insure sterility of the field and facilitate effective communication of additional supplies from the circulator to the scrub, as well as provide efficient space for other healthcare providers involved in breast surgery.

Room Prep: Basic operating room furniture in place, thermoregulatory devices, extra blankets, padding, positioning supplies to achieve optimal patient safety

Prep Solution: In room and prepared properly for procedure (review manufacturer's instructions to determine if prep solution can be warmed)

- Chlorhexidine gluconate
- Iodine and iodophors
- Alcohol (isopropyl 70%)
- Technicare

PROCEDURE CHECKLIST

Instruments

- Standard sets
- Open specialty instruments as needed; anticipate additional instruments

Specialty Suture

- As per surgeon's preference

Other Hemostatic Agents

- Mechanical
  - Staplers
  - Clip appliers and clips
  - Pressure
  - Ligatures
- Chemical
  - Absorbable gelatin
  - Collagen
  - Oxidized cellulose
  - Epinephrine
  - Thrombin
- Thermal
  - Electrosurgical unit
  - Harmonic scalpel
  - Smoke evacuator

Continued

SURGICAL TECHNOLOGY PREFERENCE CARD—cont'd

Additional Supplies: both sterile and nonsterile
- If the physician is requesting supplies, instruments, or equipment not normally used, check to be sure all have arrived to the room before opening
- Sponges
- Drapes
- Gowns and gloves for team members
- "Have ready" or "hold" supplies

Medications and Irrigation Solutions
- Follow safety precautions and manufacturer's recommendations when warming any irrigating solutions
- Appropriate-sized syringes, hypodermic needles, labels, and marking pen

Drains and Dressings
- Correct size and type for planned surgery
  - Open—Not attached to a drainage system
    - Penrose
  - Closed—Attached to a closed reservoir for fluid collection
    - Hemovac
    - Jackson-Pratt
    - Autologous blood retrieval drainage system

Specimen Care
- Proper container for each specimen
- Labels for each specimen
- Proper solution for specimen type

Before opening for the procedure, the surgical technologist should:
- Arrange furniture
- Gather positioning devices
- Damp dust lights, furniture, and surfaces
- Verify functionality of equipment
- Place items to be opened in their appropriate places

When opening sterile supplies:
- Verify exposure to sterilization
- Use sterile technique
- Open bundles in appropriate locations
- Open additional supplies onto sterile field
- Open all sterile supplies and equipment as close to the surgical start time as possible

gical setups if reconstructive surgery will be performed following a mastectomy. This prevents the potential spread of cancer cells, also known as seeding, to other regions within the body.

When scrubbing and setting up the back table, be sure to label all fluids, correctly label and identify all medications, and be neat and organized. Most facilities will have a standard back table setup, so be sure to set the back table up according to policy. Always allow enough time to be set up and ready to go before the patient enters the room. This includes all preoperative counts with the circulating nurse.

When the patient enters the room, be prepared to assist in the "time-out" procedure to correctly identify all the patient and the type of surgery they will have. All members of the team should be present and involved in this important aspect of the procedure. When the time-out has been completed, positioning the patient for surgery can be done. Do so in a way that protects the patient from injury or potential nerve damage. Pad pressure points and make sure that armboards are secure.

After the patient is positioned, the perioperative nurse will appropriately prep the surgical area for the type of procedure being done. For example, a mastectomy requires a large field. The prep extends from the neck and chest into the axilla then around the affected arm. For bilateral procedures, both arms will be prepped. Once the patient is prepped, do not apply the drapes until the prep solution has dried. Be sure that the area prepped creates an adequate field for surgery. During breast surgery, as with any other invasive procedure, in addition to maintaining the sterile field, be focused on the needs of the surgical team and anticipate the needs of the surgeons. Be ready with the ESU and be sure that there is the correct type and number of suture needed to minimize the surgical time by eliminating wasted time waiting for supplies that should already be opened on the field. When not using the ESU, be sure that it is secured in the holder so that it cannot be accidentally activated, which will create a potential fire hazard.

Breast surgery is comprised of soft tissue dissection and requires sharp blades and an assortment of clips and ligating ties readily available. Muscle dissection requires heavy clamps and large ties. Once the dissection is complete, tissue taken will need to be sent to pathology. When handling tissue that is being sent to pathology, be sure to do so carefully and confirm the type and location of specimen before handing it off of the field. Have a marking pen on the back table to assist in tracking numerous specimens. For cancer surgery, the surgeon will not generally close the wound until the pathologist calls in with the report. Once it has been determined that ade-

case cart or appropriate bins, and transport them to the decontamination area. Return to the OR suite and wipe down all surfaces with the appropriate disinfectant and prepare for the next procedure.

Surgical Interventions

BIOPSY OF BREAST TISSUE

Biopsy removes suspicious breast tissue for pathologic examination. In a *core needle biopsy (CNB)*, a disposable, cutting-type needle is introduced and advanced into the breast mass to entrap a core or plug of tissue. The needle is withdrawn, and the tissue specimen sent to a pathologist for diagnostic examination. CNB may also be performed with a vacuum-assisted core biopsy (VACB) device (Breast Health, 2006). In an *incisional biopsy*, a portion of the mass is surgically excised using a curved incision line. The tissue is sent for pathologic examination (Mulholland et al, 2006). In an *excisional biopsy*, the entire tumor mass is excised along with a small margin of normal tissue from adjacent tissue for examination as with incisional biopsy (Cornforth, 2009).

Procedural Considerations

Biopsy is usually performed after the patient has been administered a local anesthetic, a local anesthetic with IV moderate sedation/analgesia, a laryngeal mask airway (LMA), or a general anesthetic with intubation. The short delay between biopsy and further treatment has not been shown to adversely affect survival. However, when an extensive surgical procedure is anticipated in conjunction with the biopsy or when multiple lesions are to be excised and the amount of local anesthetic would exceed the maximum safe dose, general anesthesia is induced. In the instance of anticipated extensive surgery based on pathologic results, the patient must have preoperatively given informed consent to proceed with the more definitive surgery. A new surgical setup will be used. A minor instrument set is used for biopsy; the ESU is often requested. Perioperative staff should be sensitive to the fact that the patient may be alert during the procedure and use caution with oral pathology reports called over a speaker phone. Pathology reports, especially if the report confirms malignancy, should be discussed when the patient is fully awake and has a support system available.

Operative Procedure—Open Breast Biopsy

1. An incision in the direction of the skin lines (curvilinear) or along the border of the areola is made over the tumor mass. The circumareolar incision gives the best cosmetic result. If the lesion is located in an extremely lateral or medial site, a radial incision may be used.
2. Gentle traction is applied to the mass with holding forceps. If the lesion is small, the entire mass and an edge of normal tissue are removed by sharp dissection. If a large lesion is present, a small incisional biopsy of the main mass is done. The specimen should not be placed into a formalin solution if a frozen section is to be done at the time of surgery; instead, it is sent fresh, as exposure to formalin prevents frozen-section examination. The specimen may be marked with a sterile marker as to its orientation in the breast and/or may be placed on a sterile towel that is marked with a sterile marker to orient the specimen. This assists the sur-

quate margins have been accomplished, the wound is irrigated and closed. During the closure, drains will be placed. Closing counts are completed and verbally reported to the surgeon when completed.

After the surgery is complete, prepare the instruments for processing and be sure that all sharps have been removed and disposed of properly. Place all instrument trays and sets in the

RESEARCH HIGHLIGHT

Understanding "Chemobrain"

Chemobrain refers to a wide range of problems experienced by breast cancer survivors who have received treatment with chemotherapeutic agents. These changes usually first become apparent during chemotherapy (hence the name). Some literature reports that 75% of women with breast cancer experience chemobrain after therapy. These symptoms include short-term memory loss, difficulty concentrating and staying focused, reduced verbal and visual memory, difficulty managing daily activities and multitasking, fatigue, disorganization, and confusion. Some cancer-related causes could include chemotherapy, hormonal treatment, radiation therapy, and surgery; complications of cancer treatment; and emotional reactions to cancer diagnosis, treatment, and medications. The severity and duration of the symptoms differ with the individual. A recent study used magnetic resonance imaging to compare regional brain-volume differences between breast cancer survivors exposed to adjuvant chemotherapy and unexposed controls. It showed that there were physical changes in the brains of breast cancer survivors; parts of their brains were smaller. Also, in a study using positron emission tomography (PET) imaging, breast cancer survivors who had received chemotherapy in the previous 5 to 10 years used more of their brains to perform a short-term memory task than control subjects who never received chemotherapy, a sign that their brains had to work harder to complete tasks. Treatments for chemobrain are in the early stages. Some evidence suggests that central nervous system medications may ease adverse cognitive effects.

Modified from Hafner DL: Lost in the fog: understanding "chemo brain," *Nursing 2009* 39(8):42-45, 2009; Mayo Clinic Staff: *Chemobrain*, Mayo Clinic, 2009, available at www.mayoclinic.com/health/chemobrain/ncbi-n:DS01109. Accessed April 27, 2009; National Cancer Institute: Delving into possible mechanisms for chemobrain, *NCI Cancer Bull* 6(6), March 24, 2009.

▶▶ RISK REDUCTION STRATEGIES

Decreasing Lymphedema Associated with Breast Surgery

Lymphedema after breast surgery is caused by a disruption of the axillary bed by excision of lymph nodes and/or radiation therapy to the area. Patients are at a lifetime risk of edema in the upper extremity and/or in the ipsilateral upper quadrant and breast tissue. Risk factors that affect the occurrence of lymphedema include axillary node dissection, radiation therapy, tumor in the upper outer quadrant of the breast, stage of cancer at diagnosis, age, obesity, hypertension, chemotherapy, and radiation treatment. Risk reduction starts at the preoperative evaluation with education. Baseline girth and volume measurements of both upper extremities are taken and recorded. Note any factors that put the patient at increased risk for development of lymphedema. Educate the patient about arm and hand precautions. Risk reduction practices also include providing good skin care to prevent infection, preventing injury and muscle strain, avoiding limb constriction, promoting lymph drainage with elevation, using compression garments, avoiding extreme temperatures, and performing regular, light aerobic exercise. If lymphedema is diagnosed, intervention is necessary. Various approaches, including surgery, pharmacotherapy, low-level laser therapy, and complete decongestive treatment (CDT), can decrease and maintain the size of the limb. CDT is a two-phase program that consists of a treatment phase and a maintenance phase. The International Society of Lymphology considers CDT the standard of care for lymphedema. Once a diagnosis of lymphedema is made, the patient must be monitored over the course of her life. Fu's research supports provision of information about lymphedema to improve practice of risk reduction behaviors with breast cancer survivors. Compliance with the maintenance phase is related to better outcomes.

Modified from Fu MR, Ridner SH, Armer J: Post-breast cancer lymphedema, *Am J Nurs* 109(8):34-41, 2009; Johnstone PAS, Mondry TE: *Prevention and treatment of lymphedema related to breast cancer, 2007,* available at www.medscape.com/viewartcle/566471. Accessed April 14, 2008; Mulcahy N: *Recognizing lymphedema is vital in assisting oncology patients, 2009,* available at www.medscape.com/viewarticle /587127. Accessed April 15, 2009.

RESEARCH HIGHLIGHT

Cross-Cultural Relevance of Breast Cancer Survivorship Programs

Breast cancer survivorship programs to assist women in dealing with the multiple concerns they have after breast cancer treatment are important. However, few of these programs have been evaluated for cultural relevance with diverse groups. One such program, Taking CHARGE, is a theory-based self-management program developed to assist women with survivorship concerns that arise after breast cancer treatment. This research appraised both the utility and the cultural relevance of the program for African American (AA) breast cancer survivors, during which they assessed Taking CHARGE program content, format, materials, and the self-regulation process. Content analysis of audiotapes was conducted using an open, focused coding process to identify emergent themes regarding program relevance as well as topics requiring enhancement and/or further emphasis. Although findings indicated that the program's content was relevant to participants' experiences, AA women identified need for cultural enhancements in spirituality, self-preservation, and positive valuations of body image. Content areas requiring more emphasis included persistent fatigue, competing demands, disclosure, anticipatory guidance, and age-specific concerns about body image/sexuality. Suggested improvements to program materials included portable observation logs, additional resources, photographs of AA women, vivid colors, and images depicting strength. These findings can be used for program enhancements to increase the utility and cultural relevance of Taking CHARGE for AA survivors and underscore the importance of evaluating other interventions for racially/ethnically diverse groups.

Adapted from Chung LK et al: Breast cancer survivorship program: testing for cross-cultural relevance, *Cancer Nurs* 32(3):236-245, 2009.

geon in reexcision if the pathologist finds positive margins on the specimen. The tissue is examined by frozen section to determine immediate diagnosis while the patient is still anesthetized. If a 48-hour permanent section is required for definitive diagnosis, the patient is scheduled at a later time for any further surgery that may be necessary.

3. If the lesion is benign, hemostasis is checked and the subcutaneous breast tissue of the wound is approximated with absorbable suture. The skin is closed with fine sutures or skin staples, and a firm pressure dressing is applied.

4. If the lesion is malignant, the incision is tightly closed with a continuous locking suture on a cutting needle.

5. If a more extensive operation is required, it may be performed immediately. Team members regown and reglove to avoid transfer of cancerous cells to healthy tissue. The operative site is again prepped and draped. A separate sterile setup and set of instruments for a more radical procedure are then used.

Operative Procedure—Open Breast Biopsy with Needle (Wire) Localization

A radiologist performs wire placement before the patient's arrival in the OR. Care is taken during transfer to the OR bed and gown removal not to dislodge or bump the wire. Similar care is taken during positioning, prepping, and draping.

1. The skin incision is placed precisely over the expected location of the mammographically determined lesion to minimize tunneling through the breast tissue.

2. Dissection is carried out using the wire as a guide.

3. Tissue around the wire is removed en bloc with the wire and sent for specimen mammography in the radiology department.

4. The patient is kept on the OR bed with the sterile field maintained until confirmation that the lesion has been excised. It is then sent from radiology to the pathology department.

INCISION AND DRAINAGE FOR ABSCESS

Incision of an inflamed and suppurative area of the breast is performed to drain an abscess. Breast abscesses occur most frequently during the first 4 weeks of breastfeeding. Staphylococcal or streptococcal organisms enter the breast through abraded or lacerated nipple surfaces or through the lactiferous ducts. Chronic abscesses are rare. Drainage is required when the breast abscess around the nipple or in breast tissue is apparent. Biopsies may be done for additional diagnosis.

Procedural Considerations

Breast abscess is very painful and may require surgery with the patient administered a general anesthetic. Instruments are the same as those for a biopsy.

Operative Procedure

1. Generally, a radial incision extending outward from the nipple or a circumareolar incision is preferred. A short incision into the thoracomammary fold may be used for deep breast abscesses in the lower or outer quadrant.

2. After skin incision, the wound is deepened until pus is encountered.

3. A curved hemostat is directed into the cavity to determine the extent of the abscess. Specimens for aerobic and anaerobic organisms are usually taken for culture.

4. Loculations are broken up by exploring the cavity with the index finger.

5. The opening is enlarged to ensure adequate drainage, the cavity is irrigated with warm saline solution, and bleeding vessels are ligated with absorbable sutures or coagulated.

6. The wound is drained or loosely packed with gauze. Healing occurs by granulation.

LUMPECTOMY (SEGMENTAL RESECTION)

Lumpectomy is removal of a tumor mass with a margin of 1 to 1.5 mm of normal tissue. Surgical clips may be left in the operative site to assist the radiation oncologist (Lind et al, 2005). Lumpectomy, with subsequent radiation therapy, is often the treatment of choice for small tumors. It is not an option for patients who have two or more cancer sites in separate quadrants of the breast, persistent positive margins after reasonable surgical attempt, or diffuse malignant-appearing microcalcifications, as well as for patients who have undergone previous radiation to the affected breast (Mulholland et al, 2006). A lumpectomy, combined with sentinel node or axillary node dissection (Figure 8-9) and irradiation in stage I and stage II breast cancers, appears to provide results equal to a more radical procedure. If one or more axillary nodes are involved, chemotherapy also is recommended.

Procedural Considerations

In patients with large breasts, increased bleeding may occur, requiring the ESU, a smoke evacuation system, and additional hemostatic clamps.

RAPID RESPONSE TEAM

Anaphylactic shock from Lymphazurin 1% can occur 6 to 8 hours after the first episode of anaphylaxis. At this time, the patient may be in the ambulatory surgery recovery (see Patient Safety) or the medical-surgical unit. A rapid response team may be called when the symptoms of anaphylactic shock are observed, such as oxygen desaturation, systolic blood pressure in the range of 30 to 40 mm Hg, and urticaria. These teams are part of a formal interdisciplinary system to reduce death or disability through early identification, assessment, and stabilization of patients with a deteriorating medical condition before the patient's condition requires resuscitation or transfer to a higher level of care. The patient in anaphylactic shock is treated appropriately, admitted to the hospital for observation, and, when fully recovered, discharged with appropriate medications and instructions, especially with information about the allergy to Lymphazurin. The patient should inform all medical personnel of this allergy and wear a medical alert bracelet.

Modified from Liang MI, Carson WE: *Biphasic anaphylactic reaction to blue dye during sentinel lymph node biopsy, 2008,* available at www.wjso.com/content/6/1/79. Accessed April 6, 2009; Administrative Policy and Procedure Manual, Taylor Hospital, effective date April 2006.

NORMAL ANATOMY

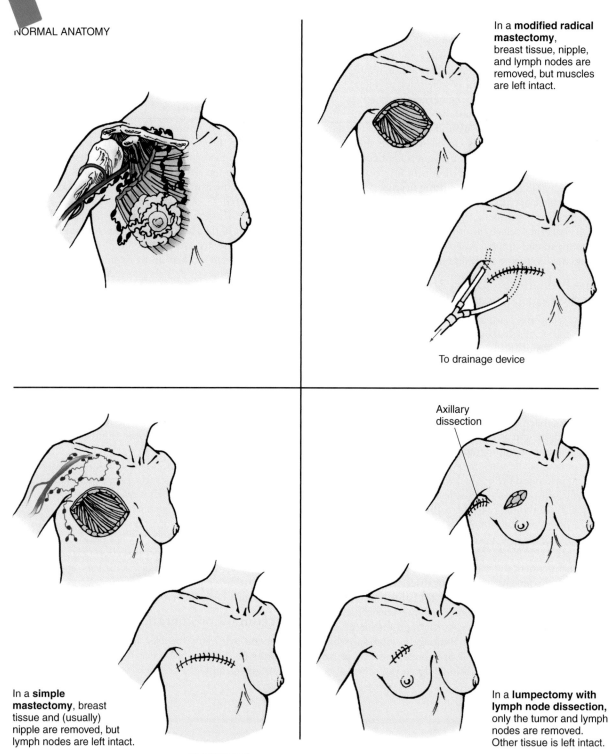

In a **modified radical mastectomy**, breast tissue, nipple, and lymph nodes are removed, but muscles are left intact.

To drainage device

Axillary dissection

In a **simple mastectomy**, breast tissue and (usually) nipple are removed, but lymph nodes are left intact.

In a **lumpectomy with lymph node dissection**, only the tumor and lymph nodes are removed. Other tissue is left intact.

FIGURE 8-9 Surgical management of breast cancer.

Operative Procedure

The procedure is as described for excisional biopsy.

SENTINEL LYMPH NODE (SLN) BIOPSY

Identification and microscopic examination of the sentinel lymph nodes (SLNs), the first lymph nodes along the lymphatic chan-nel from the primary tumor site, will help to determine the need for additional or more extensive surgeries and treatments of early-stage invasive breast cancer for patients thought to have low to moderate risk for involvement of lymph nodes (Sentinel Lymph Node Dissection, 2008). It is believed that if the cancer cells have traveled through the lymph nodes, the cells will lodge in the first nodes. The sentinel node is not located in the same site in every patient. If sentinel nodes are negative, no other nodes in the lymph node channel are likely to be involved. Evidence of a positive node requires an axillary node dissection and adjunct therapy (Sentinel Node Biopsy, 2009). Complications of SLN biopsy include risk of allergic reactions to the blue dye (Patient Safety), rare instances of sensory or motor nerve damage, and pain. Contraindications to SLN biopsy include palpable axillary nodes, large or locally advanced breast cancers, prior axillary surgery, and pregnancy or lactation (Lind et al, 2005).

Procedural Considerations

The procedure for SLN biopsy is similar to that for breast biopsy. Sentinel node identification is accomplished by injection of either isosulfan blue dye or a radiocolloid (technetium 99 [^{99m}Tc]), a gamma-emitting material. Isosulfan blue is contraindicated in patients with known hypersensitivity to the dye; careful patient monitoring and observation are mandatory, and a crash cart should be available in the instance of severe anaphylactic reaction (Rapid Response Team box). The procedure is coordinated with staff of the nuclear medicine department and requires use of a handheld detector if technetium is used. In addition to a minor instrument set, if isosulfan blue is used, a 5-ml syringe, a 25-gauge needle, an alcohol wipe, and the dye are required. For technetium, the gamma-tracer probe, counter, and sterile sleeve for the probe are required. Multiple specimen containers should be on hand along with pathology request forms. The surgeon may request that each specimen be numbered on the specimen container and the pathology request form. Safe

practices for handling surgical specimens are implemented. A combination of technetium and isosulfan blue can also be used for lymphatic mapping (Mulholland et al, 2006). SLN biopsy is quickly replacing levels I and II axillary lymph node dissection as the standard procedure for staging an axillary lymph node–negative patient (Morrow and Harris, 2009).

Operative Procedure—Using Isosulfan Blue Dye

1. Dye is injected around or near the tumor, or dye may be injected into the area of the breast mass that has been exposed as part of a breast biopsy (Sentinel Node Biopsy, 2009).
2. This may be followed by a three-stage axillary lymphatic massage (Kirby et al, 2007).
3. The sentinel nodes stained with the blue dye are identified and excised.
4. The nodes are sent fresh to the pathology department for examination.
5. Based on the results, the surgeon proceeds with the planned surgery or may elect breast conservation.

Operative Procedure—Using Technetium

1. The tumor or previous biopsy site is injected with a small amount of radioactive tracer 20 minutes to 8 hours before the surgery. It can also be injected after anesthesia is induced (Sentinel Node Biopsy, 2009).
2. This may be followed by massage.
3. A handheld detector is passed over the top of the patient's chest to identify the area of the sentinel node by a positive reading. The probe may also be used with the addition of a sterile sleeve during excisional biopsy. Isosulfan blue dye may be used in conjunction with technetium during a procedure to enhance visibility of nodes.
4. The surgeon marks the skin with a skin scribe to indicate the reactive area.
5. The area is prepped, and the surgeon proceeds with the planned procedure for excisional biopsy of the sentinel lymph node.

AXILLARY NODE DISSECTION

Axillary node dissection (Figure 8-10) is removal of axillary nodes through an incision in the axilla after determining that the sentinel node is malignant. Removal and examination of the axillary nodes allow staging (see Figure 8-7) of the disease. Adjunct treatment can be more accurately planned when the pathologic stage is determined.

Procedural Considerations

The patient is placed supine on the OR bed with the operative side near the bed edge. The arm on the operative side is extended to less than 90 degrees on an armboard. The skin is prepped and draped as previously described.

Operative Procedure

1. An incision is made slightly posterior and parallel to the upper lateral border of the pectoralis major muscle or transversely across the axilla.
2. The fascia is incised over the pectoralis muscle and the pectoralis minor muscle is exposed. Major blood and lymphatic vessels are clamped and ligated. The use of electrosurgery is avoided around the axillary vessels and nerves to reduce the

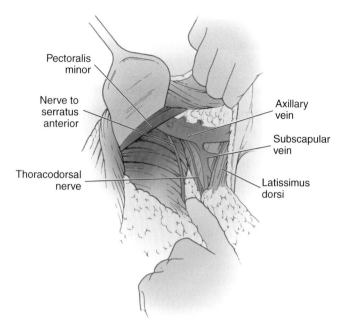

FIGURE 8-10 Axillary dissection.

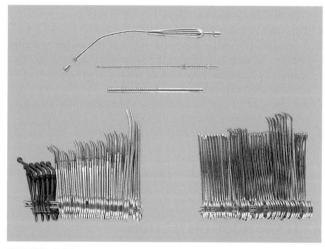

FIGURE 8-11 *Top to bottom:* Yankauer suction tube and tip; Poole abdominal suction tube and shield. *Bottom, left to right:* First instrument stringer: 6 paper drape clips; 2 Backhaus towel forceps; 8 Halsted mosquito hemostatic forceps, curved; 12 Crile hemostatic forceps, 5½ inch; 8 Crile hemostatic forceps, 6½ inch; 2 Mayo-Péan hemostatic forceps, long; 2 Halsey needle holders, serrated, 5 inch; 2 Crile-Wood needle holders, 7 inch. Second instrument stringer: 12 Allis tissue forceps; 4 Babcock tissue forceps; 4 Ochsner hemostatic forceps, straight, short; 8 Adair breast clamps, short; 4 tonsil hemostatic forceps; 4 Westphal hemostatic forceps; 4 Lahey traction forceps.

risk of inadvertent injury and subsequent impaired muscle function.

3. The tissue over the axillary vein is incised.
4. Lymph nodes between the pectoralis major and pectoralis minor muscles are removed. Care is taken not to injure the medial and lateral nerves of the pectoralis major muscle.
5. Axillary fat and lymph nodes are freed from the axillary vein and chest wall. The long thoracic nerve is identified along the chest wall near the axillary vein, and the thora-

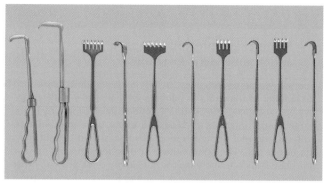

FIGURE 8-12 *Left to right:* 2 Richardson retractors, small and medium; 2 Volkmann retractors, 6 prong, sharp, front view and side view; 2 Volkmann retractors, 6 prong, dull, front view and side view; 2 Volkmann retractors, 4-prong, dull, front view and side view; 2 Volkmann retractors, 4 prong, sharp, front view and side view.

codorsal nerve posteriorly is dissected free from the specimen.
6. The fat and nodes are removed. The incision is closed with sutures and staples, and a dressing is applied. A closed wound drainage system is usually placed through a separate stab incision for lymphatic drainage.

SUBCUTANEOUS MASTECTOMY

Subcutaneous mastectomy is removal of all breast tissue with the overlying skin and nipple left intact. This procedure is recommended for patients who have central tumors of noninvasive origin, chronic cystic mastitis, hyperplastic duct changes, or multiple fibroadenomas or who have undergone several previous biopsies. Breast reconstruction may be undertaken at the time of mastectomy or at a later date if desired.

Procedural Considerations

The patient is positioned as for a biopsy. If reconstruction is to be undertaken, appropriate equipment and supplies are also required. Common instrument sets used for mastectomies are shown in Figures 8-11, 8-12, and 8-13.

Operative Procedure

1. An incision is usually begun in the inframammary crease and may be made on the medial or the lateral aspect of the breast. Some surgeons initially remove and preserve the nipple-areola complex by employing lateral extensions of wide circumareolar incisions.
2. Blunt dissection is performed to elevate the breast from the pectoral fascia.
3. The breast tissue is separated from the skin with an attempt made to remain in a plane between the subcutaneous tissue and the breast. Dissection is carried out toward the axilla. With care, 90% or more of the breast tissue, including the tail of Spence, can be removed. Some lymph nodes in the axillary area also may be removed. Bleeding vessels are clamped and ligated.
4. If a preoperative decision was made for immediate reconstruction, that procedure follows at this time. Provided that the subareolar tissue shows no signs of tumor, as verified by a pathologist, the salvaged areolar complex is placed on a deepithelialized dermal bed.

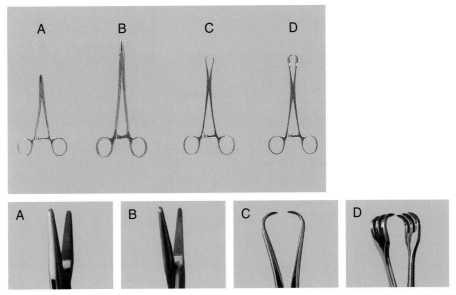

FIGURE 8-13 *Left to right:* **A,** Halsey needle holder, serrated, 5 inch, and tip; **B,** Crile-Wood needle holder, 7 inch, and tip; **C,** Adair breast clamp and tip; **D,** Lahey goiter vusellam forceps and tip.

5. A closed-wound suction catheter typically is inserted. The wound is closed, and a light pressure dressing is applied.

SIMPLE MASTECTOMY

Simple mastectomy is removal of the entire involved breast without lymph node dissection (see Figure 8-9). A simple mastectomy is performed to remove extensive benign disease, if malignancy is believed to be confined only to the breast tissue, or as a palliative measure to remove an ulcerated advanced malignancy.

Procedural Considerations

The patient is positioned as for a biopsy.

Operative Procedure

1. Through a transverse elliptic incision, using a knife, curved scissors, and the ESU, the skin edges are freed from the fascia. Bleeding vessels are clamped with hemostats and ligated with sutures or electrocoagulated.
2. The skin edges of the wound can be protected with warm, moist laparotomy pads; the breast tissue is grasped with Allis forceps and is dissected free from the underlying pectoral fascia with curved scissors, a knife, or an ESU.
3. The tumor and all breast tissue are removed. Bleeding vessels are clamped and ligated or electrocoagulated.
4. A closed-wound drainage catheter is inserted and anchored to the skin with a fine suture. The wound is closed with fine sutures or staples; a dressing is applied.

MODIFIED RADICAL MASTECTOMY

Modified radical mastectomy is performed after a tissue biopsy with a positive diagnosis of malignancy and removes the involved breast and axillary contents (all three levels of nodes—axillary, pectoral, and superior apical) (see Figure 8-9). The underlying pectoral muscles are not removed before or after removal of axillary nodes. A modified radical mastectomy is done to remove the involved area with the hope of decreasing the spread of the malignancy. This surgery's elliptic incision encompasses the nipple-areolar complex, a biopsy scar if an open biopsy has been performed, and excess skin of the breast. If skin is needed for reconstruction (see Chapter 13), it can be preserved and exposure obtained through incision rather than excision (Mulholland et al, 2006).

Procedural Considerations

The patient is placed supine on the OR bed with the operative side near the bed edge. The arm on the operative side is extended to less than 90 degrees on a padded armboard. The skin is prepped and draped as previously described. Tissue removed during surgery will be submitted for microscopic analysis to further classify it (type, tumor size, grade, invasion, lymphocytic response, clean margin size). Additional analysis such as hormone receptor status (estrogen and progesterone positive or negative) and HER-2/neu (human epidermal growth factor receptor 2) expression may also be performed. This information assists the oncologist in planning subsequent adjuvant therapies (Ignatavicius and Workman, 2010).

Operative Procedure

1. An oblique elliptic incision with lateral extension toward the axilla is made through the subcutaneous tissue (see Figure 8-14, *A*). The bleeding points are controlled with hemostats and ligatures or electrocoagulation.
2. The skin is undercut in all directions to the limits of the dissection by means of a #3 knife handle with a #10 blade, curved scissors, or the ESU. Knife blades need to be changed frequently to ensure precise dissection.
3. The margins of the skin flaps are covered with warm, moist laparotomy pads and then retracted. The fascia and breast are resected from the pectoralis major muscle (Figure 8-14, *B*), starting near the clavicle and extending down to the

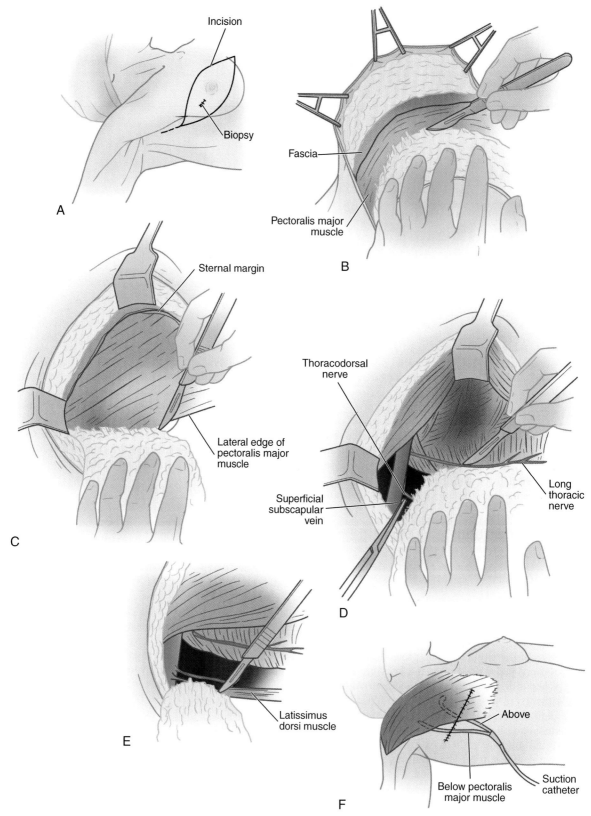

FIGURE 8-14 Modified radical mastectomy. **A,** Lines of incision. **B,** Resection of breast from lateral edge of pectoralis major muscle. **C,** Dissection of breast from lateral edge of pectoralis major muscle. **D,** Thoracodorsal and long thoracic nerves identified. **E,** Resection from latissimus dorsi muscle. **F,** Incision is closed, and closed-wound drainage systems are placed.

GERIATRIC CONSIDERATIONS

The Elderly Patient—Breast Surgery

As in most countries of the world, older women outnumber older men in the United States, and the proportion that is female increases with age. In 2006, women accounted for 58% of the older population and for 68% of the population age 85 years and older. The United States is fairly young by comparison with other countries, with just more than 12% of its population age 65 years and older. In most European countries, the older population comprised more than 15% of the population, and it included nearly 20% of the population in both Italy and Japan in 2006 (Ebersole et al, 2008).

As women age, breast tissue flattens and elongates; the breast becomes suspended loosely from the chest wall. When the breast is palpated, it has a finer, more granular feel than the breast tissue of a younger woman (Ignatavicius and Workman, 2010). Breast cancer in older women is an increasing problem, as its incidence and prevalence increase with age. Breast cancer screening is more widespread, and the death rate due to breast cancer has been declining since the early 1990s. Nonetheless, breast cancer is the leading cause of death in women aged 55 to 74 (Meiner, 2011). In addition to mammographic discovery of a breast lesion, other presenting signs and symptoms include asymptomatic nodules discovered on self breast exam or clinical breast examination by a physician, nipple discharge, or enlarged lymph nodes. Depending upon the stage of the breast cancer, mastectomy or breast preservation surgery with sentinel node biopsy will be performed. Controversy exists regarding the benefits of adjuvant chemotherapy or postoperative irradiation of the breast in women over 70. In general, management is guided by how lethal the carcinoma is and the life expectancy and functional reserve of the individual woman (Fillit et al, 2010). As with younger women, the older female may fear treatment outcomes and effects on her functional status.

Modified from Ebersole P et al: *Toward healthy aging: human needs and nursing response*, ed 7, St. Louis, 2008, Mosby; Fillit HM et al, *Textbook of geriatric medicine and gerontology*, ed 7, Philadelphia, 2010, Saunders; Ignatavicius DD, Workman ML: *Medical-surgical nursing: patient-centered care*, ed 6, Philadelphia, 2010, Saunders; Meiner SE: *Gerontologic nursing*, ed 4, St. Louis, 2011, Elsevier.

midportion of the sternum. The pectoralis muscle is left intact.

4. The intercostal arteries and veins are clamped and ligated.
5. The axillary flap is retracted for dissection of the axilla. Careful attention is directed to preventing injury to the axillary vein and to the medial and lateral nerves of the pectoralis major muscle.
6. The fascia is dissected from the lateral edge of the pectoralis muscle (Figure 8-14, *C*). Vessel ligation is performed in the axilla and adjacent to the sternum. The fascia is then dissected from the serratus anterior muscle. The thoracic and thoracodorsal nerves are preserved (Figure 8-14, *D*).
7. The breast and axillary fascia are freed from the latissimus dorsi muscle and suspensory ligaments (Figure 8-14, *E*). The specimen is then passed off the field.
8. The surgical area is inspected for bleeding sites, which are ligated and electrocoagulated. The wound is irrigated with normal saline. Closed-wound suction catheters are inserted into the wound through stab wounds and secured to the skin with a nonabsorbable suture on a cutting needle (Figure 8-14, *F*).
9. A few absorbable sutures may be used in the subcutaneous tissue to approximate the skin edges. The incision is closed with interrupted nonabsorbable sutures, staples, or a running subcuticular stitch for a better cosmetic result.
10. The dressing can be a simple gauze dressing, a bulky dressing held in place by a Surgi-Bra, or a gauze or elastic bandage wrap.

BREAST SURGERY SUMMARY

Understanding and a working knowledge of the anatomy and physiology of the breast provide a solid foundation for understanding the disease processes and anomalies of this part of the body. Having a thorough understanding of the basic anatomy is a very practical starting point to understanding the many surgical procedures that are performed. As a surgical technologist, it is important to also understand the basis for diagnosing the diseases of the breast. After reading this chapter the surgical technologist is now aware of and able to identify some of the procedures utilized in the surgical care for patients as well as steps taken to identify and reduce surgical wound infection. At this point it is always a good idea to review what has been presented and re-read any sections that remain unclear. Always be prepared to ask questions so that the information learned is reinforced and therefore retained.

REVIEW QUESTIONS

1. Describe the anatomy of the breasts.

2. What is a sentinel node biopsy?

3. What is the difference between simple and radical mastectomy?

4. Describe potential sources of surgical site infection. How can this risk be reduced?

5. Why is proper patient positioning important?

6. Each breast is made up of _____ glandular lobes.
   a. 12 to 20
   b. 1 to 6
   c. 16 to 25
   d. 30 to 50

7. Sentinel lymph node biopsy (SLNB) is the standard procedure for staging of the axilla in patients with clinically node-negative breast cancer. The sentinel lymph node is located by:
   a. x-ray
   b. fluoroscopy
   c. injection of blue dye
   d. needle aspiration

8. A simple mastectomy is removal of:
   a. involved breast and lymph nodes
   b. breast tissue with overlying skin
   c. lymph nodes on affected side
   d. involved breast without lymph nodes

Critical Thinking Question

We know that surgical site infections (SSIs) are a concern in any surgical procedure. How are they classified? Describe steps that can prevent SSIs in breast surgery.

9. Symptoms of fibrocystic breast disease are:
   a. bilateral fullness and tenderness
   b. solid mass
   c. nipple discharge
   d. mass in a duct

10. _____% of all breast cancers appear in women.
    a. 85
    b. 99
    c. 100
    d. 75

11. Define and briefly describe the following surgical procedures:
    Sentinel lymph node (SLN) biopsy
    Lumpectomy
    Modified radical mastectomy

REFERENCES

American Cancer Society: What are the risk factors for breast cancer? 2009, available at www.cancer.org/docroot/CRI/content/CRI_2_4_2X_what_are_the_risk_factors_for_breast_cancer_5asp?sitearea. Accessed April 2, 2009.

Association of periOperative Registered Nurses: Recommended practices for a safe environment of care. In *Perioperative standards and recommended practices,* Denver, 2009, The Association.

Bland KL et al: Radiofrequency, cryoablation and other modalities for breast cancer ablation, *Surg Clin North Am* 89:539–550, 2009.

Boon HS et al: Trends in complementary/alternative medicine used by breast cancer survivors: comparing survey data from 1998 and 2005, *BMC Womens Health*, 2007; 7:4. Published online.

Breast Health: *Diagnostic procedure options (clinical study guide),* Washington, DC, 2006, AORN 53rd Congress.

Cornforth T: Breast Biopsy-excisional-incisional-fine needle aspiration-core needle, 2009, available at www.womenshealth.about.com/cs/breastlumps/a/brstlumpbiopsy.htm. Accessed May 18, 2009.

Fearmonti RM et al: Integrating partial breast irradiation into surgical practice and clinical trials, *Surg Clin North Am* 87:485–498, 2007.

Hormonal therapy changes, 2007, available at www.breastcancer.org/search.jsp?terms=estrogen+receptor+%28ER%29+down-regulators+. Accessed August 7, 2009.

Hulvat M et al: Multidisciplinary care for patients with breast cancer, *Surg Clin North Am* 89:133–176, 2009.

Ignatavicius DD, Workman ML: *Medical-surgical nursing: patient-centered collaborative care,* ed 6, St Louis, 2010, Saunders.

Kassam F et al: Survival outcomes for patients with metastatic triple-negative breast cancer: implications for clinical practice and trial design, *Clin Breast Cancer* 9(1):20–33, 2009.

Kirby RM et al: Three stage axillary lymphatic massage optimizes sentinel lymph node localisation using blue dye, International Seminars in Surgical Oncology, 2007, available at www.issoonline.com/content/4/1/30. Accessed May 15, 2009.

Lind DS et al: Breast procedures, ACS surgery principles and practice, 2005, available at www.medscape.com/viewarticle/503006. Accessed May 27, 2009.

Martinez-Cecilia D: Preoperative MRI can change surgical approach to breast cancer. 6th European Breast Cancer conference (EBBC), 2008. Medscape Medical news online at www.medscape.com/viewarticle/573066. Accessed August 9, 2009.

Mikula C: Mammography and biopsy, *Adv Nurses* 10(9):21–23, 2008.

Morrow M, Harris JR: Comprehensive management of regional breast lymph nodes, 2009, available at cme.medscape.com/viewarticle/590749. Accessed August 8, 2009.

Mulholland M et al: *Greenfield's surgery,* ed 4, Philadelphia, 2006, Lippincott Williams & Wilkins.

National Cancer Institute: What you need to know about breast cancer, 2007, available at www.cancer.gov/cancertopics/wyntk/breast. Accessed April 5, 2009.

Nelson R: Women with BRCA mutation most likely opt for prophylactic mastectomy, 2009, Medscape Medical News, available at www.medscape.com/viewarticle/589280. Accessed May 6, 2009.

O'Shaughnessy J et al: Efficacy of BSI-201, a poly (ADP-ribose) polymerase-1 (PARP1) inhibitor, in combination with gemcitabine/carboplatin in patients with metastatic triple negative breast cancer: results of a randomized phase 11 trial, *J Clin Oncol* 27(155), 2009:Abstract 3.

Re-excision for close margins? 2008, available at www.breastcancer.org/symptoms/path_report/ask_expert/question_03.jsp. Accessed August 7, 2009.

Sentinel Lymph Node Dissection, 2008, available at www.breastcancer.org/treatment/surgery/lymph_node_removal/sentinel_dissection/index.jsp. Accessed August 7, 2009.

Sentinel Node Biopsy, 2009, e-Medicine Health, Web MD, LLC. available at www.emedicinehealth.comsentinel_node_biopsy/page6_em.htm. Accessed May 18, 2009.

Stephan P: Stereotactic breast biopsy for breast abnormalities, 2009, available at www.breastcancer.about.com/od/breastbiopsy/p/stereotactic.htm. Accessed May 18. 2009.

U.S. Department of Health and Human Services: New screening catches more breast cancers, 2008, available at www.hhs.gov/diseases/indexhtml. Accessed April 10, 2009.

Weaver C: Caring for a patient after mastectomy, *Nursing* 39(5):44–48, 2009.

Winkeljohn DL: Oncology nursing 101 triple negative breast cancer, *Clin J Oncol Nurs* 12(6):861–863, 2008.

Zuckerman D: 2007 Update: when should women start regular mammograms? 40? 50? National Research Center for Women & Families 2007, available at www.center4research.org/wmnshlth2007/mam04.07.html. Accessed May 25, 2009.

Ophthalmic Surgery

After studying this chapter the reader will be able to:

- Describe the anatomy of the eye
- Correlate physiology to conditions requiring surgical intervention
- Describe the risk factors associated with ophthalmic surgery
- Compare diagnostic methods for determination of surgical interventions
- Understand and explain ophthalmic surgical procedures
- Identify potential sources of surgical site infection
- List the pharmacologic and hemostatic agents utilized during ophthalmic surgery
- Explain the purpose and expected outcomes of ophthalmic surgical procedures

CHAPTER OUTLINE

Overview

Statistics about vision loss are staggering: throughout the world, more than 161 million people have significant vision loss and that number is expected to double by 2020; more than 37 million people are completely blind, with someone going blind every 5 seconds. Ninety percent of eye accidents, thousands of which occur daily, are preventable with the use of proper safety eyewear (Prevent Blindness America [PBA],

2005). Preventable or treatable conditions cause 80% of blindness worldwide (Lighthouse International, 2007).

Early detection of eye disease through regular eye exams can provide the most effective treatment and ultimately preserve vision (Figure 9-1). However, a national telephone survey of more than 3000 adults found that most Americans are not aware of risks and warning signs of the diseases that could blind them. Over 70% said that losing their eyesight would have the greatest impact on their daily life. Many considered losing their eyesight to be worse than losing an arm or leg, or losing hearing or the ability to speak (National Eye Institute [NEI], 2008a). As a result of the survey, the National Eye Institute is increasing its efforts to educate healthcare professionals about methods of communicating with patients to better maintain eye health (NEI, 2008a). At the same time, outpatient surgeries have been increasing: cataract is the leading diagnosis for ambulatory surgery visits, with more than 3 million lens extractions performed yearly (Cullen et al, 2006). The surgical technologists must keep abreast of changes in technology, procedural techniques, safety issues, and patient education resources to provide optimal care to ophthalmic surgery patients.

Surgical Anatomy

The major eye structures and normal eye function will be reviewed here; conditions requiring surgery will be discussed under Surgical Interventions. The surgical technologist uses this combined knowledge to understand the surgeon's plan of treatment and to prepare the patient, instrumentation, supplies, and equipment for the procedure.

Bony Orbit

The two orbital cavities are situated on either side of the midvertical line of the skull between the cranium and the skeleton of the face. The seven bones that form the orbit are the maxilla, palatine, frontal, sphenoid, zygomatic, ethmoid, and lacrimal bones.

Each orbit is in the shape of an irregular, four-sided pyramid, with its base at the front of the skull and its axis pointing posteromedially toward the apex. The orbit contains the globe; orbital fat; extraocular muscles, nerves, and blood vessels; and part of the lacrimal apparatus. The orbit also acts as a distribution center for certain vessels and nerves that supply the facial areas around the orbital aperture.

The *orbital septum* is a sheet of connective tissue that descends from the periosteum of the orbital margin to the eyelid retractors near the skin surface. The septum protects the contents of the bony orbit, and divides the area into anterior (preseptal) and posterior (postseptal) spaces.

Lacrimal Apparatus

The lacrimal apparatus effectively functions like a sink, with a faucet (main and accessory lacrimal glands) and drain (lacrimal puncta, canaliculi, sac, and nasolacrimal duct). The lacrimal gland produces tears and secretes them through a series of ducts onto the anterior ocular surface, thereby keeping the cornea moist and washing away any debris. The tears then flow inward to the puncta, from which they are conducted by the canaliculi to the lacrimal sac and finally pass into the nasolacrimal duct (Figure 9-2).

Eyelids

The palpebral fissure refers to the space between the margins of the two eyelids (Figure 9-3). When the eye is closed, the fissure becomes a mere slit and the cornea is completely covered by the upper eyelid. The upper eyelid is more mobile and larger than the lower. The upper and lower lids meet at the medial and lateral angles (canthi) of the eye. The eyelids are closed by the orbicularis oculi muscle, innervated by the seventh cranial nerve. The upper lid is opened by the levator muscle, which is innervated by the third cranial nerve.

The anterior eyelid layers contain the eyelid skin, ocular adnexa (eyelashes and associated glands), and subcutaneous tissue, lymphatics, and muscles.

The tarsus is a plate of dense fibrous tissue that forms the main scaffolding of the eyelids. The tarsus is anchored to the walls of the orbit by the medial and lateral palpebral ligaments.

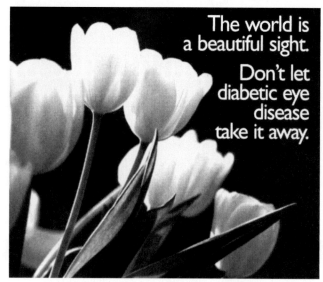

FIGURE 9-1 Public service announcement on prevention of diabetic eye disease.

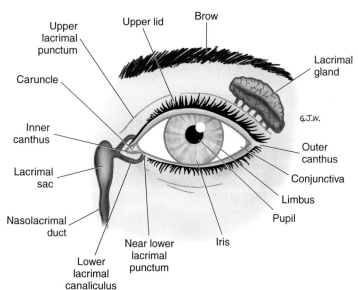

FIGURE 9-2 Lacrimal apparatus.

Within the tarsus are the meibomian glands, which secrete the oily component (sebum) of the tear film. The orifices of these sebaceous glands are found at the eyelid margin just posterior to the eyelashes.

Conjunctiva

The conjunctiva is a thin, transparent mucous membrane divided into a palpebral portion (lining the inside of the eyelids) and a bulbar portion (lining the surface of the globe) (see Figure 9-3). The junction between the palpebral and bulbar conjunctivae forms a forniceal sac.

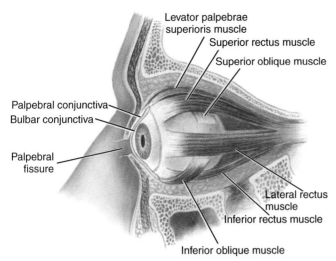

FIGURE 9-3 Orbit and muscles. Medial rectus is located on nasal side of globe.

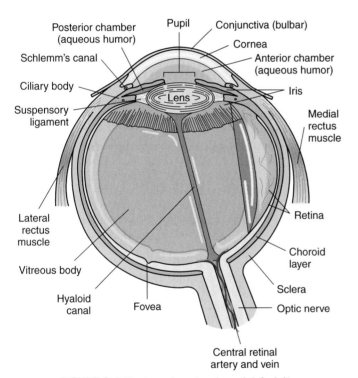

FIGURE 9-4 Horizontal section through left globe.

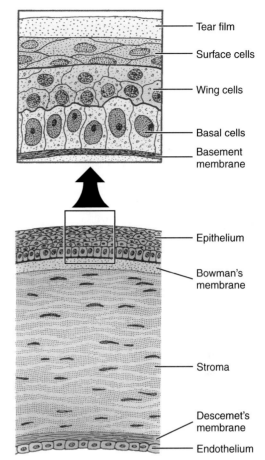

FIGURE 9-5 Five layers of cornea. *Inset,* Layers of epithelium.

Muscles

Named according to their relative position on the eyeball, the extraocular muscles of the eyeball include the four recti (the *superior rectus, inferior rectus, medial rectus, and lateral rectus*) and two oblique muscles (the *superior oblique and inferior oblique*) (see Figure 9-3). Except for the inferior oblique muscle, these muscles originate from the back of the orbit. The muscles work in yoked pairs, with ocular movements generated by an increase in the tone of one set of muscles and a decrease in the tone of the antagonistic muscles. The extraocular muscles are supplied by cranial nerves III (oculomotor,

supplying the superior, inferior, and medial recti), IV (trochlear, supplying the superior oblique), and VI (abducens, supplying the lateral rectus).

Globe

The eyeball (globe) is supported in the orbital cavity on a cushion of fat and fascia. The fibrous external layer includes the clear cornea and white sclera; the middle, vascular pigmented layer comprises the iris, ciliary body, and choroid; and the internal layer is the sensory retina. The globe is filled with two clear liquids: the aqueous humor (anterior to the lens) in the *anterior segment* and the vitreous humor (behind the lens) in the *posterior segment*. Light and images are focused (*refracted*) by the lens, suspended behind the pupillary opening of the iris, and the cornea (Figure 9-4).

Refractive Apparatus

Cornea. The *cornea* is the transparent, avascular window through which light rays pass to the retina; it joins the sclera at a transitional zone called the *limbus*. Corneal sensation is provided via ophthalmic branches of the fifth cranial nerve. The cornea is composed of five layers: the epithelium, Bowman's membrane, the stroma, Descemet's membrane, and the endothelium (Figure 9-5). The epithelium consists of constantly renewing cell layers with many nerve endings, accounting for the cornea's great sensitivity to foreign bodies and abrasions. Bowman's membrane is connective tis-

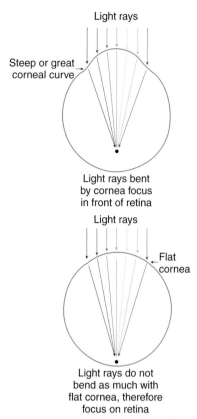

FIGURE 9-6 Variations in the curvature of the cornea change its refractive power.

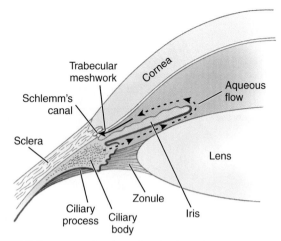

FIGURE 9-7 Anterior chamber, ciliary body, and aqueous circulation.

sue thickening that forms a barrier to trauma and infection under the epithelium. If damaged, Bowman's membrane does not regenerate and a permanent scar is formed. The stroma accounts for 90% of the corneal thickness and is composed of precisely layered fibers. If this layering is disrupted (for example, by edema), the corneal clarity decreases. Descemet's membrane is a thin layer between the endothelial layer of the cornea and the stroma. The corneal endothelium is a single layer of hexagonal cells that acts as a fluid pump to keep the cornea clear by maintaining the proper level of stromal dehydration. Because corneal endothelial cells do not regenerate, damage to this layer may cause persistent corneal edema and loss of transparency.

The *sclera* is the opaque "white" part of the external layer, and is made up of collagenous fibers loosely connected with fascia. The sclera receives attachments of the extraocular muscle tendons, and is pierced by the ciliary arteries and nerves posteriorly by the optic nerve.

Visual images are refracted (focused) by the cornea, the aqueous humor, the lens, and the vitreous body. The cornea has the greatest refractive power of the ocular structures. Variations in the curvature of the cornea change its refractive power (Figure 9-6).

Lens. The biconvex lens is suspended behind the iris and connected to the ciliary body by delicate collagenous strings called *zonules* (Figure 9-7). The lens changes shape and focus (accommodation) by relaxation and tightening of the zonular fibers. Over time (particularly after age 40), the lens and lens zonules become progressively less elastic, resulting in *presby-*

opia. This loss of accommodative power is typically corrected with reading glasses or bifocals.

Vitreous. The vitreous body is a glasslike, transparent, gelatinous mass composed of 99% water and 1% collagen and hyaluronic acid. It fills the posterior four fifths of the eyeball and is adherent to the retina at the vitreous base.

The eye functions similarly to a camera. Light rays from an object pass through the system of refractory devices—the cornea, aqueous humor, lens, and vitreous—and are refracted (bent) so that the rays strike the retina. For information to be received correctly and sent to the cerebral cortex, all structures must function together to focus the light rays. The lens must be able to bend the light waves correctly and bring an object into clear focus. Refractive errors, or errors in focusing ability, occur when the cornea is misshapen or when the lens cannot appropriately change shape to focus images.

Nerve and Blood Supply

The optic nerve (second cranial nerve) extends between the posterior eyeball and the optic chiasm. This cranial nerve carries visual impulses, as well as the sensations of pain, touch, and temperature, from the eye and its surrounding structures to the brain. The third cranial nerve (oculomotor) is the primary motor nerve to the inferior oblique as well as all rectus muscles except the lateral rectus, which is innervated by the sixth cranial nerve (abducens). The fourth cranial nerve (trochlear) innervates the superior oblique muscle.

The ophthalmic artery, the main arterial supply to the orbit and globe, is a branch of the internal carotid artery. It divides into branches supplying the globe, muscles, and eyelids. The central retinal artery and central retinal vein travel through the optic nerve and provide a separate blood supply for the retina.

Physiology of Vision

Clear vision requires all of the following: healthy, functioning eye structures; adequate light; intact neurovascular communication with the brain; and the brain's effective interpretation of the images relayed. Since the eye is similar to a camera with a lens system, the following cycle, if completed in the full sequence, leads to accurate visual images:

1. Light rays emanate from an object in the field of vision and transmit to the eye.
2. Iris muscles control the size of the pupil, thereby determining the intensity of light (similar to the shutter of a camera).
3. These light rays pass through the optical system (cornea—"window of the eye"), aqueous fluid, lens, vitreous to reach the retina (which is similar to the film in a camera). The flexible lens bends the light rays to form the image on the retina, ideally striking at the macula, the area of highest sensitivity for details.
4. The visual sensory nerve endings of the retina pass the images as nerve impulses through nerve fibers of the optic nerve to the brain, where the occipital area interprets the images.

Since early treatment for various eye diseases can potentially save sight, people 60 years of age or older should have a comprehensive dilated eye exam every 2 years as a minimum (NEI, 2008b). Any condition that disrupts eye health or the process of these steps impairs vision. Other structures within the eye exist, but it is beyond the scope of this chapter to adequately cover all details of the complex organ of sight. Specific conditions requiring surgical intervention will be explained under Surgical Interventions.

Surgical Technologist Considerations

With surgical refraction an option, the field of optometry is ever changing. Of the many surgical specialties, ophthalmic surgery can seem overwhelming to many new surgical technologists. The apprehension to this type of surgery may be related to the delicate and specialized instrumentation required or the uncomfortable image of part of the patient's face being exposed as well as invasive work being performed on parts of the globe.

Preparation for Surgery

Preparing for eye surgery involves a great deal of planning to ensure a successful surgical day. There are numerous specialty blades and irrigating tips, suture, and an assortment of implants available to the surgeon. Planning for surgery begins well in advance of the actual surgery date. Some specialty packs require several weeks to be ordered, built, and delivered. When ordering lenses for cataract surgery, several types are needed for each eye. Generally, a surgeon will require a primary and a secondary lens. When ordering lenses, two of each type should be ordered for each eye. In other words, four lenses will be ordered for each cataract patient. Imagine what would happen if only one lens was ordered and it was damaged or otherwise rendered unusable during surgery.

Depending on where the surgical technologist is employed, he or she will have varied levels of responsibility in ordering supplies and equipment for surgical days. In some facilities, only registered nurses order the supplies and lenses.

Because of the fast pace of the surgical day, on the morning of surgery the surgical technologist will have supplies for numerous procedures prepared and ready to open for each surgical procedure. It is very important to have everything ready to go and to develop a system to do so.

Specialized equipment such as the phacoemulsification unit and the operative microscope must be in the room and checked for proper operation before the first procedure. Check that there is a back-up bulb for the microscope available so that surgery is not delayed, which can have serious consequences for the patient. Special positioning equipment must be ready for the day and any other equipment requested by the surgeon should be ready and operationally checked.

Most surgeons have a specific arrangement for the equipment and foot pedals. Be sure to look at the preference cards and confirm placement of these items with the surgeon if time allows.

Surgical instruments for ophthalmic surgery are very small and delicate. Extra care should be taken when handling these instruments. Care should also be taken to protect the blade edges because they are easily damaged.

When scrubbed for surgery, be sure to wipe any residual powder from the surgical gloves and restrict the use of linen to prevent small fibers from contaminating the eye as well as the various fluids on the field. These small particles are irritating to the eye and can potentially scratch the cornea or the lens implant.

Intraoperative Considerations

Make sure that lint from the surgical towels and drapes is controlled and that any powder is rinsed from the surgical gloves. During surgery, be aware of your equipment at all times so that it does not get bumped or jarred. Most patients are awake for these procedures and any sudden movement will startle them. Sudden movement under the microscope, especially when the surgeon has instruments in the eye, can be very dangerous. Be sure all medications and solutions are properly labeled and easily recognized. This is very important since the room lights are normally dimmed to very low levels during the procedure.

When handling implants, especially the intraocular lenses, be sure of the orientation so that it can be inserted correctly. There are newer lenses that do not have a specific orientation.

Have all ointments and dressings ready for the surgeon. It is good to develop a set routine to provide a consistent pace for each procedure.

Postoperative Considerations

Assist with the patient as needed. After the procedure, be sure to rinse all instruments thoroughly with water, especially any cannulated tips or handles. If this is not done, salt crystals from the irrigating solution can crystallize in the instruments, making them malfunction on future procedures. Be very careful to protect the tips of delicate instruments and dispose of any single-use items on the field. If an item is labeled for single use, that means per patient not per day.

Safety Measures in Administering Medications. Medications used in the perioperative period are extremely important to the outcome of the procedure and the safety of the patient. Drugs for diagnosing and treating eye disorders are potent. One error could result in total, irreversible blindness.

The patient's medical and ocular histories determine the selection of an appropriate ophthalmic agent. The surgical technologist should be knowledgeable about specific medication and contraindications.

The nurse checks the medication label for name, strength, and expiration date during preparation and before medication administration. This precaution is especially important because many ophthalmic drugs are distributed in single-dose units that closely resemble one another. The patient must be

SURGICAL TECHNOLOGY PREFERENCE CARD

Ophthalmic surgery is specialty surgery. It is essential to understand what procedure is being done in order to facilitate the surgical team.

Arrive to the procedure room early to acquaint yourself with its layout and the supplies and equipment. Discuss special needs with the perioperative team, taking into consideration additional equipment that may be needed for ophthalmic surgery such as the phacoemulcification equipment, microscope, and other special equipment. Understanding the room layout before setting up for the procedure allows the traffic pattern in the room to be maximized. Controlling room traffic helps in infection prevention, keeps noise levels down, facilitates communication between the surgical technologist and circulator, and allows for efficient placement of equipment. Check for specific settings for the surgeon for the microscope and phaco machine as well as for specific placement of foot pedals, positioning requirements, and other requirements listed on the surgeon's preference card.

Room Prep: Basic operating room furniture in place, specialized equipment (microscope, phaco, etc.), extra blankets, padding, positioning supplies to achieve optimal patient safety

Prep Solution: Check for the proper prep; ophthalmic iodine solution is typical

PROCEDURE CHECKLIST

Instruments
- Ophthalmic set, plastic set, specialty muscle and micro sets
- Anticipated additional instruments

Specialty Suture
- As per surgeon's preference

Other Hemostatic Agents
- Thermal
  - Electrosurgical unit (monopolar or bipolar)
  - Laser
  - Eye cautery
  - Smoke evacuator

Additional Supplies: both sterile and nonsterile
- If the physician is requesting supplies, instruments, or equipment not normally used, check to be sure all have arrived to the room before opening
- Sponges
- Drapes
- Gowns and gloves for team members
- Have ready or hold supplies

Medications and Irrigation Solutions
- Local anesthetic agents (topical or injectable, per planned procedure)
- Other medications according to planned procedure (see Surgical Pharmacology box)

Dressings
- Sterile eyepad
- Eye shield
- Other per planned procedure (collagen shield, pressure dressing)

Specimen Care
- Proper container for each specimen
- Labels for each specimen
- Proper solution for specimen type

Before opening for the procedure, the surgical technologist should:
- Arrange furniture
- Gather positioning devices
- Damp dust lights, furniture, and surfaces
- Verify functionality of equipment
- Place items to be opened in their appropriate places

When opening sterile supplies:
- Verify exposure to sterilization
- Use sterile technique
- Open bundles in appropriate locations
- Open additional supplies onto sterile field
- Open all sterile supplies and equipment as close to the surgical start time as possible

positively identified, and the site of the administration must be clearly translated from the physician's orders. Abbreviations should not be used. The words "right eye," "left eye," or "both eyes" should be used in writing orders. Handwashing between patients when administering eyedrops is imperative, and Standard Precautions should be followed.

All solutions on and off the sterile field must be clearly labeled. To meet The Joint Commission's *2009 National Patient Safety Goals*, medications in a procedural setting must have labels that include drug name, strength/concentration, and amount (TJC, 2009). Medication errors are the most common medical errors. Compliance with requirements can be an issue. One facility found that staff are more likely to label medications when preprinted labels are provided (Jennings and Foster, 2007). Preprinted labels are commercially available. Sterile waterproof pens and labels are also available to avoid smearing from liquids.

Instillation of Eyedrops. Hand hygiene should be performed before administering eyedrops. The patient may be supine or sitting, with the head tilted back slightly. The patient will then look upward while the lower eyelid is pulled to expose the lower conjunctival sac (Figure 9-8). The prescribed number of drops is then administered without touching the tip of the dropper to the eye or the administer's fingers. The natural blinking of the lids distributes the drug evenly onto the eye surface. When anesthetic eyedrops are instilled for topical anesthesia, they are placed on the cornea.

To minimize systemic absorption of certain eyedrops, such as atropine, the nurse may instruct the patient to press on the nasolacrimal duct for 1 minute to prevent absorption into the circulatory system.

Ophthalmic Pharmacology. Numerous medications are used during ophthalmic surgery. See the Surgical Pharmacology table on pp. 337-339 for the purpose and description of each.

Anesthesia

GENERAL ANESTHESIA. Youth, deafness, language barriers, dementia, severe anxiety, specific systemic diseases, known sensitivity to local anesthetics, potential of blood entering the airway (such as in tear duct procedures), and long duration of the operative procedure are among the conditions that may dictate use of general anesthesia.

LOCAL ANESTHESIA. Local anesthesia or monitored anesthesia care (MAC) is used for most eye surgery. Consideration must be given to the patient's age, systemic condition, and discharge plan in determining whether to use preoperative sedation, such as sublingual or oral midazolam hydrochloride (Versed). Intraoperative sedation, when indicated, may be prescribed and managed by either the anesthesia provider or the surgeon. The perioperative nurse, however, is often accountable for monitoring the patient's response to the sedation and the local anesthetic in the perioperative period.

The perioperative nurse assembles the sterile local anesthesia setup as required by the surgeon before the patient enters the OR, checking to ensure correct medications, proper concentrations and dosages, and appropriate sizes and gauges of needles and syringes. Local anesthetics should not be mixed far in advance of the time of intended use, because they may deteriorate, producing a reduced effect for the patient. The addition of epinephrine prolongs the duration of action of most local anesthetics and the vasoconstrictive effect can reduce bleeding, often present in eyelid procedures.

Administration Methods of Local Anesthesia. The *topical method* of local anesthesia has gained popularity for cataract-extraction procedures. A combination of anesthetic eyedrops is instilled into the eye and may be supplemented with infiltration of preservative-free anesthetic into the anterior chamber. Selection of patients for the topical method requires that they can cooperate and follow verbal commands to keep their eyes open and look up or down. Conditions that render the patient a poor candidate for topical anesthesia include inabil-

ity to tolerate eyedrops, Alzheimer's disease, extreme anxiety, and communication problems (e.g., language barriers, hearing impairment, auditory aphasia).

The *infiltration method* involves the surgeon injecting the anesthetic solution beneath the skin, beneath the conjunctiva (subconjunctival), or into Tenon's capsule, depending on the type of surgery.

The most common technique for regional anesthesia in eye surgery is a *peribulbar block.* The anesthetic is injected around the soft tissue of the globe after the needle is directed to the floor (inferior) or roof (superior) of the orbit (Figure 9-9).

Retrobulbar block is injection of anesthetic solution into the base of the eyelids at the level of the orbital margins or behind the eyeball to block the ciliary ganglion and nerves (Figure 9-10). The surgeon administers the retrobulbar injection 10 to 15 minutes before surgery to produce temporary paralysis of the extraocular muscles. Since the tip of the needle cannot be visualized, training and experience are key. Potential complications of retrobulbar injection are brainstem anesthesia and death, oculocardiac reflex, perforation of the globe,

AMBULATORY SURGERY CONSIDERATIONS

Ophthalmic Surgery in Elderly and Team Communications/Hand-Off

Anesthetic management impacts the success of eye surgeries. Safe outpatient surgery, especially in the elderly population, depends on patient selection, preoperative evaluation, preparation, monitoring, and local anesthesia techniques. In addition to standard preoperative evaluation, special considerations apply for anesthesia in ophthalmic surgery. For example, elderly patients scheduled for eye surgeries may have co-morbidities of congestive heart failure, hypertension, diabetes, angina, chronic lung disease, senility, parkinsonism, and/or arthritis, any of which may disrupt the surgical procedure. Some patients with Alzheimer's disease, head tremor in Parkinson's disease, claustrophobia, chronic cough, or shortness of breath while lying flat may benefit from general anesthesia because of difficult management with regional anesthesia and light sedation. Patients may benefit from leaving dentures in place since they may even breathe easier.

It is essential that the patient understand the procedure and routine. Thorough explanations (technique, monitoring, and safety precautions) regarding regional anesthesia for eye surgery can relieve patient anxiety and enhance cooperation. Most importantly, the preoperative anesthesia interview can set the tone and obtain patient acceptance. Premedication can serve as an adjunct to decrease anxiety and provide amnesia during injection of the block. Monitoring and titration of IV medications selected should achieve proper sedation levels and effect. Narcotic doses must be adjusted (decreased) in the elderly because increasing age alters pharmacodynamics.

Established regimens of cardiac medications should be continued in the perioperative period with beta-blocker use considered to prevent complications associated with increased heart rate; regional anesthesia is generally safe, even for elderly patients with a history of myocardial infarction. Following outpatient surgery, the patient needs to have the services of a responsible adult (assistance with walking, eating, and home care) for up to 24 hours after discharge.

Amato-Vealey and colleagues (2008) state, "Care provided in all phases of the perioperative process is driven by the need for rapid turnover; for increased volume and efficiency; to improve physician satisfaction; and to accelerate throughput for the surgical patient." Such a hurried environment can lead to communication errors and mistakes that could be fatal. Errors can occur throughout multiple phases of perioperative care. Active communication should be used to verify and clarify accurate exchange of information (e.g., correct person, correct site, correct procedure, special concerns) between all healthcare personnel, such as at the following transition of care points:

◆ Between the surgeon's office scheduling and the healthcare facility
◆ Between the healthcare facility scheduling and the preoperative area
◆ Between preoperative and intraoperative areas
◆ From intraoperative to phase I PACU
◆ From phase I to phase II recovery and discharge

"Effective and standardized communication between care providers at hand-off points during the perioperative process will help them facilitate safety and anticipate and limit complications. Communication that is timely, accurate, complete, unambiguous, and understood by the recipient reduces error and results in improved patient safety" (Amato-Vealey et al, 2008).

Modified from Amato-Vealey EJ et al: Hand-off communication: a requisite for perioperative patient safety, *AORN J* 88(5):763-770, 2008; Donlon JV et al: Anesthesia for eye, ear, nose and throat surgery. In Miller RD, editor: *Miller's anesthesia,* ed 4, Philadelphia, 2005, Churchill-Livingstone.

---

and retrobulbar hemorrhage (Bollinger and Langston, 2008). Additional risks include ptosis, conjunctival or eyelid bruising, optic nerve damage, and central vein and artery occlusion. A systematic review found no evidence of difference in pain perception in surgery with retrobulbar or peribulbar anesthesia; both were largely effective. Similarly, the review found no evidence of difference in complete akinesia or need for further injections of the local anesthetic. Retrobulbar hemorrhage was uncommon; severe local or systemic complications were rare in both approaches. Overall, retrobulbar and peribulbar anesthesia were found to be equal in efficacy and safety, including acceptability to patients (Alhassan et al, 2008).

For eyelid repairs, the surgeon injects the solution through the upper or lower lid. For operations on the lacrimal apparatus, the anesthetic is injected at the level of the anterior ethmoidal foramen to anesthetize the internal and external nasal nerves. Injection of local anesthetic into the lateral adipose compartment from an inferior temporal needle insertion blocks the nasociliary, lacrimal, frontal, supraorbital, and supratrochlear branches of the ophthalmic division of the trigeminal nerve and infraorbital branch of the maxillary division; this may be used before retrobulbar block.

Positioning. Positioning the patient for ophthalmic surgery generally requires additional devices for stabilizing the head, protecting bony prominences, and providing appropriate alignment to prevent peripheral neurovascular injury. The

ophthalmology stretcher, which is a combination transport device and OR bed, is often used for convenience and comfort as the surgical bed. This special bed, with a tapered head end, allows for closer access to the patient's face and eliminates sev-

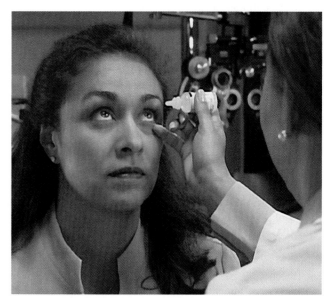

FIGURE 9-8 An eye care professional applies eyedrops to dilate a patient's pupils.

SURGICAL PHARMACOLOGY

Medications Used During Ophthalmic Surgery

Drug/Name	Purpose/Description
MYDRIATICS	
Phenylephrine (Neo-Synephrine, Mydfrin), 2.5%, 10%	Mydriasis (dilates pupil but permits focusing); used for objective examination of retina, testing of refraction, easier removal of lens; used alone or with a cycloplegic
CYCLOPLEGICS	
Tropicamide (Mydriacyl), 0.5%, 1%	Cycloplegia (paralysis of accommodation; inhibits focusing); dilates pupil; anticholinergic, used for examination of fundus, refraction
Atropine, 1%	Anticholinergic, dilates pupil, inhibits focusing; potent, long duration (7-14 days)
Cyclopentolate (Cyclogyl), 0.5%, 1%, 2%	Anticholinergic, dilates pupil, inhibits focusing
Scopolamine hydrobromide (Isopto Hyoscine), 0.25%	Anticholinergic, dilates pupil, inhibits focusing
Homatropine hydrobromide (Isopto Homatropine), 2%, 5%	Anticholinergic, dilates pupil, inhibits focusing
Epinephrine (1:1000) preservative free (PF)	Dilates pupil; added to bottles of balanced salt solution for irrigation to maintain pupil dilation during cataract or vitrectomy procedure
MIOTICS	
Carbachol (Miostat), 0.01%	Potent cholinergic, constricts pupil, used intraocularly during anterior segment surgery
Carbachol (Isopto Carbachol), 0.75%, 1.5%, 2.25%, 3%	Potent cholinergic, constricts pupil, used topically for lowering intraocular pressure in glaucoma
Acetylcholine chloride (Miochol-E), 1%	Cholinergic, rapidly constricts pupil, used intraocularly during anterior segment surgery; reconstitute immediately before using
Pilocarpine hydrochloride, 1%, 4%	Cholinergic, constricts pupil, used topically for lowering intraocular pressure in glaucoma
TOPICAL ANESTHETICS	
Tetracaine hydrochloride (Pontocaine), 0.5%	*Onset:* 5-20 sec; *duration of action:* 10-20 min
Proparacaine hydrochloride (Ophthaine), 0.5%	*Onset:* 5-20 sec; *duration of action:* 10-20 min
INJECTABLE ANESTHETICS	
Lidocaine (Xylocaine), Lidocaine MPF,* 1%, 2%, 4%	*Onset:* 4-6 min; *duration of action:* 40-60 min, 120 min with epinephrine; MPF solution is preservative free
Bupivacaine (Marcaine, Sensorcaine), Bupivicane MPF, 0.25%, 0.50%, 0.75%	*Onset:* 5-11 min; *duration of action:* 480-720 min with epinephrine; often used in 0.75% combination with lidocaine for blocks; MPF solution is preservative free
Mepivacaine (Carbocaine), 1%, 2%	*Onset:* 3-5 min; *duration of action:* 120 min; duration of action greater with epinephrine
Etidocaine (Duranest), 1%	*Onset:* 3 min; *duration of action:* 300-600 min
ADDITIVES TO LOCAL ANESTHETICS	
Epinephrine 1:50,000-1:200,000	Combined with injectable local anesthetics to prolong anesthesia and reduce bleeding
Hyaluronidase	Enzyme mixed with anesthetics (75 units/10 ml) to increase diffusion of anesthetic through tissue, improving effectiveness of block; contraindicated if skin inflammation or malignancy present
VISCOELASTICS	
Sodium hyaluronate (Healon, Amvisc, Provisc, Vitrax) in a sterile syringe assembly with blunt-tipped cannula	Lubricant and support; maintains separation between tissues to protect endothelium and maintain anterior chamber intraocularly; removed from anterior chamber to prevent postoperative increase in pressure; should be refrigerated (except Vitrax); allow 30 min to warm to room temperature
Sodium chondroitin/sodium hyaluronate (VisCoat) in a sterile syringe assembly with blunt-tipped cannula	Maintains a deep chamber for anterior segment procedures, protects epithelium of cornea, and enhances visualization; may be used to coat intraocular lens before implantation; should be refrigerated
DuoVisc	Packages of separate syringes of Provisc and VisCoat in same box
VISCOADHERENTS	
Hydroxypropyl methylcellulose 2% (Occucoat) in a sterile syringe assembly with blunt-tipped cannula	Maintains a deep chamber for anterior segment procedures, protects epithelium of cornea, and may be used to coat intraocular lens before implantation; removed from anterior chamber at end of procedure; stored at room temperature
Hydroxyethylcellulose (Gonioscopic Prism Solution); Hydroxypropyl methylcellulose 2.5% (Goniosol)	Used as coupling solution for gonioscopy; stored at room temperature

Continued

SURGICAL PHARMACOLOGY

Medications Used During Ophthalmic Surgery—cont'd

Drug/Name	Purpose/Description
IRRIGANTS	
Balanced salt solution (BSS, Endosol)	Used to keep cornea moist during surgery; also used as internal irrigant into anterior or posterior segment
Balanced salt solution enriched with bicarbonate, dextrose, and glutathione (BSS Plus, Endosol Extra)	Used as internal irrigant into anterior or posterior segment; need to reconstitute immediately before use by addition of part I to part II with transfer device
HYPEROSMOTIC AGENTS	
Mannitol (Osmitrol)	Intravenous osmotic diuretic; increases osmolarity of plasma, causing osmotic pressure gradient to pull free fluid from eye to plasma, and reduces intraocular pressure
Glycerin (Osmoglyn, Glyrol)	Oral osmotic diuretic given in chilled juice or cola; increases osmolarity of plasma, causing osmotic pressure gradient to pull free fluid from eye to plasma, and reduces intraocular pressure
ANTIINFLAMMATORY AGENTS	
Betamethasone sodium phosphate and betamethasone acetate suspension (Celestone)	Glucocorticoid; injected subconjunctivally after surgery for inflammation prophylaxis; also used to treat severe allergic and inflammatory conditions
Dexamethasone (Decadron)	Adrenocortical steroid; injected subconjunctivally after surgery for inflammation prophylaxis; also used to treat severe allergic and inflammatory conditions and intraocularly for endophthalmitis
Methylprednisolone acetate suspension (Depo-Medrol)	Glucocorticoid; injected subconjunctivally after surgery for inflammation prophylaxis; also used to treat severe allergic and inflammatory conditions
ANTIINFECTIVES	
Polymyxin B/bacitracin (Polysporin ointment)	Topical treatment of superficial ocular infections of conjunctiva or cornea; used prophylactically after surgery
Polymyxin B/neomycin/bacitracin (Neosporin ointment)	Topical treatment of superficial infections of external eye; used prophylactically after surgery; potential hypersensitivity to neomycin
Neomycin and polymyxin B sulfates and dexamethasone (Maxitrol ointment or suspension)	Topical treatment of steroid-responsive inflammatory ocular conditions or bacterial infections of external eye; potential hypersensitivity to neomycin
Tobramycin/dexamethasone (TobraDex)	Topical treatment or prevention of superficial infections of external part of eye; also has antiinflammatory properties
Cefazolin (Ancef, Kefzol)	Prophylactically injected subconjunctivally after procedure; also topically, intraocularly, and systemically for endophthalmitis
Gentamicin sulfate (Garamycin)	Prophylactically injected subconjunctivally after procedure; also topically, subconjunctivally, and intraocularly for endophthalmitis
Ceftazidime (Fortaz, Tazicef, Tazidime)	Injected subconjunctivally and intraocularly for treatment of endophthalmitis
MISCELLANEOUS	
Cocaine, 1%-4%	Topical use, never injected; used on cornea to loosen epithelium before debridement and on nasal packing to reduce congestion of mucosa
5-Fluorouracil (5-FU)	Antimetabolite used topically to inhibit scar formation in glaucoma-filtering procedures; handle and discard in compliance with Occupational Safety and Health Administration (OSHA) and facility policies for safe use of antineoplastics
Mitomycin (Mutamycin)	Antimetabolite used topically to inhibit scar formation in glaucoma-filtering procedures and pterygium excision; handle and discard in compliance with OSHA and facility policies for safe use of antineoplastics
Tissue plasminogen activator (TPA) (Activase)	Thrombolytic agent; used to treat fibrin formation in postvitrectomy patients; lysis of clots on retina
Fluorescein	Yellowish-green fluorescence of this IV diagnostic aid is used in fluorescein angiography to diagnose retinal disorder; topical stain—fluorescein strip temporarily stains cornea yellow-green in areas of denuded corneal epithelium

SURGICAL PHARMACOLOGY

Medications Used During Ophthalmic Surgery—cont'd

Drug/Name	Purpose/Description
Timolol maleate (Timoptic)	Beta-adrenergic receptor blocking agent; treatment of elevated intraocular pressure in ocular hypertension or open-angle glaucoma
Acetazolamide sodium (Diamox)	Carbonic anhydrase inhibitor; given IV to decrease secretion of aqueous humor and results in a drop in intraocular pressure; diuretic effect

MPF, Methylparaben free.
Modified from Hodgson BB, Kizior RJ: *Saunders nursing handbook 2009,* St Louis, 2009, Saunders; Epocrates online, available at https://online.epocrates.com. Accessed May 28, 2009.

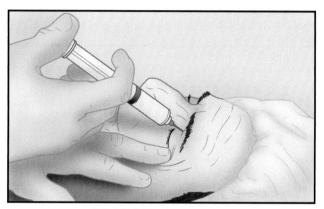

FIGURE 9-9 Peribulbar block.

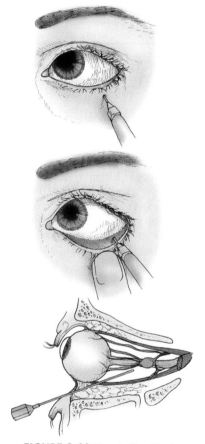

FIGURE 9-10 Retrobulbar block.

eral transfers for the patient. The surgical technologist positions the patient with a foam donut or headrest under the head and a pillow under the knees. The nurse tucks the patient's arms at the side, padding the elbows to protect the ulnar nerve, facing the palms inward and maintaining the wrists in a neutral position (Denholm, 2009). A drape secures the arms. It should be tucked snuggly under the patient, not under the mattress. This prevents the arm from shifting downward intraoperatively and resting against the OR bed rail.

If patients are to be sedated, the nurse asks if they are comfortable and offers reassurance that there are ways to increase comfort. Some elderly patients prefer not to discuss their discomfort for fear of being bothersome.

Intraocular surgery is usually carried out with the use of a microscope. A special wrist rest may be used to stabilize the surgeon's hands and may include a perforated tubing or bar to provide oxygen under the drapes. The nurse or surgical technologist should attach it to the bed and secure it approximately 2.5 cm below the patient's lateral canthus before draping. The wrist rest may be placed unilaterally or may encircle the head. A strip of tape may be placed over the patient's forehead (avoiding the eyebrows) and secured to the operative bed to stabilize the head.

Prepping. The operative site is prepped under aseptic conditions, usually after the anesthetic is administered. A sterile prep tray commonly contains sterile normal saline solution, irriga-

tion bulb, basins, gauze sponges, cotton-tipped applicators, towels, and antimicrobial skin disinfectant.

Some surgeons order one or two drops of 5% povidone-iodine solution administered to the eye surface before the prep of the face and eyelids to decrease the number of surface microbes. Unless the patient has been administered a general anesthetic, a topical anesthetic drop is placed to minimize the stinging sensation. Povidone-iodine solution may be contraindicated in patients with allergic reactions to *topical* iodine. For these patients, hexachlorophene can be used as the agent for the facial prep; however, it is not applied directly to the ocular surface because of its surface toxicity.

RAPID RESPONSE TEAM

The goal of a rapid response team is to intercede in a clinical situation before the patient deteriorates and requires advanced life support. The underlying principle of the rapid response team, proactive intervention, has applicability in the care of patients undergoing ophthalmic procedures.

The oculocardiac reflex (OCR) is a trigeminal-vagal response that can occur during eye surgery in response to traction on extraocular muscles, pressure on the globe, or retrobulbar block. The most common symptom of OCR is sinus bradycardia, which can lead to asystole. The patient may become hypotensive and may experience a wide range of other dysrhythmias attributable to negative inotropic and conduction effects. The incidence of OCR reported ranges from 32% to 90%; in as many as 1 in 2200 strabismus surgeries, transient cardiac arrest may ensue.

The goal in treating OCR is to prevent progression to sinus arrest, which coincides with the philosophy of the rapid response team—intervening before the patient becomes critical and requires cardiopulmonary resuscitation. Heightened awareness of the patient's overall status is imperative for safe eye surgery.

Gentle surgical technique in traction on eye muscles is one method of preventing OCR. When OCR develops and treatment is required, the surgeon should immediately stop stimulating the eye and release the traction. The surgeon may also inject lidocaine near the eye muscle in an effort to block the response. Depending on the dysrhythmia noted, the anesthesia provider may administer atropine 0.007 mg/kg IV, ensure adequate depth of anesthesia and adequate ventilation (as hypoventilation and hypercarbia significantly increase the incidence of bradycardia in strabismus surgery), and request that the surgeon stop all operative manipulation. The surgical technologist provides supportive assistance as required by the situation. Teamwork and communication during critical times (such as during an episode of cardiac dysrhythmia) in conjunction with prevention, vigilance, and early intervention can help avoid a more urgent emergency rescue.

Modified from Donlon JV et al: Anesthesia for eye, ear, nose and throat surgery. In Miller RD, editor: *Miller's anesthesia*, ed 4, Philadelphia, 2005, Churchill-Livingstone; McGoldrick KE, Gayer SI: Anesthesia and the eye. In Barach PG et al, editors: *Clinical anesthesia*, ed 5, Philadelphia, 2006, Lippincott Williams & Wilkins.

The nurse or surgical technologist cleans the patient's lid margins by everting the lids and cleaning with cotton-tipped applicators moistened with antimicrobial skin disinfectant, taking care to prevent the solution from entering the patient's ears. The eye or eyes may be then irrigated with normal saline solution using an irrigating bulb. When toxic chemicals or small particles of foreign matter must be removed, the eye surface and conjunctival sac are thoroughly flushed with tepid sterile normal saline solution using an irrigation bulb or an Asepto syringe. The prep area is dried so the drape will adhere.

Draping. Special concerns for eye surgery draping include repelling water, eliminating lint and fiber particles, and providing adequate air exchange for patients receiving local anesthetics. A cardboard bridge that adheres to the sides of the patient's face may be used to support the drape above the patient's mouth and nose. The surgeon may request that the nurse place a Mayo stand above the patient before the draping process to provide a platform to decrease the weight of the drapes and surgical handpieces/tubing on the patient. The use of a one-piece disposable drape, with a self-adherent, fenestrated plastic section for the eye, eliminates the need to lift the patient's head during draping and facilitates drape removal at the end of the procedure. The eyelids may be separated when applying the self-adherent plastic eye drape to keep the eyelashes out of the operative eye. A fluid drainage bag with wicking strip may also be adhered to the plastic eye drape.

In an alternative method, the surgeon may drape the head with a half-sheet and two towels, use a large sheet or U-drape/split sheet to cover the patient and OR bed, and place a fenestrated plastic eye drape over the operative site.

Instrumentation. Basic eye instruments are shown in Figures 9-11 through 9-20. Additional instruments, depending on the type of procedure, can be added to the basic instrument set. Special surface finishes are used to reduce light reflection. Instruments are designed with round handles for

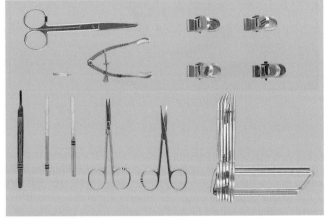

FIGURE 9-11 *Top, left to right:* 1 plastic scissors, straight, sharp, 5½ inch; 1 Lancaster speculum; 4 Edwards holding clips. *Bottom, left to right:* 1 Bard-Parker knife handle #9; 2 Beaver knife handles, knurled, one insert above; 1 iris scissors, straight, 4½ inch; 1 Stevens tenotomy scissors; 4 Halsted mosquito hemostatic forceps, curved; 2 Halsted mosquito hemostatic forceps, straight.

smoother motion and rotation under the microscope. The instruments to be placed on the Mayo stand and the order of their use can also be listed on the preference card or computerized picklist.

A variety of ophthalmic forceps are designed for specific use with different tissues of the eye. Fixation forceps, used to hold tissue firmly in place or provide traction before incision, have an angled tooth that overlaps for secure fixation. Suturing forceps, used to pick up wound edges for dissection or suturing, are single-toothed forceps with the tooth at a right angle to the shank of the forceps. Tying forceps have a flat platform for holding suture as it is tied. The tips of the most commonly used forceps are illustrated in Figure 9-21.

CARE AND HANDLING. To maintain the quality and precision of all ophthalmic instruments, including microsurgi-

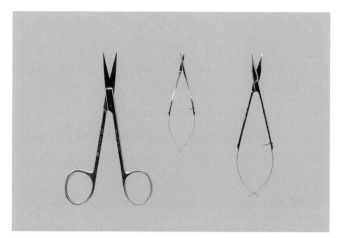

FIGURE 9-12 *Left to right:* 1 suture scissors, straight; 1 Vannas capsulotomy scissors; and 1 Westcott tenotomy scissors.

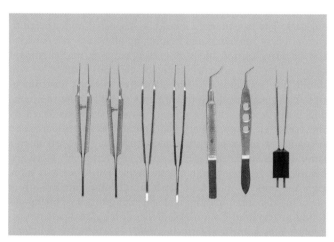

FIGURE 9-13 *Left to right:* titanium tying forceps, 1 straight, 1 curved; 2 Castroviejo suturing forceps, wide handles, 0.12 mm and 0.5 mm; 1 Lehner Utrata forceps; 1 Kelman-McPherson tying forceps, angled; and 1 Codmen cautery forceps.

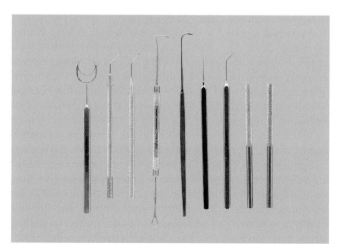

FIGURE 9-14 *Left to right:* 1 Thornton fixation ring; 1 Nagahara nucleus manipulator; 1 Drysdale nucleus manipulator; 1 Kirby hook and loop; 1 Von Graefe strabismus hook; 1 Sinskey iris and IOL hook; 1 Elschnig cyclodialysis spatula; and 2 Beaver knife handles.

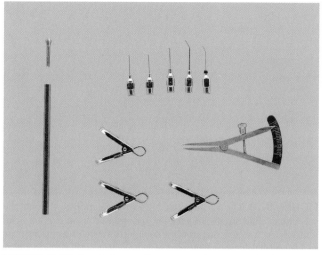

FIGURE 9-15 *Top, left to right:* 1 insert for Beaver knife handle; 5 needle cannulas, 2 27-gauge, 1 Chang, 1 19-gauge, and 1 30-gauge. *Bottom, left to right:* 1 Beaver knife handle; 3 Edwards holding clips; and 1 Castroviejo caliper.

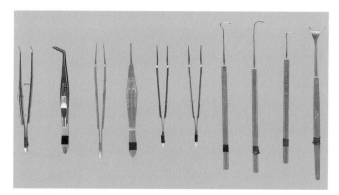

FIGURE 9-16 *Left to right:* 2 Jameson muscle recession forceps, right, front view and side view; 2 Castroviejo suture-tying forceps, wide handles, without tying platforms, 0.5 mm teeth (1 × 2), front view and side view; 2 McCullough utility forceps, cross-serrated; 1 Jameson muscle hook; 1 Von Graefe strabismus hook; 1 Stevens tenotomy hook; 1 Desmarres lid retractor.

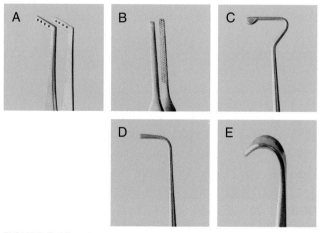

FIGURE 9-17 *Left to right:* enlarged tips: **A,** Jameson muscle recession forceps, right; **B,** McCullough utility forceps, cross-serrated; **C,** Jameson muscle hook; **D,** Stevens tenotomy hook; **E,** Desmarres lid retractor.

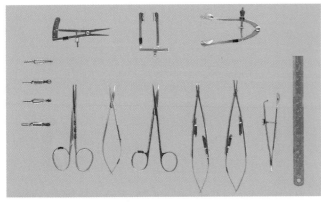

FIGURE 9-18 *Top, left to right:* 1 Castroviejo caliper; 1 Cook eye speculum, child-sized; 1 Lancaster speculum. *Bottom, left to right:* 4 serrefines; 1 strabismus scissors, straight; 1 Westcott tenotomy scissors, curved; 1 Stevens tenotomy scissors, curved; 1 Castroviejo needle holder with lock, curved; 1 Castroviejo needle holder with lock, straight; 1 Erhardt chalazion clamp; 1 metal ruler, small.

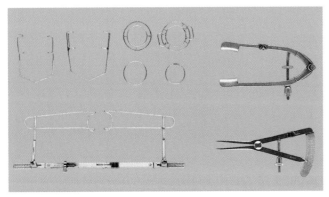

FIGURE 9-19 *Top, left to right:* 2 Barraquer wire speculums, 1 Flieringa fixation ring (double ring); 1 McNeil-Goldman scleral ring (with wings); 2 single-wire Flieringa fixation rings; 1 Lancaster speculum. *Bottom, left to right:* 1 Schott eye speculum; 1 Castroviejo caliper.

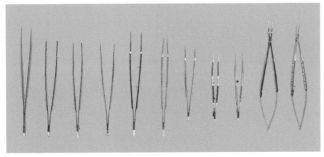

FIGURE 9-20 *Left to right:* 1 jeweler's forceps, straight; 1 Elschnig fixation forceps; 1 Lester fixation forceps; 1 serrated forceps, fine; 1 Castroviejo suturing forceps, 0.5 mm; 1 Castroviejo suturing forceps, 0.12 mm; 1 McPherson tying forceps, angled; 1 Troutman-Barraquer forceps (Colibri type); 1 Polack double-tipped, corneal forceps (Colibri type); 1 Maumenee corneal forceps; 1 Clayman lens-holding forceps.

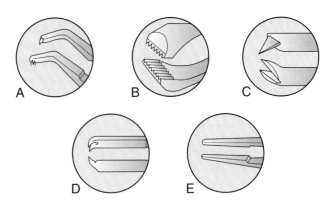

FIGURE 9-21 Close-up of tips of micro instruments used in phacoemulsification procedures and for inserting intraocular lenses (IOLs). **A,** Colibri forceps. **B** and **C,** Fixation forceps. **D,** Suturing forceps. **E,** Tying forceps.

cal instruments, strict criteria for care and handling must be followed. Storage cases protect instrument tips and cutting surfaces. The instruments should be inspected under magnification when purchased and before and after each use, observing for burrs on tips, nicks on cutting surfaces, and alignment of jaws. Eye instruments should be cleaned during use with nonfibrous sponges to avoid damaging delicate instrument tips. Personnel handling instruments should know the name and purpose of each instrument. Tissue can be damaged by the use of an inappropriate instrument, and instruments can be damaged by inappropriate use. After use, the instruments should be cleaned, thoroughly dried, and terminally sterilized before storage in protective containers. A broader and more rigorous look at the entire flash sterilization process—from cleaning, decontaminating, and sterilizing to transporting—is found in The Joint Commission's focus on optimal patient outcomes. This coincides with the *AORN Perioperative Standards and Recommended Practices* (AORN, 2009) in that "flashing or abbreviated cycles should not be performed for convenience, as an alternative to purchasing additional instrument sets or to save time" (Mitchell, 2009).

It is recommended that microsurgical instruments undergo ultrasonic cleaning with distilled water and an appropriate enzymatic cleansing agent. They can be individually handheld or immersed together in the ultrasonic cleaner as long as they are not touching each other. Instruments should be rinsed with distilled water and thoroughly dried. A hot air blower (never a towel) should be used for drying instruments. Instrument lubricant should not be used on irrigating cannulae because residue can be introduced into the eye and cause damage (Risk Reduction Strategies).

In addition to basic care and handling, a routine preventive maintenance program should be established for sharpening, realigning, and adjusting the precision eye instruments. Keeping an instrument in good repair is much less expensive than buying a new one. Disposable instruments (Figure 9-22) are becoming popular with surgeons because of accessibility and quality assurance; for example, forceps are properly aligned for each use because they have not been used on other procedures. Benefits for the institution include elimination of costs related to repairs. Knives are available that have safety features of retractable blades to be in compliance with the Needlestick Safety and Prevention Act, requiring implementation of

▶▶ RISK REDUCTION STRATEGIES

Prevention of Toxic Anterior Segment Syndrome

Toxic anterior segment syndrome (TASS), also known as sterile endophthalmitis, is a sterile noninfectious form of acute inflammation that occurs after eye surgery (typically cataract surgery). The onset of the syndrome typically begins within 24 hours after surgery and is characterized by decreased vision, significant corneal edema, and moderate to severe inflammation in the anterior chamber of the eye. Patients may report blurred vision, eye pain, and eye redness. The cornea is most often affected by TASS because the corneal epithelium is the most sensitive tissue in the anterior chamber. Complications of TASS may include permanent iris damage, in which the pupil does not dilate or constrict appropriately, or ocular hypertension or glaucoma. Overall, TASS can be a very serious and sight-threatening condition.

TASS is thought to be a response to the introduction of a noninfectious, toxic substance into the anterior segment of the eye during surgery. Substances that have been implicated include irrigating solutions and other agents such as anesthetics and antibiotics. TASS may also be related to the improper cleaning or sterilization of instruments.

The surgical technologist plays a key role in implementing risk reduction strategies for TASS, not only in prevention through the vigilant implementation of recommended practices for the use, cleaning, disinfection, and sterilization of equipment and instrumentation, but also in the provision of effective patient education. Timing is critical with TASS, and treatment must be initiated quickly to prevent permanent damage; therefore the perioperative nurse must ensure that discharge instructions for the patient include a directive to contact the surgeon immediately at the first indication of visual disturbance, no matter how mild.

Members of professional organizations (including cataract surgeons and ophthalmic and surgical nurses), infection control personnel, manufacturers of cataract surgical instruments, the Centers for Disease Control and Prevention (CDC), and the U.S. Food and Drug Administration have provided the following recommendations for the prevention of TASS:

- Basic principles for cleaning and sterilization must be followed to prevent TASS.
- Manufacturer directions for use should be followed. For example, directions for use of many intraocular instruments require or recommend sterile distilled or sterile deionized water

for most cleaning steps. Sterile distilled or sterile deionized water is required for final rinsing. Rinsing serves the purpose of removing all cleaning solutions along with debris loosened during the cleaning process. (Note: Agitation in a basin of water is not considered a final rinse.)

- Manufacturer recommendations for sterilizer maintenance must be followed.
- All steps of cleaning and sterilization should be completed; adequate time should be allotted for the task.
- Sufficient numbers of instrument sets (including phacoemulsification, irrigation and aspiration handpieces, and lens inserters) should be available to allow sufficient time for cleaning and sterilization between procedures.
- Precise measurements of water and detergent should be used in mixing cleaning solutions.
- Disposable cannulae and tubing should be used if possible and discarded after use.
- Instruments used in the eye should be cleaned separately from nonophthalmic surgical instruments.
- Ultrasonic cleaning machines must be emptied, cleaned, disinfected, rinsed, and dried daily at minimum, but preferably after each use.
- Cleaning tools (e.g., syringes, brushes) should be discarded after each use.
- Cleaning solutions should be discarded after each use.
- Rinse water flushed through an instrument should be discarded and not reused.
- Only lint-free materials should be used in cleaning/drying and on the sterile field.
- Surgeons should check instruments under the microscope before use and reject any with notable debris or defect.
- The minimum interval for verifying quality of water used in a facility's steam sterilizing system is yearly.
- Staff involved in the cleaning and sterilization process of ophthalmic instruments should undergo competency testing and performance evaluation through direct observation and with a competency checklist so that all staff are evaluated consistently.
- Each healthcare facility should develop and write specific procedures for instrument cleaning and sterilization.

Modified from American Society of Cataract and Refractive Surgery, Ad Hoc Task Force on Cleaning and Sterilization of Intraocular Instruments: *ASCRS, ASORN Special Report: Recommended practices for cleaning and sterilizing intraocular surgical instruments,* Fairfax, Va, 2007, Author; Conner RL: Clinical issues: Toxic anterior segment syndrome, *AORN J* 84(5):841-844, 2006; Forster DJ: Phacogenic uveitis. In Yanoff M, Duker JS, editors: *Yanoff & Duker: Ophthalmology,* ed 4, St Louis, 2008, Mosby; Johnston J: Toxic anterior segment syndrome—more than sterility meets the eye, *AORN J* 84(6):969-984, 2006.

safer medical devices to minimize occupational exposure to bloodborne pathogens from accidental sharps injuries, which remains a serious problem (Harris, 2008).

RANGE OF EQUIPMENT USED. A wide range of equipment is used in ophthalmic surgery. The perioperative team's knowledge of proper functioning and troubleshooting should be confirmed through inservice education and training specific to new equipment. For safety, all items must be used according to the manufacturer's directions and tested for proper performance before the patient enters the OR. Although the products and manufacturers may vary, the following are some of the typical pieces of equipment and accessories used in ophthalmic surgeries:

- *Phacoemulsification machines:* Similar to the action of a jackhammer, these machines use ultrasound to break up the cata-

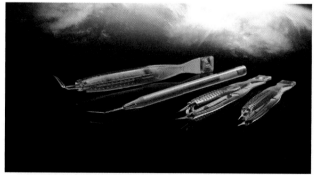

FIGURE 9-22 Disposable ophthalmic (cataract) instruments.

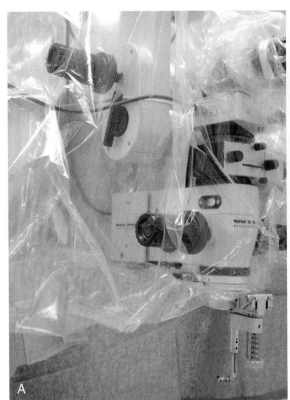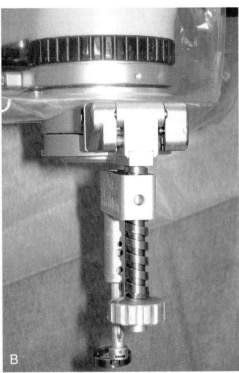

FIGURE 9-23 **A,** Draped microscope with attachment for wide-angle view inside the eye. **B,** Close-up of wide-angle attachment that can swing out of the way to use contact lens on eye.

ract. Irrigation and aspiration ("I&A") handpieces are used as well. Bipolar electrosurgical unit (ESU) and anterior vitrectomy handpieces may also be attached when needed. The surgeon controls the foot pedal and chooses one of the following modes by depressing the pedal to a certain position: irrigation alone; irrigation and aspiration; and irrigation, aspiration, and phacoemulsification combined. Some machines also have an anterior vitrector. As the surgeon manipulates the handpiece and operates the foot pedal to emulsify the lens nucleus, the perioperative nurse is responsible for monitoring the function of the instrument and operating the console controls to change settings such as irrigation bottle height. Displays may show cumulative density of energy and other settings, even video input of the procedure.

♦ *Posterior vitrectomy machines:* Functions on these machines may include vitrectomy with cutter handpieces for removal of vitreous; extrusion for gentle aspiration near sensitive retina and macula; oil infusion; bipolar electrosurgery/diathermy; and motorized cutting with electric scissors attachment. Foot pedal or manual control can set eye pressure and cut and suction rates.

♦ *Cryotherapy machine:* The cryotherapy machine is generally used to cause an inflammatory reaction in the retinal tissue that seals a break or tear. The unit uses nitrous oxide as the freezing agent. Adequate pressure settings are needed for acceptable levels of freeze. Either external or intraocular handpieces are available.

♦ *Lasers:* Lasers are used for various applications in eye procedures, whether for clearing an opacified posterior cap-

sule after cataract surgery, for reshaping or creating a flap of the cornea, or for direct use inside the eye during posterior vitrectomy. Settings must be confirmed with the surgeon. All persons present in the OR when the laser is in use must wear appropriate protective eyewear according to the laser's wavelength. Warning signs are posted on doors and windows are covered to avoid scatter outside the room.

♦ *ESU units:* Bipolar or monopolar ESU may be used. The return electrode monitor placement must follow manufacturer guidelines. Fire precautions must be observed, especially in the presence of oxygen.

♦ *Operating microscope:* Proper care and maintenance of the operating microscope are essential to ensure optimal functioning and durability of this sophisticated, expensive piece of equipment typically used for intraocular procedures (Figure 9-23). The surgical technologist must be familiar with how to adjust pupillary distance (PD—distance between pupils of the user's eyes) and diopter settings on the oculars (eyepieces) for operator vision correction to work without eyeglasses (Figure 9-24). Users who have astigmatism should wear their eyeglasses and set the oculars at zero. Some microscopes used for other applications such as plastic surgery may utilize light sources that are so bright they can damage the retina. The surgical technologist must ensure that the microscope used in ophthalmic surgery is specifically intended and safe for use in eye surgery.

Ophthalmic Sutures. Sutures used in ophthalmic surgery are very fine and range in size from 4-0 to 10-0. Handling and

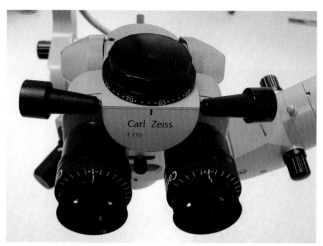

FIGURE 9-24 Oculars of microscope set for surgeon's pupillary distance and diopter adjustments for clear viewing.

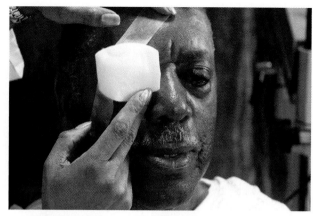

FIGURE 9-25 A patient wearing a protective eye patch.

arming these sutures can be a challenge for the surgical technologist with uncorrected presbyopia. Fine eye sutures produce minimum reaction and discomfort for the patient. They should be handled as little as possible to avoid weakening and fraying. Ophthalmic needles also are very delicate and must be handled with extreme care and inspected for evidence of burrs before use.

Ophthalmic Dressings. At the completion of the operation, the operative eye area is cleansed with saline sponges. After plastic procedures on the lids or lacrimal ducts, antibiotic ointment may be thinly spread over the skin and eyelashes to prevent adhesion of the bandage.

The initial dressing is a sterile eye pad secured with nonallergenic tape (Figure 9-25). After intraocular operations, when external pressure on the eyes might be harmful, the initial dressing is covered with a protecting, perforated aluminum plate or plastic eye shield. Postcataract dressings range from traditional eye pads, to collagen corneal shields rehydrated in an antiinfective-antiinflammatory solution, to no dressing at all. A pressure bandage, consisting of a folded eye patch covered with a second single-layer eye patch, may be used when a compression effect is desired.

Surgical Interventions

SURGERY OF THE GLOBE AND ORBIT

Surgery of the globe (eyeball) and orbit is usually performed because of trauma. Rupture of the eyeball may be direct at the site of injury or, more frequently, indirect from an increase in intraocular pressure that causes the wall of the eyeball to tear at weaker points, such as the limbus. When the intraocular contents have become so deranged that useful function is prohibited or the blind eye becomes painful, removal of the eye contents (evisceration procedure) or of the entire eyeball (enucleation) is indicated. If either procedure is required, an inert globe or a coralline hydroxyapatite (coral) implant may

be inserted as a space filler and to aid in the movement of a prosthesis (artificial eye).

Enucleation

Enucleation is removal of the entire eyeball, with the severing of its muscular attachments and optic nerve. This life-altering procedure is indicated for a blind, painful eye; intraocular tumors; and as a last resort after trauma (Dodge-Palomba, 2008). Usually, a round implant is inserted into the socket to replace the globe and provide support for a prosthetic eye. Sphere implants may be coralline (hydroxyapatite) or synthetic though glass and silicone implants are still commonly used. Hydroxyapatite, a lightweight, coral-like material, may be used as the foundation for a prosthetic eye because its porous structure encourages fibrovascular ingrowth. The hydroxyapatite implant is wrapped in human donor sclera or Silastic sheeting before insertion into the orbital space. New porous polyethylene implants have the advantage of allowing the rectus muscles to be sutured directly to the implant, thus eliminating the wrapping and expense of donor sclera. Suturing rectus muscles to the orbital implant enables improved postoperative movement of the ocular prosthesis.

The patient typically consults with an ocularist 4 to 6 weeks after enucleation or evisceration surgery for a prosthetic eye. A temporary prosthesis may be inserted while a custom-made prosthesis is fabricated. Ocularists may belong to an international professional and educational organization for professionals who specialize in fabricating and fitting custom-made ocular prosthetics (artificial eyes). The American Society of Ocularists (ASO) promotes research in the development of ophthalmic prosthetics and advancement of the methods, techniques, and skills of its members, thereby providing the public with continual improvements (ASO, 2009). Figure 9-26 provides examples of patients using ocular prostheses made by an ocularist certified by the National Examining Board of Ocularists. Medicare and most insurance companies in the United States provide benefits for prosthetic devices. Ready-made or mass-produced eyes are for short-term use (less than 3 months) only. After the prosthesis is created and fitted, the patient will follow up with the ocularist every 1 to 6 months to evaluate its size and to resurface (polish) the prosthesis to maintain the health

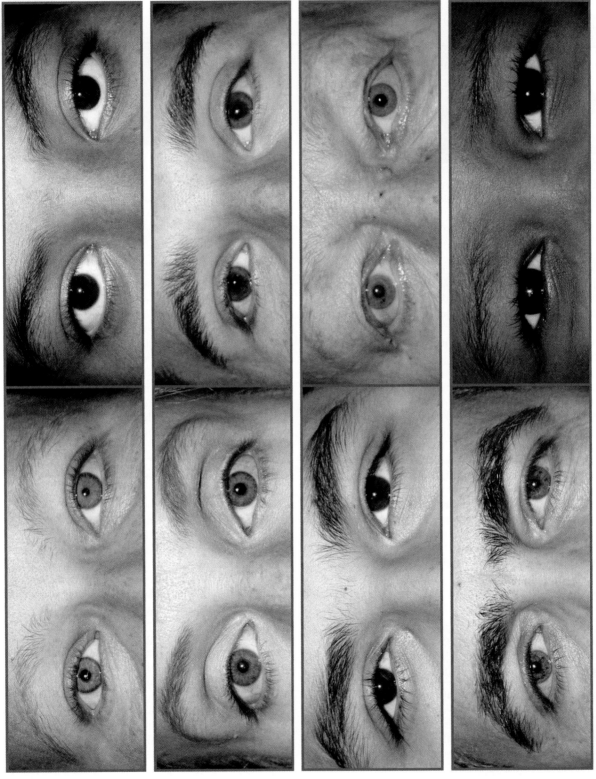

FIGURE 9-26 Patients who have an enucleation can have excellent cosmetic results when fitted with an ocular prosthesis designed by a board certified ocularist.

of surrounding socket tissue. An appointment is warranted if the prosthesis becomes uncomfortable, feels rough to the touch, or changes in appearance, such as the lids appearing droopy or the eye turning in, out, up, or down (Nichols, 2009). The nurse should stress the importance of protecting the visually viable eye, such as using safety eyewear when participating in sports (Dodge-Palomba, 2008).

Operative Procedure

1. The surgeon places a speculum retractor into the palpebral fissure.
2. The conjunctiva is divided around the cornea with sharp and blunt dissection.
3. The medial, lateral, inferior, and superior rectus muscles are divided, leaving a stump of medial rectus muscle. If a coralline hydroxyapatite implant with donor sclera will be used, the four rectus muscles and two oblique muscles are identified and secured with 6-0 suture (to be used to reattach muscles to cut-out areas in donor sclera) before the muscles are disinserted. The two oblique muscles are similarly detached, but are often not subsequently secured to the orbital implant.
4. Using blunt-pointed curved scissors, retractors, hemostats, and forceps, the surgeon separates the globe from Tenon's capsule. The eye is rotated laterally by grasping the stump of the medial rectus muscle.
5. A large, curved hemostat is passed behind the globe, and the optic nerve is clamped for 60 seconds. The hemostat is removed, the enucleation scissors are passed posteriorly, and the optic nerve is transected. The oblique muscles are severed as the eye is lifted out of the socket by the stump of the medial rectus muscle.
6. Hemostasis is provided with either pressure via a sterile test tube or packing with saline-soaked sponges.
7. The muscle cone is filled with an implant, and the rectus muscles may then be sutured to the surface. Tenon's capsule and the conjunctiva are carefully closed over the implant in separate layers.
8. A plastic socket conformer is placed into the cul-de-sac.
9. A pressure dressing is applied.

Evisceration

Evisceration is removal of the contents of the eye, leaving the sclera and the attached muscles intact.

Operative Procedure

1. The conjunctiva is not separated from the sclera as it is for enucleation. A sharp-pointed knife is inserted through the limbus anterior to the iris.
2. The surgeon removes the contents of the eye (iris, vitreous, lens).
3. The choroid adhering to the sclera is removed with curettes.
4. Bleeding is controlled with delicate hemostatic forceps, electrocoagulation, and sutures.
5. A plastic or coral implant is placed within the empty shell.
6. Using nonabsorbable 4-0 or 5-0 sutures, the surgeon approximates the conjunctival and scleral edges.
7. A pressure dressing is applied.

Exenteration

Exenteration is removal of the entire orbital contents, including the periosteum, for certain malignancies of the globe or orbit. The procedure may also include removal of the external structures of the eyelids.

Procedural Considerations. General anesthesia is usually administered.

Operative Procedure

1. Depending on circumstances, exenteration of the eye may include the removal of the lids. An incision is made down to the orbital rim, through the periosteum, and around the entire orbit.
2. The surgeon frees the periosteum from the orbital walls and apex of the orbit with periosteal elevators.
3. The optic nerve is clamped, and the entire contents of the orbit are removed en bloc.
4. Hemostasis is obtained using the ESU and bone wax.
5. A skin graft or temporal muscle implant may be used to fill the orbital cavity or iodoform gauze is used to fill the cavity.
6. A pressure dressing is applied. The cavity is allowed to granulate.

SURGERY OF THE LACRIMAL GLAND AND APPARATUS

Surgery of the lacrimal gland is usually performed for treatment or diagnosis of tumors of the lacrimal fossa or to correct epiphora, which is abnormal overflow of tears related to a congenital or acquired obstruction of the lacrimal drainage system.

Surgery of the Lacrimal Fossa

Surgery of the lacrimal fossa is performed for biopsy of any structure in the lacrimal fossa.

Operative Procedure. The lacrimal fossa, which is in the upper temporal quadrant of the orbit, may be approached directly through the lid or through the conjunctiva by everting the upper lid. The lacrimal gland is divided into a palpebral and an orbital part by the orbital septum. Surgery on the palpebral portion may produce a dry eye.

Nasolacrimal Duct Procedures

Operative Procedure
SIMPLE PROBING

1. Using a punctual dilator the surgeon widens the tear duct opening along the medial aspect of the upper and lower eyelids.
2. A lacrimal probe (sizes vary from 00 to 4) is passed through the punctum, canaliculus, lacrimal sac, and nasolacrimal duct into the nasal cavity (under the middle meatus).
3. Adequacy of the duct opening is confirmed via metal-on-metal contact with the probe within the nasal cavity or via irrigation of fluorescein-tinged saline through the tear duct, aspirated in the nose.

PROBING WITH INTUBATION

1. After opening the duct as described in the previous procedure, the surgeon may place a Silastic tube or stent in one or both canaliculi to reduce the chance of postoperative reobstruction.
2. The surgeon threads the polyglactin leader on the stent through a stylet inserted in the punctum and retrieves it

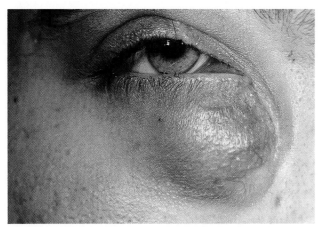

FIGURE 9-27 Chronic infection of lacrimal sac (dacryocystitis) causes swelling of inner lower corner of eye socket.

from the nasal cavity in the nose with a hook. Bicanalicular stents may employ a pliable metal rod attached to the Silastic tube. Such Crawford tubes require a special hook to engage the terminal bulb within the nose before removal.

Dacryocystorhinostomy

Dacryocystorhinostomy (DCR) is the establishment of a new tear passageway for drainage directly into the nasal cavity. The minimally invasive approach to DCR surgery includes the use of a transconjunctival incision, lasers, and endoscopic techniques.

Dacryocystitis (Figure 9-27) is an infection in the lacrimal sac, which may result in a localized cellulitis. Chronic or recurrent dacryocystitis in adults may necessitate probing or DCR because of resistant obstruction of the nasolacrimal duct related to infection-associated scarring, dacryolith (calculus in the duct), or trauma. Another indication for DCR surgery may be intolerable epiphora (tearing) resulting from tear duct laceration following medial orbital wall fracture.

Procedural Considerations. The nasal cavity is anesthetized topically with cocaine just before surgery. The surgery is performed after the patient has been administered a local or general anesthetic.

Operative Procedure

1. An external incision is made in the medial canthal area or inside the nose when an internal approach is used (Figure 9-28).
2. Blunt dissection is carried through the orbicularis down to the nasal bone. The orbicularis is separated from the bone with a Freer elevator. The lacrimal fossa sac is exposed.
3. The surgeon uses a hemostat to press an opening through the lacrimal bone. If this is unsuccessful, the anterior lacrimal crest is perforated with a power burr or mallet and chisel. The opening is enlarged to a 10-mm circle with a Kerrison rongeur, and hemostasis is obtained with bone wax if necessary.
4. The inferior punctum is dilated, and a probe is passed into the lacrimal sac.
5. The lacrimal sac and nasal mucosa are incised with H flaps. The surgeon sutures the posterior nasal mucous membrane flap to the posterior lacrimal sac flap with 4-0 absorbable sutures.

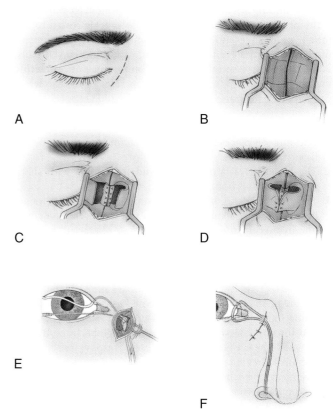

FIGURE 9-28 Dacryocystorhinostomy. **A,** Skin incision for dacryocystorhinostomy or dacryocystectomy. **B,** Lacrimal sac and lacrimal bone exposed. Opening made in lacrimal bone and lacrimal crest. **C,** Posterior flap of wall of sac sutured to posterior flap of nasal mucosa. **D,** Anterior flap of wall of sac sutured to anterior flap of nasal mucosa (drawing is somewhat distorted for visualization of relative positions). **E,** Canaliculi are intubated with Silastic tubes. **F,** Tubes are secured to lateral nasal wall and allowed to slide back into nose.

6. The surgeon passes the first end of the wire stylet of a Silastic lacrimal duct intubation set through the upper canaliculus, through the opening, and out through the nose (under the inferior meatus). The procedure is repeated for the lower canaliculus.
7. The anterior nasal mucous membrane flap is sutured to the anterior lacrimal sac flap with 4-0 absorbable sutures to create a bridge over the Silastic tubing. The tubing remains in place until the sutures become absorbed, thereby acting as a stent around which epithelial union between the lacrimal and nasal mucosa can occur.
8. The orbicularis is closed with 6-0 absorbable sutures. Skin margins are approximated and closed with nonabsorbable 6-0 sutures. Antibiotic ointment is applied to the incision.
9. The surgeon cuts the wire stylets off the Silastic tubing, and ties the ends of the tubing together. The tubing is sutured to the lateral nasal wall with 6-0 nonabsorbable suture. The tubing is cut so that it retracts into the nostril. An absorbent sponge may be taped under the nostrils.

SURGERY OF THE EYELIDS

Oculoplastic procedures performed on the eyelids include treatment of chalazion, entropion, ectropion, dermatochala-

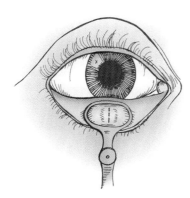

FIGURE 9-29 Transconjunctival approach. Clamp everts eyelid during surgery for chalazion. Viscous contents of chalazion will be removed with curette.

sis, and ptosis; biopsy and excision of eyelid tumors; and repair and reconstruction of eyelid trauma or post-biopsy damage.

Removal of Chalazion

Obstruction of meibomian gland secretion may lead to a chalazion, manifesting as a variably firm bump in the eyelid. Although chalazia can become infected, this is not primarily an infectious process. If persistent, incision of the chronic chalazion may be warranted.

Procedural Considerations. Incision of chalazion is often performed in an office setting, but pediatric and very anxious patients may require intravenous sedation. Local anesthesia, with 1:100,000 epinephrine in the local anesthetic, is usually employed. The majority of chalazia are surgically approached from the conjunctival side of the tarsal plate, but cutaneous incisions or repair of friable cutaneous tissue may be required (Figure 9-29).

Operative Procedure (Transconjunctival Approach)

1. Using a chalazion clamp, the surgeon everts the affected lid to expose the chalazion.
2. A vertical incision is made on the inner lid surface with a sharp blade; the small lesion is curetted, or the chalazion wall is excised, in part or in toto.
3. Hemostasis is achieved through use of the bipolar ESU.
4. The wound is left open for drainage. Cutaneous sutures are placed when needed. Pressure eye patching may be performed.

Repair of Entropion

Entropion occurs when the eyelid margin inverts. It may cause significant corneal irritation, attributable to rubbing of inturned eyelashes against the ocular surface. The most common type is *involutional entropion,* when laxity and degeneration of facial attachments between the pretarsal muscle and the tarsus permit the pretarsal muscle to override the lid margin during contraction. *Cicatricial entropion* is attributable to contraction of either the upper or the lower tarsus and its conjunctiva, causing inturned lashes (trichiasis) to abrade the cornea. Commonly employed surgical techniques

for entropion repair include lateral tightening of a lax eyelid via either a *tarsal strip* procedure or a *pentagonal wedge resection,* and suture eversion (via either a *Wies* or a *Quickert suture technique*).

Procedural Considerations. The causes of entropion vary, and corrective procedures also vary depending on the pathologic process. Local anesthetic is typically used, and antiinfective ointment is applied postoperatively.

Operative Procedures
BLEPHAROPLASTY OF LOWER LID FOR INVOLUTIONAL ENTROPION

1. The surgeon injects local anesthetic into the lower lid through the conjunctiva using an angled needle.
2. The skin is marked, and an incision is made in the lateral canthus.
3. The orbicularis is dissected off the orbital septum.
4. The skin excision is extended across the lower lid.
5. The orbital septum is incised to expose fat pockets.
6. The surgeon removes extra fat, and hemostasis is achieved.
7. After incising the lateral canthus, the surgeon pulls the lower lid laterally and shortens (tightens) it to correct entropion.
8. The tarsus is reattached to the lateral canthal tendon, and the lower lid fascia is reattached to the orbicularis.
9. The excess skin is pulled up, marked, and excised.
10. The skin incisions are closed.

WIES PROCEDURE FOR CICATRICIAL ENTROPION

1. A marking pen is used to draw a parallel line 4 mm below the lower lid margin; the local anesthetic is then injected.
2. The surgeon places a double-armed 4-0 nonabsorbable retraction suture through the conjunctiva and lower lid 4 mm from the lateral canthus and 4 mm from the medial canthus.
3. A lid plate retractor is placed behind the lower lid as it is pulled up with the traction suture. The surgeon uses a #15 blade to make the skin incision on the marked line.
4. The lid plate retractor is placed in front of the lid, and the lower lid is everted using the traction suture. The conjunctiva is incised with the #15 blade.
5. A full-thickness blepharotomy is extended laterally and medially with scissors.
6. The surgeon passes one end of the double-armed 4-0 suture through the conjunctiva and lower lid tendons and between the orbicularis and tarsus on the medial aspect of the lower lid. This process is repeated approximately 4 mm laterally with the other end of the 4-0 suture.
7. Six mattress sutures are placed and tied to evert the lower lid (Figure 9-30).
8. Excess skin is excised, and the skin incision is closed with 7-0 nonabsorbable sutures.

Repair of Ectropion

Ectropion (sagging and eversion of the lower lid), usually bilateral, is common in older persons (Figure 9-31). Ectropion may be caused by the relaxation of the orbicular muscle and canthal tendons. Symptoms include tearing, conjunctival infection, irritation, and inadequate corneal protection leading to injury to the cornea. Surgery is indicated when facial paralysis is permanent or when scarring follows lacerations, lesions, or penetrating injuries and the cornea becomes exposed, resulting in ulceration and photophobia.

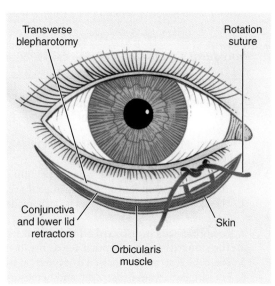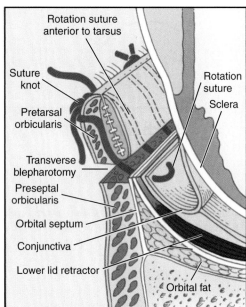

FIGURE 9-30 Wies procedure for entropion. Placement of an everting mattress suture across a transverse blepharotomy.

Procedural Considerations. The causes of ectropion vary, and corrective procedures also vary depending on the pathologic process. Local anesthetic is typically used, and antiinfective ointment and ice compresses are applied postoperatively.

Operative Procedure
LATERAL CANTHAL SLING PROCEDURE

One method of correction for ectropion is the lateral canthal sling procedure (Figure 9-32), which repositions and tightens the lower lid in a horizontal direction.

1. The lateral canthus is incised, and a strip of tarsus and lateral canthal tendon is isolated.
2. The surgeon sutures the tarsus/tendon to the periosteum along the inner surface of the lateral wall of the orbit, thereby tightening the lid and correcting the ectropion.

Plastic Repair for Dermatochalasis

Dermatochalasis is a condition of drooping skin and herniated fat of the upper and lower lids that causes the skin of the upper eyelids to hang down over the palpebral fissure, sometimes obscuring vision. It may occur in older persons who have lost normal elasticity in the skin of their upper lids or in persons who have persistent angioneurotic edema with stretching of the skin of the eyelids. If ptosis is present, it accentuates the condition.

Procedural Considerations. Dermatochalasis is corrected with blepharoplasty of the redundant skin of the upper or lower eyelids. A segment of skin and fat is removed. In the lower lid, a transconjunctival excision that leaves no external incision may be performed. Brow droop, or ptosis, may also be corrected alone or in combination with blepharoplasty to correct dermatochalasis. Procedures for correcting brow ptosis include direct brow lift, coronal brow lift, and endoscopic brow lift. Most procedures are performed using a local anesthetic with IV sedation.

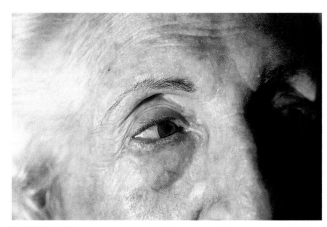

FIGURE 9-31 Ectropion, or eyelid eversion (turning out of lid), is most commonly caused by relaxation of eyelid framework.

Operative Procedure
BLEPHAROPLASTY OF UPPER LID
FOR DERMATOCHALASIS

1. The surgeon marks the amount of skin to be excised in the upper lid above the lid crease and injects local anesthetic.
2. Stretching the skin of the upper lid tautly, the surgeon incises along the predrawn lines.
3. The skin between the marked lines is excised, the orbicularis between the incision edges is excised, and hemostasis is achieved.
4. The surgeon incises the septum; applies finger pressure on the globe; and clamps, cuts, and electrocoagulates the bulging fat.
5. If fat is found in the temporal pocket, it may contain a prolapsed lacrimal gland. The lacrimal gland should be resuspended with 5-0 nonabsorbable suture.
6. The surgeon restores the lid crease by suturing the lower skin muscle incision line to the levator at the upper edge of the tarsus.

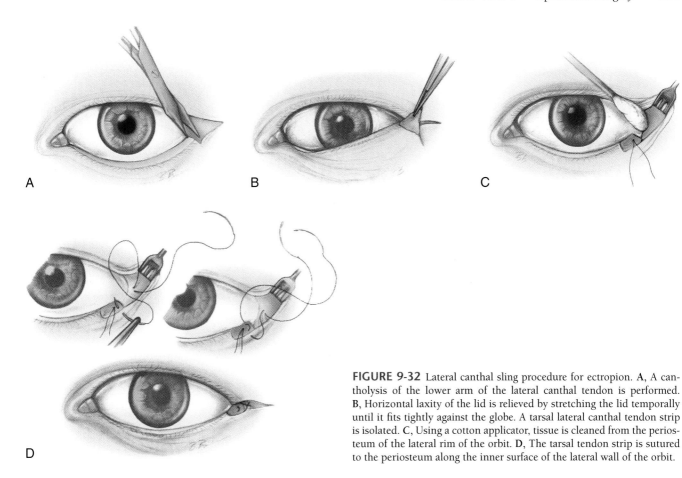

FIGURE 9-32 Lateral canthal sling procedure for ectropion. **A,** A cantholysis of the lower arm of the lateral canthal tendon is performed. **B,** Horizontal laxity of the lid is relieved by stretching the lid temporally until it fits tightly against the globe. A tarsal lateral canthal tendon strip is isolated. **C,** Using a cotton applicator, tissue is cleaned from the periosteum of the lateral rim of the orbit. **D,** The tarsal tendon strip is sutured to the periosteum along the inner surface of the lateral wall of the orbit.

7. The skin is closed with 6-0 nonabsorbable suture in a continuous running fashion.

TRANSCONJUNCTIVAL BLEPHAROPLASTY OF LOWER LID
1. The surgeon injects local anesthetic into the lower lid through the conjunctiva using an angled needle.
2. Finger pressure is placed on the upper lid while the lower lid is being retracted to expose the conjunctiva of the inferior cul-de-sac.
3. The surgeon incises the conjunctiva and exposes the fat pockets. Prolapsed fat is clamped and removed, and hemostasis is achieved.

Surgery for Unilateral or Bilateral Ptosis

Ptosis is true drooping of the upper lid and may be congenital or acquired. In congenital ptosis there usually is developmental weakness of the levator muscle. The condition may be unilateral or bilateral. The child often compensates by raising the eyebrow or tilting the chin upward.

Acquired ptosis can be neurogenic, myogenic or involutional, which is manifested by a gradual stretching or dehiscence of the levator aponeurosis. The eyelid crease may be high or absent.

Procedural Considerations. The objective of ptosis surgery is to achieve a good cosmetic result, expand the superior visual field, and restore function with elevation of the lid. Many surgical procedures have been devised, directed at the levator aponeurosis, frontalis muscle, or the levator-Müller muscle complex. These muscles are the elevating forces of the

upper lids. Local anesthesia may be preferred in cooperative individuals so that intraoperative adjustments can be made. Frontalis suspension uses fascia lata or synthetic materials to attach the tarsus to the frontalis, bypassing the ineffective levator muscle. Harvesting fascia lata requires an additional incision in the leg.

Operative Procedure
LEVATOR APONEUROSIS REPAIR
1. The surgeon marks the existing or potential eyelid crease. With the skin of the upper lid held taut, the skin incision is made (Figure 9-33).
2. An incision is made through the orbicularis. The surgeon dissects the orbicularis off the orbital septum and the levator aponeurosis anterior to the tarsus.
3. The aponeurosis is incised across the tarsus and dissected off the orbicularis. The levator is reattached to the tarsus with interrupted 6-0 suture.
4. If the patient is awake, he or she is asked to look forward and the sutures are adjusted as needed.
5. The pretarsal orbicularis is sutured to the aponeurosis to reconstruct the lid crease.
6. The surgeon closes the skin incision with a running 6-0 nonabsorbable suture.

FRONTALIS SUSPENSION
1. The upper lid is marked, one incision is made in the lid crease, and two incisions are made above the eyebrow (Figure 9-34, *A* and *B*).

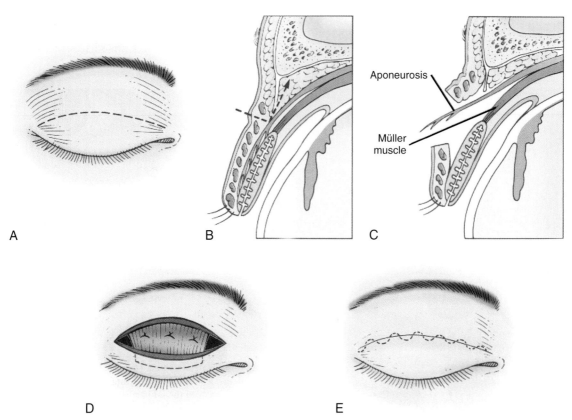

FIGURE 9-33 Levator aponeurosis repair for ptosis. **A**, Eyelid crease is marked. **B**, Skin incision is made, and the orbicularis and orbital septum are divided while dissection proceeds toward the orbital rim. **C**, The anterior surface of the tarsus is exposed, and the aponeurosis is separated from the Müller muscle. **D**, The aponeurosis is reattached to the tarsus with partial-thickness permanent sutures. Lid contour and position are adjusted. **E**, The eyelid crease is created by suturing the pretarsal orbicularis muscle to the aponeurosis, and the skin is closed.

2. The surgeon places a lid plate behind the upper lid, exposes the tarsus, and secures the suspension material (fascia graft or a synthetic implant) to the tarsus with nonabsorbable sutures (Figure 9-34, *C*).
3. Using a Wright needle, the surgeon passes the suspension material away from the globe deeply into the orbital septum and out through one eyebrow incision (Figure 9-34, *D*).
4. The remaining end of the suspension material is passed in the same manner.
5. The surgeon sutures the pretarsal orbicularis to the tarsus to form the lid crease (Figure 9-34, *E*).
6. The lid incision is closed with a running 6-0 nonabsorbable suture (Figure 9-34, *F*).
7. The surgeon passes the long end of the suspension material under the skin between the brow incisions to complete the loop, and sutures the ends of the material together.
8. The brow incisions are closed with interrupted 6-0 nonabsorbable suture.

Excisional Biopsy

Excisional biopsy is removal of lesions for diagnostic examination. Basal cell carcinomas account for 95% of neoplastic lesions of the lid; the treatment of choice is excision with frozen-section analysis or Mohs' technique.

Operative Procedure. Through-and-through excision of skin, muscle, tarsus, and conjunctiva is followed by careful structural closure of anatomic spaces. Depending on the type, extent, and location of the lesion, rotation flaps or free grafts may be necessary.

Plastic Repair for Traumatic Injuries

Lacerations of the lids, including damage to the inferior canaliculus, are repaired surgically. Paramount for success is the careful approximation of the borders of the lid margin and the ends of a torn canaliculus.

Operative Procedure. Lacerations of the lid margin are closed with a 6-0 silk suture to align the gray line of the lid that lies between the lash follicles and the orifices of the meibomian glands. Once this anatomic line has been approximated, all other sutures are placed, maintaining the approximation. If the canaliculus has been lacerated, the lacrimal drainage system is intubated with a silicone tube and the canaliculus and lid are reconstructed around the tube.

SURGERY OF THE CONJUNCTIVA

The conjunctiva of the eye is a transparent and elastic membrane that lines the inner surface of the eyelids and covers

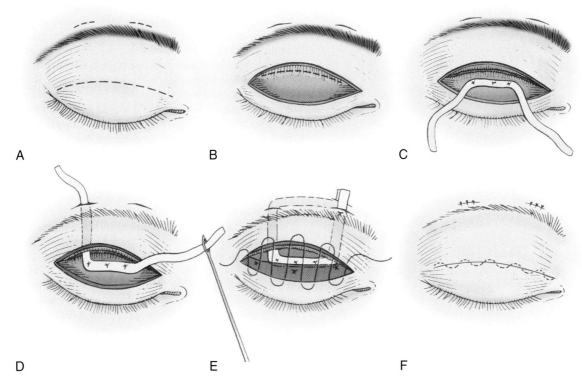

FIGURE 9-34 Frontalis suspension for ptosis. One method used to suspend the eyelid from the brow.

the sclera. Lacerations caused by injury as well as deficits resulting from excision of tumors, cysts, nevi, or pterygia can usually be repaired by simple undermining and suturing.

Pterygium Excision

A pterygium is a fleshy, triangular encroachment of conjunctiva onto the peripheral area of the cornea. Because pterygia tend to recur, surgery is delayed until vision is affected by encroachment on the visual axis.

Operative Procedure. The major steps in the McReynolds technique are illustrated in Figure 9-35. A pterygium can also be excised totally and the limbus treated with an eye cautery or bipolar ESU. The conjunctiva can then be closed, or the sclera can be left bare.

Surgery may be combined with beta-radiation, application of mitomycin, conjunctiva autologous grafts, and lamellar corneal grafts, and more recently with amniotic membrane graft.

Excisional Biopsy

Any suspect lesion of the conjunctiva can be removed by simple elliptic excision and sent for pathologic examination. The conjunctiva may or may not be closed, depending on the surgeon's particular technique.

Strabismus Surgery

Strabismus refers to ocular misalignment. Although often neurogenic rather than muscular in origin, surgery on the extraocular muscles may be indicated to improve this misalignment. Strabismus surgery is described in Chapter 17.

SURGERY OF THE CORNEA

Surgery of the cornea is indicated for a variety of conditions in which cosmetic, therapeutic, restorative, and refractive outcomes are desired.

Repair of Lacerations

Corneal lacerations may be closed with direct appositional suturing with 10-0 suture viewed through an operating microscope or with a tissue adhesive, such as cyanoacrylate monomers. The sterile tissue adhesive is applied to well-dried tissue that has been properly oriented anatomically. It polymerizes and seals the wound on contact with the tissue.

Culture specimens are usually obtained at the time of surgery. Antibiotics are injected subconjunctivally before the dressing is applied.

Corneal Transplantation (Keratoplasty)

A corneal transplantation (keratoplasty) is performed when the patient's cornea is thickened or opacified by disease and degeneration. The transparency of the cornea may be impaired as a result of scars, infection (bacterial, fungal, or viral), thermal or chemical burns, Fuchs' dystrophy, edema after cataract surgery, or keratoconus (abnormal steepening). Ocular surgery such as phacoemulsification, vitrectomy, or intraocular lens implant can potentially damage the corneal endothelium. Corneal transplantation, in which corneal tissue from one human eye is grafted to another, is done to improve vision when the retina and optic nerve are functioning properly; it was first performed in 1905. Because the cornea is tissue that lacks blood vessels, it can be transplanted with less rejection and at a 90% suc-

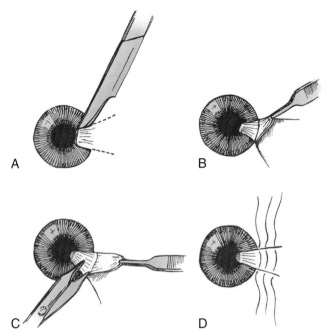

FIGURE 9-35 McReynolds technique for pterygium excision. **A,** Cornea around head of pterygium is incised. **B,** Pterygium flap is dissected upward, leaving clear cornea. **C,** Lower margin of pterygium is dissected, and whole pterygium is freed from sclera. **D,** Sutures are placed for closure of conjunctiva.

cess rate. Keratoplasty may be performed as a lamellar (partial-thickness) graft or a penetrating (full-thickness) graft. Over 50,000 grafts were made available in 2007. Corneal transplant is one of the most frequently performed human transplant procedures, with more than 700,000 performed since 1961 (Eye Bank Association of America [EBAA], 2009.)

Phototherapeutic keratectomy (PTK) procedures use excimer laser ablation to remove superficial corneal lesions and smooth the corneal surface. PTK can be used on conditions that would require corneal transplant and may delay or replace the occurrence of penetrating keratoplasty in some cases.

Procurement of Corneas. The eye bank may be a central community agency or may be owned and operated by a hospital. Eye banks help coordinate the procurement of eyes from recently deceased persons under the Eye Bank Association of America (EBAA) guidelines. Persons of any age can be eye donors, and poor eyesight or cataracts do not influence eye viability (EBAA, 2009). The donor's family, medical, and social histories are reviewed. It is not necessary to perform antigen matching as with other tissue or organ transplants, but blood serum tests for human immunodeficiency virus (HIV) and hepatitis B virus are performed on the donor. The procurement team removes donor eyes within 6 hours of death in accordance with legal regulations. Tissue, such as a cornea, must be recovered, processed, and transplanted in controlled surgical environments. If the donor eye is unsuitable for the cornea to be transplanted, the eye can be used for research or education.

Many individuals have signed donor cards or eye-donor designation on their drivers' licenses. A special consent form is required and should be signed by the authorized next of kin and by a hospital representative designated by institutional

policy. Federal regulations require hospitals to report all deaths and imminent deaths to organ procurement organizations. With the collaboration of hospitals, organ procurement organizations, and eye and tissue banks, the family of every potential donor is informed about the option to donate organs or tissues.

The enucleations may be done in the hospital morgue or emergency department under aseptic conditions. The procured cornea is placed in Optisol GS sterile buffered tissue culture medium within 12 hours of death and transplanted within 3 to 7 days. Optisol GS sterile buffered tissue culture medium contains polypeptides, dextran, and antibiotics (gentamicin and streptomycin) and can preserve a donor cornea for 14 days under refrigeration. It is best if corneal transplantation is performed in 2 or 3 days because the cornea may become boggy from constant exposure to the tissue culture solution.

PROCEDURAL CONSIDERATIONS. Postmortem preparation includes elevating the donor's head with a pillow to minimize edema in the face or near the eye. The eyes are irrigated and lightly taped closed to avoid pressure on the eye. A small ice pack may be applied to the forehead or over the eyes if the donor is not in a refrigerated morgue within 1 hour of death.

For the procurement procedure, the eyes are washed and irrigated in the routine manner of preparation for eye surgery. The sterile field, drapes, and instruments are essentially the same as those for an enucleation on a living patient. For the transplant procedure, the patient is positioned and prepped in the same fashion as a cataract procedure.

OPERATIVE PROCEDURES

Donor Tissue Procurement

1. Eye specimen jars are labeled for right and left eyes.
2. The speculum is inserted, and after routine enucleation the donated eye is placed with the cornea up and secured in a metal eye cage or on gauze in the sterile specimen jar.
3. The eye sockets are packed with cotton, and the lids are closed.
4. Specimen jars are sealed with tape and labeled with the donor's name or identification number, time of death, time of enucleation, and date. The jars are placed on wet ice in an insulated carrier and transported to the eye bank. The entire cornea with a scleral rim will be placed in Optisol GS before transplant.

Penetrating Keratoplasty

1. After insertion of the eye speculum the surgeon places superior rectus and inferior rectus bridle sutures if a Flieringa ring is not to be used. If a ring is used, the surgeon secures it in place with four 5-0 sutures (Figure 9-36).
2. A corneoscleral button that has been refrigerated and stored in tissue culture medium (Optisol GS) is removed from its container.
3. The surgeon places the donor corneoscleral button on a sterile Teflon block with the epithelial (outside) surface down. Using the corneal trephine as a punch, the surgeon presses out the button. A drop of Optisol GS may be used to cover the donor button until it is implanted.
4. Using a handheld trephine or a disposable suction trephine, the surgeon excises a corneoscleral button from the recipient's cornea. The section of cornea removed from the recipient's eye is usually 0.25 mm in diameter smaller than the graft taken from the donor's eye.
5. Peripheral iridectomies or iridotomies may be performed at this time at the surgeon's discretion, or a cataract extraction with IOL implantation may also be performed if the lens is opaque.

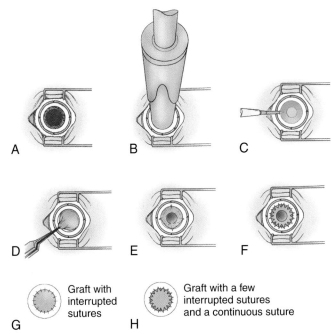

FIGURE 9-36 Corneal transplantation. **A,** Eye of patient who will undergo corneal transplantation. Flieringa fixation ring is sutured in place with 5-0 nonabsorbable sutures. **B,** Corneal trephine is placed on recipient cornea, and partial penetration is made approximately three fourths through stroma. **C,** Anterior chamber is entered through groove, and the remainder of button is excised with right and left corneal microscissors. **D,** Corneal button is removed. **E,** Donor cornea graft is sutured in place with four sutures. **F,** Donor cornea graft is sutured in place with interrupted or continuous 10-0 nonabsorbable suture (**G** and **H**).

6. The surgeon places the graft into the opening of the recipient's eye and anchors it in place by means of four single-armed sutures placed at the four cardinal meridians, viewed through an operating microscope. Some surgeons preplace sutures in the graft. The surgeon sutures the graft to the host with either continuous or interrupted 10-0 nonabsorbable sutures.

7. Air or sodium hyaluronate (Healon) may be injected into the anterior chamber of the recipient's eye to keep the iris from adhering to the suture line. Mydriatic or miotic solutions are used at the surgeon's discretion.

8. A subconjunctival injection of antibiotic solution or a topical application of antibiotic drops may be used at the completion of the procedure. Antibiotic ointment is applied, followed by an eye pad and a protective shield.

Lamellar Keratoplasty

1. The surgeon inserts the eye speculum and then places the superior rectus and inferior rectus bridle sutures (if needed).

2. The perioperative nurse presents the donor eye from the eye bank to the sterile field; the surgical technologist washes it in balanced salt solution.

3. The surgeon wraps the donor eye in a surgical dressing and makes a groove at the desired depth in the cornea with the trephine. The Castroviejo keratome is set at the desired depth, and the lamellar sheet of cornea is removed and placed into a petri dish.

4. The recipient cornea is grooved with the same trephine to the appropriate depth. Using the operating microscope, the surgeon performs a lamellar resection, that is, removes the anterior part of the cornea at a predetermined depth with a Gill knife, Beaver knife blade #64, or other corneal splitter.

5. The surgeon sutures the donor tissue in place with a continuous 10-0 nonabsorbable suture.

6. A mydriatic agent and subconjunctival or topical antibiotics may be used.

7. The eye is patched.

DEEP LAMELLAR ENDOTHELIAL KERATOPLASTY. Deep lamellar endothelial keratoplasty (DLEK) is an emerging technique. It consists of replacing the endothelium without transplanting the cornea to restore vision. This technique offers the potential for highly predictable corneal power for extended periods without the astigmatism that often occurs with penetrating keratoplasty. The transplanted endothelium is inserted into the host through a small incision, greatly reducing the risk of infection.

Keratorefractive Procedures

Keratorefractive procedures are corneal procedures designed to correct myopia, hyperopia, astigmatism, and aphakia. These procedures require reshaping the cornea with relaxing incisions or cryolathing corneal tissue to change the refractive power of the cornea. They include photorefractive keratectomy (PRK), which uses the excimer laser to treat myopia (nearsightedness), and laser-assisted in-situ keratomileusis (LASIK), which uses the excimer laser for photoablation of the corneal stroma bed to alter the curvature of the cornea and correct myopia or hyperopia (farsightedness).

PRK is a surface ablation technique that involves manual scraping, alcohol, and a brush. Surface ablation avoids the complications of flap formation and provides excellent visual results. A major drawback, however, is delayed visual rehabilitation and pain, though it can be controlled with topical and oral therapy. Epi-LASIK, another form of surface ablation, mechanically separates the epithelial layer from Bowman's membrane with the use of a mechanized keratome but without alcohol. After ablation the epithelial flap is positioned on the cornea followed by a bandage contact lens. Some strategies to promote healing include careful preoperative testing for dry eye and using nontoxic antibiotics (Donnenfeld, 2008).

More than 800,000 Americans underwent LASIK surgery in 2007. Excimer laser technology was introduced in 1975 and exploration of ophthalmic applications began in 1983. Stuart (2008) notes that improvements in performance and reliability, combined with a host of complementary techniques and innovations, have turned excimer refractive surgery into the most popular elective surgical procedure worldwide. Thus it is especially important for the surgical technologist to keep updated with emerging technologies and techniques as they develop.

LASIK Surgery.

With the LASIK procedure, the curvature of the cornea is reshaped using an excimer laser. The purpose is to permit the individual to see well at a distance without glasses. For nearsighted patients the central curvature of the cornea is flattened. To flatten the cornea, the surgeon removes stromal tissue from the center of the cornea (Figure 9-37, *A*). For farsighted patients the central curvature of the cornea is steepened. To steepen the cornea, stromal tissue is removed from the periphery of the cornea, leaving the center untreated (Figure 9-37, *B*).

PROCEDURAL CONSIDERATIONS. An extensive preoperative evaluation (refraction, topography, wavefront analysis, and determination of targets for desired refraction) is necessary to be sure that the patient is a candidate for the LASIK procedure. Before surgery, a topical antibiotic and topical anesthetic are placed in the patient's eye. If the patient has astigmatism, he or she is taken to a slit lamp and a mark is made on the conjunctivae to assist in the correction of the astigmatism. Circular corneal markers (3 mm and 4 mm) may be used. The LASIK complication rate has been dramatically reduced by the development of new-generation microkeratomes and the improvement in the femtosecond laser. The three basic steps in LASIK are: (1) prepare stroma or create flap, (2) perform photoablation to change refraction, and (3) reposition flap (Donnenfeld, 2008).

OPERATIVE PROCEDURE

1. The patient is positioned supine, and the surgeon positions a locking lid speculum. The patient's head position is adjusted to account for the astigmatism.
2. The surgeon marks the cornea to assist in the placement of the "corneal cap" after the procedure. A suction device is placed on the eye to immobilize it.
3. A microkeratome (e.g., Hansatome, ACS, Moria, Amadeus) is used to create a lamellar keratectomy of 0.130 to 0.180 micrometers in thickness. This piece of cornea is reflected out of the way with a flat cornea spatula, and the laser treatment is applied to the base of the lamellar keratectomy.
4. The surgeon replaces the corneal cap on the stromal bed using a Slade irrigating cannula on a 3-ml syringe with saline. The corneal cap is permitted to dry for several min-

utes. The corneal cap stays in position because of capillary attraction.
5. Antibiotic drops and nonsteroidal antiinflammatory drops are placed in the eye. A goggle is placed over the eye to prevent slippage of the corneal cap for the next 24 hours.

LASEK Surgery. Laser epithelial keratomileusis (LASEK) is similar to PRK, because the procedure is performed on the surface of the cornea. After numbing the eye with topical anesthetic drops, the surgeon loosens the epithelium with a diluted alcohol solution and pushes it aside. A laser is then used to treat the corneal surface, similar to PRK and LASIK procedures. The epithelial flap is then returned to its original position, and a bandage contact lens is placed for the duration of the healing process, which may last several days.

SURGERY OF THE LENS
Cataract Extraction

A cataract is defined as any opacification of the lens. Cataracts may be congenital, posttraumatic, or induced by medications (particularly corticosteroids), but are most commonly the result of age-related changes.

Normally, light passing through a clear lens projects a sharp image onto the retina. When the lens becomes cloudy (cataractous) through the aging process, vision becomes blurred. A cataract can be compared to a window that is frosted or yellowed (Burlew-Quartey, 2008). More than half of all Americans over age 80 have a cataract or have undergone surgery for it. The lens is made of mostly water and protein; over time, some of the protein may clump together, leading to clouding of the lens (cataract). The vision gradually gets worse as the lens changes from clear to a yellow/brown color (Figure 9-38); the

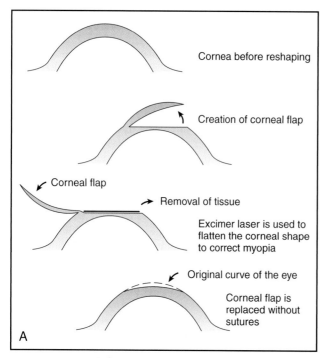

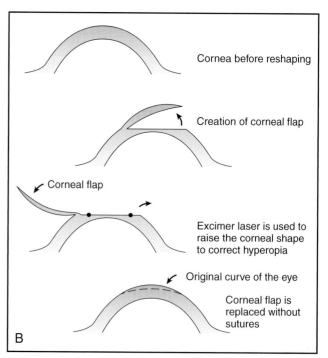

FIGURE 9-37 Laser-assisted in-situ keratomileusis (LASIK) surgery. **A,** Diagram of LASIK correction for nearsightedness. **B,** Diagram of LASIK correction for farsightedness.

pupil may appear gray. The tinting eventually makes it difficult to differentiate certain colors like purple or blue, and difficult to read or perform routine activities. Cataract removal is warranted when there is interference with everyday activities such as driving, reading, and watching television (NEI, 2008b). Other symptoms include having poor night vision, noticing glare from headlights or lamps, and perceiving that sunlight is too bright. Halos may be noticed around lights as well. Double vision might also be noticed. These symptoms may indicate other eye problems so an eye exam would be warranted to determine the exact cause. See Figure 9-39 for a depiction of a person's view with normal vision, cataract, glaucoma, and diabetic retinopathy.

Besides age-related cataracts, the following other types of cataracts exist:
◆ *Congenital*—Children may be born with cataracts or develop them throughout their youth.
◆ *Traumatic*—After eye injury or electric shock, cataracts may develop even years later.
◆ *Secondary*—After eye surgery for other conditions, cataracts may develp, or they may be associated with other health problems such as diabetes, steroid use, smoking, and prolonged exposure to sunlight (NEI, 2008b).

A cataract extraction is removal of the opaque lens from the interior of the eye and can be accomplished by several methods. The *intracapsular cataract extraction* (ICCE) method of cataract removal consists of removing the lens within its capsule with a cryoprobe and is rarely performed today except in the event of a dislocated lens. If an ICCE is scheduled, alpha-chymotrypsin (Catarase, Chymar), an enzyme that acts on the zonules of the lens, and a cataract cryoprobe need to be procured.

In the extracapsular method (ECCE), the anterior portion of the capsule is first ruptured in a controlled manner and removed. The surgeon expresses the lens cortex and nucleus from the eye, leaving the posterior capsule behind. Restoration of functional vision is necessary after removal of the crystalline lens (aphakia). Contact lenses can be used to correct aphakia. They offer an excellent option for visual correction and can be used for monocular aphakia.

Over the past years numerous microsurgical techniques have been developed for lens removal through a small self-sealing incision and most recently through a clear corneal

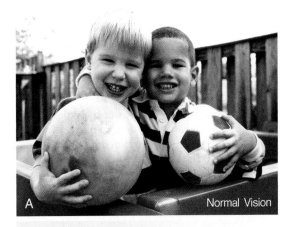
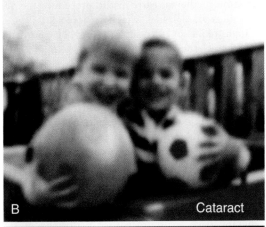
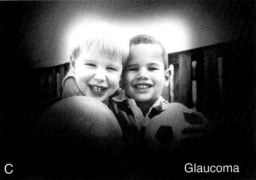
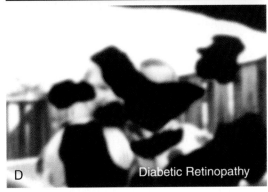

FIGURE 9-39 Comparative views with (**A**) normal vision, (**B**) a scene as it might be viewed by a person with cataract, (**C**) a scene as it might be viewed by a person with glaucoma, and (**D**) a scene as it might be viewed by a person with diabetic retinopathy.

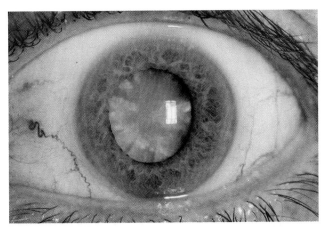

FIGURE 9-38 A hypermature age-related cortico-nuclear cataract with a brunescent (brown) nucleus.

incision. ECCE with phacoemulsification is still performed, especially with very mature or hard cataracts, and may be performed in combination with trabeculectomy for patients with glaucoma. Patients receiving long-term glaucoma therapy (which causes pupil constriction) may not dilate well and may need iris retractors during surgery. Adequate pupil dilation is necessary for safe visualization of all affected intraocular structures.

Basically, each technique involves opening the lens capsule and using a phacoemulsification unit with irrigation and aspiration (I/A). Pressures in the anterior and posterior chambers are generally equal. Once the surgeon makes the incision into the anterior chamber, aqueous fluid leaks from it. Pressure in the anterior chamber falls below that in the posterior chamber, and vitreous from the back of the eye tries to push forward and could carry other structures with it. To minimize the risk from these pressure gradients, early in the procedure the surgeon will inject thick viscoelastics, which do not leak.

The high-frequency ultrasonic energy of phacoemulsification fragments the hard lens material (similar to a jackhammer), which can then be aspirated from the eye. Some phacoemulsification units utilize oscillating movements (side-to-side). All perioperative personnel using specialized instruments and equipment must have thorough knowledge of the operation as well as problems that may be encountered and actions to correct them.

Roughly 90% of people who have cataract surgery have better vision afterward. Cataract surgery not only is one of the most common surgeries performed in the United States but also is one of the safest and most effective surgeries (NEI, 2008b). Patients with cataracts in both eyes that need surgery will generally have their procedures performed at separate times, usually 4 to 8 weeks apart. Months or years after cataract surgery, cells may grow back, causing opacification of the posterior capsule and a haze in the vision. The YAG laser may then be indicated for capsulotomy, creating a hole in the center of the capsule to allow light to pass through and restore clear vision (Burlew-Quartey, 2008).

Potential complications, though rare, are discussed as part of informed consent. In a patient with vision in only one eye, the risks/benefits of surgery must be carefully evaluated. The potential problems include infection, bleeding, inflammation, loss of vision, double vision, and high or low eye pressure (NEI, 2008b). The American Society of Cataract and Refractive Surgery and the American Academy of Ophthalmology (AAO) have issued a joint clinical *Information Statement and Patient Advisory*, recommending that "patients taking alpha-blockers to treat prostate enlargement or other conditions inform their ophthalmologist about these medications before undergoing eye surgery. Prior to being started on this class of drugs, patients with cataracts should be informed that alpha-blockers, in general, and Flomax (tamsulosin), in particular, may increase the difficulty of cataract surgery" (AAO, 2009). The condition of intraoperative floppy iris syndrome (IFIS), first reported in 2005, is explained: "The iris, the part of the eye that gives it its color, opens and closes in response to varying light levels. Because the iris is located in front of the cataract, the pupil (opening in the iris) must be widely dilated to perform the surgery. A large pupil is obtained, in part, by using dilating drops that stimulate the iris dilator muscle. Alpha-blockers, such as Flomax, block this iris muscle, leading to poor dilation and sometimes causing the pupil to suddenly constrict during surgery." The patient advisory emphasizes the importance of communicating any history of Flomax use as the complication may occur even if the drug has been discontinued. This communication for proper medical judgment for each individual patient is essential for positive outcomes: "The overall risk of serious cataract surgical complications is low, and when the ophthalmologist is informed of the patient's history of alpha-blocker use, the success rate of cataract surgery remains very high."

Although various manufacturer's systems and platforms exist for cataract surgery, basic considerations remain. Parameters are not interchangeable between formats; power and vacuum settings are measured differently in different machines. Even the height of the irrigation bottle may be measured differently. The nurse and surgical technologist must challenge themselves to new ideas in evaluating new technology and adjusting to varied practice settings. Foot pedals also are different; for example, positions 1, 2, and 3 have different functions in each machine. Overall, through teamwork and adequate training and monitoring for competency, the surgical team can optimize technology for safety and efficiency in cataract surgery regardless of the equipment used.

Intraocular Lens. Extraction of the cataractous lens removes one of the major refractive components of the eye. Three options for replacing this lost refractive power are (1) use of aphakic glasses, (2) use of aphakic contact lenses, and (3) intraocular lens (IOL) implantation. IOLs offer many advantages to patients, including reduced dependence on spectacles, reduced thickness of any spectacle correction needed, and elimination of aberrations produced by aphakic glasses or contact lenses.

Current generation IOLs are made of silicone or acrylic resin. Foldable and injectable designs and new implantation techniques challenge perioperative nursing personnel to keep abreast of changes in techniques for IOL implantations. Posterior chamber lenses (PCLs) can be implanted only when the cataract was removed by extracapsular cataract extraction (ECCE). Placement behind the iris is the most physiologic position for an artificial lens (posterior chamber lens) and is the most common method. Anterior chamber lenses (ACLs), placed in front of the iris, are used in the absence of capsular support, including after vitreous loss or ICCE and for secondary lens implantation (when the cataract was previously removed without lens replacement) (Burlew-Quartey, 2008).

IOLs are available in various diopter powers. The necessary power customized for each patient is determined by measuring the curvature of the patient's cornea (keratometry) and the axial length (length from cornea to retina). A mathematical formula is then used to calculate the correct lens power. IOLs are also available in bifocal and multifocal types. Some feature ultraviolet protection.

Sutureless cataract techniques have become increasingly popular because of rapid visual rehabilitation. Clear corneal microincisions (3 mm wide or less) with the use of topical anesthesia and insertion of foldable IOLs have produced even better visual results with the opportunity to fully correct refractive errors.

Procedural Considerations. Instrumentation varies with surgeon's preference but usually includes forceps to insert the lens and lens haptics and a hook to aid in rotating and positioning the lens. Perioperative personnel must be familiar with institutional policies pertaining to IOLs and their use. For example, the American Academy of Ophthalmology (AAO, 2008) developed recommendations to minimize the occurrence of preventable errors such as wrong IOL implant (i.e., to ensure the highest level of patient safety in surgery). The tenets encompass the importance of communication with surgery staff. The recommendations emphasize the importance of heightened communication and verifications of preoperative calculations of lens style and power ordered, and documenting it as a written order. Besides verifying the implant during the time-out, it is recommended that the surgeon have some form of written documentation regarding the case and IOL (white board, or copy of operative plan taped to microscope) available to view when scrubbed, gowned, and gloved and seated at the surgical microscope.

Surgical techniques vary based on surgeon training and experience. Some surgeons sit at the head of the bed whereas others use a temporal approach (Figure 9-40). Some use topical drops, and others use anesthetic gel. Regardless, the surgery follows certain basic steps.

TOPICAL CLEAR CORNEAL CATARACT PROCEDURE. Developments with the use of topical anesthetics, new materials for foldable IOLs, and diamond knives for self-sealing or no-stitch wounds led to clear cornea incisions and new techniques for phacoemulsification and lens implantation for cataracts. Clear cornea microincisions create the opportunity for full correction of refractive errors during the surgical procedure.

Topical anesthesia replaces retrobulbar anesthesia for cataract surgery, and because the patient can fixate, this allows for refractive surgical techniques. Patients must be able to hear and follow directions so that they can cooperate with verbal instructions to fixate on the microscope light. Various medications and protocols are used for administering topical anesthetics before cataract surgery.

Procedural Considerations. The nurse administers a drop of topical tetracaine 0.5% into the operative eye before the patient enters the OR. The patient is instructed to keep this eye closed to prevent the cornea from drying. As the patient is being positioned, the nurse administers another drop of tetracaine. An armrest is positioned on the operative side, and the patient's head and the microscope are adjusted. The patient is instructed to look at the light of the microscope and told where to fixate. If the patient cannot open his or her eye, a facial nerve block should be considered. If the patient cannot fixate on the light at all, a retrobulbar block should be considered.

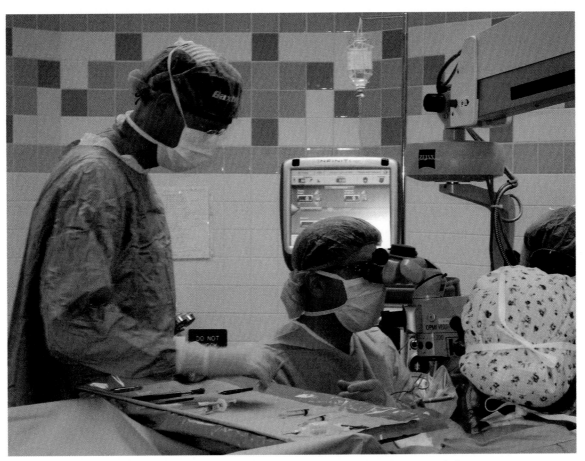

FIGURE 9-40 Cataract surgery in progress. Note irrigation bottle and phacoemulsification unit in background; surgeon sitting at side of patient (temporal approach); scrub person ready to anticipate surgeon's needs; anesthesia provider at patient's side for reassurance and comfort. Circulating nurse, not shown, is coordinating all activities and monitoring for safety.

Operative Procedure

1. The surgeon places an eyelid speculum with an open temporal area.
2. A 1-mm-wide stab incision (paracentesis, tiny incision in cornea opposite the main incision) is made at 5 o'clock in the left eye or at 11 o'clock in the right eye into the anterior chamber.
3. Intercameral anesthesia may be used: 1 ml of unpreserved lidocaine is slowly injected into the anterior chamber through a 30-gauge cannula using a tuberculin syringe.
4. The surgeon injects viscoelastic material into the anterior chamber to deepen the chamber and widen the pupil.
5. The temporal cornea incision is made with a (diamond or single-use) keratome. Some surgeons may use a caliper to mark the incision width, and may use a second knife to make a vertical cut before the horizontal pass with the keratome (Figure 9-41, *A*).
6. A capsulotomy and capsulorrhexis are performed with a capsulorrhexis forceps (Figure 9-41, *B*). This step of tearing the capsule in a controlled manner is critical in creating a round, stable opening into the capsular "bag."
7. Using a 30-gauge cannula and saline, the surgeon performs hydrodissection (and sometimes hydrodelineation) to separate the center/nucleus from the capsule and maneuver the lens within the capsule (Figure 9-41, *C*).
8. The surgeon uses a phacoemulsification tip to sculpt the nucleus with the ultrasound vibration.
9. A second instrument is inserted through the left-handed paracentesis incision to help rotate and divide the cataractous nucleus into quadrants (Figure 9-41, *D*).

10. Cataractous nucleus removal usually proceeds in two phases: nuclear sculpting, wherein the nucleus is cracked or sculpted into smaller fragments, and quadrantic emulsification of those fragments.
11. Following removal of the lens nucleus, the surgeon places an irrigation/aspiration (I/A) tip into the eye and uses it to remove the remaining cortical material (Figure 9-41, *E*). This combination of irrigation and aspiration intends to maintain equilibrium within the eye. Removing the cortex minimizes postoperative inflammation.
12. Some surgeons may polish the posterior capsule or aspirate anterior lens epithelial cells.
13. The surgeon injects viscoelastic material to inflate the anterior chamber and capsular bag.
14. A posterior chamber IOL is folded and placed into the eye with an injector or forceps and then into the capsular bag (Figure 9-41, *F* and *G*). The IOL is positioned with a Sinsky hook or the I/A tip. Some surgeons may need to widen the corneal incision before placing the IOL.
15. The surgeon uses the I/A tip to remove any remaining viscoelastic material. Leaking of the wound may be controlled or prevented by hydrating the wound edges. Occasionally a 10-0 nylon suture is necessary.
16. Topical antibiotics or combination antibiotic-corticosteroid ointment or drops are placed on the eye. The eye is not patched, but a shield is commonly used.

EXTRACAPSULAR METHOD WITH PHACOEMULSIFICATION

Operative Procedure

1. After a superior rectus bridle suture is placed, a small limbus-based flap is dissected superiorly.
2. Using sharp dissection with a Beaver knife blade the surgeon cleans the surgical limbus. Hemostasis is obtained with the bipolar ESU.
3. A 3-mm or smaller incision is made into the eye with either a keratome or a sharp microknife.
4. The surgeon opens the lens capsule with capsulorrhexis forceps or a cystotome. The anterior chamber may be kept formed with air or an irrigating solution.
5. The lens nucleus is loosened from the cortex with the cystotome or a blunt cyclodialysis spatula.
6. The surgeon checks the ultrasonic handpiece for appropriate vacuum control and introduces it into the eye. *The vacuum control check is critical and must be performed before the handpiece is introduced into the eye.*
7. When the lens nucleus has been emulsified and removed, the surgeon removes the lens cortex with the I/A handpiece.
8. If a foldable IOL is to be implanted, the surgeon may use a keratome to widen the incision to 3.2 mm before folding and inserting the lens. If a rigid IOL is to be implanted, the wound is extended to 5.1 mm to accommodate the lens diameter. Acetylcholine may be introduced to constrict the pupil.
9. The corneoscleral wound is closed with a 10-0 nonabsorbable suture.
10. The conjunctival flap is closed with a suture or using the bipolar ESU.
11. An eye pad and shield are applied.

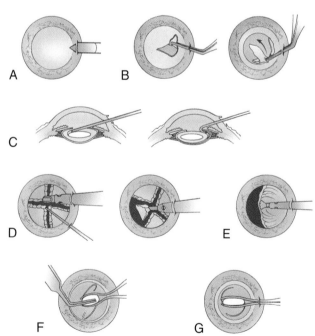

FIGURE 9-41 Clear cornea cataract extraction. **A,** A 2.6-mm incision is made into the cornea. **B,** Capsulorrhexis is performed on anterior capsule of lens. **C,** Nucleus of lens is loosened by hydrodissection. **D,** Nucleus of lens is "cracked" into four quadrants and removed with phacoemulsification. **E,** Irrigation and aspiration (I/A) handpiece is used to strip the remaining cortex from the capsule. **F,** Intraocular lens (IOL) is folded. **G,** IOL is placed into the capsular bag.

Anterior Segment Vitrectomy

The main indications for vitrectomy in the anterior segment are as follows:

- Vitreous loss during cataract extraction
- Opacities in the anterior segment
- Complications associated with vitreous in the anterior chamber
- Miscellaneous causes, such as hyphema, pupillary membranes, and residual soft lens material

Procedural Considerations. The procedure varies according to the surgeon's preference. A pathologic condition in the anterior segment can be approached through a limbal incision, as in lens extraction with vitreous loss, or through an "open sky" approach, after trephine incision for penetrating keratoplasty. Most phacoemulsification equipment has a vitrector that can be quickly attached if needed.

Operative Procedure
ANTERIOR VITRECTOMY FOR VITREOUS LOSS DURING CATARACT EXTRACTION

1. The surgeon introduces the vitreous cutter into the eye through the cataract wound. Infusion may be through the handpiece or a separate cannula and infusion line.
2. The cutter is placed in the middle of the pupil, posterior to the iris, and enough vitreous is removed to ensure that no vitreous remains in the anterior chamber and that the iris has fallen back into its normal position.
3. The pupil is constricted with acetylcholine. The anterior chamber may be re-formed with balanced salt solution (BSS).
4. The procedure is completed as for a lens extraction.

ANTERIOR VITRECTOMY FOR ANTERIOR SEGMENT OPACITIES, HYPHEMA, PUPILLARY MEMBRANES, AND RESIDUAL SOFT LENS MATERIAL

1. Appropriate fixation sutures or a lid speculum is placed.
2. The surgeon makes an incision at the limbus either through clear cornea or under a conjunctival flap. One to three incisions are made, depending on the vitreous cutter chosen and the technique.
3. If a multifunction probe is not used, the surgeon places an infusion cannula into one incision and the vitreous cutter into another incision. A third incision may be used for an accessory instrument. The vitreous, blood, or other material is removed.
4. The incisions are closed, and the eye is patched.

SURGERY FOR GLAUCOMA

Iridectomy

Peripheral iridectomy is removal of a section of iris tissue (Figure 9-42). Peripheral iridectomy is usually performed as part of a trabeculectomy procedure or may be performed when laser iridotomy is not feasible because of cloudy cornea or uveitis. Peripheral iridectomy is done in the treatment of acute, subacute, or chronic angle-closure glaucoma when extensive peripheral anterior synechiae have not formed. This operation is performed to reestablish communication between the posterior and anterior chambers, thus relieving pupillary block

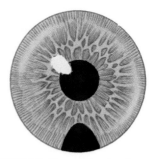

FIGURE 9-42 Peripheral iridectomy.

and permitting the iris root to drop away from the trabecular meshwork to reestablish the outflow of aqueous fluid through Schlemm's canal.

Operative Procedure

1. The speculum is introduced. The globe is fixed with a 4-0 traction suture passed under the superior rectus and fastened to the drape with a hemostat.
2. A small beveled incision is made at the superior limbus, or a perpendicular incision is made in the clear cornea.
3. The surgeon grasps the peripheral iris with forceps, pulls it through the incision, and excises it.
4. The iris is repositioned by gently stroking the cornea with a blunt spatula or muscle hook. The iris can also be repositioned by irrigating with BBS.
5. A clear corneal incision is closed with 10-0 nonabsorbable suture, and a limbal incision is closed with absorbable suture. Subconjunctival antibiotics may be administered, and an eye pad is applied.

Trabeculectomy

Trabeculectomy is a filtering procedure accomplished by incising a conjunctival flap and a scleral flap, creating a fistula, performing an iridectomy, and creating the filtering bleb. Trabeculectomy is often combined with cataract removal (phacoemulsification) and insertion of an IOL.

Procedural Considerations. Adjunctive medical therapy to decrease postoperative fibrosis includes application of an antimetabolite-soaked sponge (5-fluorouracil [5-FU] or mitomycin C) placed under the conjunctival flap. Because 5-FU and mitomycin C are antimetabolites, nursing precautions for handling hazardous waste must be carried out. The perioperative nurse must wear gloves while drawing up the antimetabolite from the vial to transfer to the operative field. All items used with the medication should be disposed as hazardous waste. Instruments that contact antimetabolites should be washed separately.

Operative Procedure

1. Incisions are made into the conjunctiva and Tenon's capsule, dissection is done, and a conjunctival Tenon's capsule flap is created. Hemostasis is obtained with bipolar coagulation (Figure 9-43).
2. If antimetabolite is to be used, the surgeon applies it to the sclera before making any incision into the sclera. A small

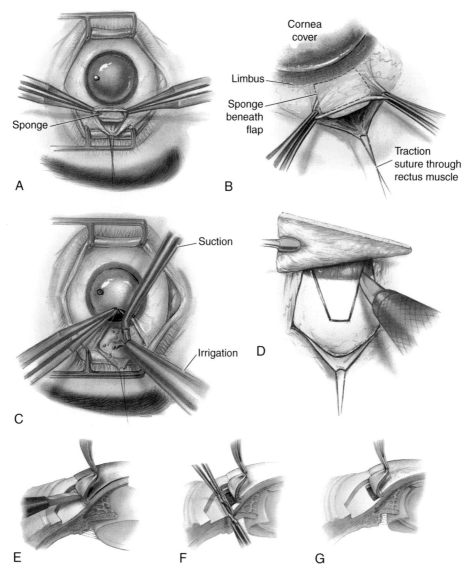

FIGURE 9-43 Trabeculectomy. **A,** Sponge soaked in antimetabolite is placed on sclera and (**B**) held in place for 3 to 5 minutes. **C,** Area is thoroughly irrigated. **D,** Scleral flap is formed. **E,** Incision is made into anterior chamber. **F** and **G,** Fistula is created by removing a flap of limbal tissue.

piece of sponge is saturated in the antimetabolite (5-FU or mitomycin C) and placed between the conjunctival Tenon's capsule flap and the sclera. The sponge is left in place for 3 to 5 minutes, and then the site is irrigated vigorously with copious amounts of BSS.

3. The surgeon creates a square or triangular partial-thickness scleral flap.

4. The scleral flap is retracted, and the surgeon makes an incision into and through the limbus into the anterior chamber with the tip of the blade. The limbal incision is extended to a rectangular flap of deep limbal tissue, which is then excised to create the fistula.

5. An iridectomy is performed. The eye cautery is applied to bleeding sites and to the ciliary processes.

6. The surgeon replaces the scleral flap and closes it with interrupted 10-0 nonabsorbable sutures. The conjunctival Tenon's capsule flap is closed with a running suture, and the conjunctiva is closed.

7. BSS is injected through a cannula into the anterior chamber to deepen the anterior chamber and elevate the conjunctival bleb.

8. An eye pad and shield are applied.

Glaucoma Drainage Devices

Several types of drainage devices (Figure 9-44) have been implanted into the posterior subconjunctival space with varying success when filtering procedures have been unsuccessful. These include the Molteno implant, Krupin valve, Ahmed device, Baerveldt device, and Schocket implant. Complications have been reduced through modifications in design and technique (Evidence for Practice).

Procedural Considerations. The glaucoma drainage device may be soaked in an antibiotic solution, and the pericardium or donor patch graft will also need to be hydrated or soaked. The drainage device and graft are documented as implants per facility procedure.

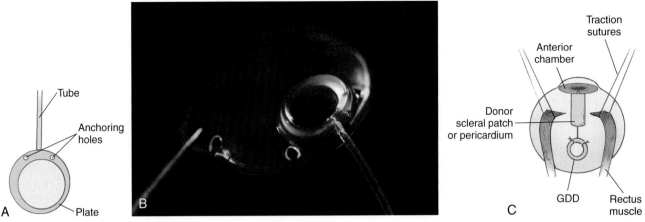

FIGURE 9-44 Glaucoma drainage devices (GDDs). **A,** Components of GDD. **B,** Photo of Molteno3 implant. **C,** GDD in place. Tip of drainage tube in anterior chamber. Donor scleral patch or pericardium covering tube from plate to edge of cornea.

EVIDENCE FOR PRACTICE

Systematic Review of Aqueous Shunts in Glaucoma Surgery

When surgeons are unable to control primary or secondary glaucoma with medication, laser treatments, or standard surgical techniques (e.g., trabeculectomy), they may have to utilize an aqueous shunt. A variety of commercially produced shunts are available for use. Shunts lower intraocular pressure (IOP) by providing a passageway for aqueous fluid to drain from the eye and be absorbed via the capillaries into the general circulation.

Numerous studies and clinical trials have been conducted to determine which type of shunt is most effective and if shunts are more effective than other forms of therapy aimed at reducing IOP. A Cochrane Database Review examined 15 trials with a total of 1153 participants with mixed diagnoses. Other researchers reported findings to the American Academy of Ophthalmology after examining 17 previously published randomized trials, 1 prospective nonrandomized comparative trial, 1 retrospective case-control study, 2 comprehensive literature reviews, and published English language, noncomparative case series, and case reports. Both groups concluded that at this time there is no demonstrable evidence of superiority of one type or brand of shunt over another but stated that aqueous shunts do offer benefits comparable to trabeculectomy; they agree that further long-term, comparative studies are necessary to determine efficacy and note that the physician's judgment should be the key factor when making treatment decisions for patients with IOP.

Modified from Mickler DS et al: Aqueous shunts in glaucoma, *Cochrane Database Syst Rev* 19(2):CD004919, 2006; Mickler DS et al: Aqueous shunts in glaucoma: a report by the American Academy of Ophthalmology, *Ophthalmology* 115(6):1089-1098, 2008.

Operative Procedure

1. The surgeon incises the conjunctiva and exposes the sclera.
2. Two rectus muscles are isolated using silk ties as traction sutures.
3. The surgeon takes measurements for placement of the plate of the device. The plate is then sutured to the sclera.
4. After the patency of the device is checked, the surgeon inserts an occluding suture into the drainage tube.
5. With a needle, a tunnel is created into the anterior chamber for the tube and paracentesis tract.
6. The tube is trimmed and inserted into the anterior chamber. The surgeon sutures the tube to the sclera with 9-0 nonabsorbable suture.
7. The tube is covered with patch graft of donor sclera or pericardium.
8. The occluding suture is passed through Tenon's capsule and the conjunctiva into the inferior cul-de-sac, secured with absorbable suture, and trimmed.
9. The surgeon removes the traction sutures from around the rectus muscles, and closes the conjunctiva with a continuous 7-0 absorbable suture.
10. Antiinfective agents are injected subconjunctivally. The eye is dressed with an eye pad and shield.

VITREORETINAL SURGERY

Vitreous fluid fills about two thirds of the eye, helps keep the round shape of the eyeball, and is originally attached to the retina. The vitreous slowly liquefies, atrophies, and shrinks as we age. The vitreous then can become stringy, and shadows can be cast onto the retina, causing "floaters" ("cobwebs" or specks that float in the field of vision). They may look like spots, threadlike strands, or squiggly lines. Floaters are more noticeable when looking at bright objects, such as a white piece of paper. Floaters are more common in patients who have diabetes, have undergone cataract surgery, or are nearsighted. Over time, the floaters usually settle below the line of sight but do not completely disappear. Floaters in and of themselves generally do not require treatment. However, if a patient experiences a sudden increase in the number of floaters, retinal examination is warranted to rule out a retinal tear, break, or hole (NEI, 2008c).

The retina, the light-sensitive layer of tissue lining the eye, sends visual signals via the optic nerve to the brain. Attached to the retina are millions of fine fibers intertwined with the vitreous. The shrinking vitreous in an aging eye causes the fine fibers to pull on the retinal surface. When the fibers break, the vitreous separates and shrinks from the retina, causing traction on the retina. Normally, the vitreous detaches from the retina (a posterior vitreous detachment). However, sometimes the vitreous can create traction on the retina and pull a piece of the retina with it, creating a retinal tear. Fluid can then leak under the retina into the subretinal space, leading to a retinal detachment; symptomatic breaks (manifested as new floating objects or flashing lights) are likely to progress to a retinal detachment.

Posterior vitreous detachments (PVDs) are usually not sight-threatening and, like floaters, typically do not require treatment. Patients at risk for the development of PVD are those who are nearsighted and more than 50 years of age. The condition is very common after age 80. Again, it may not be noticeable, or will simply be annoying because of an increase in floaters. A small but sudden increase in new floaters is a symptom of vitreous detachment. Flashes of light in side vision may also occur (NEI, 2008d).

Occasionally, some of the vitreous fibers pull so hard on the retina that it causes a retinal detachment (RD)—that is, the sensory retina (neural layer) is separated from the underlying retinal pigment epithelium layer. RD is considered an emergency and should be treated immediately. Anyone who has a sudden increase in floaters or an increase of lightning flashes in peripheral vision (a result of separation of the retina) should see a retinal specialist as soon as possible for an eye exam. The dilated eye exam is the only way to diagnose the exact cause of the vision problem; potentially, permanent loss of vision can occur without timely treatment (NEI, 2008e).

An additional symptom of retinal detachment is the appearance of a "curtain" in the field of vision, from above, below, or the side. Retinal detachment may occur because of the presence of intraocular neoplasms originating in the retina or choroid (exudative type) or, more commonly, as a result of retinal tears or holes associated with injury, degeneration, or vitreous contraction. One in 10,000 people develops a retinal detachment each year; 1 in 3 patients who have undergone cataract surgery develop it. Males are more likely to develop retinal detachment than females (Gutierrez and Peterson, 2007). The most common cause is diabetic retinopathy. Retinal detachment is more common in people older than 40 years. Caucasians are affected more than African Americans. Other risk factors include history of nearsightedness or retinal detachment in the other eye, family history of RD, presence of lattice degeneration (thinning of the retina in nearsighted people), and occurrence of an eye injury.

Other retinal diseases can be grouped into categories. Treatment of specific conditions partly depends on the category, such as surgical repair for structural disorders or laser repair for vascular conditions. Retinal disease categories and examples include the following:

- *Traumatic/structural:* retinal detachment, intraocular foreign body
- *Neoplastic:* choroidal melanoma, retinoblastoma
- *Immune/infectious:* endophthalmitis (infection inside the eye including pus)
- *Vascular:* diabetic retinopathy, retinal vein occlusions
- *Toxic:* systemic tamoxifen retinal toxicity

Prevention is a key emphasis to avoid the need for treatments. Studies show that optimal management of systemic disease can potentially and dramatically prevent vision loss. For example, one study demonstrated strict glucose level control over 5 to 10 years reduces the onset of diabetic retinopathy by 75% and reduces progression of retinopathy by 50%; another study showed a 35% reduction in the need for retinal laser treatment through strict control of high blood pressure (Gariano, 2008).

Microvascular disease is related to the eye's vulnerability as a result of its dense network of capillary vessels. Diabetes leads to retinal changes (diabetic retinopathy). The presence of diabetes for more than 15 years significantly increases the likelihood of developing some form of retinopathy, typically bilaterally. However, the severity may be different between eyes. Retinopathy is classified in either of the following ways:

- *Background, or nonproliferative:* In this form of retinopathy disease is confined to the retinal surface. Retinal capillary walls develop microaneurysms (bulges) that can lead to leakage and the development of exudates under the retina. Hemorrhages occur within the retina and are reabsorbed. Capillary membrane changes result in blocked capillaries and, thereby, retinal ischemia. Eventually deterioration progresses to the next stage.
- *Proliferative:* Neovascularization, or the formation of new retinal blood vessels, can develop within the retina in an attempt to relieve ischemic anoxia secondary to microvascular damage caused by diabetes. These new vessels are fragile and can rupture spontaneously, causing bleeding, and they are very permeable, causing leakage. Hemorrhage into the retina and/or vitreous can consequently ensue, leading to severe visual loss (Phillips, 2007).

The presence of retinopathy predisposes the patient to retinal detachment. In retinal detachment, pigment or blood cells are freed in the vitreous, causing the previously mentioned symptoms of flashes and floaters. Fluid from the vitreous cavity can seep through the retinal tears into the subretinal space and progressively detach the retina. The part of the retina that has separated from its nutritional source becomes damaged and relatively nonfunctional. On occasion, inflammatory/scar tissue can develop on the retinal surface, leading to an epiretinal membrane that can distort vision. As the inflammatory/scar tissue, which is firmly attached to the retina, contracts, the retina can wrinkle or "pucker." When the wrinkle is over the area of the macula, the central vision becomes blurred and distorted. Diabetic retinopathy can also lead to the macular pucker.

In the same manner, as the shrinking vitreous pulls the retina, it can cause microscopic damage. The retina heals itself by scarring, and the macular pucker can result. If the shrinking vitreous pulls too hard, the retina can tear at any location. When the macula is affected, it is more serious because of the effect on central vision, and is called a macular hole. Both macular pucker and macular hole have the same symptoms—distorted, blurred vision (NEI, 2008f). Additionally, a macular hole may present with distortion of straight lines, and difficulty reading. Vision ranges from 20/25 to 20/400 (the latter for untreated macular hole). Fifty percent of very early macular holes close on their own. Vision recovery potential is better for patients who had a macular hole for 6 months (American Society of Ophthalmic Registered Nurses [ASORN], 2007).

Various types of retinal detachment exist:

- *Rhegmatogenous:* This is the most common type. Fluid exudate from a tear or break in the retina leaks under the retina, separating it from the retinal pigment epithelium (RPE).
- *Tractional:* This form of retinal detachment is often secondary to diabetic retinopathy, especially if untreated. The retina

also separates from the RPE, but this time it is attributable to the contraction of scar tissue on the retina's surface.

♦ *Exudative or serous:* In inflammatory retinal disease or trauma, fluid exudate leaks under the retina. In this type, however, there are no breaks or tears in the retina.

Location of the pathology on the retina affects visual symptoms. Macular pucker, for example (also called epiretinal membrane, preretinal membrane, retina wrinkle, or internal limiting membrane disease), generally affects the macula, located in the center of the retina. The macula normally provides sharp, central vision needed for reading, driving, and fine detail work, and when puckered can cause blurred, distorted central vision.

Various modalities for surgical treatment include laser treatments, scleral buckling, vitrectomy, and retinopexy. In addition to any of these therapies, freeze treatment (cryopexy) may be performed in the surgeon's office for small holes and tears to help "weld" and reattach the retina (NEI, 2008d).

LASER TREATMENT IN DIABETIC RETINOPATHY

Laser energy is used to apply burns to peripheral retinal tissue to help neovascularization regress. The pathophysiologic mechanism for regression of neovascularization is not completely understood, but is thought to occur as a result of the reduced retinal oxygen requirement as a result of the scarred retinal tissue. This method of eliminating abnormal vascularization is called panretinal photocoagulation (PRP). Again, in principle, early diagnosis and control of blood glucose levels are paramount, as laser treatment does indeed partially destroy the retina in order to help arrest neovascularization. Thus surgeons use the laser before excess damage occurs, electrocoagulating minute hypoxic areas to prevent the new vessels from forming (Phillips, 2007) (Figure 9-45). Laser treatments may initially begin in an office setting or later within the OR in conjunction with surgeries. The laser may be applied through the slit lamp, with the indirect ophthalmoscope, or directly during vitrectomy surgery using an intraocular endolaser probe.

VITRECTOMY

Vitrectomy is narrowly defined as removal of all or part of the vitreous gel (body). In the broader clinical sense of the term, vitrectomy surgery can also include the excision and removal of fibrotic membranes, removal of epiretinal membranes, and electrocoagulation of bleeding vessels. In its normal state, the vitreous gel of the eye is transparent. In certain disease states, bleeding from damaged or newly formed vessels may cause the vitreous to become opaque, which may severely decrease vision. In addition to the patient's inability to see, the surgeon is unable to visualize the retina and therefore treat the underlying pathologic condition before permanent damage can occur. In these cases, vitrectomy surgery is indicated to restore the patient's vision and to allow the surgeon to institute treatment if indicated.

Formation of membranes may block the visual axis and may cause decreased vision. Contraction of these membranes may produce traction-type or rhegmatogenous retinal detachment. In these cases, vitrectomy surgery is indicated to relieve the underlying pathologic processes leading to decreased vision.

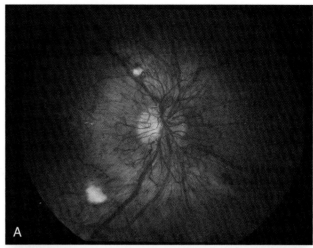

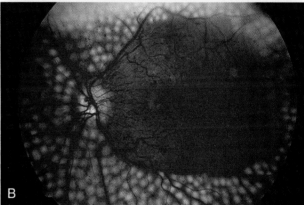

FIGURE 9-45 **A,** Proliferative retinopathy, an advanced form of diabetic retinopathy, occurs when abnormal new blood vessels and scar tissue form on the surface of the retina. **B,** Fundus photo showing scatter laser surgery for diabetic retinopathy.

Posterior Segment Vitrectomy

A pathologic condition in the posterior segment is usually approached through the pars plana, which is tissue that is anterior to the anterior attachment of the retina, typically located 3 to 4 mm from the limbus (corneoscleral junction). Since the pars plana has no retinal tissue, entry at this site poses little risk for retinal detachment (Phillips, 2007). The main indications for posterior segment vitrectomy through the pars plana are as follows:

♦ Long-standing vitreous opacities
♦ Advanced diabetic eye disease
♦ Severe intraocular trauma
♦ Retained foreign bodies
♦ Proliferative vitreoretinopathy
♦ Retinal detachment from giant tears
♦ Endophthalmitis
♦ Diagnostic vitreous biopsy

Essentially, vitrectomy vacuums any pooled blood to enhance clarity. Complications of vitrectomy include retinal detachment, retinal tears, cataract, and infection. Of course, the risk of no treatment can be total loss of vision.

Procedural Considerations. Vitrectomy of the posterior segment is a microsurgical procedure requiring a viewing system (operating microscope with an X-Y coupling, zoom lens,

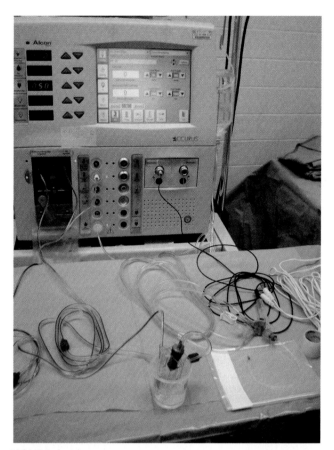

FIGURE 9-46 Mayo stand setup for posterior vitrectomy. *Left to right:* Extrusion tubing for aspiration with soft-tip cannula; vitrectomy cutter handpiece tested in BSS; infusion cannula; intraocular light pipe; bipolar electrosurgery cord. Note bottle hangs at level of patient's eye.

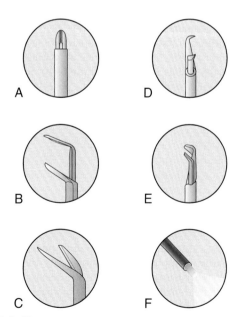

FIGURE 9-47 Tips of micro instruments used in vitrectomy procedures. **A** and **B**, Peeling forceps. **C**, Horizontal scissors. **D**, Vertical scissors. **E**, Membrane peeler and cutter (MPC). **F**, Lighted pick.

and fine focus), contact lens system or noncontact wide-angle viewing system (e.g., Biom), an illumination system, a cutting-suction-infusion system, and accessory instruments.

The surgeon can hold the contact lens in place by hand or can suture it for stabilization. Another option to a sew-on lens is the use of a noncontact panoramic wide-angle viewing system. This system allows a wide, noncontact view of the macula and is mounted to the microscope and swings out of the way for extraocular phases of the vitrectomy. Other advantages are that it provides a good view under air, eliminates the time needed to sew on a lens, and does not require an assistant to hold the lens. The eye may be rotated freely to view the extreme periphery. The image is inverted by a manual knob, foot pedal, or hand control.

The infusion system consists of a 500-ml bottle of buffered BSS, such as BSS Plus or Endosol Extra, a standard IV administration set, and an infusion needle or sleeve. The level of intraocular pressure can be varied by elevating or lowering the infusion bottle in relation to the patient's eye and by adjusting the digital readout of the nitrogen gas–forced infusion.

The suction and cutting systems vary in sophistication and technology. All cutters engage tissue into a port and then cut it by the shearing action between the edges of a moving and a nonmoving part. Guillotine cutters have a linear, back-and-forth action, whereas reciprocating or oscillating cutters rotate in a clockwise-counterclockwise fashion. Suction is operated with a pump controlled by a foot switch to maintain the level of aspiration. The cutter may be part of a single-use multifunction handpiece.

An endolaser or indirect laser delivery system is usually available for photocoagulation. Illumination for vitrectomy is *external*, using the operating microscope for anterior segment vitrectomy; and *internal*, using a fiberoptic light pipe (endoilluminator) for posterior segment vitrectomy. A special light pipe (cannonball) that illuminates a wider area is needed if a wide-angle viewing system is used on the microscope. See Figure 9-46 for the Mayo stand setup of vitrectomy machine attachments.

Replacement of the vitreous with air is facilitated with a special air-exchange unit that may be incorporated into the multifunction vitrectomy machine. Other substances for intraocular tamponade are liquid perfluorocarbons, silicone oil, perfluoropropane gas (C_3F_8), and sulfur hexafluoride gas (SF_6).

Accessory instruments originally had a 20-gauge diameter so that they can be interchanged throughout the procedure. Several accessory instruments may be used for pars plana vitrectomy, depending on the extent of the procedure. Microhooks, picks, and subretinal forceps and scissors (Figure 9-47) are used for dissection, peeling, and removal of membranes. These instruments can be manually operated with a thumb control or run with compressed air from the automated vitrectomy console. Even smaller 23-gauge and 25-gauge trocars allow for finer instrumentation without the need for suturing the trocar sites. This microincisional sutureless surgery has become increasingly prevalent with retinal surgeons. Foreign-body microforceps and various magnetic devices are used to retrieve foreign objects of glass, metal, or other substances. An intraocular cryoprobe for cryocoagulation directly on the retina surface can be attached to the cryotherapy device. Flute needles or disposable soft-tipped cannulae are handheld or

RESEARCH HIGHLIGHT

Patient Perspective of Extended Facedown Positioning Revealed through Journaling

Facedown positioning is required after certain ophthalmic procedures, such as macular hole surgery, to optimize retinal reattachment. Adherence is often difficult because of physical and psychologic challenges. The experience according to a patient's perspective is rarely documented in research literature.

In a separate study on functional outcomes of macular hole surgery, a self-motivated patient presented to researchers the diary that she had written during her 77-day recovery period. When the researchers requested a qualitative analysis of her journal, she consented.

Seven categories of content emerged: emotional state, quality of sleep, nutritional considerations, visual functioning, physical status, social support, and entertainment needs. Overall, this study gives patients and their caretakers a better understanding of what facedown positioning means to an individual during the extended recovery period. This patient's successful coping can provide hope for other potential patients. Guidelines can be developed and refined for overcoming both physical and psychologic barriers.

Modified from Wittich W, Southall K: Coping with extended facedown positioning after macular hole surgery: a qualitative diary analysis, *Nurs Res* 57(6):436-443, 2008.

attached to an extrusion or aspiration line for evacuating pools of blood or for fluid-gas exchange. The soft silicone tips can come into close proximity to the retina without scratching or damaging the tissue.

To prepare for a vitrectomy procedure, the surgical technologist must know the location of the ocular problem, the surgeon's plan to address the problem, the instrumentation to be used, and the anticipated extent and length of the procedure. Instrument and equipment functioning should be thoroughly checked before the patient is transferred into the OR. When preparing for pars plana vitrectomy in the posterior segment, the surgical technologist must be aware that a combined scleral buckling procedure may be necessary. Clear communication with surgeons paves the way for effective preparations.

In the case of giant retinal tears, C_3F_8, SF_6, liquid perfluorocarbons, and silicone oil can be used to provide retinal tamponade. Intraocular expansible gases (C_3F_8, SF_6) can be used to provide retinal tamponade, but usually require the patient to be positioned facedown for several weeks in order to help reattach the retina. The expansible gas will slowly be absorbed by the body (usually over a period of 2 to 3 months) as aqueous humor produced by the ciliary body slowly displaces it (Research Highlight). Silicone oil can be used for complicated cases and when positioning would be difficult for patients. The disadvantage of silicone oil is that the patient will require another surgery to remove the silicone oil in the future as the index of refraction of silicone oil is significantly different than that of vitreous, giving patients the impression that they are "looking through a crystal ball."

Liquid perfluorocarbons such as perfluorooctane (PFO) or Perfluoron, being heavier than BSS, will allow the retina to be pushed posteriorly and so are used as a tamponade to help repair a giant retinal tear. The liquid is then removed from the posterior segment. Silicone oil is a highly viscous oil with a high surface tension that mechanically limits fibrovascular proliferation. The oil may be left in place, but it is recommended that it be removed within 1 year if the retina is reattached and stable. Silicone oil may cause increased intraocular pressure and secondary glaucoma. The National Eye Institute supported a nationwide clinical trial comparing treatment of proliferative vitreoretinopathy with silicone oil or long-acting intraocular gas. The results indicate that either treatment is effective and surgeons thus have options in treating such cases (NEI, 2008d).

Vitrectomy procedures vary in length from less than 1 hour to more than 3 hours. When a long procedure is anticipated, care must be taken to protect the patient's skin and reduce pressure areas. A foam mattress pad, heel and elbow protectors, and elasticized stockings may be used. A wrist support may be placed around the patient's head to support the surgeon's wrist during manipulation of the intraocular instruments.

Because of the amount of fluid used in the operative field during this procedure the surgical technologist carefully assists with draping to allow for removal of infusion fluid from the field and ensures the electric foot pedals are protected from fluid damage.

Operative Procedure
PARS PLANA VITRECTOMY

1. The eye is prepped and draped using standard sterile conditions for ophthalmic surgery. The surgeon places a lid speculum and incises the conjunctiva (Figure 9-48).
2. The surgeon sutures the infusion line in place with a purse-string suture (for 20-gauge surgeries) and checks it for proper placement.
3. Generally, three incisions are made through the pars plana: one for infusion, one for endoillumination, and one for a vitreous cutter or other instrumentation (e.g., pick, forceps, scissors, laser probe, extrusion needle). In the right eye, these incisions are placed at clock hours 8, 10, and 2; for the left eye, this corresponds to 2, 4, and 10. An illuminating chandelier can also be placed (typically at the 6 o'clock position) for bimanual surgery.
4. The operating microscope is aligned. A wide-angle viewing system is swung into position, or a fundus lens is fixed on the anterior surface of the cornea.
5. The perioperative nurse confirms that the proper infusion rate, cutting rate, and aspiration rate are set on the machine console. If a dense cataract or retained lens material blocks the view of the retina, a lensectomy may be performed with a Fragmatome or other ultrasonic handpiece at this time.
6. The surgeon removes the vitreous under direct visualization. Once the medium has been removed and the retinal condition visualized, the necessary injections or treatments (endolaser photocoagulation, repair of macular pucker, insertion of silicone oil, gas-fluid exchange) (Figure 9-49) are completed. A scleral buckling procedure may also be performed.
7. The trocars are removed from the pars plana incisions. Cultures from the vitreous washings are taken if necessary.
8. Subconjunctival injections of steroids or antibiotics are given. An eye pad and shield may be applied for protection of the eye, although some surgeons opt not to use them.

Scleral Buckling

Procedural Considerations. In the treatment of retinal detachment, the aim is to return the retina to its normal anatomic position. For this specific procedure, repair is done from outside the

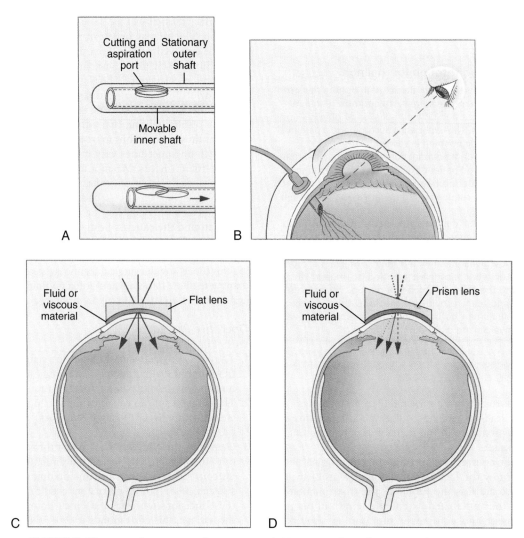

FIGURE 9-48 Essential components for vitrectomy. **A,** Vitrector probe with its cutting/aspirating port close to the tip of the intraocular portion of the handpiece. **B,** Infusion cannula, placed in pars plana, is viewed for correct position. **C,** Flat contact lens, resting on cushion of fluid or viscoelastic material on the cornea, is used for viewing posterior half of the vitreous cavity and retina. **D,** Prism contact lens used for viewing anterior structures in the vitreous cavity.

globe. The purpose of the scleral buckling procedure for retinal detachment is to cause an intrusion or push into the eye at the site of the pathologic source. Treatment by diathermy or cryotherapy causes an inflammatory reaction that leads to a permanent adhesion between the detached retina and underlying structures. The surgery also involves sealing off the area in which the tear or hole is located and may include drainage of the subretinal fluid.

The procedure may be performed using general anesthesia or MAC with local blocks. The scleral buckling may be done using episcleral (working outside of the sclera) technique or by scleral dissection (making a partial-thickness incision into the sclera and creating flaps to expose the underlying tissue). Both techniques may use drainage of subretinal fluid, encircling bands, diathermy, light coagulation, or cryotherapy. Cryosurgery or light coagulation may be used alone or in combination with a buckling procedure.

Operative Procedure

1. A detailed drawing of the retina may be made before surgery and is displayed in the operating suite accord-

ing to surgeon preference. On the basis of this drawing, the surgeon opens the conjunctiva to a previously determined extent, for example, 90 degrees for a simple horseshoe tear or 360 degrees for an aphakic detachment (Figure 9-50).

2. The inferior, superior, lateral, and medial rectus muscles are isolated using 0 silk ties as traction sutures.

3. Using the indirect ophthalmoscope, the surgeon locates the detachment and tear and marks the site with nonpenetrating diathermy by indentation or with a methylene blue marking pen.

4. Under direct visualization, the surgeon applies the retinal cryoprobe to the external surface of the globe in the area of the pathologic condition and treats the area. An ice ball is seen to form in the proper areas until the entire lesion has been treated.

5. The buckling component of the procedure secures silicone bands, sponges, plates, or tires to the sclera. The surgeon places nonabsorbable sutures (4-0 or 5-0) into the sclera sur-

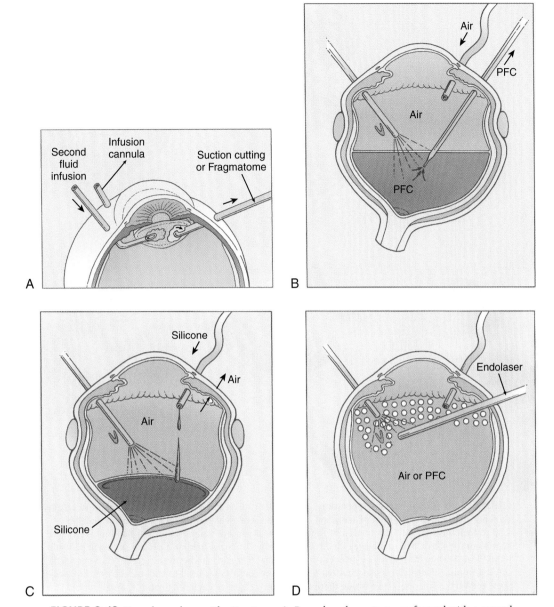

FIGURE 9-49 Procedures done with vitrectomy. **A,** Pars plana lensectomy performed with a second infusion line. **B,** Air/perfluorocarbon (PFC) exchange. The PFC has been placed in the vitreous cavity for removal of subretinal fluid and anatomic reattachment of the retina. Air under positive pressure is then placed through the infusion cannula as the PFC is simultaneously extruded through the tapered needle. **C,** Silicone/air exchange. Silicone is inserted through the infusion cannula as a temporary intraocular tamponade. Silicone is heavier than air and fills the globe from the bottom up, and the air escapes through the sclerotomy site. In silicone/fluid exchange, the silicone floats on the fluid and the fluid is removed with an extrusion needle. **D,** Endolaser photocoagulation is performed after the retina is returned to its normal position.

rounding the lesion and ties them over the silicone sponge, causing the outer shell of the eye to be pushed toward the elevated retina.

6. If an encircling band is to be used, the surgeon places mattress sutures into the sclera in four quadrants. A silicone band is passed 360 degrees around the eye under the sutures and the rectus muscles. The sutures are tied, and a self-holding Watzke sleeve is applied to the band to maintain a predetermined circumference. This causes a 360-degree constriction of the outer coats into the eye.

7. If drainage of subretinal fluid is desired, the surgeon chooses an area under direct visualization in which a significant fluid level exists under the retina, and places a diathermy mark on the sclera. The sclera is split to the choroid, and a small amount of diathermy is applied to the choroid bed. A 27-gauge ½-inch needle is then used to puncture the choroid into the subretinal space to permit drainage of fluid.

8. Air or replacement fluids may be introduced into the eye after the drainage of subretinal fluid. This is usually done through the pars plana under direct visualization.

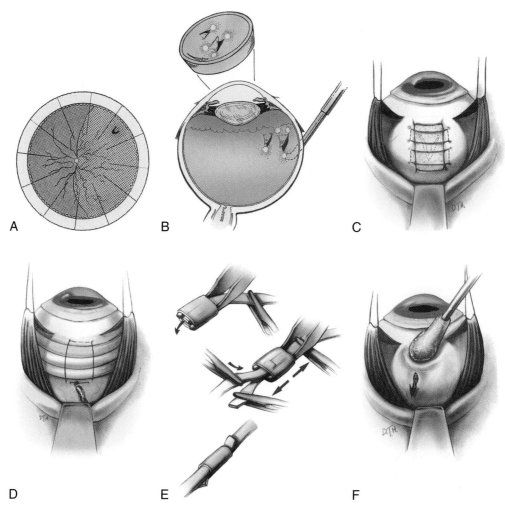

FIGURE 9-50 Scleral buckling operation for treatment of retinal detachment. **A,** Diagram of retina showing detachment of retina of temporal half of left eye, with retinal tear at equator of globe at 1:30 o'clock position. **B,** Examination of fundus by means of ophthalmoscope and handheld lens and depression of sclera with diathermy electrode. Surgeon visualizes field and places electrode beneath retinal tear; burn mark is made on sclera at site of retinal tear with diathermy electrode. **C,** A sponge is sutured in place over treated site of retinal tear. **D,** Band and tire are used to encircle the eye. **E,** Placement of Watzke silicone sleeve is one method to secure edges of encircling band. **F,** Small incision is made through sclera, and choroid is finely incised to allow subretinal fluid to drain.

9. The surgeon removes the traction sutures from around the muscles and closes the conjunctiva with 7-0 absorbable suture. A subconjunctival injection of an antibiotic, steroid, or both may be given, and an eye pad is applied.

Retinopexy

In pneumatic retinopexy (Figure 9-51) an intraocular injection of a bubble of air or therapeutic gases provides pressure against retinal breaks, allowing the detached retinal breaks to approximate the pigment epithelium. Retinopexy may be used in combination with scleral buckling and posterior vitrectomy; it may be performed as part of an ambulatory procedure for treatment of certain retinal detachments, using laser photocoagulation with injection of the gas bubble followed by specific postoperative positioning. The gases are drawn through a Millipore 0.22-micrometer filter and may be mixed with filtered air so that the concentration may be varied. The gas bubble is a ratio mixture of gas and air. The higher the concentration of gas to air, the longer the bubble remains in the eye before being "absorbed." Patient positioning after retinopexy is often facedown for several days to weeks but may include tilting the head to one side or the other as well. The head position is determined by the location of the retinal tear/hole. For example, if the retinal tear/hole is located superior temporal in the right eye, the patient would be instructed to tilt the head down and to the left, so the bubble will float upward and to the right where the tear/hole is located. The larger the tear/hole, the longer the bubble needs to be in contact with the area to be reattached.

Sulfur hexafluoride gas (SF_6) is colorless, odorless, and nontoxic. It increases 2.5 times in volume within 48 hours after injection by drawing other gases, specifically nitrogen and oxygen, from the surrounding tissues. SF_6 bubbles remain for at least 10 days (Donlon et al, 2005).

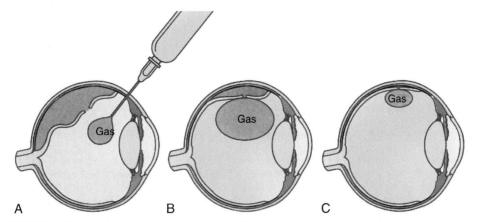

FIGURE 9-51 Pneumatic retinopexy. **A,** Gas bubble is injected through the pars plana. **B** and **C,** The bubble closes and supports the retinal break. After a 7- to 10-day healing period and when the retina is returned to normal position, laser surgery or cryotherapy can be performed to seal the break.

Perfluoropropane gas (C_3F_8) is colorless, odorless, and non-toxic. It quadruples its volume within 48 hours after injection. A 1-mm bubble can remain up to 30 to 50 days.

Because SF_6 and C_3F_8 are expansible gases, certain precautions are required. Patients are given a wristband to wear that states what kind of gas bubble is in their eye and when it was instilled. If they would require surgery, they need to alert the anesthesia provider of the presence of the gas bubble. The intent of instilling a gas bubble is to sustain its size and hold the retina in place. SF_6 and C_3F_8 are inert, very insoluble in water, and poorly diffusible. Since nitrous oxide (N_2O) is 117 times more diffusible than SF_6, it rapidly enters the gas bubble. With continued administration of N_2O the injected gas bubble can increase to three times its original size. Intraocular pressure (IOP) can increase from 14 to 30 mm Hg; 18 minutes after discontinuation of N_2O, IOP will decrease along with the smaller bubble size. Such quick and wide variations in bubble size can negatively affect the surgical outcome. Therefore N_2O should be discontinued at least 20 minutes before an intravitreal gas injection to ensure stable bubble size and IOP. Some anesthesia providers avoid using N_2O for any case where intravitreal gas injection is anticipated. Patients are instructed to avoid air travel until the gas bubble is completely resolved or decreased to a level of 5% of the vitreous volume. Cabin pressurization in air travel will cause severe enlargement of the gas bubble with an increase in intraocular pressure and eye pain. Car or train travel to high elevations should also be avoided unless the change in altitude is done gradually. N_2O should be avoided for 3 to 4 weeks after intravitreal gas injection. The exposure to N_2O could reexpand the bubble, increase IOP, and thereby occlude the retinal artery with loss of vision (Donlon et al, 2005).

Overall, 90% of patients with retinal detachment can now be successfully treated. This is a great advance considering some of the same conditions were inoperable 40 years ago. Visual outcomes, however, are not always predictable, and additional treatment may be necessary. A successful anatomic result of retinal reattachment unfortunately does not always correlate with improvement in visual function. It may take up to several months to evaluate the final visual result. Occasionally, even with the best efforts and multiple attempts at repair, treatment may fail; sight may not be able to be restored. This discussion is part of informed consent. Repairing a detachment before the macula detaches provides the best visual results.

OPHTHALMIC SURGERY SUMMARY

The human eye is an amazing organ. Sight is important to everyday life, and when traumatic injury, aging, or disease decreases or perhaps even destroys the ability to see clearly, the results can be very devastating. As a surgical technologist, there will be opportunity to be a part of correcting and restoring vision. There will be times when that will not be possible, but there is a need to look "normal" and a cosmetic implant is placed. No matter what the situation, a thorough knowledge of the structures of the eye and the physiology of the eye are important to understanding the reason for the surgical procedures performed on the eyes.

In this chapter, special considerations were presented as well as many of the surgical interventions in current use today. There are many options to correct vision today and to restore function after traumatic injury. Take the time to review this chapter and the many procedures explained to provide the best service to the clients being cared for. Ask questions to enhance learning of this material. Review the procedures and the anatomy of the eye to reinforce learning.

GERIATRIC CONSIDERATIONS

The Elderly Patient—Ophthalmic Surgery

There are well-recognized age-related changes in vision. The eyelid loses tone and becomes more lax. Eyebrows often turn gray and outer edges thin. The conjunctiva thins, yellows, and may become drier. The cornea develops a noticeable surrounding ring (the arcus senilis) made up of fat deposits. The pupil and iris decrease in size and limit the amount of light entering the eye. As the lens becomes more dense and rigid, the eye is less able to focus and transmit light. Information that is helpful for aging patients about their eyes includes:

1. Use bright light when performing tasks such as sewing, reading, and cooking; avoid fluorescent light.
2. Use a magnifying glass, if necessary, for close work.
3. See your healthcare provider regularly to detect health problems (e.g., diabetes, hypertension) that might affect your eyes.
4. Have your eyes examined and a glaucoma test performed by a qualified specialist every 1 to 2 years. Have your eyes examined more frequently if you have a disease or condition that is known to affect your vision.
5. Symptoms that require an immediate call to your healthcare provider or eye care specialist include pain, discharge, redness or swelling, and loss of vision (no matter how slight).
6. The use of a humidifier in the home or artificial tears may relieve dry eyes, which is a common condition. Check with your healthcare provider or eyecare specialist before using any over-the-counter preparations.
7. Excessive tearing can be a benign condition or it may reflect a more serious problem. See your healthcare provider or eyecare specialist if you are troubled by this problem.
8. Floaters, a common occurrence in older persons, are just spots or flecks that literally "float" across your field of vision. They usually occur gradually and are most noticeable in a brightly lit environment. If they occur in association with light flashes in your visual field, call your healthcare provider or eyecare specialist.
9. Cataracts are a normal part of the aging process. They develop gradually and without pain. However, when tasks become increasingly difficult and fatiguing because of the vision changes that cataracts produce, see your healthcare provider or eyecare specialist to discuss treatment options.

Because of elders' long life span, undergoing eye surgery (most commonly for cataracts) is more likely than other surgical procedures. Most ophthalmic procedures are minimally invasive and have a high success rate. Because elderly patients may have concurrent systemic disease, even a low-stress procedure should not be treated lightly. Age-related changes, such as hearing loss and musculoskeletal disease, may pose a challenge during ophthalmic surgery because the patient must lie still for long periods and be able to follow verbal instructions. Patients with chronic lung disease lying in the supine position may experience coughing, which can increase intraocular pressure and jeopardize the outcome of the surgery.

Data from US Department of Health and Human Services: Aging and your eyes, Bethesda, Md, 2009, National Institute on Aging.

REVIEW QUESTIONS

1. Entropion is best described as:
   a. inward turning of one or both eyes
   b. an opacity of the lens
   c. outside of the globe
   d. outward turning of one or both eyes

2. Extropion is best described as:
   a. inward turning of one or both eyes
   b. an opacity of the lens
   c. outside of the globe
   d. outward turning of one or both eyes

3. A cataract is:
   a. inward turning of one or both eyes
   b. an opacity of the lens
   c. outside of the globe
   d. outward turning of one or both eyes

4. Aqueous humor is a:
   a. vasoconstrictor
   b. transparent liquid in the posterior
   c. transparent liquid in the anterior chamber of the eye
   d. viscous jelly used in the anterior chamber of the eye

5. Which of the following is NOT a surgical procedure to treat glaucoma?
   a. Trabeculectomy
   b. Iridectomy
   c. Molteno drain
   d. Anterior vitrectomy

6. An anterior vitrectomy is performed for:
   a. vitreous loss
   b. opacities in the anterior chamber
   c. complications associated with vitreous in the anterior chamber
   d. all of the above

7. Obstruction of meibomian gland secretion may lead to a _____.

8. A _____ is a fleshy, triangular encroachment of conjunctiva into the peripheral area of the cornea.

9. Strabismus refers to _____.

10. A corneal transplant is performed when the patient's cornea is thickened or _____ by disease or degeneration.

11. Define and briefly describe the following surgical procedures:
    Dacryocystorhinostomy
    Corneal transplantation
    Topical clear cataract extraction

Critical Thinking Questions

1. During certain ophthalmic procedures the patient will be awake for the duration of the procedure, thus causing increased sensitivity to noise and activity within the room. What can the room staff do to ensure a peaceful surgical suite?

2. Ophthalmic surgical supplies differ from that of most other types of supplies. Discuss the differences in managing patient safety with specialized ophthalmic surgical supplies.

REFERENCES

Alhassan MB et al: Peribulbar versus retrobulbar anaesthesia for cataract surgery, *Cochrane Database Syst Rev 2008* (Issue 3), 2008, Art. No.: CD004083.

American Academy of Ophthalmology (AAO): Clinical statements: Flomax patient advisory, San Francisco, June 2009, available at http://one.aao.org/CE/PracticeGuidelines/ClinicalStatements_Content.aspx?cid=21255f9c-6e66-4684-a3ca-5aa1f4f13ad3. Accessed June 11, 2009.

American Academy of Ophthalmology (AAO): Patient Safety: Recommendations of American Academy of Ophthalmology Wrong Site Task Force 2008, available at http://one.aao.org/CE/PracticeGuidelines/Patient_Content.aspx?cid=d0db838c-2847-4535-baca-aebab3011217&popup. Accessed May 10, 2009.

American Society of Ocularists (ASO): *The American Society of Ocularists: 50+ years of excellence in the field of ocular prosthetics: research, education, standards*, Coralville, IA, 2009, ASO.

American Society of Ophthalmic Registered Nurses (ASORN): The aging retina, *Insight* (4):1–11, 2007.

Association of periOperative Registered Nurses (AORN). *Perioperative standards and recommended practices*, Denver, 2009, The Association.

Bollinger KE, Langston RH: What can patients expect from cataract surgery? *Cleve Clin J Med* 75(3):193–200, 2008.

Burlew-Quartey J: Anterior Segment Surgery and the Nurse's Role, Atlanta, November 2008, Presentation at ASORN Conference.

Cullen KA et al: Ambulatory surgery in the United States, 2006, Centers for Disease Control and Prevention, National Center for Health Statistics, Division of Health Care Statistics, Hyattsville, MD, available at www.cdc.gov/nchs/data/nhsr/nhsr011.pdf. Accessed April 19, 2009.

Denholm B: Tucking patient's arms and general positioning, *AORN J* 89(4):755–757, 2009.

Dodge-Palomba S: Providing compassionate care to the pediatric patient undergoing enucleation of the eye, *Insight* 33(1):10–12, 2008.

Donlon JV et al: Anesthesia for eye, ear, nose and throat surgery, In Miller RD, editor: *Miller's anesthesia*, ed 4, Philadelphia, 2005, Churchill-Livingstone.

Donnenfeld E: Refractive surgery update—2008, Atlanta, November 2008, Presentation at ASORN Annual Meeting.

Eye Bank Association of America (EBAA): Frequently asked questions: corneal transplant, available at www.restoresight.org/aboutus/faqs.htm. Accessed May 8, 2009.

Gariano R: Medical and Surgical Treatment of Retinal Diseases, Presentation at ASORN Annual Meeting, Atlanta, November 2008.

Gutierrez KJ, Peterson PG: Alterations in visual and auditory function. In Peterson PG, Gutierrez KJ, editors: *Saunders nursing survival guide: Pathophysiology*, ed 2, St. Louis, 2007, Saunders.

Harris J: Sharps safety in the ophthalmic setting, Franklin Lakes, NJ, 2008, BD Medical Ophthalmic Systems, p. 26.

Jennings J, Foster J: Medication safety: just a label away, *AORN J* 86(3):618–625, 2007.

Lighthouse International: The Lighthouse for the 21st century: helping millions with vision loss, San Francisco, CA, 2007.

Mitchell S: Sterilization: practicing the complete sterilization process, *AORN Connections* 7(5):10, 2009.

National Eye Institute (NEI, 2008a): 2005 Survey of Public Knowledge, Attitudes, and Practices (KAP) related to eye health and disease, available at www.nei.nih.gov/kap/. Accessed on April 19, 2009.

National Eye Institute (NEI, 2008b): NEI health information: facts about cataracts, available at www.nei.nih.gov/health/cataract/cataract_facts.asp. Accessed March 25, 2009.

National Eye Institute (NEI 2008c): NEI health information: facts about floaters, available at www.nei.nih.gov/health/floaters/index.asp. Accessed April 22, 2009.

National Eye Institute (NEI 2008d): NEI health information: facts about retinal detachment, available at www.nei.nih.gov/health/retinaldetach/index.asp. Accessed April 22, 2009.

National Eye Institute (NEI 2008e): NEI health information: facts about vitreous detachment, available at www.nei.nih.gov/health/vitreous/index.asp. Accessed April 22, 2009.

National Eye Institute (NEI 2008f): NEI health information: facts about macular pucker, available at www.nei.nih.gov/health/pucker/index.asp. Accessed April 22, 2009.

Nichols JR: Taking care of your scleral cover shell ocular prosthesis, June R.R. Nichols, Ocularist Ltd.; ASO diplomate, Board Certified, Des Plaines, IL, 2009.

Pagana KD, Pagana TJ: *Mosby's diagnostic and laboratory test reference*, ed 9, St Louis, 2009, Mosby.

Phillips N: *Berry & Kohn's operating room technique*, ed 11, St Louis, 2007, Mosby.

Prevent Blindness America (PBA): The Vision Learning Center: Eye safety: prevent eye injuries at home, at work, and at play! 2005, available at www.preventblindness.org/safety/. Accessed April 19, 2009.

Stuart A: "Birthday for a Beam of Light: Happy 25! A Quarter Century of the Excimer Laser." In Academy News: Eye Net Magazine: Scientific Highlights of Atlanta 2008, available at www.aao.org/publications/eyenet/upload/01AN.pdf. Accessed May 31, 2009.

The Joint Commission: NPSG.03.04.01: Labeling in procedural areas, available at www.jointcommission.org/AccreditationPrograms/Office -Based-Surgery/Standards/09_FAQs/NPSG/Medication_safety/NPSG.03.04.01/Labeling+in+procedural+areas.htm. Accessed April 27, 2009.

CHAPTER 10

Otorhinolaryngologic Surgery

LEARNING OBJECTIVES

After studying this chapter the reader will be able to:
- Identify relevant anatomy in select otorhinolaryngology surgery
- Correlate physiologic conditions necessitating surgical intervention
- Identify tissue layers and incisional approaches used in otorhinolaryngologic surgery
- List the pharmacologic and hemostatic agents utilized during otorhinolaryngologic surgery
- Identify specialized instruments, equipment, and supplies used for otorhinolaryngologic surgery
- Describe diagnostic studies used to determine the need for surgical interventions
- Compare minimally invasive with invasive surgical options for otorhinolaryngologic surgery
- Apply broad otorhinolaryngologic concepts and knowledge to clinical practice for enhanced surgical patient care

CHAPTER OUTLINE

Overview

Otorhinolaryngology is the study and science of the human ear (oto), nose (rhino), and throat (laryngo). It is a specialty that continues to evolve as a result of cutting-edge technology; high-powered surgical microscopes; narrower, flexible endoscopes; computer imaging; wound care improvements; and navigation systems that communicate with radiologic imaging. Such advances yield significant gains in improving the health and surgical outcomes of patients with physical ailments of the head and neck. This chapter comprehensively and respectively reviews perioperative care of patients undergoing surgical procedures to the ear, nose, head, and neck.

Surgical Anatomy

EXTERNAL, MIDDLE, AND INNER EAR

The ear is a sensory organ for the identification, localization, and interpretation of sound as well as for the maintenance of equilibrium. Hearing is the sense by which sounds are appreciated. Referred to as the "watchdog of the senses," hearing is the last sense to disappear when one falls asleep and the first to return when one awakens. The physical nature of sound results from the compression and rarefaction of pressure waves and moving molecules, but the sensations humans actually experience are the product of complex mechanical, electrical, and psychologic interactions in the ear and central nervous system. Three anatomic segments—the external ear, middle ear, and inner ear—work together to provide hearing and balance (Figure 10-1).

This chapter was originally written by Troy J. DeRose, CRNP, RNFA, and Gregory J. Artz, MD, for the 14th edition of Alexander's Care of the Patient in Surgery and has been revised by Barbara Krukemeier, CST, for this text.

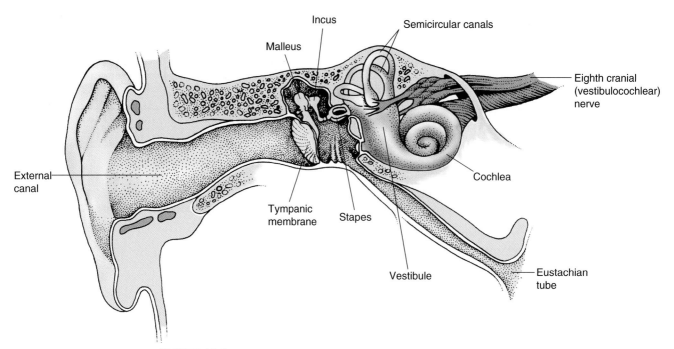

FIGURE 10-1 Anatomic structures of external ear, middle ear, and inner ear.

RIGHT TYMPANIC MEMBRANE

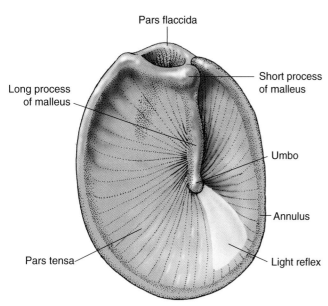

FIGURE 10-2 Structural landmarks of tympanic membrane.

The *external ear* includes the auricle (or pinna) and external auditory canal, and is composed of cartilage covered with skin. The auricles are fixed in position and lie close to the head; they concentrate incoming sound waves and conduct them into the external auditory canal. Both ears provide stereophonic hearing that gives us very specific sound localization capabilities. Without binaural hearing, determining where sounds emanate can be difficult; this is a common problem for patients with unilateral or asymmetric hearing loss.

The external auditory canal, an S-shaped pathway leading to the middle ear, is approximately 2.5 cm in length in adults and shelters the tympanic membrane. Its skeleton of bone and cartilage is covered with very thin, sensitive skin. The canal lining is protected and lubricated with cerumen, a waxy substance secreted by sebaceous glands in the distal third of the canal. Cerumen helps to trap foreign material, and has a mildly acidic pH that reduces bacterial levels in the outer ear.

Located at the end of the external auditory canal is the *tympanic membrane* (eardrum) (Figure 10-2). It is a thin structure with three distinct layers: an outer squamous epithelial layer in continuity with the skin of the external ear canal, a fibrous middle layer for strength and support, and a medial mucous membrane layer that is continuous with the lining of the middle ear.

The *middle ear* is filled with air, which flows from the nasopharynx through the eustachian tube. It is divided into three areas: the epitympanum (upper), mesotympanum (middle), and hypotympanum (lower). Posteriorly, the epitympanic portion of the middle ear communicates with the mastoid air cells of the temporal bone via the mastoid antrum. The mucous membrane of the middle ear is continuous with that of the pharynx and the mastoid cells, making it possible for infection to travel to the middle ear (otitis media) and mastoid cells (mastoiditis). The eustachian tube serves to aerate the air-filled spaces of the temporal bone and to equalize pressure in the middle ear with atmospheric pressure. It is normally closed at rest and actively opens during yawning, sneezing, or swallowing. A chain of three small articulated bones (ossicles) extends across the middle ear cavity and conducts vibrations (airborne sound waves) from the tympanic membrane across the middle ear into the oval window and the fluid-filled inner ear (Figure 10-3).

The *malleus* (hammer) consists of a head, neck, handle, and short process. The handle and short process are attached to the undersurface of the eardrum, and the head articulates with

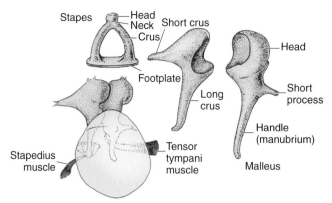

FIGURE 10-3 Articulated ossicles of right middle ear.

the body of the incus in the upper segment of the middle ear called the epitympanum or "attic." The *incus* (anvil) consists of a body and long and short processes (see Figure 10-2). The distal end of the long process of the incus is called the lenticular process and articulates with the capitulum (head) of the stapes, which is the third, innermost bone. The *stapes* (stirrup) consists of a head, neck, anterior and posterior crura, and a mobile footplate that is secured to the oval window by an annular ligament. The movable joints between these ossicles contribute to a lever system that amplifies the received sound and transmits and converts vibrations from ambient air to the fluid of the inner ear.

The inner ear is protected from loud noise by the *tensor tympani* muscle, which draws the drum inward to increase tension and restricts its ability to vibrate, and the *stapedius* muscle, which contracts and tightens the stapes in the oval window to reduce the intensity of vibrations passing through the ossicles into the inner ear. The middle ear and mastoid are supplied with blood from the branches of the internal and external carotid artery systems.

The *inner ear* is a membranous, curved cavity located in the petrous portion of the temporal bone; it contains hair cell receptors that provide us with both hearing and balance. The inner ear consists of a bony labyrinth filled with a watery fluid (perilymph) that surrounds and bathes a membranous labyrinth filled with another fluid with distinct electrolyte characteristics, called the endolymph. The bony labyrinth includes the cochlea and the vestibular labyrinth.

The *cochlea* resembles a snail shell. It is divided into three compartments: the scala vestibuli, which is associated with the oval window; the scala tympani, which is associated with the round window; and the cochlear duct. The scala vestibuli and scala tympani are filled with perilymph, whereas the cochlear duct contains endolymph. On the basilar membrane of the cochlea lies the organ of Corti—the neural end organ for hearing. Its neuroepithelium projects thousands of hair cells that are set into motion by vibrations passing through the ossicles and oval window to the perilymph. The hair cells convert the mechanical energy of wave movement from vibration in the perilymph into electrochemical impulses. The *vestibular labyrinth* is composed of the utricle, the saccule, and three semicircular canals, referred to as the *lateral, superior,* and *posterior canals.* They are positioned at right angles to one another and are responsible for detecting angular acceleration that can be

elicited with any head or body movement. Each canal contains a sense organ (crista) that responds to fluid movement in the endolymph, which triggers impulses in the vestibular branch of the acoustic nerve. Cristae are stimulated by angular accelerations and movements, such as head turning. The maculae of the utricle and saccule of the vestibular labyrinth are gravity-oriented. Linear accelerations are detected by the utricle and saccule; they both have a mat of sensory cells (*otoconia*) imbedded in a gelatinous material covered with calcium deposits. The weight of these otoconia constantly orients us to the direction of gravity. Their inertia gives information about linear accelerations. The combined signals from the cristae of the semicircular canals and the sensory cells of the utricle and saccule provide a sense of balance and orientation in space. The internal auditory branches of the basilar artery supply the inner ear.

NASAL ANATOMY

The nose is covered with skin and is supported internally by bone and cartilage. The two external nares provide openings for the passage of air through the nasal cavity. These openings contain internal hairs for the filtration of coarse particles that are sometimes carried by air. The nose is divided into the prominent external portion and the internal portion known as the *nasal cavity* (Figure 10-4). The chief purpose of the nose is to prepare air for use in the lungs.

The nasal bones and the frontal process of the maxilla form the upper portion of the external nose, and the lower portion is formed by a group of nasal cartilages and connective tissue covered with skin (Figure 10-5). The nostrils and the tip of the nose are shaped by the major alar cartilages. The nares are separated by the *columella,* which is formed by the lower margin of the septal cartilage, the medial parts of the major alar cartilages, and the anterior nasal spine, all of which are covered with skin. The nasal cavity is divided medially into right and left portions by the *nasal septum.*

The *nasal septum* is composed of three structures: the nasal cartilage, the perpendicular plate of the ethmoid bone, and the vomer bone. The septum is covered by mucoperichondrium on either side that contains blood vessels and mucus-secreting cells. The rich blood supply warms and moistens the air while the sticky mucus traps dust, pollen, and other small particles.

The nasal cavity communicates with the outside by its external openings, called the *nares.* The nares open into the nasopharynx through the choanae. The nasal cavity is also associated with each ear, sharing the torus tubarius (opening of the eustachian tube in the nasopharynx) with the paranasal sinuses (frontal, maxillary, ethmoidal, sphenoidal) through their respective orifices (meatus). The nasal cavity also communicates with the conjunctivae through the nasolacrimal duct. The nasal cavity is separated from the lingual cavity by the hard palate and soft palate (see Figure 10-4) and from the cranial cavity by the ethmoids. It is held together by periosteal covering over bone and by perichondrium, which extends over the cartilages. The turbinate bones of the nasal structure are arranged one above the other, separated by grooves that are comprised of pseudostratified columnar ciliated respiratory epithelium. The turbinates act as drainage passages of the accessory sinuses and also increase the turbulence of airflow to humidify the air that is nasally inspired. This area is commonly referred to as the *sphenoethmoidal recess* and contains

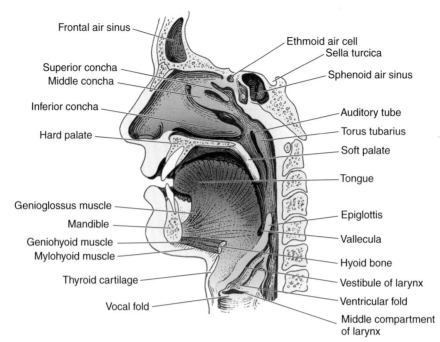

FIGURE 10-4 Sagittal section of face and neck.

Frontal air sinus
Superior concha
Middle concha
Inferior concha
Hard palate
Genioglossus muscle
Mandible
Geniohyoid muscle
Mylohyoid muscle
Thyroid cartilage
Vocal fold

Ethmoid air cell
Sella turcica
Sphenoid air sinus
Auditory tube
Torus tubarius
Soft palate
Tongue
Epiglottis
Vallecula
Hyoid bone
Vestibule of larynx
Ventricular fold
Middle compartment of larynx

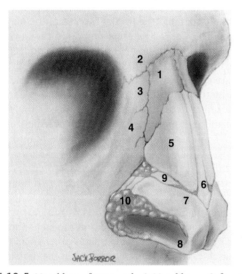

FIGURE 10-5 Nasal bony framework. *1,* Nasal bone; *2,* frontal bone; *3,* lacrimal bone; *4,* maxillary bone; *5,* upper lateral cartilage; *6,* nasal septum; *7,* lower lateral cartilage, lateral crus; *8,* lower lateral cartilage, medial crus; *9,* sesamoid cartilage; *10,* fibrofatty tissue.

these bony shelves known as the *superior, middle,* and *inferior meatus* or *turbinates* (Figure 10-6).

The nasal sinuses serve as air spaces and communicate with the nasal cavity through the meatus. Anteriorly, on each side of the skull, the frontal sinus, the anterior ethmoidal sinus, and the maxillary sinus (antrum of Highmore) drain into the middle meatus; posteriorly, the ethmoidal and the sphenoidal sinuses drain into the superior meatus and the sphenoethmoidal recess (see Figure 10-6). A passageway for the flow of air is provided by the irregular air spaces between these structures.

THROAT ANATOMY

Oral Cavity

The *oral cavity* is comprised of the mouth and salivary glands. The mouth is formed by the cheeks, the hard palate, the mandible, and the tongue. It extends from the lips to the junction of the hard and soft palates. The portion of the mouth outside the teeth is the buccal cavity, and that on the inner side of the teeth is the lingual cavity. The hard palate forms the upper boundary of the oral cavity. The hard palate is formed by the maxilla and palatine bones. The mandible and floor of the mouth form the lower boundary of the oral cavity (Figure 10-7).

The *salivary glands* consist of three paired glands: the sublingual, the submandibular, and the parotid. They communicate with the mouth and produce saliva, which serves to moisten the mouth and initiate digestion of carbohydrates. The minor salivary glands exist in the submucosa of the cheeks, tongue, palates, and floor of the mouth, pharynx, lips, and paranasal sinuses.

The *sublingual gland* lies on the undersurface of the tongue beneath the mucous membrane on the floor of the mouth and the side of the tongue, on the inner surface of the mandible. The many tiny ducts of each gland separately enter the oral cavity on the sublingual fold.

The *submandibular gland* lies partly above and partly below the posterior half of the base of the mandible and on the mylohyoid and hyoglossus muscles. Its duct (Wharton's duct) runs superficially beneath the mucosa of the floor of the mouth and enters the oral cavity behind the central incisors.

The *parotid gland,* the largest of the salivary glands, lies below the zygomatic arch in front of the mastoid process and behind the ramus of the mandible; it is divided into a superficial portion and a deep portion. The parotid duct (Stensen's duct) pierces the buccal pad of fat and the buccinator muscle, finally opening into the oral cavity opposite the crown of the upper second molar tooth.

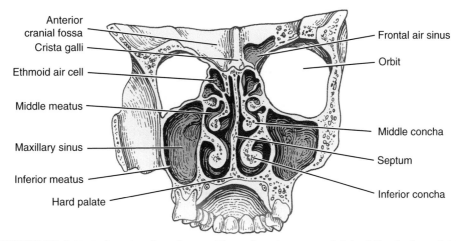

Anterior cranial fossa
Crista galli
Ethmoid air cell
Middle meatus
Maxillary sinus
Inferior meatus
Hard palate

Frontal air sinus
Orbit
Middle concha
Septum
Inferior concha

FIGURE 10-6 Vertical section through nose. Plane of section passes slightly obliquely through left first molar tooth and behind second right premolar tooth. Posterior wall of right frontal sinus removed.

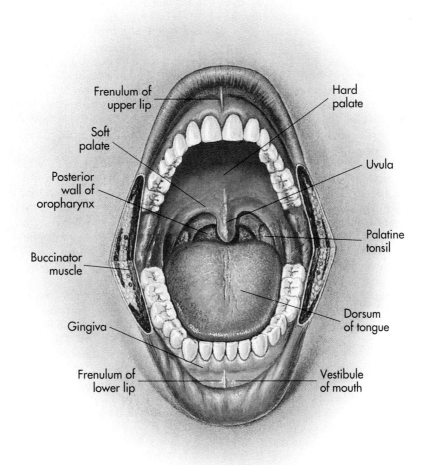

Frenulum of upper lip
Soft palate
Posterior wall of oropharynx
Buccinator muscle
Gingiva
Frenulum of lower lip

Hard palate
Uvula
Palatine tonsil
Dorsum of tongue
Vestibule of mouth

FIGURE 10-7 Anatomic structures of the oral cavity.

Pharynx

The pharynx extends from the posterior portion of the nose to the esophagus and larynx and serves as a channel for both the digestive and respiratory systems (Figure 10-8). It is composed of muscular and fibrous layers with a mucous membrane lining. It is approximately 13 cm long and lies anterior to the cervical vertebrae and posterior to the nasal and oral cavities. The pharynx is associated above with the sphenoid sinus and the basilar part of the occipital bone, and it joins the esophagus below. Seven cavities communicate with the pharynx: the two nasal cavities, the two tympanic cavities, the mouth, the larynx, and the esophagus. The pharynx comprises three groups of constrictor muscles. Each muscle fits within the one below, and each inserts posteriorly in the median line with its mate from the opposite side. The constrictor muscles provide constriction of the pharynx for swallowing. Between the origins of the constrictor muscle groups are so-called *intervals,* through which ligaments, nerves, and arteries pass. The pharynx is divided anatomically into three sections: the nasopharynx, the oropharynx, and the hypopharynx.

Nasopharynx. The nasopharynx lies posterior to the nasal cavity and extends over the soft palate. It communicates with the oropharynx through the pharyngeal isthmus, which is closed by muscular action during swallowing. Infection can spread from the nasopharynx to the middle ear through the eustachian tube.

Oropharynx. The oropharynx lies posterior to the oral cavity and extends from the palate to the level of the hyoid bone. The tonsils are situated on each side of the oropharynx, lodged in a tonsillar fossa that is attached to folds of membrane-containing muscle. The palatine tonsils (a pair of oval structures) are the only lymphatic organs covered with stratified squamous epithelium. The lateral surface of each tonsil is usually covered with a fibrous capsule. The anterior and posterior tonsillar pillars join to form a triangular fossa, with the posterior lateral aspects of the tongue at its base. The lingual tonsils are lodged in each fossa. The adenoids, or pharyngeal tonsils, are suspended from the roof of the nasopharynx and consist of an accumulation of lymphoid tissue.

Hypopharynx. The hypopharynx extends from the hyoid bone and empties into the esophagus posteriorly and the larynx anteriorly. The piriform sinuses are bound medially by the arytenoepiglottic fold and laterally by the thyroid cartilage and hypothyroid membrane. The fossae are involved in speech.

Larynx and Associated Structures

Larynx. The larynx is a cartilaginous box that lies midline in front of the fourth, fifth, and sixth cervical vertebrae between the trachea and the root of the tongue, at the upper front part of the neck. The location of the larynx between the gastrointestinal (GI) and respiratory systems is strategic in protecting the airway during swallowing and breathing. The larynx has three main functions: as a passageway for respiration, as a valve to prevent aspiration, and as a vibratory source for vocalization.

The larynx can be divided into three portions: *supraglottis* (or upper portion above the true vocal cords), *glottis* (level of the true vocal cords), and *subglottis* (below the true vocal

cords). The upper portion of the larynx is continuous with the pharynx above and includes the epiglottis, vallecula, and the laryngeal cartilages. Its lower portion joins the trachea. The skeletal structure provides for patency of the enclosed airway. The complex muscle action and arrangement of tissues within the larynx provide for closure of the lumen, to protect against trauma and entrance of foreign bodies, and for speech.

Laryngeal Cartilages. The skeletal framework of the larynx consists of cartilages and membranes. Of the nine separate cartilages, three are single and six are arranged in pairs. The main cartilages of the larynx include the thyroid, the cricoid, the epiglottis, two arytenoid, two corniculate, and two cuneiform. The thyroid cartilage, or Adam's apple, forms the anterior portion of the voice box. The cricoid cartilage is a complete cartilaginous ring that resembles a signet ring; it rests beneath the thyroid cartilage and supports the airway (see Figure 10-8). The epiglottis is a slightly curled, leaf-shaped, elastic, fibrous membrane that is attached in the midline to the upper border of the thyroid cartilage. The epiglottis helps to protect the larynx during swallowing. Contraction of the cricothyroid muscle pulls the thyroid cartilage and the cricoid cartilage to tighten the vocal cords and close the glottis. The arytenoid cartilages, which rest above the signet-ring portion of the cricoid cartilage, support the posterior portion of the true vocal cords.

Laryngeal Ligaments. The extrinsic ligaments of the larynx are those connecting: (1) the thyroid cartilage and epiglottis with the hyoid bone and (2) the cricoid cartilage with the trachea. The intrinsic ligaments of the larynx are those connecting several cartilages of the organ to each other. They are considered the elastic membrane of the larynx.

The mucous lining of the larynx blends with fibrous tissue to form two folds on each side of the larynx. The upper set is known as the *false vocal cords.* The lower set is called the *true vocal cords* because they are concerned primarily with the speaking voice and protection of the lower respiratory channels against the invasion of food and foreign bodies. The region of the larynx at the true vocal cord level is called the *glottis,* a triangular space between the vocal cords. During swallowing, the rising action of the muscular larynx, the closure of the glottis, and the doorlike action of the epiglottis all serve to guide food and fluid into the esophagus.

Laryngeal Muscles. The laryngeal muscles perform two distinct functions: the extrinsic muscles (Figure 10-9) regulate the degree of tension on the vocal cords, and the intrinsic muscles open and close the glottis. The spoken voice also depends on the sphincter action of the soft palate, tongue, and lips. The muscle action of the larynx permits the glottis to close either voluntarily or involuntarily by reflex action. The closure of the inlet by this mechanism protects the respiratory passages. The closure of the glottis and the action of the vocal cords are precisely coordinated to produce the voice.

Trachea. The trachea is a cartilaginous tube about 15 cm in length and 2 to 2.5 cm in diameter. It begins in the neck and extends from the lower part of the larynx, on a level with the sixth cervical vertebra, to the upper border of the fifth thoracic

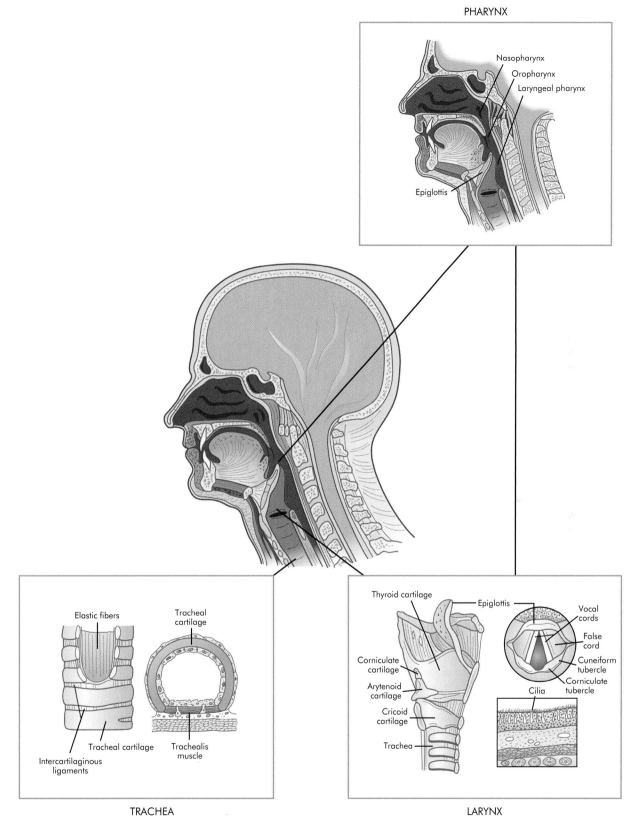

FIGURE 10-8 Structures of the upper airway.

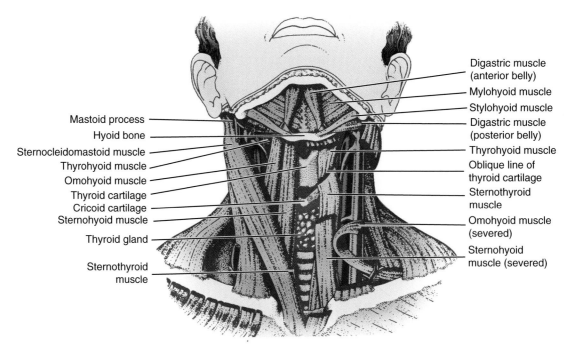

Mastoid process
Hyoid bone
Sternocleidomastoid muscle
Thyrohyoid muscle
Omohyoid muscle
Thyroid cartilage
Cricoid cartilage
Sternohyoid muscle
Thyroid gland
Sternothyroid muscle

Digastric muscle (anterior belly)
Mylohyoid muscle
Stylohyoid muscle
Digastric muscle (posterior belly)
Thyrohyoid muscle
Oblique line of thyroid cartilage
Sternothyroid muscle
Omohyoid muscle (severed)
Sternohyoid muscle (severed)

FIGURE 10-9 Extrinsic muscles of larynx.

vertebra. It descends anteriorly to the esophagus, enters the superior mediastinum, and divides into right and left main bronchi. The trachea is composed of a series of C-shaped rings of hyaline cartilage. The posterior surface of the trachea is flattened rather than round because the cartilaginous rings are incomplete. The carina is a ridge on the inside of the bifurcation of the trachea. It is a landmark during bronchoscopy and separates the upper end of the right main branches from the upper end of the left main branches of the bronchi. Branches from the arch of the aorta—the brachiocephalic (innominate) and left common carotid arteries—are in close relation to the trachea. The cervical portion of the trachea is related anteriorly to the sternohyoid and sternothyroid muscles and to the isthmus of the thyroid gland.

Musculature of the Neck

A layer of deep cervical fascia surrounds the neck like a collar and is attached to the trapezius and sternocleidomastoid muscles. The sternocleidomastoid muscle extends from the upper part of the sternum and medial third of the clavicle to the mastoid process. The trapezius muscle extends from the scapula, the lateral third of the clavicle, and the vertebrae to the occipital prominence. The relationship of these muscles to each other and to the adjacent bone creates triangles used as anatomic landmarks.

The pretracheal fascia of the neck lies deep in the strap muscles (sternothyroid, sternohyoid, thyrohyoid, and omohyoid) and partially encloses the thyroid gland, trachea, and larynx. The pretracheal fascia is pierced by the thyroid vessels. It fuses with the front of the carotid sheath on the deep surface of the sternocleidomastoid muscle. The carotid sheath consists of a network of areolar tissue surrounding the carotid arteries and vagus nerve.

Laterally the carotid sheath is fused with the fascia on the deep surface of the sternocleidomastoid muscle; anteriorly it is fused with the middle cervical fascia along the lateral border of the sternothyroid muscle. Lying between the floor and roof of this triangular formation of muscles are the lymph glands and the accessory nerve. Arteries and nerves traverse and pierce this triangle.

PROXIMAL STRUCTURES

Cranial Nerves

The trigeminal (fifth cranial) nerve supplies sensory innervation to the face, oral cavity, nose, nasal cavity, and maxillary sinuses. It provides motor innervation to the muscles of mastication.

The right and left facial (seventh cranial) nerves are responsible for all the movements of the facial muscles. Both nerves have a very complex and tortuous course from the brainstem to the motor endplates of the facial musculature. The facial nerve enters the internal auditory meatus along with the eighth (vestibulocochlear) cranial nerve and travels through the internal auditory canal, passing through the labyrinthine portion of the temporal bone to the geniculate ganglion, where it turns sharply and passes superior to the oval window. It then turns inferiorly through the mastoid and exits through the stylomastoid foramen. There are three primary branches of the facial nerve in the temporal bone: the greater superficial petrosal nerve controls lacrimation; the stapedial branch controls the stapedius muscle; and the chorda tympani nerve carries the taste sensation to the anterior two thirds of the tongue.

The vestibulocochlear (eighth cranial) nerve connects the inner ear to the brain through its brainstem nuclei and ascending neural pathways. The recurrent laryngeal branch of the vagus (tenth cranial) nerve is the important motor nerve of the intrinsic muscles of the pharynx and larynx.

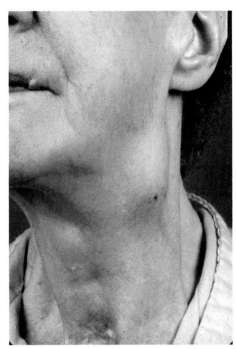

FIGURE 10-10 Advanced cancer of the mouth with metastasis to the neck.

Lymphatic System

The lymphatic system serves both immunologic and circulatory functions. Interstitial fluid, which may contain bacteria, viruses, or tumor cells, is returned to the blood circulation through the lymphatic channels. As the lymph nodes trap the foreign matter, the nodes may become enlarged, infected, or the focus of metastatic cancer (Figure 10-10).

The nasal cavity, the paranasal sinuses, and the pharynx drain into the retropharyngeal nodes. The mouth, lips, and external nose are drained by the submandibular nodes. The lymphatics of the tip and lateral aspects of the tongue drain to the submental nodes, and the posterior tongue lymphatics drain to the cervical nodes.

The lymphatic drainage of the neck can be divided into superficial and deep nodes (Figure 10-11). Lymph nodes of the neck can be further classified into subzones. Level Ia nodes are submental nodes; level Ib nodes are submandibular nodes. Level IIa nodes are upper jugular nodes anterior to cranial nerve IX. Level IIb nodes are upper jugular nodes posterior to cranial nerve IX. Level III nodes are middle jugular nodes. Level IV nodes are lower jugular nodes. Level Va nodes are posterior triangle nodes of the spinal accessory group, and level Vb nodes are posterior triangle nodes of the transverse cervical artery and supraclavicular group. Level VI nodes are anterior tracheal nodes. Level VII nodes are superior mediastinum nodes.

Surgical Technologist Considerations

Familiarity with otorhinolaryngologic conditions is essential. The surgical technologist should understand the patient's his-

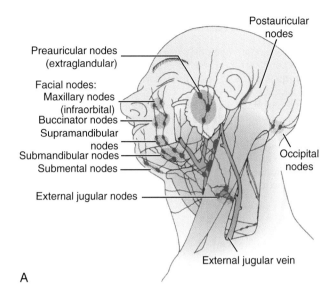

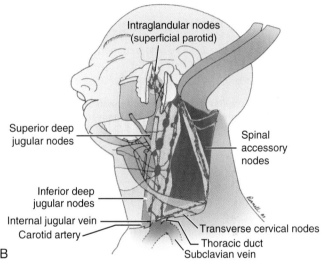

FIGURE 10-11 Lymphatic drainage of neck. **A,** Superficial cervical and facial nodal drainage patterns. **B,** Deep cervical lymphatic drainage patterns. Note that sternocleidomastoid muscle is reflected.

tory and diagnosis related to the head and neck. Communication skills might be affected by loss of hearing or loss of voice. OR personnel must provide alternate means of communication (e.g., pen and paper, erasable board).

The surgical technologist should have an understanding of local and general anesthesia agents as well as an understanding of the anatomy, instrumentation, and specialized equipment used in head and neck surgery to provide the best patient care.

Diagnostic Studies

Computed Tomography. CT scans are radiographic studies that visualize structures by producing serial sections, many times clinically referred to as "cuts," through planes of the head and neck. CT imaging provides visualization of bone, soft tissue, and adjacent intracranial and extracranial pathologic conditions. Intravenous (IV) injection of iodine contrast agents produces

SURGICAL TECHNOLOGY PREFERENCE CARD

For all otorhinolaryngologic procedures, be aware of OR size and where equipment will be located. For ear and some neck procedures where the microscope is used, the head of the OR bed will need to be turned to the foot in order to accommodate the microscopes and surgeon's legs. In some procedures the entire OR bed will be turned 90 to 180 degrees with the foot section toward the anesthesia provider.

Room Prep: Basic operating room furniture, thermoregulatory devices, sequential compression devices (SCDs), extra blankets, padding/positioning devices, safety belt/restraining devices are required

Prep Solutions: In room
- Baby wash/shampoo
- Ivory soap
- Iodine/iodophor
- Chlorhexidine gluconate (CHG) (Note: CHG must not be used in the inner ear)

PROCEDURE CHECKLIST

Instruments
- Standard sets
- Specialty instruments
  - Drill/saw
  - Irrigation accessories
  - Nerve monitoring device

Equipment
- Microscope
- Video equipment
- Laser
- Electrosurgical units (ESU) (both monopolar and bipolar)
- Suction
- Smoke evacuator
- Headlights

Additional Supplies: both sterile and nonsterile
- Check with physician for any other requested supplies, instruments, or equipment not normally used before the start of the procedure
- Ear drainage tubes
- Prosthetic devices
- Tracheotomy tubes
- Nasal splints
- Sponges
- Drapes
- Gowns and gloves for team members
- "Have ready" and "hold" supplies

Medications and Irrigation Solutions
A sterile table or Mayo stand will be required for local anesthesia administration. The "local" will be used before prepping or draping. The remainder of the local anesthesia is kept on the sterile field, labeled appropriately, with medication safety practices followed.
- Lidocaine with epinephrine
- Decongestant such as phenylephrine
- Cocaine (nasal procedures)
- Topical adrenaline for hemostasis
- Absorbable gelatin
- Oxidized cellulose
- Silver nitrate
- Epinephrine
- Thrombin

Drains and Dressings
- Cottonoids
- Packing
- Sterile rubber band (ear procedures)
- Penrose drains (ear and neck procedures)
- Jackson-Pratt (neck procedures)

Specimen Care
- Proper container for each specimen
- Labels for each specimen
- Proper solution for specimen type

Types of Hearing Loss

Classification	Definition	Causes
Conductive	Loss of hearing acuity resulting from failure to conduct sound from external ear to middle ear	Blockage of external canal with cerumen or foreign bodies Edema Trauma Infection Tympanic perforation Otosclerosis, ossicular chain fixation
Sensorineural	Loss of hearing acuity resulting from failure to conduct sound to inner ear (cochlea or acoustic nerve)	Ototoxic medications Exposure to loud noise Trauma Meniere's disease Tumor Presbycusis Infectious disease (measles, mumps, meningitis)
Mixed	Loss of hearing acuity resulting from combination of conductive and sensorineural factors	Develops secondary to either conductive or sensorineural loss (e.g., patient with presbycusis and impacted cerumen)

visual enhancement of some anatomic structures and pathologic tissues, including highly vascularized tumors. CT is the study of choice to assess intratemporal bone pathologic conditions and to evaluate the paranasal sinuses and adjacent structures. It is also used in the assessment of the oral cavity and neck.

Magnetic Resonance Imaging. Magnetic resonance imaging (MRI) is an imaging modality using powerful magnetic and radiofrequency waves to reproduce cross-sectional images of the human body without exposing the patient to ionizing radiation. On an MRI scan, fat and fluid produce high-intensity signals, which appear as bright areas, whereas bone and air emit weak signals and appear as darkened areas on the scan. MRI is often used with CT imaging in a complementary fashion when evaluating lesions in and around bone for a variety of head and neck conditions including tumors in the oral cavity, external auditory canal, middle ear, and mastoid.

Audiogram. Patients scheduled for otologic surgery may have undergone evaluation of their hearing through audiograms to determine whether they have normal hearing, conductive hearing loss, or sensorineural hearing loss (see table above). Two types of audiometric testing, pure tone and speech audiometry, are performed on patients with suspected hearing loss.

EVIDENCE FOR PRACTICE

Strategies for Communicating with a Hearing-Impaired Patient

Hearing deficits in patients must be considered when performing assessment, planning and implementing interventions, and providing education. Preexisting and postoperative hearing deficits can present a communication challenge for patients, their families, and OR team. Recommended strategies for communicating with a hearing-impaired patient include the following:

◆ Position yourself directly in front of the patient. Most people who have hearing loss rely heavily on seeing the speaker's face (best distance is about 3 feet).
◆ Ensure that the room is well lighted, making sure the light is shining at the speaker and not in the eyes of the patient.
◆ Get the patient's attention before beginning to speak.
◆ Ask the patient what you need to do so that he or she can best understand you.
◆ If one ear is better than the other, move closer to the less-affected side.
◆ Speak clearly and slowly using a good elocutionary style (do not exaggerate mouth movements).
◆ Do not shout. Shouting raises the frequency of sound and makes understanding more difficult.
◆ Try not to mumble or lower the sound intensity of words at the end of sentences.
◆ Decrease background noise as much as possible when attempting communication with the patient.
◆ Do not chew gum and speak at the same time.
◆ Keep hands and other objects away from your mouth and the speaker's mouth when talking to the patient.
◆ When family members are present, speak directly to the patient. Do not refer to the patient in the third person.
◆ Minimize distractions.
◆ Rephrase rather than repeat—the patient may not have understood a particular word or phrase.
◆ Have the patient repeat back, in his or her own words, your statements to assess understanding.
◆ Use appropriate hand motions.
◆ Be patient and relax. By working together, you can help maximize effective communication.
◆ Write messages on paper if the patient is able to read.

Modified from Russek JA: Care of patients with ear and hearing problems. In Ignatavicius DD, Workman ML, editors: *Medical-surgical nursing: patient-centered collaborative care,* ed 6, Philadelphia, 2010, Saunders; Medwetsky L: Hearing loss. In Duthie EJ et al, editors, *Practice of geriatrics,* ed 4, Philadelphia, 2007, Saunders.

Planning

The development of a plan of care is based on the preoperative assessment, expected outcomes, and the surgery being performed. Patients undergoing otolaryngologic procedures may have special communication needs that must be considered in planning effective care. The OR team should determine the best way to communicate with patients who have hearing deficits or impaired vocalization. Information given to the patient should be reinforced as needed throughout the perioperative experience. The OR environment must be quiet and free of any loud noise. Intraoperative noises, such as those from suction, electrosurgical units (ESUs), and other equipment, should be explained to the locally anesthetized patient before they are generated. This will help avoid startling the patient and adversely affecting the success of the surgery. Patients receiving local anesthetics need to remain still during the procedure, so providing for comfort measures becomes especially important. The room temperature should be regulated at a comfortable setting, and the patient should be adequately covered to maintain normal body temperature.

Preparation of the OR includes checking the availability and functional capacity of suction, the surgeon's headlight and light source, and the ESU. It is essential that the x-ray view box is in working order and appropriately located so that scans may be easily viewed by the surgeon during the procedure. In endoscopic procedures, the navigation tower and monitor should be rolled to the head of the table and tested to ensure proper functioning of the light source for the camera wands and suction. If the surgeon plans on video-recording the procedure, assurance that the video recorder is adequately working is needed before the start of the procedure.

Implementation

The following interventions should be instituted by the OR team:

1. Use the institutional verification process immediately before surgery to identify the correct surgical site. This should include verifying the operative side and site with the patient or family and confirmation through review of the medical record, informed consent, diagnostic test reports, and other members of the surgical team during the time-out.
2. Verify that the patient has maintained nothing-by-mouth (NPO) status as directed and that requested laboratory studies are on the medical record.
3. Provide calm, careful, and comforting measures to reduce the patient's anxiety. Allow the patient time to comply with requests, and explain the sequence of perioperative events.
4. Allow patients who wear hearing aids to wear them to the OR. Properly remove them at the time of or after anesthesia induction, or leave them in place if local anesthesia is used. Prescription eyewear should be brought into the holding area because hearing-impaired patients may require them to assist in lip reading when instructions and procedures are explained. If the patient has impaired vocalization, the OR personnel should ensure that the patient's preferred method of communication (e.g., pen and paper, artificial larynx) is available. Disposition of any assistive devices brought into the OR must be documented on the record.
5. Protect patients with impaired communication from injury. The OR must be a controlled environment because excess stimulation interferes with the patient's ability to hear, vocalize, and comply with instructions and explanations.
6. Carefully review instructions for patients receiving local anesthetics. Remind the patient of the need to remain immobile during the procedure and report any adverse symptoms related to the anesthetic. Symptoms of adverse drug reactions include skin changes, such as rash or itching; restlessness; unexplained anxiety or fearfulness; diaphoresis; and complaints of blurred vision, tinnitus, dizziness, nausea, palpitations or acute changes in heart rate, disturbed respiration, pallor or flushing, and syncope. Emergency drugs,

suction apparatus, and resuscitation equipment, including a defibrillator should be readily available.
7. The circulator will remain with the patient throughout the induction phase of anesthesia.
8. Perform any hair removal by clipping. Protect the patient's eyes during skin preparation.
9. Promote normothermia through the use of thermal warming blankets, forced-air warming units, and warm IV and irrigating solutions.
10. Use sequential compression devices (SCDs) to decrease the risk of deep venous thrombosis (DVT) and pulmonary embolism (PE) during long surgical procedures.
11. Document the serial number and lot numbers of any implanted materials according to institutional policy.
12. Initiate and document laser safety precautions if the laser is used.

Preoperative Room Preparation. Before the patient enters the OR, the perioperative nurse and surgical technologist gather the equipment and supplies for the scheduled procedure. A well-organized surgical environment can significantly reduce anesthesia time and enable the perioperative nurse to spend more time attending to the preoperative and intraoperative needs of the patient. Planning includes identifying equipment, instrumentation, furniture, and positioning accessories necessary to perform the surgery. Such equipment may include the operating microscope, video system, monopolar and bipolar ESUs, suction, nerve integrity monitors, specialty instrument sets, prosthetic devices, drill and irrigation accessories, and the laser. A dedicated otorhinolaryngologic specialty storage cart centrally houses assorted prostheses, drill burrs and accessories, and dressing and packing materials, which contributes to efficiency when providing intraoperative care.

Positioning. The supine position with modifications is used during otorhinolaryngologic procedures. The OR personnel gather the supplies necessary to ensure comfort of the patient in a supine position. These usually include a foam headrest or a pillow for under the knees, and warm blankets. The patient's extremities at pressure points and at major nerves should be padded. A pillow should be placed under the thighs and the legs should be slightly angled to decrease pressure on the patient's back; this positioning should be carried out before the patient is anesthetized to ensure comfort. Arms are placed on padded armboards with the palms up and fingers extended. Armboards are maintained at less than a 90-degree angle to prevent brachial plexus stretch. If there are surgical reasons to tuck the arms at the side, the elbows are padded to protect the ulnar nerve, the palms face inward, and the wrist is maintained in a neutral position (Denholm, 2009). A drape secures the arms. It should be tucked snugly under the patient, not under the mattress. This prevents the arm from shifting downward intraoperatively and resting against the OR bed rail. The placement of IV lines in an arm that is to be tucked at the side should be avoided, but in cases where this is not avoidable, patency of those lines must be ensured.

OTOLOGIC SURGICAL POSITIONING. Microscopes are used for most otologic procedures. Based on the design of the microscope and the OR bed used, the patient may be placed on the bed in the reverse position—with the patient's head at the foot of the bed—to facilitate proper placement of the microscope mounted on a floor stand and to allow adequate space for the surgeon and assistant to be positioned on sitting stools near the surgical site.

The patient is placed supine with the operative side as close to the edge of the OR bed as possible, with the head turned and the operative ear upward. This positioning gives the surgeon access in viewing all areas of the middle ear and mastoid. One or more safety/restraining belts are used to secure the patient on the OR bed to ensure safety when turning or rotating the bed. During some procedures, such as mastoidectomy, the patient's head may be secured in position by placing tape across the head and attaching it to the frame of the OR bed. For other procedures, such as myringtomy, the patient's head may be immobilized and supported on a foam headrest. A donut-shaped foam head support helps to immobilize the head and permits easy adjustment of the angle while the operating microscope is being used.

To protect the nonoperative ear, ensure that it is in the center of the donut hole and that the headrest does not cause any pressure on the ear. The dependent arm on the nonoperative side must also be well padded and properly positioned to minimize pressure injury; the patient's body weight could cause injury when the OR bed is rotated laterally to optimize surgical access. Special consideration must be given when the patient's head is positioned for surgery, especially when general anesthetics are used. Extremes in neck extension and head torsion can cause injury to the brachial plexus or cervical spine. Other options to assist in patient positioning are determined by the otologic procedure to be performed and by the surgeon's preference. They may include ophthalmic headrests with a crescent-shaped pad, a padded horseshoe-shaped headrest, or a headrest with skull pins such as the Mayfield, which is used in certain neurologic procedures.

Positioning of the surgeon is equally important to the success of the surgery. The surgeon's chair should be positioned at a height and distance that allow comfortable access to the operative site. The use of hydraulic or electric chairs enables the surgeon to adjust the position to meet these needs.

RHINOLOGIC SURGICAL POSITIONING. A standard headrest may be used to maintain the head in normal position but is not necessary. The entire bed is turned 90 degrees to allow the right-handed surgeon to work from the patient's right side, and the right arm is tucked in at the patient's side. Pad the elbows to protect the ulnar nerve; place the palms facing inward and the wrist in a neutral position. Depending on the procedure, the left arm may be maintained by the anesthesia provider and usually has the IV line placed in it for easier access. The anesthesia provider will be at the patient's head. Raising the head of the bed greater than 45 degrees uses gravity to help minimize intraoperative bleeding. The scrub person may stand at the patient's head or near the patient's waist next to the surgeon's right arm (Figure 10-12). The Mayo stand can be positioned at the head and to the side of the bed; however, it is most commonly positioned over the patient's chest, depending on where the scrub person is standing. If indicated for the procedure, the perioperative nurse assists with setting up the navigation towers and video monitor equipment at this time.

ORAL CAVITY/LARYNGOLOGIC/NECK SURGICAL POSITIONING. The patient is usually placed in the supine

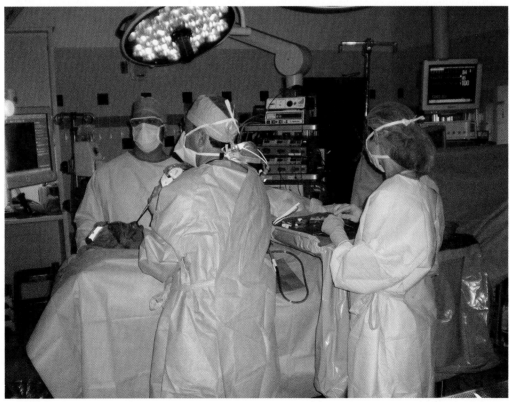

FIGURE 10-12 Nasal procedure with scrub person on right side of surgeon.

BOX 10-1

Nitrous Oxide and the Middle Ear

The middle ear and paranasal sinuses are normal body air cavities and consist of open, nonventilated spaces. The middle ear cavity is vented periodically when the eustachian tube opens. During general anesthesia, inhaled nitrous oxide diffuses into the middle ear space through the capillaries of the middle ear mucosa. This results in increased middle ear pressure. Rapid increases in middle ear pressure proportional to inhaled levels of nitrous oxide and abnormal eustachian tube function may cause nausea, vomiting, and rupture of the tympanic membrane in susceptible patients. This includes patients having previous ear surgery, otitis media, sinusitis, upper respiratory tract infections, enlarged adenoids, or other disorders of the nasopharynx.

When nitrous oxide is discontinued, the gas is rapidly reabsorbed and strong negative pressure in the middle ear may occur. This negative pressure may result in nausea, vomiting, serous otitis, hemotympanum, disarticulation of the stapes, and impaired hearing. Some practitioners believe the use of nitrous oxide as an anesthetic inhalation agent is hazardous to hearing in patients who have undergone previous reconstructive middle ear surgery.

Modified from Donlon JV et al: Anesthesia for eye, ear, nose, and throat surgery. In Miller RD, editor: Miller's anesthesia, ed 6, Philadelphia, 2005, Churchill Livingstone.

position. A shoulder roll may be used for hyperextension of the neck. The headrest should allow easy movement of the head from side-to-side yet should maintain support. The patient's arms are often tucked at the sides as described earlier in this section to allow access of the surgical team to the operative site. If a microscope or video equipment is used, the OR bed may be turned to accommodate this equipment.

Anesthesia. Both the use of general anesthesia and the infiltration of a local anesthetic agent (local anesthesia) have advantages during otorhinolaryngologic surgery. General anesthesia provides airway control and allows the patient to remain still throughout the procedure, thereby making surgery technically easier to perform, but requires particular attention to extremes in head positioning, possible air emboli, the control of bleeding, and, for otologic procedures, the effects of nitrous oxide in the middle ear (Box 10-1). All anesthetics create an oxygen-rich atmosphere and the perioperative team must consider the patient's safety in this environment (Risk Reduction Strategies).

Local anesthesia is used alone or as an adjunct to many procedures. Safe administration of medication is essential for achieving optimal outcomes (Surgical Pharmacology). Lidocaine is frequently combined with epinephrine. A concentration of 1:200,000 provides maximum vasoconstriction, but some surgeons prefer a concentration of 1:100,000. Cocaine 4% topical solution is the second medication that is used commonly for rhinologic procedures. It is a good vasoconstrictor with the added benefit of anesthetic properties. Some surgeons use a nasal decongestant instead of cocaine for nasal vasoconstriction. These decongestants do not produce some of the cardiac effects seen with cocaine. Because nasal and sinus surgeries are performed in such a confined space, vasoconstriction becomes crucial for appropriate visualization of the surgical field. Hypertension can increase bleeding despite the use of vasoconstrictive agents and may need to be managed medically by the anesthesia provider intraoperatively if the visual field becomes compromised and surgery is impaired.

For rhinologic procedures, before the patient arrives in the OR the surgical technologist prepares a separate prep table, which includes a labeled container of the vasoconstrictor solution, x-ray–detectable cottonoid sponges (usually ½ inch × 3 inches with attached strings), bayonet forceps, and a small nasal speculum. The surgeon soaks the cottonoid sponges with the vasoconstrictor solution and usually packs the nose with the sponges before prepping and draping, to allow time for the vasoconstrictive properties to take effect. The cottonoids are left in place. Some surgeons will also inject local anesthetic at this time, but others may wait to inject at the time of surgery. Maximum vasoconstriction occurs in approximately 10 to 12 minutes after the administration of epinephrine. If a local anesthetic is to be injected next, the prep table should also include a 10-ml Luer-Lok syringe, appropriate-size needle (usually 25 gauge, 1½ inches), and labeled lidocaine (0.5% to 2%, according to surgeon's preference). Additional syringes, needles, and labeled local anesthetic solution should be available on the sterile field for additional administration intraoperatively. Additional labeled cocaine solution and cottonoids should be available on the sterile field as well. The nurse and scrub person ensure that the cottonoids are counted before and at the end of the procedure. (If a cottonoid is placed extremely posterior along the nasal floor, it can slide past the palate and may be swallowed or aspirated by the patient.)

Topical agents used in laryngeal surgery include epinephrine, phenylephrine hydrochloride, or cocaine. These agents may be applied on a cottonoid or sprayed directly on the vocal cords. Lidocaine 4% (Xylocaine) may be instilled into the trachea to decrease the cough reflex when it becomes an obstacle to a thorough physical assessment.

Local anesthesia combined with sedation or monitored anesthesia care is often employed for surgery in the premeatal region and for stapedectomy and uncomplicated middle ear procedures of less than 2-hours' duration, some rhinologic procedures, and some excisional neck procedures. Sedation should render the patient calm, comfortable, cooperative, and able to understand and communicate. Patients should not be overmedicated to the point of demonstrating obtunded reflexes or being out of touch with their surroundings. Documentation should follow institutional policy for recording intraoperative medications administered (AORN, 2009a).

Preparation of the Operative Site. If hair removal is absolutely necessary, clipping is preferred because shaving may injure the skin and increase the risk of infection. Postauricular and endaural incisions extending upward from the meatus require hair to be about 1 to 2 cm away from the proposed

▶▶ RISK REDUCTION STRATEGIES

Managing the Risk of Fire in Oxygen-Rich Environments

Some estimates suggest that between 50 and 200 OR fires occur in the United States every year, with as many as 20% of reported fires resulting in serious injury or death (Caplan, 2008). Three elements must be present for fire to occur: heat, fuel, and oxygen. All elements are present in the OR.

Patients undergoing otorhinolaryngologic procedures are at greater risk for fire injury because of the proximity of the surgical field to high concentrations of oxygen. Devices used in this specialty (e.g., lasers, fiberoptic light cables, ESU, high-speed surgical drills and burrs) further contribute to risk by providing heat and fuel.

Specific recommendations include:

◆ Awareness of risk factors. Oxygen vents into the atmosphere from facemasks, nasal cannulae, and uncuffed endotracheal tubes, accumulating under surgical drapes. This creates an oxygen-enriched atmosphere within the proximity of the surgical site for otorhinolaryngologic procedures.

◆ Discussion of risk. The perioperative nurse and scrub person should collaborate before procedures to plan for risk and ensure that sterile saline is available on the surgical field, the holster is used for the active ESU electrode, and the volumes of music, conversation, and ambient room noise are reasonable so that the audio from the ESU or laser can be heard. A careful review of the facility protocol for handling fire in the OR, including verification of the location of fire pull alarms, extinguishers, and evacuation routes, is essential and should not be minimized.

◆ Implementation of specific safety protocols for the use of the laser and the ESU in the airway:

  • Use only air for open delivery on the face for spontaneous breathing sedated patients who can maintain safe blood oxygen saturation without supplemental oxygen.

• A laser-resistant endotracheal tube should be used, specific to the laser used for the procedure (e.g., CO_2, Nd:YAG). The cuff of the laser tube should be filled with saline and colored with an indicator dye such as methylene blue. Before activating the laser the surgeon should inform the anesthesia provider so that the oxygen concentration delivered to the patient can be safely reduced. Additionally, the surgeon should wait a few minutes before activating the laser to allow the oxygen concentration to diminish.

• Cuffed endotracheal tubes should be used whenever possible for airway procedures. Before activating the ESU inside the airway, the surgeon should give the anesthesia provider adequate notice that the ignition source is about to be activated. The anesthesia provider should reduce the oxygen concentration to the minimum required to prevent hypoxia and the surgeon should wait a few minutes before using the ESU to allow the oxygen concentration to diminish.

• Scavenging with the wound suction may be used to reduce the oxygen concentration in the operative field.

• Sponges and cottonoids (and cottonoid strings) should be moistened when used in oxygen-rich environments to reduce the ignition potential from sources such as the laser or ESU.

• If an uncuffed endotracheal tube must be used, moistened sponges should be used around the field to minimize leakage and reduce potential heat buildup.

◆ An immediate halt to the procedure when early warning signs of a fire are noticed. For fire in the airway or breathing circuit, the endotracheal tube should be removed and all flammable and burning materials should be removed from the airway. Delivery of all airway gases should stop, and saline should be poured into the patient's airway to extinguish any residual embers and cool the tissues.

Modified from Association of periOperative Registered Nurses: Guidelines for fire prevention in the operating room. In *Perioperative standards and recommended practices*, Denver, 2009, The Association; Caplan RA: Practice advisory for the prevention and management of operating room fires: a report by the American Society of Anesthesiologists task force on operating room fires, *Anesthesiology* 108:786-801, 2008; Everson CR: Fire prevention in the perioperative setting: perioperative fires can occur everywhere, *Periop Nurs Clin* 3:333-343, 2008; Richter GT, Willging JP: Suction cautery and electrosurgical risks in otolaryngology, *Int J Pediatr Otorhinolaryngol* 72:1013-1021, 2008; (no author): Fire prevention: avoid oxygen to face, *OR Manager* 261 (1) 18, 2010.

---

incision site so that hair will not be in the operative field. Long hair is easily managed and kept out of the way with tape or lubricant. It is good practice to pull the top hair out of the way and only clip under the hair, to help maximize normal hair aesthetics postoperatively. Plastic adhesive drapes can be applied circumferentially around the proposed incision site, or a clear sterile drape laid over the entire surgical area. Parotid surgery may require hair removal from just below the temple to a line even with or slightly behind the pinna of the ear. Head and neck surgeries may require removal of hair on the chest to the nipple area on both sides. Thorough drying of the surgical area after the prep has been applied is critical for proper adhesion of the drapes to the skin so sterility is maintained throughout the operative procedure.

A povidone-iodine solution is generally used (unless the patient is allergic to iodine) to prep the surgical site for otologic and head and neck procedures. Povidone-iodine 10% (i.e., Betadine) is generally considered safe for the middle ear space and has not been found to be ototoxic in animal studies; however, in the presence of a tympanic membrane perforation, swabbing of

the ear canal skin is preferred to gross spillage in the ear canal to prevent large volumes of prep solution from entering the middle ear space. All other surgical prep solutions, such as chlorhexidine and alcohol, are considered ototoxic and should be strictly limited to the outer ear and surrounding skin. Head and neck procedures may involve extensive skin preparation and usually include the entire area from the chin to the nipples; it may also include a donor skin graft site if a defect or large flap coverage is anticipated. Some surgeons prefer the patient's face to be included in the prep, depending on the type of surgery anticipated and the site of the lesion. If a flap may be raised to reconstruct a defect, saline should be available to remove the discoloration from the skin to allow the surgeon to check for flap viability.

Prepping of the nose and face may or may not be done for rhinologic and laryngeal/oral cavity procedures, depending on the surgical procedure and institutional policy. These areas are considered "dirty" and not possible to prep as effectively as other surgical sites, such as an abdomen. The surgical field is maintained in sterile fashion, and these procedures usually have a "clean contaminated" wound classification.

SURGICAL PHARMACOLOGY

Medications Commonly Used in Otorhinolaryngologic Surgery

Category	Dose/Route/Mechanism	Purpose/Action	Adverse Reactions
LOCAL ANESTHETICS			
Lidocaine, 0.5% or 1%	Local injection	Blocks pain and temperature fibers, used as medium to dilute epinephrine	Cardiovascular, hypotension, confusion, dizziness, headache, somnolence, tremor, injection site pain, cardiac arrest, cardiac dysrhythmia, seizure
Tetracaine (Pontocaine)	Topical; 0.25%-0.5% by nebulization or direct application	Blocks pain, suppresses gag reflex	Pain, redness, irritation on initial contact
Benzocaine/tetracaine/ butamben (Cetacaine)	Topical; available in gel, liquid, and spray	Blocks pain, suppresses gag reflex	Dry mouth, dizziness
Benzocaine	Topical; available in 20% gel and 20% spray	Blocks pain, suppresses gag reflex	Dry mouth, dizziness
Lidocaine hydrochloride	Available as 4% solution, 2% viscous solution	Local anesthetic	High doses may cause cardiac dysrhythmias, minor burning and stinging of mouth and throat on initial contact
Cocaine hydrochloride	4% topical swab, packing instilled into cavity or spray, may be applied directly to vocal cords or other laryngeal structures on pledgets to promote vasoconstriction	Local anesthetic (also used as vasoconstrictor)	CNS depression, CNS stimulation, anxiety, tachydysrhythmia, seizures; may interact with cannabis, promethazine (Phenergan), and St. John's wort
VASOCONSTRICTORS			
Oxymetazoline hydrochloride (Afrin Nasal Spray, Neo-Synephrine 12 Hr, Nasacon)	0.05% nasal spray	Nasal decongestant used for vasoconstriction	Headache, insomnia, nervousness, nasal congestion, rebound congestion, dry nasal mucosa, nasal stinging/burning, sneezing, cardiac dysrhythmia, hypertension, tachydysrhythmia
Epinephrine	1:100,000 to 1:200,000	Used for vasoconstriction	Palpitations, tachydysrhythmia, paleness and sweating, nausea and vomiting, asthenia, dizziness, headache, tremor, pain in eye, anxiety, apprehension, nervousness, dyspnea, cardiac dysrhythmia, hypertensive crisis, pulmonary edema
ANTIBIOTICS			
Mupirocin (Nasal Bactroban)	2% topical	Antibacterial and lubricant for nasal packing, applied topically to skin incisions	Dermatologic, nasal stinging and burning, disorder of taste, headache
Bacitracin	Topical ointment, 500 units/g	Antibacterial, antibiotic	Swelling, contact dermatitis, pruritus
STEROIDS			
Triamcinolone acetonide (Aristocort, Kenalog)	Topical	Used topically to lubricate packs or expand packing	Hypertension, atrophic condition of skin
Cortisporin Otic suspension (neomycin and polymyxin B sulfates/ hydrocortisone)	Topical	Used after otologic surgery as an antiinflammatory/ antibiotic agent	Itching, pain, stinging, burning, ototoxicity

CNS, Central nervous system.

Modified from Dimmitt P: A review of topical anesthetics and decongestants, *ORL Head Neck Nurs* 23(2):21-24, 2005; Skidmore-Roth L: *Mosby's drug guide for nurses with 2010 update,* ed 8, St Louis, 2010, Mosby; Hodgson BB, Kizior RJ: *Saunders nursing drug handbook 2010,* St Louis, 2010, Saunders; Chow AW: Infections of the oral cavity, neck, and head. In Mandell GL et al, editors: *Principles and practice of infectious diseases,* ed 6, Philadelphia, 2005, Churchill Livingstone.

Facial Nerve Monitoring. Audible facial nerve monitors are used intraoperatively during procedures in which the facial nerve is at risk. The purpose of this monitoring technique is to assist in the early identification of the nerve, to increase the possibility of its preservation by minimizing trauma, and to assess its integrity after dissection (Mahlan et al, 2005). Electrodes are placed into the facial muscles before the patient is draped. Consultation and communication with the anesthesia provider are essential because the use of muscle relaxants and long-term paralyzing agents must be avoided. In the setting of a tympanic membrane perforation, lidocaine should not be allowed to spill into the middle ear space when injecting the ear canal, as temporary facial paralysis can ensue from topical anesthesia of a dehiscent facial nerve in the tympanic segment. Facial nerve monitoring is commonly used during acoustic neuroma and mastoid surgery (Figure 10-13).

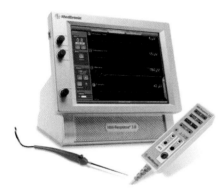

FIGURE 10-13 NIM-Response 3.0 Nerve Integrity Monitor System.

Draping. Barrier draping minimizes the risk of postoperative infection. Draping technique is based on the surgeon's preference and the procedure to be performed.

OTOLOGIC DRAPING. Draping may be minimal for procedures such as myringotomy. For major otologic procedures, plastic adhesive drapes are applied around the ear to keep the patient's hair out of the surgical field. Sterile, plastic, aperture drapes may be placed over the surgical site with the ear exposed through the opening. The surgeon may elect to expose a portion of the face on the affected side to observe facial movement.

Three or four towels are draped over the aperture drape around the ear and may be secured with nonpenetrating towel clips. A fenestrated drape is unfolded over the patient, with the opening centered over the operative site. An alternative method is the use of a split sheet with the split end secured at the base of the ear and the open flaps wrapped around the patient's head. Disposable drapes with adhesive backing may be used to secure the sheet to the patient.

During mastoid surgery and for resections of acoustic tumors, fluid-collection pouches may be attached to the drape. These pouches will catch fluid runoff when drilling and irrigation are planned. The operating microscope is draped to extend the sterile field (Figure 10-14).

Special consideration must be given to the selection of draping material used during ear surgery and to the technique for removing powder from surgical gloves. Powder and lint cling to gloves and can be transferred to instruments and introduced into the ear. They act as a foreign body in the wound, causing the formation of granulomas in the middle and inner ear, and may contribute to irreversible hearing loss. Therefore gloves

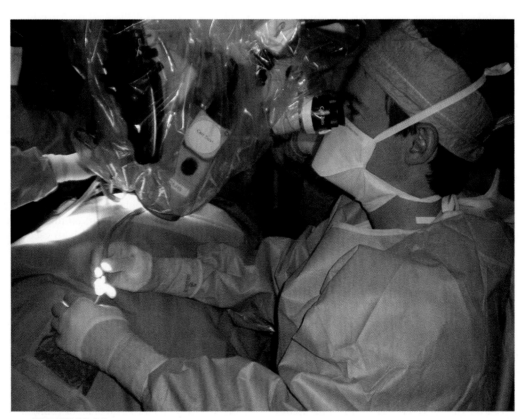

FIGURE 10-14 Draped microscope for otologic surgery with surgeon in correct sitting position.

worn by the surgical team should be rinsed to remove powder and lint. Lint-free drapes should be used.

RHINOLOGIC DRAPING. Draping is done for most rhinologic procedures. A small sheet with a towel on top of it is placed under the patient's head, and the towel is secured around the hairline with a nonpenetrating towel clip. A split sheet is then placed around the head. It is good practice to place a towel over the endotracheal (ET) tube if one is in place; this helps prevent the adhesive portion of the split sheet from sticking to the ET tube and inadvertently pulling on the tube once the procedure is completed and drapes are removed. Except during certain endoscopic procedures, the patient's eyes should be covered with moist gauze or towels if the patient is awake or taped closed if the patient has received a general anesthetic, protecting the eyes from nasal drainage or injury from instruments.

ORAL CAVITY/LARYNGOLOGIC/NECK PROCEDURE DRAPING. Draping of the patient for a laryngeal procedure for a benign lesion (intraoral approach) is minimal, with the primary focus being protection of the patient's eyes and face. This may be accomplished by (1) placing ointment in the patient's eyes, (2) taping the eyelids closed with a nonabrasive, nonirritating tape, (3) applying moist padding over the tape (if use of a laser is anticipated), and (4) placing self-adhering eye pads over the moistened pads. A head drape may be placed over the patient's face to expose only the lips and chin.

Draping for neck procedures often varies according to surgeon preference and is similar to the draping procedures described for rhinologic surgery. Additional drapes may be needed if skin grafts or flaps will be used for reconstructive procedures.

Surgical Microscope. The surgical microscope is often used to provide illumination and magnification for complex procedures to the ear, laryngeal surgery, or reconstructive free flap procedures following neck surgery. Several kinds of surgical microscopes with different attachments are available for otologic and laryngologic surgery. The microscope may be floor- or ceiling-mounted. Optimal light is provided by a xenon or halogen light source. Numerous types of monocular and binocular heads are available for the microscope. These heads may be fixed in a straight or angled plane, or they may be designed to be adjustable in an inclinable plane. For operations through an ear speculum, the microscope provides direct light and permits the surgeon to select a magnification of ×6, ×10, ×16, ×25, or ×40. A common eyepiece magnification for an otologic microscope is ×12.5, and the usual objective (lens) is 250- or 300-mm focal length (f). A 400-mm lens is used for laryngeal surgery. The total magnification is determined by multiplying the magnification of the eyepiece times that of the microscope body times that of the objective. The type of head and objective selected is based on the surgeon's preference. Microscopes equipped with a variable distance feature allow the surgeon to adjust the focal length from 200 mm to 400 mm without changing the lens objective. Video equipment may be attached to the microscope, which allows other team members to follow the procedure and to anticipate the necessary instrumentation. Before lenses are placed into the microscope, they should be checked to ensure that they are free from lint, dust, fingerprints, and soil. The surgeon adjusts the microscope before it is draped for surgery and manipulates it during the

procedure. The microscope is draped with a sterile cover for otologic surgery, but is often left undraped for laryngeal procedures. It is necessary to keep the drape material away from the light source fan of the microscope. Doing so will allow cool air to continue to circulate and will avoid overheating of the fan, which could prematurely burn out the lamp and possibly cause a fire. When micromanipulators are secured to transmit laser energy to tissue through the operating microscope, special microscope laser drapes must be used. These drapes have an opening in the plastic at the base of the micromanipulator covering the objective, allowing laser energy to pass through the opening of the drape without risk of burning the drape.

Care should be taken when removing the drapes from the microscope to avoid discarding the eyepieces with the drapes or dropping them on the floor. Eyepieces have been lost or damaged in this manner, necessitating costly repair or replacement.

When the microscope is not in use, it should be kept in a locked, upright position and stored in an area that is away from traffic, free from dust, and properly ventilated. Ideally, a set of eyepieces should be left in the scope to prevent the inside of the scope from becoming dusty. The microscope may also be covered with either a protective cover or a plastic bag.

Equipment and Instrumentation. Equipment that may be used in otorhinolaryngologic surgery includes an ESU (both monopolar and bipolar), a forced-air warming unit or other device to maintain normothermia, and headlights. Lasers assist in vaporization of scar tissue, granulomas, and cholesteatomas without damaging surrounding tissue and may be used for select otolaryngologic procedures. Lasers used in this specialty include the carbon dioxide (CO_2), potassium titanyl phosphate (KTP), erbium:yttrium-aluminum-garnet (Er:YAG), and neodymium:yttrium-aluminum-garnet (Nd:YAG) lasers. Lasers can be secured to the operating microscope and laser energy delivered to the tissue by means of a micromanipulator. Laser energy is delivered directly to tissue by fiberoptic probes, which can be navigated around obstructing structures.

For complex reconstructive procedures in the neck, a Doppler unit (to determine the viability of blood vessels) and an electromyographic nerve monitor (to determine the location and quality of nerves) may be employed.

Specimen cups, labels, and a marking pen should be available on the sterile field because often several specimens are obtained. Institutional procedure for correct patient and specimen identification should be followed (AORN, 2009b).

The instrumentation used in otorhinolaryngologic surgery is quite specific and is discussed with each surgical intervention. Head and neck instrumentation combines general surgical instruments and procedure-specific instruments. Many otolaryngologic procedures use delicate microinstruments that should be handled individually and should not be allowed to physically contact each other (Figure 10-15). Fine tympanoplasty and stapedectomy instrumentation should be kept in special storage and sterilization trays. These trays help separate instruments, aid in quick identification, protect the instruments from damage, and facilitate handling during surgery. Instruments used in the path of the operating microscope may have an ebony glare-reducing finish. Handles of assorted knives and dissectors may be flat, hexagonal, or round for better gripping or handling during surgery (see Figure 10-15). The shaft of

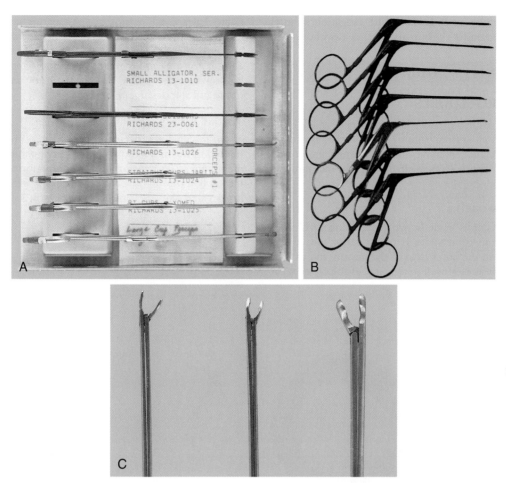

FIGURE 10-15 A, Microsurgical ear forceps including various sizes of cup forceps and alligator forceps. **B**, Forceps out of tray. **C**, Close-up of types of forceps tips. *Left to right*, Straight cup forceps, right cup forceps, large cup forceps.

these instruments may be straight, angled, or bayonet-shaped. Other commonly used instruments are shown in Figures 10-16 through 10-21.

Powered Equipment. A powered sagittal saw is used for complex neck procedures. A power drill and assorted rotating burrs are essential for middle ear surgery and some sinus procedures. Many drills are commercially available that are pneumatically or electrically driven. Pneumatic drills must have high torque (power) and more than 20,000 revolutions per minute (rpm) (speed). Some surgeons believe electrically powered drills offer equal torque but better control of the drill tip.

A selection of burrs including assorted sizes of round cutting burrs and diamond polishing burrs should be available. A diamond burr cuts slowly and grinds the bone away rather than tearing into it; it is commonly used around vital structures. Cutting burrs assist in quickly removing bone from areas not close to vital structures. The grooves or teeth of burrs must be clean of bone dust. Bone-cutting burrs tend to clog more easily than coarse-toothed burrs. A sterile wire brush may be used to keep burrs clean intraoperatively. Bone dust must be prevented from settling in areas such as those in stapedectomy, tympanoplasty, endolymphatic sac, or fenestration surgery.

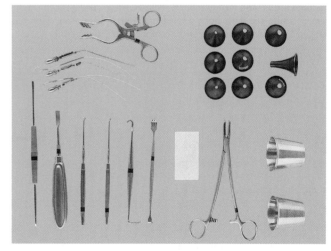

FIGURE 10-16 *Left, top to bottom:* 1 Weitlaner retractor, dull prongs, angled; 3 Baron ear suction tubes with finger valve control: 3, 5, and 7 Fr; 2 stylets. *Right, top to bottom:* 9 Richards ear speculums, assorted sizes, 4 to 8 mm, one side view. *Bottom, left to right:* 1 Cottle elevator, double-ended; 1 Lempert elevator (converse periosteal); 2 Johnson skin hooks; 2 Senn-Kanavel retractors, side view and front view; 1 House Teflon block; 1 House Gelfoam press or Sheehy fascia press; 2 metal medicine cups, 2 oz.

A sterile field continuously flooded with irrigation solution helps to lessen clogging of the burr and washes away bone dust.

Surgical Interventions

OTOLOGIC PROCEDURES

The majority of otologic procedures are performed either through the ear canal or from behind the ear. Incisions through the ear canal include endaural and transcanal approaches. The postauricular approach is made through an incision from behind the ear.

Endaural Approach

The endaural incision is made in two steps, using a #15 blade scalpel. The first incision starts at the superior meatal wall about 1 cm in from the outer edge of the meatus and extends down the posterior meatal wall to the edge of the conchal car-

tilage. The second incision on the superior meatal wall extends upward to a point halfway between the meatus and upper edge of the auricle. This approach offers direct access to the external auditory meatus and tympanic membrane and may be used for meatoplasty, canalplasty, selected tympanic membrane perforations, and stapes surgery.

Transcanal Approach

The transcanal approach is used for those procedures that are limited to the mesotympanum, hypotympanum, and tympanic membrane. The incision entails a superiorly based tympanomeatal flap through the ear canal and involves making a semilunar canal skin incision anywhere from 2 to 10 mm lateral to the tympanic membrane. For exposure, the skin, fibrous

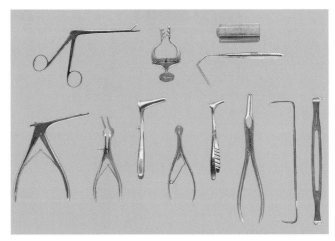

FIGURE 10-19 *Top, left to right:* 1 Ferris-Smith fragment forceps; 1 mastoid articulated retractor; 1 Cottle bone crusher, closed; 1 Aufricht retractor. *Bottom, left to right:* 1 Kerrison rongeur, upbite; 1 Killian nasal speculum, 2 inch, front view; 1 Killian nasal speculum, 3 inch, side view; 1 Vienna nasal speculum, 1⅜ inch, front view; 1 Vienna nasal speculum 1⅛ inch, side view; Asch septal forceps; 2 Army-Navy retractors, side view and front view.

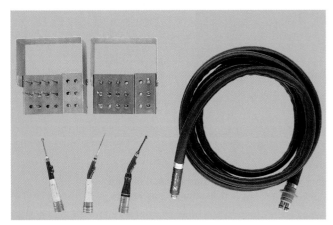

FIGURE 10-17 *Left, top:* Ototome drill bits and burrs in cases, diamond, cutting, and air microburrs. *Bottom, left to right:* straight high-speed handpiece with burr; angled high-speed handpiece with bit; angled low-speed handpiece with diamond burr; power cord.

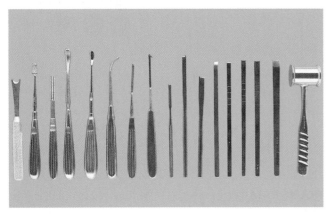

FIGURE 10-18 *Left to right:* 1 Bauer rocking chisel; 1 Lewis rasp; 1 Maltz rasp; 1 Aufricht rasp, large; 1 Aufricht rasp, small; 1 Wiener antrum rasp; 2 Ballenger swivel knives; 1 Ballenger chisel, 4 mm; 2 Converse guarded osteotomes; 1 Cottle osteotome, round corners, curved, 6 mm; 4 Cottle osteotomes, straight: 4, 7, 9, and 12 mm; 1 mallet, lead-filled head.

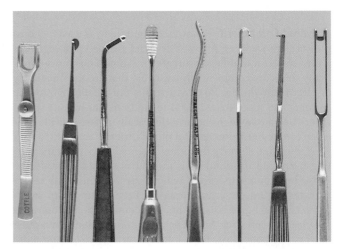

FIGURE 10-20 *Left to right:* Tips: 1 Cottle columella forceps; 1 Freer septum knife; 1 Joseph button-end knife; 1 Aufricht rasp, small, front view; 1 Aufricht rasp, large, side view; 1 Cottle knife guide and retractor, side view; 2 Ballenger swivel knives, side view and front view.

annulus, and tympanic membrane are elevated as a unit. Posterior tympanomeatal flaps may be used in stapedectomy, labyrinthectomy, myringoplasty, tumor biopsy, ossiculoplasty, and removal of glomus tympanicum tumors. Congenital cholesteatomas are best approached by superior tympanomeatal flaps, whereas perforations of the tympanic membrane may be accessed through an inferior tympanomeatal flap (Chole and Suddath, 2005).

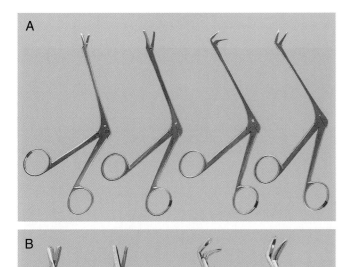

FIGURE 10-21 A, *Left to right:* Gruenwald nasal forceps, size 2: 1 straight, cutting; 1 Struycken nasal cutting forceps; 1 90-degree upward-bent; 1 upward-bent. **B,** *Left to right:* Gruenwald nasal forceps, size 2, tips: 1 straight, cutting; 1 Struycken nasal cutting forceps; 1 90-degree upward-bent; 1 upward-bent.

Postauricular Approach

The postauricular incision is made 2 to 5 mm behind the ear as the surgeon follows the curve of the posterior auricular fold, providing wide-field exposure and a versatile and adaptable incision. It is commonly used for tympanoplasty procedures and it is also used to expose the mastoid process for a mastoidectomy, endolymphatic sac procedure, labyrinthectomy, or translabyrinthectomy resection of an acoustic neuroma.

Myringotomy

A standard myringotomy is an incision in the pars tensa of the tympanic membrane. Myringotomy is often accompanied by the aspiration of fluid under pressure in the tympanum, and the subsequent placement of small, hollow, pressure equalization tubes (PETs) (also known as *tympanostomy* or *myringotomy tubes*). It is indicated for acute otitis media in the presence of an exudate that has not responded to antibiotic therapy. Acute otitis media (AOM) occurs in 84% to 93% of all children. Otitis media with effusion (OME) occurs in 80% of children under the age of 10 years. The majority of children with AOM have spontaneous resolution. Hearing loss is the main concern when fluid is present in the middle ear (OME) (Thrasher, 2009). If left untreated, hearing loss can affect language development. If the fluid persists more than 8 to 12 weeks and is accompanied by hearing loss, removal of the fluid and placement of ventilating tubes in the eardrum are necessary.

Otitis media, although more common in the pediatric population, is also seen in adults. Tympanic fibrosis is common in adults and is a result of repeated infections that occurred in childhood. Acute otitis media is a collection of infected pus in the middle ear. The patient may have severe pain and bulging of the tympanic membrane (Figure 10-22). Failure to respond to oral antibiotics and analgesics or other complications, such as facial nerve paralysis, may require a myringot-

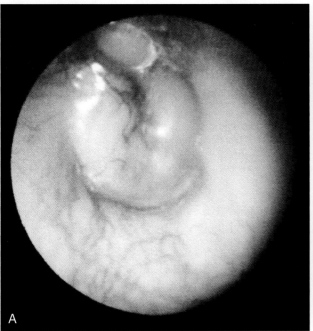
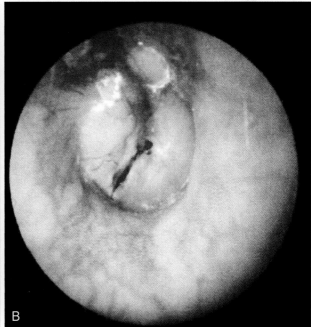

FIGURE 10-22 A, In purulent otitis media, pus under pressure pushes eardrum outward, resulting in bulging tympanic membrane. **B,** Radial myringotomy incision.

omy. By release of the pus or fluid, hearing is restored and the infection can be controlled. The procedure may be performed for chronic serous otitis media in which the presence of fluid in the middle ear produces a hearing loss. Frequently, tubes are inserted into the tympanic membrane (Figure 10-23) to allow ventilation of the middle ear. Myringotomy tubes may be used for the treatment of colds and fluid in the ear on a short-term basis (a few months), on an intermediate basis (6 to 18 months), and in long-term treatment (years) for chronic situations. Tubes may also be placed in patients undergoing hyperbaric therapy to prevent ear pain and tympanic rupture while in the hyperbaric chamber. Care must be taken to avoid getting water in the ears while the tubes are in place. Myringotomy is usually performed on an ambulatory surgery basis. A recent alternative to tube placement is CO_2 laser–assisted myringotomy, in which the laser energy is used to create a precise hole in the tympanic membrane. This remains open for 4 to 6 weeks. Laser-assisted myringotomy is done using a topical anesthetic and may be performed in the physician's office.

Procedural Considerations. Myringotomy with tube placement is considered a clean procedure. In adult patients, the procedure may be performed using a topical anesthetic. Pediatric patients generally require general anesthesia. The surgeon may wear gown and gloves or gloves only, depending on the policy related to Standard Precautions at the institution in which the procedure is performed. Myringotomy procedures require a sharp knife for making incisions into the tympanic membrane. Sterile, disposable, single-use blades are supplied with integrated handles or as single blades that may be secured into reusable handles. Myringotomy blades are spear-, lancet-, and sickle-shaped and are a matter of the surgeon's preference. The instrument setup includes a myringotomy knife and disposable blade, assorted sizes of aural specula, ear curettes, suction tip and tubing, a delicate Hartmann forceps, metal aural applicators, a curved needle, a culture tube (if cultures are to be taken), and myringotomy tubes (as applicable). Several types of disposable myringotomy tubes are available for implantation, depending on the length of time the surgeon wishes the tube to remain in place (see Figure 10-23). Once the tube falls out, the tympanic membrane incision usually heals.

Operative Procedure

1. With the head and microscope in position, the surgeon inserts the aural speculum into the ear canal. The external canal is cleaned of excess cerumen using a wire loop curette. With a sharp myringotomy knife, the surgeon makes a small, curved or radial incision in the anterior inferior quadrant of the pars tensa (see Figure 10-22).
2. A culture may be taken to determine the type of organism present. Pus and fluid are suctioned from the middle ear.
3. A tube may be inserted into the incision with alligator forceps or a tube inserter. Care should be taken to consult the manufacturer's directions for handling the tube.
4. Antibiotic drops may be instilled after positioning the tube. Ofloxacin 0.3% otic drops may be instilled to 10 drops per ear.
5. A cotton ball may be placed in the external canal at the end of the procedure.

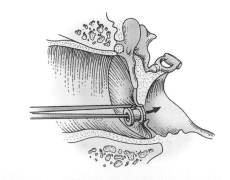

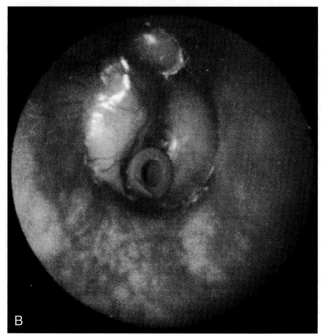

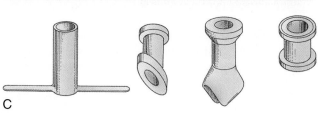

FIGURE 10-23 **A,** Tube (placed on end of alligator forceps) being inserted into tympanic membrane. **B,** Tube in place. **C,** Several types of plastic tubes that may be inserted into tympanic membrane. Purpose of tubes is to aerate middle ear and reduce middle ear infections.

Tympanoplasty

Tympanoplasty is the surgical repair of the tympanic membrane and the tympanum and the reconstruction of the ossicular chain. It is indicated for conductive hearing losses caused by perforation of the tympanic membrane as a result of trauma or infection; for ossicular discontinuity; for chronic or recurrent otitis media; for progressive hearing loss; and for the inability to safely bathe or participate in water activities as a result of perforation of the tympanic membrane with or without hearing loss.

Perforation of the tympanic membrane is the most common ear injury necessitating surgical intervention. Perforations may result from (1) direct injury (e.g., cotton applicators, pencil), (2) blow to the ear, and (3) injury from temporal bone fractures. Early diagnosis is the key to proper management.

Conductive hearing loss is caused by an obstruction in the external canal or middle ear, which impedes the passage of sound waves to the inner ear. It may be attributable to disease of the middle ear or tympanic membrane. Occasionally the tympanic membrane does not heal after myringotomy.

Ossicular discontinuity may result from chronic otitis media, trauma, or cholesteatoma—a skin cyst that erodes bone. Various methods and materials are presently used in constructing a closed, air-contained middle ear cavity and restoring a sound-pressure transforming action. Among these materials are high-density polyethylene, silicone, hydroxyapatite, and titanium prostheses.

Procedural Considerations. The ear is prepped and draped as previously described. An endaural or postauricular approach may be used. Both approaches provide similar functional results. The procedure most often is performed after the patient has been administered a general anesthetic.

Operative Procedure
1. The following three approaches may be used when performing a tympanoplasty:
   a. When an *endaural approach* is used, a Lempert speculum is introduced into the external meatus of the ear canal, and the microscope is appropriately positioned. The surgeon injects lidocaine with epinephrine postauricularly and into the external meatus and external auditory canal. The endaural incision is made as detailed previously and then the tympanomeatal incision is made using a sharp, round knife.
   b. When a *postauricular approach* is used, the surgeon injects lidocaine with epinephrine postauricularly. An ear speculum is introduced, and the microscope is appropriately positioned. Additional lidocaine is injected into the external auditory canal. The microscope head is moved from directly over the patient's ear. The surgeon incises the skin behind the fold of the ear with a #15 knife blade. Bleeding vessels are coagulated. An incision is then made into the periosteum down to the bone, and the periosteum is elevated from behind the incision with a Lempert elevator.
   c. During the *transcanal approach,* the surgeon injects the four quadrants of the fibrocartilaginous canal with a 1% or 2% lidocaine solution with 1:100,000 epinephrine. An endaural speculum gently compresses the tissue edema resulting from the injection and assists in the placement of a speculum within the confines of the bony canal. A 30-gauge needle is used to inject the skin of the bony canal. There are various canal incisions that can be made, all of which accomplish the same goal of lifting the posterior ear canal skin and the tympanic membrane in continuity. Once the incisions have been made, the skin is elevated to the tympanic annulus, subcutaneous tissue at the tympanomastoid suture is dissected, and bleeding is controlled before the middle ear is reached.
2. At this point, the surgeon or the assistant harvests a section of temporalis fascia for the graft material used in the repair of the tympanic membrane. Lidocaine with epinephrine may be injected under the fascia to separate it from

the temporalis muscle. The surgeon uses a narrow Shambaugh elevator or duckbill elevator to separate the fascia and excises the amount needed using small, sharp scissors or a knife blade. The fascia is trimmed of excess tissue with small, sharp scissors and set aside to dry on a Teflon cutting block that is standard in most otologic instrument trays. Some surgeons prefer to thin the fascia by using a House Gelfoam press before placing the graft on the cutting block.
3. The canal skin may be elevated from the canal with a duckbill elevator, curved needle, gimmick, or similar microinstrument, or it may be removed (lateral/overlay tympanoplasty), depending on the size and location of the tympanic membrane perforation.
4. The surgeon uses a sickle knife, curved needle, 45- or 90-degree pick, or cup forceps to remove all the epithelium from the drum surrounding the perforation edges of the tympanic membrane in preparation for receiving the graft. This is referred to as "freshening the edges" and is a critical step in promoting reepithelialization of the graft.
5. If an edge of the perforation or tympanic membrane cannot be visualized because of the bony canal, the surgeon uses a microcurette or drill to remove the overhang of bone.
6. The middle ear is explored with a pick or similar instrument, and any epithelium present is removed with an alligator, or cup, forceps. The surgeon inspects each ossicle to ensure that it is intact and mobile.
7. If the malleus or incus is diseased or eroded, it may be removed and replaced with a partial ossicular replacement prosthesis (PORP). Ossicles that are removed may be reshaped with the aid of a drill and small burr and replaced. If all ossicles are diseased or eroded, they may be removed and replaced with a total ossicular replacement prosthesis (TORP). This step is accomplished with microinstrumentation, such as Bellucci scissors, cup forceps, malleus nipper, incudostapedial joint knife, sickle knife, picks, and a curved needle.
8. The surgeon prepares the graft for insertion. The edges are trimmed with a #15 knife blade or sharp scissors to fit the shape of the ear canal and the size of the perforation. The surgical site is suctioned with a microsuction device. Hemostasis may be achieved by applying very small, epinephrine-soaked Gelfoam balls with an alligator forceps.
9. Different tissues—such as temporalis fascia or loose connective tissue, tragus perichondrium, and vein grafts—have been used for a tympanoplasty procedure. The most common tissue used is temporalis fascia. Most surgeons prefer to use autograft tissue, although homograft tympanic membranes have also been used. The risk of transmission of infectious disease has reduced homograft use. For easier manipulation, the graft may be dipped in water or saline before its insertion with alligator forceps. A gimmick, sickle knife, pick, curved needle, or similar microinstrument is used to position the graft into place. Small pieces of absorbable gelatin sponge may be packed below the graft in the middle ear space to ensure support and position. The graft and tympanomeatal flap are then laid back into place and Gelfoam packing is used to secure the flap, remnant tympanic membrane, and graft in the proper position. This outer ear canal packing is left in place for 1 to 2 weeks postoperatively and removed in the surgeon's office.

10. The external ear canal is then packed with MeroGel; moistened, absorbable, gelatin sponge pledgets; or antibiotic ointment.
11. The incision is closed with suture of the surgeon's preference.
12. A pressure dressing consisting of fluffed gauze placed around the ear and an elastic gauze wrapped around the affected ear and the head may be applied for the first 24 hours to reduce swelling. Commercially prepared postauricular incision dressings are available.

Mastoidectomy

Mastoidectomy is the removal of diseased bone of the mastoid process and mastoid space. Before the introduction of antibiotic therapy, mastoidectomy was commonly performed for infection. Although occasionally still performed for eradication of infection, it is more frequently used in the treatment of cholesteatoma. Cholesteatoma is the result of accumulation of squamous epithelium and its products in the middle ear and mastoid. It occasionally forms a cystlike mass (Figure 10-24). As it expands, it is destructive to the middle ear and mastoid. As a result, the diseased bone (ossicles and mastoid bone) must be removed to prevent recurrence of the cholesteatoma.

There are three types of mastoidectomy. A *simple mastoidectomy* is removal of the diseased bone of the mastoid with preservation of the ossicles, eardrum, and canal wall. This procedure is performed to eradicate chronic infections unresponsive to antibiotics or to remove cholesteatoma. A *modified radical mastoidectomy* is removal of the diseased bone of the mastoid along with some of the ossicles and the canal wall. The eardrum and some of the ossicles remain, leaving a mechanism for the patient to hear. A canal-wall-up mastoidectomy is similar to the modified mastoidectomy without removing the posterior ear canal wall. The benefit of a canal-wall-up mastoidectomy is that the patient's ear canal will appear and function normally. Canal-wall-down mastoid cavities require maintenance with debridement of aculeate debris at least yearly.

A *radical mastoidectomy* is removal of the canal wall along with the ossicles and tympanic membrane. It is rarely performed except for unresectable disease. With either the modified radical or the radical mastoidectomy, a meatoplasty is performed to enlarge the ear canal opening. This facilitates cleaning the mastoid bowl that has been created.

Procedural Considerations. The patient is prepped and draped as for a tympanoplasty. An endaural or postauricular incision may be used (Figure 10-25), but most surgeons believe that the postauricular incision offers better exposure to all areas of the mastoid and middle ear. A drill is used to remove diseased bone and tissue. Facial nerve monitoring is used to alert the surgeon to the proximity of the nerve within the surgical field.

Operative Procedure. Steps 1 through 6 from the tympanoplasty procedure are performed.
7. The surgeon uses a drill with a large cutting burr to drill the mastoid bone under direct vision. As the mastoid cavity is created, the scrub person should be able to anticipate changes needed in burr size. Once the vital structures have been identified, diseased bone is removed by use of diamond burrs of the appropriate size. The surgeon may interrupt drilling to explore areas of the mastoid with a pick,

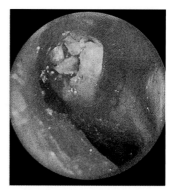

FIGURE 10-24 Cholesteatoma.

curved needle, or annulus elevator, or with other microinstruments to identify surrounding structures.
8. On completion of the mastoidectomy, the surgeon focuses on the middle ear. Diseased ossicles are removed, middle ear mucosa is inspected and removed if necessary, and all evidence of cholesteatoma is removed. Depending on the extent of the disease and the reliability that the patient will be available for follow-up care, the surgeon then reconstructs the ossicular chain or prepares the cavity created by a radical mastoidectomy. Some surgeons do not reconstruct at the time of mastoidectomy but reconstruct as a second-stage operation, which serves the added purpose of reexploring the middle ear and mastoid for residual or recurrent cholesteatoma.
9. The mastoid cavity and middle ear may be packed with an absorbable gelatin sponge or MeroGel. The external auditory canal may be packed with MeroGel, an absorbable gelatin sponge, or antibiotic ointment.
10. The incision is closed and dressing applied in similar fashion to that used for postauricular tympanoplasty (as detailed previously).

Stapedotomy

Stapedotomy is removal of the stapes superstructure and creation of a fenestra (opening) in the fixed stapes footplate for treatment of otosclerosis and placement of a prosthesis to restore ossicular continuity and alleviate conductive hearing loss. Otosclerosis is the formation of abnormal bone around the stapes footplate, resulting in immobility of the footplate. Sound waves cannot be transmitted adequately through the oval window and round window to be changed into electrochemical impulses in the cochlea.

There are two types of procedures for replacing the immobile stapes. In *stapedotomy*, the footplate of the stapes is not removed; only the superstructure is removed. A hole is made in the stapes footplate, and the prosthesis is secured laterally to the long process of the incus and positioned medially over the hole created in the footplate. The carbon dioxide (CO_2) laser may also be used for stapedotomy—to create (drill) a hole in the footplate of the stapes for insertion of a prosthesis or to vaporize the stapedial tendon. Ideally, laser energy should be completely absorbed by the footplate and should not heat the perilymph or damage the inner ear (House and Cunningham, 2005). The laser stapedotomy offers improved postoperative hearing results while reducing postoperative

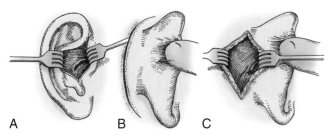

FIGURE 10-25 Mastoidectomy incision. **A,** Endaural. **B,** Postauricular. **C,** Postauricular incision retracted.

dizziness and sensorineural hearing loss. An older procedure that is still used today, however not as frequently as in years past, is the *stapedectomy*. In stapedectomy, the entire stapes (superstructure and footplate) is removed, a graft is placed over the oval window, and a prosthesis is attached laterally to the long process of the incus and positioned medially on the graft over the oval window. Both of these procedures may be performed using monitored anesthesia care (MAC) or local anesthesia for adults, enabling the surgeon to test hearing before the conclusion of the surgery. Certain patient populations, such as children, patients with anxiety, and non–English-speaking patients, may find it difficult to remain immobile during the procedure, and general anesthesia is recommended in these populations to facilitate surgery and patient comfort.

Procedural Considerations. Various materials are used as the prosthesis for the stapes; the most common are stainless steel, titanium, platinum, nitinol, and Teflon. The most common types are either bucket-handle or piston prostheses (Figure 10-26). Both are secured to the incus and extend to the stapes footplate to reconstitute the ossicular chain. The use of stainless-steel materials may present a risk for prosthesis displacement and subsequent sensorineural hearing loss if the patient undergoes MRI studies in the future.

The prosthesis of choice is determined by the surgeon's experience and preference. The scrub person must be aware of each step in the procedure and hand the instruments to the surgeon expediently. Because the oval window is left uncovered, some perilymph may leak from the inner ear into the middle ear. This leak subjects the patient to the possible complication of a sensorineural hearing loss postoperatively.

Microsuction tips (18- to 26-gauge) are used in this procedure because large suction tips may suction perilymph from the oval window, resulting in permanent hearing loss as well as promoting bleeding in the middle ear. After the incision and reflection of the flap, footplate hooks are used because the tips on picks are too large and long and may cause damage rather than assist in the procedure.

Operative Procedure—Stapedotomy

1. The surgeon or the assistant may harvest a temporalis fascia, fat, perichondrium, or vein graft at the start of the procedure to cover the oval window. Depending on the surgeon's graft preference, the ear, hand, or a portion of the abdomen may be prepped for the graft. Most surgeons use temporalis fascia or postauricular subcutaneous tissue as it is within the surgical field and easily accessible.

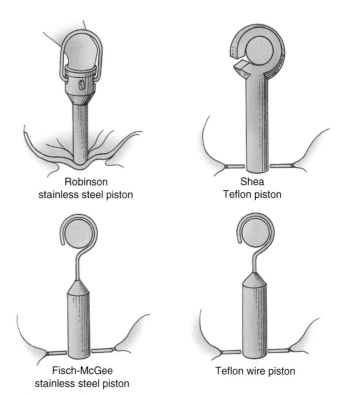

Robinson
stainless steel piston

Shea
Teflon piston

Fisch-McGee
stainless steel piston

Teflon wire piston

FIGURE 10-26 Stapedectomy prostheses. *Top left,* Prostheses used after the footplate has been removed. *Top right and bottom,* Footplate had been "drilled" to accept a prefabricated piston precisely.

2. The ear speculum is introduced, and the microscope is appropriately positioned. The surgeon cleans any cerumen or debris from the ear canal and may gently wash the canal with physiologic irrigating solution.
3. The surgeon injects lidocaine with epinephrine into the ear canal.
4. An ear speculum is inserted, the tympanomeatal flap is created, and the tympanic membrane is reflected forward, exposing the middle ear.
5. If visualization of the ossicles is inadequate because of the overhang of bone, the surgeon may use microcurettes or a drill to remove enough bone to allow proper visualization. Attempts to save the chorda tympani nerve are made because it controls taste from the anterior two thirds of the tongue. If this nerve obstructs the view of the stapes, it may on rare occasion be divided for exposure, and at the conclusion of the procedure the neural ends are reapproximated.
6. The surgeon may measure the distance from the incus to the stapes footplate at this time or after the removal of the stapes. It is accomplished with a depth gauge and done to ensure the proper fit of the prosthesis.
7. The incudostapedial joint is disarticulated to allow fracture and subsequent removal of the stapes, usually accomplished through the use of a joint knife or right-angle hook.
8. Both crura of the stapes are treated with a laser or fractured laterally, usually with a footplate pick or curved needle, and the superstructure is removed with alligator forceps. The surgeon may take this opportunity to ensure hemostasis,

using tiny sponges soaked in epinephrine and applying suction with a microsuction tip. The laser helps coagulate middle ear vessels, thus improving hemostasis.

9. An opening is created in the footplate with a laser or a sharp footplate pick. If the footplate is extremely thick, a microdrill may be used. If a stapedectomy is to be carried out, each half of the footplate is removed using a Hough hoe, footplate pick, or footplate hook.

10. The oval window is inspected to ensure that it is long enough, and then a measuring stick is used to approximate the correct size prosthesis required for reconstruction.

11. Holding the prosthesis with alligator forceps, the scrub person passes it to the surgeon. The prosthesis is introduced into the middle ear with the shaft resting against the oval window graft.

12. The wire is positioned over the long process of the incus using picks, Hough hoes, or footplate hooks. Once it is in proper position, the surgeon crimps the wire onto the long process of the incus to ensure its attachment.

13. The surgeon may test the patient's hearing by softly whispering to the patient (if the procedure is performed with the patient administered a local anesthetic) or by touching the malleus with a pick and observing for mobility of the malleus, incus, and stapes prosthesis (if performed with the patient administered a general anesthetic).

14. Tiny pieces of the previously harvested graft tissue are then placed around the base of the prosthesis to ensure its stability. Alligator forceps, picks, a gimmick, and similar instruments may be used for this step.

15. The tympanomeatal flap is returned to its original location. The external ear canal may be packed with an antibiotic gel or ointment or a moistened, compressed gelatin sponge.

16. Cotton is placed in the concha of the ear, and a Band-Aid or small dressing is usually applied to the graft site.

Ossicular Chain Reconstruction

Ossicular reconstruction may be required for long-standing recurrent ear infections. It is commonly performed for the replacement of the incus portion of the ossicular chain. There are many surgical techniques for ossicular reconstruction.

Natural and synthetic prosthetic materials are available for ossicular reconstruction or replacement. The autologous ossicle (incus or head of malleus) taken from the patient's ear is often used, particularly in children who do not have a cholesteatoma. A synthetic PORP (partial ossicular reconstruction prosthesis) or TORP is indicated for reconstitution of the ossicular chain.

Alloplastic materials for partial and total ossicular reconstruction prostheses are available. Hydroxyapatite is used in many prostheses because its mineral content is very similar to that of bone and it is well tolerated by the middle ear, thereby decreasing extrusion rates. Because it is brittle, it is often combined with other materials to allow it to be more easily trimmed for a precise fit in the middle ear. Titanium is another material being used more frequently in middle ear prostheses. Titanium is ideal for ossicular reconstruction because of its properties of being rigid and lightweight. Regardless of the type of prosthesis used, the surgeon must sculpt/trim it to bridge the ossicular gap by simulating the ossicular configuration and preserving the lever mechanism of the middle ear.

Procedural Considerations. Minor columella is a term that refers to an ossiculoplasty with a strut from the head of the stapes to the tympanic membrane (or graft) or manubrium. *Major columella* refers to a strut extending from the footplate to the tympanic membrane (or graft) or manubrium. The patient is prepped and draped as for stapedotomy or tympanoplasty.

Operative Procedure. The procedure steps are similar to those for stapedotomy, except that the stapes footplate is not removed or opened.

Endolymphatic Sac Decompression or Shunt

An endolymphatic shunt procedure is the creation of an opening into the endolymphatic sac and the insertion of a shunt to allow drainage of excess endolymph into the cerebrospinal fluid (CSF) or into the mastoid cavity. In Meniere's disease, the endolymphatic sac cannot resorb endolymph, resulting in an overaccumulation. This surplus leads to vertigo, in which patients feel a spinning sensation. Movement usually increases the vertigo, which may be accompanied by severe nausea and vomiting. The vertigo attacks occur unpredictably and may last from several minutes to several hours. Most patients with Meniere's disease complain of tinnitus, pressure or fullness in the affected ear, and a fluctuating hearing loss that begins in the lower frequencies. Diagnostic audiometry reveals the hearing loss to be sensorineural. The vertigo may be so severe that it disrupts the patient's lifestyle. With a medical regimen of tranquilizers, diuretics, vasodilators, and a low-sodium diet, the majority of patients are able to adequately control their symptoms. About 10% to 15% of persons eventually fail medical therapy and may seek surgical intervention (Furman, 2008).

Procedural   Considerations. Preoperative   assessment should confirm that the patient's electrolyte levels (especially potassium) are adequate; this provides a basis for the support system to be carried out intraoperatively and postoperatively. Because Meniere's disease may develop bilaterally in some patients, conservative therapy is often employed (Schessel et al, 2005). The patient is prepped and draped as for a mastoidectomy.

Operative Procedure. The procedure that follows describes decompression with a shunt. Some surgeons perform endolymphatic sac decompression only, without the shunt. The majority of the bone overlying the sac is removed to allow for more compliance of the sac and the membranous labyrinth.

Steps 1 through 7 of the decompression with shunt are the same as those for mastoidectomy.

8. The surgeon continues drilling with a diamond burr over the posterior fossa dura until the endolymphatic sac is identified.

9. Using a microknife, such as a sickle, Beaver blade, or Ziegler, the surgeon incises the lateral wall of the sac.

10. A shunt (commercially prepared tube, Silastic tubing, or Silastic sheeting) is inserted with microforceps and manipulated into place using microinstruments, such as a curved needle, fine pick, or gimmick (Figure 10-27).

11. The incision is closed and a pressure dressing applied to the affected ear.

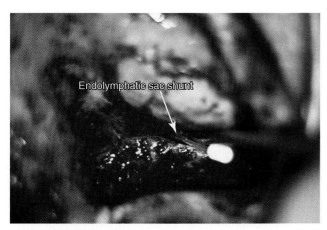

FIGURE 10-27 Endolymph Silastic shunt in place.

Labyrinthectomy

Labyrinthectomy is a procedure that eliminates the vestibular and auditory function of the labyrinth to relieve severe vertigo. The procedure is usually performed when the disease is unilateral, a shunt/decompression procedure has been ineffective, and the affected ear has severe or total loss of hearing. Because the inner ear is removed, the patient may be very dizzy for several days until the brainstem begins to compensate for the destroyed labyrinth. The operation also leaves the ear with no residual hearing.

Procedural Considerations. The procedure is most commonly performed via the transmastoid approach. The patient is prepped and draped as described for the tympanoplasty/mastoidectomy procedure.

Operative Procedure
1. The surgeon creates a postauricular incision and performs a simple mastoidectomy.
2. The vertical segment of the facial nerve is identified, and the incus is disarticulated and removed.
3. The horizontal, posterior, and superior semicircular canals are drilled and removed. The neuroepithelium is completely removed from the ampullae of the three semicircular canals. The vestibule is exposed and the neuroepithelium from the utricle and saccule is removed.
4. The incision is closed in layers. An external pressure dressing of elastic gauze is applied.

Vestibular Neurectomy

Vestibular neurectomy is the division of the vestibular portion of the eighth cranial nerve (acoustic nerve) with preservation of the cochlear portion of the eighth cranial nerve. It may be performed for a unilateral ear disorder, including classic Meniere's disease, recurrent vestibular neuronitis, traumatic labyrinthitis, or vestibular Meniere's disease. It may also be performed when attacks of vertigo severely affect a patient's lifestyle. Vestibular neurectomy is performed when a patient has adequate hearing and accepts elimination of vestibular function on the affected side.

Procedural Considerations. Vestibular neurectomy is most commonly performed through a retrosigmoid craniotomy.

Refer to Chapter 12 for procedural considerations related to craniotomy.

Operative Procedure
1. The surgeon creates a 4-cm curvilinear incision 4 cm behind the postauricular sulcus.
2. A craniotomy is drilled posterior/inferior to the junction of the transverse and sigmoid sinuses.
3. The surgeon incises the dura, retracts the cerebellum, and identifies the seventh and eighth cranial nerve complex.
4. The vestibular and cochlear portions of the nerve are correctly identified and the surgeon divides the vestibular portion.
5. The dura is closed with suture and the craniotomy reconstructed with hydroxyapatite cement or titanium mesh plating.

Facial Nerve Decompression

Facial nerve decompression is a procedure designed to identify and relieve an area of compression of the facial nerve. Damage to the facial nerve may occur from trauma, infection, or tumors and may result in a facial nerve palsy, but the most common form of facial paralysis is Bell's palsy. The cause is unknown, although clinical and laboratory evidence indicates a virus of the herpes simplex group may be involved. The patient experiences multiple problems, such as decreased tearing, inability to close the affected eye, and drooping of the affected corner of the mouth with pooling of oral secretions. The facial nerve may be decompressed by a translabyrinthine approach when trauma has destroyed hearing and caused facial nerve paralysis. The narrowest segment of the bony canal compressing the facial nerve is deep in the temporal bone and may also be accessed through the middle cranial fossa approach when hearing is to be preserved. Both approaches may be useful under selected circumstances.

Transmastoid, Translabyrinthine Approach
PROCEDURAL CONSIDERATIONS. The patient is prepped and draped as described for mastoidectomy. Neurologic intensive care is required for the first 24 hours. Preoperatively, ointments protect the eye and the eyelid is taped closed, or an adhesive bubble is placed over the eye to trap moisture. This protection is continued into the postoperative period unless a tarsorrhaphy (suturing the eyelid closed) is performed intraoperatively.
OPERATIVE PROCEDURE. Steps 1 through 7 are the same as those for mastoidectomy.
8. After completing the mastoidectomy, the surgeon continues the dissection using cutting and diamond burrs until the internal auditory canal and the posterior fossa bone are removed.
9. The bone immediately over the facial nerve is removed by the use of nerve excavators and picks.
10. Using a facial nerve knife, neurectomy knife, sickle knife, neurectomy scissors, or micropick, the surgeon incises the facial nerve sheath. The majority of surgeons do not incise the epineurium of the facial nerve, and decompression only is felt to be equally efficacious and less traumatic to the nerve itself.
11. Hemostasis is achieved by the use of moistened, absorbable gelatin sponge; cottonoids; oxidized cellulose; bipolar ESU; or a combination of these.

12. The incision is closed and a pressure dressing of elastic gauze applied.

Middle Cranial Fossa Approach

PROCEDURAL CONSIDERATIONS. The patient's hair is clipped almost to the midline on the affected side. Povidone-iodine solution generally is used for the prep, which includes the portion of the head that has been clipped, the affected side of the face, and the neck. Lidocaine with or without epinephrine usually is injected subcutaneously above the ear to assist in hemostasis. The patient's eye on the affected side is protected as previously described.

OPERATIVE PROCEDURE

1. The surgeon incises the temporalis muscle and elevates it with a Lempert, Shambaugh, or similar type of elevator.
2. Hemostasis is achieved by clamping and tying vessels or by electrocoagulation.
3. The surgeon drills a square of bone from the temporal bone to expose the middle cranial fossa dura. (The bone is saved for replacement at the end of the procedure.)
4. A self-retaining retractor with a blade for retraction of the middle fossa (e.g., Fisch middle fossa retractor, House-Urban retractor) is inserted.
5. The microscope is positioned appropriately, and the surgeon elevates the dura from the floor of the middle fossa with a Freer elevator, a gimmick, or similar instruments.
6. Once hemostasis is achieved and the blade is inserted over the dura to expose the middle fossa, drilling may proceed.
7. When the bone becomes quite thin, the surgeon may remove the remaining bone with excavators to avoid damaging the nerve sheath.
8. The facial nerve sheath can be incised with a facial nerve knife, neurectomy knife, neurectomy scissors, or microknife.
9. The retractor is removed when hemostasis is achieved, and the bone flap is replaced.
10. The temporalis muscle is approximated and sutured, the incision closed, and a pressure dressing applied.

Removal of Acoustic Neuroma (Vestibular Schwannoma)

Acoustic neuromas arise from the Schwann cells of the vestibular portion of the eighth cranial (acoustic) nerve and are therefore more appropriately termed *vestibular schwannomas*. These tumors are benign but may grow to a size that produces symptoms of cerebellar and brainstem origin. Bilateral vestibular schwannomas are a common finding in patients with neurofibromatosis type 2 (NF2) (Gantz and Meyer, 2005).

Most patients experience unilateral tinnitus and hearing loss—the main symptoms of a possible acoustic neuroma. However, depending on the rate and direction of tumor growth, signs and symptoms may include hearing loss, tinnitus, vertigo, headaches, double vision, diplopia, decreased corneal reflex, decreased blink reflex, impaired taste, reduced lacrimation, facial paralysis, diminished gag reflex, vocal cord paralysis, atrophy or fasciculation of the tongue, weakness of the sternocleidomastoid and trapezius muscles, disturbance in balance and gait, hydrocephalus, lethargy, confusion, drowsiness, and coma.

Several surgery centers have developed great expertise in acoustic neuroma surgery, which requires the combined team of a neurologist and a neurosurgeon.

Procedural Considerations. The translabyrinthine approach for the removal of an acoustic tumor reduces mortality and morbidity and offers a good chance of saving the facial nerve if the tumor has not directly invaded it. The patient should be informed about the presence of a Foley catheter, arterial line, temperature probe, clipped hair, and graft-site incision. The patient's hair is clipped to the midline of the affected side. Some patients prefer to have the entire head clipped to facilitate wearing a wig. This option should be presented preoperatively to enable the patient to make a decision before surgery. The patient is prepped and draped as described for labyrinthectomy. Lidocaine with or without epinephrine may be injected subcutaneously behind the ear. A facial nerve monitor is routinely used in the excision of cerebellopontine angle tumors. A sequential compression device (SCD) is used intraoperatively and for the first 24 to 48 hours postoperatively or until the patient is ambulatory to decrease the risk of deep vein thrombosis (DVT) and pulmonary embolism (PE).

Operative Procedure

1. The surgeon makes a postauricular incision slightly longer and more posterior than the incision for mastoidectomy and elevates the periosteum from the mastoid bone with a Lempert, Shambaugh, or similar type of elevator.
2. Self-retaining retractors are inserted, and the cortical mastoidectomy is begun with a large cutting burr.
3. The microscope is positioned, and the attic is opened to visualize the ossicles. The sigmoid sinus, middle fossa dura, and superior petrosal sinus are left in place with a thin covering of bone. The semicircular canals are exposed. The incus is removed with alligator forceps or cup forceps and suction.
4. The surgeon excises the semicircular canals with the drill. The utricle and saccule are removed, and the aqueduct of the vestibule is drilled out to expose the internal auditory canal 270 degrees circumferentially.
5. Using nerve excavators, Fisch dissectors, or picks, the surgeon removes the remainder of bone from the dura of the internal meatus, posterior fossa, middle fossa, and petrosal angle. The wedge of bone between the facial and superior vestibular nerves (Bill's bar) is removed.
6. The dura is opened with microscissors or a dura knife. The surgeon dissects the tumor with a gimmick, Freer microelevator, microinstrument, and bipolar forceps (with or without suction). Hemostasis is achieved with a moistened, absorbable gelatin sponge; cottonoids; oxidized cellulose; or the bipolar ESU.
7. The tumor is removed by the use of pituitary cup forceps, long alligator forceps, and similar instruments.
8. Graft material (e.g., fat, fascia, or muscle) is obtained to pack the mastoid cavity created from the drilling. The packing is performed meticulously to avoid a cerebrospinal fluid leak.
9. The wound is closed and a thick pressure dressing applied.

Assistive Hearing Devices

A variety of assistive devices are available to patients with hearing loss, including phone amplifiers, closed captioning broadcasts, Telecommunication Device for the Deaf (TDD), and electronic devices, such as hearing aids. Technology has evolved tremendously in the field of otology, enabling surgeons

Evaluating Language Outcomes in Children After Cochlear Implantation

The impact of hearing loss on the pediatric population is significant. Of every 1000 children in the United States, 1 is born with profound hearing loss. Before the availability of cochlear implants, children with hearing loss were treated with hearing aids. While hearing aids do provide sound amplification, children who use them often display delays in written and spoken communication. Language and cognitive development are closely related and language is a known predictor of academic success in children.

Cochlear implants provide an improved auditory experience for children with hearing loss, and the positive impact on speech perception and development is well documented in the literature. This study sought (1) to assess receptive language scores in children after cochlear implantation and compare them with scores from normal hearing children and children with hearing loss that use hearing aids, and (2) to determine how demographic factors, such as age of implantation, impact language outcomes. Researchers hoped to identify factors that impact language skills and gain a better understanding of language development in pediatric patients after cochlear implantation.

A group of 56 pediatric patients aged 6 months to 12 years were evaluated. Participants were educated in the oral communication mode after implantation and were administered language tests at intervals varying from 6 months to 5 years after implantation. Analysis of the data showed that more than 50% of children with cochlear implants had receptive language scores that were within the average range for normal hearing children, and scores that exceeded language skills of children who used conventional hearing aids.

This research serves to validate existing knowledge about the impact of cochlear implantation on pediatric language skills.

Modified from Baldassari CM et al: Receptive language outcomes in children after cochlear implantation, *Otolaryngol Head Neck Surg* 140: 114-119, 2009.

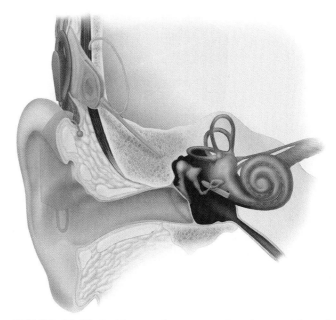

FIGURE 10-28 Cochlear implant system. Sound is transformed into electrical signal in speech processor. Signal is transmitted from external to internal induction coil, which is connected to electrode implanted near cochlear nerve.

scores on open-set sentence tests of less than 50%, (4) no evidence of central auditory lesions or lack of an auditory nerve, and (5) no evidence of contraindications for surgery in general (Wackym et al, 2005). Pediatric candidates (1) are 12 months through 17 years of age, (2) have profound sensorineural hearing loss, (3) experience minimal benefit from hearing aids, (4) have no evidence of central auditory lesions or lack of an auditory nerve, and (5) have no evidence of contraindications to surgery (Wackym et al, 2005). Appropriate auditory training and psychologic counseling are needed after appropriate selection of candidates.

OPERATIVE PROCEDURE

1. A *modified postauricular incision is used.* The posterior flap, including the temporalis muscle, is elevated, exposing the underlying bone. The site of the internal receiver is identified, and with a special drill a circular depression in the squamous portion of the temporal bone is made to house the receiver.
2. A mastoidectomy is performed with preservation of the bony ear canal and opening of the facial recess.
3. The surgeon secures the internal receiver in the depressed area in the temporal bone, and introduces the intracochlear electrode through the facial recess via a cochleostomy into the cochlea. It is secured in place with a piece of temporalis fascia.
4. The wound is closed. The patient is observed for 2 to 4 weeks until the wound is completely healed. Then the external signal processor is fitted and programmed. This allows transmission of an electrical signal, picked up at an ear-level microphone and processed in a microprocessor worn on the body.

Implantable Hearing Aids. Conventional hearing aids transmit sound using air conduction and bone conduction. Tradi-

to use surgically implantable devices in the treatment of hearing loss. These devices have greatly benefited the recipients, allowing some to distinguish sounds for the first time. Research continues in this field to develop applications for conditions previously considered untreatable and to refine and improve existing technology.

Cochlear Implantation. Technologic advances have given the deaf patient new hope in the area of cochlear implantation (Research Highlight). The device is implanted in the cochlea, with the receiver resting in the mastoid (Figure 10-28). As the device receives sound through the receiver, it emits electrical impulses through the transmitter into the cochlea and along the acoustic nerve. These impulses are interpreted as sound in the auditory area of the brain, which is in the temporal/parietal area of the cerebral cortex. The patient must be taught to interpret these sounds, which requires extensive training. Adult candidates for cochlear implantation generally possess the following characteristics: (1) severe or profound hearing loss with pure-tone average of 70-dB hearing loss, (2) use of appropriately fitting hearing aids or a trial with amplification, (3) aided

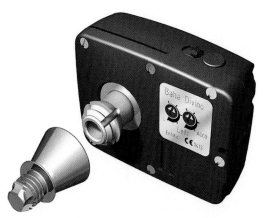

FIGURE 10-29 Bone-anchored hearing aid (BAHA) components. *Top to bottom,* External processor, abutment, fixture.

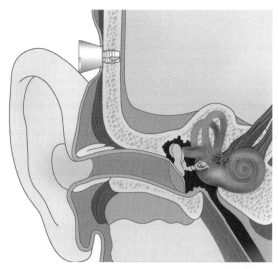

FIGURE 10-30 Cross section showing fixture and abutment.

tional bone-conduction hearing aids are external and secured to the head with a spring device. Their design makes them uncomfortable and obtrusive, causing headaches and skin abrasions. The quality of sound is inferior, and they often require a higher battery consumption. Air-conduction devices use an ear mold that fits into the ear canal. These devices may be contraindicated for patients with physical abnormalities that prevent the insertion of the ear mold into the canal and for those who have chronic eczema, ear drainage, or inflammation in the ear canal. Implantable hearing devices are designed for patients with moderate to severe conductive and sensorineural hearing loss (unilateral or bilateral). Ideally, implantable hearing devices should improve sound quality, provide comfort, improve appearance, and reduce the risk of chronic ear infections. Surgical implantation of hearing devices may be performed on an ambulatory basis using local or general anesthetics. The device is usually implanted in the ear with the best cochlear function.

BONE-ANCHORED HEARING AIDS. Conventional bone-conduction hearing aids transmit sound vibrations transcutaneously to the skull, bypassing a diseased or impaired external or middle ear and going directly to the cochlea. Disadvantages to using traditional bone-conduction hearing aids include discomfort, poor sound quality, poor aesthetics, and shifting of the transducer, which affects speech recognition (Palmer and Ortmann, 2005).

The bone-anchored hearing aid (BAHA, by Cochlear Corp., NSW, Australia) eliminates many of the disadvantages associated with traditional external bone-conduction hearing aids. It is designed for patients 5 years of age and older with moderate to severe conductive hearing loss (unilateral or bilateral) caused by congenital malformations but who maintain good cochlear function (down to 45-dB hearing loss) and for patients with otitis media, cholesteatoma, otosclerosis, microtia, and canal atresia who are unable to benefit from conventional amplification. More recently it has been approved and increasingly used in patients with single-sided deafness, most commonly from sudden profound hearing loss or after surgical excision of an acoustic neuroma. The BAHA system consists of a conventional microphone and amplifier, a specially designed transducer, and a coupling device to attach the device to the skin-penetrating and bone-anchored implant (Figure 10-29). The area behind the

ear is prepped and draped, and the implant site is marked. It is important to ensure that the hearing aid does not touch the pinna, which may cause acoustic feedback. A semicircular incision is made around the proposed fixture site. A titanium fixture is permanently implanted (tapped) into the mastoid bone, and a permanent skin penetration is made with a titanium snap coupler (Figures 10-30 and 10-31). A sound processor is fitted and adjusted to the patient's hearing loss 8 to 12 weeks after the implantation, depending on the age of the patient and ensuring the osseointegration process has taken place (Santina and Lustig, 2005) (Figure 10-32). When the BAHA is placed in young children, the sound processor is fitted in 3 to 6 months to ensure adequate osseointegration.

SEMI-IMPLANTABLE HEARING AIDS. Semi-implantable hearing aids are used in the middle ear and provide sound through direct stimulation of the ossicles; they allow for comfort because the external ear canal remains open. They consist of a microphone speech processor connected to a transmitter with an external coil that transmits electrical energy transcutaneously to an internal device. The internal device consists of an internal receiving coil connected to a receiver, which provides electrical energy to a mechanical driver connected to the ossicular chain. The driver vibrates the ossicles, mimicking the normal vibrations that occur as a result of acoustic sound input (Santina and Lustig, 2005). The internal receiver is implanted in the temporal bone, and the driver is attached to the incus. The external processor is fitted approximately 3 to 6 weeks after the surgery.

Research is ongoing in the development of semi-implantable and fully implantable hearing devices, which are currently considered experimental.

RHINOLOGIC (NASAL) PROCEDURES

Rhinologic surgery is performed to correct structural issues of the nose and to treat sinusitis and other conditions; it is also used an as adjunctive procedure to treat other disorders (e.g., pituitary neoplasms). Procedures that involve both internal

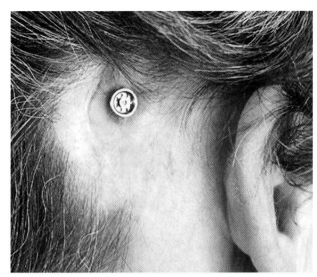

FIGURE 10-31 Bone-anchored hearing aid (BAHA) abutment.

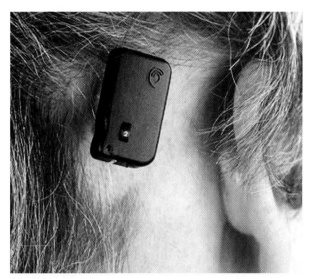

FIGURE 10-32 Patient with implanted bone-anchored hearing aid. The implant is positioned to avoid contact with the pinna, which could cause acoustic feedback if the device is driven at maximum output.

and external nasal reconstruction can be done with local anesthetics, usually supplemented with IV sedation and analgesia. If the patient is particularly apprehensive or anxious, a general anesthetic may be more appropriate.

Nasoseptoplasty or Submucous Resection of the Septum (SMR)

A nasoseptoplasty is straightening of either the cartilaginous or the osseous portions of the septum that lie between the flaps of the mucous membrane and the perichondrium. When the nasal septum is deformed, fractured, or injured, normal respiratory and nasal function may be impaired, interfering with airflow and sinus drainage. Deviations of the septum involving cartilage, bony parts (spurs), or both may block the meatus and compress the middle turbinate on that side, thereby resulting in an obstruction of the sinus opening. Septal deviations tend to produce sinus disease and nasal polyps.

The objective of the procedure is to establish an adequate partition between the left and right nasal cavities, thereby providing a clear airway through both the internal and external cavities of the nose.

Procedural Considerations. The procedure may be performed using local anesthesia, MAC, or general anesthesia. Regardless of the method chosen, the surgeon will use topical and injected anesthetics to aid in hemostasis. In most cases, the surgeon will opt to wear a headlight to improve visualization of the intranasal structures.

Operative Procedure

1. The surgeon opens the nostril with a nasal speculum and incises through the mucoperichondrium of the septum with a #15 blade. Using a Freer elevator, the tissues are separated and elevated (Figure 10-33).
2. The cartilage is incised with a knife, and the mucous membrane is elevated with a septal elevator.
3. Deviated cartilage and bony, thickened structures are trimmed or removed with a septum punch and a nasal cutting forceps.

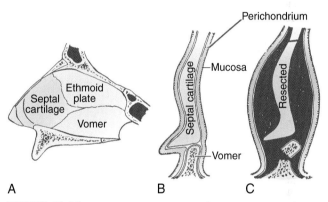

FIGURE 10-33 **A,** Primary components of septum. Incision line is for Killian type of submucous resection. **B,** Septum with deviated cartilage and spur at junction of vomer and septal cartilage. **C,** Resection of obstructive parts after careful elevation of mucoperichondrium and mucoperiosteum.

4. The surgeon trims the bony septal spurs with a punch forceps or chisel, gouge, and mallet. Suction is used to expose the field. Bleeding is controlled by insertion of additional cottonoids soaked with a topical hemostatic agent or by using the ESU.
5. The perpendicular plate of the ethmoid as well as the vomer may be removed by means of a suitable septum-cutting forceps.
6. The incision is sutured with 4-0 absorbable atraumatic suture on a small, straight needle.
7. Nasal splints made of plastic or Silastic may be inserted to prevent adhesions and maintain the septum. Some surgeons use mattress sutures to provide a patent airway while maintaining support for the septum.
8. A mustache dressing (i.e., a piece of 2-inch × 2-inch gauze folded and placed below the nose and secured with tape across the face or bridge of the nose) is applied. A small ice bag (e.g., a surgical glove filled with ice) may be applied to the nose.

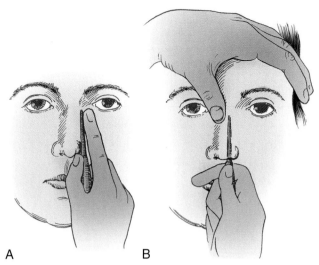

FIGURE 10-34 Reduction of nasal fracture. **A,** Boies elevator is placed along lateral wall of nose to point below nasofrontal angle. Distance to ala is marked with thumb. **B,** Elevator is then placed under depressed nasal bone, lifting it into position; opposite thumb carefully exerts downward pressure on elevated contralateral bone.

Closed Reduction of Nasal Fracture

The nose is the structure most susceptible to trauma because it is seated midface. The paired nasal bones are thin and project like a tent on the frontal process of the maxilla. If the trauma is caused by a direct frontal blow, usually both nasal bones are fractured, displaced outward, and depressed into the ethmoid sinus, and the septal cartilages become displaced. Noncontrast CT scans of the sinuses may be performed with protocols compatible with endoscopic navigation systems to have an accurate sense of extension of deviation or possible injury to surrounding sinuses and structures.

Procedural Considerations. Simple nasal fractures often can be managed with topical and local anesthesia. However, as with most nasal procedures, if the patient is significantly anxious, general anesthesia may be necessary. Topical and local anesthetics are used with a general anesthetic to provide vasoconstriction and enhance visualization for the procedure. The patient is prepped and positioned for nasal surgery.

Operative Procedure

1. The nose is packed with nasal cottonoids saturated with 4% cocaine. The local anesthetic is injected as previously described. When epinephrine is used, 10 minutes is the optimum time to wait for the effects of the hemostatic agent. This period of time will vary with other agents.
2. A Boies elevator is inserted into the nostril, and the nasal bones are elevated and molded into place by external manipulation (Figure 10-34).
3. Nasal packing or a Denver splint may be used to stabilize the reduction because sometimes the bony fragments tend to return to a depressed status.

Treatment of Epistaxis

The treatment of patients with epistaxis dates back more than two centuries (History box). Patients with nasal bleeding

usually control the problem themselves with direct pressure application. When their efforts fail, they seek help from their physician or an emergency department. When more conservative measures (which involve vasoconstrictive agents and nasal packing) taken in the emergency department fail, surgical intervention becomes necessary.

When epistaxis occurs, it is an important first step to spray oxymetazoline nasal spray in both nares and apply direct pressure to the nose. An initial hold of 15 minutes is recommended. Thereafter, inspection of the anterior nose and posterior oral pharynx should be performed to determine if the site of bleeding is anteriorly based in the nose or posteriorly located deep in the nasal cavity. Evidence of a posterior bleed is usually demonstrated by a trickling flow of blood from the nasopharynx running down along the posterior pharyngeal wall during an oral inspection. Blood may also appear on the tongue and the patient may complain of swallowing blood. Anterior epistaxis characteristically trickles down the front of the face upon the upper lip. If oxymetazoline spray and direct pressure fail to arrest the bleed, packing with nasal tampons or posterior packs should be considered.

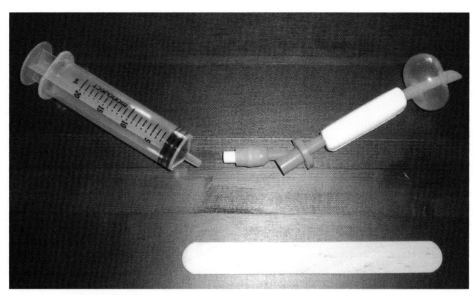

FIGURE 10-35 Posterior nasal packing with syringe for balloon inflation.

The length of the pack should be based upon the suspicion of where the bleed originates. Longer packing (8- or 10-cm packing) is considered when bleeds are more posterior in the nasopharynx. More anterior bleeds can be packed with 4.5-cm packing. Packing should be generously coated with antibiotic ointment and inserted in a horizontal angle following the floor of the nose. The packing is then sprayed with saline or oxymetazoline spray and expands. The patient should receive broad-spectrum antibiotics, such as oral third-generation cephalosporins, and instructed to follow up in 3 to 5 days for removal of packing.

Posterior nasal packing has an exterior balloon along the tube length as well as an anchoring balloon on the end (Figure 10-35). The anchoring balloon is first inflated to keep the tubes in place, and then the pressure balloons are inflated to compress bleeding vessels. If packing is used, it is placed directly against the bleeding site. Posterior nasal packing is placed by inserting a catheter-based tube, usually surrounded with packing, through the nostril. The tube is expanded with saline or oxymetazoline spray and 3 to 5 ml of air is pushed into the port, inflating a distal balloon. The proximal end of the catheter is pulled through the oral cavity with a Kelly clamp (while the distal end remains extending from the nostril).

If this fails to stop the oozing and other hemostatic agents, such as gelatin-based packing, silver nitrate sticks, or oxidized cellulose, fail to halt the bleed, an endoscopic approach to control the epistaxis is warranted. The endoscopy is performed in the OR with the use of general anesthesia or conscious sedation. Occasionally, ligation or embolization of the ethmoid, carotid, or maxillary artery is necessary and should be considered for persistent bleeds.

The setup for endoscopic control of epistaxis is the same as that for all nasal case prepping and draping. Once the navigation mask is applied to the patient and the video monitor is calibrated and functional, attention should be focused on Kiesselbach's plexus in the anterior nasal cavity and on the sphenopalatine artery as these are common sites of persistent bleeds. Suction electrosurgery should be used to electrocoagulate any visual bleeding and to clear the nasal passages of any clot or oozing. Other surgical options include transmaxillary internal maxillary artery ligation, transoral internal maxillary artery ligation, anterior/posterior ethmoid ligation, external carotid ligation, transnasal endoscopic sphenopalatine artery ligation, and submucosal supraperichondrial septoplasty.

Sinus Surgery

Sinusitis can be either recurrent, acute, or chronic. It is caused by bacteria and/or fungi and may be associated with anatomic abnormalities of the nose, such as a deviated septum or poor drainage pathways from the sinuses. Medical management of acute bacterial sinusitis involves a course of appropriate antibiotic therapy for 10 days to 2 weeks. If a patient does not respond to medical treatment for acute bacterial sinusitis or if sinus complaints persist, surgical drainage of the sinuses is indicated. Sinus procedures can be performed intranasally with or without the aid of endoscopes and video or through an open approach determined by which sinus cavity is involved. Generally, surgical treatment involves endoscopy to create a nasal window in acute maxillary sinusitis; a Caldwell-Luc procedure for chronic maxillary sinusitis; ethmoidectomy for ethmoid or sphenoidal sinusitis; and creation of an osteoplastic flap to drain the frontal sinus. Acute fungal sinusitis is treated by serial endoscopic debridements followed by a prolonged course of antifungals.

Functional Endoscopic Sinus Surgery (FESS). The field of FESS provides a more physiologic type of drainage by reducing trauma to normal tissues. Using direct endoscopic visualization, the surgeons' experience has expanded as technology and instrumentation have improved. Procedures performed endoscopically decrease trauma to normal structures and reduce morbidity. Fewer traumas mean a shortened healing process for the patient (Research Highlight). Many procedures that were once done with an open approach are now performed endoscopically and are considered safer because they are performed under direct visualization by means of an endoscope. Dedicated endoscopic sinus and skull base suites present a popular option for FESS because of the ease of setup and the comfort of multiple monitors, improving exposure (Figure 10-36).

FESS involves the endoscopic resection of inflammatory and anatomic defects of the sinuses. Because of the anatomic relationship to multiple systems, this procedure has many risks, which should be incorporated into the informed consent process. It is considered to be a technically demanding surgery, and techniques vary significantly. Most surgeons now prefer the endoscope to be attached to a video monitor, but some prefer to look directly through the eyepiece. The operative instruments are introduced into the nose alongside the endoscope.

The purpose of FESS is to ensure adequate ventilation and restore mucociliary clearance in the sinuses. If there is contact between the mucosa and the sinus, mucociliary clearance is inhibited and secretions are retained in the sinus. This predisposes the patient to sinus infections and mucocele.

The following sections are discussed with the understanding that they are more commonly performed endoscopically but may be done with an open approach as necessary.

PROCEDURAL CONSIDERATIONS. FESS can be performed after induction of general anesthesia or MAC, depending on the surgeon's and patient's preference. The setup for FESS is the same as the setup for any nasal surgery in terms of prepping, draping, and positioning. The instruments required are the basic nasal set, video equipment including monitor, and light source with the appropriate light cord adapted to the type of endoscope used. The endoscopes used in sinus surgery are much like endoscopes used in other procedures. They are 4 to 5 mm in diameter and have different directions of view: 0, 30, 70, 90, or 120 degrees. Depending on which sinus will be the operative site, the appropriate lens will be requested. Often if work is to be done in several sinus cavities, the surgeon may change lenses intraoperatively to obtain the optimal view in each cavity.

In addition to endoscopes, other instruments that may be used in FESS include endoscopic suction tips and suction elevators, biopsy forceps, forceps for retracting and cutting/excising tissue, and scissors. Patients undergo preoperative CT studies to determine the specific areas affected by the sinusitis. These CT scans should be available in the OR and will be referenced by the surgeon during the surgery (Figure 10-37).

The video equipment is located at the head of the bed. The surgeon operates from the right side of the patient, the scrub person stands at the right of the surgeon, and the first assistant usually stands across from the surgeon on the opposite side of the table. More commonly, the surgeon, the first assistant, and the scrub person stand during the procedure. With the use of a navigational system, the surgical procedure can also be viewed on a computer monitor by the rest of the surgical team.

Navigational systems are especially useful in revision sinus surgery, in which the familiar anatomy of the sinuses has been altered by previous surgery and the typical landmarks of the sinuses are now changed. Unfortunately, because of the nature of sinus disease itself in terms of allergic tendencies and mucous membrane irritation that are often chronic conditions, sinus disease can recur. Some patients may decide that their symptoms have recurred to the troublesome point where they elect to undergo surgery more than once. From a safety standpoint and to reduce the risk of a revision surgery, many

---

RESEARCH HIGHLIGHT

Endoscopic Sinus Surgery and Symptom Relief

Functional endoscopic sinus surgery (FESS) is an established treatment for a variety of sinus disorders. FESS offers the advantage of targeting and removing small areas of disease in very specific regions, thereby opening the sinuses for better aeration. Multiple studies have demonstrated the efficacy of FESS in reducing symptoms related to sinus disease, but no reports (including a large-scale evaluation of specific symptom response) existed before the meta-analysis conducted by researchers from Georgetown University and St. Louis University School of Medicine.

Researchers evaluated 21 relevant studies involving a total of 2070 patients with chronic rhinosinusitis who were followed for a mean of 13.9 months after surgery. The study dates evaluated ranged from 1980 through 2008. Inclusion criteria included studies with 20 or more adult participants, studies published in the English language, and studies in which the participants had three or more symptoms as defined by the American Academy of Otolaryngology–Head and Neck Surgery Rhinosinusitis Task Force. Individual meta-analyses were conducted for each symptom reported to compare preoperative and postoperative scores of symptom severity.

Results of the study demonstrated that nasal obstruction, facial pain, headache, smell, and postnasal discharge improved by approximately 59%, 61%, 53%, 49%, and 47%, respectively, providing a large body of evidence that symptom improvement is noted generally after FESS.

Modified from Chester AC et al: Symptom-specific outcomes of endoscopic sinus surgery: a systematic review, *Otolaryngol Head Neck Surg* 140:633-639, 2009.

---

surgeons will not attempt a revision sinus procedure without having an image-guided system available.

Several navigational systems are available, and many of these systems have applications for different types of surgeries, so the initial expense of the machine itself can be defrayed if it is shared with different surgical specialties, such as neurosurgery. Also, technical components to facilitating this type of sinus surgery must be mastered by the perioperative nursing staff, who must develop competence in system setup, transfer of the CT scan data into the system, and maintenance procedures.

To avoid possible injury, instruments should be passed to the surgeon or first assistant in the closed position and never over the patient's face. They should be passed smoothly and carefully so that the surgeon's or practitioner's eyes do not leave the endoscope or video monitor, limiting distractions. Some surgeons will request a suction-irrigation device that provides visualization of the sinus recesses by allowing simultaneous suction and irrigation of the operative field.

An antifog solution can be used to treat the lens of the endoscope. The solution should not be wiped off the lens; it should be applied to the lens in a thin layer. Another consideration that is crucial to a successful outcome in FESS is to maintain the integrity of the patient's periorbital cavities. The patient's eyes must be visible to the surgeon at all times to avoid injury to the orbit or to immediately recognize injury if it occurs. The surgeon will monitor for movement of the eyeball or appearance of an intraorbital hematoma.

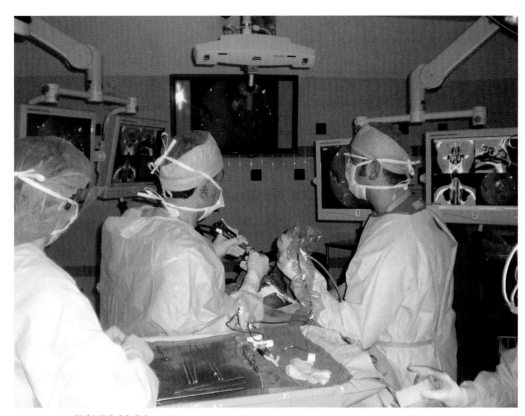

FIGURE 10-36 Endoscopic suites demonstrating navigation systems and monitors.

Encroachment of the orbit can be recognized if yellow tissue is seen because orbital fat is yellow. This finding should be communicated immediately to the surgeon. Another good technique is for the scrub person to place all tissue removed by the surgeon into a small labeled container of normal saline or lactated Ringer's solution on the surgical field. If any of the tissue "floats," the surgeon should be notified immediately. The surgeon will push the tissue in question with an instrument and rotate it a few times to release any small air bubbles that may be trapped in it, which could be causing it to float. If this is the case, the tissue will then sink to the bottom of the container; it should then be considered diseased tissue that needs to be removed. However, any tissue that continues to float naturally is presumed to be fat or brain tissue. In this case, it is presumed that the orbit has been encroached, and the situation is treated as a potentially serious complication.

OPERATIVE PROCEDURE

1. The surgeon applies topical anesthetic and administers the local anesthetic.
2. The lens of the endoscope is treated with antifog solution before the endoscope is introduced into the nose.
3. The natural ostium of the maxillary sinus is enlarged with a Lusk probe to provide physiologic drainage through the middle meatus. This creates a maxillary antrostomy and allows a larger drainage pathway into the ostiomeatal complex (Figure 10-38).
4. The diseased tissue is visualized through the endoscope, and straight or angled true-cuts are used to remove it.
5. If an anterior ethmoidectomy is indicated, the surgeon inserts the endoscope into the ostiomeatal complex and performs the ethmoidectomy by taking small bites of the honey-combed bones with straight true-cuts and removing

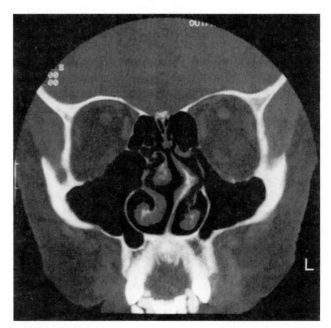

FIGURE 10-37 Computed tomography (CT) scan of maxillary and ethmoid sinuses. Note septal deviation, maxillary sinus ostia, turbinates, and ocular muscles.

them manually and/or with suction. This reduces the many-celled ethmoid labyrinth into one large cavity to ensure adequate drainage and aeration.

6. A sphenoidotomy is created by biting an opening into one or both of the sphenoidal sinuses with a straight true-cut. It is usually performed only if sphenoid sinus disease is present

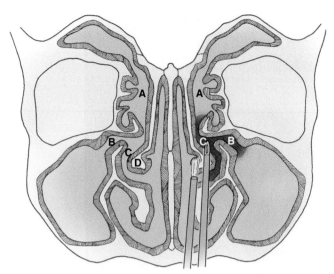

FIGURE 10-38 Surgery is performed using endoscope and forceps by intranasal approach. Diseased tissue is being removed from shaded areas depicting ethmoid sinus area (*A*), maxillary sinus ostia (*B*), and middle meatus (*C*). Middle turbinate is unaffected (*D*).

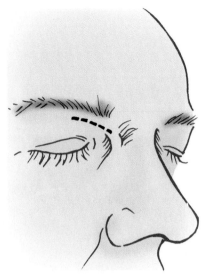

FIGURE 10-39 Incision to expose ethmoidal and frontal sinuses. Resulting scar is almost invisible.

on CT. Sphenoidotomies are often done with ethmoidectomies because once the ethmoid labyrinth is removed, the surgeon has excellent access through a lateralized middle turbinate exposing the sphenoidal sinuses.

7. Because no incisions are made, no sutures are required. Epistaxis should be controlled endoscopically until it becomes a slow ooze.
8. Absorbable gelatin film may or may not be placed into the patient's middle meatus to maintain patency and reduce stenosis. If used, it is rolled into a cylindric splint and set in place with bayonet forceps. An antibiotic ointment may be applied to the splint first, according to the surgeon's preference. The gel splints dissolve gradually, or they may be removed with irrigation.
9. A mustache dressing is applied.

Frontal Sinus Trephination and Obliteration

Frontal sinus trephination is the creation of a hole in the frontal sinus to drain pus or fluid accumulation. It is performed to treat the signs and symptoms of frontal sinusitis, which may include fever and headaches. A catheter may be surgically sewn into place at the incision site of the opening made into the affected frontal sinus; this serves as a drain and medium with which to irrigate the sinus until the disease resolves. If chronic suppuration with repeated acute attacks of frontal sinusitis persists, further surgery via a coronal craniotomy may be performed to remove the diseased lining of the sinus, obliterate the cavity with a fat graft, and reconstruct the nasofrontal duct to provide the necessary drainage. The procedure for a frontal sinus trephination follows.

   PROCEDURAL CONSIDERATIONS. The patient's face is prepped according to the surgeon's preference. The head is draped as in nasal procedures. Local anesthetic may be injected in the skin under the eyebrow. Culture tubes should be available as should drainage catheters.

OPERATIVE PROCEDURE
1. The incision is made medially below the eyebrow, along the same contour of the brow (Figure 10-39).

2. The periosteum is elevated from the bone, and a small diamond or cutting burr is used to drill a hole into the sinus.
3. Cultures may be taken of any pus present in the sinus, followed by irrigation.
4. A large Silastic or Teflon tube or appropriate-size catheter may be placed through the incision into the sinus.
5. The incision is closed with suture of the surgeon's preference.
6. A small dressing is usually applied to absorb drainage from the incision and catheter.

Endoscopic Transnasal Repair of Cerebral Spinal Fluid Leak

Cerebral spinal fluid (CSF) leaks are usually created by surgery or trauma. Although rare, spontaneous CSF leaks do occur. Patients usually complain of clear rhinorrhea with a salty taste from the nose, worse when either leaning forward or lying flat. Headache may accompany the rhinorrhea because of low spinal column pressures. Diagnosis is confirmed by sending the nasal fluid to the laboratory to test for β_2-transferrin, a protein specifically found in cerebrospinal fluid. A CT cisternogram assists with diagnosing the leak and often helps locate the site of dehiscence. Prepping and draping of the patient are performed in the same sterile fashion as for an endoscopic transsphenoidal approach to resection of pituitary mass, including prepping one lateral thigh and abdomen for potential graft use. All steps are followed as in a transsphenoidal resection of mass while paying close attention to the location of the carotids on the navigation system. Once the leak is found, a decision on what type of closure to use will be made by the otolaryngologist.

Caldwell-Luc with Radical Antrostomy

The purpose of a radical antrostomy is to establish a large opening into the wall of the inferior meatus, which ensures adequate gravity drainage and aeration. This large opening allows removal of the diseased tissues in the sinuses under direct vision. The Caldwell-Luc approach is also used to access the maxillary artery in cases of extreme epistaxis. The procedure requires an incision into the canine fossa of the upper jaw and

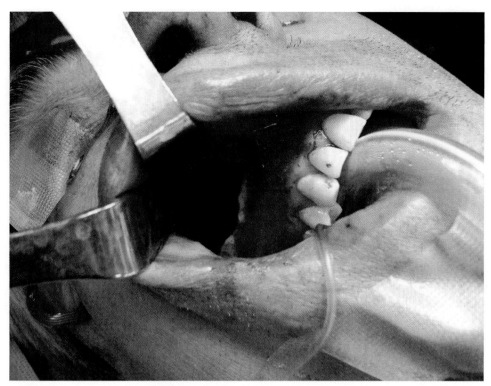

FIGURE 10-40 Caldwell-Luc operation.

exposure of the antrum for removal of bony diseased portions of the antral wall and contents of the sinus (Figure 10-40).

FESS can be used to treat patients with chronic sinusitis, obviating the need for radical procedures, such as Caldwell-Luc. FESS allows the surgeon to target the ostiomeatal complex (OMC) in the anterior ethmoid sinus region, where thickened and diseased tissue often blocks the OMC. Obstruction in this area leads to subsequent infection in the maxillary, frontal, and sphenoidal sinuses. FESS permits removal of only the diseased tissue; recovery is more rapid, with minimal and usually temporary effects on the patient's appearance.

Nasal Polypectomy

A nasal polypectomy is the removal of polyps from the nasal cavity (Figure 10-41). Nasal polyps are benign, grapelike clusters of mucous membrane and connective tissue. When the polyps become large, they obstruct the free passage of air, make breathing difficult, and cause a change in speech quality. Performed endoscopically, nasal polypectomies are often done with other sinus procedures that also require removal of diseased tissue. Because of the viscous nature of polyps, microdebriders are particularly helpful in these procedures. They can greatly shorten surgical time by their mechanism of morcellating the polyp and removing it by immediate suctioning while controlling bleeding, as opposed to each polyp being manually extracted with an instrument in small pieces. Procedures involving inverting papilloma may recur and may require repeat polypectomies as symptoms recur.

Procedural Considerations and Operative Procedure. Nasal polypectomy setup is as for any intranasal procedure, with the addition of endoscopic equipment. Additional instruments may

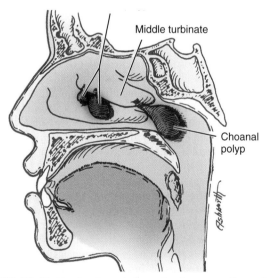

FIGURE 10-41 Nasal polyps. A choanal polyp is usually single and originates in the maxillary sinus; however, most polyps are found in the middle meatus.

include a nasal polyp snare if a microdebrider is not used. Packing is typically not needed or used.

ORAL CAVITY/LARYNGOLOGIC/ NECK PROCEDURES

Surgery of the Oral Cavity and Pharynx

The oral cavity is susceptible to both benign and malignant lesions, in part because of environmental risk factors. It is estimated that in 2009 (ACS, 2009) 35,720 men and women

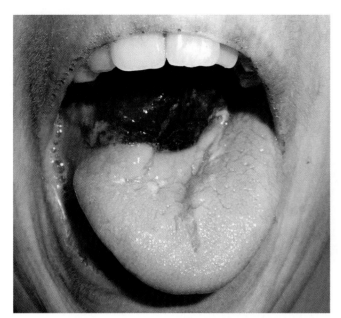

FIGURE 10-42 Carcinoma of the dorsal tongue.

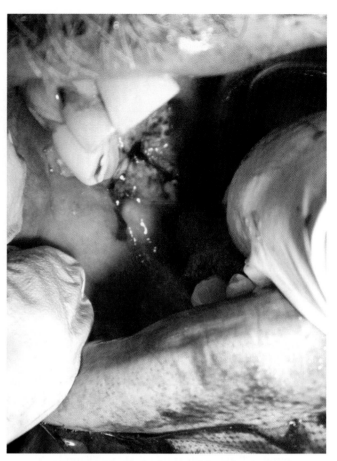

FIGURE 10-43 Carcinoma of the right tonsil.

(25,240 men and 10,480 women) will be diagnosed with cancer of the oral cavity and pharynx, and 7600 will die. Oral malignancies can be linked to specific carcinogens, the most important one being tobacco use. Incidence rates are more than twice as high in men as in women and are greatest in men who are older than 50 years.

Benign or malignant lesions of the tongue, floor of the mouth, alveolar ridge, buccal mucosa, or tonsillar area are excised depending on extensiveness of disease, involvement of surrounding vessels and nerves, and candidacy for surgery (Figures 10-42 and 10-43). Benign or small malignant tumors of the oral cavity may be excised without a neck dissection, though in the presence of diagnosed or highly suspicious metastatic disease, a selective neck dissection may be performed in an effort to control a cancerous growth in the upper jugular lymphatic chain of the neck.

In the treatment of carcinoma of the floor of the mouth with involvement of the mandible, a CT scan and/or MRI of the face and neck should be obtained to evaluate extension of the disease. A portion of the tongue is resected and may require a combined operation with reconstructive surgeons. A tracheostomy, percutaneous endoscopic gastric tube, neck dissection, and composite resection of both the mandible and the tongue with free flap reconstruction must be considered for extensive disease. When the primary intraoral lesion is confined to the tongue, a neck dissection and a hemiglossectomy are performed without resection of the mandible. In the presence of a lesion of the tonsil or an extensive lesion of the base of the tongue with pharyngeal wall involvement, resection of the mass may require removal of portions of the base of the tongue, pharyngeal wall, and soft palate to secure an adequate margin of normal tissue around the lesion. In recent years nonsurgical management with chemoradiotherapy has advanced for select oropharyngeal tumors. A free flap may be considered to fill a soft tissue defect if one is created from surgical resection. Psychologic preparation of the patient is extremely important because these procedures may be done for a minor lesion in the oral cavity or may be the first stage of much more extensive surgery in the head and neck area. A supportive and accepting family is important to the patient because of the possibility of disfigurement after surgery.

Procedural Considerations. The patient is placed in a supine position with shoulders elevated. Generally, endotracheal anesthesia is used and a pharyngeal pack of moist gauze may be inserted in the mouth. Instruments and supplies vary, depending on the surgical intervention.

Operative Procedure. Although the procedure may be scheduled as a local excision, frequently lesions of the oral cavity require more extensive excision. The setup should be designed to include the instruments for a neck dissection, or they should be readily available. For some tumors of the oral cavity, a tracheostomy is performed to ensure a patent airway after surgery. A laser may be used to excise locally confined lesions of the oral cavity.

Salivary Gland Surgery

Disorders of the salivary glands typically fall into one of three categories: inflammatory, obstructive, and neoplastic. Inflammatory conditions, such as bacterial or viral infections, can lead to salivary gland abscesses and ductal stone formation. Obstructive conditions can be a secondary consequence of inflammatory processes. Masses of the salivary glands may be benign or malignant, and 70% of them occur in the parotid gland. Three fourths of these parotid masses are benign (Elluru and Kumar, 2005). Perioperative surgical technologists will facilitate surgical care for patients experiencing any of these conditions.

Excision of the Submandibular Gland. Excision of the submandibular gland is performed to remove mixed tumors and calculi associated with extensive chronic inflammation. An incision is made below and parallel to the mandible and extending to beneath the chin to remove the gland and tumor.

PROCEDURAL CONSIDERATIONS. The patient is placed on the OR bed in a supine position, with the affected side up and is prepped for neck surgery. The instruments include a minor neck dissection setup. A set of lacrimal probes should also be added to the instrument setup if exploration of the submandibular (Wharton's) duct is necessary during surgery. No local anesthetic agents should be on the sterile field if identification of major nerves is anticipated. A nerve stimulator and bipolar ESU may be requested.

OPERATIVE PROCEDURE

1. The surgeon makes a small skin incision below and parallel to the mandible, extending forward to beneath the chin (Figure 10-44, *A*). The platysma is incised with scissors; the skin flaps and undersurface of the platysma and cervical fascia covering the gland are undermined with fine hooks, tissue forceps, and Metzenbaum scissors (Figure 10-44, *B*).
2. The mandibular branch of the facial nerve is retracted with a small loop retractor or nerve hook.
3. The submandibular gland is elevated from the mylohyoid muscle (Figure 10-44, *C*). The edge of the muscle is retracted anteriorly to expose the lingual veins and nerve and the hypoglossal nerve, which is identified and preserved.
4. The gland is freed by blunt dissection, and the submandibular duct is clamped, ligated, and divided with care to prevent injury to the lingual nerve.
5. The facial artery is clamped, ligated, and divided. The submandibular gland is removed (Figure 10-44, *D*).
6. The wound is closed with interrupted absorbable sutures. The skin edges are approximated with nonabsorbable sutures. A drain is inserted into the submandibular bed and secured to the skin. Dressings are applied.

Parotidectomy. Parotidectomy may be performed to treat recurrent parotiditis, but it is more commonly performed as part of the management of parotid gland tumors. In parotidectomy for tumor removal, the tumor and a portion of or the entire parotid gland are removed through a curved incision in the upper neck, in front of the earlobe, or through a Y type of incision on both sides of the ear and below the angle of the mandible. Even when a mass in the parotid gland is benign, the closeness of the facial nerve makes removing the entire mass surgically challenging (Figure 10-45). The facial nerve exits the stylomastoid foramen, enters the substance of the salivary gland, and then bifurcates into the temporofacial and cervicofacial branches, variably communicating with the gland. These branches then further divide into the temporal, zygomatic, buccal, and marginal mandibular and cervical branches near the edge of the parotid. The gland is divided artificially into a *superficial* and a *deep* lobe according to its relationship to the facial nerve. The possibility of damaging the facial nerve (resulting in facial nerve weakness or paralysis)

during the dissection of the gland should be considered carefully by all patients contemplating parotidectomy. Therefore the surgeon must understand that the most definitive way of avoiding damage to the facial nerve is to identify it early in the procedure. In addition, the patient should understand that a more radical procedure might be required if a malignant tumor is discovered to involve adjacent structures.

PROCEDURAL CONSIDERATIONS. The patient is placed on the OR bed in a supine position with the entire affected side of the face up. The entire side of the face, the mouth, the outer canthus of the eye, the ear, and the forehead are prepped and left exposed.

The instrument setup is a neck dissection set. A nerve stimulator or nerve integrity monitor should be available. A set of lacrimal probes should be included in the setup if exploration of the ductal system of the parotid is necessary during the course of surgery. Bipolar ESU may also be required.

OPERATIVE PROCEDURE

1. The incision (Figure 10-46) may extend from the posterior angle of the zygoma downward in front of the tragus of the ear and behind the lobule of the ear backward; the incision continues over the mastoid process and then downward and forward on the neck parallel to and below the body of the mandible. (A chin incision may also be used.) Bleeding vessels are controlled by hemostats and fine ligatures or with the ESU.
2. Using fine-toothed tissue forceps and scissors, the surgeon elevates the skin flaps as described for thyroidectomy (see Chapter 7) and retracts the flap with silk sutures fastened to clamps.
3. The upper portion of the sternocleidomastoid muscle is exposed and retracted, the auricular nerve is identified, and the lower part of the parotid gland is elevated with curved hemostats.
4. The superficial temporal artery and vein and external jugular vein are identified by means of blunt dissection. The parotid tissue is dissected from the cartilage of the ear and the tympanic plate of the temporal bone. The temporal, zygomatic, mandibular, and cervical branches of the facial nerve are identified and preserved.
5. The diseased portion of the parotid gland is removed, which can be superficial or deep.
   a. The *superficial portion* of the parotid gland containing the tumor is removed. In some cases the entire superficial portion is removed, followed by ligation and division of the parotid duct (Figure 10-47).
   b. When the *deep portion* of the parotid gland must be removed, the facial nerve is gently retracted upward and outward and then the parotid tissue is removed from beneath the nerve. Kocher retractors are used to retract the mandible. The external carotid artery is identified. In many cases the internal maxillary and superficial temporal arteries are clamped, ligated, and divided.
6. The wound is closed in layers with absorbable suture. If a divot is observed or anticipated overlying the resected portion of the parotid gland, abdominal fat may be harvested. A small drain is inserted, the skin is closed with fine nonabsorbable suture, and a pressure dressing may be applied depending on the surgeon's preference.

Uvulopalatopharyngoplasty. Uvulopalatopharyngoplasty (UPPP) is performed primarily to relieve obstructive sleep

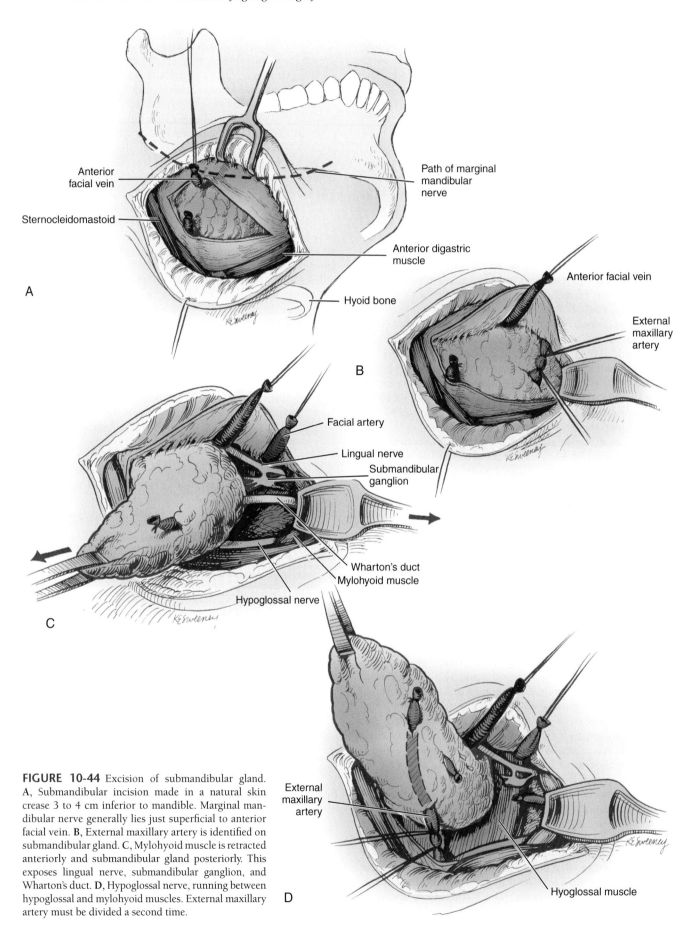

FIGURE 10-44 Excision of submandibular gland. **A,** Submandibular incision made in a natural skin crease 3 to 4 cm inferior to mandible. Marginal mandibular nerve generally lies just superficial to anterior facial vein. **B,** External maxillary artery is identified on submandibular gland. **C,** Mylohyoid muscle is retracted anteriorly and submandibular gland posteriorly. This exposes lingual nerve, submandibular ganglion, and Wharton's duct. **D,** Hypoglossal nerve, running between hypoglossal and mylohyoid muscles. External maxillary artery must be divided a second time.

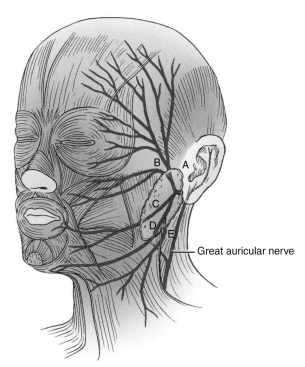

FIGURE 10-45 Branches of facial nerve. *A,* Temporal; *B,* zygomatic; *C,* buccal; *D,* mandibular; *E,* cervical.

apnea (OSA) and snoring (Figure 10-48) (Research Highlight). UPPP is not a substitution for the use of continuous positive airway pressure (CPAP), though the procedure may be considered when conventional use of CPAP fails. Two or more of the following indications are reason to perform the operation:

♦ An O_2 saturation that drops below 80%
♦ Apnea index worse than 20
♦ Significant daytime sleepiness
♦ Heroic snoring, producing social or marital problems
♦ Cardiac dysrhythmias, other than tachycardia or bradycardia, during sleep

PROCEDURAL CONSIDERATIONS. On occasion, tracheostomy may be performed with UPPP because of postoperative edema with subsequent risk of airway obstruction. The tracheostomy tube is removed and the incision is closed when the danger of postoperative edema and bleeding has passed. Because some of these patients are obese (causing the tissue of the pharynx to sag during sleep), preoperative planning should include obtaining an assortment of tracheostomy tubes, including extra long tubes, before the start of the procedure. Care must be taken in positioning the obese patient to ensure proper body alignment. Emergency tracheotomy or bronchoscopy should be anticipated in the event of airway obstruction after anesthesia induction. The surgeon may choose to administer a local anesthetic with the anesthesia provider monitoring the patient. The ease of intubation should have already been determined by this time, choosing the safest method of intubation (i.e., fiberoptic intubation, GlideScope). Once the method of intubation has been established and an airway is secured, a general anesthetic may be delivered. If the tonsils are present, a tonsillectomy is performed along with the UPPP.

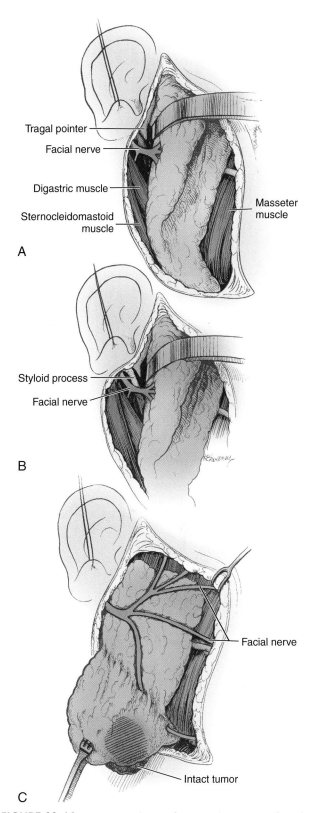

FIGURE 10-46 Operative technique for parotidectomy. **A,** Blunt dissection of parotid gland from external auditory canal cartilage exposes tragal pointer. Facial nerve lies approximately 1 cm deep and slightly anteroinferior to pointer and 6 to 8 mm deep to tympanomastoid suture line. **B,** Facial nerve exits stylomastoid foramen to run anteriorly between styloid process and attachment of digastric muscle to digastric ridge. **C,** Nearly completed process with tumor within intact superficial parotidectomy specimen.

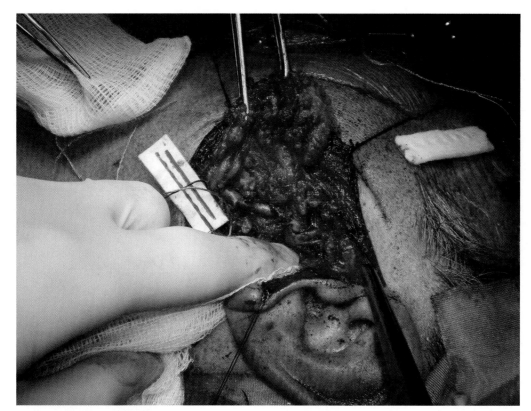

FIGURE 10-47 Surgical removal of superficial parotid mass.

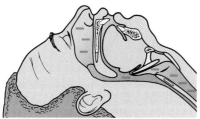

Patient predisposed to OSA

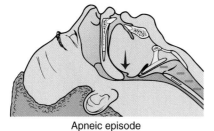

Apneic episode

FIGURE 10-48 Sleep apnea syndrome is a condition in which airflow is temporarily obstructed during sleep. Airflow obstruction occurs when the tongue and the soft palate fall backward and partially or completely obstruct the pharynx. The obstruction may last from 10 seconds to as long as 2 minutes. During the apneic period, the patient experiences severe hypoxemia (decreased PaO_2), hypercapnia (increased $PaCO_2$), and acidosis. These changes interrupt sleep and cause the patient to partially awaken. When the patient begins to awaken, the tone of the muscles of the upper airway increases. The tongue and soft palate move forward, and the airway opens. Apnea and arousals occur repeatedly during the night, separated by several normal breaths. The cause of sleep apnea is not definitely known. However, three factors appear to be involved: (1) shape of the upper airway, (2) neural control of the respiratory muscles, and (3) hormonal balance. *OSA,* obstructive sleep apnea.

OPERATIVE PROCEDURE

1. The McIvor mouth gag is inserted.
2. The tissue to be resected may be outlined by an electrosurgical blade. A #3 knife handle with a #15 blade or a #7 knife handle with a #12 blade may be used to make the incision, though surgical technique has changed from resection with scalpel to completing the entire resection with the ESU. The incision is made in the soft palate and anteriorly to the tonsillar pillar (if the patient has not previously undergone a tonsillectomy) or posteriorly to the tonsillar pillars (if the patient has undergone a tonsillectomy) (Figure 10-49).
3. Larger blood vessels may be clamped until the tissue is removed, or a suction coagulator or hand-controlled electrosurgical pencil may be used to obtain hemostasis as the tissue is excised.
4. Once the tissue is removed and hemostasis is achieved, absorbable sutures are used to approximate the edges of the mucosa. Depending on the surgeon's preference, 2-0 and 3-0 absorbable suture should be available. Needle holders should be long enough to allow the surgeon ease in delivering the atraumatic needle to the edges of the mucosa.
5. The oral cavity should be rinsed of blood and debris and the incision inspected before the patient is transferred from the OR.

   When inspecting the incision in the postoperative period, care should be taken not to disturb it with a tongue blade, if one is used to provide access for inspection. The patient must not use a straw for fluid intake because it might disturb the suture line. Gentle oral cavity rinsing is recommended several times daily to decrease the chance of postoperative infection and to increase patient comfort.

Obstructive Sleep Apnea and Surgical Risk

Obstructive sleep apnea (OSA) is the most prevalent sleep disorder. An estimated 82% of men and 92% of women with moderate-to-severe sleep apnea have not been diagnosed. Patients with undiagnosed OSA may have increased perioperative complications. The goal of this study was to determine whether a simple screening protocol for OSA-related signs and symptoms performed at the time of preoperative assessment for elective surgery, followed by home nocturnal oximetry in selected cases, could identify patients who were at increased risk of perioperative complications.

Participants for the study were identified during preanesthetic evaluation based on at least two clinical features suggestive of OSA as determined by a standardized screening questionnaire and physical examination (e.g., snoring, excessive daytime somnolence, witnessed apneas, or crowded oropharynx). Based on the initial screening, 172 patients, ranging in age from 27 to 85 years, were selected for home nocturnal oximetry testing. The oximetry results were interpreted by sleep medicine–trained physicians before the scheduled surgery and they established a baseline for the incidence of oxygen desaturation episodes at 4% or more.

Analysis of the data showed correlation between documented oximetric preoperative oxygen desaturation episodes and postsurgical complications. A complication was defined as an adverse event affecting a major organ system that required further monitoring, additional diagnostic testing, or direct therapeutic intervention. A significantly higher rate of complications was noted in patients who experienced five or more desaturation levels based on preoperative screening as compared to patients who had fewer than five episodes. The patients who had experienced 5 to 15 episodes of desaturation had a complication rate of 13.8% and those who had more than 15 episodes had a complication rate of 17.5%. The majority of complications were respiratory in nature, followed by cardiovascular, bleeding, and gastrointestinal complications.

While nocturnal oximetric testing does not confirm the presence of OSA, it may have usefulness as a screening tool for patients with this disorder. Effective screening will allow physicians to identify patients who are at risk for complications related to OSA and better plan their perioperative course to improve outcomes.

Modified from Hwang D et al: Association of sleep-disordered breathing with postoperative complications, *Chest* 133:1128-1134, 2008; Chung F, Elsaid H: Screening for obstructive sleep apnea before surgery: Why is it important? *Curr Opin Anaesthesiol* 22(3):405-411, 2009.

Laryngeal Surgery

Laryngeal surgery may be performed for diagnostic reasons or as a means of treatment for both benign and malignant conditions. This type of surgery involves both endoscopic and traditional "open" approaches and always has the potential to alter the patient's ability to communicate verbally in the postoperative period. As is the case with oral cavity malignancies, cancerous lesions within the laryngeal structures are often attributed to environmental factors, such as tobacco and alcohol use (Figure 10-50). Benign conditions, such as vocal cord polyps and nodules, are often treated with laryngeal surgery.

ENDOSCOPIC PROCEDURES

Laryngoscopy

Laryngoscopy is direct visual examination of the interior of the larynx by means of a rigid, lighted speculum known as a *laryngoscope* (Figure 10-51) to obtain a specimen of tissue or secretions for pathologic examination. Vocal cord visualization may also be accomplished in the office setting with a flexible, fiberoptic nasopharyngoscope.

Procedural Considerations. Most rigid laryngoscopies are performed with the patient receiving a general anesthetic. If the patient is unable to tolerate general anesthesia, a local or topical anesthetic of lidocaine, tetracaine, cocaine, or benzocaine/tetracaine will be administered. The patient should be sufficiently relaxed by reassurance and by pharmacologic preparation if the procedure is performed using local anesthesia. Sedatives may be administered before surgery. Immediate preoperative assessment should include the presence of any dental appliances and loose teeth and the condition of dental work. Any stiffness or immobility of the neck or shoulders should be evaluated. Respiratory problems such as asthma must receive careful attention. The patient should be cautioned about not eating or drinking after surgery until the gag reflex has returned and swallowing occurs without difficulty.

The setup includes the following:

- Labels for all medications and solutions used in the sterile field
- Local anesthesia setup
- Gauze sponges, 4 × 4 inches
- Laryngeal mirror
- Cotton balls
- Small cup of hot water (to warm the laryngeal mirror so that it does not fog when inserted into the mouth to view the vocal cords) or an antifog solution
- Emesis basin
- Syringe, 5 ml; and Abraham cannula
- Medication cup
- Jackson laryngeal application forceps
- Anesthetic spray, with angulated tip, or other topical anesthetic for the oral mucosa
- Instrument setup:
  - One laryngoscope
  - Two laryngeal suction tubes
  - One light carrier, fiberoptic
  - Two laryngeal biopsy forceps, one straight and one up-biting
  - Two sponge-carrier forceps with extra sponges
  - One tooth guard
  - One fiberoptic light cord
  - Zero-degree telescope: may be requested for close visualization or attached to the camera for photographs of specific areas
  - One laryngeal probe: may be used to retract tissue or assess mobility of tissue

Accessory items include suction tubing, a specimen container, a basin with sterile saline, gauze sponges, sterile towels, and gloves.

If the surgeon wishes to perform a suspension laryngoscopy, a self-retaining laryngoscope holder is added to the instrument table, as well as microlaryngeal instruments, which include scissors, cup forceps, and alligator forceps. A special platform may be mounted onto the OR bed or a Mayo stand may be placed above the patient's chest and over the

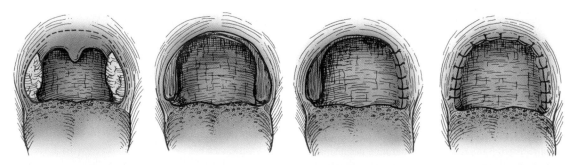

FIGURE 10-49 Technique of palatopharyngoplasty as advocated by Simmons and associates.

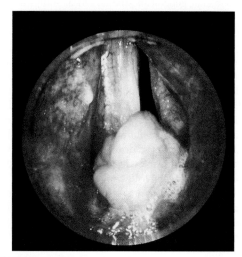

FIGURE 10-50 Large granular tumor on the true cord.

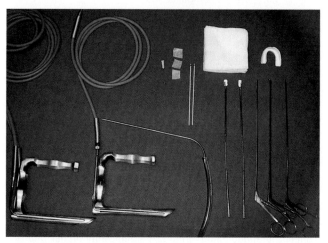

FIGURE 10-51 Instrument setup for direct laryngoscopy includes Jako and Dedo laryngoscopes, laryngeal suction, assorted laryngeal forceps, and sponge carriers.

OR bed to provide a place for the laryngoscope holder to rest. The surgeon normally uses the operating microscope with a 400-mm lens during suspension laryngoscopy. The patient is placed in a supine position to facilitate visualization of the vocal cords. A shoulder roll should be available if slight hyperextension of the neck is necessary to assist in visualization of the larynx.

Operative Procedure

1. Moist gauze pads or tape should be placed over the patient's eyes to protect them from the instrumentation and to prevent injury and irritation from secretions during the procedure. The head may also be wrapped in a sterile towel. A sterile drape may be used to cover the patient. A tooth guard or moist 4-inch × 4-inch gauze sponge is placed to protect the patient's teeth.
2. The surgeon introduces the spatula end of the laryngoscope into the right side of the patient's mouth and directs it toward the midline; then the dorsum of the tongue is elevated so that the epiglottis is exposed.
3. The patient's head is first tipped backward and then lifted upward as the laryngoscope is advanced into the larynx.
4. The larynx is examined, a biopsy is taken, secretions are aspirated, and bleeding is controlled.
5. The patient's face is cleansed.

Laryngoscopy instrumentation should remain set up in the room until the patient is transferred because the equip-

ment may be needed if the patient experiences laryngospasm postoperatively.

Microlaryngoscopy

Microlaryngoscopy facilitates improved diagnosis and allows the laryngologist to view with relative ease areas that previously were inaccessible or difficult to visualize. It may also be used for minor surgery of the larynx, especially for the removal of polyps or nodules on the vocal cords (Figure 10-52). Intralaryngeal surgery using the laryngoscope is often referred to as *phonosurgery*. Instrumentation may vary according to surgeon preference. Research is currently under way to determine the feasibility of using robotics for laryngeal surgery.

Procedural Considerations. If the procedure is done to remove polyps or nodules from the vocal cords, the patient must be cautioned to observe complete voice rest or to whisper postoperatively. The patient should be provided with a pencil and paper or erasable slate to aid in communication. The patient's restriction on speaking should be noted on the nursing plan of care and on the front of the chart.

The basic instrument setup for laryngoscopy is used. Microlaryngeal instruments are added to the setup and include the following:

- Self-retaining laryngoscope holder
- Jako microlaryngeal grasping forceps

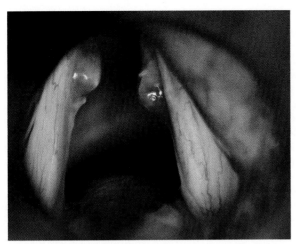

FIGURE 10-52 Bilateral vocal cord polyps.

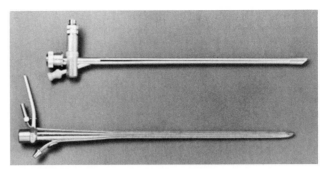

FIGURE 10-53 Pediatric and adult esophagoscopes.

- Jako microlaryngeal cup forceps, straight and up-biting cups
- Jako microlaryngeal scissors, straight, angled, and up-biting
- Jako microlaryngeal knives, straight and curved
- Laryngeal probe
- Microlaryngeal mirror
- Open-ended microlaryngeal suction tube
- Laryngoscope (dual light channel)

The aforementioned instruments are 22 cm long to allow use with the microscope, and are long enough to keep the surgeon's hands out of the visual field. The patient's head is adjusted to allow visualization of the larynx. The surgeon usually adjusts the microscope. The microscope lens should have a 400-mm focal length. Focal length is the distance from the lens to the operative area and is the point at which the field can be clearly viewed through the microscope. Beyond this point the field becomes fuzzy. The 400-mm lens gives the surgeon a 40-cm focal length, or working distance.

Carbon Dioxide Laser Surgery of the Larynx

Laryngologists often use the CO_2 laser to treat lesions of the larynx and vocal cords. This laser is efficient and has a high power output. The beam destroys tissue at a precise point with minimal destruction of the surrounding tissue. It is especially useful in surgeries such as removal of webs in the larynx, vocal cord papillomas, and carcinoma in situ of the larynx, as well as benign endobronchial lesions.

Procedural Considerations. The basic setup for laryngoscopy and microlaryngoscopy is used. All instrumentation used for laser laryngoscopy should be ebonized. A general anesthetic is usually administered. The operating microscope with a 400-mm lens is used, with the laser micromanipulator attached to the microscope head. The beam should also be tested for proper working order before use on the patient. Extreme care should be used when handling this delicate piece of equipment. A smoke evacuator should be used to remove the laser plume—a smokelike steam rising from the impact site; high-filtration laser masks should be worn by personnel. Where minimal plume is generated, a central wall suction with an in-line filter may be used for plume evacuation (AORN, 2009c). All other laser precautions apply.

Adjunctive Procedures

Although the following procedures do not technically involve the larynx, they are often performed by otorhinolaryngologists in conjunction with laryngeal surgery and are of particular use in the diagnostic arena.

Bronchoscopy. The trachea, bronchi, and lungs are visualized directly with a rigid or flexible bronchoscope that has a fiberoptic lighting system. A rigid scope gives a larger viewing area, whereas a flexible scope is easily inserted into the patient and manipulated. Bronchoscopy is fully described in Chapter 14. The Nd:YAG laser may be used for lesions of the trachea or bronchi, depending on the type of lesion. Most diagnostic bronchoscopies are performed using topical anesthetics and moderate sedation, requiring careful patient monitoring by the perioperative nurse.

Esophagoscopy. Esophagoscopy is the direct visualization of the esophagus and the cardia of the stomach. This procedure is used to observe the area for extension of tumor, to remove tissue and secretions for study, or to evaluate for second primary tumor sites.

PROCEDURAL CONSIDERATIONS. Esophagoscopy facilitates the diagnosis of esophageal carcinoma, diverticula, hiatal hernia, stricture, benign stenosis, and varices. Patients with suspected obstruction, symptoms of bleeding, or regurgitation may require endoscopy. The Nd:YAG laser may be used in the treatment of some of these lesions. Esophagoscopy may also be used for therapeutic manipulations, such as removal of a foreign body or insertion of an esophageal bougie to treat esophageal stenosis.

The setup includes the following:
- Esophagoscopes of desired type, size, and length (Figure 10-53)
- Suction tubing
- Fiberoptic light source and light cords
- Bougies, if desired
- Forceps of desired type and length
- Specimen containers
- Water-soluble lubricating jelly
- Gauze sponges
- Basin with sterile saline
- Suction tips (with velvet-eyed tips to avoid suctioning the mucosa of the esophagus into the tip)

OPERATIVE PROCEDURE
1. The fiberoptic light carrier is inserted into the esophagoscope and the fiberoptic light cord attached. A thin layer of lubricant is applied to the scope. The scope is passed into the mouth. The tongue, epiglottis, laryngeal inlet, and cri-

copharyngeal lumen are identified. If necessary, a person holding the patient's head may be required to tip the head backward while extending the neck anteriorly. Usually the esophagoscope is passed to the right side of the tongue, and the patient's head is turned slightly to the left.

2. When the scope has passed the inferior constrictors, the patient's head is moved in various directions so that all areas of the esophageal wall may be examined.

3. Specimens of secretions from the esophageal lumen may be obtained with an aspirating tube and suctioning apparatus. In some cases, saline may be injected through the esophagoscope's aspirating channel and the fluid is withdrawn immediately for histologic study. A tissue biopsy may be taken. After biopsy, the area is assessed for bleeding and the esophagoscope is then removed.

Triple Endoscopy. When laryngoscopy, bronchoscopy, and esophagoscopy are performed in a single session on a patient, the procedure is termed *triple endoscopy* or *panendoscopy.* The order in which the procedures are performed depends on the surgeon's preference. The purpose of triple endoscopy is usually diagnostic. While inspecting for a malignancy, the surgeon views the structures, takes specimens for biopsy, and possibly makes smears or washings of the suspect areas. For any of the aforementioned endoscopy procedures, all equipment or instrumentation should be set up and be in working order (i.e., light carriers in place; light cables connected and working). Instrumentation to be used through the various scopes (i.e., suction tips, telescopes, biopsy forceps) should be checked for appropriate length. Specimens taken during endoscopic procedures should be labeled and removed from the back table as soon as possible. In some instances, it may be helpful to indicate on the label that the specimens are microscopic.

OPEN NECK AND LARYNGEAL PROCEDURES
Tracheostomy

Tracheostomy is the opening of the trachea and the insertion of a cannula through a midline incision in the neck, below the cricoid cartilage. A tracheostomy may be permanent or temporary. It is used as an emergency procedure to treat upper respiratory tract obstruction, which can be caused by bilateral vocal cord paralysis, swelling of the neck or airway caused by trauma, allergic reactions, or neoplasms. It is also used as a prophylactic measure in the presence of chronic lung disease, in extensive neck resections where massive upper airway edema is anticipated, or if radiation-induced edema is expected during the treatment of cancers involving the tongue and neck. Tracheostomy is also considered the "gold standard" in treating sleep apnea in which obstruction may occur. Tracheostomy may be performed to permit easy and frequent pulmonary toileting on patients having a difficult time managing and expectorating their own secretions. Additionally, tracheostomy should be performed on patients experiencing prolonged intubation to avoid overgrowth of granulation tissue and subsequent subglottic stenosis.

The patient's psychologic status should be carefully evaluated because of the altered body image, which may be either temporary or permanent, depending on the disease entity involved. Tracheostomy care should be explained carefully

and thoroughly so that the patient will understand why self-care should be performed frequently. Reinforcement should be given regarding the ability to communicate with others by means of a pencil and paper or message board. As recovery progresses and secretions diminish, the patient can be shown how to occlude the opening of the tube for brief periods to be able to speak a few words. The patient also must be taught the mastery of tracheostomy self-care. If a tracheostomy tube with a disposable inner cannula is inserted, the patient must have a replacement cannulae in the event occlusion or blockage occurs in the immediate postoperative period

Procedural Considerations. Before tracheostomy tube cuffs are inserted, they should be tested for air leaks by inflating and then deflating the balloon. Cuffed tracheostomy tubes are used on patients at risk for aspiration, patients receiving positive-pressure ventilation, or patients who have undergone skull base surgeries involving open communication of the sinuses into the intracranium, where it is desirable to avoid pneumocephalus. The patient is placed in a supine position, with the shoulders raised by a small rolled sheet to slightly hyperextend the neck and head. Using a skin marker the surgeon marks a midline incision site, halfway between the sternal notch and the cricoid cartilage, between the second and third tracheal rings. The neck is prepped, and sterile drapes are applied. A soft suction catheter should be available on the sterile field for suctioning after the tube is inserted.

Operative Procedure

1. The surgeon injects lidocaine with epinephrine into the subcutaneous tissue across the tracheotomy site previously marked with a surgical marker.

2. A horizontal incision is made with a #10, #15, or #11 blade. Soft tissues and muscle are divided, using blunt hemostats and sharp dissection through the platysma and the overlying strap muscles. The thyroid gland is identified; attention is directed to the isthmus with the intention of transecting this area of the gland. Occasionally, the isthmus can be retracted from the surgical site without transection (Figure 10-54).

3. The plane between the isthmus and the trachea is separated by the surgeon with a blunt hemostat, exposing the thyroid gland so the surgical assistant can carefully transect it with the ESU knife. This exposes the underlying tracheal rings—usually the second and third. In some cases, two curved clamps may be inserted through this incision across the isthmus and then the isthmus is transected.

4. The transected ends of the isthmus are oversewn or suture-ligated with absorbable sutures.

5. Once the trachea is identified, a horizontal incision is made with a #11 blade through the second and third tracheal rings. The incision is extended and the tracheotomy tube is inserted. Two 2-0 silk sutures are then sewn into the trachea for future use during the first tracheostomy change. In two motions, one silk suture is inserted into the trachea, and then retrieved with the needle driver through the horizontal incision. This is then repeated with another silk suture through the bottom half of the horizontal incision. Air knots are tied into each of the sutures and secured with tape onto the chest so they are ready for easy retrieval for retraction during the first tracheostomy change, about 5 to 7 days later.

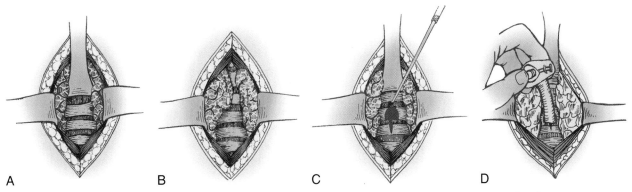

A   B   C   D

FIGURE 10-54 Operative technique for elective tracheostomy. **A,** Retractor exposing trachea by drawing isthmus of thyroid upward. **B,** Alternative method to that shown in (**A**). Isthmus of thyroid is divided to expose trachea. **C,** Two tracheal rings are cut, and upper ring is partially resected. Tracheal hook pulls trachea from depth of wound nearer surface. **D,** Insertion of tube.

By tradition, one air knot is placed in the upper stay suture and two air knots are placed in the lower stay suture to allow for easy identification and proper retraction at the time of tracheostomy tube change or in the event of tracheostomy tube dislodgement. The air knots are cut and removed once the first tracheostomy change takes place.

An additional tracheostomy tube of the same size and the obturator should be kept with the patient at all times, in the event the tube becomes dislodged or plugged with secretions. This practice expedites changing the tracheostomy tube with minimal potential for complications to the patient.

Laryngofissure

Laryngofissure is an opening of the larynx for exploratory, excisional, or reconstructive procedures that cannot be accomplished endoscopically.

Procedural Considerations. A laryngofissure may be performed when access to the intrinsic larynx is necessary. The thyroid cartilages are split in the midline, and the true vocal cords and false vocal cords are incised at the midline anteriorly. A neck dissection instrument set is required, plus an oscillating power saw.

Operative Procedure
1. A tracheotomy is performed, and an endotracheal tube is inserted. A general anesthetic is administered.
2. A transverse incision is made through the skin and first layer of the cervical fascia and platysma muscles, approximately 2 cm above the sternoclavicular junction or in the normal skin crease. The upper skin flap is undermined to the level of the cricoid cartilage, and the lower flap is undermined to the sternoclavicular joint.
3. Bleeding vessels are clamped with mosquito hemostats and ligated. The strap muscles are elevated and incised in the midline.
4. The thyroid cartilages are cut with an oscillating saw, and the true vocal cords are visualized through an incision into the cricothyroid membrane. The true vocal cords are divided in the midline (anterior commissure), and the interior of the larynx is exposed.
5. The tracheostomy tube must be left in place after surgery to ensure an airway.

Phonosurgery

Phonosurgery refers to various operations on the laryngeal framework to improve phonation for patients with communication disorder. Type I thyroplasty is used to change or improve the voice. Thyroplasty types II and III are used to alter vocal cord tension and voice pitch.

Thyroplasty. Type I thyroplasty is a form of phonosurgery for the treatment of unilateral vocal cord paralysis, which may be caused by trauma, neoplasms, paralysis from thyroidectomy, paralysis after extensive aortic and mediastinal vascular surgery, and mechanical and central nervous system dysfunctions. A window is created surgically in the thyroid cartilage, into which a silicone implant is placed. The implant pushes the paralyzed cord medially, which allows the moving cord to touch the paralyzed cord and close the opening.

The procedure is done using monitored local anesthesia to allow the patient to speak during surgery. This allows the surgeon to evaluate the quality of the patient's voice in an effort to attain the best result.

OPERATIVE PROCEDURE
1. The patient is positioned on the OR bed in a semisitting position. A laryngoscopy is done by means of a flexible fiberoptic laryngoscope.
2. As the patient is asked to speak, the surgeon determines the extent of approximation of the vocal cords as well as the patient's breath control. After a thorough evaluation, the patient is then prepped and draped.
3. A local anesthetic is injected into the surgical site. A horizontal incision is made at the middle level of the thyroid ala. Gelpi retractors are used to maintain exposure as dissection to the thyroid cartilage is completed. Measurements for the placement of the window are taken and marked with a marking pencil. A #15 blade is used to create a window in the thyroid cartilage. In some cases, a power drill with a cutting burr may be used. A periosteal elevator may be used to displace the vocal cords during phonation in an effort to determine voice quality.
4. When voice quality is satisfactory, the implant is placed into the window. Final laryngoscopy is done to view approximation of the vocal cords with the implant in place. The incision is then closed, and a dressing is applied.

Partial Laryngectomy

Partial laryngectomy is removal of a portion of the larynx. It is done to remove superficial neoplasms that are confined to one vocal cord or to remove a tumor extending up into the ventricle or the anterior commissure or a short distance below the cord. A cancer confined to the intrinsic larynx is generally a low-grade malignancy and tends to remain localized for long periods. The patient should be prepared for an altered voice quality postoperatively as well as for the possibility of total laryngectomy if the tumor proves too extensive for partial resection (Table 10-1). Types of partial laryngectomies include a vertical hemilaryngectomy, supraglottic laryngectomy, and supracricoid laryngectomy. With the advancements of cancer treatment (including the surgical excision of the tumor along with postoperative administration of chemotherapy concurrently with external beam radiation therapy), cure rates have increased while preserving some function of the larynx. The goal of partial laryngectomy is to avoid removing the entire larynx and to preserve the patient's natural swallowing ability. A successful partial laryngectomy should leave the patient with the ability to phonate, though usually with a more hoarse voice quality. The otolaryngologist must carefully stage the laryngeal cancer via a panendoscopy with biopsy and determine the overall candidacy of the patient who may receive a partial laryngectomy. If tumor extension does not warrant a partial laryngectomy, a total laryngectomy must be performed. Steps and procedural considerations for a total laryngectomy are described next.

Total Laryngectomy

Total laryngectomy is the complete removal of the cartilaginous larynx, the hyoid bone, and the strap muscles connected to the larynx and possible removal of the preepiglottic space with the lesion. A wide-field laryngectomy is done when there is a loss of mobility of the cords and to treat cancer of the extrinsic larynx and hypopharynx (Figure 10-55). Malignant tumors of the extrinsic larynx are more anaplastic and tend to metastasize. When laryngeal carcinoma involves more than the true cords, a prophylactic (preventive) modified, or selective, neck dissection is done to remove the lymphatics. Depending on the extent and severity of disease in the neck, a radical neck dissection may be warranted though rarely routinely performed.

Laryngectomy presents many psychologic problems. The loss of voice that follows total laryngectomy is traumatic for the patient and family. The patient may be taught to talk by using either an esophageal voice or an artificial larynx. The esophageal voice is produced by the air contained in the esophagus rather than by that in the trachea. Speech requires a sounding air column. With instruction and practice, the patient is able to control the swallowing of air into the esophagus and the reintroduction of this air into the mouth with phonation. The sounding air column is then transformed into speech by means of the lips, tongue, and teeth. A tracheoesophageal fis-

---

TABLE 10-1

Surgical Procedures for Laryngeal Carcinomas and Predictions of Vocal Quality after Surgery

Structures Removed	Structures Remaining	Postoperative Condition
TOTAL LARYNGECTOMY		
Hyoid bone	Tongue	Loses voice
Entire larynx (epiglottis, false cords, true cords)	Pharyngeal walls	Breathes through tracheostoma
Cricoid cartilage	Lower trachea	No problem swallowing
Two or three rings of trachea		
SUPRAGLOTTIC OR HORIZONTAL LARYNGECTOMY		
Hyoid bone	True vocal cords	Normal voice
Epiglottis	Cricoid cartilage	May aspirate occasionally, especially liquids
False vocal cords	Trachea	Normal airway
VERTICAL LARYNGECTOMY (OR HEMILARYNGECTOMY)		
One true vocal cord	Epiglottis	Hoarse but serviceable voice
One false cord	One false cord	Normal airway
Arytenoid	One true vocal cord	No problem swallowing
Half thyroid cartilage	Cricoid	
PARTIAL LARYNGECTOMY		
One vocal cord	All other structures	Hoarse but serviceable voice; occasionally almost normal voice
		No airway problem
		No swallowing problem
TRANSORAL CORDECTOMY		
Portion or all of one vocal cord	All other structures	May have normal/hoarse voice
		No other problems
LASER SURGERY		
Tumor only removed	All other structures	Normal/hoarse voice

From Workman ML: Interventions for clients with noninfectious problems of the upper respiratory tract. In Ignatavicius DD, Workman ML, editors: *Medical-surgical nursing: patient-centered collaborative care*, ed 6, Philadelphia, 2010, Saunders.

tula facilitates insertion of a Blom-Singer duckbill prosthesis for the purpose of speech (Figure 10-56, *A*). This fistula may be created during the initial surgical procedure (primary tracheoesophageal puncture [TEP]) or at a later date when healing has occurred (Figure 10-56, *B*).

Because the stump of the trachea is exteriorized to the skin of the neck to form a permanent stoma, all the patient's breathing is done directly into the trachea and no longer through the nose and mouth. The nose no longer moistens this air. Drying and crusting of the tracheal secretions occur. Humidification may be provided with a humidified tracheostomy collar or a humidified moisture exchange system later during the healing process. The patient will be anxious to know about postoperative voice quality, which depends on the specific procedure performed.

Procedural Considerations. The patient is placed on the OR bed in a supine position with the neck extended and shoulders elevated by a shoulder roll or folded sheet. A general anesthetic is administered. Airway considerations are paramount when approaching a patient with laryngeal cancer. An awake tracheostomy may be performed initially to control the airway, and occasionally patients have previously placed tracheostomy tubes. If the tracheostomy is performed initially or is preexisting, the use of a cuffed, wire-reinforced, flexible endotracheal tube will ensure effective delivery of the anesthetic and give the surgical team flexibility as the larynx and trachea are manipulated during the surgical procedure. An effective suction apparatus is essential. The proposed operative site, including the anterior neck region, the lateral surfaces of the neck down to the outer aspects of the shoulders, and the upper anterior chest region, is prepped and draped in the usual manner. The instrument setup is a neck dissection set.

Operative Procedure
1. The surgeon makes a midline incision from the suprasternal notch to just above the hyoid bone. Skin flaps are undermined on each side. The sternothyroid, sternohyoid, and omohyoid muscles (strap muscles) on each side are divided by means of curved hemostats and a knife.
2. The suprahyoid muscles are severed from the portion of the hyoid to be divided. The hyoid bone is skeletonized with care to preserve the hypoglossal nerves. Bleeding vessels are clamped and ligated.
3. The superior laryngeal nerve and vessels are exposed and ligated on each side with long, curved fine hemostats and fine ligatures.
4. The isthmus of the thyroid gland is divided between hemostats. Each portion of the thyroid gland is dissected from the

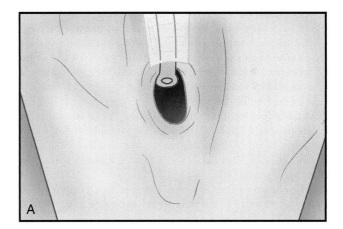

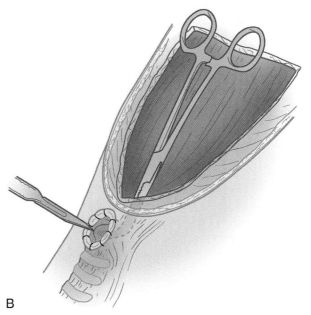

A

B

FIGURE 10-56 Artificial larynx to facilitate speaking. **A,** Speech valve in place. **B,** Primary tracheoesophageal puncture technique. Note preliminary repair of stoma to allow accurate positioning of puncture site before pharyngeal closure. Feeding tube (14F) is inserted through puncture down esophagus to the stomach.

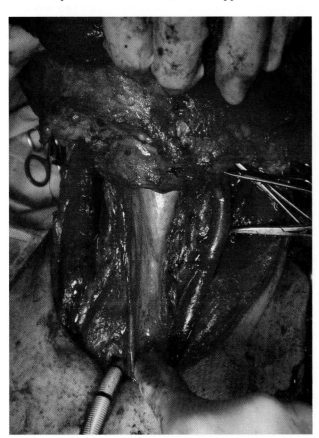

FIGURE 10-55 Wide-field defect following removal of the larynx.

trachea with Metzenbaum scissors and fine tissue forceps. The superior pole of the thyroid is retracted. The superior thyroid vessels are freed from the larynx by sharp dissection. Sometimes, one or both lobes of the thyroid gland are included in the resection for oncologic purposes.

5. The larynx is rotated. The inferior pharyngeal constrictor muscle is severed from its attachment to the thyroid cartilage on each side.

6. The endotracheal tube is removed. The trachea is transected with care to keep an adequate margin from the tumor. The upper resected portion of the trachea and the cricoid cartilage are held upward with Lahey forceps. A balloon-cuffed, wire-reinforced endotracheal tube is inserted into the distal portion of the trachea.

7. The larynx is freed from the cervical esophagus and attachments by sharp and blunt dissection. A moist pack is placed around the endotracheal tube to help prevent leakage of blood into the trachea.

8. The pharynx is entered. In most cancers of the intrinsic larynx, the pharynx is entered above the epiglottis. The mucous membrane incision is extended along either side of the epiglottis; the remaining portion of the pharynx and cervical esophagus is dissected well away from the tumor by means of fine-toothed tissue forceps, Metzenbaum scissors, knife, and fine hemostats. The specimen is removed en bloc (Figure 10-57).

9. A nasal feeding tube is inserted through one naris into the esophagus; closure of the hypopharyngeal and esophageal defect is begun with continuous inverting fine 3-0 absorbable sutures. The nasal tube is guided down past the pharyngeal suture line.

10. The pharyngeal suture line is reinforced with running horizontal or vertical mattress Vicryl sutures; the suprahyoid muscles are approximated to the cut edges of the inferior constrictor muscles.

11. The diameter of the tracheal stoma is increased by means of a knife and heavy scissors. The two portions of the thyroid behind the tracheal opening are approximated with interrupted nonabsorbable sutures, thereby obliterating dead space posterior to the upper portion of the trachea.

12. Using a scalpel, the surgeon makes a small puncture wound through the neck, lateral to the incision, using the tips of a hemostat inserted on the inner wound bed as a guide.

13. The hemostat is then switched into the puncture wound, grasping the distal drain tubing and pulling it through until the fluted portion of the drain is visible in the wound bed. The drain is trimmed and measured to fit into the wound.

14. The drain is secured to the skin just lateral to where the puncture wound was made and an air knot is tied using square knots.

15. The edges of the deep cervical fascia and the platysma are closed separately.

16. A laryngectomy tube of desired size is inserted into the tracheal stoma; a pressure dressing may be applied to the wound and neck, although some surgeons prefer leaving the wound without dressings to observe the skin flaps.

Radical Neck Dissection

In a radical neck dissection, the tumor, all soft tissue from the inferior aspect of the mandible to the midline of the neck to the clavicle end posterior to the trapezius muscle, and lymph nodes are removed en bloc from the affected side of the neck. This procedure is done to remove the tumor and metastatic cervical nodes present in malignant lesions as well as all nonvital structures of the neck (Figure 10-58). Metastasis occurs

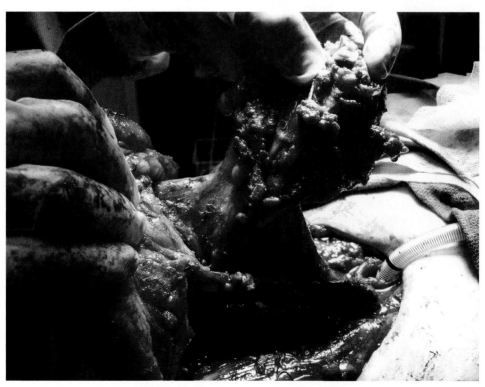

FIGURE 10-57 Removal of the larynx en bloc.

through the lymphatic channels by way of the bloodstream. Diseases of the oral cavity, lips, and thyroid gland may spread slowly to the neck. Radical neck surgery is done in the presence of cervical node metastasis from a cancer of the head and neck that has a reasonable chance of being controlled. Sentinel node biopsy may also be performed in conjunction with a neck dissection (Box 10-2).

A prophylactic neck dissection implies an elective neck dissection when there is no clinical evidence of metastatic cancer in the cervical lymph nodes.

Procedural Considerations. The patient is placed on the OR bed in a supine position. General endotracheal anesthesia is induced before the patient is positioned for surgery. A shoulder roll may be placed to slightly hyperextend the neck with the head slightly turned to the contralateral side. The head of the bed may be slightly elevated to reduce venous bleeding.

During the operation the anesthesia provider works behind a sterile barrier at the patient's unaffected side. The preoperative skin prep is extensive, including the neck, lower face, and upper chest. The patient's neck is draped so as to leave a wide operative field. On occasions, local muscle flaps are harvested to cover and protect the carotid artery (as when a patient has received extensive previous radiation therapy). If this is the case, the thigh area is also prepped and draped with sterile towels in readiness for obtaining a dermal graft before closure of the neck wound. It is usually more convenient to use the thigh on the same side as the neck dissection. Patient and family education includes tracheostomy care (if applicable), pain management, care of the surgical incision, reportable signs and symptoms, healthful behaviors, and review of physical therapy exercises.

BOX 10-2

Sentinel Lymph Node Mapping and Biopsy

In many oral cancers, the nearby lymph nodes are routinely removed during surgery (known as a lymph node dissection). The sentinel node procedure can help the surgeon determine whether the cancer has already spread to these nodes, which may allow the patient to avoid more extensive surgery if the cancer has not metastasized. Sentinel node mapping and biopsy allow the surgeon to identify and examine the "sentinel node(s)"—the first node(s) affected by the cancer before metastasis to other lymph nodes. If the sentinel node does not contain cancer, it is very unlikely that any other nodes would contain cancer.

In this procedure, the surgeon injects a radioactive material around the tumor, usually the day before surgery. The material will travel the same route that any cancer cells would likely have taken if they had spread to the lymph nodes. On the day of surgery a blue dye is injected into the tumor site, which will also travel to the nearby lymph nodes.

During surgery, the surgeon can use a radiation detector to identify the lymph node region that is the source of radioactivity (and presumably cancer). The surgeon then cuts into the area to look for radioactive or blue-stained lymph nodes. These are removed and examined by a pathologist. If there is no cancer, then no further surgery is needed. If there is cancer, then all the lymph nodes in the area will be removed.

This procedure is still experimental, and more work is needed to determine if this can replace routine lymph node removal.

Modified from *What's new in oral cavity and oropharyngeal cancer research and treatment?*, available at www.cancer.org/docroot/CRI/content/CRI_2_4_6X_Whats_new_in_oral_cavity_and_oropharyngeal_cancer_research_and_treatment_60.asp. Accessed June 27, 2011.

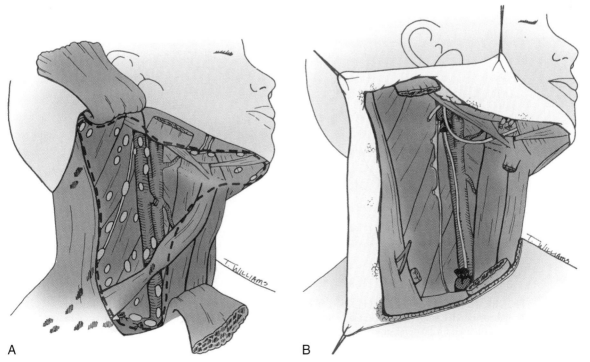

FIGURE 10-58 Radical neck dissection. **A,** Diagram of extent of operation. **B,** Diagram of operation.

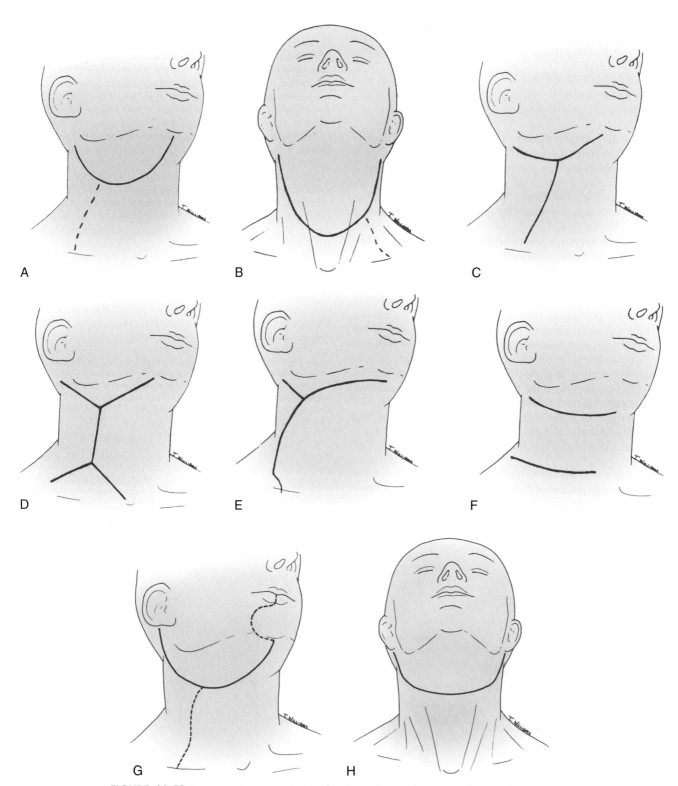

FIGURE 10-59 Dissection incisions. **A,** Latyshevsky and Freund. **B,** Freund. **C,** Crile. **D,** Martin. **E,** Babcock and Conley. **F,** McFee. **G,** Incision used for unilateral supraomohyoid neck dissection. **H,** Incision used for bilateral supraomohyoid neck dissection.

Operative Procedure

1. One of several types of incisions may be used, including the Y-shaped, H-shaped, or trifurcate incision (Figure 10-59), all of which aim for complete lymphadenectomy while preserving good, viable skin flaps.

2. The upper curved incision is made through the skin and platysma with a knife, tissue forceps, and fine hemostats; ligatures are used for bleeding vessels. The upper flap is retracted; then the vertical portion of the incision is made, and the skin flaps are retracted anteriorly and posteriorly with retractors. The anterior margin of the trapezius muscle is exposed by means of curved scissors. The flaps are retracted to expose the entire lateral aspect of the neck. Branches of the jugular veins are clamped, ligated, and divided.

3. The sternal and clavicular attachments of the sternocleidomastoid muscle are clamped with curved Péan forceps and then divided with a knife. The superficial layer of deep fascia is incised. The omohyoid muscle is severed between clamps just above its scapular attachment.

4. By sharp and blunt dissection, the carotid sheath is opened. The internal jugular vein is isolated by blunt dissection and then doubly clamped, doubly ligated with medium silk, and divided with Metzenbaum scissors. A transfixion suture is placed on the lower end of the vein.

5. The common carotid artery and vagus nerve are identified and protected. The fatty areolar tissue and fascia are dissected and removed using Metzenbaum scissors and fine tissue forceps. Branches of the thyrocervical artery are clamped, divided, and ligated.

6. The tissues and fascia of the posterior triangle are dissected, beginning at the anterior margin of the trapezius muscle and continuing near the brachial plexus and the levator scapulae and scalene muscles. During the dissection, branches of the cervical and suprascapular arteries are clamped, ligated, and divided.

7. The anterior portion of the block dissection is completed. The omohyoid muscle is severed at its attachment to the hyoid bone. Bleeding is controlled. All hemostats are removed, and the operative site may be covered with warm, moist laparotomy packs.

8. The sternocleidomastoid muscle is severed and retracted. The submental space is dissected free of fatty areolar tissue and lymph nodes, from above downward.

9. The deep fascia on the lower edge of the mandible is incised; the facial vessels are divided and ligated.

10. The submandibular triangle is entered. The submandibular duct is divided and ligated. The submandibular glands with surrounding fatty areolar tissue and lymph nodes are dissected toward the digastric muscle. The facial branch of the external carotid artery is divided. Portions of the digastrics and stylohyoid muscles are severed from their attachments to the hyoid bone and on the mastoid. The upper end of the internal jugular vein is elevated and divided. The surgical specimen is removed.

11. The entire field is examined for bleeding and then irrigated with warm saline solution. Although rarely necessary, a skin graft may be placed to cover the bifurcation of the carotid artery, extending down approximately 4 inches, and sutured with 4-0 absorbable suture on a very small cutting needle.

12. Closed-wound suction drains are placed into the wound.

13. The flaps are carefully approximated with interrupted fine nonabsorbable sutures or with skin staples. A bulky pressure dressing may be applied to the neck, depending on surgeon preference.

Modified Neck Dissection

Modified neck dissection (Figure 10-60) is removal of neck contents, except for the sternocleidomastoid muscle, internal jugular vein, and eleventh cranial nerve.

Procedural Considerations. This modified type of neck dissection facilitates removal of a tumor and lymph nodes suspected of metastases and allows the patient a minimal defect and minimally impaired shoulder function. With radical and modified neck dissection, the surgeon and medical and radiation oncologists may decide on a course of postoperative radiation therapy or chemotherapy. The decision depends on the type and location of tumor, stage of disease, and condition of the patient. Research on chemotherapy protocols to avoid extensive surgical dissection is ongoing.

Reconstructive Procedures

Depending on the surgical defect, head and neck surgical procedures to remove malignant tumors also involve reconstructive procedures. The wound may be closed primarily, or local flaps and split-thickness skin grafts (as for facial and intraoral defects) or full-thickness skin grafts (as for nasal and facial defects) may be used. Regional flaps (e.g., pectoralis major musculocutaneous flap), microvascular tissue transfer (e.g., radial forearm, latissimus dorsi, anterior lateral thigh free flap), or microvascular osteocutaneous flaps (e.g., fibula free flap) may be used to restore function as well as cover defects. Combinations of these grafts and flaps are often necessary when large defects are created. Skin grafts and flaps are discussed in Chapter 17.

If microvascular flaps are used, surgical and anesthesia time is extended significantly (approximately 8 to 12 hours); since veins and arteries are microscopically connected, nerve grafts may be used, and bone must be connected with the use of plates and screws.

The use of a Doppler unit (intraoperatively and postoperatively) and thorough nursing assessment skills are paramount in detecting occlusions or spasms of the vessels and subsequent survival of the transplanted flap.

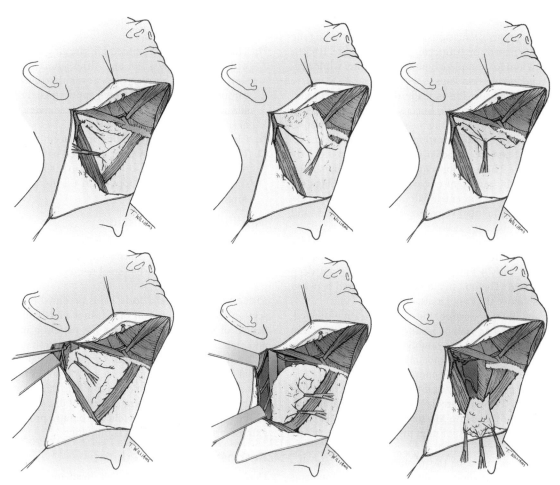

FIGURE 10-60 Steps of modified radical neck dissection with preservation of spinal accessory nerve, internal jugular vein, and sternocleidomastoid muscle.

OTORHINOLARYNGOLOGIC SURGERY SUMMARY

As with any surgical service, in otorhinolaryngologic surgery it is imperative to know the anatomy and physiology of the surgical area, including the head, neck, nose, and ear, as well as facial and optic nerves. Understanding the anatomy and physiology will allow the surgical technologist to think several steps ahead in the procedure.

The surgical technologist will need to be prepared for a difficult airway with these types of procedures; a difficult airway cart in the operating room may prove to be helpful in this situation.

Specialty equipment such as nerve monitoring devices, microscopes, and lasers may be necessary in some cases; having them readily available is key to the success of the procedure.

The surgical technologist should also be prepared for intraoperative bleeding, with sponges, suture, vascular clamps, and specific retractors to gain the necessary exposure. Hemoclips and other hemostasis adjuncts such as thrombin and absorbable gelatin should be rapidly available.

Because there may be several specimens, the surgical technologist should have the proper specimen containers and supplies to store and label each specimen to avoid specimen errors. Having the appropriate drains and dressing ready will facilitate an efficient and effective closure of the procedure.

GERIATRIC CONSIDERATIONS

Sensory changes in hearing and smell may influence the patient's response to care. If preadmission communication is done, the patient should be asked about any problems with hearing and reminded to bring the hearing aids to the facility (Clayton, 2008). Hearing impairment is a major chronic condition in the aging population; about 30% of those over 60 years of age are affected, and this rises to about 40% to 50% in those over 65 years (Fillit et al, 2010). Approximately 11% of adults with hearing impairment also experience tinnitus (ringing in the ears), which compounds hearing difficulty.

Presbycusis, or loss of hearing sensitivity, is irreversible, bilateral, and primarily sensorineural, although metabolic and mechanical causes are also possible. It is the most frequent cause of hearing loss in the geriatric patient. Hearing loss, which appears to be greater in men than in women, is mostly within the higher frequencies (above 1000 Hz). In addition, cerumen thickens and the eardrum becomes less pliable, and such changes also contribute to diminished hearing. Often geriatric patients are labeled "confused" or "senile" because they respond inappropriately to questions they did not hear.

When communicating with elderly adults who have sensory impairments, perioperative nurses and surgical technologists should consider the following strategies (Wold, 2008):
- Try not to startle the person when starting a communication.
- Approach from the front, knock, or announce your presence by calling the person's name.
- Approach patients who have a left-sided hemiparesis from the right side.
- Identify yourself.
- Communicate when the person is most alert.
- Eliminate or reduce noise and distractions.
- Make sure you have the person's attention before speaking.
- Try to use a variety of words or descriptions until meanings are clear.
- Ask clear, specific questions.
- Ask only one question at a time.
- Pay attention to the emotional context of conversation.
- Use pictures and gestures in addition to words.
- Have the person sit up for conversation whenever possible. Keep messages simple and repeat as needed.
- Be patient and do not interrupt. Slow down the pace of communication.
- Treat the person as normally as possible.

Changes in taste and smell begin to occur at approximately 60 years of age and become more pronounced with advanced age. Older adults have two to three times more difficulty in detecting flavors than do young adults. Oral hygiene, dental disease, and decreased salivary function may also alter tasting ability. There is a close association between the sense of smell and human behavior. Smell can affect emotions when a person recalls a particular odor. Other functions include protection of the individual by warning of danger in the air, such as smoke or gas fumes; assistance in digestion; and helping a person to remember or recollect. In elders, the sense of smell can be reduced, as well as the ability to identify odors (Wold, 2008).

Modified from: Clayton JL: Special needs of older adults undergoing surgery, *AORN J* 87(3):557-570, 2008; Fillit HM et al: *Textbook of geriatric medicine and gerontology*, ed 7, Philadelphia, 2010, Saunders; Wold GH: *Basic geriatric nursing*, ed 4, St Louis, 2008, Mosby.

REVIEW QUESTIONS

1. The microscope lens focal length used in ear surgery is _____ and in laryngeal surgery is _____.
   a. 250–300 mm; 400 mm
   b. 400 mm; 250–300 mm
   c. 300 mm; 100–250 mm
   d. 100–250 mm; 300 mm

2. Which bone is not part of the middle ear?
   a. malleus
   b. incus
   c. humerus
   d. stapes

3. Which elevator is most commonly used in closed nasal reduction surgery?
   a. House
   b. Cottle
   c. Boises
   d. Adson

4. _____ is a term used in these three surgeries: laryngoscopy, bronchoscopy, and esophagoscopy.
   a. Triscopy
   b. LBE
   c. Triple endoscopy
   d. All of the above

5. Which is not a primary component of the septum?
   a. eardrum
   b. septal cartilage
   c. ethmoid plate
   d. vomer

6. The _____ is used because the malleus and incus are diseased or eroded.
   a. PORP
   b. TORP
   c. laser
   d. none of the above

7. The _____ is used because all ossicles are diseased or eroded.
   a. PORP
   b. TORP
   c. laser
   d. none of the above

8. Name the three incisional approaches used in otologic surgery.

9. In otologic surgery during general anesthesia, which gas should not be used?

10. List instruments that should be included in a setup for laryngoscopy.

11. Define and briefly describe the following procedures:
    Tympanoplasty
    Frontal sinus trephination and obliteration
    Tracheostomy

Critical Thinking Question

During FESS, a number of potential injuries can occur. The patient's eyes are visible so the surgeon can monitor for movement of the eyeball of appearance of an intraorbital hematoma. Another potential injury is "encroachment of the orbit." Discuss what findings the surgical technologist would immediately communicate to the surgeon. What is a technique the surgical technologist can use when handling specimens to also monitor for this injury?

REFERENCES

American Cancer Society (ACS): *Cancer facts and figures 2009*, Atlanta, 2009, The Society.

Association of periOperative Registered Nurses: Recommended practices for documentation of perioperative nursing care, *Perioperative standards and recommended practices*, Denver, 2009a, The Association.

Association of periOperative Registered Nurses: Recommended practices for the care and handling of specimens in the perioperative environment, *Perioperative standards and recommended practices*, Denver, 2009b, The Association.

Association of periOperative Registered Nurses: Recommended practices for laser safety in practice settings, *Perioperative standards and recommended practices*, Denver, 2009c, The Association.

Chole RA, Suddath HH: Chronic otitis media, mastoiditis and petrositis. In Cummings CW et al, editors: *Otolaryngology: head and neck surgery*, ed 4, Philadelphia, 2005, Mosby.

Denholm B: Tucking patient's arms and general positioning, *AORN J* 89(4):755–757, 2009.

Elluru RG, Kumar M: Physiology of the salivary glands. In Cummings CW et al, editors: *Otolaryngology: head and neck surgery*, ed 4, St Louis, 2005, Mosby.

Furman JM: Episodic vertigo. In Rakel RE, Bope ET, editors: *Conn's current therapy 2008*, ed 60, Philadelphia, 2008, Saunders.

Gantz BJ, Meyer TA: Auditory brainstem implants, In Cummings CW et al, editors: *Otolaryngology: head and neck surgery*, ed 4, Philadelphia, 2005, Mosby.

House JW, Cunningham CD: Otosclerosis. In Cummings CW et al, editors: *Otolaryngology: head and neck surgery*, ed 4, Philadelphia, 2005, Mosby.

Mahlan ME et al: Neurologic monitoring. In Miller RD, editor: *Miller's anesthesia*, ed 6, Philadelphia, 2005, Churchill Livingstone.

Pagana KD, Pagana TJ: *Mosby's diagnostic and laboratory test reference*, ed 9, St Louis, 2009, Mosby.

Palmer CV, Ortmann A: Hearing loss and hearing aids, *Neurol Clin* 23: 901–918, 2005.

Santina CC, Lustig LR: Surgically implantable hearing aids. In Cummings CW et al, editors: *Otolaryngology: head and neck surgery*, ed 4, Philadelphia, 2005, Mosby.

Schessel DA et al: Meniere's disease and other peripheral disorders, In Cummings CW et al, editors: *Otolaryngology: head and neck surgery*, ed 4, Philadelphia, 2005, Mosby.

Thrasher RD: Middle ear, otitis media with effusion, August 2009, available at: http://emedicine.medscape.com/article/858990-overview. Accessed August 5, 2009.

Wackym PA et al: Patient evaluation and device selection in cochlear implantation. In Cummings CW et al, editors: *Otolaryngology: head and neck surgery*, ed 4, Philadelphia, 2005, Mosby.

Orthopedic Surgery

After studying this chapter the reader will be able to:

- Identify the main parts of the skeletal system including the bones, muscles, ligaments, tendons, cartilage, and joints
- Correlate physiologic conditions with the surgical interventions that treat them
- Discuss purposes and potential problems and risks associated with orthopedic surgery
- Demonstrate a working knowledge of perioperative considerations in orthopedic surgery
- Discuss diagnostic methods for determination of surgical interventions and approaches
- Identify specialized instruments, equipment, and supplies
- Differentiate among types of fracture fixations sets and traction devices for fractures beds
- List the pharmacologic and hemostatic agents used during orthopedic surgery
- Apply broad orthopedic surgical concepts and knowledge to clinical practice for enhanced surgical patient care

CHAPTER OUTLINE

Overview
Surgical Anatomy
Surgical Technologist
   Considerations
Surgical Interventions
   Allografts/Autografts
   Electrical Stimulation

Fractures and Dislocations
Surgery of the Shoulder
Surgery of the Humerus, Radius,
   and Ulna
Surgery of the Hand
Surgery of the Hip and Lower
   Extremity

Surgery of the Lower Leg (Distal
   Femur, Tibia, and Fibula)
Surgery of the Ankle and Foot
Pelvic Fracture and Disruption
Total Joint Arthroplasty
Arthroscopy
Surgery of the Spine

Overview

The word *orthopédie* is derived from the Greek *orthos*, meaning "straight," and *paideia*, meaning "rearing of children." It was first used by Nicholas Andry in 1741 in the title for a book addressing the prevention and correction of skeletal deformities in children. Orthopedic surgery has been defined by the American Association of Orthopaedic Surgeons' Board of

This chapter was originally written by Barbara A. Bowen, RN, MSN, CRNP, CRNFA, for the 14th edition of Alexander's Care of the Patient in Surgery and has been revised by Michelle Whitlow, CST, BS, for this text.

Orthopaedic Surgery as "a broad based medical and surgical specialty dedicated to the prevention, diagnosis, and treatment of diseases and injuries of the musculoskeletal system" (American Board of Orthopaedic Surgeons [ABOS], 2009).

Orthopedic surgery is an ever-changing field that is a challenge for the surgical technologist. Technologic advances in the multitude of systems and hardware used have resulted in improved treatment of orthopedic disorders. In addition to understanding anatomic and physiologic responses, the surgical technologist should have a general understanding of the concepts and purposes of these systems to provide the most safe and efficient care. Knowledge of the principles of bone fixation and healing and the relationship of bone and soft tissues will provide a strong basis to ensure continued understanding of the care required for the orthopedic patient.

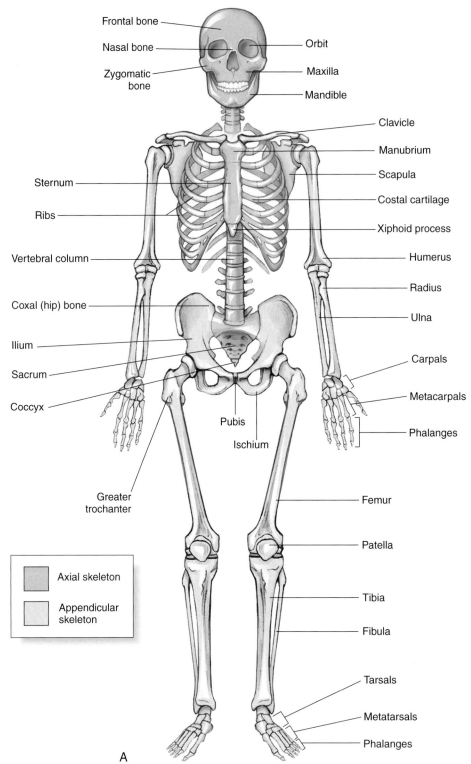

Frontal bone

Nasal bone

Zygomatic bone

Orbit

Maxilla

Mandible

Clavicle

Manubrium

Scapula

Costal cartilage

Xiphoid process

Humerus

Radius

Ulna

Carpals

Metacarpals

Phalanges

Sternum

Ribs

Vertebral column

Coxal (hip) bone

Ilium

Sacrum

Coccyx

Pubis

Ischium

Greater trochanter

Femur

Patella

Tibia

Fibula

Tarsals

Metatarsals

Phalanges

Axial skeleton

Appendicular skeleton

A

FIGURE 11-1 A, Anterior view of the skeleton.

Surgical Anatomy

Anatomic Structures

The 206 bones of the body form the appendicular or axial framework that supports soft tissues, provides storage areas and reservoirs for minerals, and serves as a site for formation of blood cells (Figure 11-1). The skeletal system is composed of varied elements, including bone, muscle, and associated structures.

Bone remains in a constant state of formation and resorption, preventing development of excessive thickness or thin-

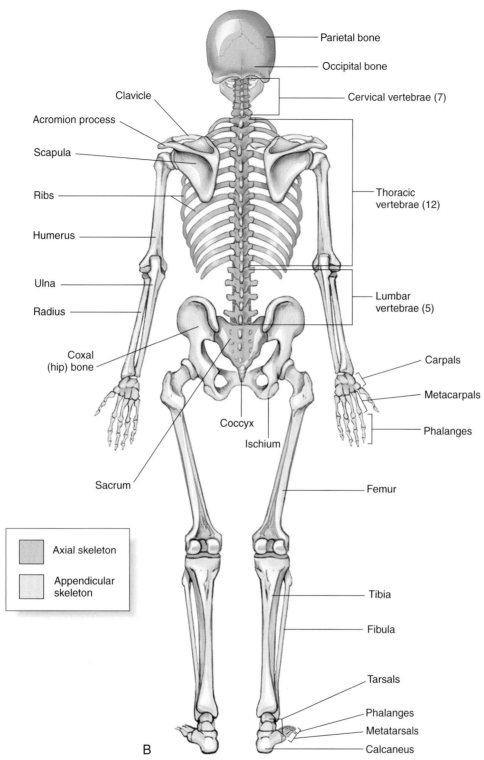

Parietal bone
Occipital bone
Clavicle
Acromion process
Cervical vertebrae (7)
Scapula
Ribs
Thoracic vertebrae (12)
Humerus
Ulna
Radius
Lumbar vertebrae (5)
Coxal (hip) bone
Carpals
Metacarpals
Phalanges
Coccyx
Ischium
Sacrum
Femur

Axial skeleton
Appendicular skeleton

Tibia
Fibula
Tarsals
Phalanges
Metatarsals
Calcaneus

B

FIGURE 11-1, cont'd B, Posterior view of the skeleton.

ness. These processes are related to individual metabolism and absorption of calcium, vitamin D, and phosphorus. Levels of minerals affect disease processes, causing bone changes. A layer of connective tissue called *periosteum* covers all bone.

Muscles are masses of tissue that cover bones and provide movement to the skeletal system. Muscles interact with nerves, minerals, skin, and other connective tissue to contract and

extend. Individual muscles are short or long and vary in diameter, depending on their position on a specific bone.

Ligaments, tendons, and cartilage also form the skeletal structures. Ligaments are bands of dense connective tissue that hold bone to bone. They provide stability to a joint by encircling or holding ends of bone in place. Tendons are tough, long strands of fibers that form the ends of muscles. They transmit forces to bone or cartilage without being damaged. Cartilage is a layer of elastic, resilient supporting tissue found at the ends of the bones. It forms a cap over the bone end to protect and support the bone during weight-bearing activities and provides a smooth gliding surface for joint movement. Cartilage is aneural (without nerves), alymphatic (without lymph tissue), avascular (without blood vessels), and high in water content. The lack of vascularity and loss of water from cartilage during a lifetime are causes of resulting degenerative disease, such as arthritis. Weight bearing and joint movements keep cartilage from becoming thin or damaged and help prevent degenerative conditions.

Joints are articulations where bones are joined to one another or where two surfaces of bones unite. Joints are classified by the type of material between them or according to movement. Material between joints is fibrous, cartilaginous, or synovial. The type of movement is synarthrotic (immovable), amphiarthrotic (slightly movable), or diarthrotic (freely movable). Synarthrotic joints are connected by fibrous tissue or ligaments (e.g., the suture type of joints holding the bones of the skull; connections between two bones, such as the radius and ulna). Amphiarthrotic joints are connected by cartilage. Joints of this type include the symphysis pubis, intervertebral joints, and manubriosternal joint. The majority of joints are diarthrotic; these are the only joints with one or more ranges of motion. These joints are lined with a synovial membrane and are called *synovial joints*. Examples include the knee, cervical vertebrae 1 and 2 (C1 and C2), the radius articulating on the wrist bones, the hip, and the shoulder.

The two types of bone tissue are *cortical* and *cancellous*. Cortical bone is the hard bone forming the outer shell—the main supporting tissue. Cancellous bone is soft and spongy—located at the iliac crest, tibia, sternum, and ends of long bones. It contains the red bone marrow for hematopoiesis.

Bones are divided according to their shape: long, short, flat, irregular, and round (Figure 11-2). Long bones are present in the limbs and consist of a shaft and two ends; the ends generally flare out, are covered with articular cartilage, and provide a surface for articulation and musculotendinous attachment. Short bones, such as the carpals and tarsals (in the wrist and midfoot areas, respectively), are present where the structure is strong but limited movement is required. Flat bones are the scapula, the sternum, and the pelvic girdle. Irregular bones are found in the skull and vertebral column. Round bones, or sesamoid bones (resembling a sesame seed), are found within tendons. The patella is a large sesamoid bone; however, most are small, such as the two found on the head of the first metatarsal, which form the "ball" of the foot.

Long bones consist of a shaft (diaphysis) and two ends (epiphyses). The shaft is composed of compact bone. The epiphyses flare out and consist of cancellous bone. They are covered by cartilage, which provides a cushion and offers protection during weight bearing and movement. Until skeletal maturity, a line of cartilage called the *epiphyseal plate* separates the epiphysis from the diaphysis. Fractures in this region by children can be devastating because they often lead to malformation and permanent limb shortening.

Trabeculae are located within cancellous bone and consist of an interconnecting network of bone oriented along the lines of stress. These structures are important for weight bearing,

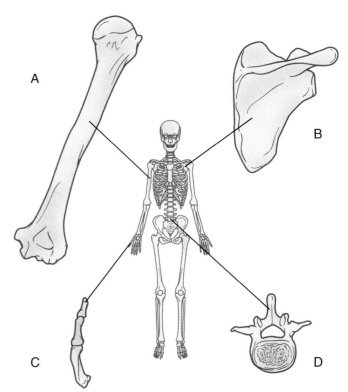

FIGURE 11-2 Types of bones, as examples. **A**, Long bones (humerus). **B**, Flat bones (scapula). **C**, Short bones (phalanx). **D**, Irregular bones (vertebra).

providing strength to withstand stress placed on the bone. The periosteum is a thin, outer covering of bone containing nutrient arteries for nourishment of bone cells. Disruption of these periosteal vessels after bone trauma can influence the ability of bone to heal. The haversian system consists of thousands of microscopic units found in the cortical bone. These units of matrix cells, canals, and conduits allow flow of nutrients and facilitate calcium absorption.

Vertebrae

Vertebrae form the longitudinal axis of the skeleton. The vertebral bodies are connected by several cartilaginous joints, which enable the vertebrae to flex, extend, or rotate while being held together. Intervertebral discs and ligaments connect the bodies of adjacent vertebrae. The ligamenta flava bind the laminae of adjacent vertebrae together. Other ligaments connect the spinous processes and vertebral bodies.

Seven cervical vertebrae form the skeletal framework of the neck. Twelve thoracic vertebrae support the thoracic region, and five lumbar vertebrae support the small of the back. Below the lumbar vertebrae lie the sacrum and coccyx. Each of these bones is composed of fused vertebrae—five for the sacrum and four for the coccyx.

The vertebral column is curved. After birth, there is a continuous posterior convexity. As development occurs, secondary posterior concavities develop in the cervical and lumbar regions, resulting in improved balance.

Each area of the vertebral column has specific bony structures. General features include a body (except the first two cervical vertebrae) on the anterior part. The posterior portion of

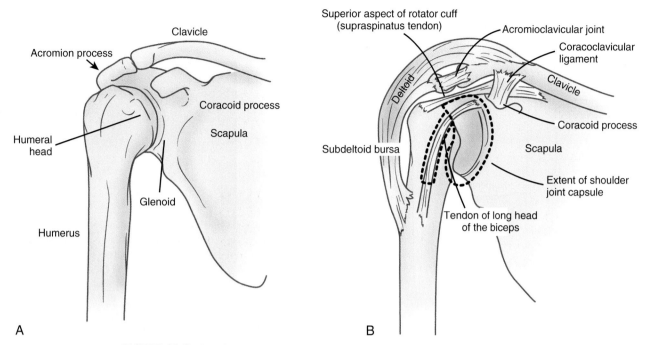

FIGURE 11-3 Shoulder. **A,** Joint showing anterior view. **B,** Girdle showing articulations.

the vertebrae consists of a neural arch formed by pedicles and laminae and the spinous and transverse processes.

Shoulder and Upper Extremity

The clavicle, which is a long, doubly curved bone, serves as a prop for the shoulder and holds it away from the chest wall. The clavicle rests almost horizontally at the upper and anterior part of the thorax, above the first rib. It articulates medially with the manubrium of the sternum and laterally with the acromion of the scapula; it is tethered to the underlying coracoid process of the scapula by the coracoclavicular ligaments.

The scapula (shoulder blade) is a flat, triangular bone that forms the posterior part of the shoulder girdle, lying superior and posterior to the upper chest. The glenoid cavity on the lateral side of the scapula provides a socket for the humerus (the bone of the upper arm). The acromion process articulates with the clavicle medially. The scapula is attached to the thorax by muscles.

The shoulder (pectoral) girdle consists of the glenohumeral, sternoclavicular, and acromioclavicular (AC) joints (Figure 11-3). The glenohumeral joint has a multidirectional range of motion, whereas the latter two joints have limited motion. The AC joint, located at the top of the shoulder, is the articulation between the outer end of the clavicle and a flattened articular facet situated on the inner border of the acromion. The muscles immediately surrounding the shoulder joint are the supraspinatus, infraspinatus, teres minor, and subscapularis muscles; together they are referred to as the *rotator cuff*. These muscles stabilize the shoulder joint, whereas the powerful deltoid, pectoralis major, teres major, and latissimus dorsi muscles move the entire arm. Shoulder girdle strength and stability are maintained by the soft tissue integrity—not the bony structures. A pathologic condition in this area can be the result of bone, soft tissue, or combined injury.

The humerus is the longest and largest bone of the upper extremity. It is composed of a shaft and two ends. The proximal end, or head, has two projections—the greater and lesser tuberosities (Figure 11-4). The circumference of the articular surface of the humerus is constricted and is termed the *anatomic neck*. The anatomic neck marks the attachment to the capsule of the shoulder joint. The constriction below the tuberosities is called the *surgical neck* and is the site of most fractures.

The greater tuberosity is situated at the lateral aspect of the humeral head. Its upper surface has three impressions where the supraspinous, infraspinous, and teres minor tendons insert. The lesser tuberosity is situated in the anterior neck and has an impression for the insertion of the tendon of the subscapular muscle. The attachment sites for the rotator cuff, the tuberosities, are separated from each other by a deep groove (bicipital groove), in which lies the tendon of the long head of the biceps muscle of the arm. The tendon of the pectoralis major inserts on the lateral margin of the bicipital groove, and the latissimus dorsi and teres major insert on the medial margin.

The distal humerus flattens and ends in a broad articular surface. The surface is divided into the medial and lateral condyles, which are separated by a slight ridge. On the lateral condyle, the rounded articular surface is called the *capitulum*, which articulates with the head of the radius. On the medial condyle, the articular surface is termed the *trochlea*, which articulates with the ulna.

The ulna is located medial to the radius. The proximal portion of the ulna, the olecranon, articulates with the trochlea of the humerus at the elbow. The radius rotates around the ulna. At the proximal end is the head, which articulates with the capitulum of the humerus and the radial notch of the ulna. The tendon of the biceps muscle is attached to the tuberosity just below the radial head. The distal end of the radius is divided into two articular surfaces. The distal surface articulates with

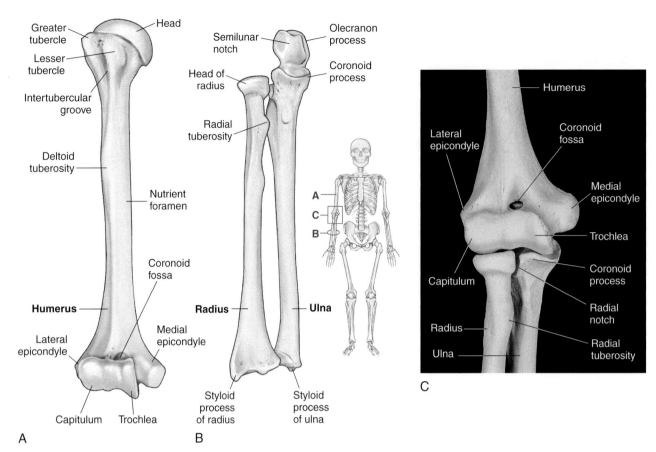

FIGURE 11-4 Bones of the arm, anterior view, showing the humerus, radius, and ulna.

the carpal bones of the wrist, and the surface on the medial side articulates with the distal end of the ulna.

Wrist and Hand

The skeletal bones of the wrist and hand consist of three distinct parts: (1) the carpals, or wrist bones; (2) the metacarpals, or bones of the palm; and (3) the phalanges, or bones of the digits (Figure 11-5).

The eight carpal bones are arranged in two rows. The distal row, proceeding from the radial to the ulnar side, includes the trapezium, trapezoid, capitate, and hamate; the proximal row consists of the scaphoid (also called the *navicular*), lunate, triquetrum, and pisiform. Functionally, the scaphoid links the rows as it stabilizes and coordinates the movement of the proximal and distal rows. Each carpal bone consists of several smooth articular surfaces for contact with the adjacent bones, as well as rough surfaces for the attachment of ligaments. The five metacarpal bones (long bones) are situated in the palm. Proximally they articulate with the distal row of carpal bones, and distally the head of each metacarpal articulates with its proper phalanx. The heads of the metacarpals form the knuckles. The phalanges, or fingers, consist of 14 bones in each hand—2 in the thumb and 3 in each finger. Each phalanx consists of a shaft and two ends.

Pelvis, Hip, and Femur

The pelvis (Figure 11-6) is a stable circular base that supports the trunk and forms an attachment for the lower extremities.

It is a massive, irregular bone created by the fusion of three separate bones. The largest and uppermost of the three bones is the ilium, the strongest and lowermost is the ischium, and the anterior-most is the pubis. Together these are termed the *os coxae*, or innominate bone.

The acetabular portion of the innominate bone and the proximal end of the femur (Figure 11-7) form the hip, which is a ball-and-socket joint. The hip joint is surrounded by a capsule, ligaments, and muscles that provide stability. The iliofemoral ligament connects the ilium with the femur anteriorly and superiorly, and the ischiofemoral and pubofemoral ligaments attach the ischium and pubis to the femur, respectively. The acetabulum is a deep, round cavity that articulates with the head of the femur. The proximal end of the femur consists of the femoral head and neck, the upper portion of the shaft, and the greater and lesser trochanters (Figure 11-8).

The greater trochanter is a broad process that protrudes from the outer, upper portion of the shaft and projects upward from the junction of the superior border of the neck with the outer surface of the shaft. It serves as a point of insertion for the abductor and short rotator muscles of the hip.

The lesser trochanter is a conical process projecting from the posterior and inferior portion of the base of the neck of the femur at its junction with the shaft. It serves as a point of insertion for the iliopsoas muscle. The lower end of the femur terminates in the two condyles. Anteriorly, the condyles are separated from one another by a smooth depression, called the *intercondylar*, or *patellar*, *groove*, forming

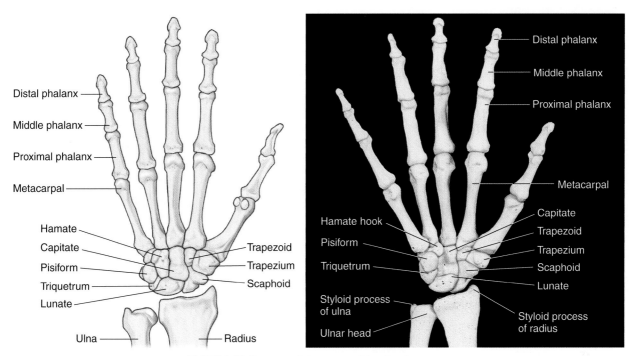

FIGURE 11-5 Bones of the wrist and hand, palmar view.

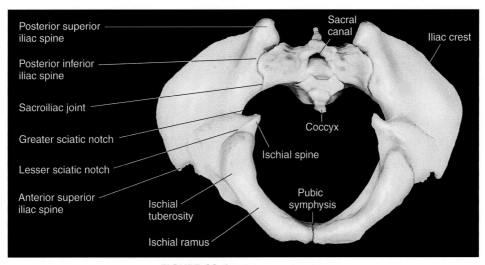

FIGURE 11-6 Pelvis, superior view.

an articulating surface for the patella. Posteriorly, they project slightly, and the space between them forms the intercondylar fossa—a supporting structure for neurovascular structures.

The upper or condylar end of the tibia presents an articular surface corresponding with those of the femoral condyles. The articular surface of the two tibial condyles forms two facets, which are deepened by the semilunar cartilage into fossae for the femoral condyles.

Knee, Tibia, and Fibula

The knee joint (Figure 11-9) consists of two articulations. One articulation is between each condyle of the femur and the tibial plateau; the other is between the patella and the femur. These areas are subject to degenerative changes, often requiring

reconstructive surgery. The bones of the knee joint are connected by extraarticular and intraarticular structures. The extraarticular attachments consist of the joint capsule, multiple muscular attachments, and two collateral ligaments. The intraarticular ligaments consist of the two cruciate ligaments and the attachments of the menisci.

The patella, or kneecap, is anterior to the knee joint in the intercondylar groove, or trochlea, of the distal femur. It is a sesamoid bone contained within the quadriceps tendon. The anterior surface of the patella is united with the patellar tendon as the tendon originates and inserts above and below the knee joint. The posterior surface of the patella articulates with the femur.

The capsule of the knee joint is attached proximally to the femoral condyles, and it is attached distally to the con-

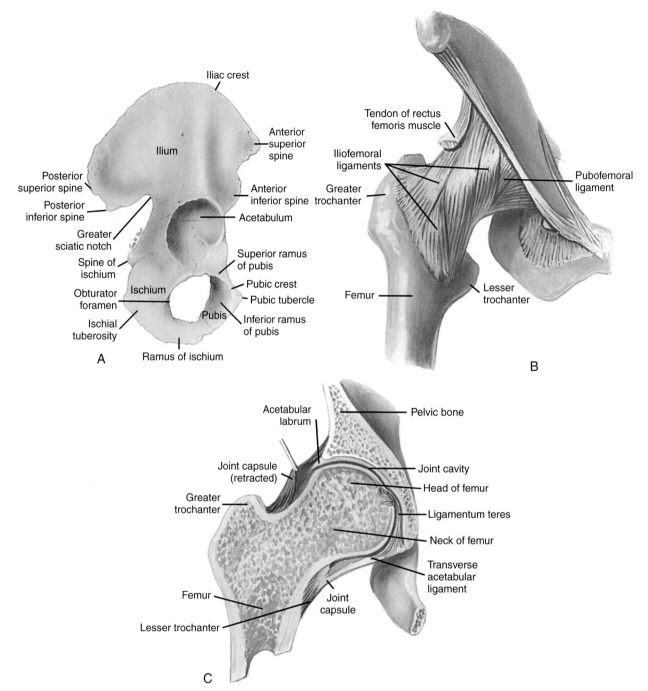

FIGURE 11-7 Hip joint. **A,** Coxal bone disarticulated from the skeleton. **B,** Ligamentous structure. **C,** Bone structure.

dyles of the tibia and to the upper end of the fibula. The capsule is reinforced anteriorly by the patellar and quadriceps tendon, on the sides by the medial and lateral collateral ligaments, and posteriorly by the popliteus and gastrocnemius muscles.

The cruciate ligaments (Figure 11-10), consisting of two fibrous bands, extend from the intercondylar fossa of the femur to attachments anterior and posterior on the intercondylar surface of the tibia.

The menisci are interposed between the condyles of the femur and those of the tibia (see Figure 11-10). Each meniscus is attached to the joint capsule. The ends of the cartilage are

attached to the tibia in the middle of its upper articular surface. These structures are almost totally avascular, and degenerative changes are usually permanent.

Synovial membrane lines the capsule of the joint and covers the infrapatellar fat pad, parts of the cruciate ligaments, and portions of the bone. The portion of the knee joint cavity that extends upward in front of the femur is called the *suprapatellar pouch,* or *bursa* (Figure 11-11).

The tibia is the larger and stronger of the lower leg bones. The fibula is smaller and located more laterally, articulating at the proximal end with the lateral condyle of the tibia. The proximal end of the tibia articulates with the femur to form the

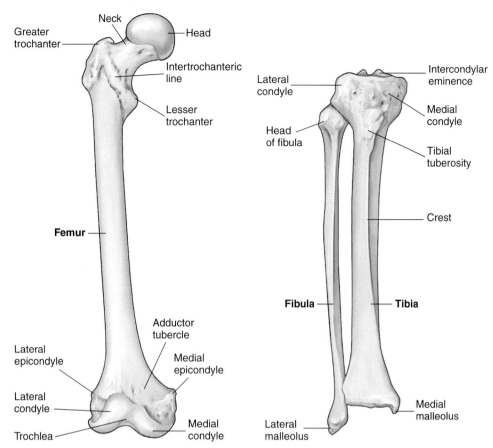

FIGURE 11-8 Bones of the upper and lower leg.

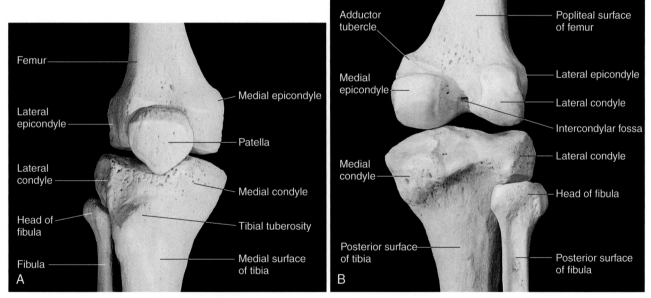

FIGURE 11-9 Bones of the knee showing the tibia and fibula. **A,** Anterior aspect. **B,** Posterior aspect.

knee joint. Distally the tibia articulates with the fibula and with the talus, forming the ankle joint.

Ankle and Foot

The ankle is a hinge joint, formed by the distal end of the tibia and fibula and the proximal end of the talus. The tibia (medial and posterior malleoli) and fibula (lateral malleolus) form a mortise (notch) for the reception of the upper surface of the talus and its facets. The talus is an irregular bone consisting of a body, neck, and head. The bones are connected by ligaments, which spread out from the malleoli to attach to the talus, calcaneus, and navicular bones (Figure 11-12). A thin capsule surrounds the joint.

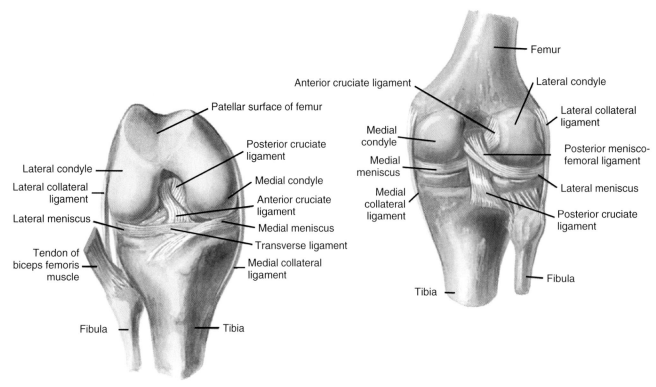

FIGURE 11-10 Bony structures of the knee joint.

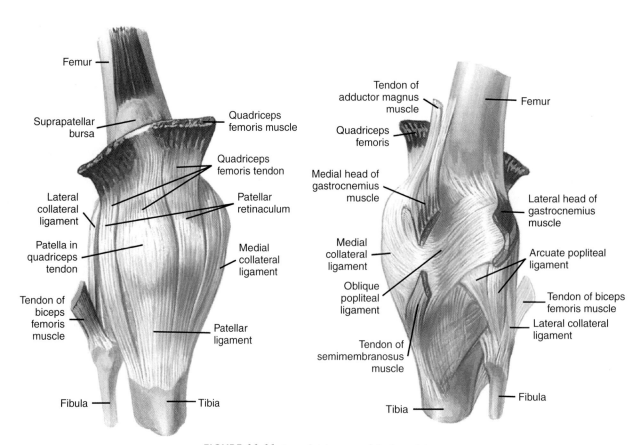

FIGURE 11-11 Superficial aspect of the knee joint.

The bony framework of the foot (Figure 11-13) comprises 7 tarsal bones, 5 metatarsal bones, and 14 phalanges. The calcaneus forms the heel and gives support to the talus. The cuboid bone articulates proximally and posteriorly with the calcaneus and distally with the fourth and fifth metatarsals and the third cuneiform bones.

The navicular bone articulates with the cuneiform bones, which lie side by side just anterior to it. The metatarsal bones articulate proximally with the tarsal bones and distally with the bases of the first phalanges of the corresponding toes. There are two phalanges for the great toe and three for each of the other toes.

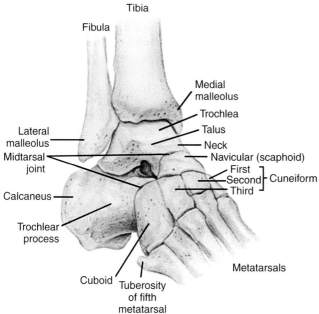

FIGURE 11-12 Anatomy of the ankle.

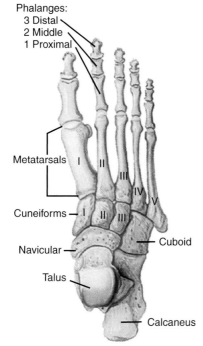

FIGURE 11-13 Bones of the foot viewed from above.

Surgical Technologist Considerations

Measures that should be undertaken to verify the correct operative side and site include marking the surgical site and having the patient verify the site with the surgeon during the marking process; using a verification checklist (which includes documents such as the medical record, x-ray films, imaging studies); using verbal verification by the patient of his or her identity, surgical site/side, and planned surgical procedure; confirming this information during the time-out by each member of the surgical team; and monitoring safe site protocol compliance with these procedures (Evidence for Practice).

Planning

The care of surgical patients undergoing any type of surgery requires planning for routine procedures that are always followed, as well as anticipating the unexpected. The surgical team should be consistent and systematic in the planning process to expedite actual steps required to facilitate the surgical

---

EVIDENCE FOR PRACTICE

Universal Protocol for Preoperative Site Verification as Indicated for Orthopedic Surgery

The Joint Commission's Universal Protocol for correct patient, procedure, and surgical side and site as well as the AORN Position Statement on correct site surgery both emphasize verification and marking of the surgical site (or invasive procedure site), especially when it involves laterality, levels, or multiples. As part of this process, protocols are used to verify the correct patient, correct procedure, correct patient position, and availability of necessary equipment, implants, imaging studies/equipment, or other special requirements. These protocols are part of the preoperative verification process as well as the time-out before the start of the surgical procedure.

For surgery, a recommended protocol may involve these additional steps:

◆ Preoperative skin marking of the procedure site is present.
◆ Preoperative films or images are present in the OR or procedure room.
◆ The time-out includes patient identity (using two unique identifiers); procedure to be performed; correct patient position; correct procedure side, level, or site; and presence of necessary implants, imaging, equipment, or other special requirements.
◆ If there are any discrepancies by any members of the surgical team the procedure will not proceed until the institution's reconciliation procedure is initiated and the results of the reconciliation should be documented.
◆ Should intraoperative imaging be necessary, opaque instruments marking the specific bony landmarks are placed accordingly and x-rays are taken and compared with the preoperative films or images by the surgeon performing the procedure.

Modified from Institute for Clinical Systems Improvement: *Health care protocol—safe site protocol for all invasive, high-risk, or surgical procedures,* January 2006, available at www.icsi.org/perioperative_protocol_36011/perioperative_protocol.html. Accessed June 23, 2009; The Joint Commission: *Universal protocol UP.01.01.01,* available at www.jointcommission. org/NR/rdonlyres/E5943278-3B89-469F-A265-E5AFB8729AD0/0/NPSG_UniversalProtocol_AHC_20090512.pdf. Accessed March 15, 2009.

procedure. Care of the orthopedic patient presents unique challenges because of the psychosocial, physical, and technical aspects of patient care. Planning includes attention to environmental factors, positioning, transfusion supplies, equipment, and instrument needs, in addition to practices that will prevent complications.

The optimal environment is comfortable for the patient and surgical team. The patient should feel relaxed and secure enough to allow the surgical team to become his or her advocates during the procedure. Physical preparation of the environment changes with individual patients. At the time the procedure is posted in the OR, traffic flow is considered to determine room location. The temperature is selected for the procedure with consideration given to the age and general health of the patient, attire worn by the operative personnel (body exhaust suits), or use of polymethylmethacrylate (PMMA) (bone cement). Temperature should be monitored for all but very brief surgical procedures, such as those lasting less than 30 minutes.

Equipment and instrumentation needed for the procedure are planned before the patient's arrival in the OR; orthopedic procedures may vary significantly because of the patient's physical condition or age. It may be necessary to communicate with the manufacturer's representative to facilitate obtaining items needed for the procedure. It is common for healthcare industry representatives to bring requisite orthopedic instruments to the OR or to act as a product resource regarding new equipment. However, industry representatives must comply with all institutional policies and AORN standards defining requirements and procedures and restrictions that govern their presence in the OR (AORN, 2006).

Aseptic technique is essential in the perioperative environment and should be considered a priority when caring for the orthopedic patient. Osteomyelitis is an infection of the bone that can remain unrecognized for a long time and requires expensive, intensive treatment. Osteomyelitis can lead to severe bone loss and possible loss of a limb. Preventive measures, including administration of antibiotics within 60 minutes of the initial incision, have been demonstrated to be efficacious in preventing surgical site infection.

OR equipment such as defibrillators and resuscitative equipment must always be available, functional, and familiar to staff. This includes supplies needed for emergency treatment of a patient condition, such as malignant hyperthermia or unanticipated blood loss. All medications and solutions along with their containers should be labeled both on and off the surgical field. Equipment alarms should be activated with appropriate settings and should be sufficiently audible. Orthopedic procedures may also require a change in the plan of care in the event of a fracture, damage to vascular integrity, or changes in the patient's condition, requiring an understanding of methods and equipment needed to manage these situations.

Implementation

Implementing care for the orthopedic surgical patient requires an understanding of anatomic, physiologic, psychologic, cultural, spiritual, and technical patient needs. Orthopedic surgical procedures demand special equipment, instruments, and psychomotor skills that differ from those required by other specialties. Implementation includes an understanding of the procedures, patient needs, and perioperative practices to protect the patient while delivering care.

An explanation should be provided to the patient about the intraoperative phase, including the anticipated sequence of events, personnel, environment, required positioning, and procedures such as administration of a regional anesthetic and application of a tourniquet. The patient may be alert during the procedure; therefore noise from power equipment and activities that will occur should be explained. Immobilization devices, such as splints, casts, braces, and drains, should also be explained.

Positioning and Positioning Aids. The orthopedic patient requires proper positioning on the OR bed or specialty bed to provide adequate exposure of the operative area, maintain body alignment, minimize strain or pressure on nerves and muscles, allow for optimal respiratory and circulatory function, and provide adequate stabilization of the body. Selection of position depends on several factors, including the type of procedure, the location of the injury or lesion, and the preference of the surgeon. Guidelines for placing the patient in the supine or recumbent position are followed, with modifications to facilitate the specific orthopedic procedure.

Procedures performed in lateral, prone, or modified positions require use of positioning aids and devices to support these positions. Patients undergoing surgical procedures risk neuromuscular and skin injury. Preoperative assessment should be thorough to plan the position, taking into consideration the prevention of neurovascular compromise, the potential for impaired chest excursion, and the danger of falls. The safety strap does not always provide adequate security, and other methods of securing the patient on the OR bed may need to be implemented. The surgeon is responsible for selecting the position and ensuring that adequate exposure can be obtained. The perioperative staff must understand the meaning of terms such as *flexion, extension, abduction,* and *adduction* when positioning the patient. The staff must also be thoroughly familiar with the function of the orthopedic surgical bed and its various attachments (e.g., the leg attachment for arthroscopy, the three-point positioner for lateral position, and positioning devices for shoulder procedures).

Many orthopedic operations require a device for holding the extremities. Various holders are available for both upper and lower extremities. Positioners used intraoperatively can be sterilized for the procedure, resulting in the ability to reposition as needed throughout the procedure. These types of positioners include the shoulder positioner (Figure 11-14), Alvarado foot holder (Figure 11-15), and ankle distractor (Figure 11-16). Many other orthopedic positioning devices are also available.

The lateral position is sometimes used for a total hip arthroplasty. Padded anterior and posterior supports may be positioned at the umbilicus and lumbar regions, respectively, to hold the patient in the lateral position. A vacuum beanbag can also achieve this position. Pressure points on the lateral area of the skull, ear, axilla, hip, knee, and ankle should be adequately padded. The feet are placed in the neutral position to prevent excessive plantar flexion or dorsiflexion. A conscientious effort should be made by the surgical team to avoid leaning on the patient during the procedure.

The patient is positioned prone for surgery on the posterior aspect of the body, including the back; posterior portion of the shoulder, arms, and legs; and Achilles tendon; and for posterior iliac bone graft harvesting. This position presents a

SURGICAL TECHNOLOGY PREFERENCE CARD

The first thing you need to think about with orthopedic surgery is what extremity you are working on, on which side, and in what position, so that you know what side to set up on. You also must know whether the surgeon plans to use fluoroscopy, laminar flow, or any other specialty equipment. What type of OR bed will they need? Common OR beds that could be used for an orthopedic procedure are a fracture table, a Jackson table, and a regular OR bed. OR beds with special positioning devices such as a hand table, beach chair, or the peg board with a bean bag and gel pad for lateral position are also utilized in certain procedures.

In orthopedic surgery you often have other healthcare personnel in the operating room, such as radiology technologists and sales representatives, so arriving to the room early to get a feel for the room layout and room stored supplies and equipment will be beneficial. Discuss the surgical bed position with the perioperative team, taking into consideration additional equipment that may be needed for orthopedic surgery. Understanding the room layout before setting up for the procedure allows the traffic pattern in the room to be maximized. This step can help insure sterility of the field and facilitate effective communication about the transfer of additional supplies from the circulator to the scrub, as well as provide efficient space for other healthcare providers involved in the orthopedic procedure.

Room Prep: Basic operating room furniture in place, thermoregulatory devices, extra blankets, padding, positioning supplies to achieve optimal patient safety

Prep Solution: In room
- Chlorhexidine gluconate (CHG)
- Iodine and iodophors

Catheter: In room and correct size
- Catheter set and tray
  - Latex/rubber
  - PVC
  - Silicone
- Sizing
  - French
- Nonretaining
  - Red rubber (Robinson)
- Retaining
  - Foley
    - 2-way
    - 3-way
  - Mushroom/Pezzer/Malecot
- Other urine collection devices

PROCEDURE CHECKLIST
Instruments
- Standard sets according to extremity
- Bone sets according to extremity
- Surgeon-indicated implants and bone reduction clamps
- Anticipated additional instruments

Specialty Suture
- As per surgeon's preference

Hemostatic Agents
- Mechanical
  - Staplers
  - Clip appliers and clips
  - Pressure
  - Ligatures
  - Bone wax
  - Pledgets
- Chemical
  - Absorbable gelatin
  - Collagen
  - Oxidized cellulose
  - Epinephrine
  - Thrombin
- Thermal
  - Electrosurgical unit
  - Laser
  - Smoke evacuator

Additional Supplies and Equipment: both sterile and nonsterile
- If the physician is requesting supplies, instruments, or equipment not normally used, check to be sure all have arrived to the room before opening
- Sponges
- Drapes
- Gowns and gloves for team members

Continued

SURGICAL TECHNOLOGY PREFERENCE CARD—cont'd

- Cement supplies, if necessary
- Pneumatic tourniquet
- "Have ready" or "hold" supplies

Medications and Irrigation Solutions
- Do these need to be warmed?
- Appropriate-sized syringes, hypodermic needles, labels, and a marking pen

Drains
- Correct size and type for planned surgery
  - Open—Not attached to a drainage system
    - Penrose
    - Cigarette
  - Closed—Attached to a closed reservoir for fluid collection
    - Hemovac
    - Jackson-Pratt
    - Autologous blood retrieval drainage system

Dressings
- Soft padding
- Cast materials
- Splints
- Immobilizers

Specimen Care
- Proper container for each specimen
- Labels for each specimen
- Proper solution for specimen type

Before opening for the procedure, the surgical technologist should:
- Arrange furniture
- Gather positioning devices
- Damp dust lights, furniture, and surfaces
- Verify functionality of equipment
- Place items to be opened in their appropriate places

When opening sterile supplies:
- Verify exposure to sterilization
- Use sterile technique
- Open bundles in appropriate locations
- Open additional supplies onto sterile field
- Open the sterile supplies as close to the surgical start time as possible

---

challenge for the anesthesia team to monitor and manage the airway because of the potential for impaired chest excursion and gas exchange. Extremities need to be moved through a normal range of motion when transferring and positioning into the prone position. Vascular integrity is always assessed before the patient is moved into position and reassessed after the patient is positioned; the nurse should note the quality of pulses, extremity warmth, and capillary refill.

The prone position is often attained with the use of adjunctive frames, such as the Wilson, Hastings, Canadian, Relton-Hall, Cloward saddle, or Andrews, or with the Andrews bed (Figure 11-17). Each frame has qualities that meet the patient's or physician's needs. The Hastings and Andrews frames and the Andrews bed maintain the patient in a modified knee-chest position. The frames require assembly and are labor-intensive when positioning; some can be used only with certain beds. The Andrews bed is similar to the Andrews frame but has the attachments built in and is used exclusively for this position.

On an OR fracture bed (Figure 11-18), generally used for femoral neck and shaft fixation, the team places the patient in supine or lateral position to allow exposure of the surgical site while maintaining alignment. The patient's legs are positioned on outriggers, allowing access by the image intensifier to obtain multiple radiographic views. Applying or releasing traction can be done to reduce the fracture or aid in intramedullary surgical techniques. Like all positioning devices, the fracture bed must be set up by experienced personnel and padded adequately. There are several moving parts, which can lead to injury if not operated properly.

If the patient is positioned supine, special attention must be paid to the arms. Arms are placed on padded armboards with the palms up and fingers extended. Armboards are maintained at less than a 90-degree angle to prevent brachial plexus stretch. If there are surgical reasons to tuck the arms at the side, the elbows are padded to protect the ulnar nerve, the palms face inward, and the wrist is maintained in a neutral position (Denholm, 2009). A drape secures the arms. It should be tucked snugly under the patient, not under the mattress. This prevents the arm from shifting downward intraoperatively and resting against the OR bed rail.

Surgical Prep. A primary concern in orthopedic surgery is the prevention of infection. The orthopedic surgical prep must be meticulously carried out using aseptic technique. Physi-

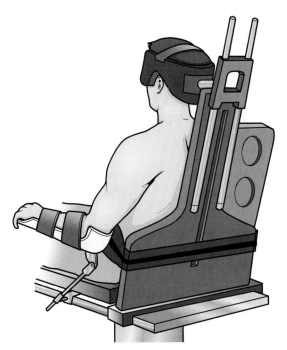

FIGURE 11-14 Shoulder positioner allows distraction of the joint for visualization.

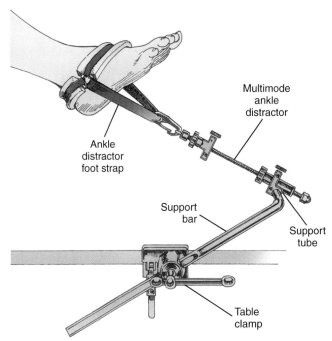

FIGURE 11-16 Ankle distractor, noninvasive, for distraction of the joint and visualization.

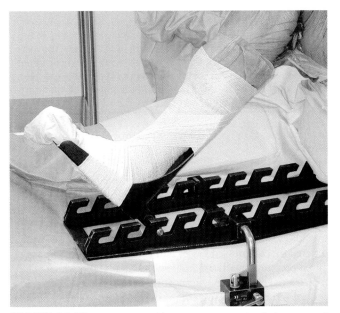

FIGURE 11-15 Innomed's Robb Leg Positioner used during total joint procedures to position the extremity for exposure.

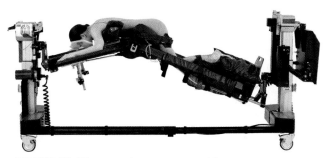

FIGURE 11-17 Axis Jackson System used for prone positioning.

cians often instruct patients to complete a scrub prep with an antimicrobial agent before arrival for surgery. The surgical prep for the orthopedic patient may include preoperative removal of hair from the surgical site. Surgical shave preps contribute to the possibility of infection caused by abrasion and cutting of the skin. If hair removal from the incisional site is ordered, it should occur immediately before surgery, using clippers or a depilatory. If a razor is required, the site should be lathered with soap before shaving. Trauma patients require precau-

tions during the skin prep to prevent further injury caused by solution contact with membranes or injury to the bone and soft tissue from movement.

Skin preparation is performed to remove microorganisms from the operative site. The site should be prepped with a broad-spectrum antimicrobial agent. The prep proceeds from the incision site to the periphery. Pooling of the prep solution beneath the patient or tourniquet must be avoided. Prep solutions should be allowed to dry before draping; this is a fire safety precaution and may be included in the time-out. The groin and anal areas should be isolated when the surgical site is on the upper third of the leg.

Devices such as leg stirrups may help support an extremity to complete a circumferential prep. When multiple extremities or other areas, such as a bone graft site, are prepped, cross-contamination of previously prepped areas must be prevented. Knowledge of aseptic technique and the ability to organize the activity are important in proper preparation of the surgical site.

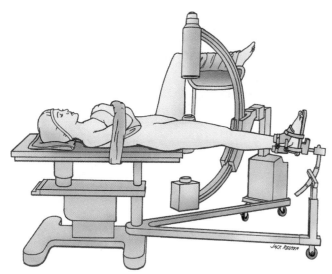

FIGURE 11-18 Patient positioned on the orthopedic fracture bed for femoral neck, femoral shaft, or tibial fixation, with image intensifier in position.

Draping. Application of sterile drapes is the final step in preparing the patient for the operation. The surgeon and surgical technologist cover the patient's extremities with a cloth or water-impervious stockinette—a cylindric drape that is rolled up the arm or leg. Impervious sheets are essential when large amounts of fluid are used, such as during arthroscopy and wound irrigation. Prefabricated disposable drapes with fenestrations for the upper and lower extremities are available.

Antimicrobial incise drapes can be used to isolate the surrounding area from the incisional site. Many of these drapes contain iodophor-impregnated adhesive, which slowly releases iodine during the procedure, inhibiting proliferation of organisms from the patient's skin. They are contraindicated for patients with an allergy to iodophors. An alcohol skin wipe may be done before placement of the antimicrobial incise drape.

Equipment and Supplies. Orthopedic ORs require a variety of special equipment and accessories in addition to routine OR equipment. Nitrogen-powered, battery-powered, and electrically powered equipment, video systems, pneumatic tourniquets, laminar airflow systems, x-ray equipment, lasers, and special orthopedic tables are included in the operative armamentarium. Manufacturers' pamphlets with illustrations and directions on equipment use and sterilization should be readily available for reference.

RADIOGRAPHIC INTERVENTION. Radiographic intervention is widely used in orthopedic surgery (History box). Many procedures require portable x-ray or fluoroscopy machines. Fluoroscopy, also known as *image intensification* or *C-arm,* allows the team to view the progression of the procedure, confirming fracture reduction or intramedullary reaming of the humerus, femur, or tibia. A radiologic technologist operates radiographic equipment. An understanding of equipment placement, function, and safety precautions is necessary. X-ray cassettes brought onto the sterile field are draped with a sterile plastic cover. Lead aprons and thyroid shields are to be worn by all personnel in proximity to the x-ray equipment, and personnel should be monitored for exposure to radiation. Measures

should be taken to protect patients from direct and indirect radiation exposure.

PNEUMATIC TOURNIQUETS. Pneumatic tourniquets are frequently used for procedures involving the extremities (Figure 11-19). A tourniquet is a fabric-covered cylindric bladder inflated by compressed gas or ambient air. It applies circumferential pressure on arterial and venous circulation, which results in a relatively bloodless surgical field; this promotes visualization of structures during the procedure. Limb exsanguination is achieved by elevating the limb or by wrapping it, distally to proximally, with an Ace or Esmarch rubber bandage before tourniquet inflation. The majority of tourniquets used today are run by a microprocessor for regulation of pressure and time setting, providing both auditory and visual feedback for the user.

Tourniquet safety should be a priority; the surgical team should understand recommended parameters and precautions. Safety guidelines for the use of tourniquets include preventive measures and evaluation (AORN, 2009). Preoperative assessment of the patient includes determining contraindications for use, including compartment syndrome, McArdle disease (e.g., glycogen storage disease), hypertension, or other vascular problems. If the tourniquet must be used for patients with these conditions, specific guidelines must be observed.

HISTORY

History of Medical Imaging

As humans became more aware of injuries and how to treat them, certain people in each culture accepted the responsibility and honor of healing. In some tribal cultures, that person was a medicine man, or bonesetter. Neolithic people may have had fractures splinted—probably with bark and sticks. Other tribes used clay, soaked strips of rawhide, and linen. Hippocrates described using a wooden rack to treat a fracture of the femur and using techniques such as traction and countertraction. However, bone healing as we know it today depended much on the development of imaging techniques.

The era of medical imaging began with the publication of *De Humani Corporis Fabrica* in 1543 by Andreas Vesalius. This comprehensive, detailed, and accurate set of anatomic illustrations set new standards in the art of medical observational science and research. Through direct observation, Vesalius conveyed his knowledge of the anatomy of the human body. These works were undisputed and stood the test of time until 1895, when Wilhelm Konrad Roentgen accidentally discovered x-rays (roentgenograms). Composed of high-energy electrons, x-rays are absorbed in varying degrees by structures in the body, based on their density and mass. The image is produced in two dimensions on photographic film and allows for indirect observation through a noninvasive technique. For the next 70 years, x-rays remained the standard in medical imaging until computerized axial tomography, or CAT scan, was introduced in 1972 by Godfrey Hounsfield. Detailed images of the body could be created by directing narrow x-ray beams at various angles. This was the first technique that incorporated computers into medical imaging. Since then, medical imaging has dramatically expanded, facilitating the surgical team's understanding of anatomy, physiology, and pathophysiology.

Modified from Gray JE, Orton CG: Medical physics: some recollections in diagnostic x-ray imaging and therapeutic radiology, Radiology 217(3):619-625, 2000.

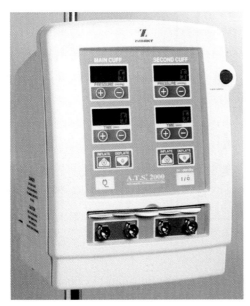

FIGURE 11-19 Pneumatic gauge.

Before application, the tourniquet equipment should be checked for proper functioning. Inflation pressures are established based on the systolic blood pressure, age of the patient, and circumference of the extremity. Duration of tourniquet inflation should be kept to a minimum. It is recommended in the average, healthy 50-year-old person to apply continuous tourniquet pressure less than 1 hour on the upper extremity and less than 2 hours on the thigh. Tourniquet pressure should not exceed the recommended maximum cuff pressure limits of 300 to 350 mm Hg for the thigh and 250 to 300 mm Hg for the arm and the lower leg. Kleinert and colleagues (2007) notes the interval between inflation and deflation should be 5 minutes for every 30 minutes of tourniquet ischemia to minimize effects on muscle and nerves.

The tourniquet should be placed on the extremity without compression on bony structures and superficial neurovascular structures. The person placing the cuff should ensure it is positioned as high as possible without pinching skinfolds. Soft padding or stockinette is wrapped around the extremity and kept free of wrinkles and gatherings beneath the cuff. Cuffs should overlap a minimum of 3 inches and a maximum of 6 inches; excess overlap can pinch skinfolds. A tourniquet cuff that is too short can loosen after inflation. Care must be taken to ensure that the line from the air supply to the cuff is not kinked.

Tourniquet equipment should be checked periodically and serviced when problems arise. Injury from tourniquets may result from inadequate precautions, faulty preparation, or use of inaccurate equipment. The gauges and other related equipment should be checked with commercially available test equipment. Patient evaluation requires assessment of the extremity (skin color, temperature, pulses, movement, sensation) after removal of the tourniquet. Abnormal findings need to be reported to the surgeon and documented (Evidence for Practice).

TRACTION. The surgeon uses traction preoperatively, intraoperatively, or postoperatively for prevention or reduction of muscle spasm, immobilization of a joint or body part, reduction of a fracture or dislocation, and treatment of a joint disorder. Traction alignment must be constant.

Various traction techniques can be used, including manual, skin, and skeletal (Figure 11-20). In manual traction, the hands provide the forces pulling on the bone being realigned. Skin traction uses strips of tape, digital straps, moleskin, or an elastic bandage applied directly to the skin. Common forms of skin traction are Buck's extension and Russell traction. Skeletal traction applies forces directly to the bone, using pins. Manual and skin traction can be applied in the emergency department or patient room, whereas skeletal traction is applied preoperatively in the emergency department or in the OR.

Skeletal traction is often used in conjunction with the OR fracture bed, using the traction attachment to aid in reduction of a long bone fracture. Postoperatively the patient may be confined to bed with balanced skeletal traction using a Thomas splint (Figure 11-21) and a Pearson attachment. Some cervical spine fractures or injuries may require Crutchfield or Gardner-Wells tongs or a cervical halo inserted directly into the skull to stabilize the vertebrae and reduce spinal cord damage or further injury. Application of skeletal traction requires the use of sterile supplies, including a traction bow, pins, and drill.

POSTOPERATIVE IMMOBILIZATION. Postoperative immobilization may require use of a cast, splint, or other supplies designed for the specific anatomic part. A cast is a common method of immobilizing a fractured bone during healing (Patient and Family Education). The forces of distraction, rotation, and malalignment can be overcome with the application of a cast. Closed reduction with a cast may be an option, thus minimizing the disadvantages and complications of open reduction, such as infection and tissue damage.

The surgeon uses plaster or synthetic materials such as fiberglass for casting. Plaster is less expensive, with a greater weight/strength ratio (it requires a greater weight of plaster

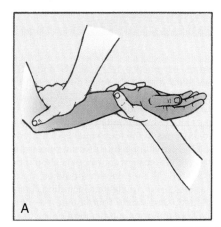
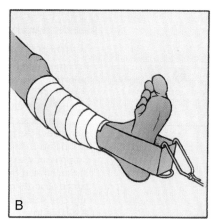
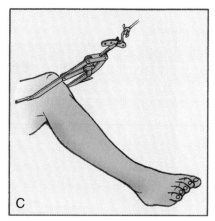

FIGURE 11-20 Traction techniques. **A,** Manual. **B,** Skin. **C,** Skeletal.

to produce the same strength of fiberglass). Plaster casts may be burdensome if the casts are too heavy. They are routinely used as the primary cast after surgical procedures and are replaced later with a lighter fiberglass cast to promote patient mobility.

Casting material sets up and hardens rapidly once activated with water, and such a property necessitates that it be prepared with all necessary materials. Soft padding or stockinette should be applied to the extremity before the cast is applied to protect the skin from thermal injury while the plaster sets, as well as to protect the skin from undue abrasion and pressure. The plaster must be prepared, applied, and handled carefully and safely.

Figure 11-22 shows types of casts. After wrist fractures, the surgeon applies a short arm cast from below the elbow to the metacarpal heads. A long arm cast extends from the axilla to the metacarpal heads, immobilizing forearm or elbow fractures. The surgeon uses a short leg cast, applied from the tibial tuberosity to the metatarsal heads, to immobilize the ankle and foot. The long leg cast is used for fractures involving the femur, tibia, or fibula or for complicated ankle fractures. The femoral cast brace is used in the treatment of femoral shaft fractures. A snug-fitting thigh cast and short leg cast are hinged at the knee joint. The cast brace is generally used after 4 to 6 weeks

of skeletal traction after initiation of callus formation at the fracture site. A cylinder cast incorporates the leg from the groin to the ankle and is applied when complete knee immobilization is required. This is often required after surgery involving soft tissue reconstruction around the knee.

The hip spica cast is used when complete leg immobilization is desired. The patient's trunk, affected side, and unaffected side may all be incorporated into the cast. Spinal immobilization is accomplished with a body jacket.

Splints may also be employed for postoperative immobilization but are not circumferential and allow for swelling and closer observation of the surgical site.

Another immobilization device is the abduction pillow, used after total joint replacement. This prevents the patient's leg from adducting, or rotating internally, and the hip from flexing, which could cause dislocation of the hip. Further discussion of this and other devices is included with the description of various surgical interventions.

LASERS. Laser application has been increasing in the field of orthopedics. Their use mandates safety precautions, certification, patient consent, and protective attire. Laser types include carbon dioxide, holmium:yttrium-aluminum-garnet (Ho:YAG), neodymium:YAG (Nd:YAG), potassium titanyl phosphate (KTP), erbium:YAG (Er:YAG), and excimer. Laser technique differs for use on bone, muscle, tendon, and cartilage. Lasers have been used successfully for osteotomy, revision arthroplasty (removal of polymethylmethacrylate), nerve and tendon repair, arthroscopy, and discectomy.

AIRFLOW CONTROL. Airflow control in the orthopedic OR is critical to prevent introduction of microorganisms. Surgical site infections may result from airborne bacteria or transient bacteria from the patient or surgical team (AORN, 2009). Laminar airflow is a system designed to provide highly filtered air and continuous air exchange for reducing airborne bacteria. Body exhaust suits are also used as a defense against airborne bacteria (Figure 11-23). Aseptic practices, sterile technique, and conscientious behaviors in ORs using conventional airflow can be used to maintain low rates of surgical site infections.

Instruments and Accessory Items. Orthopedic surgical procedures require an extensive inventory of instruments and

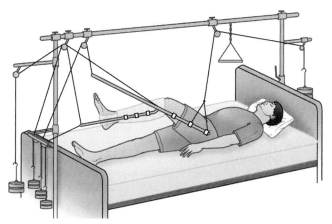

FIGURE 11-21 Thomas splint balanced suspension.

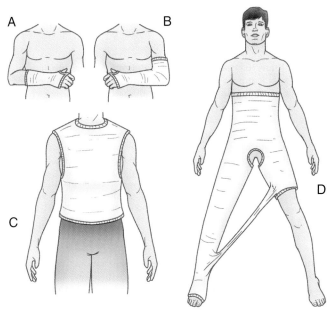

FIGURE 11-22 Types of casts. **A,** Short arm cast. **B,** Long arm cast. **C,** Plaster body jacket cast. **D,** One and one half hip spica cast.

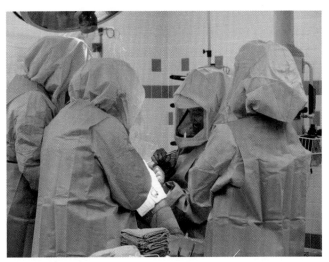

FIGURE 11-23 Body exhaust system used in arthroplasty.

implants and specific instruments to implant and apply hardware. Revision surgery requires that the perioperative staff be prepared with the appropriate tools and extractors needed to remove an old implant and an understanding of equipment use.

IMPLANT INVENTORIES. Implant inventories include plates and screws, intramedullary nails and rods, total joint implants, and a host of accessory items. Surgeon preference, patient population, and equipment cost are considered when selecting stock items. The surgical team must ensure these items are stocked in a timely fashion to prepare for consecutive implant use.

Inventory should be organized by manufacturers, type of implants (e.g., total hip, knee), and comparative sizes. Some may be provided on a loaner or consignment basis. Staff must be familiar with the varied types and refer to manufacturer's information pertaining to each implant. Practices should ensure that the correct implant is opened on the operative field to prevent unnecessary expense or error in placement.

Many different alloys are used in the manufacturing of implants. However, all devices implanted in a patient must be of the same metallic composition to prevent galvanic corrosion; internal fixation implants used during an orthopedic procedure should be of the same metal. Screws, for example, should be of the same composition as the metal plate affixed to the bone. Alloys that are used most frequently include stainless steel, cobalt-chromium, and titanium-vanadium-aluminum.

Internal fixation devices should never be reused. Resulting imperfections, such as abrasions or scratches, increase the potential for corrosion and weakening of the implant. Bending implants to conform to the contour of the bone should be avoided whenever possible to prevent loss of strength. When bending is necessary, the proper bending press should be used. Once an implant is bent, it should not be reshaped or straightened; doing so may weaken the implant.

Orthopedic equipment and implants require special care, storage, and handling. When possible, implants should be individually wrapped and processed. Today's implants, excluding some plates and screws, are packaged separately by the manufacturer. During sterilization, implants should not be placed in a position in which knocking or bumping might occur. Appropriate sterilizing cases and trays should be used, and implants should be sterilized according to the manufacturer's instructions. An internal fixation device that has become damaged as a result of improper storage or handling must be discarded.

The perioperative team assigned to orthopedic patients should have a working knowledge of the general types and sizes of implants that might be selected. Templates of radiographs are often made preoperatively, providing a general idea of the size of the implants needed.

The U.S. Food and Drug Administration (FDA) requires strict guidelines in properly documenting and tracking implant devices. Documentation should include, but not be limited to, the patient's permanent record, the operative record, and an implant registry maintained by the OR. Many manufacturers now include mailers to return information to the company for data collection. Information to be recorded includes the lot and serial numbers of those implants used and the manufacturer, size, type, and anatomic position of the implants.

ORTHOPEDIC INSTRUMENTATION. Orthopedic instrumentation varies from very small to large instruments. Some procedures require multiple instrument containers (sets). Organization of instrument sets for multiple uses prevents the need for duplication and requires thoughtful consideration of anatomic and physiologic needs. When preparing for a procedure, the surgical technologist should open the minimum number of instruments yet be prepared for unexpected or untoward events. Careful planning and preparation of instrumentation ensure efficient use of time and equipment.

Instruments that do not function properly (as a result of dullness, poor adjustment, lack of lubrication, damage, improper fit, or incomplete cleaning) are primary sources of complaints and problems in the OR. Instrument maintenance is vital to ensure availability for the procedure and ease in com-

▶▶ RISK REDUCTION STRATEGIES

Deep Vein Thrombosis Prevention in Orthopedic Procedures

Prevention of venous thromboembolism is a major consideration for patients undergoing orthopedic surgery, especially total joint arthroplasty. The *American College of Chest Physicians Evidence-Based Clinical Guidelines* for use of antithrombic and thrombolytic agents and therapy contain review of the literature, expert opinions, and recent clinical trial evaluations. Approximately 40% to 60% of orthopedic hip and knee arthroplasty patients develop deep vein thrombosis postoperatively. Additional risk factors for orthopedic patients include age greater than 75, malignancy, immobilization, and the use of certain medications. Currently, surgeon preference influences which anticoagulation therapy is initiated after surgery (see Surgical Pharmacology, p. 452). The ACCP recommendations include that all hospitals have a formal, institutional-wide written policy addressing thromboprophylaxis. The policy would include dividing patients into categories of low, moderate, or high risk. Thromboprophylaxis would be provided when its benefit outweighs the risk. Regular reassessment is necessary.

From Geerts WH et al: Prevention of venous thromboembolism: American College of Chest Physicians evidence-based clinical practice guidelines, *Chest* 133:381S-453S, 2008; *Joint Commission National Patient Safety Goals, NPSG.03.05.01*, available at www.jointcommission.org/NR/rdonlyres/31666E86-E7F4-423E-9BE8-F05BD1CB0AA8/0/HAP_NPSG.pdf. Accessed June 16, 2009.

pletion of the procedure. Instruments should be used for the intended purpose during the procedure. Movable parts should be lubricated after each cleaning and checked for cracks or damage after each use. The perioperative team is responsible for instrument maintenance and familiarity with sterilization and packaging procedures.

The following basic bone instrument sets should be available in the orthopedic OR. Soft tissue instrument sets appropriate for the size of the anatomic site are used for procedures not requiring bone instruments or in addition to the sets. Additional instruments and special equipment are mentioned with the discussion of various surgical interventions.

- *Incision hip set:* total hip arthroplasty or fractures of the neck and proximal femur
- *Total knee set:* total knee arthroplasty or supracondylar and distal femoral fractures
- *Shoulder set:* shoulder arthroplasty and other shoulder procedures
- *Large bone set:* bone work on the large bones, including hip, knee, upper arm, and elbow
- *Extremity or small bone set:* bone work on the hand or foot
- *Fusion or bone graft instruments:* additional instruments necessary for an autograft

POWERED SURGICAL INSTRUMENTS. Powered surgical instruments (Figure 11-24) used in the OR have eliminated the need for many hand-operated tools, thereby reducing operative time and improving technical results. They are available as air-driven, battery-driven, or electrically driven equipment. Fingertip control provides the surgeon speed and power. Variable-speed saws, drills, and reamers offer wide flexibility. Power equipment has a safety control that prevents inadvertent activation; this should be engaged when passing the instrument to the surgeon or assistant. The perioperative nurse and surgical technologist should monitor the sterile field to make certain that powered instruments are not rested on the patient when they are not in use.

It is important to follow the manufacturer's recommended cleaning, sterilizing, and lubricating instructions. With proper care, powered surgical instruments have a long life span and many uses.

SUTURE MATERIAL. Suture material requires increased tensile strength and minimal degradability for the select type of tissue. Tendons and ligaments are fibrous, avascular tissues, resulting in a slower healing process than that occurring in tissues rich in blood supply. Absorbable suture may be used for sewing tendon or ligaments to bone. Nonabsorbable sutures, including polyester and surgical steel, are also used. For various ligament replacement grafts, a harvested tendon may be customized with multiple strands of suture material, increasing tensile strength and length of time until fibrous union occurs.

POLYMETHYLMETHACRYLATE. PMMA (bone cement) is an acrylic, cementlike substance composed of a liquid methylmethacrylate monomer and a powder methylmethacrylate-styrene co-polymer. The powder component is 10% barium sulfate, U.S. Pharmacopoeia (USP), which provides radiopacity to the finished product. The liquid monomer is highly flammable, and the OR should be properly ventilated. Caution should be exercised during mixing of the two components to prevent excessive exposure of OR personnel to the vapors of the monomer. This exposure can cause irritation of the respiratory tract and eyes. Personnel in a room where methylmethacrylate is being mixed should not wear soft contact lenses. Many special hoods and mixing devices are available to minimize staff exposure to the fumes. It is common practice in many ORs that pregnant perioperative team members may step out of the room while PMMA is being mixed because of possible risks to the fetus.

Adverse patient reactions with PMMA include transitory hypotension, cardiac arrest, cerebrovascular accident, pulmonary embolus, thrombophlebitis, and hypersensitivity reaction. Cardiac arrest and death, although uncommon, have resulted after insertion of bone cement. Adverse reactions have been attributed to a combination of factors, including a rise in intramedullary canal pressure causing embolic phenomena, a possible chemical and blood reaction causing sudden hypotension, and certain pre-existing patient conditions. More research is needed to discover the exact cause of adverse reactions. Patient care should include collaborating with the anesthesia provider before insertion of PMMA and then monitoring for side effects after insertion.

Medications. Antibiotics, hemostatics, and antibacterial agents are used commonly. Antibiotics are delivered both intravenously and locally in irrigation solutions. Common antibiotics used in irrigation include polymyxin and bacitracin. Irrigation may also be delivered using pulsatile lavage, with anti-

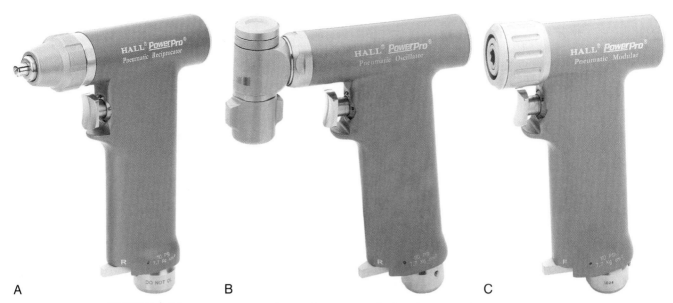

FIGURE 11-24 Pneumatic-powered surgical instruments for large bone procedures. **A,** Reciprocating saw. **B,** Oscillating saw. **C,** Single-trigger modular handpiece.

biotics added to the solution. Hemostatic agents may include bone wax, gelatin foam, thrombin, microfibrillar collagen, and parecoxib sodium. Parecoxib sodium is a liquid, sprayable hemostatic agent consisting of collagen, thrombin, the patient's own platelets, and fibrinogen. Antibacterial ointments are pre-impregnated in gauze dressings from the manufacturer or are applied before the application of the dressing. Other medications used during orthopedic procedures include steroids, local anesthetics, and normal saline. Local anesthetics are often injected near the end of the surgical procedure to minimize postoperative pain.

Protective Measures. Orthopedic procedures require caution as a result of the use of fluids for irrigation or bloody procedures. Personnel protective measures include handling items (blades, sharp instruments, bone) cautiously to prevent inadvertent punctures or cuts and wearing protective masks, eyewear, or a face shield as well as protective attire, including gowns and boots. Sharp bone edges are a hazard and can puncture gloves and skin. Double-gloving or use of protective gloves should be employed to protect the patient and personnel.

Bone Banking. The American Association of Tissue Banks (AATB) accredits and periodically inspects bone-banking programs to ensure that specific standards are followed in the retrieval, processing, storage, and distribution of bone allografts (AATB, 2008). Allografts are frozen until use. Vacuum-sealed freezers are monitored with an alarm. When requested for a procedure, the bone allograft is delivered to the field, slightly thawed, cultured, and washed with an antibiotic solution. Banked bone is available in many shapes of cortical and cancellous tissue.

Records are maintained on both donors and recipients. Donor records provide the donor identification, medical history (with circumstances of death if applicable), labora-tory results, and graft description. Recipient records include recipient identification, surgeon and organization implanting the graft, surgical procedure, culture results, and any adverse reactions. Like other implants, the recipient's operative record should include the name of the bone bank from which the allograft was received, type of allograft, tissue number, and expiration date if applicable.

Surgical Interventions

ALLOGRAFTS/AUTOGRAFTS

Bone grafting using allografts or autografts may be used (1) to fill cavities after removal of large amounts of bone that might result in instability, (2) to fill bony defects, and (3) to promote union of fractures at the time of open reduction. The type of graft used depends on the location of the fracture or defect, the condition of the bone, and the amount of bone loss as a result of injury. Bone grafts may be used for procedures involving revision of joints if there is significant bone loss caused by resorption or mechanical destruction after removal of bone cement.

The bone graft may be the patient's own bone (autogenous in origin and referred to as *autograft*) or bone obtained from a tissue bank (homogeneous in origin and referred to as *allograft*). Autografts are often harvested from the iliac crest, where there is cortical and cancellous bone. Various harvesting techniques are used. Struts of cortical bone from the iliac crest can be fashioned to the desired shape and used in areas needing structural strength. The amount of cancellous bone is plentiful. It is used to promote bone growth in areas of defect. Local bone graft material may be taken from the site of injury. Allografts are used when bone is not available from the patient because of the lack of sufficient quantity or because a secondary procedure is undesirable for the patient.

Procedural Considerations

Cancellous grafts may be taken from the ilium, olecranon, or distal radius; cortical grafts may be taken from the tibia, fibula, iliac crest, or ribs. When the recipient site of an autogenous graft is diseased, instruments used for the recipient site must be separated from donor graft site instruments. The operating team must change their gowns and gloves to take the bone graft and again follow the procedure to prevent cross-contamination. The patient is positioned to allow exposure to the surgical site. A sandbag may be placed beneath the area for easier access.

The instrumentation for taking a bone graft includes soft tissue instruments and a bone graft set. Grafts may be harvested with hand instruments, power tools such as an oscillating saw, or high-speed tools such as the Midas Rex. Power tools may be necessary if a uniformly shaped graft is needed to fill a defect. Because hemostasis is sometimes difficult to achieve as a result of the vascular nature of bone, wound drains may be desirable.

Operative Procedure

Harvest of Bone Graft. A cancellous bone graft consists of spongy bone usually taken from the anterior or posterior crest of the ilium. A cortical bone graft, consisting of hard, dense bone, is removed from the crest of the ilium or the tibia. The location of the crest of the ilium is subcutaneous, allowing exposure without difficulty.

1. The surgeon makes an incision along the border of the iliac crest, and strips, elevates, and retracts the muscles on the outer table of the ilium.
2. Strips of the iliac crest can be removed with an osteotome or oscillating saw.
3. A cortical window may also be made in the outer table, and the surgeon may use curettes or gouges to remove cancellous bone chips.
4. A drain may be inserted. The surgeon closes the wound in layers and applies a pressure dressing.

SURGICAL PHARMACOLOGY

Anticoagulation Therapy

Venous thromboembolism (VTE), including deep vein thrombosis (DVT) and pulmonary thromboembolism (PE), is one of the most common preventable causes of hospital death. More than 900,000 Americans experience DVT each year, and 500,000 of these persons develop PE, which causes approximately 300,000 deaths. Analysis of related data has suggested that fewer than 50% of patients diagnosed and hospitalized with DVT had received prophylaxis. In 2003, recognizing that the incidence of DVT/VTE was a significant patient safety issue, the National Quality Forum (NQF) endorsed Safe Practice 17: *Evaluate each patient upon admission, and regularly thereafter, for the risk of developing DVT/VTE. Utilize clinically appropriate methods to prevent DVT/VTE,* and Safe Practice 18: *Utilize dedicated anticoagulation services that facilitate coordinated care management.*

In addition, the Surgical Care Improvement Project (SCIP) targeted DVT as a key area for improvement in surgical patient care. SCIP is a national partnership of organizations committed to improving the safety of surgical care through the reduction of postoperative complications, with a goal of reducing the incidence of surgical complications nationally by 25% by the year 2010. SCIP identified two process measures in the reduction of VTE: (1) that surgery patients have the appropriate VTE prophylaxis ordered and (2) that it be administered within 24 hours before their surgery or within 24 hours after it.

More than 50% of major orthopedic procedures are complicated by DVT, and up to 30% by PE, if prophylactic treatment is not instituted. DVTs in the perioperative period involve several components, including venous stasis, acquired hypercoagulable state, endothelial injury, and the positioning of the limb intraoperatively. Despite the well-established efficacy and safety of preventive measures, studies show that prophylaxis is often underused or used inappropriately. Both low-dose unfractionated heparin (LDUH) and low-molecular-weight heparin (LMWH) have similar efficacy in DVT and PE prevention.

Some common drugs used to prevent DVT and their mechanisms of action are as follows:

◆ *Ardeparin*—LMWH; prevents conversion of fibrinogen to fibrin and prothrombin to thrombin by enhancing inhibitory effects of antithrombin III; used for preventing DVT after total knee arthroplasty (TKA)
◆ *Danaparoid*—glycosaminoglycan; prevents conversion of fibrinogen to fibrin and prothrombin to thrombin by enhancing inhibitory effects of antithrombin III; used for DVT prevention in total hip replacement or hip fracture surgery
◆ *Desirudin (Iprivask)*—thrombin inhibitor; prevents thrombin, resulting in prolongation of clotting time; used for DVT prophylaxis in hip replacement surgery
◆ *Enoxaparin (Lovenox)*—LMWH; prevents conversion of fibrinogen to fibrin and prothrombin to thrombin by enhancing inhibitory effects of antithrombin III and produces higher ratio of anti–factor Xa to anti–factor IIa; used for prevention of DVT and PE in hip and knee replacement surgery
◆ *Heparin (Calcilean, Calciparine, Hepalean, heparin sodium, Heparin LEO, heparin lock, Hep-Lock)*—anticoagulant and antithrombotic; prevents conversion of fibrinogen to fibrin and prothrombin to thrombin by enhancing inhibitory effects of antithrombin III; used for prevention of DVT and PE
◆ *Warfarin (Coumadin, Sofarin, warfarin sodium, Warfilone Sodium)*—anticoagulant; interferes with blood clotting by indirect means; depresses hepatic synthesis of vitamin K–dependent coagulation factors (II, VII, IX, X); DVT and PE prevention

Patient education should include the reason for DVT prophylaxis, the name (both generic and trade) of the drug, dosage, time of administration, and side effects. Because bleeding is a dangerous complication, signs and symptoms of both minor bleeding and major bleeding should be reviewed. Patients should receive both oral and written information along with the name of a physician or nurse to call if complications or questions arise.

Modified from Canobbio MM: *Mosby's handbook of patient teaching,* ed 3, St Louis, 2006, Mosby; SCIP: *A national quality partnership,* available at www.qipa.org/shared/content/pa_documents/Patient%20Safety%209SOW. Accessed June 23, 2009; Skidmore-Roth L: *Mosby's drug guide for nurses with 2010 update,* ed 8, St Louis, 2009, Mosby.

ELECTRICAL STIMULATION

The healing process in bone involves several stages (Figure 11-25). When a bone is damaged, such as during a surgical procedure or fracture, bleeding occurs. The amount of extravasated blood depends on the vascularity of the fracture site. The blood exudate infiltrates the surrounding area, where a clot is formed. Fibroblasts invade the hematoma and form a fibrin meshwork.

As osteoblasts invade the fibrin meshwork, blood vessels develop to build collagen. After several days, calcium deposits may form in the granulation tissue. These deposits eventually form new bone, known as *callus*. Within the callus, cartilage cells develop a temporary semirigid tissue that helps stabilize the bone fragments. The callus is immature bone that is remodeled by new connective tissue cells (osteoblasts) of the periosteum and the inner membrane of the bone cavity. Through this process, mature bone is formed, excess callus is resorbed, and trabecular bone is placed.

After several months, depending on the age and physical condition of the individual, the bone becomes firmly united, although the ossification process is not yet completed. Complete union of the fractured bone or joint is determined by means of clinical and radiologic examination.

Healing of bone is classified by degree. *Delayed union* signifies that healing has not occurred within the average time. The average time depends on many factors, and delayed unions must not be considered nonunion until the healing process has ceased without bony union. *Malunion* signifies that the fracture has united with deformity sufficient to cause impairment of the function or a significant angulation of the extremity. *Nonunion* signifies that the process of healing has ended without producing bony union; in this case, electrical stimulation may be used.

Electrical stimulation is artificially applied electrical current that induces or influences the formation of new bone. Various types of stimulators (Figure 11-26) are available for treatment of nonunion, including invasive (implantable) and noninva-

sive (capacitance coupling). The bone stimulator of choice depends on the patient, pathologic condition, and the physician's comfort with the device.

The bone-growth stimulator is used in patients with high risk of nonunion. It can be used to provide electrical stimulation for treatment of nonunion, delayed union, congenital pseudarthrosis, and bone defects. It may be used with or without internal fixation devices, external fixation devices, or bone grafting. Patients who have undergone previous surgery, who have sustained significant tissue loss, or in whom bone grafting is contraindicated are candidates. Electrical stimulation requires long periods of immobilization of the site. This prolonged immobilization may impede rehabilitation.

Procedural Considerations

Instructions for implanting and components selected vary according to the type. The position of the patient depends on the implant site.

In addition to the implant of the surgeon's choice and the implant-specific instrumentation, a soft tissue set is used. Curettes, osteotomes, or bone rasps are used for bony debridement and to scarify the donor bed. Power drills with drill bits may be necessary to create access through the bone for the electrical leads.

Operative Procedure

1. The surgeon exposes the site and debrides it as necessary. A stimulator may be implanted after the surgical procedure.
2. A bone slot is fashioned, spanning the nonunion site.
3. The surgeon makes a second incision about 8 to 10 cm from the first one and dissects the tissue. Before the generator is implanted, hemostasis must be achieved. The use of electrosurgical equipment may interfere with function of the bone-growth stimulator.
4. Using blunt or sharp dissection, the surgeon creates a subcutaneous channel for the cathode.
5. The surgeon guides the long cathode lead through the channel.
6. The generator is carefully implanted near the skin surface. The generator should be inserted into soft tissue—not against bone or metal fixation devices; it should not create a bulge beneath the skin.
7. The surgeon places the electrical coils in the prepared bone slot in equal lengths above and below the fracture site.
8. Cancellous bone grafts are placed between the coils if large bony defects are being treated.
9. Routine closure of the subcutaneous and skin tissue is carried out.

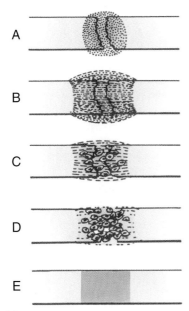

FIGURE 11-25 Bone-healing process. **A,** Hematoma formation. **B,** Fibrin network formation. **C,** Invasion of osteoblasts. **D,** Callus formation. **E,** Remodeling.

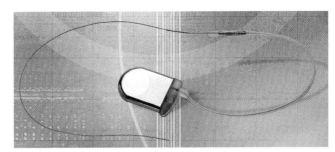

FIGURE 11-26 Bone-growth stimulator used after procedures to induce bone formation.

Once union has occurred (5 to 6 months), the surgeon removes the generator after a local anesthetic has been administered.

FRACTURES AND DISLOCATIONS

A fracture is a break in the continuity of a bone. The care of fractured bones or dislocation of a joint is complicated when there is trauma to the soft tissues, including muscles, nerves, ligaments, and blood vessels. Bone diseases, which can increase the risk of a fracture, can be metabolic, infectious, or degenerative. Metabolic diseases are disorders of bone remodeling. The most common are osteoporosis, osteomalacia, and Paget's disease, all of which may result in bone fractures. The most common infectious process is osteomyelitis. Degenerative musculoskeletal conditions are associated with aging. Osteoarthritis is the most common degenerative change.

Osteoporosis is one of the most common and serious of bone diseases and is responsible for more than 2 million fractures a year. Osteoporosis-related fractures most commonly occur in the hip, spine, and wrist, but any bone can be affected. The number of fractures caused by osteoporosis is expected to rise to more than 3 million by 2025 (National Osteoporosis Foundation [NOF], 2009).

Osteoporosis is characterized by excessive loss of calcified matrix, bone mineral, and collagenous fibers, causing a reduction of total bone mass. Decreasing levels of estrogen and testosterone in the older adult result in reduced new bone growth and maintenance of existing bone. Inadequate intake of calcium or vitamin D; lack of weight-bearing activities, exercise, and physical activity; smoking; and caffeine intake are other contributing factors. Osteoporotic bone is porous, brittle, and fragile, fracturing easily under stress. This results in susceptibility to spontaneous fractures and pathologic curvature of the spine (Barclay et al, 2008).

Osteomalacia is a metabolic bone disease characterized by inadequate mineralization of bone as a result of vitamin D deficiency, which leads to a reduced absorption of calcium and phosphorus. Risk factors for development of osteomalacia include malabsorption problems, vitamin D and calcium deficiencies, chronic renal failure, and inadequate exposure to sunlight. Medical treatment includes dietary supplements and exposure to sunlight.

Paget's disease is a disorder affecting older adults. It is characterized by proliferation of osteoclasts and compensatory

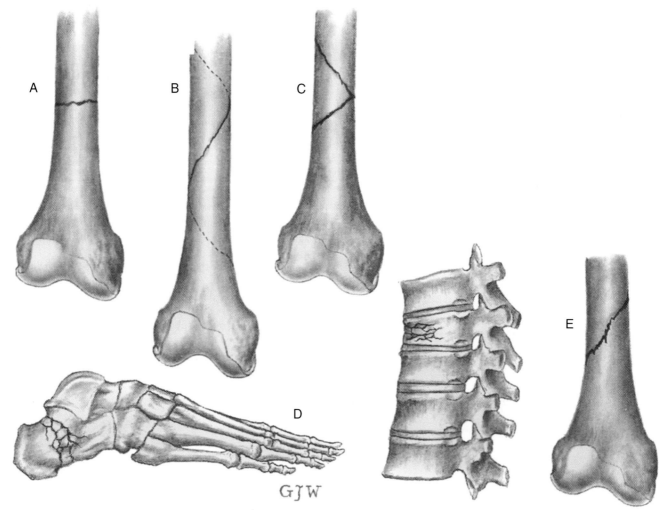

FIGURE 11-27 Fracture types, which may be open or closed. **A,** Transverse. **B,** Longitudinal or spiral. **C,** Comminuted. **D,** Compression. **E,** Oblique.

increased osteoblastic activity, resulting in rapid, disorganized bone remodeling. The bones are weak and poorly constructed.

Types of Fractures

Fractures are classified into two main groups: closed fractures and open or compound fractures. *Closed fractures* are those in which there is no communication between the bone fragments and the skin surface. *Incomplete closed fractures* are those in which the whole thickness of the bone is not broken but is bent or buckled, such as in greenstick fractures, which commonly occur in prepubertal children. *Open fractures* exist when the break in the bone communicates with a wound in the skin. These fractures are usually considered contaminated, requiring measures to control potential infection.

The many varieties of fracture architecture (Figure 11-27) include (1) transverse fracture, in which the fracture line runs at a right angle to the longitudinal axis of the bone; (2) longitudinal fracture, which runs along the length of the bone; (3) oblique fracture and spiral fracture, in which bone is twisted apart (similar except that oblique is shorter than spiral); (4) comminuted fracture, in which the bone fragments splinter into more than two pieces; (5) compression fracture, in which one fragment is driven into the other end and is relatively fixed in that position; and (6) pathologic fracture, in which a bone will fracture easily because it is weakened by disease. A fracture in the shaft of a long bone is described as being in the proximal, middle, or distal third or at the junction of one of these two divisions. A fracture of one of the bony prominences of the end of a long bone is described as a fracture of that prominence by name. Examples include a fracture of the olecranon, medial malleolus, or lateral condyle of the femur.

An epiphyseal separation occurs when a fracture passes through or lies within the growth plate of a bone. When this occurs in a child with immature bone, retardation of limb length and growth may occur. These injuries require immediate and expert treatment.

An avulsion fracture results in a ligamentous attachment remaining intact on a separated bone fragment. This may occur after joint dislocation or rotational injury, such as the femoral condyle separating from the tibial plateau. A dislocation (luxation) is a complete displacement of one articular surface from another. This injury can disrupt neurovascular structures, requiring immediate attention. A subluxation is a partial dislocation, often indicated by ligamentous instability.

Principles of Treatment

The purpose of fracture treatment is to reestablish the length, shape, and alignment of the fractured bones or joints and restore anatomic function. Acute fracture treatment is necessary to alleviate neurovascular compromise. The surgical team should consider the following principles when providing care for the patient: (1) the patient's extremity or fracture site must be handled gently; (2) initial general medical treatment must be provided; (3) equipment and personnel must be readily available to treat impending or existing shock and to control hemorrhage; (4) aseptic technique must be maintained; (5) positioning must allow adequate circulatory and respiratory function with adequate exposure; and (6) patient comfort must be considered.

The primary goal in treatment of an upper extremity fracture is to preserve mobility and restore range of motion, enabling the individual to perform skilled and delicate work. In fractures of a lower extremity, the objectives of surgery are to restore alignment and length and provide stability of the extremity for weight bearing.

In the presence of open fractures involving soft tissues, several associated conditions may arise, including (1) secondary hemorrhage, (2) infection, (3) severe damage to soft tissues, (4) damage to blood vessels and nerves, and (5) Volkmann's contracture (ischemic paralysis).

Basic Treatment Techniques

Closed Reduction. The surgeon may treat fractures with closed reduction—manipulating the fragments into position without incising the skin. When possible this is the treatment of choice because it decreases the opportunity for infection, improves results (including bone union of the fracture), and minimizes the recovery period. Significant bone comminution, periosteal damage, or soft tissue entrapped within the fracture site may result in complications.

PROCEDURAL CONSIDERATIONS. The choice of anesthesia depends on the site of fracture and the patient's condition. A closed reduction can be performed with (1) infiltration of local anesthetic agent into the fracture site (hematoma block), (2) intravenous regional anesthesia (Bier block), (3) regional or spinal nerve block, or (4) general anesthesia. Closed reduction may take place before an open procedure to reduce the fracture site. Skeletal traction may also be applied to the fracture site (Figure 11-28), requiring a surgical skin prep and application of drapes. The team consults with the surgeon to determine the appropriate casting or brace materials and makes certain they are readily available to prevent loss of fracture reduction. Instrumentation and supplies should be available in the event it is necessary to open the fracture site and apply fixation.

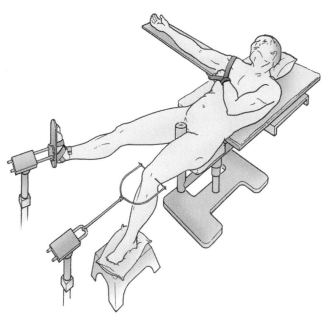

FIGURE 11-28 Application of skeletal traction with the patient positioned supine on the OR fracture bed.

OPERATIVE PROCEDURE

1. The surgeon uses manual traction to manipulate the fragments into alignment.
2. Reduction is confirmed using radiography (x-ray or fluoroscopy).
3. After reducing the fracture the surgeon immobilizes it with casting material or bracing techniques.

External Fixation. External fixation of fractures provides rigid fixation and reduction with the ability to manage severe soft tissue wounds. Because of the increased chance of infection in patients with an open fracture, external fixation is often the preferred treatment. Advantages of external fixation include the absence of casting material, fracture stabilization at a distance from the injury site, ability to perform subsequent procedures such as skin grafts or vascularized grafts, minimal joint interference, early mobilization, and the ability to use internal fixation or other skeleton-fixation devices at the same time or sequentially.

Indications for external fixation include (1) severe open fractures, (2) highly comminuted closed fractures, (3) arthrodesis, (4) infected joints, (5) infected nonunion, (6) fracture stabilization to protect arterial or nerve anastomoses, (7) major alignment and length deficits, (8) congenital deformities, and (9) static contractures. External fixation provides a bridge between fracture reduction and insertion of an internal fixator such as an intramedullary nail, allowing time for vascular recovery. Internal fixation can take place at a later date.

Many improvements have been made in the design and articulations of external fixation devices. The fixators can be applied to most anatomic sites. The available external fixators vary greatly in design; however, all contain three main components: (1) bone-anchoring devices (threaded pins, Kirschner wires), (2) longitudinal supporting devices (threaded or smooth rods), and (3) connecting elements (clamps and partial or full rings). Improvements have resulted in the use of lightweight and stronger materials, which are radiopaque, for use as connecting rods. The radiopaque feature prevents postoperative radiographic interference when viewing the fracture site for progress in healing.

The Ilizarov device uses principles of tension-stress and distraction to correct bone defects and limb-length discrepancies. It is not routinely used for acute fracture fixation; however, the principles and technique are similar. Limb length may be adjusted with gradual bone distraction of bone ends, stimulating new bone formation.

PROCEDURAL CONSIDERATIONS. External fixators are applied using sterile technique after the patient has been administered a general or regional anesthetic. Radiographic imaging ensures fracture reduction after closed manipulation; it also ensures proper pin placement. Because the incision site is small to allow introduction of pins, a soft tissue set appropriate to the site will be necessary. Many different external fixators are available for use. Some examples are shown in Figures 11-29 to 11-32. Irrigation and debridement at the fracture site and surrounding soft tissue may be necessary if soft tissue is damaged, so pulsatile lavage with 3000 ml of normal saline solution should be available. The surgeon will use a power drill at the pin sites, and a periosteal elevator if necessary for blunt or sharp dissection. An appropriate-size pin cutter should also be available to shorten the pins if the need arises. The dressing consists of an antibacterial ointment, antibiotic-impregnated gauze, or nonadherent gauze with gauze overwrap.

OPERATIVE PROCEDURE

1. The fracture is reduced manually.
2. The surgeon incises the skin.
3. Using a periosteal elevator, the surgeon dissects the periosteum from the bone if necessary.
4. The surgeon predrills the cortex, using a drill sheath to protect surrounding soft tissue.
5. Hand drilling or low-speed power drilling is used to insert the half pins above and below the fracture.
6. Universal joints are slipped over the pins and joined with a connecting rod.
7. The surgeon tightens the frame using the appropriate wrenches.

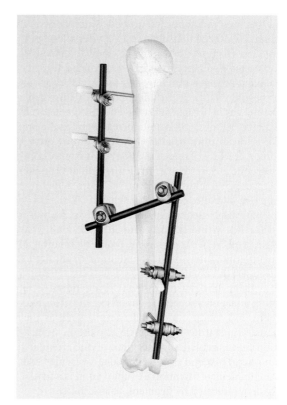

FIGURE 11-29 Synthes external fixator.

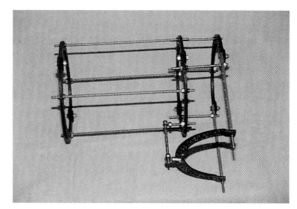

FIGURE 11-30 Ilizarov tibial external fixator.

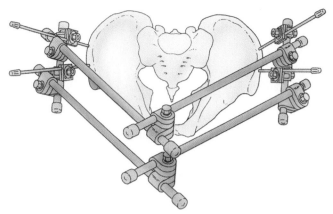

FIGURE 11-31 Pelvic external fixator, double frame using tube-to-tube clamps.

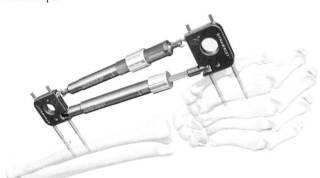

FIGURE 11-32 Dynawrist dynamic wrist external fixator.

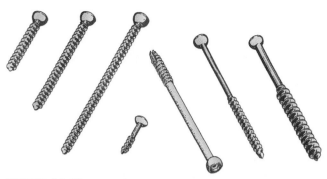

FIGURE 11-33 Types of screws used for fixation with or without plating systems.

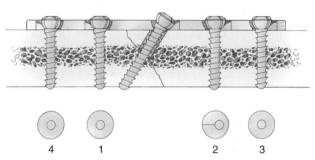

FIGURE 11-34 Plating a closed forearm fracture using dynamic compression showing final position of the screw insertion.

8. Radiography or fluoroscopy is used to confirm reduction and alignment.
9. Dressings are applied to the pin sites.

Internal Fixation. Internal fixation is often the treatment of choice for correction of fractures of long bones or those in the hip region. Application of compression plates and screws and insertion of pins, intramedullary rods, nails, or wiring are methods of internal fixation. Fractures of most anatomic parts in adults can be repaired using internal fixation.

Many principles and techniques apply when using internal fixation. Types of screws (Figure 11-33) include cortical, cancellous, lag, pretapped, and self-tapping. Cortical bone screws have threads that are closer together and narrower than other types of threads. These threads run along the entire length of the screw and transfix bone, gaining purchase (grab) of bone cortex.

Cancellous bone screws feature threads that are broader and farther apart than those of cortical screws. Cancellous screws are used in cancellous bone, which is less dense than cortical bone; the bone accumulates within the threads to provide the purchase for fixation. Like cortical screws, cancellous screws can traverse fracture sites and hold plates onto bone. The screw threads do not completely traverse the bone through the opposite cortex. Cancellous screws are commonly used when fractures occur at the condylar ends of the shaft.

Plating of a fracture may occur with or without dynamic compression (Figure 11-34). Dynamic compression uses screw and plate configurations to apply forces through the fracture site. Semitubular plates are less rigid and do not have the ability to produce dynamic compression. This type of plate is used in the forearm and fibula, where weight bearing, which could break the plate, is not a factor.

CLOSED REDUCTION METHOD. The surgeon may reduce fractures using closed reduction methods of manipulation and traction combined with percutaneous insertion of pins, intramedullary nails, or rods. Pins can be placed percutaneously (Figure 11-35) to fix fractures involving the digits, wrist, elbow, and foot. A rod or nail is placed percutaneously (Figure 11-36) in a large bone such as the humerus or femur. Closed reduction is, however, a misnomer, since small openings in the soft tissue and bone are made to facilitate introduction of the devices. These incisions are considerably smaller than those created when repairing the fracture using open reduction. The advantages of closed reduction over open reduction and internal fixation are (1) a lower incidence of infection and (2) absence of additional soft tissue or vascular damage.

OPEN REDUCTION AND INTERNAL FIXATION. Open reduction and internal fixation is a method of providing exposure of the fracture site and using pins, wire, screws, a plate and screw combination, rods, or nails to correct the fracture (Figure 11-37). Surgeons use open reduction and internal fixation when they are unable to reduce a fracture by closed methods and skeletal traction is not indicated. The advantage is that anatomic alignment of the fracture can usually be obtained and verified through direct observation. Fractures that are comminuted or difficult to reduce can be more effectively treated using this technique. The incidence of infection and nonunion, however, is increased when the wound is opened.

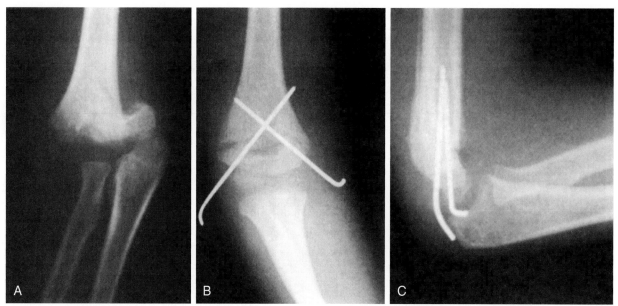

FIGURE 11-35 Percutaneous pinning of a supracondylar fracture. **A,** Severely displaced supracondylar fracture. **B** and **C,** Treated by closed reduction and percutaneous pinning.

The procedure varies for each anatomic site, using the principles for specific fixation devices. Several procedures described in the text identify steps for completion of open reduction and internal fixation. Reference examples include the following:

- *Pin fixation:* application of a unilateral frame
- *Wire fixation:* reduction of patellar fracture, tension banding of the olecranon
- *Screw fixation:* correction of scaphoid fractures
- *Plate and screw fixation:* repair of a comminuted distal humeral fracture
- *Rod or nail fixation:* correction of fractures of the shaft of the humerus, femoral shaft, or tibial shaft

SURGERY OF THE SHOULDER

Correction of Acromioclavicular Joint Separation

Acromioclavicular joint separation (Figure 11-38), a common occupational and athletic injury, results from a force applied downward, most commonly from a fall, directly to the top of the shoulder. The ligamentous support of the distal clavicle in the form of the coracoclavicular, coracoacromial, and acromioclavicular ligaments is disrupted. The result is either a posterior or a superior displacement of the lateral end of the clavicle.

The purpose of surgery in an acutely injured patient is to reestablish the proper relationship between the clavicle and the acromion, thereby reducing long-term shoulder pain and increasing function. This is accomplished by replacing the coracoclavicular ligaments with heavy suture or Mersilene tape or by inserting a screw through the clavicle and into the coracoid process. It may also be necessary to stabilize the acromioclavicular joint by placing a smooth Steinmann pin across the acromion and into the clavicle. Sometimes the distal end of the clavicle is also resected. If resection of the clavicle is the only treatment required, this may be completed arthroscopically. Shoulder arthroscopy is detailed in the Arthroscopy of the Shoulder section of Arthroscopy, p. 514.

Procedural Considerations. The patient is positioned in the supine or semisitting position with a sandbag or folded sheet under the affected shoulder. The patient's shoulder is positioned slightly off the OR bed (Figure 11-39) to allow full range of motion, or if mobility of the arm is unnecessary, a shoulder positioner is used. The head is turned to the opposite side, taking care not to overstretch the nerves of the brachial plexus. The surgical technologist assists with draping the patient's arm with a stockinette to the midhumeral level.

A soft tissue set and bone instrumentation specific for the shoulder (Figure 11-40) are required. Depending on the technique used, bone screws and their instrumentation, free-cutting needles, bone-anchoring devices, and power instruments may be necessary.

Operative Procedure
CORACOCLAVICULAR SUTURE FIXATION

1. A curved incision is made to expose the acromioclavicular joint, the distal end of the clavicle, and the coracoid process.
2. The surgeon exposes the acromioclavicular joint and removes any loose fragments or debris.
3. Mattress sutures are placed in the ruptured coracoclavicular ligaments but not tied.
4. The surgeon places drill holes in the clavicle above the coracoid in the anteroposterior (AP) plane.
5. A #5 nonabsorbable suture is placed beneath the base of the coracoid and superiorly through the two holes in the clavicle. With the joint reduced, the sutures are tied.
6. If instability is still a concern, the surgeon places small Kirschner wires across the acromioclavicular joint, through

the lateral border of the acromion. The ends of the wires are bent 90 degrees at the lateral border to prevent proximal migration.

7. The surgeon ties the sutures previously placed in the coraco-clavicular ligaments.
8. The acromioclavicular joint capsule and the origins of the deltoid and trapezius muscles are repaired.
9. A sling-and-swathe bandage is then applied to the extremity.

Correction of Sternoclavicular Dislocation

Traumatic dislocation of the sternoclavicular joint usually occurs from an indirect blow on the anterior shoulder while

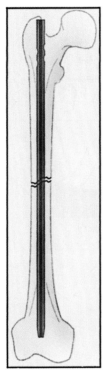

FIGURE 11-36 Rod placement for femoral fracture.

the arm is abducted. The clavicle most frequently is displaced anteriorly, but posterior or retrosternal dislocations can occur. Posterior dislocation can be more severe because injury to the trachea, esophagus, thoracic duct, and large vessels of the mediastinum is possible. Except in severe cases, dislocation of the sternoclavicular joint is treated nonoperatively with manual traction and immobilization bandages.

Clavicular Fracture

Fractures of the clavicle are some of the most common bony injuries. These injuries rarely require surgical intervention. The majority of clavicular fractures are the result of an indirect or direct blow on the clavicle or shoulder. The most common site of clavicular fractures is the middle-third portion of the bone, mainly at the middle- and outer-third junction.

Clavicular fractures are usually treated by immobilization in a figure-of-eight splint. The chances of nonunion are greatly increased when open reduction is used for a clavicular fracture. The outcome may result in a bony prominence, which may be disturbing to the patient; the overriding fragments are resorbed with time.

Clavicular fractures may require open reduction and internal fixation after nonunion, neurovascular compromise that cannot be resolved with reduction, distal clavicular fracture with torn coracoclavicular ligaments in the adult, or persistent wide separation of the fragments with soft tissue entrapment. Surgery is necessary when the fracture is displaced enough to cause underlying damage to the vessels and brachial plexus. Open reduction is accomplished with a tubular plate and screws or intramedullary pin fixation.

Procedural Considerations. The patient is positioned in the supine or semisitting position with a sandbag or folded sheet under the affected shoulder. The patient's head is turned to the opposite side, and care is taken to not stretch the nerves of the brachial plexus. The surgical technologist assists the surgeon with draping the entire extremity after it is prepped. Soft tissue instruments and bone instruments are used for dissection. Bone-reduction forceps and clamps will be used to obtain

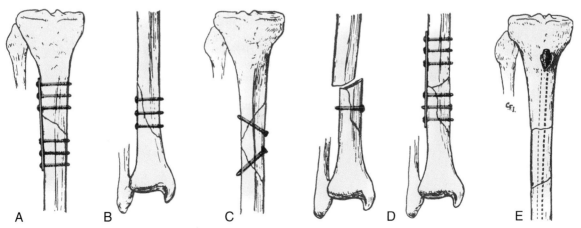

FIGURE 11-37 Types of internal fixation for fracture repair. **A,** Plate and screws for transverse or short oblique fracture. **B,** Transfixion screws for long oblique or spiral fractures. **C,** Transfixion screws for long butterfly fragment. **D,** Fixation for short butterfly fragment. **E,** Medullary fixation.

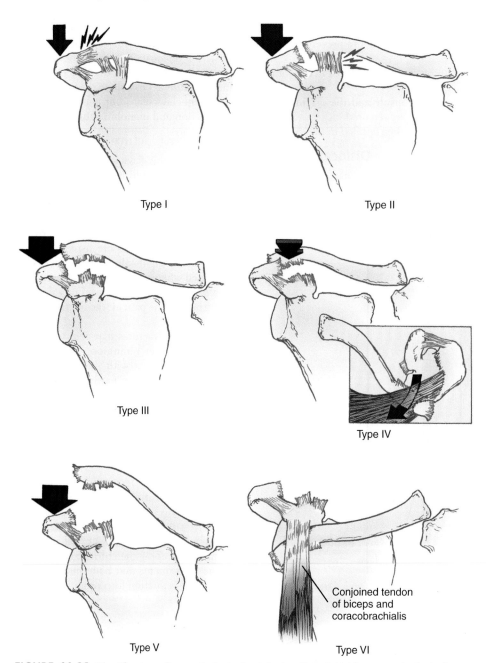

Type I

Type II

Type III

Type IV

Type V

Type VI

Conjoined tendon
of biceps and
coracobrachialis

FIGURE 11-38 Classification of acromioclavicular injuries. *Type I,* Neither acromioclavicular nor coracoclavicular ligaments are disrupted. *Type II,* Acromioclavicular ligament is disrupted, and coracoclavicular ligament is intact. *Type III,* Both ligaments are disrupted. *Type IV,* Ligaments are disrupted, and distal end of clavicle is displaced posteriorly into or through trapezius muscle. *Type V,* Ligaments and muscle attachments are disrupted, and clavicle and acromion are widely separated. *Type VI,* Ligaments are disrupted, and distal clavicle is dislocated inferior to coracoid process and posterior to biceps and coracobrachialis tendons.

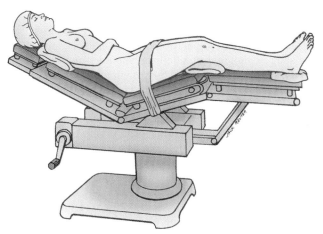

FIGURE 11-39 Positioning for a surgical procedure on the shoulder with the patient in a semisitting position and support beneath the affected shoulder.

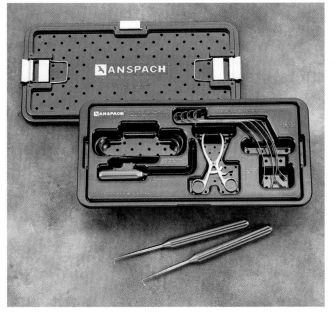

FIGURE 11-40 Shoulder instrumentation set including humeral head retractors, glenoid neck retractor, modified Gelpi retractors, Goulet retractors, conjoined tendon retractor, subscapularis retractor, and glenoid awl.

reduction, and Kirschner wires may be used to temporarily hold the reduction. Permanent reduction will be held with either Steinmann pins or plate and screws. A power drill will be necessary to apply these. In the case of a nonunion, bone grafting will be used.

Operative Procedure

1. The surgeon makes a 2.5-cm incision over the fracture site. The incision may need to be extended for comminuted fractures.
2. Dissection is carried down to the clavicle, taking care not to strip periosteum or disrupt vessels or nerves.

3. The surgeon exposes the fracture site and reduces the fracture with bone-holding forceps.
4. If pinning the clavicle is to be done, a Steinmann pin is passed into the medial fragment medullary canal and removed.
5. The pin is then passed in the same manner into the distal fragment.
6. The surgeon reduces the fracture again, and uses a threaded Steinmann pin across the fracture site through both fragments to transfix it.
7. If plating the clavicle is to be done, a small semitubular plate is used with at least two screw holes on each side of the fracture site.
8. The surgeon strips a small portion of the periosteum from the clavicle so that a plate can be applied to the anterior surface.
9. Extreme care must be taken when drilling screw holes to avoid damage to the subclavian vein and thoracic contents.
10. After closure, an immobilization sling is applied.

Correction of Rotator Cuff Tear

Most rotator cuff tears occur through the insertion of the tendinous fibers of the supraspinatus muscle that attaches onto the greater tuberosity of the proximal humerus. In severe tears, the remaining tendons of the cuff, the subscapularis, infraspinatus, and teres minor, may also be involved. Supraspinatus syndrome, also known as *impingement syndrome,* can involve multiple pathologic conditions, such as calcium deposits, bicipital tendonitis, subacromial bursitis, tenosynovitis, and other nonarticular lesions along with a cuff tear. The approach to diagnosis and treatment is similar for both partial and complete rotator cuff tears.

Partial rotator cuff tears and impingement usually affect people in the middle decades of life or later and are often attributable to a long-term degenerative process. Complete tears of the rotator cuff occur after accidental injury of younger patients, such as pitchers and football quarterbacks. Patients with rotator cuff tears may not be able to initiate abduction of the shoulder because the stabilizing forces of the ruptured tendons on the humeral head are lost. Many rotator cuff tears can be treated conservatively with physical therapy and nonsteroidal antiinflammatory drugs (NSAIDs).

A variety of procedures may be performed for these conditions when conservative treatment is unsuccessful. Methods of repair depend on the size and shape of the tear. The common goal is to restore joint stability, alleviate pain, and allow the patient to return to normal activities. In some instances a significant reduction in preinjury activity may be permanent.

Procedural Considerations. The patient is positioned in the supine or semisitting position with a sandbag or folded towel under the affected shoulder. The patient's head is gently turned to the opposite side, taking care to avoid undue stretch to the brachial plexus. A shoulder positioner can be used if intraoperative mobility of the arm is not a factor. In addition to a bone set and a soft tissue set, shoulder instruments will be required. The remaining equipment needs will depend on the severity of the tear. Minor tears may require no more than heavy nonabsorbable suture. Major tears will require a power drill and burr and possibly a microsagittal saw. Fixation may be gained with bone-anchoring devices. Free needles will be necessary if these are used.

Operative Procedure

1. The surgeon makes an anterosuperior deltoid incision and divides the coracoacromial ligament at the acromial attachment.

2. A subacromioplasty (resection of the undersurface of the acromion) is completed. This is also primary treatment for impingement syndrome.

3. Small, simple tears can be repaired by suturing the torn edges with heavy nonabsorbable sutures.

4. Massive tears may require attaching the torn edges to the greater tuberosity using bone-anchoring devices.

5. If the defect cannot be bridged, the surgeon may transpose a flap from the subscapularis tendon and suture it to the supraspinatus and infraspinatus muscles.

6. If impingement is involved or solely the cause of a rotator pathologic condition, other measures involving the same approach are taken.

7. The surgeon excises any calcium deposits encased in the tendon to alleviate mechanical obstruction or performs an acromioplasty.

8. After closure, a sling is applied.

Patients with small tears may begin motion on the third to fourth postoperative day. Larger tears may require immobilization for 2 to 8 weeks.

Correction of Recurrent Anterior Dislocation of the Shoulder

The anterior fibers of the shoulder capsule are stretched and weakened as a result of frequent dislocations of the shoulder joint. More than 150 operations or modifications have been devised to treat recurrent anterior dislocation. The goals are to (1) prevent recurrence, (2) prevent surgical complications, (3) prevent creation of arthritic changes, (4) maintain joint motion, and (5) correct the problem. The surgeon selects the procedure appropriate for the patient's condition that will satisfy the conditions necessary for correction of the problem. A stapling procedure was once common treatment of recurrent dislocation, but it has been replaced by other accepted procedures.

Procedural Considerations. The patient is positioned in the supine or semisitting position with a sandbag or folded sheet under the shoulder. The patient's arm is draped free so that the extremity can be manipulated. The surgeon will make an anterior curved incision or a longitudinal incision in the anterior axillary fold over the shoulder joint, depending on the location of the tear and procedure planned. A soft tissue set and a bone set will be required, as well as a set of instruments specific to shoulder surgery, power drill and burr, bone-anchoring devices, and free needles.

Operative Procedure

BANKART PROCEDURE. For the Bankart procedure (Figure 11-41), the scapula is not elevated with a sandbag or folded sheet. The surgeon reattaches the attenuated anterior capsule to the rim of the glenoid fossa with heavy sutures. The glenoid fossa rim is decorticated with a curette to provide a raw surface to which the capsule is attached. Special instruments designed for the Bankart procedure, such as the curved awl and humeral head retractor, facilitate the surgery, although the capsule may be attached with bone anchors, obviating the use of the awl. If

the coracoid process is to be removed to obtain better operative exposure, a drill, bone screws, and washer should be available for reattachment. Postoperatively the extremity is immobilized in a sling or shoulder immobilizer. Shoulder motion is begun at 3 days postoperatively, and the patient may return to contact sports or heavy labor after approximately 6 months.

PUTTI-PLATT PROCEDURE. The steps of the Putti-Platt procedure are similar to those of the Bankart procedure in that the joint capsule is sutured to the glenoid rim. In addition, the Putti-Platt procedure requires the lateral advancement of the subscapularis. This produces a barrier against dislocation of the shoulder. This procedure is rarely useful when the anterior capsular mechanism is of poor quality.

The surgeon divides the subscapularis tendon 2.5 cm medially to its insertion. The glenoid and humeral head are inspected using palpation to assess osteochondral changes. The lateral portion of the subscapularis is sutured to the anterior glenoid rim. The medial portion of the subscapularis is sutured to the rotator cuff at the greater tuberosity. The layers of the shoulder joint are imbricated (overlapped), a technique used often in soft tissue reconstruction. The incision is closed, and a shoulder immobilizer is applied. The immobilizer is worn for approximately 3 weeks. External rotation of the arm should be avoided immediately after the repair.

BRISTOW PROCEDURE. In the Bristow procedure, the coracoid process, along with the attached muscles, is detached and inserted onto the neck of the glenoid cavity, where it is attached with a screw through the subscapularis muscle. This stabilizes the anterior joint capsule and prevents recurrent dislocation. A Bristow procedure is considered an appropriate alternative when the anterior capsular mechanism is of poor quality. Disadvantages of this procedure are (1) internal rotation contracture, (2) inattention to labrum or capsule disorders, (3) potential for injury to the musculocutaneous nerve, (4) reduction of internal rotation power by shortening of the subscapularis muscle, (5) possible limitation of external rotation, (6) possible penetra-

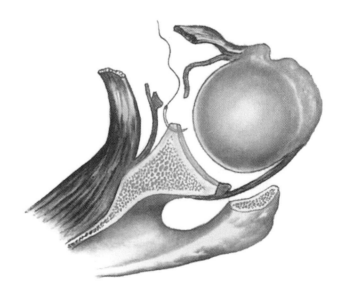

FIGURE 11-41 Bankart procedure for restoration of shoulder stability. Holes are made in the rim of the glenoid, and the free lateral margin of the capsule is sutured to the rim of the glenoid. The medial margin of the capsule is sutured to the lateral surface.

tion of the screw into the articular surface of the glenoid, and (7) later development of early joint disease of the shoulder.

Correction of Humeral Head Fracture

Comminuted fractures of the humeral head (Figure 11-42) with displacement may require open reduction and internal fixation with screws or pins or closed reduction with a humeral nail or rod. However, if the fracture is badly comminuted, a prosthetic replacement is indicated. Traumatic or degenerative arthritic shoulder joints may be so painful or dysfunctional that a total shoulder joint replacement is necessary.

Extensive rehabilitation for the shoulder is required. Surgery should be performed as soon as possible as delay can allow time for increasing scar formation, contracture of the muscles, and increasing osteoporosis of the bone fragments. The shoulder is the most difficult joint in the body to rehabilitate because it has (1) the greatest range of motion, (2) a second space beneath the acromion that must be mobilized, and (3) many muscles that enter into complex movements.

SURGERY OF THE HUMERUS, RADIUS, AND ULNA

Fractures of the Humeral Shaft

Closed manipulation and immobilization usually reduce a fractured humerus as well as minimize the risk of nonunion and infection. When closed reduction is impossible or when non-union of the fracture has occurred, surgery is indicated. The fracture is reduced and held with intramedullary fixation, a compression plate, a lag screw, or a rigid locking nail, with distal and proximal bone screws that will transfix the rod within the canal. This last device can control rotation of the fracture fragments and prevent distraction at the fracture site (Figure 11-43). Multiple flexible nails may be used if more rigid nails are not available. A bone graft may be used, depending on both the extent of the fracture and the length of time since injury. Compression plating of shaft fractures is usually reserved for supracondylar involvement or when other treatment has failed.

Procedural Considerations. Fluoroscopy and permanent radiographs are required to ensure proper alignment, reduction, and placement of implants. The perioperative team arranges for intraoperative radiology support and a radiolucent OR bed before the patient's arrival in the OR suite. The surgeon and team position the patient supine with the body near the edge of the bed to facilitate moving the arm. The extremity is prepped and draped from the middle of the chest to below the elbow.

A soft tissue set and a large bone set are required. In addition, the intramedullary fixation device of choice and the required instruments for its insertion will be needed. PMMA may be used in the case of pathologic fractures. Instruments that are required for harvesting bone graft might be needed as well. A traction tray could be used to gain reduction. A power drill will be necessary if screws are used to lock the device. Sterile x-ray cassette covers will be needed for permanent intraoperative films.

Operative Procedure

MEDULLARY FIXATION: ANTEGRADE TECHNIQUE

1. Proper length and alignment of the fracture must be attained with traction. Nail length should ensure proximal burying to avoid subacromial impingement and be 1 to

2 cm proximal to the olecranon fossa. The surgeon makes a skin incision from the lateral point of the acromion over the tip of the greater tuberosity. The fascia is incised, and the greater tuberosity is palpated.

2. Using a small awl, the surgeon enters the greater tuberosity and confirms placement with fluoroscopy in both antero-posterior (AP) and lateral views.

3. The surgeon removes the awl and inserts a ball-nosed reamer guidewire, advancing it down the medullary canal (periodically verified with fluoroscopy). Confirmation is made with each step to ensure that the wires, reamers, or implant has not fractured through the cortex along the shaft.

4. The guidewire is advanced to within 1 to 2 cm of the olecranon fossa, avoiding distraction or shortening.

5. If Enders nails are being used, each one is advanced in the same fashion as the guidewire.

6. Nail length can be determined by using a second guidewire of the same length held against what remains extended from the humerus. The difference between the length protruding and the length remaining on the second rod is the approximate length requirement of the humeral nail. Another

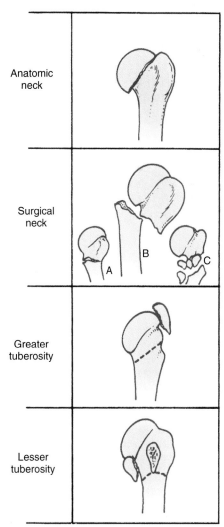

FIGURE 11-42 Fractures and fracture-dislocations relate to the pattern of displacement. Fractures can occur in two, three, or four parts.

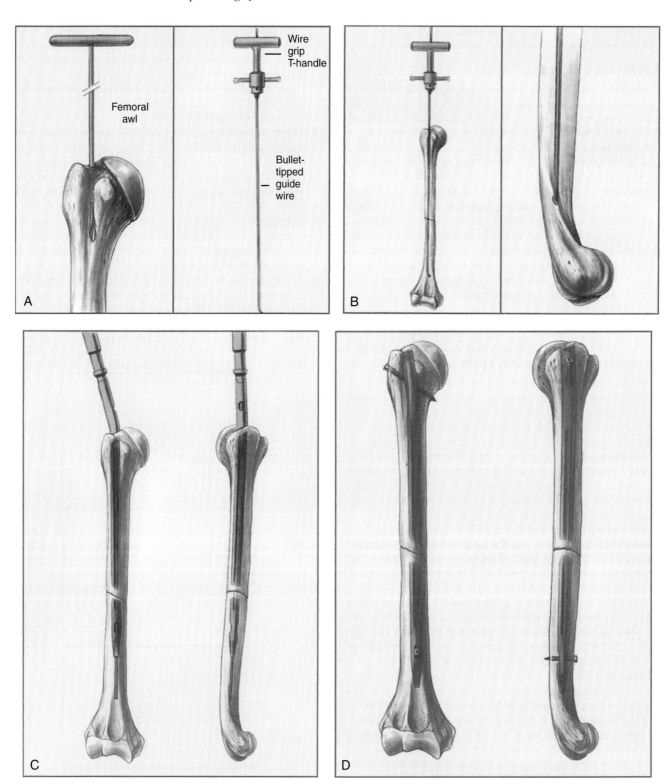

FIGURE 11-43 Placement of the humeral rigid locking nail with distal and proximal screws. **A,** After incision and exposure, a femoral awl is used to make an entry portal. **B,** Guidewire is advanced into the center of the epicondylar region. **C,** After reaming, the nail is advanced over the fracture site and seated. **D,** Proximal and distal locking takes place after the correct screw placement is determined.

method uses a nail-length gauge that is held directly against the upper arm, viewed with fluoroscopy, and read directly on the gauge.

7. Enders nails may be held directly against the arm and viewed with fluoroscopy to determine proper length. If Enders nails are used, the surgeon drives two or three nails down the shaft, across the fracture site, and into the distal fragment. Fluoroscopy is used to confirm proper placement and reduction.

8. If intramedullary nailing is to be accomplished, the surgeon may use a cannulated reamer over the guidewire to ream the humerus. Reaming of the canal is completed in 0.5-mm increments. The humerus becomes smaller in diameter. Reaming is gentle to ensure that protrusion through the bone does not occur. The bone is reamed 0.5 to 1 mm larger than the selected nail diameter.

9. The surgeon uses a medullary exchange tube to maintain fracture reduction.

10. The ball-tipped guidewire is replaced with a non–ball-tipped guidewire.

11. The medullary nail is assembled for impaction with the appropriate outrigger and drill guides.

12. The nail is guided into the proximal end of the humerus, and the humeral nail driver is used to impact the nail within the canal. Care must be taken to avoid splitting the humerus or creating a supracondylar fracture by wedging the tip of the nail.

13. As the nail approaches and crosses the fracture site, manual reduction must be maintained.

14. The surgical technologist attaches the proximal drill guide to the nail impactor with the nail coupled; the surgeon makes a stab wound in the skin and pushes the nail to reach the bone.

15. An 8-mm drill sleeve is inserted through the drill guide, followed by a 2.7-mm drill guide into the first guide.

16. The surgeon scores the cortex with the 2.7-mm trocar, and transfixing of the hole is completed with a 2.7-mm drill from the lateral to distal areas of the cortex.

17. The humeral screw-depth gauge is inserted and read directly to determine the appropriate screw size.

18. A 4-mm fully threaded humeral screw is inserted to the selected length. The surgeon confirms the screw position by inserting a guidewire down the end of the nail, where it is impeded by the transfixing screw.

19. Fluoroscopy is used to target the distal humeral locking screw.

20. The surgeon creates a second percutaneous access from the anterior to posterior cortex of the bone to the bone surface of the humerus.

21. With the freehand technique, the cortex of the bone is scored followed by insertion of the 8-mm handheld drill sleeve and the 2.7-mm drill bit.

22. The selected size of humeral screw is gauged and inserted. Placement is confirmed with fluoroscopy, and the impactor assembly is removed from the nail.

23. Full-view radiographs are obtained in both dimensions, and the wound is irrigated and closed.

NOTE: Many variations of approach and technique are used, depending on the complexity of the fracture and any associated injury. Often the fracture site may have to be opened if it is comminuted or will not reduce properly through closed techniques.

The radial nerve or other neurovascular structures may become entrapped or traumatized, requiring exploration and repair.

Although this type of antegrade fixation, using locked rods, is preferred for this type of fracture, it is not the only method. Often a retrograde technique is used, with the patient in the prone or lateral decubitus position. The retrograde technique, used more commonly in the care of femoral shaft fractures, is described on p. 476.

Distal Humeral Fractures (Supracondylar, Epicondylar, and Intercondylar)

Distal humeral fractures are classified into several types, depending on location and the presence or absence of articular involvement (Figure 11-44). Supracondylar fractures of the humerus do not involve the articular surface and can generally be treated with closed reduction and casting. Transcondylar fractures may or may not have articular involvement, and this will dictate treatment. Intercondylar fractures involve both condyles with a comminution of injury, are intraarticular, and present the greatest challenge for the surgical team. Fractures of the articular components—the capitulum and the trochlea—are usually the result of a fall on an outstretched arm. The force drives the radial head to shear off the capitulum, producing an intraarticular fragment. The lateral or medial condyles and epicondyles are also subject to fracture by various mechanisms.

Patients may present with a single isolated fracture or any combination, as previously mentioned. Neurovascular and other soft tissue trauma is considered in selecting the type of reduction and fixation. Screws, pins, a variety of different plates, and dynamic compression technique can be used for internal fixation. Certain fixation techniques of the distal portion of the humerus may require an osteotomy of the olecranon (proximal ulna) to properly align and affix hardware (Figure 11-45). The general goals of treating these injuries are to (1) maintain neurovascular integrity, (2) restore normal joint articulation, (3) preserve motion of the joint, and (4) correct other soft tissue injuries.

Procedural Considerations. Regional anesthesia can be used for procedures on the distal end of the humerus. Bone graft harvesting may require use of general anesthesia. The patient may be prone with the elbow flexed over a small table, supine with the arm over the chest, supine with the arm on a hand table, or in the lateral position. A tourniquet is placed before the surgical prep and inflated during surgery as needed.

A soft tissue set, a large bone set, and a bone graft set are needed, in addition to a compression set, bone-holding clamps, reconstruction plates, and smooth Kirschner wires. A power drill and Kirschner wire driver will be needed to apply the hardware.

Operative Procedure
COMMINUTED DISTAL HUMERAL FRACTURE
(Figure 11-46)

1. The surgeon makes an incision over the distal humeral fracture site.

2. The fracture is exposed and reduced using bone-reduction clamps and temporary small, smooth Kirschner wires, driving them across the fracture site with the power drill.

3. A cancellous bone screw is placed using drill and tap to transfix from one condyle to the other. The surgeon is careful not to violate the joint surface with the threads of the screw.
4. If the reduction is maintained, the surgeon removes the Kirschner wires.
5. A one-third tubular or reconstruction plate is contoured to the shape of the distal humeral fracture and applied to bridge the fracture fragments.
6. Throughout the entire procedure, the articular surface is periodically inspected to ensure integrity. The plates are held in place by hand while the patient's elbow is moved through its range of motion. The plates should not encroach on the olecranon or coronoid fossa (distal end of the ulna), since this will limit flexion and extension of the arm.
7. The bone is drilled and tapped from one cortex to the other with the appropriate drill and tap. The screw is inserted and

seated to the bone surface on the plate. This is done for all subsequent screws, observing the fracture site and articular surface.
8. Interfragmentary screws may be used in addition to the cortical screws spanning the condyles. If osteotomy of the olecranon was previously done for exposure, it is reattached using the tension band technique with a cancellous bone screw and heavy-gauge (18 or 20 gauge) wire (Figure 11-47).
9. The surgeon irrigates the wound, places a drain (as needed), and closes the incision. A long arm posterior splint is applied.

Olecranon Fracture

If the olecranon fracture fragment is small, it may be excised and the triceps tendon reattached to the ulnar shaft. This does not result in loss of stability of the elbow joint. However, larger fragments must be reduced and held with internal fixation. Osteotomy of the olecranon is often done electively for surgi-

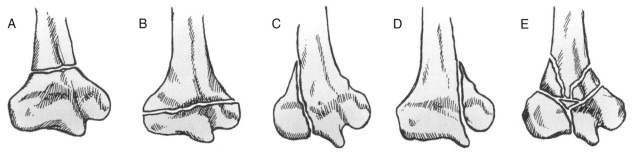

FIGURE 11-44 Classification of distal humeral fractures. **A,** Supracondylar. **B,** Transcondylar. **C,** Lateral condyle with trochlea. **D,** Medial condyle. **E,** Intercondylar with comminution.

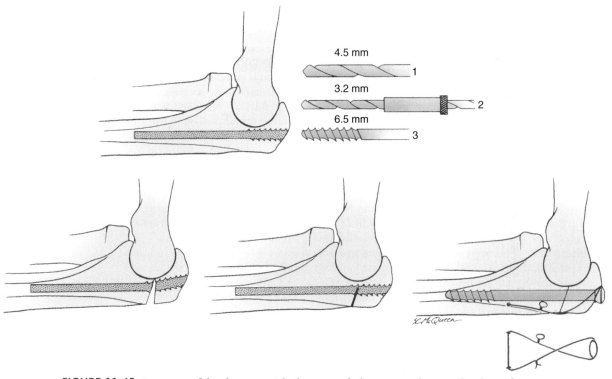

FIGURE 11-45 Osteotomy of the olecranon with placement of a lag screw and tension band wire fixation.

cal exposure (see previous section) and repaired in the same fashion as for a traumatic fracture.

Procedural Considerations. The patient is placed in the prone position with the arm on an armboard or hand table. A soft tissue set, a bone set, AO/ASIF instrumentation (AO/ASIF is the abbreviation for Swiss Association of Osteosynthesis/ Association for the Study of Internal Fixation), heavy stainless-steel wire (16 and 18 gauge in long lengths), a wire tightener, Kirschner wires, bone-reduction clamps, a power drill, and Kirschner wire driver will be needed.

Operative Procedure

TENSION BANDING (Figure 11-48)

1. The surgeon makes an incision over the olecranon and exposes the fracture.
2. A drill hole is made in the distal fragment, traversing the bone.
3. Stainless-steel wire is passed through the drilled holes, crossed over, and pulled toward the tip of the olecranon.

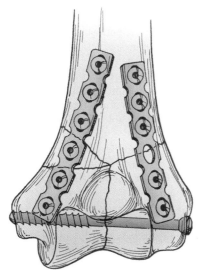

FIGURE 11-46 Repair of the distal comminuted humeral fracture with 3.5-mm reconstruction plates.

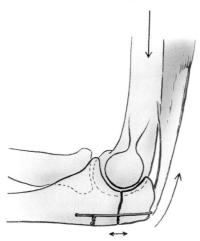

FIGURE 11-47 Tension band technique used for repair of the olecranon.

4. After using the drill and tap, the surgeon uses a cancellous bone screw to attach the proximal fragment to the distal, stopping short of totally seating the screw.
5. The surgeon pulls the wire and loops it around the exposed shaft of the screw while reduction is maintained manually or by using a reduction clamp. The wire can be tightened using the wire tightener. Two smooth Steinmann pins, bent over the exposed portion to hook the loop of wire, can substitute for the cancellous screws.
6. The remaining screw is threaded into the bone; the fracture site is observed for opposition.
7. The wound is irrigated and closed. Drains are generally not necessary. A long arm posterior splint is placed.

NOTE: Using this technique requires early active motion of the arm. Compression of the fracture site is achieved by moving the elbow through its range of motion and applying force by the hardware.

Transposition of the Ulnar Nerve

Transposition of the ulnar nerve involves freeing the nerve from a groove at the back of the medial epicondyle of the humerus and bringing it to the front of the condyle. The ulnar nerve is frequently divided or damaged after fracture or wounds to the elbow caused by trauma. Dislocation of the elbow may also cause ulnar nerve damage. Late traumatic neuritis may occur after an old injury, resulting in stretching of the ulnar nerve. The hand appears atrophied, and sensory loss is extensive. In severe cases, a clawhand deformity develops.

Procedural Considerations. The patient is placed in the supine position with the extremity slightly flexed on a hand table or over the chest. A tourniquet is applied to the upper arm, and the entire arm (fingers to tourniquet) is prepped and draped. A soft tissue set is required. Bone instruments may be required.

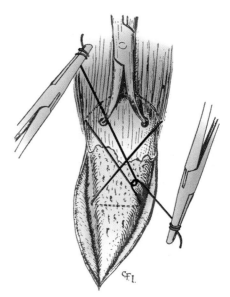

FIGURE 11-48 Operative procedure: tension banding with stainless-steel wire passed through drill holes; figure-of-eight adds stability to the fracture.

Operative Procedure

1. The surgeon makes an incision on the lateral aspect of the elbow near the epicondyle.
2. The fascia and the flexor carpi ulnaris muscle are divided.
3. The surgeon frees the ulnar nerve and dissects the medial intermuscular septum.
4. The nerve is then drawn anteriorly and placed deep into the brachialis flexor muscle origin.
5. The wound is irrigated and closed. A drain is not necessary. A short arm posterior splint is applied to the elbow postoperatively.

Excision of the Head of the Radius

Fractures of the radial head can be displaced or nondisplaced, segmental, or comminuted. Complications can arise when treatment is delayed, causing limitation of motion, pain, and posttraumatic arthritis. A congruous radial head is essential for proper rotation of the forearm at the elbow. Consequently, in an adult it is necessary to excise the radial head if a severely comminuted fracture with angulation interferes with rotation. The radial head should never be excised in children. The outcome for the patient undergoing radial head excision may result in some permanent loss of pronation and supination of the forearm. Noncomminuted fractures that are easily reduced can be treated using closed reduction and casting.

Procedural Considerations. The patient is supine with the arm over the chest or on a hand table. A tourniquet is applied. A soft tissue set, a small bone set, and an oscillating microsaw with blades are needed.

Operative Procedure

1. The surgeon makes an incision on the shaft of the radius from 5 cm distal to the radial head, extending proximally over the lateral humeral condyle.
2. Dissection is continued between the extensor carpi ulnaris and extensor digitorum muscles onto the joint capsule.
3. With the head and neck of the radius exposed through the joint capsule, the surgeon irrigates the joint to clear bone debris and blood clots.
4. The surgeon excises the radial head just proximal to the radial tuberosity, and removes all the periosteum to limit new bone formation. The remaining annular ligament is also excised. The fragments of the radial head should be saved and readily available so that they may be reassembled to ensure that all fragments have been retrieved.
5. The wound is closed, and a long arm posterior splint is applied with the elbow at 90 degrees.

Fractures of the Proximal Third of the Ulna with Radial Head Dislocation (Monteggia)

The Monteggia type of fracture presents with a proximal ulnar fracture and dislocation of the radial head. The fracture is rarely treated with open reduction in children. The open technique is often used to treat adults. A direct blow to the ulnar aspect or a fall while the arm is hyperextended produces this type of injury. If the open reduction approach is chosen, closed reduction of the radial dislocation is attempted and often is successful. At times the annular ligament may prevent reduction of the radial head dislocation, and open reduction becomes necessary. Deforming forces of the forearm vary, depending on the location of the fracture in relation to the insertion of muscles. These forces are often encountered when treating forearm injuries. The dynamic compression technique uses compression plates that are stockier and stronger than the semitubular plates mentioned earlier for distal humeral fractures. They are used to plate shaft fractures, where stress forces on the shaft are greater and stronger plates are required.

Procedural Considerations. The patient is placed in the supine position with or without a hand table. A tourniquet is applied and inflated as needed. A soft tissue set and a large bone set are required, as well as bone-reduction clamps and bone-grasping forceps, AO/ASIF instrumentation, plates and screws, and a power drill.

Operative Procedure

FIXATION WITH DYNAMIC COMPRESSION PLATE
(Figure 11-49)

1. The surgeon performs a closed reduction to reduce the radial head dislocation.
2. An incision is made; the ulnar fracture site is dissected.
3. The surgeon strips the periosteum and reapproximates the fragments using bone-reduction and bone-grasping forceps.
4. The bone is assessed for placement of a small- or large-fragment dynamic compression plate (DCP), with at least three screw holes proximal and three distal to the fracture site.
5. A concentric (neutral) hole is drilled into the ulna (through one of the screw holes on the plate) to the opposite cortex.
6. After the hole is gauged, the selected size of screw is inserted, with purchase of the opposite cortex ensured. A second screw is inserted on the opposite fragment in the neutral position.
7. On either side of the fracture site, an eccentric (loading) hole is drilled in the same fashion to the opposite cortex. The hole is gauged and tapped, and the screw is inserted.
8. The selected screw is entered eccentrically into the plate. As the screw seeks the center of the screw hole while riding the bevel of the screw hole, it compresses the fracture site. This screw should be tightened completely, and the other screws should be slightly loosened.
9. The fracture site is now visualized radiographically as the action of the screw in the plate compresses the fracture site.
10. The remaining bone screws are inserted following the same procedure.
11. The wound is irrigated and closed; a drain may or may not be inserted.
12. A long arm posterior splint is placed with the arm in 110 to 120 degrees of flexion.

Correction of Colles' Fracture with External Fixation

Colles' fracture is a dorsally angulated fracture of the distal end of the radius. Most of these fractures can be managed successfully with closed reduction and immobilization, but external fixation is especially useful in the case of a comminuted intraarticular fracture. Internal fixation is indicated when the distal end of the radius is severely comminuted and

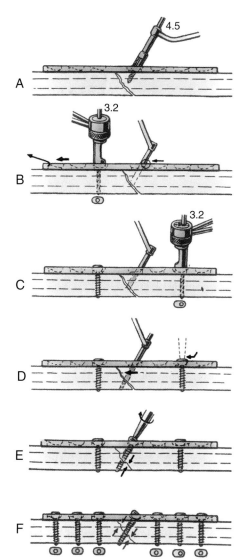

FIGURE 11-49 Fixation with dynamic compression plate. **A,** Gliding hole with drill bit. **B,** Fracture is reduced, drill sleeve is inserted, the fracture is drawn together, a hole is drilled, and a screw is inserted in the neutral position to correct the fracture. **C** and **D,** One screw is inserted in load position (eccentric) into the other fragment; as the screw is tightened, axial compression is generated. **E,** Lag screw inserted across the fracture site. **F,** Remaining screws inserted in the neutral position.

displaced. In these cases, Kirschner wires are used for internal fixation.

Procedural Considerations. The patient is in the supine position with the arm extended on a hand table and may require traction by means of finger traps. A soft tissue set and a small bone set are required, along with a power drill, small elevator, and the external fixation device of choice. Fluoroscopy is necessary.

Operative Procedure
1. Small incisions are made, and the surgeon places two pins through the second metacarpal—one at the base and the

other distalward a distance equal to the span between the openings in the fixator.
2. Two pins are placed in the radius 8 cm from the styloid.
3. The surgeon confirms pin placement radiographically in both the AP and lateral views.
4. A frame is constructed to incorporate all four pins.
5. Reduction of the fracture is obtained, and the surgeon secures the frame.
6. Postreduction films are obtained to check alignment and pin position.

SURGERY OF THE HAND

Hand surgery has become highly specialized. The surgical technologist encounters numerous procedures for treating bone, soft tissue, or both. Many of the techniques and principles used to treat large bone defects are used in the treatment of hand injuries. Hand procedures range from carpal tunnel release to complex digit reimplantation.

Tourniquets and regional anesthetics are often used for hand surgery. The OR team usually sits down at a hand table but may move to areas such as the iliac crest for bone grafting. The instruments for hand surgery are common to orthopedics but on a smaller scale. Many instruments and reconstruction systems have been developed primarily for hand surgery. Air- or battery-powered drills and saws are frequently used. The surgery often requires the use of eye loupes (glasses for magnification) or the microscope.

Carpal Tunnel Release

Carpal tunnel syndrome results from entrapment of the median nerve on the volar surface of the wrist; it is caused by thickened synovium, trauma, or aberrant muscles. Carpal tunnel syndrome is frequently seen in patients with rheumatoid synovitis or malaligned Colles' fracture and is associated with obesity, Raynaud's disease, pregnancy, and occupational injuries. The symptoms are pain, numbness, tingling of the fingers, and weakness of the intrinsic thumb muscles. These symptoms are usually reversible after the flexor retinaculum is incised so that the compressed median nerve is relieved. Carpal tunnel release may be completed endoscopically or by open incision.

Procedural Considerations. The patient is placed in the supine position with the arm extended on a hand table. A tourniquet is applied to the forearm or upper arm. A hand set is required. The endoscopic approach requires use of specialized equipment.

Operative Procedure—Open Approach
1. The surgeon makes a curvilinear, longitudinal volar incision from the proximal side of the palm, paralleling the thenar crease and extending to the crease of the wrist across the wrist joint.
2. The deep transverse carpal ligament is divided, taking care to avoid damage to the median nerve.
3. At this point the release is completed.
4. If indicated, the surgeon performs a tenosynovectomy.
5. The wound is closed, and a compression dressing and volar splint are applied.

Excision of Ganglions

A ganglion is a cystic lesion arising from a joint capsule or tendon sheath and containing glassy, clear fluid. Ganglions are most common on the dorsum of the wrist, palm of the hand, and dorsolateral aspect of the foot. Ganglions appear as firm masses that vary in size. They may resolve spontaneously but occasionally require excision because of discomfort or for cosmetic reasons.

Procedural Considerations. The patient is placed supine with the arm extended on a hand table, and the tourniquet is applied as directed by the surgeon. A hand set is required.

Operative Procedure

1. The surgeon makes a transverse incision over the ganglion.
2. The ganglion is excised with a rim of normal joint capsule or tendon sheath at its base.
3. The wound is irrigated and closed, and a pressure dressing is applied. A plaster splint may also be applied to immobilize the affected joint.

Fractures of Carpal Bones

Most fractures of the carpal bones are treated by closed reduction and immobilization. However, it is occasionally necessary to operate on a fracture because of acute instability, delayed union, or nonunion. The scaphoid is the most commonly fractured carpal bone. Internal fixation is accomplished with Kirschner wires, small compression screws, or minifragment compression plates and screws. A bone graft from the distal end of the radius or olecranon may be taken.

For displaced or unstable scaphoid fractures, the Herbert bone screw (Figure 11-50) has several advantages: (1) strong internal fixation, (2) compression at the fracture site with reversed threads at each end of the screw, and (3) reduced time required for external immobilization.

Procedural Considerations. The patient is supine with the arm extended on a hand table. A tourniquet is applied and fluoroscopy should be available. A soft tissue set and a small bone or hand set are required in addition to the Herbert screw set. If a minifragment compression set is used, a power drill and smooth Kirschner wires will also be needed. A bone graft set should also be available.

Operative Procedure
(Figure 11-51)

1. The surgeon makes a longitudinal skin incision over the palmar surface of the wrist.
2. The superficial palmar branch of the radial artery is ligated and divided.
3. The surgeon incises the flexor carpi radialis tendon sheath and retracts it to expose the capsule of the wrist.
4. The capsule is entered, and the scaphoid fracture is identified and inspected to determine the need for bone grafting.
5. The surgeon manipulates the fracture to reduce it and inserts small Kirschner wires to temporarily hold the reduction.
6. The scaphoid fracture is reduced and held with the Herbert jig.
7. A short drill bit and then a long drill bit are inserted to create a channel for the screw.

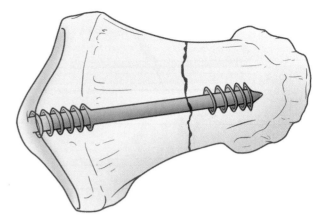

FIGURE 11-50 Herbert bone screw placement.

8. The surgeon inserts the Herbert screw and turns it until it is seated within the scaphoid.
9. Bone graft is placed around the fracture site if needed. (The loss of significant bone can often be corrected by fashioning a strut of bone from graft.)
10. The wound is irrigated and closed.
11. A splint is applied with a thumb spica or long arm cast incorporating the thumb.

SURGERY OF THE HIP AND LOWER EXTREMITY

Fractures of the Acetabulum

Fractures of the acetabulum usually result from high-energy injuries such as motor vehicle accidents and falls with a landing on the extended extremities. The fracture is directly related to the force transmitted to the femoral head through the greater trochanter or lower leg. Management of these fractures can often present the surgical team with a complex and challenging task. Indications for internal fixation of acetabular fractures include (1) greater than 2 mm of displacement, (2) presence of intraarticular loose bodies, (3) inability to reduce under closed methods, (4) unstable fractures of the posterior acetabular wall, and (5) open fractures. Internal fixation is usually delayed 3 to 10 days to allow time for the patient to be evaluated and clinically stabilized. Until internal fixation is undertaken, the fracture is reduced by means of closed methods and the patient is maintained in skeletal traction. General anesthesia may be required for closed reduction and placement of skeletal traction when the acetabular fracture is severely displaced or dislocated. The fractures are divided into five basic groups: (1) fractures of the posterior wall, (2) posterior column, or (3) anterior wall; (4) anterior column and (5) transverse fractures (Figure 11-52). Internal fixation is accomplished with reconstruction plates and screws, total hip replacement with bone grafting (see Total Hip Arthroplasty, p. 491), or fusion if the fracture cannot be reduced.

Procedural Considerations. The surgical approach depends on the type and area of the fracture and the surgeon's preference. The patient is placed on a fracture or standard OR bed in the lateral or supine position. A general anesthetic is usually administered, but the procedure can be performed solely with a regional block or concurrent epidural infusion. Procedures of this magnitude can be lengthy and involve consider-

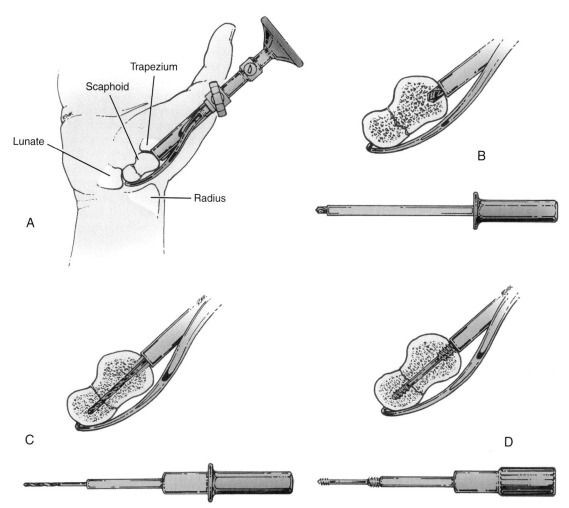

FIGURE 11-51 Repair of the scaphoid. **A,** Fracture site is exposed. **B,** Alignment guide reduces the fracture and guides all subsequent instrumentation. **C,** The screw hole is drilled by hand, and the tap is inserted. **D,** The Herbert bone screw is inserted through the drill guide.

able blood loss. Appropriate measures should be taken to avoid complications attributable to these factors. The room should remain warm, the patient protected from pressure injury, and red blood cell salvaging techniques employed.

A soft tissue set, large bone and acetabular instruments, pelvic reduction clamps, reconstruction plates and screws (both 3.5 and 4.5 mm), plate-bending irons, and a femoral distractor will be necessary. A total hip set should be available. Also needed are Kirschner wires and Steinmann pins, large-fragment bone screws, pulsatile lavage supplies, and power drill and reamer. Fluoroscopy may be used for this procedure.

Operative Procedure
POSTEROLATERAL APPROACH

1. The surgeon makes a lateral incision over the acetabular fracture site.
2. The joint is opened and the femur dislocated from the acetabulum.
3. The surgeon uses self-retaining or handheld hip retractors to maintain exposure of the acetabulum.
4. Femoral distraction or osteotomy of the trochanter may be used to improve visualization and access to the fracture.

5. The surgeon reduces the fracture using bone clamps, forceps, and a ball spike.
6. Reduction is accomplished in gradual steps using Kirschner wires to hold the fragments temporarily in place.
7. Reconstruction plates are fitted and contoured to the fracture site and secured with screws.
8. The surgeon may also use long cancellous lag screw fixation to provide interfragmentary compression, particularly in column fractures.
9. A bone graft may be needed for additional fixation. A femoral head allograft technique is sometimes used, in which the allograft is mushroomed to create a new acetabulum.
10. The surgeon uses pulsatile lavage to irrigate the wound with antibiotic solution to ensure the articular surfaces are free from loose bodies.
11. The wound is closed, drains are inserted, and pressure dressings are applied.

The leg is maintained in abduction and external rotation with traction. Once the fracture is stabilized, traction is no longer necessary.

NOTE: If there is associated traumatic dislocation of the hip with the acetabular fracture, the dislocation should be treated promptly. The dislocation should be reduced as soon as possible and skeletal traction inserted if needed to maintain reduction. Acetabular fractures often accompany femoral shaft fractures, which also need to be treated concurrently with the surgeon's desired method (see Femoral Shaft Fractures: Internal Fixation, p. 476).

Hip Fractures

Hip fractures are classified by anatomic location and can be categorized as femoral neck fractures, intertrochanteric fractures, and subtrochanteric fractures (Figure 11-53), and these can

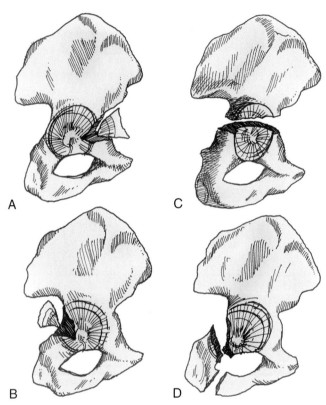

FIGURE 11-52 Acetabular fractures. **A,** Anterior wall. **B,** Posterior wall. **C,** Transverse. **D,** Posterior column.

each be subclassified. Fracture-dislocations also have a classification system and treatment protocol. Fractures of the greater or lesser trochanters alone are less common and can usually be treated nonoperatively.

Femoral neck fractures and intertrochanteric fractures commonly require open reduction and internal fixation. Neck fractures are more common in women because of several factors, including osteoporosis. Most elderly patients require a comprehensive preoperative medical evaluation to define and treat anesthetic risks. However, efforts should be made to correct the fracture as soon as possible to avoid complications related to immobility, skin pressure, pulmonary congestion, and thrombophlebitis. Avascular necrosis and degenerative changes can occur as a result of diminished blood supply to the femoral head, resulting in irreversible changes. Buck's traction may be placed preoperatively to reduce discomfort from muscle spasm caused by overriding of fracture fragments.

Manipulation, reduction, and internal fixation of these fractures are greatly facilitated by use of the OR fracture bed, which also permits adequate radiographic examination to determine placement of the internal fixation.

Intertrochanteric Fractures. Intertrochanteric fractures occur most frequently in older patients. The fractures usually unite without difficulty. However, because the lower extremity is externally rotated at the fracture site, internal fixation is necessary to prevent malunion. Internal fixation allows patients to be mobilized earlier, thereby decreasing mortality and morbidity.

PROCEDURAL CONSIDERATIONS. The patient is placed in the supine position on the OR fracture bed, and the surgeon reduces the fracture by manipulating the extremity and then confirming with fluoroscopy. Various internal fixation devices, including Ambi, Free-Lock, dynamic hip screw (DHS), and medullary fixation, may be used. Success of the procedure is determined by bone quality, fragment configuration, adequate reduction, implant design, and implant-insertion technique. Intraoperative blood loss is minimized because the hip joint is not opened.

A soft tissue set and a large bone set are required in addition to the compression hip screw instrumentation and implants,

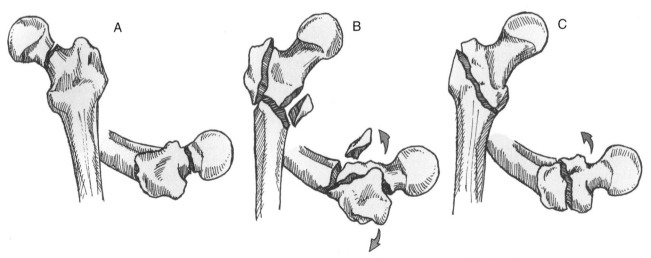

FIGURE 11-53 Proximal femur fractures. **A,** Midcervical. **B,** Comminuted subtrochanteric. **C,** Intertrochanteric.

bone-reduction and plate-holding clamps, and a power drill and reamer.

OPERATIVE PROCEDURE

Free-Lock Compression Plate and Lag Screw (Figure 11-54)

1. The surgeon reduces the fracture as previously described.
2. Reduction is checked in both the AP and lateral views with fluoroscopy.
3. The surgeon makes an incision from the greater trochanter distally to accommodate the length of the implant.
4. The dissection is completed through the fascia lata, and the vastus lateralis is exposed.
5. The reduction is visually confirmed and the surgeon inserts the guide pin after determining the angle plate to be used. A 135-degree angle plate is commonly used.
6. The pin should be centralized in the femoral head approximately 1 cm short of the femoral articular surface. Care must be taken to not enter the joint space, since this might result in arthritic changes. Further penetration of the pin through the acetabulum and into the pelvis can potentially damage large vessels or bowel. A second pin can be used to control rotation in high neck or unstable fractures.
7. The surgeon uses a conical cannulated drill bit over the guide pin to open the lateral cortex.
8. The depth gauge is placed over the guide pin. The size of the required lag screw is determined from the guide.
9. A double-barrel reamer is adjusted to correspond to the depth of the guide pin. The cortex is reamed over the guide

pin to create a channel for the lag screw and barrel of the compression plate.

10. The lag screw channel is tapped to the full distance of reaming to allow proper seating of the lag screw, particularly in young patients with firm bone. Reaming depth of osteoporotic bone is reduced 5 mm, and the tap depth is reduced approximately 1 to 2 cm to allow sufficient screw purchase.
11. The surgeon may confirm the plate angle with a trial. Once confirmed, the nurse opens the implants (plate and lag screw) to the back table.
12. The surgical technologist assembles the plate, lag screw, and insertion wrench with the centering sleeve. A screw stabilizer is passed through the center of the insertion wrench and threaded into the lag screw.
13. The surgeon places the entire assembly over the guide pin, and advances the lag screw to the desired depth with periodic verification with fluoroscopy. Penetration of the lag screw through the femoral articular surface must be avoided.
14. The insertion wrench is disassembled, and the barrel of the compression plate is placed over the lag screw. The barrel of the plate should fully cover the lag screw. The plate is seated on the lateral femoral shaft.
15. The surgeon secures the plate to the shaft of the femur with plate-holding forceps. The guide pin is removed. At this point, traction can be released to allow compression of the fracture site.

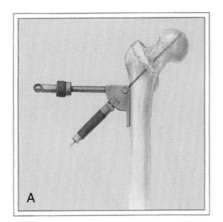

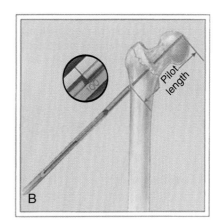

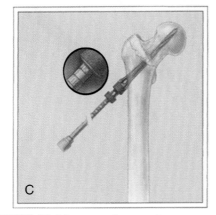

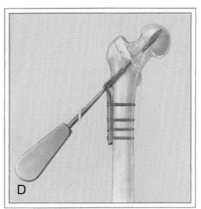

FIGURE 11-54 Intertrochanteric fracture repair with compression plate. **A,** Guide pin is inserted. **B,** Depth of guide is measured. **C,** Lag screw channel is reamed. **D,** Tube/plate is applied, and lag screw is inserted.

16. Screw holes are made using the drill guide and a 3.5-mm drill bit. The length is determined, and cortical screws are inserted through the screw hole on the plate with sufficient purchase on the opposite cortex of the shaft. The top screw hole on the plate can accept a 6.5-mm cancellous screw, which can be angled for better purchase in comminuted fractures.

17. Traction is released if not done previously. The surgeon inserts a compression screw into the barrel of the screw and threads it into the back of the lag screw, compressing the fracture site. The compression screw exerts a powerful force. The amount of compression applied should correlate with the quality of the bone.

18. The wound is irrigated and closed. Two closed suction drains may be inserted during closure.

Weight bearing may begin as early as the first postoperative day, depending on reduction and quality of bone.

NOTE: Many of the same techniques and principles of long bone fracture fixation are used in treatment of various types of hip fractures. The different screw types, dynamic compression, and lag screw effect are described throughout the chapter.

Femoral Neck Fractures: Internal Fixation. Anatomic reduction is necessary before internal fixation of femoral neck fractures because of the high incidence of associated complications, such as nonunion and avascular necrosis of the femoral head. The degree of displacement, tamponade pressure from intracapsular bleeding, and delays in reduction and fixation can affect the blood supply to the femoral head. These factors contribute to death of the femoral head and failed fixation. Growing children may sustain fractures through the epiphyseal growth plate (slipped capital femoral epiphysis). These injuries are treated by reduction and internal fixation of the femoral head, similar to

the procedures used in the adult. The Garden and AO nomenclatures are the most popular classifications for grading the fractures. Pins of various designs, such as Knowles and Hagie pins, and universal cannulated screws (Figure 11-55) are used for fixation (Figure 11-56). In cases of severe comminution or avascular necrosis of the femoral head, the patient may require a prosthetic replacement (see Total Joint Arthroplasty, p. 490).

PROCEDURAL CONSIDERATIONS. The patient is positioned on the OR fracture bed and a general or regional anesthetic (spinal or epidural) is administered. Slight traction and external rotation are adjusted on the affected side. A soft tissue set and a large bone set are required, as well as the fixation device of choice with instrumentation, Kirschner wires, Cobra retractors, a power drill, and fluoroscopy.

OPERATIVE PROCEDURE

Cannulated Screw Fixation for Nondisplaced Femoral Neck Fractures

1. The surgeon makes a 5-cm lateral incision over the greater trochanter and exposes the fracture.

2. The dissection is carried through the subcutaneous and fascial layers; the vastus lateralis is detached anteriorly and retracted, exposing the femoral neck.

3. Two guide pins are driven into the middle of the femoral head, one anterior and one posterior, within 5 mm of subchondral bone; a third pin is placed adjacent to the medial cortex at a 135-degree angle. The surgeon is careful to not violate the articular surface.

4. The guide pins are measured for correct screw length, and the cannulated screws are inserted over the guide pin without applying compression until all are seated.

5. Compression of the anterior screws is completed first and the posterior screws last to avoid collapse of the posterior aspect of the neck.

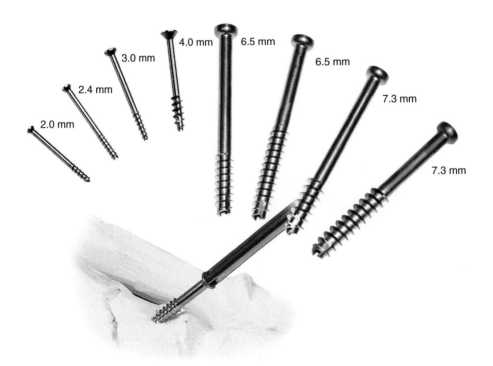

FIGURE 11-55 Cannulated screw system.

6. Traction is released, and the fracture site is visualized with fluoroscopy while the hip is rotated through a full range of motion.

7. Radiographs are taken to verify the position of the screws; the wound is irrigated and closed.

NOTE: Screw protrusion into the joint space can be disastrous to the articular surface. Radiopaque dye can be injected to rule out communication with the joint.

Femoral Head Prosthetic Replacement: Unipolar and Bipolar Implants. With the development of current cement fixation techniques and the evolution of the modular bipolar and monopolar design, the use of fixed endoprostheses such as the Austin-Moore and Thompson designs declined. During the early 1980s the bipolar system in conjunction with a cemented femoral stem became popular. Bipolar endoprostheses (Figure 11-57) were introduced to reduce the shear stresses affecting the acetabular surface, decreasing the motion and friction between the prosthetic head and the acetabulum that is seen with conventional (unipolar) endoprostheses. A femoral head prosthesis is snapped into a rotating polyethylene-lined cup that, when inserted, moves as one unit. Friction occurs between the ball and plastic instead of between the head and the acetabulum. This was a revolutionary design in the mechanics of hip motion and stresses. Current data, however, have some surgeons and engineers reevaluating the use of bipolar prostheses. It is believed that bipolar motion subsides after fibrous growth has taken place, allowing for only unipolar motion. There have also been reports of bone resorption

and subsequent prosthetic loosening in cases in which bipolar prostheses were used. Researchers are evaluating evidence of metallic head wear of the polyethylene cup, creating microscopic debris with a subsequent chemical lysis of bone. Thus there has been resurgence in the use of unipolar heads for femoral head replacement.

Trends in healthcare toward cost reduction precipitated the development of the *diagnosis-related group (DRG) prosthesis.* The modular design was retained, allowing for different combinations of head size, neck length, and stem size. Instead of being bipolar, the head is solid, or unipolar, and the stem is the result of a less costly manufacturing process. The most cost-effective prosthesis is still the original Austin-Moore design, which may be selected for those patients whose life expectancy is short and who have a minimal level of activity. If major deficiencies in the acetabular side of the joint are present, a total joint arthroplasty may be performed. In deciding between the hemiarthroplasty and total hip reconstruction, the patient's medical condition, age, and level of activity must be considered.

Current biomaterials, methods of fixation (cemented versus uncemented), prosthetic life, and modular components allow conversion of a hemiarthroplasty (reconstruction of one side of the joint) to a total hip arthroplasty, provided that the femoral component is adequately fixed. Depending on the patient's condition, the acetabulum may eventually require arthroplasty as a result of degenerative changes. Improved technology and surgical technique have increased the life span of implanted components. The portion of the implant that articulates within

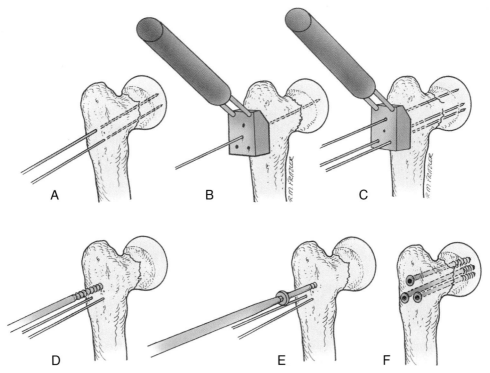

FIGURE 11-56 Internal fixation with cannulated screws (AO technique). **A,** Guidewire parallel to anteversion wire. **B,** Guidewire placed over positioning wire through diamond-patterned positioning holes. **C,** Guidewire placed through each outer triangle of holes. **D,** Cannulated tap passed over guidewire to tap near cortex. **E,** Large cannulated screw inserted over guidewire. **F,** Remaining screws inserted in same manner.

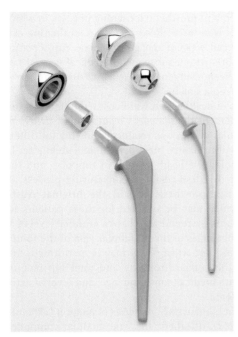

FIGURE 11-57 Modular bipolar endoprostheses.

the acetabulum can be removed and replaced with a smaller femoral head. The acetabulum is then prepared for prosthetic implantation by various means of fixation. The ability to convert from hemiarthroplasty to total arthroplasty reduces the amount of surgery required.

PROCEDURAL CONSIDERATIONS. The patient is placed in the lateral position after the administration of a general or regional anesthetic. The perioperative nurse preps the patient from the umbilicus down to and including the foot. Instrumentation for total hip replacement should be available but not opened until inspection of the resected joint is completed to determine if a total arthroplasty is required.

The soft tissue and the large bone sets are required, as well as the endoprosthesis instruments, trials, and implants. A power reciprocating or sagittal saw may be necessary. Templates or a caliper will be used to measure the size of the femoral head. Bone cement and the supplies for preparing and inserting it should also be available.

OPERATIVE PROCEDURE

Modular Austin-Moore Endoprosthesis

Both posterior and anterior approaches can be made to the hip to place an endoprosthesis. The posterior approach is quicker and generally involves less blood loss, but detractors suggest that there is a higher dislocation rate and a greater chance of infection because of the proximity of the incision to the anus. Although both approaches are widely used, the posterior approach is described as follows:

1. The surgeon makes a linear incision from 5 cm below the posteroinferior iliac spine toward the posterior aspect of the greater trochanter and distally along the posterior aspect of the proximal femur for 7 mm.
2. The capsule is entered, and the femoral head is removed and gauged with the template. Fragments that may be loose in the acetabulum or attached to the ligamentum teres are removed.

3. The surgeon inserts a trial cup into the acetabulum, and applies axial compression while checking clearance of the extremity's lateral motion.
4. The femoral neck is fashioned to achieve an accurate prosthetic fit.
5. Using a punch, the surgeon opens the medullary canal from the femoral neck. The intramedullary canal is reamed and rasped to accommodate the prosthesis.
6. Once the canal is prepared, the surgeon inserts the prosthesis of choice with or without bone cement.
7. A unipolar or bipolar assembly is snapped onto the neck of the femoral stem. The height of the head determines the neck length and is selected after trial reduction.
8. The hip is reduced, and closure is accomplished in layers over suction drains.

Femoral Shaft Fractures: Internal Fixation. Fractures involving the femoral shaft are very common in today's orthopedic OR. Prolonged immobility, with its attendant complications, and disability can result if femoral shaft fractures are not managed appropriately. The femur is the largest principal load-bearing bone in the body. Fractures of the femoral shaft can be surgically treated with several available techniques. Considerations for treatment are type and location of fracture (location on shaft), the number of segments involved, the degree of comminution (Figure 11-58), and the activity level of the patient. Femoral shaft fractures are often associated with ipsilateral (same-side) trochanteric or condylar fractures. Pathologic fractures often occur in this region.

Possible treatment methods for femoral shaft fractures are closed reduction, skeletal traction, and femoral cast bracing. External fixation has limited utility when fractures associated with surgical site infection or neurovascular compromise are treated, but it may serve temporarily until internal fixation can be performed. Although plates and screws are used for femoral shaft fractures, their use has been widely disputed because of complications such as bent or broken plates, refractures, and deep surgical site infections. Intramedullary (IM) fixation devices have become the preferred method of treatment. IM nails and rods increase the load sharing of the bone, making the implant less likely to fracture. Bone healing requires a load across the fracture site to promote osteosynthesis and prevent refracture. The open or closed method of intramedullary nailing can be used with locked and nonlocked nails. Closed methods of intramedullary fixation often minimize exposure of the surgical site and decrease surgical time, resulting in less opportunity for infection.

Intramedullary nail and rod designs vary: (1) flexible nails such as the Rusch or Enders type, (2) standard rods such as the Sampson and AO rods, and (3) interlocking nails (see Fractures of the Humeral Shaft, p. 463) such as the Grosse-Kempf and Russell-Taylor varieties. Closed reduction and intramedullary nailing with or without locking screws have become the method against which other methods are measured. Incidences of scarring, blood loss, and infection are all favorable. Fracture hematoma remains intact at the fracture site, which is important in bone healing, and the rate of bone union is increased.

PROCEDURAL CONSIDERATIONS. General or epidural anesthetics are used. The patient is placed on the OR fracture bed in the supine position, traction applied, and the fracture manually reduced and confirmed with fluoroscopy. If the fracture is profoundly unstable, the surgeon must take care dur-

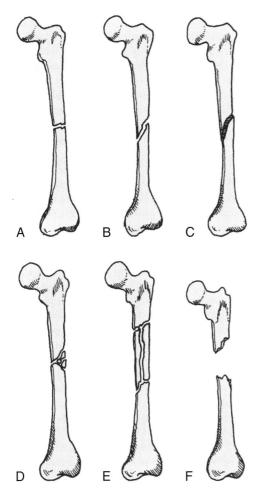

FIGURE 11-58 Femoral shaft fractures. **A,** Transverse. **B,** Oblique. **C,** Spiral. **D,** Comminuted. **E,** Longitudinal split. **F,** Complete bone loss.

ing manipulation to prevent neurovascular complications. For open IM fixation, extra retractors and bone instruments may be required. For a percutaneous reduction, a soft tissue set and a large bone set are required in addition to the IM nail implants and associated instruments, a power reamer and drill, and long guidewires for reamers. This procedure requires the use of fluoroscopy. A skeletal traction tray with Steinmann pins may be necessary.

OPERATIVE PROCEDURE

Russell-Taylor Rod With or Without Locking Screws

1. The surgeon makes an incision over the tip of the greater trochanter and continues it proximally and medially for 6 to 8 cm. The fascia of the gluteus is incised, and the piriformis fossa is palpated.
2. With a threaded guide pin followed by cannulated reamers or by use of an awl, the surgeon identifies the trochanteric fossa and penetrates the cortex. A 3.2-mm guide rod is inserted to the level of the fracture. A curved guide pin is available for more severely displaced fractures.
3. Under fluoroscopy, the surgeon advances the guidewire across the fracture site and into the distal fragment until the ball tip of the guidewire reaches the level of the epiphyseal scar. A second guidewire is held against the portion of the guidewire extending out of the proximal femur, and the length is measured. That measurement is subtracted from

90 mm (total guidewire length) to determine the length of the intramedullary nail required.

4. The cannulated reamers are placed sequentially over the guidewire. The entire femur is reamed at 0.5-mm increments. The entire shaft, and especially the fracture site, should be visualized with fluoroscopy as the reamers pass.
5. The final reamer size should be verified with the reamer gauge. The femur is reamed 1 mm over the selected nail diameter. Inserting a nail in an inadequately reamed femur or inserting a nail that is too large can cause severe bone splitting and comminution.
6. The proximal screw guide/slap hammer is assembled onto the nail. The nail is oriented to match the curve of the femur.
7. Using the handle of the inserter, the rotation of the nail is controlled and the nail is driven into the femur. The nail is fully seated when the proximal screw guide is flush with the greater trochanter. The surgeon disengages the inserter from the slap hammer.
8. Using the power drill and correct drill sleeves, the surgeon drills a 4.8-mm hole through both cortexes and measures the depth directly off the bit.
9. Through the appropriate drill sleeve, a 6.4-mm self-tapping locking screw is inserted and the drill sleeve is removed.
10. By fluoroscopy, the distal screw holes are confirmed as perfect circles on the screen. The distal targeting device is mounted on the nail, followed by the left or right adapter block. The adapter block is adjusted until the calibration reads the length of the nail. The cross hairs are aligned in the adapter to the holes in the distal nail, with confirmation by fluoroscopy.
11. The surgeon makes an incision through the adapter block over the distal femur to the lateral cortex. Following the same steps as those for placing the proximal screw, one or two distal locking screws are inserted. There are various freehand techniques for inserting distal locking screws.

SURGERY OF THE LOWER LEG (DISTAL FEMUR, TIBIA, AND FIBULA)

Many procedures on the lower leg use the same principles of fracture fixation already mentioned. Meticulous detail is required to ensure proper alignment and optimal surgical results for the patient. As in the hip, fractures around the knee require secure fixation to allow bone healing, preserve motion, and provide joint mobility as early as possible. Fracture treatment for the various described injuries is based on location and the pattern of fracture. Methods of fixation for the distal end of the femur and proximal end of the tibia include pins, wire, compression plates, intramedullary nails, supracondylar plates, and cannulated screws. Multiple-trauma patients with one or a combination of fractures may require more than one method of fixation. Open reduction and internal fixation must ensure anatomic restoration of the joint surface and rigid fixation, and allow early motion of the knee joint.

Most operations on the knee are performed with the patient in the supine position and the leg prepped and draped from the groin to the middle of the calf or including the entire foot. It is occasionally necessary for the surgeon to operate with the foot of the OR bed dropped and the patient's knee flexed to 90 degrees. Consequently, it is important for the patient to be positioned so that the knee is at a break in the bed; if it is necessary, the lower leg can then be flexed at the knee during the operation. A tourniquet is often used.

Femoral Condyle and Tibial Plateau Fractures

The joint surfaces are often involved with fractures of the distal end of the femur and proximal end of the tibia. Anatomic alignment of the articular surfaces is necessary to provide joint stability and decrease the chance of posttraumatic arthritis. Nonunion is the most common complication in supracondylar fractures, leading to failure of surgery. As with humeral head and hip fractures, it is important that the articular surfaces are reopposed as close as possible to avoid future degenerative changes. Unfortunately, these often cannot be avoided, and patients with this type of injury often face future joint arthroplasty and replacement (see Total Joint Arthroplasty, p. 490).

Distal femoral fractures result in varying degrees of comminution. Condylar fractures can be unicondylar or bicondylar, with separation of both condyles (Figure 11-59). Type A fractures are extraarticular. Type B are single condyle fractures in the sagittal or coronal planes, whereas type C fractures are T and Y configurations. Type C fractures have varying degrees of shaft and condylar comminution, presenting the greatest treatment challenge.

Simple, nondisplaced distal femoral fractures can be treated with closed reduction and immobilization by casting if anatomic reduction is achieved. Nondisplaced, extraarticular fractures can be treated with a hinged cast brace. Comminuted fractures in this region can also be treated in this manner if shortening and angulation are minimal. Traction can be used initially to augment this type of treatment. Distal femoral fractures are treated with open reduction if distal tibial traction and manipulation attempts fail. Flexible nails, locking intramedullary nails, blade plates, condylar compression screws, and condylar buttress plates are accepted methods of treating condylar fractures. Attention must be given to the attachment of the cruciate ligaments, which originate in the condylar notch and may require fixation of a partial or full disruption as a result of the injury to the knee (see "Arthroscopic Anterior Cruciate Ligament Repair," p. 513).

Tibial plateau fractures historically have been attributed to bumper or fender injuries, but a variety of falls or other traumas frequently are the cause. Compression force of the distal end of the femur on the tibia produces the various types of plateau fractures. Commonly this occurs from abduction of the tibia while the foot is planted, driving the lateral femoral condyle into the lateral tibial plateau (also called the *condyle*). There are several classification systems based on fracture and dislocation patterns. The general theme of these fracture classifications and examples of their treatment can be summarized by the following types (Figure 11-60): (1) pure cleavage, unicondylar fracture, (2) cleavage fracture combined with local depression, (3) pure central depression, (4) medial condylar wedge with depression or comminution, (5) bicondylar but with continuity of diaphysis and metaphysis, and (6) comminution with dissociation of metaphysis from diaphysis. Fractures of the tibial plateau are often associated with dislocation, which may spontaneously reduce at the time of trauma.

Special attention must be given to the possibility of neurovascular insult, which must be addressed immediately. Elevation and fixation of the depressed fracture are the focus for treatment of plateau fractures. As with distal femoral fractures, the articular surfaces and cruciate insertion require reapproximation and fixation. Repair to the menisci and ligaments should occur simultaneously to prevent knee instability.

Blade plates, buttress plates, and cannulated screws are all methods by which fractures of the tibial plateau are fixed. Severe fractures are treated using multiple buttress plates and screws (Figure 11-61). Bone graft from the iliac crest and fibular head autograft are often used when there is a significant amount of bone lost to comminution with proximal tibial fractures.

Supracondylar Fractures of the Femur

Fractures of the distal femur in the multiple-trauma patient are treated early to promote rapid ambulation, which decreases complications caused by immobility. In an effort to deliver quick fracture reduction and stabilization, many orthopedic trauma systems have been developed. Often these are the same systems used in daily orthopedic procedures with modifications to expedite implantation and fixation. Some of the intramedullary devices do not require reaming.

Procedural Considerations. Initial stabilization of the patient may immediately precede the nailing procedure. Often other team members are attending to treatment of other systems. The surgical team is challenged to control traffic, coordinate their efforts, and protect the patient from increased risk of infection by the inadvertent contamination of instruments and implants. The patient is placed in the supine position after induction of general or regional anesthesia. If possible, the patient is positioned on the OR fracture bed; if not, a radiolucent OR bed is used. A pneumatic tourniquet may be applied as high up on the femur as possible, taking care to protect the genitals during placement. The nail can be inserted using the closed or open technique.

The soft tissue set and large bone set are required, as well as the intramedullary supracondylar nail implant (Figure 11-62) and the instruments necessary for its insertion. A power drill, guidewires, intramedullary rod set, and fluoroscopy will also be needed. In addition, Steinmann pins, Kirschner wires, bone-reduction clamps, and a bone graft set should be available. Occasionally a primary total knee arthroplasty will be performed, and the appropriate instruments should be available should that possibility exist.

Operative Procedure

INTERCONDYLAR FRACTURE OF THE FEMUR, T TYPE (AIM SUPRACONDYLAR INTRAMEDULLARY NAIL)

1. The surgeon makes a standard midline skin incision with parapatellar arthrotomy. Depending on the degree of intraarticular extension, the incision may be as small as 2.5 cm or involve lateral eversion of the patella to gain visualization of the entire joint.
2. Articular fractures should be anatomically reduced and secured with 6.5-mm or 8.0-mm cannulated screws placed in the anterior and posterior aspects of the condyles to allow adequate space for the placement of the nail.
3. Using an awl, the surgeon makes an entry hole into the femoral canal just anterior to the femoral insertion of the posterior cruciate ligament. Care is taken to ensure anatomic alignment of the condyles to avoid varus or valgus femoral alignment.
4. The hole is enlarged with the nonadjustable step reamer to accept the largest diameter of the chosen nail. Further ream-

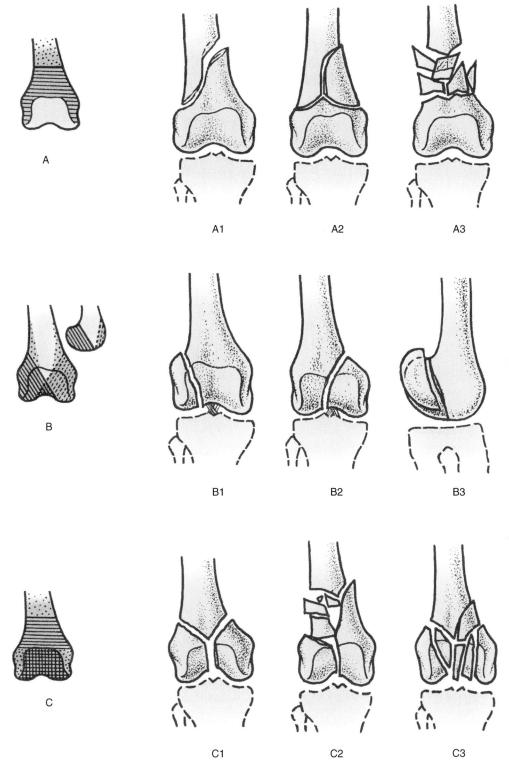

FIGURE 11-59 Classification of fractures of distal femur described by Müller and associates.

ing of the canal is necessary only in the case of nonunion, when the canal is reamed 0.5 to 1 mm larger than the size of the selected nail.

5. The selected nail is attached to the screw-targeting jig, which is then locked into place by the jig adapter. Before the nail is inserted, the alignment of the jig and nail holes is care-

fully checked by manually inserting the sheath and trocar through the selected holes.

6. The surgeon places the nail in the prepared canal and advances it retrograde either by hand or with gentle blows of a mallet on the jig adapter. The nail should be countersunk approximately 3 to 5 mm below the articular surface.

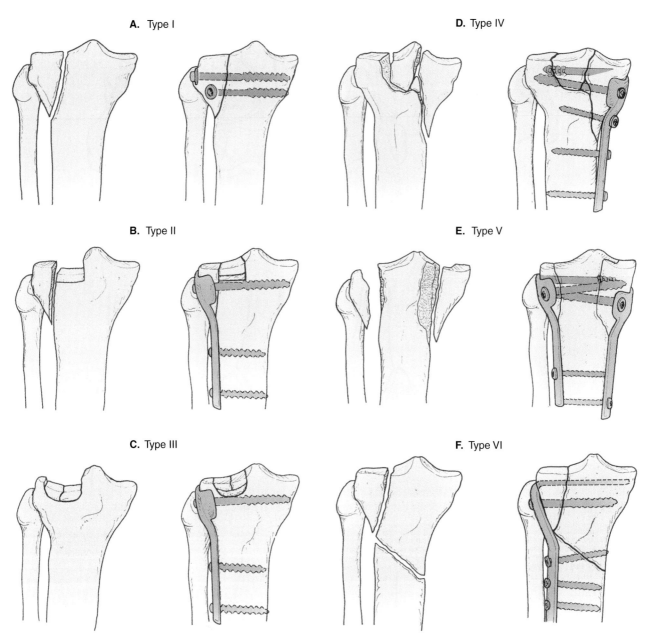

A. Type I

D. Type IV

B. Type II

E. Type V

C. Type III

F. Type VI

FIGURE 11-60 Classification of fractures of the tibial plateau. **A,** *Type I:* Pure cleavage fracture. **B,** *Type II:* Cleavage combined with depression. Reduction requires elevation of fragments with bone grafting of resultant hole in metaphysis. Wedge is lagged on lateral aspect of cortex protected with buttress plate. **C,** *Type III:* Pure central depression. There is no lateral wedge. Depression may also be anterior or posterior or involve whole plateau. After elevation of depression and bone grafting, lateral aspect of cortex is best protected with buttress plate. **D,** *Type IV:* Medial condyle either is split off as wedge or may be crumbled and depressed, which is characteristic of older patients with osteoporosis (not illustrated). **E,** *Type V:* Note continuity of metaphysis and diaphysis. In internal fixation, both sides must be protected with buttress plates. **F,** *Type VI:* Essence of this fracture is fracture line that dissociates metaphysis from diaphysis. Fracture pattern of condyles is variable, and all types can occur. If both condyles are involved, proximal tibia should be buttressed on both sides.

7. The screws may then be placed using the targeting jig, and sheath and trocar assembly. The surgeon makes a small lateral incision and advances the sheath and trocar to the femoral cortex. A 5.3-mm drill bit is advanced through the medial cortex, and the length is measured from the calibrated drill bit or by use of a depth gauge. The appropriate 6.5-mm cortical screw is inserted, and the process is repeated for placement of the second screw.

8. Proximal locking of the nail is then performed in a similar fashion, taking care to use the appropriate holes in the targeting jig

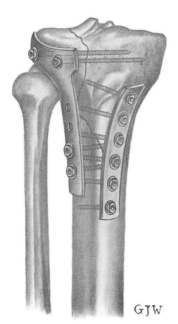

FIGURE 11-61 Severe fractures are treated by use of multiple buttress plates and screws.

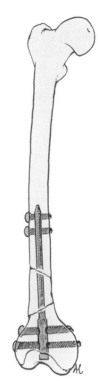

FIGURE 11-62 Supracondylar nail.

for the length of nail inserted. The 3.8-mm drill bit and 4.5-mm self-tapping screws are used to fill these holes after femoral rotation and alignment are confirmed with fluoroscopy.

9. The jig adapter and screw-targeting jig are removed, and an end cap is placed into the distal end of the nail. The surgeon irrigates the wounds and closes them in layers. A compression dressing is applied.

Range-of-motion and muscle-strengthening exercises are begun on the first postoperative day. Care is taken to protect against varus and valgus stresses. The patient is discouraged from bearing weight on the extremity until there is radiographic evidence of healing.

SUPRACONDYLAR FRACTURE (COMPRESSION PLATE)
1. The lateral area of the distal end of the femur is exposed above and below the knee joint.
2. The surgeon reduces the fracture site and inserts multiple Kirschner wires for fixation.
3. A calibrated Steinmann pin is placed transversely across the condyles parallel to the joint line. The pin must stop 8 to 10 mm short of the medial cortex.
4. The length of the lag screw is gauged when it is read directly on the calibrated Steinmann pin, and adjustable double reamers are used to ream to this depth.
5. A lag screw is inserted across the condyles, followed by the compression screw.
6. The surgeon secures the plate to the femoral shaft with cortical bone screws and confirms the repair by fluoroscopy.
7. The incision site is irrigated and closed. A knee immobilizer is placed.

MEDIAL AND LATERAL Y-TYPE TIBIAL PLATEAU FRACTURES
1. The surgeon makes a long anterolateral incision, starting 2.5 cm above the superolateral aspect of the patella and tendon and proceeding distally around the patella to the ante-

rior aspect of the tibia just below the tibial tuberosity. The distal end of the tibial shaft should be exposed.
2. The level of the prepatellar bursa is identified. The surgeon uses blunt dissection beneath the skin and retracts the proximal end of the tibia to expose it from midline medially to midline laterally.
3. Using a tibial bone plug, the surgeon detaches the patellar tendon and exposes both the medial and lateral articular surfaces. The articular surface is reconstructed using temporary Kirschner wires. A contoured T-plate is attached to the medial aspect of the tibia using cancellous screws in the proximal portion and cortical screws in the distal portion. A smaller T-plate is inserted on the lateral side and secured in the same manner. The Kirschner wires are removed. Care should be taken to ensure that the screws do not interfere with each other as they traverse from opposite sides of the tibia.
4. The surgeon reattaches the patellar tendon using a 6.5-mm cancellous screw through the bone plug.
5. The wound is closed and immobilized at 30 degrees with a posterior splint.

Patellectomy and Reduction of Fractures of the Patella

Patellectomy was a frequently performed procedure until the early 1970s. It is possible to excise a portion of the patella (for comminuted fracture) or the entire patella (for painful degenerative arthritis) without significantly affecting ordinary activities. However, patellectomy has been shown to significantly reduce power of extension as the joint extends, which is the most important function of the knee. Other complications associated with patellectomy are (1) slow return of quadriceps mechanism strength, (2) quadriceps muscle atrophy, and (3) loss of knee protection from the patella. Removal of the entire patella may result in relative lengthening of the knee extensor mechanism, which necessitates overlapping of the quadriceps tendon at the time of operation to prevent a lag in knee extension. Patellectomy should be performed only when comminution is extensive and reconstruction of the articular surface of the patella is not possible.

If the fracture consists of two large fragments that can be anatomically reduced, fixation is accomplished with a tension band, a circumferential loop technique, or bone screws. Tension band wiring produces compression forces across the fracture site and results in earlier union and immediate mobility of the knee.

Procedural Considerations. The patient is supine. The tourniquet is applied, and the leg is prepped and draped. A soft tissue set and a bone set are required, along with a power drill and bits, bone-reduction clamps, 18-gauge wire, heavy needle holders, and a wire tightener.

Operative Procedure

1. The surgeon makes a transverse curved incision over the patella.
2. Using sharp and blunt dissection the surgeon exposes the surface of the patella, the quadriceps, and the patellar tendons.
3. The joint is irrigated, and the fracture is reduced with bone-reduction clamps.
4. One length of wire is passed around the insertion of the patellar tendon and then around the quadriceps tendon. A second wire is passed more superficially through the bone fragments.
5. The fracture is overcorrected, and the wire is tightened with the wire tightener. In flexing the knee or contracting the quadriceps, the condyles press against the patellar fragments, producing compression at the fracture site.

Correction of Recurrent Dislocation of the Patella

Recurrent dislocation of the patella can be the result of violent initial dislocation or more commonly from underlying anatomic abnormalities. The underlying condition causes an abnormal excursion of the extensor mechanism over the femoral condyles. Dynamic forces, such as the vastus lateralis, and static forces, such as those arising from the shape of the patella, tend to displace the patella laterally. Dislocations occur when there are extreme displacing forces combined with internal rotation of the femur and flexion of the knee. If untreated, patellar dislocations will deteriorate the knee by causing abnormal patellofemoral articulation, chondromalacia, and meniscal tears.

Conservative treatment aimed at quadriceps strengthening may be indicated in some patients. Numerous procedures have been designed to realign the knee extensor mechanism. All the procedures include incising the lateral quadriceps tendon and shifting the insertion of the patellar tendon medially or distally to the original insertion of the tibia.

Procedural Considerations. The patient is supine. The tourniquet is applied, and the leg is prepped and draped. A soft tis-

sue set and a bone set are required, along with a large-fragment screw set, a power drill, a microsagittal saw (Figure 11-63), and osteotomes.

Operative Procedure

PATELLAR REALIGNMENT (ELMSLIE-TRILLAT)
(Figure 11-64)

1. The surgeon makes a lateral parapatellar incision beginning proximally to the patellar pole, laterally around the patella, and extending to 2 cm distally and just laterally to the tibial tuberosity.
2. A skin flap is developed and retracted medially to expose the capsule. A medial arthrotomy is completed, the joint is inspected, and any pathologic condition present is repaired.
3. The lateral retinaculum is released from the vastus lateralis proximally and the patellar tendon distally.
4. Using a ½-inch osteotome, the surgeon scores the tibial tuberosity medially and laterally, just below the fat pad and under the patella.
5. The surgeon continues the osteotomy using a microsagittal saw distally for 4 to 6 cm, and leaves the periosteum hinged at the distal-most part of the osteotomy.
6. The entire segment, with patellar tendon attached, is displaced medially and manually held in place while moving the knee through a range of motion. Tracking of the patella on the femoral groove is completed by systematically moving the knee medially in increments.
7. A cancellous bone bed is prepared at the point of reattachment of the tibial tuberosity.
8. The surgeon displaces the tuberosity medially and places a 6.5-mm cancellous bone screw.
9. The wound is irrigated and closed, and a long leg cylinder cast is applied. The cast is bivalved immediately.

Repair of Collateral or Cruciate Ligament Tears

The stability of the knee depends on the integrity of the cruciate and collateral ligaments. If any of these supporting structures is damaged, an unstable knee is likely unless properly repaired. Injuries to these supporting structures are usually not isolated. More frequently, several of the ligaments are injured at the same time. For example, the injury commonly referred to as the "terrible triad" includes a torn anterior cruciate ligament (ACL), torn medial meniscus, and torn medial collateral ligament.

The knee demonstrates grave disability with major ligamentous disruption. The *collateral ligaments* reinforce the knee capsule medially and laterally. They resist varus and valgus stresses on the knee. The *cruciate ligaments* control anterior-posterior stability. Along with the ligaments, the muscle groups stabilize the joint and control movement. Because muscle strength is the first line of defense for the knee, damage is repaired to protect the ligaments. For optimum function of the joint, damaged structures should be reconstructed as close as possible to the original anatomic structures. If the knee is left untreated, osteoarthritis will develop.

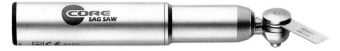

FIGURE 11-63 Microsagittal saw.

Injury to a single cruciate ligament may not significantly compromise knee function. When the injury is combined with other injuries, surgery may be warranted. Surgeons may use various types of ligament grafts to replace or augment the cruciate ligaments. Autografts, allografts, and artificial substitutes are available. Ligament substitutes act as a scaffold, stent, or augmentation of the torn cruciate ligaments. Scaffolds support the soft tissue initially to allow ingrowth of the host tissue. Stents protect the joint from excessive stress while the permanent ligament substitute is healing. Augmentation, as by the patient's own iliotibial band, protects the graft initially after repair of a partial tear. Synthetic ligaments, which are less popular, include carbon-fiber grafts, polyglycolic acid material, Dacron, polyester, and polytetrafluoroethylene.

All synthetic grafts are subject to mechanical failure from weakening with fragmentation and synovitis. These are recommended for salvage procedures only when conventional reconstruction has failed and when other autogenous tissue is unavailable for substitution. Biologic materials from animals, such as bovine xenografts, are also available for ligament substitution, although they are subject to increased risk of infection, synovitis, and rejection. Homogeneous allografts are the substitute of choice for knee reconstruction when no autogenous graft is available from the patient. Disadvantages of homogeneous allografts include long-term weakening, possible rejection, and the possibility of infectious disease transfer.

Autogenous tissues are currently the substitute of choice, with the middle third of the patellar tendon and a block of patella being the most reliable. To minimize necrosis and maintain graft strength, the fat pad with its blood supply may be preserved along with the patellar tendon. Using this graft and other soft tissue autografts, the cruciate-deficient knee can be reconstructed arthroscopically (see Operative Arthroscopy, p. 512). A combination of a torn ACL, medial meniscus, and medial collateral ligament in the past often indicated the need for an open procedure (arthrotomy). With developing technology, many of these procedures can now be done arthroscopically. When reconstructing the cruciate ligament, the surgeon must have the graft biomechanically correct to maintain proper function. Many devices and systems are used to provide placement assistance and gauge appropriate graft tension. These devices are used either separately or in some combination. Though the variations are many, the principles are the same.

Procedural Considerations. The patient is positioned supine with a tourniquet applied to the upper area of the thigh. The perioperative nurse preps the patient from the upper area of the thigh down to and including the foot. Soft tissue instruments, arthroscopy instruments, ACL reconstruction instruments, Steinmann pins, reconstruction guides (Figure 11-65), and a tension isometer are required. A power drill, microsagittal saw, and burrs are essential. The fixation device of choice should also be available. Meniscal repair instruments should be in the room.

Operative Procedure

ANTERIOR CRUCIATE REPAIR. An examination under anesthesia (EUA) is performed immediately after induction of anesthesia, when the ligaments are completely lax, to evaluate the severity of the injury.

1. The surgeon makes a straight midline or slightly medial incision across the knee.
2. Meniscus tears in the vascular zone (peripheral) are repaired with arthroscopic meniscal repair instruments or

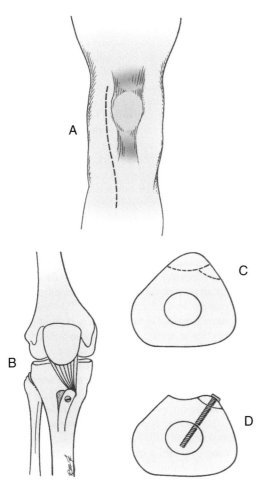

FIGURE 11-64 Elmslie-Trillat procedure as modified by Cox. **A,** Skin incision. **B,** Completed procedure. **C,** Cross section of tibia at level of tibial tuberosity to show bone cuts made to free tuberosity in center and to create new bed for transposed tuberosity to right. **D,** Cross section of tuberosity fixed with screw in new location anteromedially. Screw should not penetrate posterior aspect of cortex.

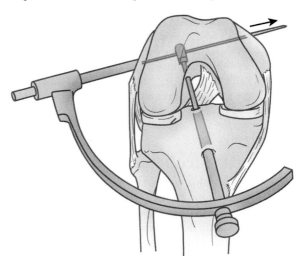

FIGURE 11-65 Reconstruction guide used for ligament repair.

cutting needles with a heavy absorbable suture to repair the meniscofemoral and meniscotibial ligaments. If the meniscus is not repairable, the surgeon will perform a partial meniscectomy.

3. Using a power saw and osteotome, the surgeon harvests patellar and tibial bone plugs from the middle third of the patellar tendon.

4. A notchplasty is then performed, debriding and smoothing the lateral intercondylar wall with a burr and curette.

5. The surgeon uses the ligament guide to develop the femoral and tibial osseous tunnels and passes guidewires from the lateral area of the femoral condyle and tibial tubercle into the intercondylar notch at isometric points near the anatomic attachment site of the ACL.

6. The pins are then overdrilled with cannulated drills as close to the size of the patellar tendon graft as possible. The tunnels are smoothed with a curette.

7. Sutures are placed through drill holes at both ends of the graft to pass the graft through the tunnels.

8. The surgeon passes the graft through the femoral and tibial osseous tunnels and fixes it at both ends with interference screws, staples, or polyethylene buttons.

9. The medial collateral ligament and posterior oblique ligament are then individually repaired at their insertion sites with bone screws and spiked washers.

10. Additional extraarticular repair is done if necessary.

11. The surgeon closes the wound over intraarticular and subcutaneous drains, and a locking knee brace or knee immobilizer is applied.

Popliteal (Baker) Cyst Excision

Baker cysts occur in joints, frequently affecting the popliteal fossa. Baker cysts are often painful and can become very large, especially when associated with rheumatoid arthritis. Cysts in the popliteal fossa occur without a precipitating cause in children; in adults they often indicate an intraarticular disease process, such as rheumatoid arthritis, or a torn meniscus.

Procedural Considerations.   In contrast to many other operative procedures on the knee, the patient is placed in the prone position. A soft tissue set and a bone set are required.

Operative Procedure

1. The surgeon makes an oblique incision in the popliteal area over the mass and divides the fascia to expose the mass.

2. Using blunt dissection, the surgeon frees the cyst and clamps it at the base of its attachment to the joint capsule.

3. The cyst is divided, and the pedicle is inverted and closed.

4. After the mass has been removed, the surgeon irrigates and closes the wound.

   Postoperatively, the knee may be immobilized in extension with a posterior splint.

Fractures of the Tibial Shaft

The location of the tibia results in frequent exposure to injury. Open fractures are more common in the tibia than in other major bones because one third of its surface is subcutaneous. Tibial shaft fractures are difficult to treat. The blood supply to the tibia is more precarious than that of other long bones because of its lack of enclosure by heavy muscle. The presence of hinge joints at the knee and ankle allows no adjustment for rotational deformity

after fracture, so special care is required to correct for rotation during reduction and fixation. Rotational deformities are often seen. Delayed union, nonunion, and infection are fairly common complications. Closed reduction and casting provide excellent healing without significant complications, but this treatment can require casting for 6 months or more. Surgical reduction and internal fixation generally allows for earlier weight bearing and a shortened period of casting; however, the rate of complications is higher.

In general, torsional fractures seem to heal better and are more amenable to treatment than transverse fractures. It is theorized that twisting injuries cause less damage to endosteal vessels than that caused by transverse fractures, in which periosteum and endosteal vessels are torn circumferentially. The important prognostic indicators for tibial fractures are as follows: (1) the amount of initial displacement, (2) the degree of comminution, (3) the presence or absence of infection, and (4) the severity of soft tissue injury, excluding infection. As a rule, high-energy fractures, such as those caused by motor vehicle accidents or crushing injury, have a much worse prognosis than low-energy fractures, such as those caused by falls on ice or skiing accidents.

Because intramedullary tibial nailings do not cause a significant increase in infections, external fixation of open tibial shaft fractures is less commonly performed. However, in the presence of gross contamination, severe soft tissue and vascular injury, bone infection, and delayed treatment, external fixation is the treatment of choice. The Ilizarov external fixation device is indicated when bone loss is significant and limb lengthening is required. Plate and screw fixation is another method in which tibial shaft fractures can be treated, although infection and nonunion of tibial shaft fractures are twice as likely with this method. Plate and screw fixation is indicated when intraarticular fragments of the knee and ankle are associated with the injury. Closed intramedullary nailing is the treatment of choice in tibial shaft fractures because infection is less likely to occur and the periosteal blood supply is preserved. Static locking nails (locking both proximal and distal ends of the nail) are indicated for fractures with comminution, bone loss, and lengthening osteotomies. Dynamic locking nails (locking the end closest to the fracture site) are indicated for proximal or distal tibial fractures, nonunions, and malunions. Locking tibial nails include the Russell-Taylor and the Grosse-Kempf tibial nail.

The key to successful treatment of open tibial fractures, as in all open fractures, is meticulous and systematic debridement of all foreign matter and devitalized tissue. The surgeon is careful to minimize devascularization when reducing and fixing the fracture. Systemic antibiotics and those delivered by pulsatile lavage help reduce the chance of infection.

Procedural Considerations.   The patient is usually administered a general or regional anesthetic while still on the hospital bed or in the transport vehicle and then transferred to the OR fracture bed. The patient is positioned supine with the affected hip flexed approximately 45 degrees and the knee at 90 degrees. This positioning provides a horizontal orientation of the tibia. Using a calcaneal traction pin or table foot holder, traction is applied and rotational alignment obtained. After rotational alignment is obtained, a tourniquet is applied and the leg is prepped and draped. Some surgeons prefer to use a standard OR bed, breaking it at the knee. This obviates the need to insert the calcaneal traction pin and allows for easier maneuvering of the tibia during insertion of the locking screws.

A soft tissue set and a large bone set are required, in addition to the intramedullary nail and insertion instruments of choice. A power drill and reamer-driver will be needed to use the necessary intramedullary reamers (Figure 11-66). Fluoroscopy will be needed as well. If open plating is being considered, the plates of choice and the large-fragment screws need to be available as well as bone-reduction clamps.

Operative Procedure
CLOSED OR OPEN TIBIAL INTRAMEDULLARY NAILING
(Figure 11-67)

1. If the open technique is required, the fracture site is exposed, reduced, and irrigated as necessary. Focus is then turned toward the nailing procedure.
2. The surgeon makes a 5-cm incision medial to the patellar tendon to just below the tibial tuberosity.
3. Using a curved awl, the surgeon opens the medullary canal just proximal to the tibial tuberosity.
4. A guide rod (3.2 mm) is inserted into the shaft of the tibia down to the fracture site. The proximal fragment is reduced distally and the guide rod advanced into the distal fragment. Rod types include the straight guide rod for simple fractures, a curved guide rod for displaced fractures, and a cutting tip for an obstructed canal.
5. The length of the required nail is determined by the guide rod method (see Operative Procedure under Femoral Shaft Fractures: Internal Fixation, pp. 476-477) or by using the nail-length gauge and confirming with fluoroscopy.
6. With cannulated reamers over the guide rods, the surgeon reams the entire tibia 1 mm larger than the nail to be inserted. Inserting a nail too large for the canal can have a detrimental effect.
7. The driver, proximal drill, guide, and hexagonal bolt are assembled onto the tibial nail.
8. The surgeon inserts the nail over the guide rod and, with a mallet, drives it down the proximal fragment to enter the distal fragment, crossing the fracture site. The nail is not fully seated.

9. The guide rod is removed to prevent incarceration, and the surgeon completes the seating of the nail. The proximal tip of the nail should be flush with the tibial entry site.
10. Proximal locking is accomplished with the corresponding drill and tap through the proximal drill guide for 5-mm cortical bone screws.
11. Using the distal targeting device or a freehand technique, the surgeon inserts the distal screws. The 5-mm cortical bone screws are inserted, traversing the tibia through the tibial nail.
12. The surgeon irrigates the wounds. If bone graft is to be used, the surgeon places it around the fracture site and then closes the wound. Dressings are applied, and a cast or splint for immobilization may be applied.

Dynamization, or removal of either the proximal or the distal screws, may take place after 3 months for fractures that are stable but lack callus. Dynamization produces compressive forces at the fracture, thereby promoting osteogenesis.

TIBIAL DYNAMIC COMPRESSION PLATING

1. The surgeon makes a longitudinal incision large enough to accommodate the selected plate lateral to the tibial crest and exposes the fracture site.
2. The periosteum is stripped only enough for application of the plate. Circumferential stripping can diminish blood supply.
3. The surgeon reduces the fracture, places a plate across the fracture site, and secures the plate with bone-holding and plate-holding forceps. The plate may have to be contoured with a handheld or plate-bending press.
4. Using the neutral drill guide, the surgeon drills a 3.2-mm bicortical hole into the plate screw hole close to the fracture site, gauges it, and taps to 4.5 mm. The first bone screw is inserted, ensuring purchase of the screw on the opposite cortex.
5. Using the load drill guide (eccentric), the surgeon drills a second hole next to the fracture line in the opposite fragment. Drill and tap are accomplished as in the previous step. As the screw enters the bone, it will seek the center of the screw hole (the screw is eccentric, and the screw hole is beveled). The fracture site is brought under compression as the screw seats into the hole.
6. The wounds are irrigated. If bone graft is to be used, the surgeon places it around the fracture site and then closes the wound. Dressings are applied, and a cast or splint for immobilization may be applied.

SURGERY OF THE ANKLE AND FOOT

Ankle Fractures

Ankle fractures include fractures of the medial malleolus (tibia), lateral malleolus (fibula), and posterior malleolus (posterior aspect of the articular surface of the distal end of the tibia). They may or may not be associated with ligamentous injury. Ankle fractures can be classified in anatomic lines as unimalleolar, bimalleolar, and trimalleolar. Because medial malleolar and posterior malleolar fractures involve the distal weight-bearing articular surface of the tibia, open reduction and anatomic alignment are necessary. Fixation of the lateral malleolus is also important because it forms the ankle mortise—the socket formed by the distal tibia and fibula into which the body of the talus fits.

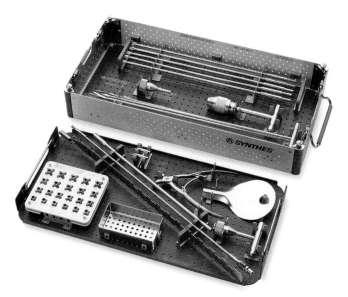

FIGURE 11-66 Intramedullary flexible reamer system.

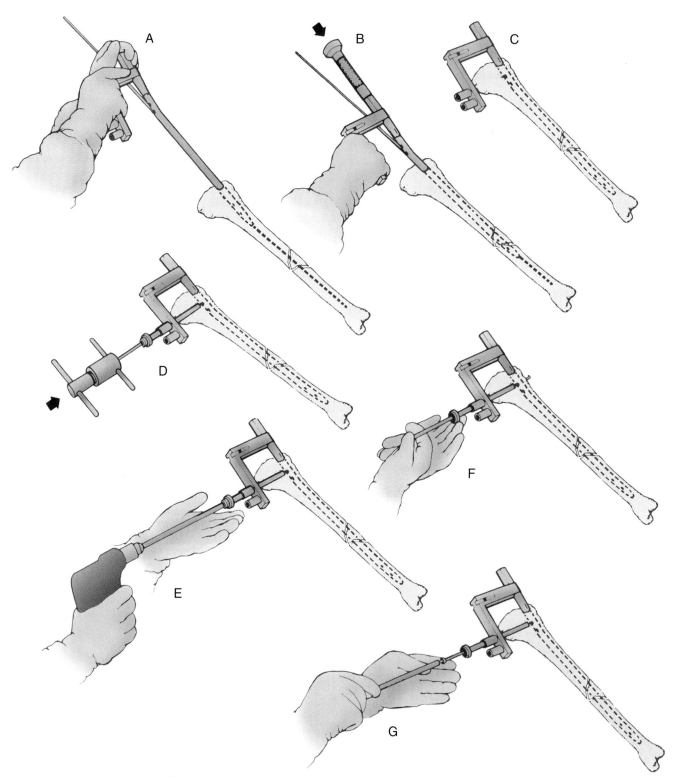

FIGURE 11-67 Tibial intramedullary nailing. **A,** Attachment of nail to proximal drill guide. **B,** Driving nail over guide rod. **C,** Final seating of nail with its tip flush with tibial entry portal. **D,** For proximal interlocking, cortex is dimpled. **E,** Depth measurements are made. **F,** Locking screw length is confirmed. **G,** Self-tapping screw is inserted through drill sleeve.

Anatomic reduction prevents the occurrence of degenerative joint disease. Displaced fractures are treated with pins, malleolar or bone screws, or plates and screws (Figure 11-68). Bimalleolar fractures can be treated with closed reduction and casting, but approximately 10% of these eventually develop a nonunion. The lateral malleolus (distal end of the fibula) is important for lateral and rotational stability of the joint. Open reduction and internal fixation using Steinmann pins or screws placed obliquely into the tibia is a common technique. Lateral malleolar fractures can be fixed with the cancellous lag technique—overdrilling the first fragment and allowing compression of the fragments. Fracture of the lateral malleolus can also be treated with a Rush rod, inserted through the fragment and into the fibular canal. Compared to the other varieties of fractures, trimalleolar fractures require surgery more frequently. The posterior lip of the articulating surface of the tibia is usually involved and needs to be anatomically reduced to minimize degenerative changes. Cannulated screws can provide efficient reduction of a posterior fragment.

Procedural Considerations. The patient is in the supine position. The affected leg is prepped and draped after application of a pneumatic tourniquet. If the lateral ankle is involved, a padded sandbag is placed beneath the hip to internally rotate it. A soft tissue set; a small bone set; a small-fragment set with plates, screws, and pins; a power drill; and bone-reduction clamps are required.

Operative Procedure
TRIMALLEOLAR FRACTURE
1. The surgeon makes medial and lateral incisions across the ankle.
2. The posterior malleolar fracture is exposed and reduced with bone-holding clamps and manipulation.
3. The surgeon inserts two Kirschner wires above the anterior tibial lip to temporarily reduce the fracture. The wires are directed anteriorly to posteriorly, to engage both fragments.
4. A drill hole is made anteriorly to posteriorly through both fragments. After measuring with a depth gauge, a malleo-

lar, small cancellous, or other preferred screw is inserted through the fracture. The wires are removed.
5. The surgeon manipulates the lateral malleolar fracture into reduction.
6. If the fracture is oblique and not comminuted, the surgeon reduces it with one or two lag screws placed anteriorly to posteriorly. If the fracture is transverse, the surgeon inserts a long screw or medullary pin across the fracture line into the canal of the proximal fragment. A small semitubular or one-third tubular plate is applied if the fracture occurs above the syndesmosis.
7. Once the posterior and lateral malleolar fractures have been fixed, the medial malleolar fracture is finally reduced using bone clamps.
8. The reduction is held with two Kirschner wires while a hole is drilled through the medial malleolus into the metaphysis of the tibia.
9. Using a depth gauge, the surgeon determines the screw length. The malleolar screw is inserted across the fracture site and the Kirschner wires are removed.
10. If rotational stability is needed, the surgeon may add an additional smaller screw or compression wiring.
11. Intraoperative radiographs are taken in AP, lateral, and mortise views.
12. The wounds are irrigated and closed, and a short or long leg cast or splint is applied.

Triple Arthrodesis

The talocalcaneal (subtalar), talonavicular, and calcaneocuboid joints must be fused in patients with pronounced inversion or eversion deformities of the foot. Such deformities occur in clubfoot, poliomyelitis, and rheumatoid arthritis. Occasionally this operation is necessary for patients who have pain resulting from degenerative or traumatic arthritis, such as that occurring after intraarticular fractures of the calcaneus. Triple arthrodesis limits motion of the foot and ankle to plantar flexion and dorsiflexion.

Procedural Considerations. The patient is in the supine position and is prepped from the midcalf down to and including the foot. The perioperative team should consult with the surgeon before the procedure to determine if bone grafting is anticipated so the patient's iliac crest area can be prepped.

A soft tissue set; a small bone set; a power saw, drill, or rasp; a bone graft set; and the AO compression plates and screws or bone staples to hold the fusion are required. Kirschner wires can be used to provide temporary fixation. A small lamina spreader is helpful in providing exposure.

Operative Procedure
1. An anterior or anterolateral approach is used.
2. The surgeon exposes the subtalar and calcaneocuboid joints and the lateral portion of the talonavicular joint.
3. The surgeon incises the capsules of the talonavicular, calcaneocuboid, and subtalar joints circumferentially to obtain as much mobility as possible. If this release allows the foot to be placed into a normal position, removal of large bony wedges is not required.
4. Using an osteotome, power saw, or power rasp, the surgeon removes the articular surfaces of the calcaneocuboid

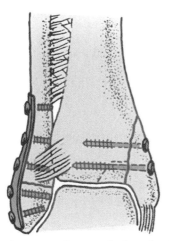

FIGURE 11-68 Plate-screw placement for lateral malleolar fragment repair using one-third tubular plate.

joint, the subtalar joint, and the talonavicular joint. The small lamina spreader is used to expose these surfaces. Care is taken to save all bone removed for later use in the fusion.

5. The removed bone is cut into small pieces to be used for bone grafting. If the quantity is insufficient, the surgeon will harvest additional bone from the anterior ilium. Most of the bone is placed around the talonavicular joint and in the depth of the sinus tarsi.

6. Smooth Steinmann pins, staples, or screws are used for internal fixation.

7. The wound is closed over a suction drain. A short leg cast or splint is applied.

Bunionectomy

A bunion (hallux valgus) is a soft tissue or bony mass at the medial side of the first metatarsal head. It is associated with a valgus deformity of the great toe (Figure 11-69). A bunion is caused by a basic structural defect of the foot, which predisposes to the development of this deformity. Ill-fitting shoes accentuate the situation and speed the development of bunions. Bunions are more common in women because of shoe styles, including high heels and pointed toes. Other factors that may contribute to this deformity are heredity, flatfeet, foot pronation, longer first toe, muscle imbalance, and inflammatory disturbances of the feet.

Symptoms include pain on the dorsomedial aspect of the first metatarsal head or directly over the medial exostosis, swelling of the big toe, painful plantar callus, and plantar keratosis. Discomfort to the entire foot occurs as the forefoot becomes more fatigued and symptomatic, with pain radiating to the leg and knee.

Hallux valgus is treated with a variety of surgical procedures (Figure 11-70). All these procedures remove the exostosis and attempt to realign the great toe by removal of bone, transfer of tendons, osteotomy of the first metatarsal shaft, or appropriate imbrication of soft tissue.

The goals of surgery are correction of the deformity (cosmesis), resection of the abnormal bony components (reconstruction), and restoration of normal or near-normal range of motion (function).

Procedural Considerations. The anesthesia provider administers a general or regional anesthetic, and a tourniquet is applied. The foot and leg are prepped and then draped using a sterile stockinette.

A soft tissue set, a small bone set, Kirschner wires, a power wire driver, and a microsagittal saw are required.

Operative Procedure
KELLER PROCEDURE

1. The surgeon makes a midline, straight, medial incision beginning at the neck of the proximal phalanx and extended proximally.

2. Using blunt and sharp dissection, the surgeon exposes the joint capsule. A flap incision is made to expose the underlying hypertrophic bone found at the dorsomedial aspect of the first metatarsal head.

3. All soft tissue attachments are removed from the base of the proximal phalanx.

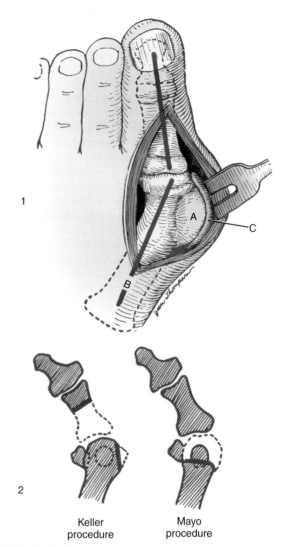

FIGURE 11-69 Bunionectomy. *1,* Bunion. *A,* Exostosis of metatarsal head; *B,* hallux valgus deformity; *C,* overlying bursa. *2,* Operations for hallux valgus.

4. The surgeon uses a power-oscillating saw to resect the proximal third of the proximal phalanx.

5. Proper alignment of the toe is maintained as one or two 0.062-inch Kirschner wires are placed in the center of the medullary canal of the phalanx and then driven into the metatarsal head, neck, and shaft.

6. The surgeon irrigates and closes the wound. A bandage is applied to maintain the toe in the correct position.

7. Postoperative convalescence requires a minimum of 6 weeks.

Correction of Hammer Toe Deformity

The term *hammer toe* is most often used to describe an abnormal flexion posture of the proximal interphalangeal joint of one of the four lesser toes. This deformity causes painful calluses to develop on the dorsal joints of the four lesser toes, since the cocked-up digits rub against the shoes. Incising the long extensor tendon to the toes and fusing the proximal interphalangeal joint treat the deformities. A smooth Kirschner wire

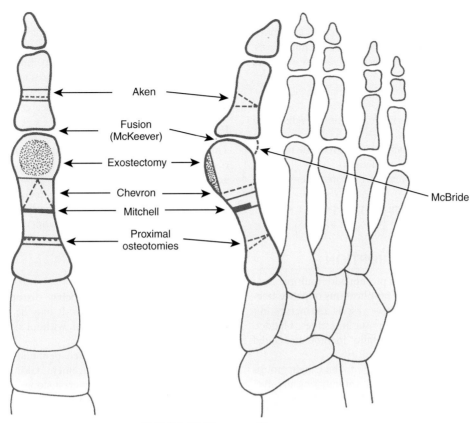

FIGURE 11-70 Types of bunionectomies.

is frequently used to stabilize the fusion and position the toe properly during the postoperative period.

Procedural Considerations. The patient is positioned supine. An ankle tourniquet is applied. The foot is prepped and draped. A soft tissue set, a small bone set, Kirschner wires, and a power wire driver are required.

Operative Procedure

1. The surgeon makes an elliptic incision over the proximal interphalangeal joint measuring 5 to 6 mm wide with a 2-mm or 3-mm lateral extension on either side.
2. The capsular tissue of the distal third of the proximal phalanx and proximal interphalangeal joint is entered to expose the defect completely.
3. Using a small rongeur or microsaw, the surgeon resects the distal third portion of the proximal phalanx. Once the capital fragment is excised, the surgeon debrides the remaining portion of the distal proximal phalanx with a rongeur or rasp.
4. Digital alignment can be maintained with small Kirschner wires.
5. The surgeon irrigates and closes the wounds. A sterile dressing and orthopedic shoe are applied for postoperative recovery.

Metatarsal Fractures

Metatarsal fractures occur in various sites. These fractures have a reduced healing potential because metatarsals consist mainly of cortical bone, which lacks vascularity. Treatment is determined by the extent of the fracture—the greater the dis-

placement, the greater the need for reduction. In general, transverse and short, oblique, midshaft fractures of the metatarsals are internally fixed because of their instability and displacement. Pins, wires, screws, and plates are used for internal fixation of metatarsal fractures. The simplest method is Kirschner wire fixation.

Procedural Considerations. The patient is placed in the supine position, a tourniquet is applied, and the foot is prepped and draped. A soft tissue set, a small bone set, Kirschner wires, and a power wire driver are required.

Operative Procedure

1. The surgeon makes a small incision over the fracture and identifies and retracts the distal fragment.
2. A smooth Kirschner wire is driven distally, exiting the skin.
3. The surgeon uses a wire driver to drive the wire proximally into the canal of the proximal fragment.
4. If the fracture is more complex or comminuted, the surgeon may cross two Kirschner wires through the fracture to transfix the fracture site.
5. The incision is closed, and a postoperative shoe is applied.

Metatarsal Head Resection

Patients with rheumatoid arthritis frequently have dorsally dislocated toes and prominent and painful metatarsal heads on the plantar surfaces of their feet. Excision of all the metatarsal heads commonly relieves the pain and corrects an associated bunion deformity.

Procedural Considerations. The patient is placed in the supine position, a tourniquet is applied, and the foot is prepped and draped. A soft tissue set, a small bone set, Kirschner wires, a power wire driver, and a power microsagittal saw are required.

Operative Procedure
CLAYTON TECHNIQUE

1. A transverse plantar incision is made, and tissue is dissected to the metatarsal heads.
2. Using a microsagittal saw the surgeon removes the metatarsal heads and half the proximal phalanges.
3. The surgeon transects the extensor tendons; they are not repaired.
4. The skin is closed, and a dressing and postoperative shoe are applied.

PELVIC FRACTURE AND DISRUPTION

Patients with multiple trauma often present with multiple fractures that can be life-threatening. Complications of pelvic fractures include injury not only to major vessels and nerves but also to major visceral organs, such as the intestines, bladder, and urethra. Factors influencing mortality include associated visceral injury, hemorrhage, and head injury.

Pelvic fracture classification is divided into three main groups (Table 11-1). *Type A fractures* are stable, without ring involvement (A1) or minimally displaced fractures of the ring (A2). *Type B fractures* are rotationally unstable and vertically stable and are also subclassified: B1 is an open book fracture, B2 has ipsilateral compression, and B3 has contralateral compression. *Type C fractures* are both rotationally and vertically unstable: C1 is unilateral, C2 is bilateral, and C3 is associated with the acetabulum. Radiographic films, computed tomography (CT) scan, and magnetic resonance imaging (MRI) all prove useful in determining the type and appropriate treatment for pelvic trauma.

Treatment is based on classification and may include closed manipulation and reduction or internal and external fixation. Internal and external fixation can be used concurrently in the treatment of some pelvic fractures.

Type A fractures are stable and can be treated nonoperatively. Type B1 fractures may be treated with external fixation or anterior plate fixation. Type C fractures usually require open procedures to fix the fractures with plates and screws, and reduction of sacral disruptions with transiliac rods or screws. Type C fractures may

TABLE 11-1

Classification of Pelvic Injuries

Type A	Stable
	A1—Fractures of pelvis not involving ring
	A2—Stable, minimally displaced fractures of ring
Type B	Rotationally unstable, vertically stable
	B1—Open book
	B2—Lateral compression: ipsilateral
	B3—Lateral compression: contralateral (bucket handle)
Type C	Rotationally and vertically unstable
	C1—Unilateral
	C2—Bilateral
	C3—Associated with an acetabular fracture

be treated with external fixation when the patient is hemodynamically unstable and a quicker, simpler procedure is prudent.

External fixation is the most widely recommended treatment for type B fractures of the pelvis. A technique similar to that of external fixation of extremity fractures is done in the OR with anesthesia and sterile conditions. If external fixation is to be used, the earlier it is attempted the greater the chance of success.

Procedural Considerations

This procedure is often done during other emergent and trauma resuscitative efforts. The patient's entire pelvic area is prepped and draped. A pelvic skeleton in the room may help the team visualize maneuvers and pin placement to be attempted to complete the reduction. A soft tissue set is needed in addition to the external fixator of choice and the instruments for its insertion, including a power drill.

Operative Procedure
AO External Fixation

1. The surgeon reduces the pelvic disruption manually and confirms it radiographically. It may be impossible to completely reduce the disruption without skeletal traction using a distal femoral pin.
2. Kirschner wires are inserted percutaneously to determine the position of the pin placement, taking into consideration the inward and downward crest slope.
3. The surgeon places parallel rows of pins into the anterior iliac crest area by drilling the outer cortex and placing 5-mm half-pins medially and distally. The pins should enter cancellous bone between the outer and inner tables of ilium.
4. Three universal frames are placed over the pins as close to the skin as possible for maximum rigidity.
5. Optimal reduction of the fracture is visualized using radiography. The surgeon applies the crossbar, and compression and distraction maneuvers are used to maintain the reduction.
6. The surgeon removes the crossbar and applies the connecting rods with couplers.
7. After the couplers are in place, the surgeon reattaches the crossbar and tightens the joints of the frame.
8. The pin sites of tented skin are released. The wounds are dressed with iodine ointment and gauze.
9. The frames are left in place generally for 8 to 12 weeks.

TOTAL JOINT ARTHROPLASTY

Arthroplasty of the joints is performed to restore motion of the joint and function to the muscles and ligaments. It is indicated in individuals with a painful, disabling arthritic joint that is no longer responsive to conservative therapy. In the past, the procedure was reserved for those with a less active lifestyle, and surgeons treated patients with reconstructive procedures such as arthrodesis or osteotomy because of the unknown life expectancy of the materials used in the manufacturing of the prostheses. Technological advances in the prostheses used today allow the younger patient, or the very active older person, to undergo joint replacement. Many total hip and knee replacements are done each year. Improvements in implant design, materials, and fixation techniques are ongoing, as is research on enhancing soft and hard tissue healing (Kolisek et al, 2007).

The classic combination of metal on polyethylene is the mainstay of joint implants. Metals used in hip and knee implants include *cobalt-chromium* (weight-bearing femoral head) and *titanium* (stems of hips and tibial components). The acetabulum and tibial articulating surfaces continue to be substituted with *ultra-high-molecular-weight polyethylene* (UHMWPE), which provides superior wear characteristics. Other designs have emerged in total hip arthroplasty, including metal on metal and the use of ceramic femoral heads.

At one time it was thought that bone cement was the weak link in the longevity of a joint implant because of a relatively high rate of loosening of cement-fixed implants, especially in younger, more active patients. In response to this belief, alternative methods of fixation have been developed. One method involves the application of a precoat of PMMA to the femoral stem to enhance bonding of the prosthesis to the cement mantle. Another method involves the attachment of a porous metal surface to parts of the femoral stem and the entire outer surface of the acetabular component. Most of the porous surfaces are composed of multiple layers sintered in place, creating interconnecting, open pores among the various particles. This allows for the ingrowth of bone to occur, ultimately anchoring the prosthesis in place. "Porous coating" was an attempt to eradicate what was termed *cement disease*—a lysis of bone around the prosthesis causing early loosening. It is now believed that this condition is caused by "wear debris"—particulate matter being shed from metal-to-polyethylene interfaces—and not necessarily from the effects of PMMA.

Bone cement, or PMMA, is an area that has received considerable attention in the search for optimal bone-to-implant fixation. Cement seems to exhibit various degrees of porosity depending on mixing methods and cement pressurization within the canal. Bone cement must prevent motion at the implant interface. Porosity can lead to fatigue and fracture, which ultimately can lead to implant loosening. Local tissue effects of PMMA may include (1) tissue protein coagulation caused by polymerization, (2) bone necrosis caused by occlusion of nutrient metaphyseal arteries, and (3) cytotoxic and lipotoxic effects of nonpolymerized monomer.

Despite the high rate of success of total joint implantation over the years, there are numerous potential complications. They are generally divided into medical complications, mechanical complications, and infections. Medical complications include, but are not limited to, cardiac dysrhythmias, myocardial infarction, hemorrhage, and pulmonary emboli. Mechanical complications are implant breakage, loosening, and wear. Infection in the patient with a total joint implant is a catastrophic complication that usually requires additional surgery and prolonged hospitalization.

Most surgeons recommend the routine use of antibiotics in primary and revision joint arthroplasty. Antibiotic coverage is initiated preoperatively, continued during lengthy procedures, and administered for 24 to 48 hours postoperatively. Pulsatile lavage systems are used to keep tissues moist, remove debris, and dilute bacteria that may be present. Additional antibiotics are often added to the physiologic saline solutions used for irrigation and to PMMA; however, data do not conclusively support or dispute this practice.

Total Hip Arthroplasty

Total hip arthroplasty is a common orthopedic procedure performed on patients with hip pain caused by degenerative joint disease, rheumatoid arthritis, or avascular necrosis. A total hip replacement can be cemented, noncemented, or hybrid. Hybrids involve cementing one component, usually the femoral stem, and then inserting a metal-backed, porous-coated acetabular component in a press-fit state. Hybrid arthroplasty is a controversial procedure for two reasons. The first relates to research that demonstrates that wear debris is increased with the larger metal-to-polyethylene interface present in the metal-backed, porous-coated acetabular component. The second relates to cost. The metal-backed, porous-coated acetabular component is significantly more expensive than the all-polyethylene component. Consequently, patient selection is very important in determining which type of component is best.

The primary function of the femoral component is the replacement of the femoral head and femoral neck after resection. The femoral head should ultimately sit where it reproduces the center of rotation of the hip. The neck length is variable and is built into several different heights of femoral heads that are eventually seated onto the Morse taper of the femoral stem. The version (implant rotation within the canal) is very important; too much anteversion or retroversion leaves the hip prone to dislocation. The normal position of the proximal femur is in 10 to 15 degrees of anteversion.

Femoral stems can be collarless or have collars that sit down on the resected femur. Collars will produce forces on the bone and may be desired in cases of osteoporotic bone, where bone genesis may be diminished because of the disease process.

Acetabular cups have also presented challenges in trying to maintain fixation within the socket. When cement techniques of the 1970s were used, femoral loosening plateaued about 5 years after surgery. Wear properties of the UHMWPE are also a concern. For this and other reasons associated with component failure, the idea of modularity was developed. Modular components, such as a polyethylene cup that snaps into a metal acetabular shell, greatly decrease the amount of surgery needed in the case of some revisions. In the case of excessive cup wear or a short femoral neck, surgery is minimized with the ability to exchange the modular components without removing the implants fixed to the bone.

Acetabular cups come with a textured back for cement fixation and may have standoff pegs to allow an appropriate cement mantle. Noncemented cups usually are porous-coated and may have screw holes present to aid in anchoring the less-than-stable cup. The presence of screw holes in an acetabular component is another controversial issue. Some believe that more wear debris is created with micromotion between the screw head and the cup as well as between the uneven surface of the screw and the polyethylene liner.

Prostheses are available for every patient's needs. Modular hip systems allow the orthopedic surgeon to choose from an array of interchangeable components that have been developed. Various femoral head sizes (22, 26, 28, and 32 mm) are available to maintain proper center of rotation. Acetabular cups may be snap fit, low profile, or deep profile, which adds additional thickness to the medial wall, where bone loss may be significant.

With modular systems, unipolar or bipolar cups are also an option when the acetabular articular surface is relatively normal. The unipolar and bipolar cups with appropriate head sizes are designed to fit on various modular system stems.

Custom prostheses or revision and extralong stems are available when bone loss is significant. These implants are employed in cases of revision where fixation is needed farther down the femoral canal or in oncologic procedures where tumor and corresponding bone have been resected.

Young, active individuals with strong, healthy bones are ideal candidates for noncemented total hip replacement arthroplasties. Elderly patients with osteoporosis and poor-quality bone are usually candidates for cemented components because their bones may lack the compressive strength to support weight-bearing forces (Boughton, 2009a) (Research Highlight).

Hip Reconstruction (Cemented). Numerous implants are available for total hip implantation. Many of the implants can be used for the same surgical indications, and one implant may not function any better than another, provided that all other conditions and techniques are the same. The instruments required to implant any one device cannot be used for another. During the preoperative verification process and time-out the perioperative nurse and surgical technologist collaborate to ensure that all the instrumentation is available.

PMMA adheres to the polyethylene and metal but not to the bone. It fills the cavity and interstices of the bone and forms a mechanical bond. PMMA is manufactured as a liquid monomer and a powder, and is mixed under sterile conditions by the surgical technologist in the OR at the time of implantation. It usually takes 10 to 12 minutes to harden. Because of the potentially harmful effects of PMMA fumes to the nasal epithelium, an exhaust system should be used during the mixing process.

PROCEDURAL CONSIDERATIONS. The patient is positioned in the lateral decubitus position and secured in place with anterior and posterior bolsters. This position is essential to ensure correct anatomic placement of the acetabular cup. The perioperative team verifies that the patient's bony prominences are adequately padded. The skin prep is completed from the level of the umbilicus down to and including the foot;

then the patient is draped. The radiographs are overlaid with the implant templates.

A soft tissue set and a large bone set are required. In addition, the total hip implants and corresponding instrumentation, acetabular reamers, hip retractor set, power reamer-driver and saw, and pulse lavage with a 3-L bag of normal saline solution (Figure 11-71) will be needed. If PMMA is used, femoral canal suction wicks, a cement restrictor and its inserter, and PMMA including its mixing supplies will be needed (Figure 11-72). If a trochanteric osteotomy is performed, the equipment of choice for its reattachment will be required.

Revision of total hip arthroplasties requires the same instrumentation as for cemented total hip reconstruction in addition to cement removal instrumentation, fluoroscopy, and the revision implants and their corresponding instrumentation.

OPERATIVE PROCEDURE

Cemented Modular Hip System, Posterior Approach

1. The surgeon makes an incision 2.5 cm distal and lateral to the anterosuperior iliac spine and curves the incision distally and posteriorly over the lateral aspect of the greater trochanter and lateral surface of the femoral shaft to 5 cm distal to the base of the trochanter.
2. The surgeon divides the tensor fasciae latae over the greater trochanter, and carries this distally to the extent of the incision. Dissection is carried proximally between the interval of the gluteus medius and the tensor fasciae latae muscles.
3. The anterior fibers of the gluteus medius tendon are tagged and detached from the trochanter. The surgeon incises the capsule longitudinally along the anterosuperior surface of the femoral neck. In the distal part of the incision, the origin of the vastus lateralis may be either reflected distally or split longitudinally to expose the base of the trochanter and proximal part of the femoral shaft.
4. After completing the capsulotomy, the surgeon dislocates the hip. Adduction and external rotation will present the femoral head anteriorly into the surgical site.
5. The surgeon places the femoral osteotomy guide over the lateral femur to identify the point on the femoral neck where the osteotomy should be made. Some femoral osteotomy guides also gauge the neck length required. The

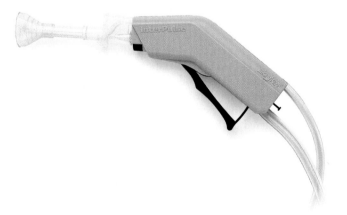

FIGURE 11-71 Pulse a vac used for pressurized irrigation when one is irrigating surgical wounds, debriding bone during a joint replacement, debriding open fractures or physically induced wounds, irrigating soft tissue injuries, or irrigating contaminated wounds.

surgeon marks the level and uses an oscillating or a recip-rocating saw to complete the femoral osteotomy.

6. The femur is retracted to expose the acetabulum, allow completion of the capsulotomy, and expose the bony rim of the entire acetabulum.

7. The surgeon inspects the acetabulum, removes any osteophytes, and reams the articular cartilage with bone-conserving reamers in a circumferential manner. The small-est reamer is progressed in a graduated method 1 or 2 mm at a time until the cartilage is reamed down to expose osteochondral bone. A hemispheric shape and bleeding bone should result.

8. Remaining soft tissue is curetted from the floor of the ace-tabulum, and cystic areas are filled with cancellous bone from the femoral canal and packed with a bone tamp. Any other bone grafting of major bony defects is accomplished using the fixation method of choice (bone screws).

9. Several 6-mm holes are drilled into the floor of the ace-tabulum, aimed into the ilium, ischium, and pubis. Holes are undercut using curettes. These prepared holes act as anchoring areas for the bone cement.

10. Trial acetabular components are placed on the positioning device and positioned in the socket. The surgeon assesses the cup for size, position within the socket, and the rela-tionship of the component compared with the bony mar-gins of the acetabulum.

11. The prepared acetabular socket is lavaged, dried with wicks, and filled with cement that has been injected and pressurized with an injection gun. The surgeon positions the acetabular shell component and holds it motionless until the cement polymerizes. Extruded cement is trimmed from around the edge of the component. A polyethylene insert is later snapped into the shell.

12. A sponge is placed in the acetabulum to protect the compo-nent from bone debris and subsequent cement as attention is turned to the femur.

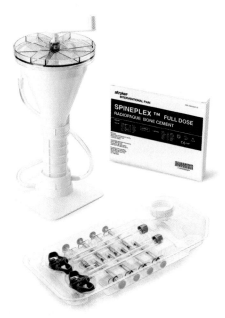

FIGURE 11-72 Polymethylmethacrylate (PMMA) and supplies for mixing and delivery in the canal.

13. Dropping the patient's foot toward the floor and internally rotating and pushing the leg proximally expose the proxi-mal femur. The surgeon accesses the femoral canal using a box osteotome or trochanteric reamer followed by the T-handle canal reamer.

14. Beginning with the smallest broach, the surgeon alternately impacts and extracts the proximal femoral canal. Progres-sively larger broaches are used to crush and remove cancel-lous bone until cortical bone is reached. A broach that is not advancing should not be used as this could result in shattering the femur.

15. With the final broach seated to the desired depth in the canal, the neck is prepared with a calcar reamer. The broach remains while the surgeon places the femoral trial compo-nent along with the various-size head, neck, and offset trial components.

16. The trial component is removed, and the canal is lavaged and brushed to accommodate the PMMA.

17. A cement restrictor is inserted into the femoral canal. The femoral components are passed and assembled on the back table.

18. The cement is injected and pressurized within the femoral canal.

19. The femoral component, with the proximal and distal cen-tralizers, is inserted into the canal with or without the fem-oral head.

20. The surgeon positions the appropriate size of femoral head onto the stem, and reduction is carried out. The joint is taken through a range of motion to check for positioning, stability, and the limit to which dislocation occurs.

21. Depending on the surgeon and the surgical approach, the greater trochanter may or may not have been removed for exposure of the hip joint. If removed, it is reattached with 18-gauge wire or a cable grip system.

22. The surgeon closes the wound in layers over suction drains. The skin is closed with staples, and a sterile dressing is applied to provide compression to the wound.

23. An abduction pillow or splint is placed between the patient's legs postoperatively if stability of the joint is of concern.

Hip Reconstruction (Noncemented). Fixation with a non-cemented prosthesis is initially accomplished by a tight fit and intimate contact of the implants within bone of substantial strength. As with all prosthetic designs, it is essential to fill the medullary canal and wedge the prosthesis in as tightly as pos-sible to provide temporary press-fit fixation. These prostheses closely follow normal anatomic shape. Only the instrumen-tation corresponding to the implant should be used. Precise machining of the femoral canal must be ensured. Acetabular components are usually press-fitted, but many systems provide holes for screw fixation if stability of the prosthesis is in doubt. Sufficient time is then allowed for the cancellous bone to heal by growing into the porous portions of the prosthesis.

The healing process requires the same amount of time as a long bone cortical fracture (approximately 3 months). The patient must be cautious after the procedure and protect the operative hip from excessive compression, rotation, and shear stresses.

PROCEDURAL CONSIDERATIONS. The position and incision are the same as those used for the cemented total hip replacement. The radiographs and implant templates are placed on the view box.

OPERATIVE PROCEDURE

Noncemented Anatomic Medullary Locking (AML) Hip System (Figure 11-73)

1. After the incision is made, the surgeon enters the capsule and dislocates the femoral head.
2. A pilot hole is established in the trochanteric fossa as an intramedullary reference point.
3. The surgeon uses progressively sized fully fluted rigid reamers to ream the intramedullary canal.
4. A femoral neck osteotomy is achieved by positioning an osteotomy template along the axis of the femur and cutting at the level of the collar.
5. The surgeon clears the soft tissue from the acetabulum and reams it with hemispheric reamers.
6. Trial acetabular sizers are placed to determine the correct position and size of the prosthetic component.
7. A hollow osteotome is used in the femoral canal to connect the pilot hole to the osteotomy site.
8. Femoral broaches are then inserted to enlarge the intramedullary space for trial insertion.
9. The surgeon may use a power calcar planer placed over the trunnion of the broach to contour the femoral neck.
10. A trial head and neck component is positioned onto the fitted broach, and a trial reduction is carried out.
11. If trial reduction is satisfactory, the surgeon removes all the trial components.
12. The appropriate size of acetabular component is inserted into the acetabulum, and a polyethylene insert is locked into place.
13. The femoral component is placed into the canal, and the modular head is seated on the trunnion.
14. Reduction of the hip is followed by standard closure with drains.
15. Abduction of the hip is maintained postoperatively with a foam abduction pillow if necessary.

Minimally Invasive Total Hip Arthroplasty. Minimally invasive total hip arthroplasty (MITHA) has resulted in minimized scarring, reduced patient morbidity, a shortened hospitalization period, and an accelerated rehabilitation process (Harby, 2005). MITHA can be performed with a single or double incision. For a single incision, the patient is placed in a lateral position; the patient is supine for a double-incision procedure. With double-incision MITHA, the acetabular and femoral components are inserted through two small incisions, one anterolateral and one posterolateral, each approximately 5 cm long. The technique spares the muscles and tendons around the hip.

PROCEDURAL CONSIDERATIONS. As with any joint replacement, templates of the x-rays preoperatively are recommended. A regular OR bed with x-ray capability is used. The team should alert the radiology department that fluoroscopy will be used. Equipment should be arranged carefully (Figure 11-74). The patient is positioned supine with a small bolster placed under the pelvis on the operative side. The patient's entire leg, from above the waist to the ankle, is then prepped and draped in the usual fashion. The time-out includes confirmation of the correct patient, site, side, procedure, position, and implants.

OPERATIVE PROCEDURE (VERSYS HIP SYSTEM)

1. The C-arm is used to define the femoral neck. The surgeon makes the anterior incision directly over the femoral neck

from the base of the femoral head. The lateral femoral cutaneous nerve is identified and located, and then carefully retracted along with the sartorius using an Army-Navy retractor. A second retractor is used for the tensor fasciae latae laterally. This exposes the lateral border of the rectus femoris.

2. The surgeon uses the electrosurgical unit (ESU) for hemostasis of the lateral femoral vessels. The Army-Navy retractors are extended deeper as the rectus femoris is dissected with a #10 blade on a long handle. A long-tipped ESU pencil may also be used.

3. The surgeon incises the femoral capsule and fat pad. A Cobb elevator is used to move the tissue medially underneath the rectus muscles and laterally off the femoral neck, allowing exposure of the capsule over the femoral neck.

4. Two curved lit retractors are placed outside the capsule around the femoral neck, perpendicular to it. If additional leverage is needed, retractor handle extenders may be attached and used. The femoral capsule is incised in line with the femoral neck lateral to the midline to facilitate future placement of the head of the femoral prosthesis. Sutures can be used to retract the capsule so that the femoral head and neck are clearly visible.

5. Fluoroscopy may then be used to verify osteotomy position. Using the oscillating saw, the surgeon places a high femoral neck cut and uses a straight, 4-cm osteotome to complete it. A second cut is then made, and a threaded Steinmann pin is inserted to remove the small wafer of bone. This allows enough room for the surgeon to make the final femoral neck cut.

6. Fluoroscopy is used to check the angle and length of resection. It is important for the surgical team to help keep the leg in neutral position, especially during these cuts. The femoral head is then removed while the surgical assistant applies gentle traction on the leg.

7. Three lit anterior retractors are placed: one superiorly in the line of the incision, over the acetabulum, and the second and third at 90-degree angles to the first. Once the acetabulum is exposed, sharp and blunt dissection is used to remove remaining tissue and synovium.

8. Reaming starts with the acetabular reamer that is close to the template size. C-arm visualization is used during the reaming. Once reaming is completed to the acceptable size, the trial components are placed to determine fit. C-arm images are used to confirm location and size. The positioning bolster is removed at this time. The appropriate-size cup and liner are then chosen. The acetabular component is then seated using the offset shell inserter, retractors are removed, and the cup is impacted into place. Multiple images are taken to check the placement and position of the cup while impacting. The inserter is then removed. If screws are used, a drill, screws, drill guide, depth gauge, and flexible screwdriver will be required. Once the cup and screws are in place, their position is again checked with fluoroscopy. The liner is inserted.

9. The second incision is found by direct palpation. The nonoperative leg is adducted. The operative leg is fully adducted, externally rotated, and flexed over the nonoperative leg. Location is verified by fluoroscopy. A stab wound is made in the posterior lateral buttock and extended to 1.5 to 3 cm as needed. Sharp dissection is

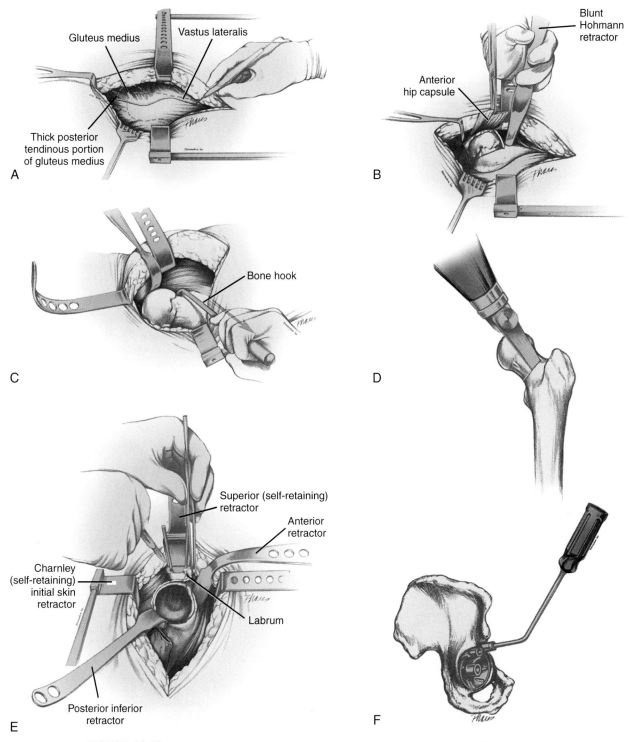

FIGURE 11-73 Noncemented hip reconstruction. **A,** After the incision, the Charnley retractor is placed, the fascia lata is incised, and the gluteus medius is detached. **B,** An anterior capsulotomy is completed. **C,** The hip is flexed, adducted, and externally rotated to dislocate from the acetabulum. **D,** The femoral neck is cut by use of an oscillating saw blade. **E,** The rim of the acetabulum is debrided of labrum, redundant capsule, and marginal osteophytes. **F,** The acetabulum is reamed; after reaming, the appropriate drill guide is inserted into the acetabulum.

Continued

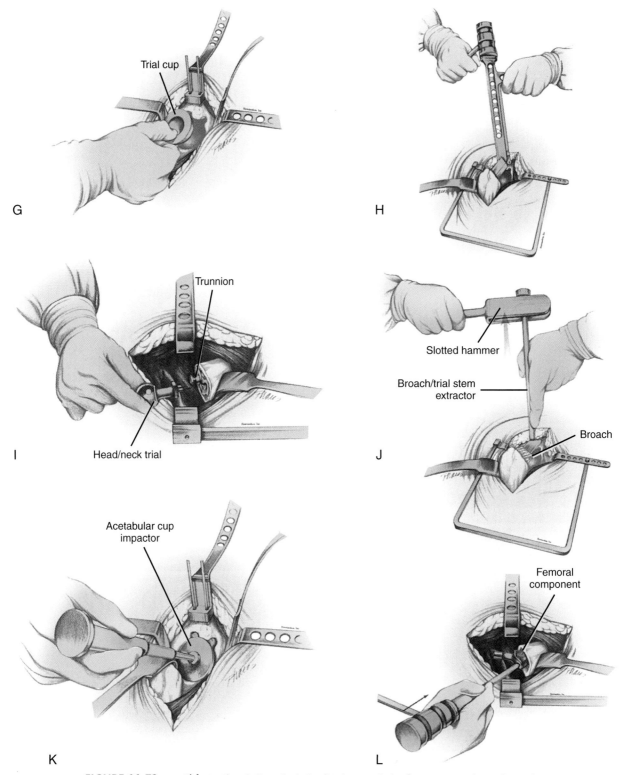

FIGURE 11-73, cont'd **G**, After drilling the holes for the acetabular fixation pegs, the trial acetabular cup is inserted. **H**, The proximal wedge of cancellous bone is removed, and the appropriate size of femoral broach is introduced down the axis of the femoral canal. **I**, The trial head is placed on the broach trunnion of trial reduction. **J**, With the slotted hammer, the femoral broach is extracted; the trial acetabular cup is removed. **K**, Acetabular fixation pegs are seated, the acetabular cup is introduced, and the component is seated. **L**, The femoral canal is irrigated with pulsatile lavage and dried with suction and sponges; the femoral canal is plugged and filled with methylmethacrylate; the femoral component is inserted.

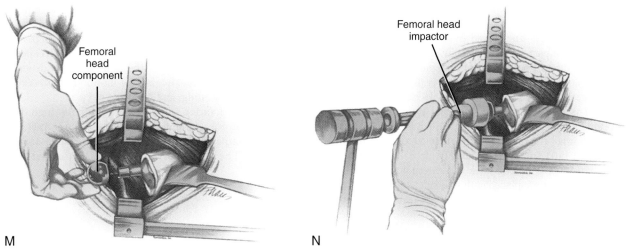

M N

FIGURE 11-73, cont'd M, The femoral head component is placed on the trunnion. N, The femoral head is impacted, the femur is reduced, and the wound is irrigated before closure.

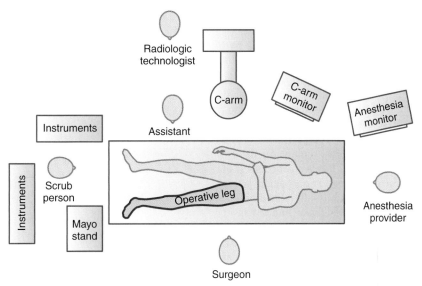

FIGURE 11-74 Illustration of room setup, including positioning of C-arm and monitor, for minimally invasive total hip arthroplasty (MITHA).

used to spread the tissue along the co-axial pathway to the piriformis fossa.

10. Downward pressure is applied to the operative knee to elevate the trochanter. The tissue protector is inserted. Reaming the femoral canal begins with the lateral reamers. All reamers should be inserted in the locked position. Once lateral reaming is complete, intramedullary reamers are used. Fluoroscopy is used at regular intervals throughout the reaming process to ensure centralization in the canal. The tissue protector is then removed.

11. The canal is rasped, with the initial rasp two to three times smaller than the template size of the canal. The rasp is tapped into place until fully seated; its position is verified with fluoroscopy. The canal is rasped until proper sizing and positioning are obtained. The C-arm is used to check the final depth, fill, and positioning of the rasp with the apex of the calcar.

12. Trial reduction is done with the final rasp in place. The provisional head is placed on the rasp, and the hip is reduced by providing longitudinal traction and internal rotation. The surgeon moves the hip through a full range of motion. Fluoroscopy may be used to check the levels of the lesser trochanters for possible leg length discrepancies. Once trial reduction is complete, the rasp is removed by way of a posterior exit and the head through the anterior incision.

13. Two lit anterior retractors are placed in the posterior incision to keep the tissue away from the stem as it is placed in the femoral canal. Once the implant is through the skin and properly rotated, the implant driver is attached. Gentle traction is placed on the leg in neutral abduction. Once the

femoral component is within the capsule of the hip, the patient's operative leg is repositioned; it is fully adducted, externally rotated, and flexed over the nonoperative leg. The stem is impacted until it is fully seated. Fluoroscopy is used to ensure proper seating and alignment.

14. The surgeon pulls the neck of the femur through the wound and places the trial head. Traction is placed on the hip, and the hip is then turned into internal rotation. Range-of-motion and leg length assessment is then done.

15. After the final trial reduction is performed, the surgeon dislocates the hip to put the final head in place. Hip dislocation is done using a dull bone hook and external rotation of the hip. Two sutures are placed in the capsule: one medially and the other laterally. This is done before the head is reduced to prevent the capsule from invaginating posteriorly. The prosthetic head can then be seated and impacted. Gentle traction and internal rotation are used to reduce the hip. A final range-of-motion and leg length assessment is performed.

16. The surgeon irrigates the incisions with antibiotic irrigation. A local anesthetic such as bupivacaine (Marcaine) may be infiltrated into the incision, the two previously placed sutures tied, and additional sutures placed to fully close the capsule. A drain may be placed.

Total Knee Arthroplasty

Total knee arthroplasty is a surgical procedure designed to replace the worn surfaces of the knee joint. Patients complain of knee pain and instability. Degenerative rheumatoid or traumatic arthritis can result in severe destruction of the entire knee joint, or only the medial or lateral compartments of the knee joint can deteriorate as a result of extreme varus or valgus deformity. Arthroplasty of the knee has been successful in relieving these symptoms. Success depends on patient selection, component design, surgical technique, and rehabilitation.

The challenge of finding the optimal knee implant is in reproducing the complicated range of motion of the knee. Motion of the knee occurs in three planes: flexion and extension, abduction and adduction, and rotation. Designs of total knees should allow preservation of the normal ligaments whenever possible while providing soft tissue balance when necessary to maintain stability.

Total knee implants may be classified into three different categories, according to the portions of the knee to be replaced. *Unicompartmental* implants are used to replace just one opposing articular surface (medial or lateral) of the femur and tibia. These implants, however, lost popularity as a result of biomechanical and technical pitfalls. *Bicompartmental* designs, mentioned only to demonstrate the progression of total knee design, replaced both the medial and lateral surfaces of the femur and tibia. Most of the total knee replacements completed today are *tricompartmental* implants, which replace not only the opposing femorotibial joint but also the patellofemoral joint.

The tricompartmental knees are further divided into three categories (Figure 11-75). *Unconstrained* prostheses have very little constraint built in between the femoral and tibial components and depend on the integrity of soft tissues to provide stability of the reconstructed joint. Where there is significant deformity and the need for soft tissue release, the surgeon may decide to use a *semiconstrained* prosthesis, which lends itself to more inherent stability necessitated by ligamentous defi-

ciency. *Fully constrained* prostheses are linked together with pure hinges, rotating hinges, and nonhinged designs. They are used in the presence of considerable bone loss, instability, deformity, and revision surgery where bone loss has been significant. Fully constrained prostheses do not provide a normal range of motion, and such a lack of motion leads to excessive wear, implant loosening, and breakage.

Methods of fixation of total knee implants include both cemented and noncemented techniques. The noncemented variety encompasses both porous bony ingrowth and press-fit designs. The choice of implant and method of fixation

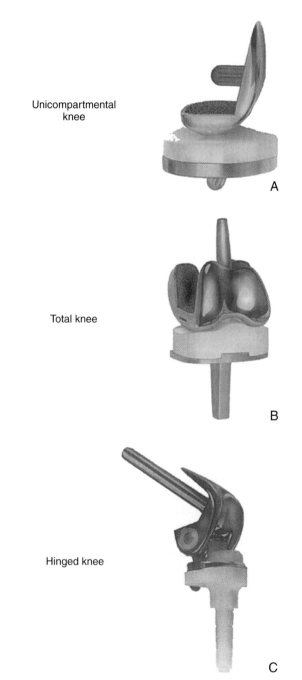

Unicompartmental knee

A

Total knee

B

Hinged knee

C

FIGURE 11-75 Knee arthroplasty implants. **A,** Unconstrained hinge. **B,** Semiconstrained hinge. **C,** Fully constrained hinge.

depend on the predisposition of the bone, the patient's age and activity level, and the surgeon's comfort with a particular technique. Previous designs did not retain the posterior cruciate ligament, which possibly led to increased joint instability. Newer designs allow the posterior cruciate to be retained. Some surgeons believe that the retention of the posterior cruciate ligament dictates the need for absolute ligament balancing beyond what may be possible in the reconstructed knee.

In the interest of more cost-effective use of medical resources, new designs have been developed for the less-active patient with a shorter expected life span. The femoral component design is a symmetric design that can be used on either the left or the right knee. The tibial component is composed entirely of UHMWPE, thereby lowering manufacturing costs. Both components are placed with the use of PMMA.

Procedural Considerations. The patient is positioned supine. A tourniquet is applied to the upper thigh. The surgical prep is completed. A soft tissue set and a large bone set; the total knee instruments, trials, and implants of choice; a power drill and saw; PMMA and cement supplies; and a pulse lavage will be required.

Operative Procedure
NEXGEN TOTAL KNEE ARTHROPLASTY (Figure 11-76)
1. With the knee flexed, the surgeon makes a straight midline incision from 3 to 4 inches above the patella, ending at the patellar tubercle.
2. The capsule is entered medially. After making a median parapatellar incision, the surgeon places Kocher clamps on both lateral and medial sides of the capsule, and reflects the patella laterally to expose the entire tibiofemoral joint.
3. Hypertrophic synovium, a portion of the infrapatellar fat pad, is excised using a toothed forceps and knife or the ESU, and then the osteophytes are removed using a rongeur. This allows easy access to the medial, lateral, and intercondylar spaces and facilitates soft tissue releases, should the need arise.
4. The knee is flexed to 90 degrees, and Hohmann retractors are placed deep to the collateral ligaments and anterior to the posterior capsule as well as laterally to the patella to protect these structures during resection of the proximal tibia. A Richardson retractor is placed medially to protect the medial collateral ligament (MCL).
5. The surgeon positions the distal cutting alignment guide extramedullary and parallel to the proximal tibial spine. Proper rotational alignment is established by positioning the appropriate malleoli wings parallel to the transmalleolar axis. The alignment rod is proximally placed just slightly lateral to the tibial tubercle.
6. The osteotomy saw is then used to resect the proximal portion of the tibia. The distal cutting guide is removed. Alignment is checked with a Gerber guide (spacer block with the alignment rod) by placing the guide on the tibia. This checks the tibial cut for valgus alignment. The tibia is then sized with templates.
7. Before proceeding further, the surgeon ensures that the extremity can be moved into normal mediolateral (ML) align-

ment in extension. If not, additional soft tissue balancing is performed until the normal mechanical axis is obtained.
8. The AP cutting guide is then used to size the femur. The guide yoke is attached to the AP block, and the yoke is slipped under the muscle anteriorly on the periosteum. The middle nail is hammered into place, while pressing down on the guide yoke. Then by pulling up on the yoke, the valgus alignment is achieved such that it is square with the tibial cut. The block is then nailed into place with two pins.
9. With the AP femoral guide in place, the surgeon positions right-angle retractors to protect the MCL and lateral collateral ligament (LCL). The anterior and posterior portions of the femur are resected. The tibial and femoral cuts are checked for balance and size at the same time with a tibial block.
10. Once the flexion balance is determined, the distal femoral cutting block is set. The tensor, placed in flexion, is then slowly moved into extension. Tension is placed on the extension gap by dialing between 30 to 40 pounds of pressure on the tensor. The amount of pressure dialed on the tensor is based on the patient's size and tightness of the ligaments. The distal cutting jig is then placed in the tensor. Once the jig is secured, the two pin holes are drilled and the tensor removed. The distal cutting guide is then placed in the exact two pin holes made by the distal cutting jig. The knee is then flexed, and the distal portion of the femur is resected.
11. The appropriate spacer block is then used to ensure equal tension in flexion and extension.
12. The knee is placed in flexion; the femoral notch and chamfer guide is centered between the epicondyles and impacted until fully seated. Three anterior fixation pins secure the guide to the femur. The surgeon drills two ¼-inch holes into the distal end of the femur, and cuts the anterior and posterior chamfers with the oscillating saw. The box osteotome is used to make the notch cut from the proximal end of the finishing guide. A power saw is used to resect the posterior femoral condyle remnants to ensure adequate flexion clearance. The femoral trial is then positioned.
13. The tibial size is reassessed using the tibial templates. The selected tibial template is then positioned rotationally and drilled, and the appropriate-size centering punch is used to cut through the subchondral bone. The tibial trial is then placed.
14. The surgeon measures the patella and places two towel clips onto the distal and proximal portions of the patella tendon, and then performs the appropriate amount of resection. The patellar template is placed over the resected surface, and the cruciate channels are created using the patellar drill through the slots in the template.
15. A trial reduction is performed. If this reduction proves satisfactory with regard to alignment and ligament laxity, the surgeon removes the trial components, irrigates with a pulsatile lavage, and places the permanent components. These can be inserted without bone cement, with bone cement, or with a combination of both.
16. Drains are placed in the joint depending on the surgeon's preference. The joint is closed in the usual fashion, and a compression dressing is applied to the leg. The tourniquet

can be released before closure or after the dressing has been applied.

Postoperative care consists of rapid mobilization and strengthening, with a target discharge of 3 to 4 days postoperatively.

Stryker Navigation Total Knee Arthroplasty

PROCEDURAL CONSIDERATIONS (Figure 11-77). During the surgical approach, the company representative will be initializing (setting up) the Smart Tools instrumentation with the surgical technologist. Healthcare industry representatives can provide valuable technical support to the perioperative team. Integration of surgical instrumentation and computers results in the ability to build a customized, digital map of the patient's anatomy and navigate the surgical instruments according to this map. Successfully executed steps are marked with a blue checkmark and are graphically visualized. Proper setup is achieved when all Smart Tools are shown inside the camera's working space. Advantages

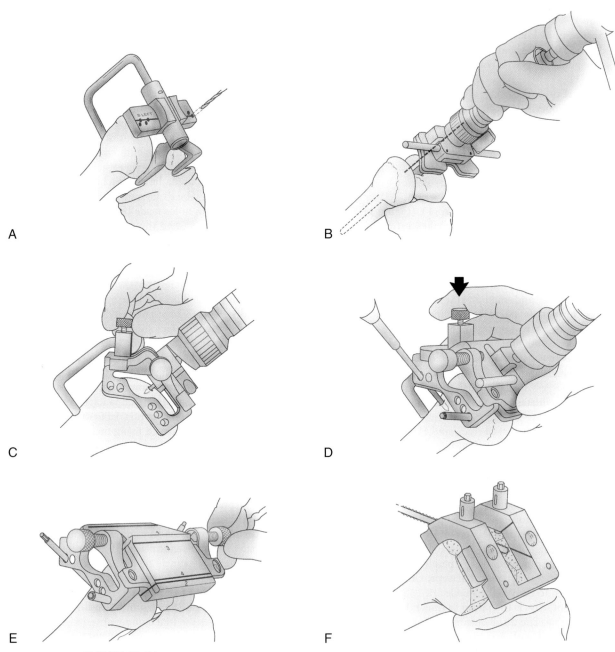

FIGURE 11-76 Total knee implant, instrumentation, and procedure. **A,** After exposure of the intercondylar notch, the femoral sizer is placed at the distal end of the femur. **B,** After the femoral canal is reamed, the femoral intramedullary alignment guide is inserted and passed up the medullary canal. **C,** Correct rotational alignment is maintained; the anterior femoral cutting guide is attached to the femoral intramedullary alignment guide. **D,** The femoral cutting guide is mounted in place. **E,** The femur is resected. **F,** Femoral cuts are completed.

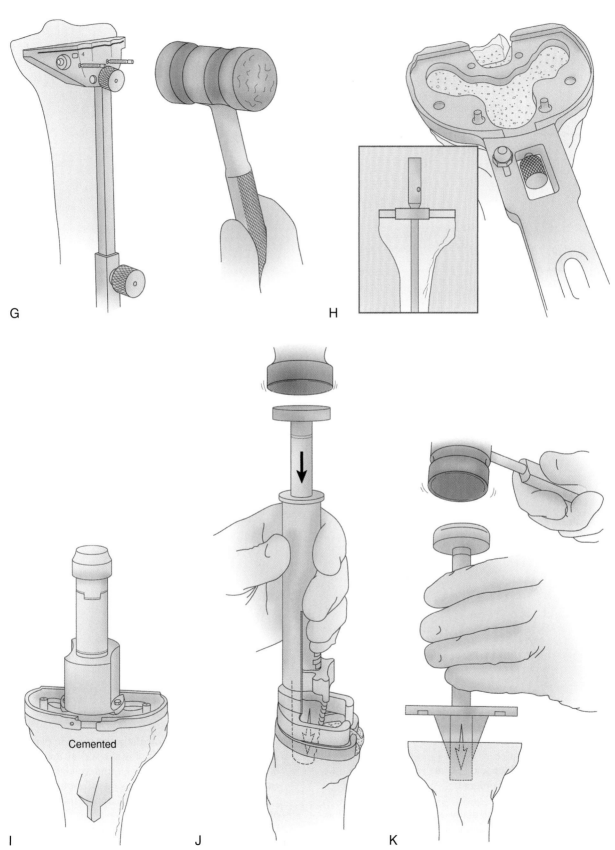

G

H

Cemented

I

J

K

FIGURE 11-76, cont'd **G**, The tibial alignment guide is placed and secured; the tibia is resected. **H**, The tibia is sized. **I**, The tibia is reamed. **J**, The tibia is impacted. **K**, The tibial trial is inserted.

Continued

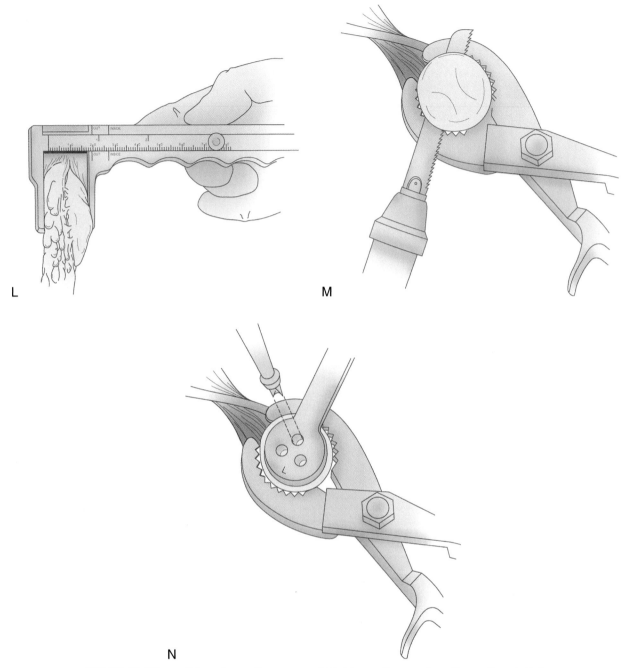

L

M

N

FIGURE 11-76, cont'd L, The patella is measured. M, The patella is sized. N, The patella is drilled.

to using a navigation system include the increased ability to verify the accuracy of cuts in less visible areas, decreased blood loss, and improved feedback to the surgeon about the patient's soft tissue balance.

A tourniquet, foot holder, and ESU are required. Antibiotics and heparin will usually be ordered.

OPERATIVE PROCEDURE

1. The capsule is entered medially. After making a median parapatellar incision, the surgeon places Kocher clamps on both lateral and medial sides of the capsule, and reflects the patella laterally to expose the entire tibiofemoral joint.

2. The surgeon begins to raise the medial flap using the ESU at the anterior tibia.

3. With a finger to retract medially, the surgeon places the tibial anchoring pin (self-tapping screws) at the distal aspect of the exposure. Drilling is then undertaken from the anterior to posterior tibial cortex using a 3.2-mm drill bit parallel to the joint line and rotated approximately 30 degrees medially.

4. Using a depth gauge, the surgeon rounds off to the size larger than measured (pins are available in 5-mm increments).

5. The surgical technologist places the pin on a T-handle for the surgeon to manually screw in the anchoring pin.

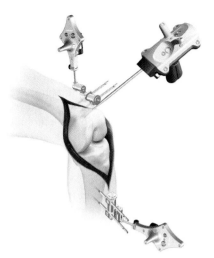

FIGURE 11-77 Stryker Navigation Tracking Equipment.

6. For the femoral anchoring pin, the surgeon next drills from the anterior to posterior femoral cortex, measures with a depth gauge, rounds up to the next larger size, and inserts the pin with a T-handle.

7. The blue tracker (B = bottom) is attached to the tibial pin and the green tracker to the femoral pin. Trackers should be placed so they are facing the camera attached to the navigation system.

8. The femoral head is registered. The hip is placed at 0 to 20 degrees of flexion and then at 45 degrees of flexion. As the leg is rotated, the LED locations yield a set of data points relative to the size of the femoral head.

9. The distal femur is then registered. The medial and lateral condyles, the center of the knee, and the AP axis of the knee are digitalized to identify the articulating surfaces.

10. The proximal tibia is then registered. The center of the tibia, AP axis, and medial and lateral tibial plateaus are traced in a similar fashion to the femur, which identifies the slope of the tibia.

11. The knee is moved through range of motion from full extension to full flexion. This kinematic datum is calculated and then recorded. Once data are recorded, the trackers are removed.

12. The surgeon excises any hypertrophic synovium and a portion of the infrapatellar fat pad using a toothed forceps and knife or ESU; the osteophytes are removed with a rongeur. This allows easy access to the medial, lateral, and intercondylar spaces and facilitates soft tissue releases, should the need arise.

13. The knee is flexed to 90 degrees, and Hohmann retractors are placed to the MCL and immediately anterior to the posterior capsule as well as laterally to the patella to protect these structures. A Richardson retractor is placed medially to protect the MCL. The surgeon uses a Kocher clamp and knife to resect the medial and lateral menisci as well as remnants of the anterior cruciate ligament (ACL) and posterior cruciate ligament (PCL).

14. The surgeon places the navigated tibial cutting guide on the proximal tibia. A cutting guide is attached to the horseshoe device and then the blue tracker to the tibial anchoring pin and the green tracker to the femoral anchoring pin. Using

two pins, the guide is anchored. The position is confirmed with the navigation system and the trackers and horseshoe device are then removed.

15. The surgeon uses a 5.5-mm round burr to open the tibial surface and then drive the keel punch slightly anteriorly. The guide and pins are then removed.

16. The horseshoe device is placed with the opening posterior on the distal femur with two pins. The distal femoral cutting guide is attached to the device, and the blue tracker is attached to the blue anchoring pins. Finally, the green tracker is attached to the femoral anchoring pins.

17. The surgeon manipulates the cutting guide to the distal femur. The first pin is driven into the guide and adjusted, and then the second and third pins are placed. The horseshoe and pins are removed. The saw is flushed with the cutting guide, the green top is attached, and the blue Gurba guide is set on the tibial surface to check the cuts.

18. The femoral 4-in-1 cutting guide is placed, and the pin is placed and cut with the saw. The LCL and MCL are protected with a finger or right-angle retractors and the pins removed.

19. The Booth retractor is then placed over the tibia. After the notch guide and pin are placed, the surgeon cuts the tibia to an appropriate depth, using a saw as well as chamfer cuts. The pins and guide are then removed.

20. Next, the patella is measured; then two towel clips are placed onto the distal and proximal portions of the patellar tendon, and the appropriate resection is performed. The surgeon places the patellar template over the resected surface, and creates the cruciate channels using the patellar drill through the slots in the template.

21. Trial components are placed, trackers attached, and the knee moved through a full range of motion. The trials and anchoring pins are then removed.

22. PMMA is prepared. Bone surfaces are irrigated with a pulsatile lavage, and the permanent components are placed. These can be inserted without bone cement, with bone cement, or using a combination of both.

23. Drains are placed in the joint depending on the surgeon's preference. The joint is closed in the usual fashion, and a compression dressing is applied to the leg. The tourniquet can be released before closure or after the dressing has been applied.

Postoperative care consists of rapid mobilization and strengthening, with a target discharge of 3 to 4 days postoperatively.

Total Knee Revision Arthroplasty. Revision arthroplasty may be indicated if the patient's original knee replacement wears out or loosens, or fails as a result of repeated dislocation, infection, or trauma. Total joint revision can be a very demanding and complicated procedure. Attention to detail, anticipation, and preparation are essential. Important patient information includes the preoperative x-rays, bone scan, laboratory results (including aspiration results), and physical findings.

PROCEDURAL CONSIDERATIONS. The patient is placed in supine position with a footrest for the affected leg. An OR bed with x-ray capability is used. Following the induction of anesthesia, the surgeon performs an EUA. Although one of the most difficult aspects of revision surgery is that there is no clear-cut sequence of events, it is best, if possible, to approach revision surgery using the same logical sequence for each procedure. This allows all members of the surgical team to anticipate the steps in the procedure and the needs of the patient. In the case of revision arthroplasty for infection, antibiotics are held, usually at the surgeon's request, to allow for one final attempt to recover an organism. Tissue and fluid cultures are obtained when the initial incision is made through the capsule and into the joint space. Once the cultures are obtained, antibiotics are given.

Instrumentation includes a basic knee set, primary total knee instrumentation, and trials (in case only one portion of the prosthesis is revised); revision instrumentation to extract the components and cement; instrumentation and trials for the revision components; cementing system and extra cement (usually double the amount of cement used in a primary total knee arthroplasty); and power equipment including saw, reamer, and burrs.

OPERATIVE PROCEDURE The previous skin incision is usually used. This maintains adequate blood flow to the skin. The skin is marked to reapproximate the skin edges after surgery. A tourniquet is used after determining that there are no contraindications based on the patient's medical and surgical history.

1. Using a #10 blade, the surgeon incises through the scar from the original surgery.
2. With heavy tooth forceps and blade, the surgeon undermines skin on each side of the incision; this allows the skin to be more easily closed at the end of the procedure.
3. Once at the capsule, a clean #10 blade is used to make a medial parapatellar incision into the joint. A Kocher is placed on the medial side of the capsule, and a towel clip is placed laterally, immediate to the patella, to aid with eversion.
4. Both tissue and fluid cultures are taken. Antibiotics are then administered by the anesthesia provider.
5. Using heavy tooth forceps or a Kocher, the surgeon performs a synovectomy with a knife or the ESU. A clean dissection is needed to allow visualization of the bone-prosthesis interface and to remove any synovitis caused by poly debris or metallosis (metallosis is a nonsuppurative osteomyelitis that occurs around metal implants as a result of corrosion or hypersensitivity reaction).
6. The surgeon uses a periosteal elevator to peel away the medial ligament, which was stripped during the original surgery.
7. The knee is dislocated with posterior placement of a Hohmann retractor immediately behind the tibia. A second Hohmann retractor is placed laterally to the patella and LCL. Medially, a Richardson retractor provides protection of the MCL.
8. If possible, the surgeon removes the poly tibia insert to allow better visualization and an increased work space.
9. Using an osteotomy saw with a small blade, the surgeon will proceed to remove the tibial plate at the bone-prosthesis interface. If the saw is unable to complete the cuts, ¼- or ½-inch curved osteotomes may be used to gain access to the posterior lateral corner. Cement is then removed from the canal using a Kocher, ¼-inch straight osteotome, chisels, mallet, and curettes. If the cement is deep, a heavy toothed alligator forceps may be required.
10. Once the tibia and cement are removed, the surgeon recuts the tibia surface using an osteotomy saw and alignment

guide. Sometimes, the tibia is completely revised before the next step. If so, the tibial template, pins, mallet, and punch will be needed.
11. With the patella everted, a Booth retractor is placed under the femur. Using a ½-inch curved osteotome and mallet, the surgeon removes the femoral component. A ¼-inch curved osteotome may be required if there are metal pegs at the distal end on the femoral component or at the posterior edge of the prosthesis. Once both sides of the prosthesis are loosened, it should fall off. If not, a femoral distractor will be used.
12. Any remaining cement is removed using osteotomes, chisels, or the saw. Any cement in the canal will be removed with a Kocher or alligator forcep.
13. Next the posterior capsule is addressed. With the leg in extension, the surgeon places a lamina spreader between the femur and tibia. Using curettes and a rongeur, the scar on the posterior capsule is removed to improve postoperative range of motion.
14. Once the capsule is released, attention is turned to rebuilding the femur. This is done by using a series of guides and trial components.
15. Augmentation of both tibia and femur components can be done using either metal augments or bone grafting. Balance between the femur and tibia is obtained first in flexion and then in extension.
16. The last component to be revised is the patella. Two towel clips are placed, distal and proximal on either side of the patella, and the button is removed, using a large-blade osteotomy saw. All poly buttons can be readily removed by this method. However, a metal-backed patella requires the additional use of a ¼-inch osteotome. Any remaining cement is removed from holes with a curette or 6.0-mm burr on a drill. The patella will be recut using a large-blade osteotomy saw.
17. The guide is placed on the patella, and the drill is used for new holes. The trial button is placed, the patella inverted, and the knee placed through a range of motion.
18. All components are removed, and the knee is irrigated with antibiotic solution using pulsatile lavage. The bone edges are dried with suction and clean sponges. This is done while the cement is being mixed.
19. Components can be cemented all at once or in stages, depending on the surgeon's preference.
20. The femur is usually cemented first. The Booth retractor is placed under the femur, and cement is put on the posterior phalanges of the femoral component and then on the distal edges of the bone. The component is placed on the end of the femur and impacted with an impactor and mallet. The cement is removed using glue knives anteriorly, laterally, and medially. Posterior glue is removed using curettes. The Booth retractor is then removed.
21. Hohmann retractors are placed posteriorly and laterally; a Richardson retractor can be placed medially if necessary. The surgeon applies cement on the tibia surface and on the tip of the tibial stem. The tibial component is then placed and impacted. Remaining cement is removed using glue knives or bayonet forceps. The retractors are removed, and the knee is relocated.
22. Cement is applied to the patella in the predrilled holes as well as on the patella button itself. The button is placed

on the patella and held with a patella clamp. Remaining cement is again removed using a glue knife or bayonets.

23. Drains are used at the discretion of the surgeon, and the wound is closed.

Total Shoulder Arthroplasty

Physically induced or accidental injury or degenerative arthritis may necessitate prosthetic replacement of the shoulder joint. The procedure may be a hemiarthroplasty with reconstruction of the humeral side or a total arthroplasty with replacement of the humeral head and glenoid (Figure 11-78).

Procedural Considerations. The patient is placed in a 30-degree semisitting position with the arm draped free on a padded armboard and the shoulder hanging slightly off the OR bed to allow movement through the entire range of motion. The perioperative team confirms that the patient's head is supported to avoid neck extension. A pad is placed beneath the scapula.

A soft tissue set and a large bone set; shoulder instruments; PMMA and cement supplies; the implants with associated instrumentation and trials; a power drill, reamer, and saw; and a pulsatile lavage system will be needed.

Operative Procedure
NEER TOTAL SHOULDER ARTHROPLASTY
(Figure 11-79)
1. The surgeon makes a 16-cm incision from the midacromion distally along the deltopectoral groove.

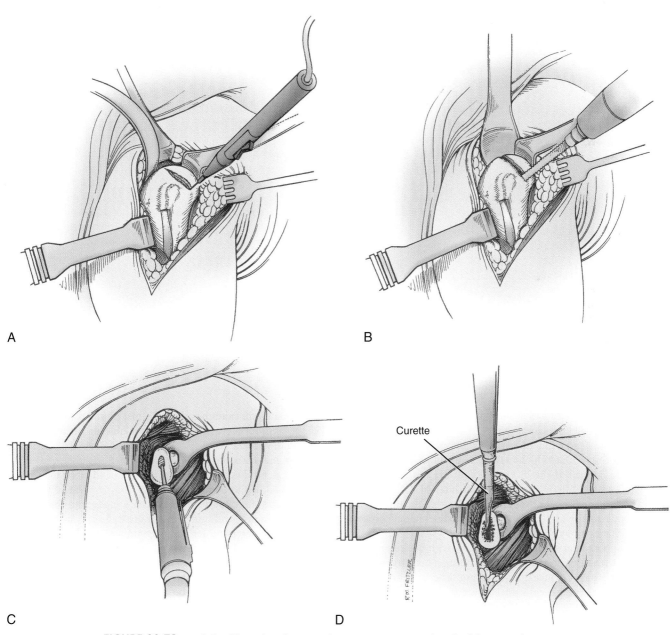

A

B

C

D

FIGURE 11-78 Total shoulder arthroplasty. **A,** The patient is positioned, and a deltopectoral incision is made to release the capsule. **B,** The humeral head is removed with a reciprocating saw. **C,** After exposure of the glenoid, a fenestration for the glenoid component is made. **D,** The glenoid bow is curetted.

Continued

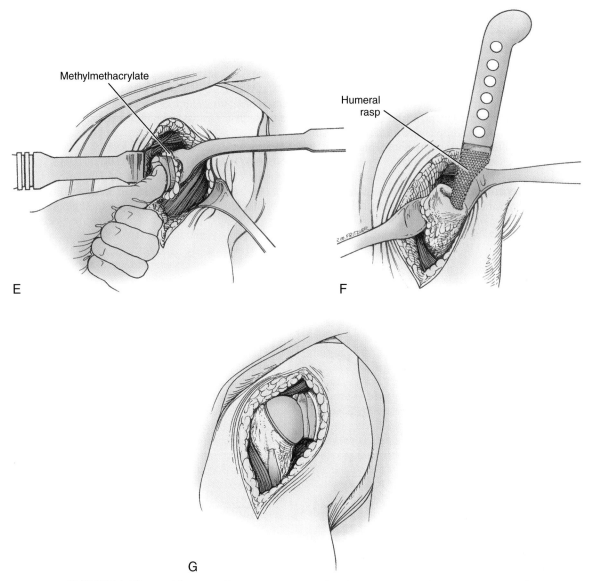

Methylmethacrylate

E

Humeral rasp

F

G

FIGURE 11-78, cont'd E, Cancellous bone is evacuated and cement impressed. F, The humeral shaft is rasped. G, The humeral component is inserted.

2. The cephalic vein is identified, and the surgeon opens and retracts the deltopectoral groove.

3. The deltoid attachment may be removed if the patient is large or muscular, which may affect rehabilitation.

4. The long head of the biceps is identified as the landmark between the tuberosities and rotator interval.

5. The surgeon elevates the subscapularis from the underlying capsule and divides it 2 cm medially to the bicipital groove, and places a stay suture.

6. The subscapularis is retracted medially with the lesser tuberosity, thereby exposing the joint and associated structures.

7. The capsule is exposed by elevation. The surgeon uses an elevator placed beneath the capsule to protect the axillary nerve. The long head of the biceps is left undisturbed and free in its groove so that it will continue to function as a depressor of the head after surgery.

8. After external rotation, the fractured humeral head is removed. The incision site is irrigated to remove blood and clots from the joint.

9. The surgeon examines the proximal humeral shaft to select the appropriately sized stem, available in various lengths and diameters.

10. Marginal osteophytes are trimmed.

11. The glenoid is inspected for integrity and sized for a prosthesis if it is to be replaced.

12. A central hole for a prosthesis fit is made into the glenoid with a high-speed burr and curette.

13. Stem diameter and length are estimated to check the prosthesis for fit. The largest stem diameter possible is used.

14. With the shaft held forward and upward, the surgeon locates the intramedullary canal with a long curette. A ¼-, ⅜-, or ½-inch drill bit is selected to correspond to the diameter of the canal; depending on the prosthesis stem length, the surgeon drills down the medullary canal 5 or 6 inches. Final preparation of the shaft is accomplished with the appropriately sized tapered reamer.

15. A heavy-gauge nonabsorbable suture is passed through holes that have been drilled on the tuberosities. The sur-

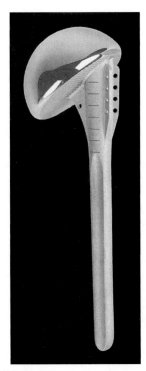

FIGURE 11-79 Neer shoulder prosthesis.

geon checks the length of the rotator cuff by pulling the tuberosities distal to the collar of the prosthesis.

16. Neck length and stability of the joint are determined before final impaction of the prosthesis.
17. A check for 35- to 40-degree retroversion is done by palpating the epicondyles at the elbow.
18. The implant is seated on the calcar with a driver and mallet, with its articular surface protected with a moist sponge. Just before final seating, further trimming of high spots with an osteotome or high-speed burr may be required. PMMA is used except in young patients, in whom a firm press-fit can be achieved.
19. Wires or sutures are passed through the holes in the neck of the prosthesis, reducing the tuberosities beneath the collar, and are secured. If wires are used, they are buried in drill holes in the bone.
20. The surgeon reduces the shoulder. The interval of the rotator cuff is closed and the biceps tendon reattached if previously detached.
21. The joint is irrigated as each compartment and layer is closed.
22. A closed-drainage system is inserted between the rotator cuff and deltoid, avoiding contact of the drainage tubes with the axillary artery. Routine closure is accomplished.
23. Dressings are placed between the body and the arm. A shoulder immobilizer is applied.

Passive range-of-motion machines may be used for patients prone to adhesion or contracture. Pendulum and gentle exercise are permitted at 10 days.

Total Elbow Arthroplasty

While not as prevalent as arthroplasty of the shoulder, knee, or hip, total elbow replacement (Figure 11-80) is indicated for patients with traumatic lesions or excessive bone loss from rheumatic or degenerative arthritis, resulting in elbow instability and

pain or bilateral elbow ankylosis. The design of implants and methods of fixation for postoperative stability have presented challenges that have been overcome in arthroplasty of other joints but remain a challenge in elbow arthroplasty. Postoperative stability of the elbow implant depends largely on the soft tissues surrounding the joint. There are devices that provide more constraint for the patient with significant soft tissue laxity or loss of bone stock. The Coonrad-Morrey, Tri-Axial, and Pritchard-Walker are just a few of the total elbow prostheses available.

The prosthesis may be used with or without PMMA, depending on the quality of the diseased bone and the design of the implant. If PMMA is not employed, bone grafting with local bone that has been resected may be used to help seat the ulnar component snugly and achieve adequate bony contact against the porous coating of the metal ulnar component. After elbow arthroplasty, patients with degenerative arthritis generally have better results than those with injury.

Procedural Considerations. The patient is placed in the supine or semi-Fowler position with the arm over the chest. A tourniquet is applied and can be inflated if needed. The arm is prepped from shoulder to fingers and draped. A soft tissue set and a small bone set; the total elbow implants and instruments; a power saw, drill, and burr; an awl; heavy-gauge wire; and a wire tightener will be needed. PMMA and cement supplies as well as a pulsatile lavage system are required if the prosthesis is placed with the use of PMMA.

Operative Procedure
1. The limb is exsanguinated, and the tourniquet is inflated to the desired pressure.
2. The surgeon makes a midline posterior incision, protecting the ulnar nerve.
3. The triceps mechanism is elevated in continuity with the periosteum, and the elbow joint is explored.
4. The surgeon explores the distal end of the humerus, proximal end of the ulna, and radial head while preserving the collateral ligaments.
5. The midportion of the trochlea is removed to allow access to the distal end of the humerus; the medullary canal is opened with a high-speed burr, and the canal is entered with a twist hand reamer.
6. The distal end of the humerus is notched with the appropriate cutting guide.
7. A high-speed burr is used to drill through subchondral bone to allow access to the medullary canal of the ulna and serially ream the canal.
8. After the humerus and ulna have been prepared for insertion of the trial prosthesis, the surgeon evaluates the elbow for flexion and extension. Bony adjustments are made where necessary.
9. The canals are cleaned of all bone fragments by irrigating with pulsatile antibiotic lavage.
10. The canal is dried before implant insertion, and the preparation is checked before the cement is mixed to ensure that the correct size of component is available.
11. The surgeon inserts the cement into the canals followed by the prosthesis. Flexion and extension of the elbow are avoided until the cement has hardened.
12. Any bone graft that may be required is secured with wire or pins.
13. The tourniquet is deflated, and hemostasis is achieved.

14. The triceps mechanism is repaired. The incision site is irrigated and closed. A drain may be inserted.
15. A long arm posterior splint is applied with the elbow at 90 degrees.

Total Ankle Joint Arthroplasty

Long-term results for total ankle arthroplasty, especially in the young population, are extremely poor. The procedure is reserved for older or more sedentary patients, especially those with subtalar or midtarsal arthritis. Ankle arthrodesis should be considered first in joint reconstruction. Indications for total ankle arthroplasty include (1) failed arthrodesis, (2) bilateral ankle arthritis when arthrodesis has already been performed on one ankle, (3) after talectomy because of avascular necrosis, and (4) revision of a previous arthroplasty. Total ankle replacement prostheses are made of high-density polyethylene and metal components.

Procedural Considerations. The patient is supine with the tourniquet placed. The leg is prepped and draped. A soft tissue set, a small bone set, the total ankle joint replacement instrumentation and implants, a power drill and saw, a pulsatile lavage system, and PMMA cement and supplies will be necessary.

Operative Procedure *(Figure 11-81)*
1. The surgeon makes an anterior incision over the ankle joint.
2. Using blunt and sharp dissection the surgeon exposes the tibiotalar joint and talus dome.
3. Once the center of the talus is identified and marked, a sizing template is used to mark the tibia.
4. A defect that is 1 inch wide by ⅜ inch deep is made using the air drill. Anchoring holes can be made in the tibia. The template is positioned in the defect while the foot is distracted.

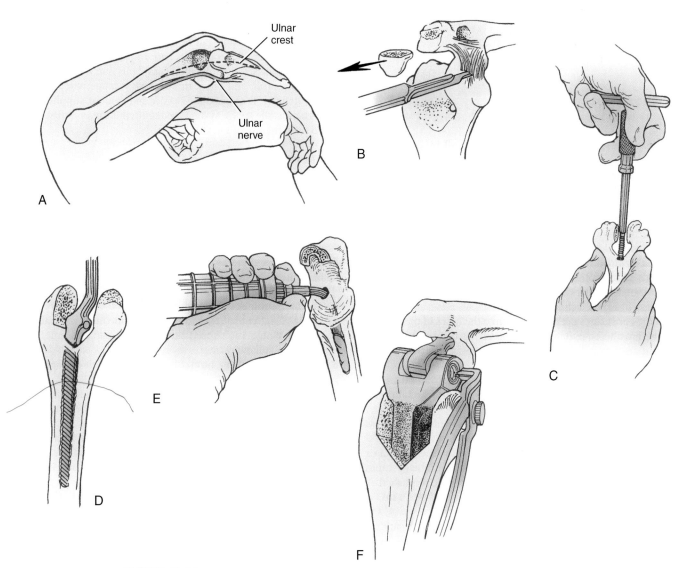

FIGURE 11-80 Total elbow arthroplasty. **A,** The arm is draped free, and the incision is made. **B,** The tip of the olecranon is excised with an oscillating saw. **C,** The canal is identified with a burr, and the canal is opened with a twist reamer. **D,** The capitellum is measured and cut. **E,** The medullary canal is cleaned and dried, and bone cement is inserted. **F,** The ulnar prosthesis is inserted, followed by cementing and inserting of the humeral components.

5. The talus is marked, and using a reciprocating saw the surgeon makes a groove that is ½ inch deep by 3/16 inch wide to accommodate the talar component.
6. A trial fit is carried out to ensure that the talar unit is in the center of the talus and that the tibial unit is parallel to the plane of the floor, both centered over the dome of the talus.
7. Once trial reduction is complete, the talar and tibial components are cemented into place.
8. The ankle joint is irrigated and closed, a drain inserted, and a posterior splint applied.

Metacarpal Arthroplasty

Metacarpal joint replacement is most often performed in patients who have pain or a disabling deformity associated with rheumatoid or degenerative arthritis of the metacarpo-

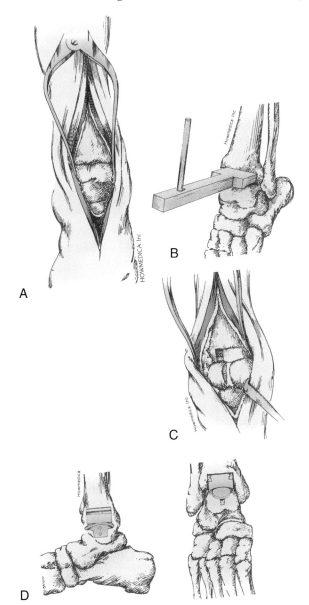

FIGURE 11-81 Total ankle arthroplasty. **A,** An anterior incision is made, and the tibiotalar joint and talus dome are exposed. **B,** The sizing template is used to mark the tibia. **C,** An air drill is used to create a defect, and anchoring holes are prepared. **D,** Trial reduction is completed, and the talar and tibial components are cemented into place.

phalangeal or interphalangeal joints. The results of rheumatoid reconstructive surgery are generally good, and pain can be eliminated and joint alignment and joint stability restored in the majority of patients. The greatest problems after surgery are weakness of grasp and pinch, and progression of the disease in adjacent joints.

Procedural Considerations. The patient is positioned supine with the arm extended on a hand table. A tourniquet is applied, and the entire extremity is prepped and draped. A hand set, instrumentation for implants, and implants are required, as well as a high-speed burr.

Operative Procedure
1. Incisions are made on the dorsum of the appropriate fingers.
2. The surgeon excises the proximal and distal portions of the joints and reams the intramedullary canals.
3. Sizers are used to facilitate a correct fit of the prosthesis.
4. Once the appropriately sized implant is determined, the surgeon positions it into the canal (Figures 11-82 and 11-83) and makes tendon and ligament repairs as indicated to improve stability.
5. The joint is irrigated and closed, and a bulky dressing is applied.
6. A short arm posterior splint is applied for immobilization.

Metatarsal Arthroplasty

Silastic implantation is indicated in the treatment of deformities associated with rheumatoid arthritis, hallux valgus, hallux rigidus, and a painful or unstable joint.

Procedural Considerations. The patient is supine. A tourniquet is applied, and the entire extremity is prepped and draped. A small bone set is required, as well as the implant instruments and implants, a power wire driver, and the microsagittal saw.

Operative Procedure
1. The incisions are made over the appropriate joints.
2. The surgeon resects the proximal phalanx and removes exostosis from the metatarsal head.
3. The medullary canal is reamed, and trial implants are fitted.
4. The surgeon determines the appropriate sized metatarsal implant and seats it.
5. The wound is irrigated and closed.

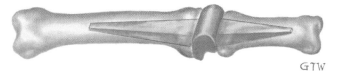

FIGURE 11-82 Metacarpophalangeal implant.

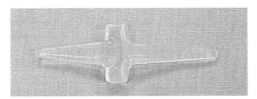

FIGURE 11-83 Silastic implant for finger joint.

6. A bulky compression dressing and orthopedic shoe are applied for early ambulation.

ARTHROSCOPY

Progress and development of arthroscopy and arthroscopic procedures have changed the approach, diagnosis, and treatment of many joint ailments. Arthroscopic techniques require skill and accomplishment in identifying three-dimensional relationships. The advantages of arthroscopic surgery surpass the disadvantages. Among the advantages are (1) decreased recovery and rehabilitation time; (2) smaller incisions; (3) less inflammatory response; (4) less postoperative pain, scar, and extensor disruption; (5) reduced complications; (6) reduced hospital stay and cost; and (7) easier, more rapid surgical procedures (Ambulatory Surgery Considerations).

Disadvantages usually relate to the size and delicacy of the instruments. Maneuverability within a joint may be difficult and produce scuffing and scoring of the articular surfaces.

Improvements in scope and camera systems, sharper scope optics, and miniaturization have made operative arthroscopy a logical extension of diagnostic arthroscopy. Surgical arthroscopy has also been aided with the development of numerous second puncture instruments and devices to repair and excise defects. There are a multitude of motorized shaving and abrader systems. Irrigation systems provide regulated disten-tion of the knee joint by infusing normal saline or lactated Ringer's solution. These systems may function by gravity flow or are mechanized with built-in microprocessors to monitor joint pressures and adjust accordingly. Lasers and ESUs can be used in tandem with arthroscopic equipment. Integrated video systems can record and store still and video images on film, tape, or digitally for education and documentation.

Arthroscopy is commonly performed on the knee, shoulder, and wrist. It is used less often in the elbow, hip, and ankle. Many corrective procedures that previously required an arthrotomy or other open procedure can be completed with the assistance of the arthroscope.

Arthroscopic equipment has certain requirements for care and handling. Fiberoptics, lenses, and cameras are heat-sensitive, requiring consideration for sterilization. Temperatures and moisture generated by steam autoclaves can damage materials used in video equipment or deteriorate the sealant, making the moisture accessible to the lens. Alternatives to steam sterilization for this equipment are ethylene oxide, cold sterilization, and high-level disinfection. Each requires consideration of patient care options for consistency. Equipment must be soaked according to the manufacturer's instructions, followed by complete rinsing and immersion in sterile water to prevent chemical burns. Cold-water sterilizing machines, which use bactericidal and sporicidal agents, can also be used to sterilize heat-sensitive equipment.

AMBULATORY SURGERY CONSIDERATIONS

Arthroscopic Surgery

Ambulatory surgery has long been part of orthopedic surgery. Recent advances in minimally invasive surgery and postoperative pain management have led to even more orthopedic procedures being performed in an ambulatory setting.

The most important factor in ambulatory surgery is patient selection. Appropriate patient selection is essential for successful orthopedic ambulatory surgery. Surgical, anesthesia, and nursing departments should work together to define the criteria used to identify suitable candidates for ambulatory surgery. Red flags should identify any patient with potential problems that indicate inability to tolerate the surgical procedure as an outpatient.

Preoperative assessment can determine which patients are the best candidates for ambulatory surgery. Careful review of health history, social history, and potential limitations postoperatively is vital in the initial assessment. Special attention to mobility both preoperatively and postoperatively is key for the orthopedic ambulatory surgery patient. Patients who will experience significant limited mobility postoperatively, live alone with no help available postoperatively, and have multiple medical co-morbidities are not ideal candidates for orthopedic ambulatory surgery. Patient education is initiated during the preoperative assessment. Gait-training, pain management, postoperative instructions, and transportation should be addressed preoperatively. Arrangements for any special equipment necessary for postoperative recovery should be made preoperatively. Attention to postoperative details before surgery will prevent delays with patient discharge postoperatively.

The anesthesia evaluation is done during preadmission testing. At that time, the anesthesia provider will develop a plan of care best suited for the patient and the anticipated surgery. Patient co-morbidities, length of procedure, and positioning during the procedure as well as the surgery itself are taken into consideration when establishing a plan of care.

KNEE ARTHROSCOPY

Knee arthroscopy is a common orthopedic ambulatory surgery procedure. New technology and approaches in surgery allow additional procedures to be done through the arthroscope. Once the patient has been identified as a candidate for ambulatory surgery, preoperative planning for preadmission testing, anesthesia evaluation, and patient education begin. The popular choice of anesthesia is one of two types based on patient history. Choices include regional or general anesthesia. Most providers prefer regional anesthesia for knee arthroscopy because of the decreased complication rates postoperatively. On the day of surgery, the history and physical are again reviewed with the patient. The surgical site is marked according to standards established by The Joint Commission and hospital policy. The patient is taken to the OR, anesthetized, prepared, and positioned for surgery. With regional anesthesia, those patients who would like to remain alert during the procedure can do so, watch the surgery on the monitor, and even converse with the surgeon about the findings. Once the surgery is over, a local anesthetic is injected into the joint to minimize pain. The length of the postoperative period depends on the regional anesthetic and the dose used. Patients will regain sensation and motion from trunk down to toes. Strength should be taken into consideration when gait-training is initiated. Patients may be discharged once discharge criteria are met, physician orders are reviewed with the patient, written discharge instructions and prescriptions are given to the patient, and the responsible adult escort is present. Phone numbers for any emergency should be listed on both physician and hospital discharge sheets.

Scopes, lenses, and fiberoptic cords should be handled carefully, and cords should never be kinked or twisted. Gradual deterioration and fiber breakage occur in mishandled cables, and light cannot be transmitted. When stored, the cords should be loosely coiled or hung.

Two types of arthroscopy may be performed. *Diagnostic arthroscopy* is for patients whose diagnosis cannot be determined by history or physical examination or whose CT or MRI findings are insufficient to warrant surgical exploration. Diagnostic arthroscopy may be performed before an anticipated arthrotomy, and surgical treatment may be modified on the basis of the findings of the arthroscopic examination. *Operative arthroscopy* is for patients presenting with an intraarticular abnormality or ligamentous injury.

Arthroscopy of the Knee

The knee is the joint in which arthroscopy lends itself to the greatest number of diagnostic and surgical procedures (Patient Safety). Arthroscopic surgery of the knee is indicated for diagnostic viewing, synovial biopsies, removal of loose bodies, resection of plicae, shaving of the patella, synovectomy, partial meniscectomy, meniscus repair, and ACL reconstruction. Anesthesia for knee arthroscopy may be general, spinal, or local. Tourniquets are often placed on the thigh but are inflated only if bleeding obscures the view. If there are no contraindications, an epinephrine solution may be injected at the portal sites or diluted into the distention fluid.

Procedural Considerations. The patient is positioned in the supine position on a standard OR bed. The surgeon may perform EUA before the patient is placed in position for the arthroscopy. The foot end of the bed may be flexed 90 degrees (Figure 11-84). A lateral post can be attached to the bed at the level of the midthigh. This post can provide a method of countertraction to open the medial side of the joint, providing better visualization of structures. After the leg is prepped, the entire

---

extremity is draped to allow complete range of motion and manipulation of the knee joint. The procedure requires specialized equipment for fluid collection and personnel protection.

Instruments and equipment needed for an arthroscopy depend on whether the procedure is diagnostic or operative. Diagnostic arthroscopy instruments include arthroscopy instrumentation (Figure 11-85); arthroscopes of 30 and 70 degrees; video with camera, light source, peripheral equipment, and arthroscopy pump (Figure 11-86); inflow and egress cannulae (Figure 11-87); 3-L bags of normal saline or lactated Ringer's solution; and a spinal needle. Operative arthroscopy instruments depend on the procedure planned. Arthroscopic powered shavers and abraders (Figure 11-88) are almost universally used. Instruments specific for ACL reconstruction or meniscal repair will be needed if those procedures are planned.

Operative Procedure
DIAGNOSTIC ARTHROSCOPY

1. The surgeon marks the anteromedial and anterolateral joint lines and portal positions with a skin marker.
2. The skin areas for portal placement are infiltrated with 1% lidocaine with 1:200,000 epinephrine. If the knee has an effusion, the surgeon aspirates it with a 16-gauge needle on a 60-ml syringe, followed by injection of a small amount of distending fluid.
3. After a small stab incision with a #11 knife blade, the surgeon inserts the irrigation cannula and trocar into the lateral suprapatellar pouch near the superior pole of the patella. Lactated Ringer's or normal saline solution is connected to the cannula, and the joint is distended using gravity or a pressure-sensitive arthroscopy pump.
4. A stab incision is then made anterolaterally or anteromedially 2 to 3 mm above the tibial plateau or patellar tendon at the joint line. A sharp trocar and sheath are inserted through the stab wound and just through the capsule.
5. A blunt trocar is used to pass the sheath into the knee joint. The surgeon removes the trocar and inserts a 30-degree scope into the sheath. The light source and video camera are connected to the scope.
6. The inflow may remain in the suprapatellar area, and the egress tubing is connected to the arthroscope, or the position may be reversed.

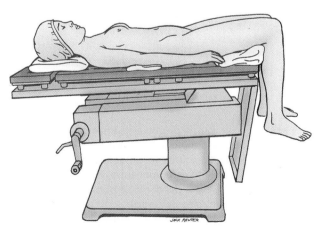

FIGURE 11-84 Positioning for a knee arthroscopy to enhance visualization.

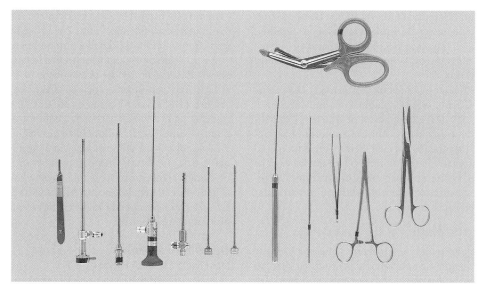

FIGURE 11-85 Arthroscopy instrumentation.

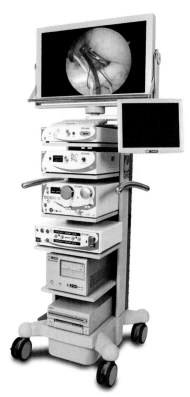

FIGURE 11-86 Arthroscopy tower with video monitor, light source, camera, and shaver system.

7. A spinal needle can be introduced under direct vision to determine the best angle for an opposite portal for insertion of probes and operative instruments. The cruciates and menisci are probed to determine integrity and tears.
8. The scope is moved to the opposite portal to allow a complete examination to be performed.
9. The joint is irrigated periodically and at the end of the procedure to maintain good visualization and clear the joint of blood and tissue fragments.

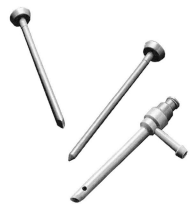

FIGURE 11-87 Cannulae.

10. The surgeon closes the portals with nylon or undyed polyglactin suture and ½-inch wound closure strips.
11. Bupivacaine (Marcaine) 0.25%, 30 ml, with epinephrine 1:200,000 may be injected intraarticularly to minimize bleeding and postoperative pain.
12. Gauze dressing, soft padding, and 4-inch and 6-inch elastic bandages are applied.

OPERATIVE ARTHROSCOPY. Operative arthroscopy includes procedures for resection of synovial plica, patellar debridement, excision of meniscal tears, partial or total meniscectomy, lateral retinacular release, removal of loose bodies, abrasion or drilling of osteochondral defects, synovectomy, treatment of osteochondritis dissecans, meniscal repairs, and ACL reconstruction.

Arthroscopic Resection and Repair of Meniscal Tear. Menisci are important structures in the knee joint that distribute load across the joint and provide capsular stability. A tear in the meniscus is the most common knee injury requiring arthroscopic surgery (Figure 11-89). Although both menisci can sustain tears, the medial meniscus is injured much more frequently than the lateral one.

Treatment of meniscus tears is aimed at preserving the structures. Some minor tears heal with cast immobiliza-

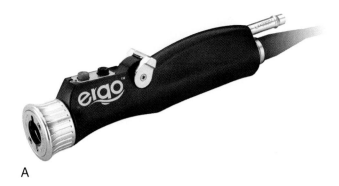

A

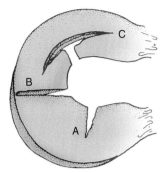

FIGURE 11-89 Meniscal tear. *A*, Incomplete. *B*, Complete. *C*, Incomplete longitudinal.

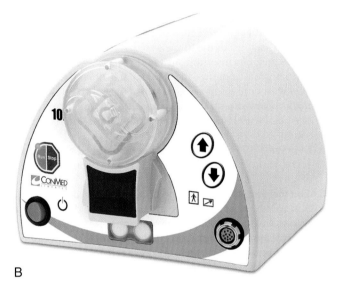

B

FIGURE 11-88 Arthroscopic shaver, **A**, with console, **B**.

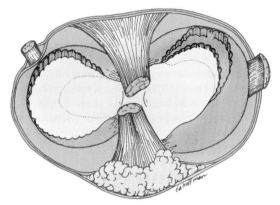

FIGURE 11-90 Lateral and medial meniscal excision.

tion, but some persist and cause symptoms. In these more severe cases, surgical intervention is necessary. A partial or complete meniscectomy may be necessary to alleviate troublesome symptoms such as locking, pain, and swelling (Figure 11-90). Partial meniscectomy is preferred, leaving a peripheral rim to share load bearing and stabilize the knee. Complete meniscectomy removes all of this load-bearing protection and also reduces knee stability. The goal is to leave an intact, balanced rim.

Arthroscopic meniscal repair is widely accepted as the standard of care. Arthroscopy provides better exposure than an arthrotomy does and enables the surgeon to approach the meniscus from the inner margin, where most tears begin. Suture repair is appropriate for meniscal tears occurring in the vascular zone (outer 10% to 25%), which heal predictably with repair and immobilization.

Operative Procedure

1. Steps 1 to 9 of the diagnostic arthroscopy procedure are repeated.
2. Working and scope portals are determined. The lateral bucket handle tear is identified, displaced, and reduced with a probe.
3. The attachment of the anterior horn of the meniscus is cut with a hook knife and clamped with a grasper.
4. An accessory portal is determined with a spinal needle.

5. The surgeon maintains traction and twisting motions on the meniscal horn to present a better edge to divide the remainder of the tear. Various scissors or push knives can be used to complete resection.
6. The motorized shaver is used to trim any frayed edges of the meniscus.
7. Limited debridement of chronic tears is completed to clean the edges.
8. When the medial meniscus is to be sutured, the surgeon places a cannula next to the inner edge of the tear. Two long meniscal-stitching needles with synthetic absorbable suture are inserted into the cannula, through the meniscus, across the tear, and through the capsule.
9. The surgeon palpates the needle tips beneath the skin, and makes a small incision to pull the suture out of the joint.
10. The sutures are tied over the capsule. Positioning the cannula enables either horizontal or vertical sutures to be placed.
11. After completing partial meniscectomy or suture repair, the surgeon irrigates the joint.
12. The incisions are closed, and the knee is lightly dressed and wrapped with soft rolled padding and elastic bandages.

Arthroscopic Anterior Cruciate Ligament Repair. The ACL is an important stabilizing structure of the knee and is the most frequently torn ligament. Injury is usually a result of simultaneous anterior and rotational stresses. Candidates for ACL reconstruction are active individuals with instability that is sufficient to interfere with their activities and that has failed to respond to bracing, rehabilitation, exercises, and other nonoperative treatment methods. The selected treatment method depends on the classification and severity of the tear, the experience and preference of the surgeon, and a history of a previous failed repair.

ACL reconstruction may be intraarticular, extraarticular, or a combination of both. Arthroscopic repair causes less patellar pain and decreased disturbance of extensor mechanisms and therefore is becoming the treatment of choice if there is no other significant capsular instability or gross disruption of the knee joint.

ACL repair most often involves replacement of the ligament with a substitute. Substitutes include autografts, allografts, and synthetic ligaments. Autografts are currently the method of choice, with a free central-third patellar tendon graft attached to patellar and tibial bone blocks used most often. The semitendinosus tendon and iliotibial band are sometimes used instead. Autografts may be used alone or augmented, although synthetic augmentation devices have fallen out of favor because of the development of chronic synovitis.

Procedural Considerations. Instrumentation for an ACL repair includes all instruments required for an operative arthroscopy. In addition, an ACL reconstruction guide system, fixation device of choice (bone screws, staples, spiked washers, or interference screws), bone tunnel plugs (Figure 11-91), a power drill, and microsagittal saw will be needed. If the surgeon believes that isometric placement of the graft is important, a tension isometer will be needed, as well as a system for finding that intraarticular position.

Operative Procedure: Reconstruction of the Anterior Cruciate Ligament with Patellar Tendon Graft

1. The surgeon performs an EUA immediately after anesthesia induction to further evaluate the stability of the knee.
2. A diagnostic arthroscopy is then carried out through the standard anteromedial and anterolateral portals.
3. Any meniscal tears or other intraarticular injuries are treated before attending to the ligament.
4. The surgeon debrides any remaining ACL tissue with a full-radius resector.
5. A notchplasty is then performed, widening the intercondylar notch with a 4.5-mm arthroplasty burr, rasp, osteotome, and curettes. Notchplasty aids in arthroscopic visualization and protects the graft from abrasion and amputation.
6. After preparation of the intercondylar area, the surgeon makes a small incision on the distal lateral aspect of the femur and extends the incision to the flare of the lateral femoral aspect of the condyle. A femoral aiming device is positioned, and a guide pin is inserted from the femoral site into the posterosuperior region of the intercondylar notch at an isometric point (Figure 11-92). Another small incision is made anteriorly, below the knee and medial to the tibial tubercle.
7. The tibial aiming device is positioned, and the surgeon inserts a guide pin from the anterior tibial incision into the intercondylar notch, anterior and medial to the center of the tibial anatomic attachment site of the ACL.
8. The pins are then replaced with a heavy suture passing through the femoral and tibial pin sites.
9. Isometric placement of the guide pins is checked with a tensioning device that is attached to the heavy suture. The knee is moved through a range of motion to determine correct isometric measurement.
10. Once isometric positioning is determined, the surgeon makes a longitudinal skin incision to the midline near the patellar tendon.

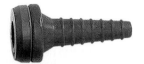

FIGURE 11-91 Example of a bone tunnel plug.

11. The central-third portion of the patellar tendon with tibial and patellar bone plugs is harvested with a mini-saw and osteotome. The graft is sized to the appropriate width, usually 10 to 12 mm, using sizing tubes (Figure 11-93).
12. Heavy nonabsorbable suture is placed through drill holes made at each end of the graft in the bone plugs (Figure 11-94).
13. The guide pins are then reinserted and overdrilled with cannulae that are close in width to the prepared graft. Overdrilling establishes the tunnels so that they are in the center of the previous insertion sites of the ACL.
14. The surgeon smoothes the femoral and tibial osseous tunnels with curettes, a rasp, or an abrader. If the tunnels are made before the graft is harvested, they are temporarily occluded with bone tunnel plugs to minimize fluid extravasation.
15. Both ends of the graft are fixed with a barbed staple, bone screw with washer, interference screw, or ligament button (Figure 11-95).
16. The incisions and joint are irrigated and closed.
17. A hinged knee brace may be applied over the dressing. The brace allows 10 to 90 degrees of motion.

Arthroscopic Posterior Cruciate Ligament Repair. Surgical procedures for tears of the PCL are considered if significant disabling instability has occurred. Patients usually return to adequate function without operative treatment. The arthroscopic procedure for repair of the PCL is similar to the technique used to repair the ACL, except that isometric placement is posterior within the joint and the femoral attachment is proximal to the medial epicondyle.

Arthroscopy of the Shoulder

Shoulder arthroscopy is a useful diagnostic and therapeutic tool in the management of shoulder disorders. It is particularly beneficial in the evaluation and management of patients with chronic shoulder problems. Arthroscopy provides extensive visualization of the intraarticular aspect of the shoulder joint and is performed for removal of loose bodies; lysis of adhesions; synovial biopsy; synovectomy; bursectomy; stabilization of dislocations; correction of glenoid labrum, biceps tendon, and rotator cuff tears; and relief of impingement syndrome.

Procedural Considerations. The patient is either in the lateral position or in a sitting position using a "beach chair" positioner. The lateral position is maintained using a vacuum beanbag positioning device or lateral rolls with a kidney rest. Three-inch adhesive tape is secured across the patient's hips. Proper padding of the uninvolved axilla and lower extremity is important to prevent soft tissue or neurovascular problems. The affected extremity is placed in a shoulder suspension system, and Buck's traction or a Velcro immobilizer is applied to the forearm to achieve adequate distraction to the glenohumeral joint. The extremity is abducted 40 to 60 degrees and forward-flexed 10 to 20 degrees, with 5- to 15-pound weights placed on the pulley system. Weight may be added to further

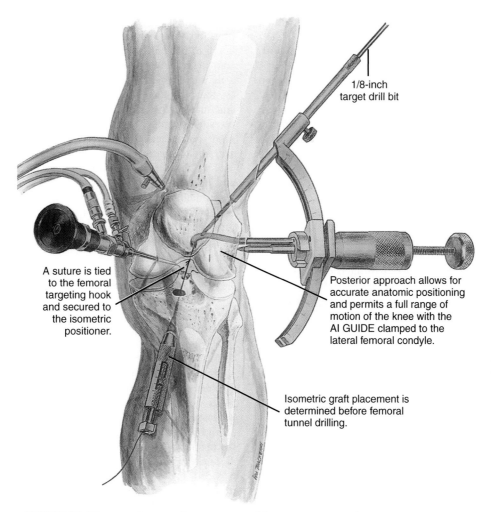

1/8-inch
target drill bit

A suture is tied
to the femoral
targeting hook
and secured to
the isometric
positioner.

Posterior approach allows for
accurate anatomic positioning
and permits a full range of
motion of the knee with the
AI GUIDE clamped to the
lateral femoral condyle.

Isometric graft placement is
determined before femoral
tunnel drilling.

FIGURE 11-92 Femoral aiming device positioned for anterior cruciate ligament reconstruction.

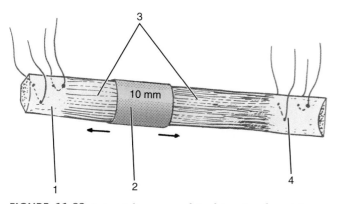

3

10 mm

1   2   4

FIGURE 11-93 Sizing tubes are used to determine the minimum diameter of tunnel necessary for passage of the graft.

distract the glenohumeral joint, taking care not to overstretch the axillary artery.

The shoulder is prepped and draped free, permitting full range of motion during the procedure.

The operative instruments and arthroscope commonly used for the knee may also be used in the shoulder, plus an 18-gauge needle, switching sticks, and a Wissinger rod. A variety of fix-

ation devices (screws and tacks) can be used to repair bony defects and tears of the labrum.

Operative Procedure (Figure 11-96)

1. An 18-gauge spinal needle is inserted through the posterior soft spot and directed anteriorly toward the coracoid process, where the surgeon's index finger has been positioned.
2. The glenohumeral joint is distended with normal saline or lactated Ringer's solution. This facilitates entry of the arthroscope.
3. Bupivacaine (Marcaine) 0.25%, 2 to 3 ml, with epinephrine 1:200,000 is injected along the needle track to minimize bleeding.
4. With the needle removed, the surgeon makes a stab incision with a #11 blade over the needle site.
5. The arthroscope sleeve and sharp trocar are then introduced through the posterior joint capsule.
6. Once the capsule has been penetrated, a blunt obturator replaces the sharp trocar to enter the joint.
7. The arthroscope is inserted and attached to inflow and outflow tubing, the video camera, and the light source.
8. Operative instruments are placed through an anterior portal that is established laterally to the coracoid process by using a Wissinger rod. A third portal can be established near

the anterior portal or supraspinous fossa portal. Switching sticks are used to change portals.

9. The surgeon moves the arm and rotates it as needed to visualize various structures in and around the joint.

10. Glenoid tears can be repaired with the insertion of an absorbable fixation tack.

11. At the conclusion of the procedure, the joint is irrigated. The surgeon may inject a long-acting local anesthetic into the joint and subacromial space through the portal to minimize postoperative discomfort.

12. The puncture wounds are closed and dressed with a sterile 4 × 4 gauze pad. The patient's arm is placed in a sling for recovery.

Arthroscopy of the Elbow

The elbow joint is accessible to arthroscopic examination, although it requires more attention to detail than the knee because instruments must be placed through deeper muscle layers and close to important neurovascular structures.

Arthroscopy of the elbow, both diagnostic and operative, has become fairly routine. Indications for its use include extraction of loose bodies, evaluation or debridement of osteochondritis dissecans of the capitulum and radial head, partial synovectomy in rheumatoid disease, debridement and lysis of adhesions of posttraumatic or degenerative processes at or near the elbow, diagnosis of a chronically painful elbow when the diagnosis is obscure, and evaluation of fractures of the capitulum, radial head, or olecranon.

Procedural Considerations. General anesthesia is preferred to local anesthesia because it affords complete comfort to the patient and provides total muscle relaxation.

The patient is placed in either the supine or the prone position. In the supine position, the forearm is flexed on an armboard or placed in a prefabricated wrist gauntlet connected to an overhead pulley device and tied off at the end of the OR bed. This provides excellent access to both the medial and lateral aspects of the elbow, allows the forearm to be freely pronated and supinated, and places the important neurovascular structures in the antecubital fossa at maximum relaxation.

A tourniquet is routinely used for hemostasis. The entire arm, including the hand, is prepped and draped.

The three portals most commonly used for diagnostic and operative arthroscopy of the elbow are the anterolateral, anteromedial, and posterolateral.

Operative arthroscopy instruments commonly used for the knee may also be used in the elbow. However, smaller-diameter scopes and instruments may be desired instead.

Operative Procedure

1. The surgeon outlines the bony anatomic landmarks with a sterile marking pen before initiation of the procedure. Lateral structures to be marked and identified are the radial head and the lateral epicondyle. The medial epicondyle is also marked.

2. An 18-gauge needle is inserted anteriorly to the radial head from the lateral side, and the joint is distended.

3. Once joint distention has been achieved with approximately 15 to 30 ml of lactated Ringer's or normal saline solution, the surgeon makes a stab wound incision with a #11 blade, and inserts the sharp trocar with cannula through the joint capsule.

4. The sharp trocar is replaced with the blunt obturator to provide safe entry of the cannula into the joint.

5. The scope replaces the blunt obturator and is attached to the video and light source.

6. A second portal and third portal are established anteromedially and posterolaterally for triangulation. With the

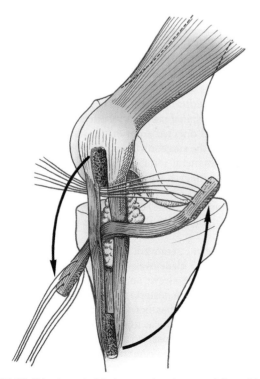

FIGURE 11-94 Three drill holes are placed into each bone block of the patellar graft, and a heavy suture is placed into each drill hole.

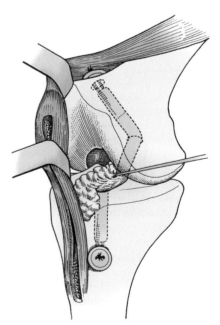

FIGURE 11-95 A patellar tendon graft is affixed by tying of sutures over bone buttons at the tibial and femoral drill holes.

patient's elbow flexed to 90 degrees and adequate distention maintained at the time of insertion of the instruments, the surgeon displaces the neurovascular structures anteriorly. This provides a greater area above the medial and lateral humeral epicondyles in which to insert the various instruments.

7. Outflow and inflow are controlled by alternating the valve on the scope or using a separate 18-gauge needle with drainage tubing.

8. After diagnostic and operative procedures have been completed, the joint is irrigated, the puncture sites are sutured, and a compression dressing is applied with soft rolled padding and elastic bandages.

Arthroscopy of the Ankle

The talocalcaneal articulations are complex and play an important role in the movements of inversion and eversion of the foot. The subtalar joints function as a single unit, but anatomically they are divided into anterior and posterior joints. The

perioperative team must be familiar with the extraarticular anatomy of the ankle to prevent neural or vascular damage.

Indications for ankle arthroscopy include osteochondral fragments or loose bodies, persistent ankle pain after trauma and despite adequate conservative treatment, biopsy, posttraumatic arthritis of the ankle joint, unstable ankle before lateral ligamentous reconstruction, and osteochondritis dissecans of the talus.

Procedural Considerations. General anesthesia is preferable because manipulation and distraction of the joint to obtain adequate arthroscopic viewing require muscle relaxation. The position of the patient is based on the surgeon's preference. The patient may be supine with the knee flexed approximately 70 degrees or supine with a sandbag under the buttock of the operative side. Ankle and thigh holders may be used; when better posterior visualization is necessary, a distractor may be used to increase the space between the tibia and talus. A tourniquet is placed around the upper thigh but is not used unless

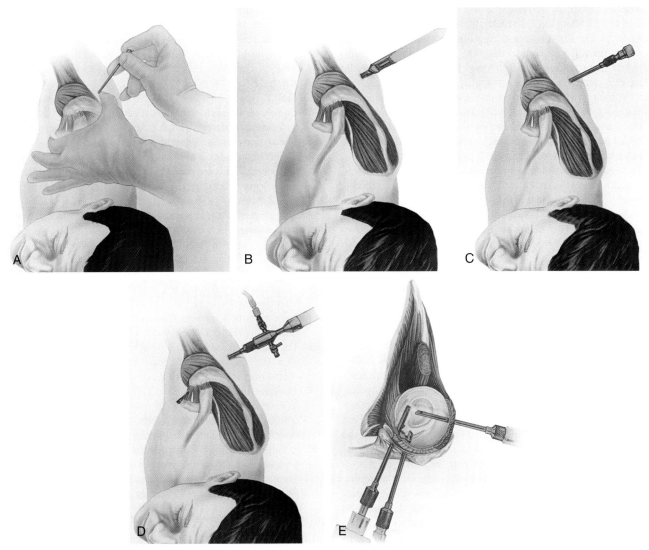

FIGURE 11-96 Shoulder arthroscopy. **A,** The spinal needle is inserted for dilation of the joint if indicated. **B,** An incision is made over the glenohumeral joint. **C,** The arthroscope sleeve and sharp trocar are inserted. **D,** The arthroscope is inserted and attached to the inflow and outflow tubing, video camera, and light source. **E,** Operative instruments are placed through the portal.

excessive bleeding, uncontrolled by irrigation, is encountered. Routine skin prepping and draping are done. Miniaturized instruments and needle scopes for the ankle are used.

Operative Procedure

1. Using a sterile marking pen, the surgeon outlines important extraarticular anatomic structures on the skin.
2. The ankle joint is then examined, using the anterolateral portal. The anteromedial joint line is palpated, and an 18-gauge, 1½-inch needle is inserted into the joint.
3. Sterile plastic extension tubing is attached to the needle, and a 50-ml plastic Luer-Lok syringe filled with normal saline is connected to the tubing to distend the joint. Approximately 15 to 20 ml is needed.
4. After intraarticular injection is confirmed by the ease with which the saline can be injected and by palpation of the joint as it is distended, the surgeon makes a small incision with a #11 blade over the site of the anterolateral portal.
5. A hemostat is then inserted and used to dissect to the capsule.
6. The sheath of the arthroscope and sharp trocar are placed into the incision, angled approximately 30 to 45 degrees laterally, and inserted with a sharp plunge as joint distention is maintained. Entrance into the joint is felt as the sleeve and trocar "pop" through the capsule and is confirmed by the rush of saline on removal of the trocar from the sheath.
7. The arthroscope is inserted into the sheath, the needle is removed, and the plastic tubing and syringe are attached to the stopcock on the arthroscope sleeve. The video camera and light source are connected to the scope. Joint distention must be maintained.
8. Triangulation through other portals is easily done by first inserting the 18-gauge needle for localization while viewing with the arthroscope. Posterior viewing is done in the same fashion except that the patient is usually placed in the prone position and instruments are inserted through the posterior portals.
9. After the procedure is completed, the surgeon irrigates the joint, closes the wounds with wound closure strips or a single suture, and covers the wound with a dressing and short leg compression elastic wrap.

SURGERY OF THE SPINE

Treatment of Back Pain

Back pain is a natural result of degenerative and arthritic change, punctuated by protrusion or rupture of a disc. It gradually progresses but may also disappear gradually. With aging, a degenerative disc-space narrowing or facet arthropathy begins to appear radiologically. The lower lumbar spine carries the burden of the body's weight, holds a person upright, and returns the body to the vertical position from sitting, lying, or a bent-over position. Degenerative changes, ruptured disc, and facet arthropathy develop at the lowest two limb segments, where the greatest weight, torsion, and shearing stress occur. This degeneration sometimes extends into the upper and middle spine.

Cervical-spine degenerative disc narrowing also develops most often at the two lowest cervical spaces, which are also the levels of greatest stress resulting from movement of the head and neck. Sometimes lumbar or cervical degenerative changes develop early from excessive repetitive movements or injury.

Epidural steroid injections, electrodes, stimulators, braces, or traction may treat back pain. A natural recovery may result after 6 or 7 days of intense pain, subsiding between 6 weeks and 4 months. Motor and sensory deficits usually disappear with resolution of pain. The ability to recover without surgery depends on fragment size and compression on the nerve root. Neural compression remains the major indication for disc excision.

Spinal fusion is a consideration, usually for patients with demonstrable posttraumatic, postsurgical, rheumatoid, infectious, or neoplastic instability.

Procedural Considerations. Radiographs are obtained. The patient's bilateral pulses and range of motion in all of the extremities are assessed. Elastic wraps or sequential compression devices may be placed. The patient is positioned prone to eliminate lordosis, reduce venous congestion, and keep the abdomen free with chest rolls or special frames after induction of general anesthesia. Depending on the extent of the procedure, blood availability may be required. The skin is prepped and the area draped. A spinal laminectomy set is used, in addition to a spinal retractor of choice and a bipolar ESU. Hemostatic adjuncts such as gelatin foam, oxidized cellulose strips, thrombin, and bone wax should be available.

Operative Procedure
LAMINECTOMY

1. The surgeon makes a midline incision over the affected disc and carries it sharply down to the supraspinous ligament.
2. The supraspinous ligament is incised, and the muscles are dissected subperiosteally from the spines and laminae of the vertebrae. These are retracted with a self-retaining retractor.
3. The surgeon denudes the laminae and ligamentum flavum with a curette.
4. A small part of the inferior margin of the lamina is removed with a rongeur.
5. The ligamentum flavum is grasped and incised where it fuses with the interspinous ligament, and this flap is then sharply removed to expose the dura.
6. The dura is then retracted medially, and the nerve root is identified.
7. Once identified, the nerve root is retracted medially so that the underlying posterior longitudinal ligament can be exposed.
8. The surgeon incises the posterior longitudinal ligament over the intervertebral space in a cruciate fashion, and enters the disc space with a pituitary grasping forceps.
9. The disc material is systematically removed, taking care not to exceed the distance to the anterior annulus. A complete search for additional fragments of nucleus pulposus, both inside and outside the disc space, is then carried out.
10. Residual bleeding is controlled with bipolar coagulation.
11. The surgeon closes the wound with absorbable sutures in the supraspinous ligament and subcutaneous tissue. Various nonabsorbable sutures or staples are used for skin closure.

Minimally Invasive Spine Surgery

Advances in technology have made minimally invasive spinal surgery (MISS) available to certain patients. Candidates for minimally invasive spine surgery are carefully selected by the surgeon. Conditions that may be amenable to MISS include disc herniation, spinal stenosis, and kyphosis. The need to con-

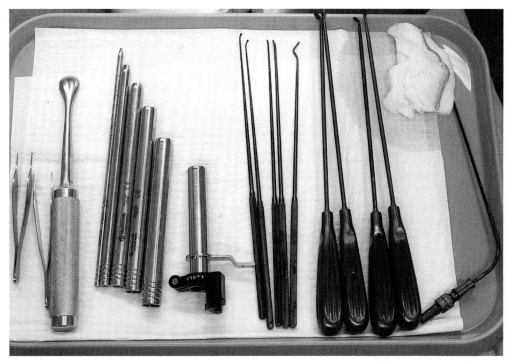

FIGURE 11-97 Instruments used for tubular microdiscectomy.

vert from MISS to the traditional incision must be discussed with the patient before the surgery and the perioperative nurse and surgical technologist must prepare for that possibility. The microdiscectomy procedure, used to treat disc herniation, is described below.

Procedural Considerations. The perioperative nurse and surgical technologist ensure that all equipment is available and assembled before the patient's arrival into the OR. Equipment needed includes the C-arm, microscope, and radiolucent spinal table. After the administration of a general anesthetic, the patient is positioned prone on the radiolucent spinal table. Care is taken to ensure proper padding of bony prominences and proper positioning of extremities. The skin is prepped and draped. Instrumentation for MISS includes the tubular microdiscectomy set and the tubular retractor (Figure 11-97). A high-speed drill and hemostatic agents such as gelatin foam, thrombin, and bone wax should be available. The perioperative nurse places sequential compression devices on the patient.

Operative Procedure

1. The surgeon inserts an 18-gauge spinal needle in the back at the level of the disc herniation and confirms the correct level with the C-arm.
2. The surgeon makes a 1- to 1.5-cm incision at the previously identified level.
3. A Cobb elevator and sequentially sized dilators are used to serially dilate the soft tissues, preserving the integrity of the muscles and ligaments.
4. The surgeon inserts a tubular retractor and connects the flex arm directly to the spinal table.
5. The tubular retractor is used as a viewing portal to visualize and operate on the spine (Figure 11-98).

6. The surgeon confirms the level again with x-ray and moves the draped microscope into position.
7. Using the long electrode on the ESU, the surgeon dissects the tissue.
8. A high-powered burr and/or assorted sizes of Kerrison punches are used to remove part of the caudal lamina.
9. Once nerve roots are identified, the surgeon enters the disc space and removes the extruded disc material with pituitary grasping forceps.
10. Gelatin foam and cotton pledgets are used to control bleeding along with the bipolar ESU.
11. The surgeon irrigates and closes the wound.

Pedicle Fixation of the Spine

Pedicle screw fixation (Figure 11-99) is a method of surgical fixation of the spinal column. Screw fixation was initially used in an attempt to avoid postoperative external immobilization and prolonged bed rest. Pedicle screw fixation has been used most often in degenerative processes, particularly iatrogenic instability after decompression, degenerative and isthmic spondylolisthesis, and discogenic disease. It is also indicated for tumor, trauma, degenerative spinal disorders, postoperative hypermobility, and infection.

Three basic approaches for fixation have been described as the procedure has evolved. Each has improved on the first, based on anatomic placement of the screw. Positioning and placement of the screw within the spine are established after direct visualization of the pedicle.

Procedural Considerations. After the administration of a general anesthetic, the patient is positioned prone. The skin is prepped, and drapes are applied. A spinal laminectomy set is used in addition to the instrumentation and implants of choice, a spinal retractor, power equipment such as a high-

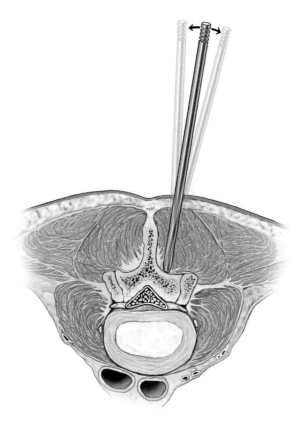

FIGURE 11-98 Wanding maneuver is used to change the position of the tubular retractor and reach different areas of the spine.

speed motorized hand tool, and hemostatic adjuncts such as gelatin foam, thrombin, and bone wax. A bone graft set will be needed to harvest graft from the iliac crest.

Operative Procedure

1. The surgeon makes a standard midline incision. The surgeon follows the steps as described in the laminectomy procedure to expose the spine.
2. The areas of the pedicles to be fixated are located using external landmarks.
3. The surgeon removes the posterior cortical wall at the entrance site using a high-speed burr.
4. A Penfield dissector is used to identify the entrance hole through the pedicle.
5. The surgeon inserts a gearshift probe to identify the path into the vertebral body.
6. The hole is tapped (5.5-mm tap) and widened.
7. The surgeon places the screw(s). Guidelines for screw sizes are 7 mm for S1, L5, and L4; 6.25 mm for L3 and L2; 5.5 mm for L1 and T12.
8. A posterolateral graft is performed, using graft strips from the iliac crest.
9. The surgeon contours the plate or rod to approximate the patient's physiologic lordosis. The longitudinal device is locked onto the screws in the appropriate position.
10. A screw-plate system may require use of the oblique and transverse washers between the screw head and plate to provide a flush fit at the screw-plate interface.

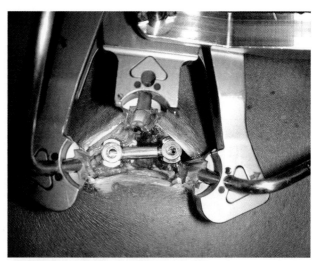

FIGURE 11-99 Pedicle screw placement using the MaXcess retractor and SpheRx fixation system by NuVasive, Inc.

11. The foramina are checked for patency before closure. The excess portion of the screw is cut close to the upper locking device.
12. A suction drain is placed; the wound is closed in layers.

Treatment of Scoliosis

Scoliosis is a three-dimensional deformity (Figure 11-100) with lateral deviation of the spinal column from the midline; it may include rotation or deformity of the vertebrae. Types are congenital, juvenile, adolescent, and adult. School screening programs provide quick and simple detection. For effective treatment of scoliosis, early detection is critical.

Scoliosis can be idiopathic (80% of the time) or congenital and may result from muscular or neurologic diseases or unequal leg lengths. Numerous posterior and anterior segmental spinal instrumentation systems are available for the treatment of idiopathic scoliosis. As a consequence, fixation strategies are more complex than they were with Harrington instrumentation. The newer systems provide better sagittal control and more stable fixation, allowing quicker mobilization of the patient. On thin patients, however, the bulk of these implants may be a problem.

Posterior Spinal Fusion with Harrington Rods. Posterior spinal fusion is most frequently performed in adolescence, when the laterally deviated curve is still flexible. Harrington rods are internal splints that help maintain the spine as straight as possible until the vertebral body fusion has become solid. Distraction rods are placed on the concave side of the curve, and compression rods are placed on the convex side. On the convex side of the curve, three to eight hooks are inserted in the transverse processes of the vertebrae and pulled together with a threaded rod. In this way the scoliotic deformity can be corrected as much as the flexibility of the spine allows.

The posterior elements of the vertebrae are denuded of soft tissue, and the bone graft is added. Blood loss can be expected, and an accurate record of the loss must be maintained. After surgery the patient is placed in an immobilizing jacket.

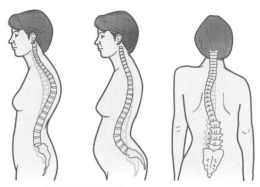

FIGURE 11-100 Scoliotic deformity.

Some disadvantages of the Harrington rod system over other systems are that there is only end-point fixation, rod breakage is increased, fixation is less, sagittal plane curves are difficult to manage, distraction for correction is not always desired, and the patient is required to wear a postoperative cast or brace. Other systems have evolved from the Harrington rods that are used for correction of some scoliotic deformities. It remains a feasible treatment of idiopathic scoliosis.

PROCEDURAL CONSIDERATIONS. The patient is placed in the prone position on a spinal table, or a spinal frame to facilitate respiration. Before the procedure begins, an x-ray cassette is placed under the patient so that a radiograph for accurate identification of the vertebrae to be fused can be taken during the operation. A single straight longitudinal incision is made down the midline of the back. Because of the amount of bleeding, the skin and subcutaneous tissues are often infiltrated with a vasoconstricting solution, such as epinephrine.

Basic spinal instrumentation and bone graft instruments are required, plus the Harrington rod instrumentation. A large pin cutter, designed to cut large pins but provided with a small end so that it will fit in the wound, should be available.

OPERATIVE PROCEDURE
1. The appropriate hooks are selected and inserted. A Harrington distraction rod of appropriate length is inserted through the two proximal self-adjusting hooks, which have been placed under the laminae.
2. A rod clamp is clamped onto the Harrington rod just below the hook, and a single regular spreader is used to obtain the first inch of distraction.
3. The Bobechko spreader is used to span over the first hook, closest to the smooth part of the rod, to apply distraction force on the most proximal hook.
4. Two C locking rings are inserted around the first ratchet immediately below the hook to prevent dislodgment of the hooks. The excessive length of protruding rod above the most proximal hook is removed with a rod cutter. The compression is tightened.

Luque Segmental Spinal Rod Procedure. The Luque segmental method employs smooth, L-shaped, stainless-steel rods, usually ³⁄₁₆ or ¼ inch in diameter, with sublaminar wires placed at every level possible. It is more secure and longer than the Harrington rod system and was the first system to employ multiple-point fixation. Luque instrumentation applies corrective forces to the spinal segments at each level, thereby spreading the corrective forces throughout the length of the deformity. Two Luque rods are wired to both sides of the spine. The rods are contoured to achieve no more than 10 degrees of increased correction beyond that exhibited on preoperative x-ray study.

PROCEDURAL CONSIDERATIONS. The patient is placed in the prone position as described for the Harrington rod procedure. Patient care is provided (see Laminectomy, p. 518). A straight midline incision is made in the back. Because of the amount of bleeding, the skin and subcutaneous tissues are often infiltrated with a vasoconstricting solution, such as epinephrine. Basic spinal instrumentation is required. In addition, Luque rods and instrumentation, a wire tightener and cutter, and bone graft instruments will be needed.

OPERATIVE PROCEDURE
1. The ligamentum flavum is detached, exposing the neural canal.
2. The surgeon passes doubled stainless-steel suture wire under the lamina. The wire loop is cut later to form two wires at each level.
3. Total bilateral facetectomies are made, forming posterolateral troughs for subsequent bone grafts.
4. Wedge osteotomies may be necessary in severe immobile curves to avoid stretching the spinal cord during correction.
5. The wire loop is cut, resulting in two separate wires at each level.
6. The L bend is secured to the base of the spinous process to prevent rod migration.
7. Initial placement of the convex rod is made.
8. Initial placement of the concave rod is made.
9. Transverse wiring is done to add increased stability to the system.
10. Stabilization of the lumbosacral joint is corrected by bending the rods distally to form sacral bars.

Cotrel-Dubousset System Procedure. The Cotrel-Dubousset system (Figure 11-101) provides three-dimensional correction of spinal deformities without sublaminar wiring and neurologic risks. This instrumentation permits distraction, compression, and derotation. The scoliotic curve is corrected by derotation and, at the same time, restores the normal sagittal contours. In addition to correction of scoliosis, the Cotrel-Dubousset system can be applied to correct kyphosis or lordosis and to stabilize and rebuild the spine after tumor resection or after injury. No external support is necessary. The Cotrel-Dubousset system has no ratchets or notches. It consists of metallic rods with diamond crosscut patterns on which hooks and screws can be positioned in any position, level, or degree of rotation. The rod is held in the open hooks with blockers. The rods are then interlocked by means of devices for transverse traction. The Cotrel-Dubousset system was the forerunner to the systems used today, such as the Texas Scottish Rite Hospital (TSRH) system and the Isola system.

PROCEDURAL CONSIDERATIONS. The patient is placed in the prone position after induction of general anesthesia. Patient assessment and precautions for the prone position are initiated. Basic spinal instrumentation is required in addition to the Cotrel-Dubousset system and instrumentation as well as the instruments used for harvesting the bone graft.

OPERATIVE PROCEDURE
1. Closed hooks are inserted at both ends of the surgical site, and open hooks are inserted at various levels between the closed hooks.

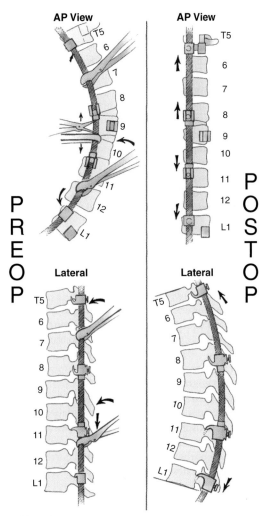

FIGURE 11-101 Cotrel-Dubousset system, representing rotation of rods.

2. Decortication and facet excision are done at the remaining interposed vertebral levels for rod placement.
3. Bone graft is placed in the areas that will be under the rod.
4. The surgeon bends the appropriate concave rod to shape for sagittal-plane correction and manipulates it into the end hooks.
5. Stabilization along the length is achieved with blockers that anchor the rod into the open hooks.
6. The spine is then derotated using the rod holders. The frontal-plane scoliosis curve becomes the sagittal-plane kyphosis.
7. Hooks are reseated for secure fixation.
8. To correct kyphosis, the surgeon bends the convex rod to shape and seats it.
9. Once the rods are placed, the surgeon applies the device for transverse traction (DTT), usually near the ends of the rods, to complete the stabilization.
10. Remaining bone graft is then applied to the fusion area.

Texas Scottish Rite Hospital (TSRH) Crosslink System. The TSRH crosslink system (Figure 11-102) is a multicomponent stainless-steel implant used to lock spinal rods together rigidly. Locking the rods increases construction stiffness and prevents rod migration. The system was originally designed for

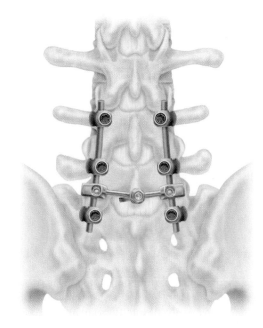

FIGURE 11-102 TSRH SILO Spinal System with an X10 CROSSLINK Plate system.

the Luque segmental system to prevent migration between the rods and wires before complete fusion occurred. By rigidly crosslinking the rods, loss of scoliotic correction was reduced. This system can also be used with the Harrington and Cotrel-Dubousset systems. Crosslinks are indicated when the rigidity of a spinal system alone is not sufficient to generate fusion in a reasonable amount of time.

PROCEDURAL CONSIDERATIONS. The patient is administered a general anesthetic and positioned prone. The skin is prepped, and drapes are applied. A spinal laminectomy set is used. Instrumentation and implants of choice, a spinal retractor, and power equipment such as a high-speed handheld tool will be necessary. Hemostatic adjuncts such as gelatin foam, thrombin, oxidized cellulose, and bone wax should be available.

OPERATIVE PROCEDURE

1. Eyebolts are placed on the spinal rods before the rods are implanted.
2. The rods are secured with hooks or wires, depending on the system used.
3. Once the rods are positioned, cross plates of varying widths accommodating different rod-to-rod distances are bolted in place between the rods and nuts.

Anterior Spinal Fusion with Isola Instrumentation. Isola instrumentation involves screw fixation into each vertebral body, complete disc excision and grafting, and segmental connection of the vertebral bodies. A semirigid rod connects the segments. The Isola anterior instrumentation is indicated in idiopathic scoliosis patients, approximately 10 to 30 years of age, with thoracolumbar or upper lumbar curves of 40 to 65 degrees.

PROCEDURAL CONSIDERATIONS. The patient is positioned in a lateral decubitus position so that posteroanterior and lateral intraoperative radiographs can be taken. The anesthesia provider should ensure incomplete pharmacologic paralysis, to allow for intraoperative neurophysiologic monitoring. In addition to a major soft tissue set and laminectomy set, the Isola instrumentation and implants, a vascular set, and power equipment will be needed.

OPERATIVE PROCEDURE

1. The surgeon approaches the spine through a transthoracic retroperitoneal (or retropleural retroperitoneal) approach, resecting the rib two vertebral levels above the upper instrumented vertebrae.

2. The sympathetic chain is mobilized laterally with the psoas.

3. The segmental vessels are temporarily occluded and, provided that there are no monitoring changes, ligated.

4. The discs are exposed to the far side to allow a full annulectomy. The bodies, however, are not exposed much beyond the midline.

5. A full 360-degree discectomy and annulectomy are done, exposing the posterior longitudinal ligament.

6. The surgeon places the screws in the vertebral body, placing the end screws first. Care is taken to place the longitudinal axis of the screw parallel to the endplate and at the apex of the vertebral body.

7. Screw placement is started with an awl and continued with a 5.5-mm tap, continuing until the tip just exits the far side of the cortex. The first one third of the hole is tapped with a 7.0-mm tap, and a 7.0-mm closed top screw with a washer is inserted. The screw must protrude through the opposite cortex by a thread or two. The same process is then repeated at the lower end vertebra.

8. The surgeon cuts the rod to the proper length and contours it to re-create the sagittal-plane angular position of the normal spine. It is then positioned in the end vertebra and used as a guide to locate the entry point for the intermediate screws.

9. Open-ended intermediate screws are inserted in a fashion similar to the end screws, taking care that their pathway is parallel to the end screws.

10. The rod is back-entered through the upper screw and then the lower screw and seated into the intermediate open screws. The open screws are capped, and the rod is rotated to place the sagittal-plane contour of the rod in the sagittal plane. An intermediate set screw is tightened to secure the new position of the rod.

11. As the remaining screws are tightened about the rod, it is essential that the disc spaces be opened completely. A Cobb elevator can be used to pry the disc space open.

12. Rib corticocancellous autograft is used to completely fill the disc spaces. The surgeon obtains the graft from the tenth rib (the usual site of entry), the twelfth rib (taken from inside the chest), and the eighth rib (taken from outside the chest).

13. The disc spaces are compressed to provide anterior column load-sharing. Care should be taken to ensure that the set screws are visited at least twice for the end-closed connections and three times for the center-capped connections.

14. Closure is in the standard manner, using chest tubes if the chest has been entered or a retropleural Hemovac if a retropleural retroperitoneal exposure has been done.

15. Postoperative care consists of an overnight intensive care stay with the patient sitting out of bed the next morning. A cast or brace is used at the physician's discretion. Activities are restricted for 6 to 12 months, until there is clear indication of graft incorporation.

Artificial Disc Replacement

Degenerative disc disease (DDD) occurs when the intervertebral disc (IVD) is worn because of aging or trauma. Discogenic back pain results from degeneration of the disc and is confirmed both by patient history and by radiographic studies. The IVD acts as the padding between the vertebrae. Once the IVD is worn out, pain, inflammation, and nerve impingement leading to numbness and muscle weakness can occur. Left untreated, nerve damage can be permanent. DDD occurs in 50% of people older than 40 years of age. Many patients are asymptomatic; however, those who are affected can be severely debilitated, changing their ability to cope with activities of daily living (ADLs) and affecting the quality of life. Artificial disc replacement (Figures 11-103 and 11-104) re-creates the natural disc

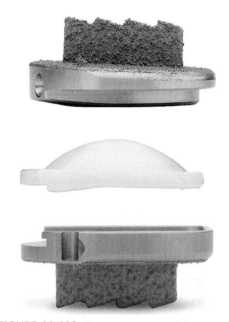

FIGURE 11-103 Three components of the ProDisc.

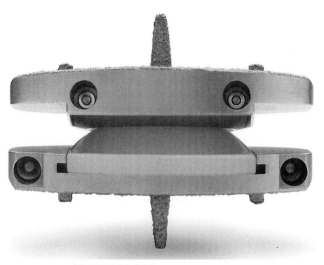

FIGURE 11-104 Assembled ProDisc.

function with preservation of spinal motion (Boughton, 2009b; Blumenthal et al, 2005; David, 2007).

Procedural Considerations. The perioperative nurse and surgical technologist collaborate to ensure the availability of implants with the manufacturer's representative and reconfirm this during the preoperative verification process. Other considerations for this procedure include the use of a blood salvaging system in both the intraoperative and postoperative periods. Templates of x-rays should be placed on the viewing box in the OR before the procedure. The patient is positioned supine on a Jackson table with the right arm draped across the body. A C-arm is used to identify the disc or discs to be replaced in the marked areas. In many institutions, laminar airflow is used.

Operative Procedure. The two general anatomic routes for anterior exposure to the lumbar spine are retroperitoneal and transperitoneal.

The *retroperitoneal approach* can proceed from a variety of incisions, including vertical midline, paramedian, oblique, and transverse. This is determined by both the spinal level and the number of lumbar levels to be exposed. An infraumbilical transverse incision can accommodate most approaches to the L4-L5 and/or S1 disc levels, whereas a more obliquely oriented incision is favored for accessing disc levels above L4.

The *transperitoneal route* is not generally used except in extenuating circumstances (e.g., prior extensive retroperitoneal surgery or revisional spine surgery).

1. The surgeon creates a midline incision and places a fixed retractor system to move the small and large bowel out of the field and facilitate direct visualization of the abdominal cavity. Trendelenburg's position can be used to assist with maintaining exposure.
2. For the L5-S1 level, the peritoneum superficial to the sacral prominence is incised.
3. The surgeon identifies the vascular structures, and uses blunt dissection to tease open the area of the facet of the disc.
4. The middle sacral vessels generally need to be divided to complete the exposure. Excessive electrocoagulation should be avoided to decrease the risk of injury to the sympathetic nerves.
5. Once the exposure is complete the surgeon will use a #3 long handle with a #15 blade to make an incision into the disc body.
6. The discectomy is completed using a rongeur and curettes to remove remaining disc tissue.
7. Correct sizing is determined using templates. Trial instrumentation is inserted and correct placement is verified with AP and lateral C-arm views.
8. The trial is centered in the AP plane, and the marker appears as a plus sign aligned with the spinous process. On the lateral x-ray, a hole in the trial represents the center of rotation.
9. Once correct placement of the trial is verified, the surgeon uses the ESU to mark the midline of the superior vertebral body and removes the trial.
10. Next, the pilot driver is aligned with the midline ESU mark.
11. The pilot driver that corresponds to the chosen footprint is then carefully impacted to verify the ability to accurately place endplates.
12. During this process, lateral C-arm imaging is used to accurately monitor the depths of the pilot driver.

13. Once the depth is achieved, the slap hammer is used, removing the pilot driver from the disc space.
14. The endplate insertion tips are then attached to the corresponding superior and inferior endplates.
15. The endplates are then carefully inserted into the disc space with the assistance of the guided impactor.
16. The insertion is monitored with fluoroscopy to accurately control the posterior depth and verify the appropriate lordotic angle.
17. With the superior and inferior endplates in place, the surgeon uses the spreading and insertion forceps to open the disc space.
18. Once the appropriate distraction is achieved, the size on the spacer can be used to select the appropriate core trial.
19. The appropriate core insertion tip is loaded into the core insertion instrument, and the sliding core is inserted between the endplates.
20. The surgeon releases the distraction on the spreading forceps, which allows the endplates to close around and engage the sliding core.
21. The core insertion instrument is removed and the final position verified using fluoroscopy (Figures 11-105 and 11-106).
22. The wound is irrigated and closed.

Vertebroplasty and Kyphoplasty

Vertebroplasty and kyphoplasty are used for the treatment of vertebral compression fractures attributable to osteoporosis or pathologic conditions. Bone cement is injected into the vertebral body to decrease back pain and prevent further vertebral body height loss. Ortiz (2008) describes the technique in the Research Highlight box.

PROCEDURAL CONSIDERATIONS. Patient selection is key in identifying appropriate candidates for this procedure. MRI is the most accurate radiologic diagnosis. Equipment includes C-arm, radiolucent OR table, and x-ray vests for staff as well as vertebroplasty system and cement injection system. Bone biopsy needles should be available. The C-arm must provide a good

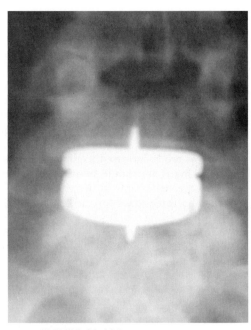

FIGURE 11-105 Implanted ProDisc.

quality image; all key bony landmarks should be clearly visible. Positioning of the patient requires careful vigilance to prevent skin breakdown and nerve damage. After the administration of anesthetic, the patient is positioned prone with hyperextension of the vertebral compression fracture on the radiolucent OR table. The patient is then prepped and draped.

OPERATIVE PROCEDURE

1. After the patient is prepped and draped, the C-arm is placed in the area undergoing surgery.
2. Confirmation of the level of the vertebroplasty (or kyphoplasty) is determined.

3. The surgeon inserts the appropriate-gauge bone needle (11- to 13-mm gauge for vertebroplasty; 8- to 10-mm gauge for kyphoplasty) at the desired level and confirms the correct level with fluoroscopy (Figure 11-107, *A*).
4. For kyphoplasty:
    a. The inflatable balloon tamp is placed. Available tamps are 10, 15, or 20 mm in length, and styles include multi-, uni-, and bidirectional (Figure 11-107, *B*).
    b. After placing the tamp, the surgeon gradually inflates the balloon to 50 pounds per square inch (psi) and then continues inflation in increments of 25 psi until the

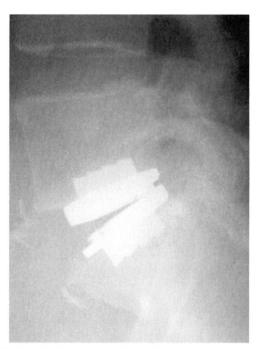

FIGURE 11-106 Implanted ProDisc with patient bending backward.

RESEARCH HIGHLIGHT

Balloon Kyphoplasty

Physical function improved and patients experienced less disability following kyphoplasty than those patients who received conservative care. Immediate improvement in pain and quality of life was reported in 149 patients with compression fractures from osteoporosis, myeloma, or metastatic disease who underwent balloon kyphoplasty. The control group consisted of 151 patients who underwent conservative treatment of back pain. Conservative care included pain medications, bracing, physiotherapy, and bed rest. Based on SF-36 scores, results showed patients assigned to the kyphoplasty group had greater improvement than those patients randomized to nonsurgical care. In addition to improved physical capabilities, kyphoplasty patients also reported less back pain, less use of analgesics and walking aids, and fewer days of limited activity. There were no statistical differences between the groups in adverse events. Kyphoplasty is a minimally invasive surgery that produces improved quality of life with little risk.

From Boughton B: American Association of Orthopaedic Surgeons 2009: Balloon kyphoplasty produces better physical function, less disability than standard care, available at www.medscape.com/viewarticle/589132. Accessed April 25, 2009.

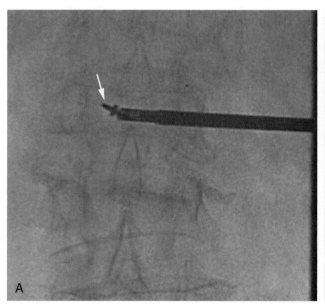

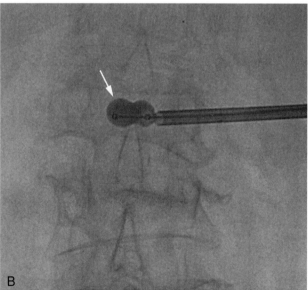

FIGURE 11-107 Vertebroplasty. **A,** Frontal fluoroscopic image shows multidirectional bone curette. **B,** Path of least resistance for subsequent balloon tamp inflation.

desired pressure is achieved and either there is height restoration of the vertebral body or the tamp is in proximity to the cortical margin. Pressure is monitored by a manometer.

   c. Once the tamp has reach maximum inflation, the surgeon deflates the balloon. A cavity is left within the vertebral body.

5. Cement is mixed and then injected through the bone needle using a 1-ml syringe (see Figure 11-107) under fluoroscopic control.

6. The needle is removed and a dressing is applied.

ORTHOPEDIC SURGERY SUMMARY

In orthopedics, it is important for the surgical technologist to know the anatomy and physiology of the surgical area since they often do not have direct visualization of the surgical procedure. A working knowledge of anatomy is needed to facilitate a smooth procedure. The surgical technologist needs to be able to think several steps ahead in the procedure to have the needed items ready when the surgeon asks for them. Planning ahead will greatly help by having the items that may be needed available. This is why it is important to know and fully understand all the aspects of positioning, equipment, supplies, and instrumentation. The surgical technologist should also know the procedural considerations of the operative procedure.

GERIATRIC CONSIDERATIONS

The Elderly Patient—Orthopedic Surgery

Osteoporosis is the most obvious skeletal change that occurs with advancing age. It leads to susceptibility to fracture, which doubles every 5 years after 50 years of age. An approximate loss of 25% to 40% of the mineral content of the bone must be present before detectable change is evident on x-ray films (Murray, 2010). To some degree, osteoporosis is related to a lessening of physical activity, but other risk factors are female gender, Northern European ancestry, multiparity, lean body build, and excessive alcohol intake (Murray, 2010). Osteoporosis is also related to decreased hormonal secretion; thus, postmenopausal women are more prone to develop the condition and therefore more likely to sustain a hip fracture.

Age-related changes in bone increase the prevalence of displaced femoral and intertrochanteric fractures of the upper femur. The prevalence of hip fracture increases with advancing age, is more common in women, and is higher in institutionalized patients. Because the usual cause of death in patients with upper femur fracture is pulmonary embolus, surgery is designed to relieve the severe pain, allow movement in and out of bed, and return the patient to his or her former environment as quickly as possible with minimal debilitation. Between 25% and 50% of individuals who sustain hip fractures are more dependent after the fracture, with deterioration occurring more often in women older than age 75, those with a poor clinical result, and those who were already dependent before the fracture. More than 60% of all joint replacements are in individuals older than 65, and females are almost twice as likely as males to have joint replacement surgery. Outcomes depend on the number of procedures the surgeon and facility have performed; the timing of the surgery; and the patient's medical status, perioperative management, and rehabilitation (Ebersole et al, 2008). A displaced femoral neck fracture must be surgically repaired or healing will not occur. In elderly patients, 70 years and older, prosthetic replacement is usually done because it allows for early ambulation and will last throughout the remaining years of the patient's life. Intertrochanteric and subtrochanteric fractures are best treated with internal fixation. These methods also allow for early mobility.

Degenerative joint disease (osteoarthritis) and inflammatory polyarticular disease (rheumatoid arthritis) are the primary indications for total joint replacement in the hip and knee. In these patients, pain that disrupts normal daily activities and interrupts sleep is the major reason for surgery regardless of the patient's age. Octogenarians and nonagenarians achieve successful pain relief and report satisfaction after the procedure. Methylmethacrylate bone cement is often used in orthopedic procedures in spite of its cardiotoxic effect. Cardiac arrest from cement insertion is a possible risk for frail patients. Supplemental inspired oxygen at the time of insertion, irrigation of the bone to remove excessive marrow elements, and retrograde insertion of the cement are methods to prevent the risk of adverse effects (Burlingame and Blanchard, 2009). Usually knee replacement procedures are elective, and patients have better functional status and a higher bone mass than those with hip fracture.

Modified from Burlingame B, Blanchard J: Bone cement implantation syndrome, *AORN J* 89(2):399–400, 2009; Ebersole P et al: *Toward healthy aging: human needs and nursing response*, ed 7, St Louis, 2008, Mosby; Murray CA: Interventions for clients with musculoskeletal problems. In Ignatavicius DD, Workman ML, editors: *Medical-surgical nursing: patient-centered collaborative care*, ed 6, St Louis, 2010, Saunders.

REVIEW QUESTIONS

1. Name four methods of verifying the operative site and side.

2. What type of device is the Alvardo Foot Holder and for what procedure is it used? What would the surgical technologist also need to have on the sterile field to attach the Alvarado?

3. Name the three techniques for traction.

4. Name three sources of power for surgical drills.

5. What is the difference between autograft and allograft?

6. Name the two main classifications of bone fractures.

7. List the varieties of fractures.

8. Name the indications for internal fixation of acetabular fractures.

9. What is the difference between cortical bone screws and cancellous bone screws and which is used more often?

10. In a total hip arthroplasty, which type of patient is more likely to require a cemented hip prosthesis versus a noncemented one?

11. Define and briefly describe the following surgical procedures:
    Repair of intertrochanteric hip fracture with plate and screws
    Repair of torn cruciate ligament
    Minimally invasive total hip arthroplasty

Critical Thinking Question

The surgical technologist is setting up for an anterior approach to an acetabular fracture on a 27-year-old male, injured in a motor vehicle accident. The patient was unrestrained in the vehicle. He has an unstable fracture with greater than 2 mm of displacement but no other critical injuries. On what type of OR bed should the patient be positioned, and in what position?

What instrument sets should be opened on the back table? What other sets should be readily available? What are some accessory items that may be needed on the sterile field? What are some of the challenges that the surgeon might face during this procedure?

REFERENCES

American Association of Tissue Banks (AATB): *Standards for tissue banking,* McLean, VA, 2008, The Association.

American Board of Orthopaedic Surgeons (ABOS): available at www.abos.org/ModDefault.aspx?module=Public. Accessed June 23, 2009.

Association of periOperative Registered Nurses (AORN): AORN position statement on the role of the health care industry representative in the perioperative/invasive setting 2006, available at www.aorn.org/PracticeResources/AORNPositionStatements/Positions_HealthCareR. Accessed March 15, 2009.

Association of periOperative Registered Nurses (AORN): AORN position statement on patient safety 2007, available at www.aorn.org/PracticeResources/AORNPositionStatements/Position_PatientSafety/. Accessed March 15, 2009.

Association of periOperative Registered Nurses (AORN): *Perioperative standards and recommended practices,* Denver, 2009, The Association.

Barclay L et al: Guidelines address drug treatments to prevent osteoporotic fractures, 2008, available at http://cme.medscape.com/viewarticle/580715. Accessed June 23, 2009.

Blumenthal S et al: A prospective, randomized, multicenter food and drug administration investigational device exemptions study of lumbar total disc replacement with the Charite artificial disc versus lumbar fusion: Part I: Evaluation of clinical outcomes, *Spine* 30(14): 1565–1575, 2005.

Boughton B: Certain factors increase risk for death after total hip arthroplasty, 2009a, available at www. medscape.com/viewarticle/588980. Accessed March 31, 2009.

Boughton B: Lumbar total disc replacement superior to spinal fusion for degenerative disc disease, 2009b, available at www.medscape.com/viewartical/588851. Accessed March 31, 2009.

David T: Long-term results of one-level lumbar arthroplasty: minimum 10-year follow-up of the Charite Artifical disc in 106 patients, *Spine,* 32(6):661–666, 2007.

Denholm B: Tucking patient's arms and general positioning, *AORN J* 89(4):755–757, 2009.

Guido GW: *Legal and ethical issues in nursing,* ed 4, Upper Saddle River, NJ, 2005, Prentice-Hall.

Harby K: Outpatient surgery in hip and knee arthroplasty requires comprehensive approach, 2005, available at www.medscape.com/viewarticle/500209. Accessed March 23, 2009.

Kleinert HE et al: Hand surgery, In Townsend CM, editor: *Sabiston's textbook of surgery,* ed 18, Philadelphia, 2007, Saunders.

Kolisek F et al: Clinical experience using a minimally invasive surgical approach for total knee arthroplasty: early results of a prospective randomized study compared to a standard approach, *J Arthroplasty* 22(1):8–13, 2007.

National Osteoporosis Foundation (NOF): Fast facts on osteoporosis, Washington, DC, National Osteoporosis Foundation, available at www.nof.org/osteoporosis/diseasefacts.htm. Accessed June 13, 2009.

Ortiz A: Vertebral body reconstruction: review and update on vertebroplasty and kyphoplasty, *Appl Radiol* 37(12):10–24, 2008.

The Joint Commission: Universal protocol UP.01.01.01, available at: www.jointcommission.org/NR/rdonlyres/E5943278-3B89-469F-A265-E5AF-B8729AD0/0/NPSG_UniversalProtocol_AHC_20090512.pdf. Accessed March 15, 2009.

CHAPTER 12

Neurosurgery

LEARNING OBJECTIVES

After studying this chapter the reader will be able to:

- Correlate the pathologic morphology of central nervous system tumors to specific cellular components
- Distinguish between structures and functions of the central nervous system (CNS) from the peripheral nervous system (PNS)
- Identify tissue layers involved in opening and closing sequences of cranial procedures
- Locate areas of the brain responsible for specific motor and sensory functions of the body
- Contrast the unique characteristics of the cranium, with regard to form and function, in the neonatal period and adulthood
- Identify internal and external anatomical landmarks of the cranium
- Discuss the properties, purpose, and problems associated with cerebrospinal fluid and the ventricular system
- Differentiate and compare the arterial and venous blood supply of the brain with other parts of the body
- Discuss the anatomical mechanism of collateral cerebral blood flow
- Identify types of vascular abnormalities within the CNS, their origin, and impact
- List the names, numbers, and specific functions of the cranial nerves
- Identify the anatomical characteristics of the spinal cord of an adult
- Examine the structural configuration of the spinal column and its individual vertebral bodies
- Discuss the impact of spinal pathological conditions on patient mobility and quality of life
- Compare diagnostic methods for determination of surgical interventions and approaches
- Identify specialized instrumentation, equipment, and supplies utilized for neurosurgical procedures
- List the pharmacologic and hemostatic agents used during neurosurgical procedures
- Compare minimally invasive or nonsurgical treatments with invasive surgical options for treatment of central nervous or peripheral nerve disorders
- Review specific procedural steps as a guide for clinical considerations
- Apply broad neurosurgical concepts and knowledge to clinical practice for enhanced surgical patient care

CHAPTER OUTLINE

This chapter was originally written by Diane L. Ferrara-Hoffman, MSN, CRNP, RNFA, APRN, BC, and Sarah J. Krizman, RN, BSN, CNOR, for the 14th edition of Alexander's Care of the Patient in Surgery and has been revised by Margaret Rodriguez, BS, CSFA, FAST, for this text.

Overview

Neurosurgery is a word that evokes a certain sense of fear, awe, or mystery among both lay people and medical providers. Neurosurgeons have some of the most extensive training and lengthiest residency requirements of all surgical specialties. Surgical technologists who participate in this specialty must be able to apply all of their skill and expertise to these highly challenging surgical interventions. Soft tissue or bone, neonates to geriatrics, anomalies to accidental injuries, superior sagittal sinus to tarsal tunnel and everything in between, the perioperative neurosurgical team must be prepared to provide the highest level of care possible. To reference an old adage, it may not be rocket science, but it is brain surgery.

A working knowledge of neuroanatomy and physiology is crucial for optimal patient care. The neurosurgeon, anesthesia provider, perioperative nurse, surgical first assistant or physician assistant, and surgical technologist are all responsible for protecting the patient from injury secondary to factors including: prolonged anesthesia, positioning, exposure and manipulation of vital structures, and other potential risks within the preoperative, intraoperative, and postoperative phases of care. Surgical interventions, or lack thereof, in cases involving neurosurgical diagnoses constitute an inherent risk of altering an individual patient in profound ways, unlike any other specialty or disease process. Patients may suffer neurological loss of function or sensation, whether transient or permanent. They may have personality changes following cranial injury or surgery that leaves family and friends bewildered. Chronic conditions rob patients of independence and society of human resources. But, in many cases, neurosurgical interventions restore function, relieve pain, maintain, and prolong the quality of life for those who put their trust in the hands of skilled perioperative personnel.

A knowledgeable surgical technologist will be able to correlate the diagnosis obtained from an intraoperative frozen section with the cellular level of neuroanatomy. An experienced surgical technologist will be able to anticipate the need for specialized equipment based on the surgical procedure scheduled. An expert and attentive surgical technologist will hand the neurosurgeon the appropriate instrumentation without being asked, based on an understanding of the procedural steps and tissue layers involved. Practitioners must have the capacity to remain focused on the surgical procedure for long periods, organize multiple setups and instrument trays, operate complex imaging and magnification systems, and be vigilant about the integrity of the sterile field in a room potentially filled with many other additional health professionals including: radiology technologists, industry representatives, neuromonitoring personnel, and autologous blood salvage unit operators. With so much at stake, it is no wonder the mention of neurosurgery can strike a nerve with the inexperienced surgical technologist and send shivers up the spine.

This chapter will provide a comprehensive blueprint of anatomy and physiology, neuropathology, procedural considerations, equipment and instrumentation, diagnostic methods, research, and history to assist the surgical technologist to build a solid foundation of knowledge. Putting the specialty of neurosurgery under the microscope will demystify its complexity and provide greater accessibility to any perioperative practitioner willing to join the surgical team.

Surgical Anatomy

The nervous system is the most complex and least understood of body systems. It is divided structurally into the central nervous system (CNS) consisting of the brain and spinal cord and the peripheral nervous system (PNS), which encompasses every neurologic structure outside the CNS, including the cranial and spinal nerves. The brain and spinal cord are protected by the skull and vertebral columns, respectively. The cranial nerves originate within the brain and emerge through openings in the skull to run peripherally. The spinal nerves that emerge from the spinal cord through the vertebral foramina also run peripherally.

The nervous system is divided functionally into a voluntary system and an autonomic, or involuntary, system. It provides a means of communication for the rest of the body. The functions of all body systems depend, in part, on nervous system function. In turn, the nervous system depends directly on circulatory system function to obtain life-sustaining glucose and oxygen. Nervous system functions include motor and sensory functions, orientation, coordination, conceptual thought, emotion, memory, and reflex response.

Nervous system tissue is composed of vast amounts of neurons and far more neuroglial cells. Neurons are intercommunicating nerve cells that encode, conduct, and transmit information to other neurons, muscle, and glandular tissue (Figure 12-1). They are composed of a body or soma with branches or extensions, called dendrites and axons, that communicate with other cells at synapses. Dendrites are short branches that conduct impulses toward the soma. Cell bodies and dendrites are mostly confined to areas of gray matter in the CNS. Axons are long branches, often encased in a white myelin sheath, that conduct impulses away from the soma. Axons pass into bundles of nerve fibers that tend to form tracts or pathways and are referred to as white matter. Tracts that cross midline to create a communication pathway from each side of the body to the opposite side of the brain are called commissures. Neuroglial cells support the neurons by creating and maintaining an appropriate environment in which neurons can operate efficiently. Glial cells include astrocytes, oligodendrocytes, ependymal cells, and microglia. The mutation of these cells can form a glioma, one of the more common brain tumors.

This chapter divides the nervous system into logical divisions within the framework of neurosurgical techniques. The brain and adjacent structures include the cranial nerves of the PNS, which are commonly encountered during brain surgery. Discussion of the spine and spinal cord includes the adjacent spinal nerves and the disks and ligaments that support the spine. Surgically significant pathology is incorporated with the normal anatomy of structures.

BRAIN AND ADJACENT STRUCTURES

Scalp

Scalp layers (Figure 12-2) include skin, subcutaneous tissue, galea, and periosteum. Scalp skin is thick. The subcutaneous tissue, which is exceptionally dense, tough, and vascular, is firmly attached to the galea. Most of the blood vessels lie superficial to the galea. The subgaleal space contains loose areolar tissue that permits mobility of the scalp. It is in this bloodless plane that the standard craniotomy scalp flap is created. The

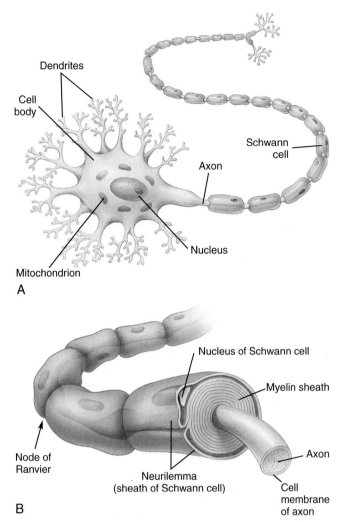

FIGURE 12-1 **A**, Many dendrites carry nerve impulses to the cell body, which then sends the nerve impulses along a single, long axon. Long axons are encased at intervals by a myelin sheath. **B**, A segment of myelinated fiber in cross section, showing myelin sheath composed of several layers of myelin, which insulate the axon.

pericranium, or outer periosteum of the skull, separates the galea from the cranium.

The arterial supply of the scalp comes from the external carotid artery through the superficial temporal, posterior auricular, occipital, frontal, and supraorbital branches. Most veins roughly follow the course of their corresponding arteries, except the emissary veins, which drain directly through the skull into the intracranial venous sinuses. The scalp, the extracranial arteries, and portions of the dura mater are the only pain-sensitive structures that cover the brain. The brain itself is insensate.

Skull

The skull provides protection for the brain. It is formed by 28 bones, most of which are paired although some in the median plane are single. Many of the bones are flat bones, consisting of two thin plates of compact bone encasing a spongy layer of cancellous bone containing bone marrow (see Figure 12-2). Infants are born with two fontanelles. These are openings in the skull that are located both anterior and posterior to the

parietal bones (Figure 12-3). The posterior fontanelle is generally closed by 2 months and the anterior by about 18 months after birth. The bones of the skull are joined by bony seams called *sutures*. Eight bones form the walls of the cranial cavity, which houses the brain. There are four single bones (frontal, occipital, ethmoid, and sphenoid) and four paired bones (temporal and parietal) (Figure 12-4). The sagittal suture lies in the medial plane and joins the two parietal bones. The coronal suture joins the frontal and parietal bones. The squamous sutures border the squamous part of the temporal bones. The lambdoid suture joins the occipital and parietal bones. Skull bones vary in thickness and tend to be thinner where they are covered in muscles, for example, in the temporal and posterior fossae. The skull articulates with the first cervical vertebra to allow for flexion and extension of the skull. The skeletal surface landmarks of the head can be palpated and are commonly used to plan surgical approaches (Figure 12-5).

The interior of the skull is anatomically divided into three cranial fossae: anterior, middle, and posterior (Figure 12-6). The anterior fossa is limited posteriorly by the sphenoid ridge, along which pituitary tumors and aneurysms of the circle of Willis are generally approached. The frontal lobes and olfactory bulbs and tracts lie in the anterior fossa. The temporal lobes lie in the middle fossa, which is shaped like a butterfly. The sella turcica, formed by the sphenoid bone, is the most central part of the middle fossa and houses the pituitary gland. The floor and lateral walls of the middle fossa are shaped from the greater wings of the sphenoid bone and parts of the temporal bone, which house the internal and middle ear structures. The posterior fossa, the largest and deepest fossa, is formed by the occipital, sphenoid, and petrous portions of the temporal bones; the cerebellum and brainstem lie here, as do many cranial nerves. The foramen magnum, the largest opening in the skull, provides passage for the spinal cord to join the brainstem in the posterior fossa. Numerous other openings exist in the base of the skull for passage of arteries, veins, and cranial nerves.

Skull Fractures. The severity of skull fractures depends on the degree of resulting brain injury. Simple skull fractures can be serious if they cross major vascular channels in the skull. If vessels are torn, epidural or subdural hematomas may form. Depressed skull fractures require a surgical procedure to elevate the depressed bone. Open skull fractures should be irrigated copiously and closed to prevent infection. Basilar skull fractures may cause cerebrospinal fluid (CSF) rhinorrhea or otorrhea. A few patients with these CSF leaks require surgical repair if they do not resolve after 2 weeks.

Deformities of the Cranium. Craniosynostosis is the most common pediatric skull deformity seen and treated by the neurosurgeon. The phenomenon is a premature closure or lack of formation of cranial sutures, leading to cosmetic abnormalities, eventual life-threatening intracranial pressure (ICP) increases, and arrested brain development unless diagnostic and surgical interventions ensue. Cranial remodeling is most often undertaken during the first year of life, when brain capacity triples (see Chapter 17).

Meninges

The brain and spinal cord are completely enveloped by the meninges, which are three membranes that provide support and

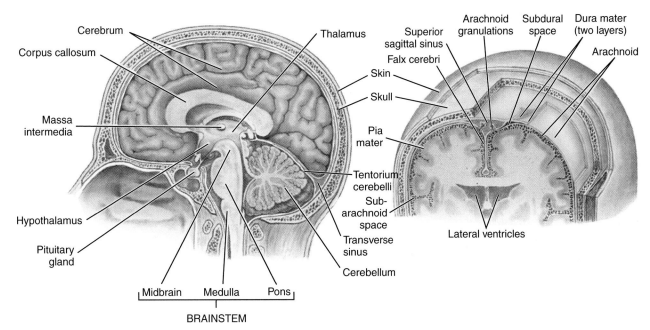

FIGURE 12-2 Scalp is composed of the following layers: skin, subcutaneous tissue, galea, and periosteum. Skull bone has three tables: outer, diploë (or spongy layer), and inner. Dura mater lies beneath skull and completely encapsulates brain. Other structures are identified for reference and are described in text.

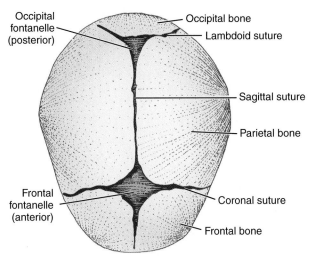

FIGURE 12-3 Skull at birth viewed from above.

protection. The meningeal layers from superficial to deep are the dura mater, arachnoid mater, and pia mater (see Figure 12-2). The space superficial to the dura is known as the epidural space. The cranial meninges are located between the skull and the brain.

The dura mater is a tough, shiny, fibrous membrane that is close to the inner surface of the skull and folds to separate the cranial cavity into compartments. The largest fold is the falx cerebri—an arch-shaped, vertically placed, midline structure separating the right and left cerebral hemispheres (see Figure 12-2). A smaller fold of dura mater, the falx cerebelli, separates the cerebellar hemispheres vertically. A transverse fold, the tentorium cerebelli, forms the roof of the posterior fossa.

The tentorium supports the temporal lobe and occipital lobes of the cerebral hemispheres. Below the tentorium lie the cerebellum and brainstem. Structures above the tentorium are referred to as *supratentorial* and those below as *infratentorial* (Figure 12-7). At margins of these dural folds lie large venous sinuses that drain blood from the intracranial structures into the jugular veins. Accidental breaching of a sinus during surgery can cause severe bleeding that is difficult to control and may put the patient at risk for a venous air embolism. Several arteries also lie within the layers of the dura. The largest is the middle meningeal, a source of serious epidural hemorrhage if torn by an overlying skull fracture. The rigid skull makes hemorrhage and swelling in the brain critical events. The volume of the intracranial cavity is fixed. Increasing the intracranial contents by a hemorrhage, tumor, or edema may lead to serious ICP problems. Pressure on brain tissue may cause irreparable damage.

Beneath the dura mater is a transparent membrane called the *arachnoid*. Although the outer layer of arachnoid closely approximates the dura mater, the space between is considered the subdural space. The inner arachnoid layer forms innumerable weblike filaments that bridge to the surface of the brain (see Figure 12-2). The arachnoid passes over the sulci and fissures of the brain, without dipping into them. The arachnoid is separated from the pia mater beneath it by the subarachnoid space, which is filled with CSF that bathes the brain. Around the base of the brain, particularly, this space becomes enlarged to form cisterns. The major intracranial nerves and blood vessels pass through these compartments. Intracranial approaches can be charted in terms of the basal cisterns.

The pia mater, the innermost membrane, closely follows the contours of the surface of the brain into the sulci and fissures. Only the microscopic subpial space separates

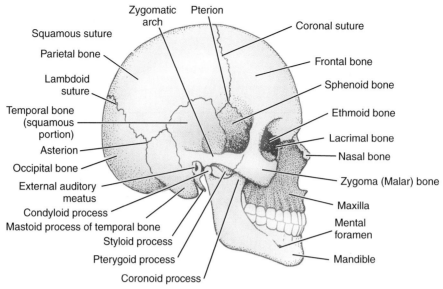

FIGURE 12-4 Skull viewed from right side.

the pia from the brain. The pia mater has a rich vascular network. Vascular fringes of pia mater project into the ventricles to form the choroid plexus of the ventricles, which produce CSF.

Brain

The anatomy of the brain, formally known as the encephalon, can be considered in multiple ways. Based on prenatal development, the principal divisions from rostral (head) to caudal (tail), descending toward the spinal cord, are the forebrain or prosencephalon, the midbrain or mesencephalon, and the hindbrain or rhombencephalon. The rhombencephalon is subdivided into the cerebellum, the medulla oblongata, and the pons. The prosencephalon includes the diencephalon and the telencephalon, or cerebrum. The medulla oblongata, pons, and midbrain are collectively referred to as the brainstem (Figures 12-7 and 12-8).

Cerebrum. The right and the left cerebral hemispheres are the largest parts of the brain and occupy the anterior and middle fossae. Each hemisphere is divided into frontal, parietal, occipital, and temporal lobes. The two hemispheres are separated by the longitudinal fissure and the falx cerebri but remain connected underneath the falx by a large transverse bundle of nerve fibers called the corpus callosum (see Figure 12-8). Each of the cerebral hemispheres controls sensation and motor activity to and receives sensory stimuli from the opposite half of the body.

The convoluted surface of the cerebrum consists of gray matter, called the *cerebral cortex*, which contains the cell bodies of the many nerve pathways of the brain. The underlying white matter contains millions of myelinated nerve axons and is relatively avascular compared with the cortex. The nerve pathways, or fiber tracts, are of three types: (1) commissural fibers, which pass from one cerebral hemisphere to the other; (2) association fibers, which connect regions of gyri and lobes longitudinally within a cerebral hemisphere; and (3) projection fibers, including the great motor and sensory systems, which run vertically to connect the cortical regions with other portions of the CNS.

The surfaces of the hemispheres form convolutions called *gyri* and intervening furrows called *sulci*, which serve as ana-

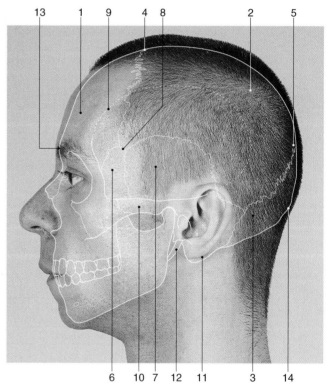

FIGURE 12-5 Lateral aspect of the head: bones. *1,* Frontal. *2,* Parietal. *3,* Occipital. *4,* Bregma (anterior fontanelle). *5,* Lambda (posterior fontanelle). *6,* Greater wing of sphenoid. *7,* Squamous temporal. *8,* Pterion. *9,* Temporal lines. *10,* Zygomatic arch. *11,* Mastoid process. *12,* Styloid process. *13,* Glabella. *14,* External occipital protuberance.

tomic landmarks. Two sulci of particular anatomic importance during surgery are (1) the lateral sulcus, or sylvian fissure, which divides the temporal lobe from the frontal and parietal lobes, and (2) the central sulcus, or fissure of Rolando, which separates the frontal from the parietal lobe. The central sulcus also separates the motor cortex (precentral gyrus) from the

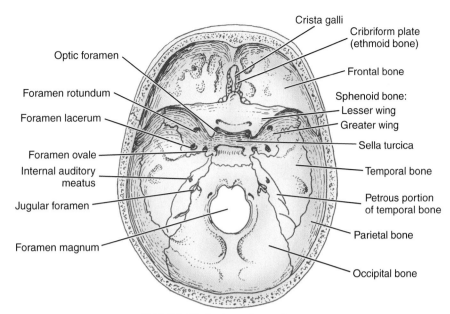

FIGURE 12-6 Floor of cranial cavity.

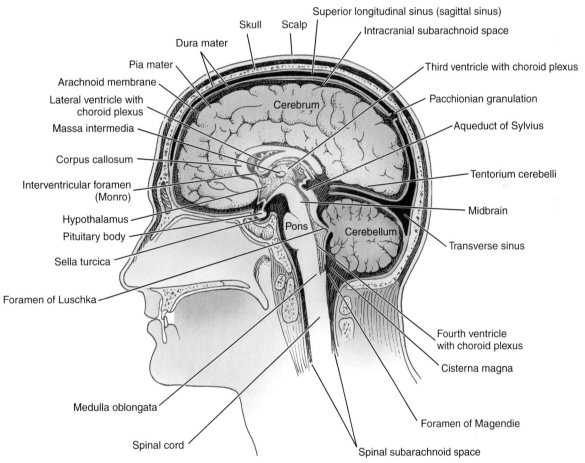

FIGURE 12-7 Sagittal section of head showing cerebrospinal fluid spaces and their relationship to venous circulation and their principal subdivision of the brain and its coverings.

sensory cortex (postcentral gyrus). The motor cortex lies anterior to the central sulcus, and the sensory cortex lies posterior to the central sulcus. Both the motor cortex and the sensory cortex can be represented by a topographically organized map called a homunculus that proportionately represents each body part at the area of the gyri that controls it. The diagrams illustrate how the number of neurons corresponds to the degree of motor and sensory control required. For example, areas that need more fine motor control, such as the fingers and face, have a higher concentration of neurons than other areas. Keep

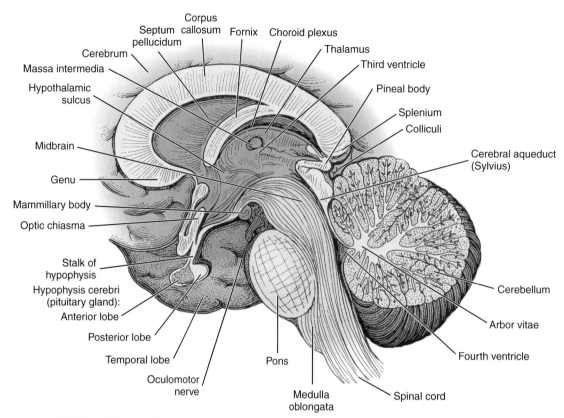

FIGURE 12-8 Sagittal section through midline of brain showing structures around third ventricle, including corpus callosum, thalamus, and hypothalamus.

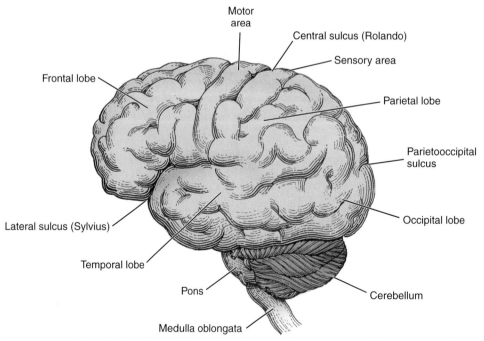

FIGURE 12-9 Lateral view of cerebral hemisphere (showing lobes and principal fissures), cerebellum, pons, and medulla oblongata.

in mind that the left motor and sensory cortices control the right side of the body and vice versa (Figure 12-9). Destruction of an area of motor cortex results in loss of voluntary motor function on the corresponding area of the opposite side of the body (Figure 12-10).

The frontal lobe is anterior to the central sulcus and controls the higher functions of intellect and abstract reasoning, along with movement, language, and personality. Posterior to the central sulcus is the parietal lobe, extending back to the parietooccipital fissure. This area contains the final

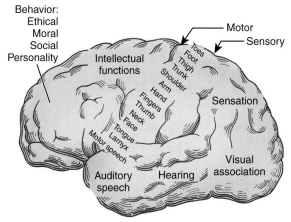

FIGURE 12-10 Principal functional subdivisions of cerebral hemispheres.

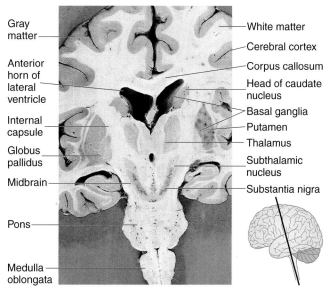

FIGURE 12-11 Oblique coronal section through the cerebral hemisphere and brainstem showing the disposition of gray and white matter, the basal ganglia, and the internal capsule.

receiving and integrating station for sensory impulses, such as pain and touch, from the contralateral side of the body. It is also involved with special relationships and object identification. The occipital lobe lies posterior to the parieto-occipital fissure. It receives and integrates visual impulses and registers them as meaningful images (see Figures 12-9 and 12-10).

Inferior to the lateral sulcus, in the middle fossa, is the temporal lobe, which is involved with memory, speech, and smell. Lesions of the left temporal lobe in right-handed persons and in many left-handed persons may affect the comprehension and verbalization of words, resulting in aphasia. The insula (island of Reil) is an area of cortex that lies deep within the lateral sulcus and can be exposed when the upper and lower lips of the fissure are separated. The insula is believed to be involved with smell, taste, touch, and possibly language.

The limbic system consists of large parts of the cortex near the medial wall of the cerebral hemisphere (cingulate and parahippocampal gyri) along with the hippocampus, amygdala, and septum. It is closely and significantly connected with the hypothalamus. It has a diffuse distribution in the brain, and many components of the limbic system have overlapping functions. The hippocampus is critical for learning and memory. The amygdala regulates the perceptive and expressive aspects of emotional and social behavior. The limbic system affects endocrine and autonomic functions of the body, recent memory, emotions, behaviors, and motivational and mood states. Restlessness and hyperactivity may result from lesions of this area.

The basal ganglia are subcortical collections of nuclei (gray matter) that include the caudate nucleus, putamen, and globus pallidus (collectively referred to as the *corpus striatum*); the substantia nigra (which is located in the midbrain); and the subthalamic nucleus (part of the diencephalon). The basal ganglia influence movement and behavior through projections to the thalamus and brainstem and subsequently the cortex (Figure 12-11). The basal ganglia function to promote and support patterns of behavior and movement that are appropriate in a given situation and to inhibit unwanted or inappropriate behavior and movements. Disorders of the basal ganglia are principally characterized by abnormalities of movement, muscle tone, and posture. Damage to these neural components

may cause rigidity of the skeletal muscles and various types of spontaneous tremors.

Diencephalon. The diencephalon is composed of the thalamus, hypothalamus, epithalamus, and subthalamus and surrounds the third ventricle. The thalamus is the major relay station for incoming sensory stimuli. Except for some olfactory impulse transmission, all sensory information transmitted to the cerebral hemispheres is relayed through the thalamus. This is also true for motor pathways from the cerebellum and basal ganglia. Because of the central role of the thalamus in perception of body sensations, surgical lesions can be made in this area in an attempt to alleviate pain.

Along the floor of the third ventricle is the hypothalamus (see Figure 12-8), which is concerned principally with the autonomic regulation of the body's internal environment and is intimately connected with the pituitary gland. It controls fluid and electrolyte balance, appetite, reproduction, thermoregulation, immune response, and many emotional responses. It influences levels of attention and consciousness. The pituitary gland is suspended from the base of the hypothalamus by the pituitary stalk. It secretes multiple hormones that are regulated by the hypothalamus. A pituitary tumor can result in a hormonal imbalance. It can also encroach on the optic chiasma, causing vision changes.

The subthalamus is a complex region of nuclear groups and fiber tracts, including the subthalamic nucleus, which is considered with the basal ganglia. The epithalamus consists of multiple nuclei and the pineal gland, an endocrine gland that regulates the circadian rhythm.

Brainstem. The brainstem consists of the midbrain, pons, and medulla oblongata. It is located in the posterior fossa and forms the floor of the fourth ventricle. It is the site of many ascending and descending fiber tracts that allow for communication among the structures of the brain and between the brain and spinal cord. All but 2 of the 12 cranial nerves attach to the brainstem. The short, stocky por-

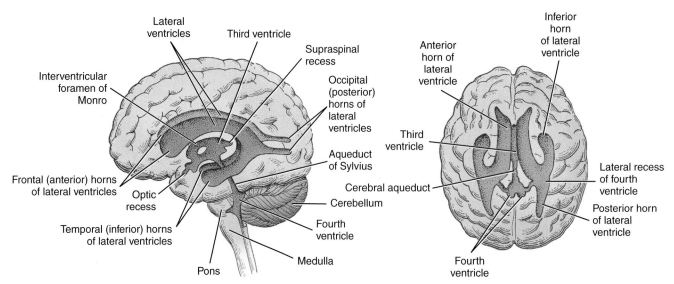

FIGURE 12-12 Ventricular system showing its relationship to various parts of brain.

tion of the brain, between the cerebral hemispheres and pons, is the midbrain (see Figure 12-7), also referred to as the *mesencephalon*. It is composed of the cerebral peduncles, the substantia nigra, numerous nerve tracts and nuclei, and association centers that control the majority of eye movements. Immediately below the midbrain is the pons, which contains control areas for horizontal eye movement and face movement. The medulla oblongata is continuous with the spinal cord at the foramen magnum. It contains the vital cardiovascular and respiratory regulatory centers (see Figure 12-9). Damage to the brainstem is often devastating and life-threatening, because it can affect movement, senses, consciousness, perception, and cognition.

Cerebellum. The cerebellum, which occupies most of the posterior fossa, forms the roof of the fourth ventricle (Figures 12-8 and 12-12). It has two lateral lobes, or hemispheres, and a medial portion, the vermis. The fissures of the cerebellum are small and run transversely. The cerebellum is concerned principally with balance and coordination of movement. It has many complex connections with higher and lower centers and exerts its influence unilaterally—in contrast to the cerebral hemispheres, which act contralaterally. By splitting the vermis in the exact midline, a satisfactory exposure of tumors that lie in the fourth ventricle is obtained without sacrificing the important cerebellar functions.

Pathologic Lesions of the Brain. An estimated new 22,070 brain and other nervous system cancers were estimated to occur in 2009 (American Cancer Society [ACS], 2009). Brain metastases outnumber primary neoplasms by at least 10 to 1, and they occur in 20% to 40% of cancer patients. Because no national cancer registry documents brain metastases, the exact incidence is unknown, but it has been estimated that 98,000 to 170,000 new cases are diagnosed in the United States each year (National Cancer Institute [NCI], 2009).

Multiple factors are suspected of playing a role in the pathogenesis of intracranial neoplasms. Early diagnosis simplifies surgical treatment because increased ICP and severe neurologic changes are not usually present. Brain tumors are

TABLE 12-1

Frequency of Primary CNS Tumors in Adults

Tumor Type	Percentage
Glioblastoma	50
Meningioma	17
Astrocytoma	10
Pituitary adenoma	4
Oligodendroglioma	3
Ependymoma	2
Medulloblastoma	2
Neurilemmoma	2
Hemangioma	2
Craniopharyngioma	1
Pinealoma	1
Sarcoma	1
Others	5

Modified from Janus TJ, Yung WKA: Primary neurological tumors. In Goetz CG: *Clinical neurology*, ed 3, Philadelphia, 2007, Saunders.

either malignant or benign, depending on the cell type. Primary tumors generally do not resemble the carcinomas and sarcomas found elsewhere in the body and rarely metastasize outside the CNS. Both primary and metastatic tumors of the brain and its membranes are included in the term *intracranial tumors*.

Traditionally, tumors are classified by cell type; however, classification of brain tumors is an evolving process. The widely used World Health Organization (WHO) system lists more than 120 types of brain tumors (NCI, 2009). Table 12-1 gives the approximate percentage of CNS tumors by histologic type. A brief description of a select list of brain tumors follows:

1. *Tumors of intraepithelial tissue* encompass gliomas, tumors believed to originate from neuroglial cells.
   a. Astrocytomas are the most common of all primary brain tumors. They usually occur in the cerebellum of children and the cerebrum of adults. They are often cystic

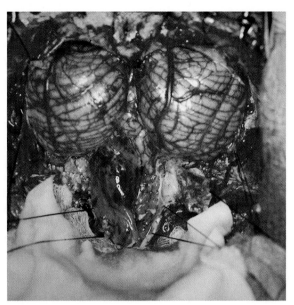

FIGURE 12-13 Ependymoma located inferior to the cerebellar tonsils.

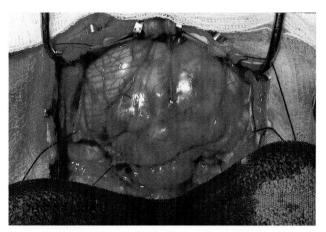

FIGURE 12-14 Medulloblastoma of cerebellum.

and discrete in children and infiltrating and ill-defined in adults. Astrocytomas are classified in the WHO system based on the principal cell type and on the degree of anaplasia as grade I to IV, with grade I being the more favorable type of tumor and grade IV being the most malignant. Glioblastoma multiforme (GBM), a grade IV astrocytoma, is an infiltrative, fast-growing, rapidly recurring cerebral tumor that occurs most frequently in the sixth and seventh decades of life. It is the most common type of primary brain tumor, accounting for about 50% of gliomas (Sloan et al, 2005). It is one of the few tumors that is capable of invading both cerebral hemispheres by crossing the midline. Areas of necrosis are characteristic. Recent studies have consistently demonstrated the benefits of radical surgical resection. Postoperative radiation therapy significantly improves survival. Even with aggressive multimodality therapy, median survival is less than 1 year and 5-year survival is less than 5% (Sloan et al, 2005).

b. Oligodendroglioma, typically found in the cerebral hemispheres, is usually infiltrating but occasionally moderately well-defined. It frequently presents in middle age with seizure. It is now believed that the true incidence of oligodendrogliomas is 5% to 15% of gliomas, much higher than previously thought. Therapy usually consists of surgery followed by radiation therapy and chemotherapy (Sloan et al, 2005).

c. Ependymoma occurs most frequently in children and is likely to arise in or near the ventricular walls. It commonly occurs in the fourth ventricle, where it abuts or involves vital medullary centers (Figure 12-13). It also frequently metastasizes into the subarachnoid spaces. This tumor accounts for 3% to 4% of gliomas. Surgical resection followed by radiation therapy is the usual treatment. The 5-year survival rate is 73% (Central Brain Tumor Registry of the United States [CBTRUS], 2007-2008).

d. Medulloblastoma is a fast-growing, rapidly recurring tumor of the vermis of the cerebellum and fourth ventricle that usually occurs in young children. It charac-

teristically metastasizes into the subarachnoid spaces, usually spreading to the base of the brain by this route. It accounts for 15% to 20% of childhood intracranial brain tumors and is the most common malignant pediatric brain tumor (Figure 12-14).

2. *Tumors of the meninges (meningiomas)* commonly occur in people in the fourth to sixth decades of life (Al-Mefty and Heth, 2005). They are usually benign, circumscribed, slow-growing tumors, arising from arachnoid cells with secondary attachment to the dura. Various factors have been implicated in the development of meningiomas. They typically involve the cortex and bone of the skull with growth. They can be very vascular and may adhere to the dural venous sinuses or major arteries, making their complete removal challenging. However, meningiomas often can be totally surgically removed.

3. *Tumors of the cranial nerves (vestibular schwannomas)* are benign; they usually arise from the neurilemma sheath cells of the vestibular portion of the eighth cranial nerve within the auditory meatus. The term *acoustic neuroma* is a misnomer. These tumors grow slowly to fill the cerebellopontine angle and may indent the brainstem. Presenting symptoms include hearing loss, tinnitus, and disequilibrium.

4. *Hemopoietic neoplasms and lymphomas:* CNS involvement with lymphoma may occur secondarily from a systemic lymphoma or may arise primarily in the CNS (CBTRUS, 2007-2008). The main role for surgery is for tumor biopsy. Stereotactic techniques are well suited for these often-deep tumors. The standard treatment after biopsy is radiation therapy, allowing for a median survival of 10 months. Adding chemotherapy can prolong survival (Greenberg, 2005).

5. *Germ cell tumors* occur in the midline (suprasellar and pineal region). Other than benign teratomas, all intracranial germ cell tumors are malignant and may metastasize by way of CSF and systemically. Tumors of the pineal region are very challenging to the neurosurgeon. Open microsurgery, endoscopy, and stereotactic biopsy are surgical options. Pineal region tumors often cause hydrocephalus. An endoscopic third ventriculostomy or a shunting procedure is routinely performed to alleviate the symptoms of hydrocephalus. Radiation therapy, chemotherapy, and radiosurgery are also treatment considerations.

a. Germinoma is a neoplasm arising from germ cells. Survival with germinomas is much better than with non-germinomatous tumors (teratoma, embryonal cell carcinoma, choriocarcinoma).

b. Teratoma is a congenital tumor containing embryonic elements.

c. Embryonal cell carcinoma consists of a highly primitive group of neoplasms that arise in childhood. Predominantly large hemispheric masses involving deep supratentorial structures, these tumors are highly vascular and have poor prognoses. The primitive neuroectodermal tumor (PNET) is one such tumor.

d. Choriocarcinoma is an extremely rare, very malignant neoplasm.

6. *Cysts and tumorlike lesions* include the following types:

a. Epidermoid and dermoid cysts are developmental, benign tumors typically located in the suprasellar region.

b. Colloid cysts are slow-growing benign tumors. They classically occur in the anterior third ventricle, blocking the foramen of Monro and causing obstructive hydrocephalus.

7. *Tumors of the sellar region* include the following types:

a. Pituitary adenomas can be classified as nonfunctioning or functioning. Nonfunctioning pituitary adenomas account for approximately 30% of pituitary tumors, usually occur in people in the fourth and fifth decades of life, and do not cause clinical hormone hypersecretion. They are typically large and cause hypopituitarism or blindness from regional compression. The usual treatment is endoscopic or microscopic transsphenoidal removal of the tumor. Following operative decompression, vision improves in approximately 80% of patients (Oyesiku, 2005). Radiation therapy or stereotactic radiosurgery may also be used. Functioning pituitary adenomas secrete excess quantities of pituitary hormones. The question of medical versus surgical treatment is ever present in the management of this group of patients. Adenomas may be further subdivided into microadenomas, which are less than 1 cm in diameter and usually discovered because of an endocrinopathy, and macroadenomas, which are larger than 1 cm and usually present with compressive effects of the tumor (Oyesiku, 2005).

(1) Chromophobe tumors are relatively common in the anterior pituitary glands of adults. They cause compression of the pituitary, adjacent optic chiasma, and hypothalamus. Compression of the hypothalamus may lead to diabetes insipidus.

(2) Eosinophilic adenomas are secretory, causing an excessive amount of growth hormone in the serum.

(3) Basophilic adenomas are responsible for the excessive secretion of corticotropic, gonadotropic, and thyrotropic hormones. Acromegaly or, less commonly, Cushing's syndrome may occur and cause the patient to seek help long before the tumor has expanded sufficiently to compromise the optic chiasma.

(4) Prolactin cell adenoma exhibits considerable differences in clinical presentation, depending on the gender of the patient. In women of reproductive age, the onset of amenorrhea and galactorrhea with associated infertility is an obvious sign. The diagnosis of a prolactinoma is established early in the course. In men, the clinical endocrine symptoms, which include decreased libido and impotence, are not as conspicuous and initially may be disregarded by the patient. As a result, male patients frequently do not seek medical attention until the tumors are large and have spread beyond the confines of the sella turcica.

b. Craniopharyngiomas account for 2.5% to 4% of intracranial tumors, with 50% occurring in childhood (Greenberg, 2005). They arise from the region of the pituitary stalk and typically contain both solid and cystic components. Calcification above the sella turcica is often seen radiographically. In addition to headache, vertigo, vomiting, and papilledema, diabetes insipidus and visual field changes are common. Although complete surgical removal is often impossible if it adheres to the carotid artery or hypothalamus, a subtotal resection with radiation offers favorable results.

8. *Metastatic tumors* are the most common brain tumor seen clinically, making up about half of brain tumors. They usually arise from carcinomas, more rarely from sarcomas, and occasionally from melanomas and retinal tumors. The most common sources are lung and breast cancer. The management of brain metastasis is complex and controversial. The current principal options for treatment include whole-brain radiation therapy, surgery, and stereotactic radiosurgery. The most important prognostic variables are the extent of systemic disease and the patient's functional status and age. These factors, along with the size, number, and location of tumors, guide treatment decisions. Median survival only increases from 3 to 6 months with radiation therapy and steroids to 9 to 12 months with surgery and stereotactic radiosurgery (McCutcheon, 2005).

A brain lesion is diagnosed by history, neurologic examination, diagnostic studies (especially computed tomography [CT] scan and magnetic resonance imaging [MRI]), and biopsy. The manifestations of an intracranial tumor fall into two classes: those resulting from irritation or impairment of function in specific areas of the brain directly affected by the tumor and those resulting from diffuse increased ICP. The most common presentation of brain tumors is progressive neurologic deficit, usually motor weakness. Headache and seizures are also common presenting symptoms (Greenburg, 2005).

Large left or bifrontal lobe tumors may cause striking personality changes and depressive symptoms. Lesions in the left frontotemporal region, where motor speech originates, lead to aphasia. Parietal lobe lesions may result in contralateral weakness and sensory changes, along with defects in the perception of objects. Occipital tumors produce hemianoptic visual defects.

Cortical tumors frequently produce focal seizures of diagnostic value. The onset of epileptiform seizures in an adult is often associated with an intracranial neoplasm. Posterior fossa tumors often manifest their presence by blocking the CSF circulation, but they may also destroy cerebellar function, resulting in incoordination, ataxia, scanning speech, and deafness.

Treatment of brain tumors, although based on the characteristics of the tumor, can involve administration of steroids or antiepileptic medications, management of hydrocephalus, surgery, radiosurgery, radiation, and chemotherapy.

OTHER ENCEPHALOPATHIES. Pathological conditions other than brain tumors may require surgical intervention either for definitive diagnosis or treatment of increased intracranial pressure or seizures. Signs and symptoms may be related to increased ICP and are similar to intracranial tumors. Diagnostic studies are usually the same. A brief description of several nontumor lesions follows.

1. *Brain abscess* is an intracerebral collection of pus. Typically, anaerobic bacteria are involved and induce an inflammatory response that encapsulates necrotic brain tissue. Etiology may remain unknown, but is usually related to history of mastoiditis, sinusitis, dental abscess, osteomyelitis, cranial trauma, neurosurgical procedures, or endocarditis (Figure 12-15).

2. *Neurocysticercosis* (NCC) is a parasitic infection caused by the pork tapeworm *Taenia solium* in its larval form. It is the most common infestation of the central nervous system (Rajshekhar, 2010) and mainly seen in developing countries. Intracranial cysticercus lesions are diagnosed following imaging studies and confirmed by antibodies in the serum. Cysts develop to encapsulate the larvae and produce symptoms based on their location within the central nervous system. Surgical management for CNS cysticercal lesions is indicated in cases of cysts located in the ventricles, cisterns, or parenchyma when imaging studies are equivocal.

3. *Encephalomalacia* is a condition of softening of brain matter or loss of brain tissue. Cerebral infarct, ischemia, and trauma are common causes. Though less a cause of increased ICP, encephalomalacia may be observed during craniotomy, noted on diagnostic imaging studies, or as a pathologic finding at autopsy (Figure 12-16).

4. *Kernicterus,* also known as *bilirubin encephalopathy,* is a rare neurological condition in neonates. Severe jaundice in the first 1 to 3 weeks of infancy may result in the excess bilirubin moving from the circulatory system and collecting in brain tissue (Figure 12-17). Swelling of brain tissues may progress to late-stage full neurological syndrome and result in permanent brain damage or death. Early detection is critical to prevent this complication. Treatment may include phototherapy or exchange transfusion.

The presentation of multiple brain lesions in a patient is of grave concern, and an infective process should be considered along with the possibility of multiple tumors. Stereotactic biopsy of the lesion is most likely to provide a diagnosis. The operative team may be required to employ precautions to prevent the spread of an unknown infective process. Identification of the infective agent and process determines proper treatment.

Neural Tube Defects

1. Encephaloceles are sac-like protrusions through skull defects in the midline. They can project anteriorly between the forehead and nose or, more commonly, posteriorly in the occipital region of the head (Figure 12-18). Meningeal membranes, CSF, and some neural tissue may be found in the sac. Posterior encephaloceles frequently present in combination with hydrocephalus, spastic quadriplegia (paralysis of all extremities), microcephaly (unusually small brain and head), ataxia (uncoordinated muscle movement affecting gait), visual difficulties, retardation, and seizures. Surgery is performed to excise the sac and close the defect. An encephalocele is a congenital anomaly that results from failure of

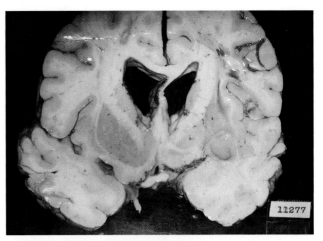

FIGURE 12-15 Multifocal brain abscesses.

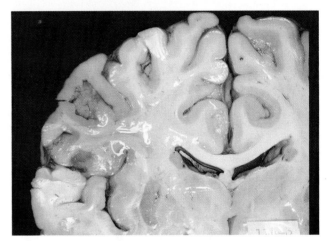

FIGURE 12-16 Encephalomalacia.

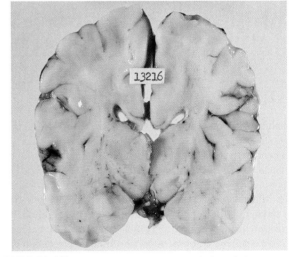

FIGURE 12-17 Kernicterus (bilirubin encephalopathy) in neonate.

the neural tube to close by the 28th day following conception, before most women realize they are pregnant. It is estimated that about 375, or 1 of every 10,000, babies are born yearly in the United States with encephaloceles (Centers for Disease Control and Prevention [CDC], 2009). Treatment of hydrocephalus secondary to neural tube defects is accom-

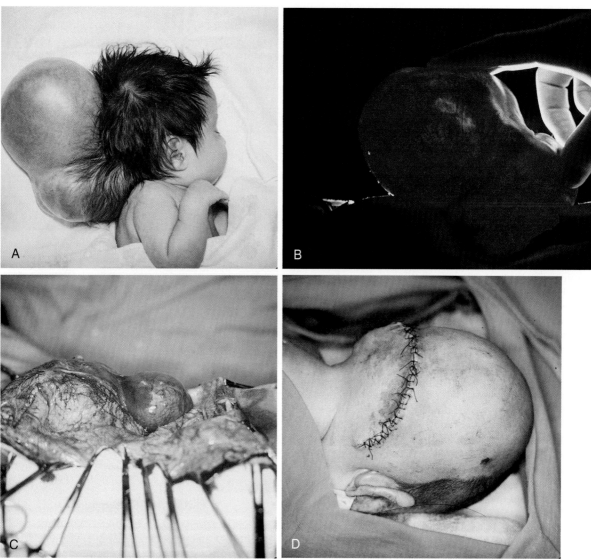

FIGURE 12-18 **A**, Occipital encephalocele, preoperative. **B**, Transillumination of occipital encephalocele filled with cerebrospinal fluid. **C**, Sac opened revealing small herniation of neural tissue. **D**, Postoperative appearance of closed occipital encephalocele.

plished with placement of a shunt to reduce intracranial pressure.

2. Anencephaly and spina bifida are more common neural tube defects (NTDs) and occur in approximately 1 of every 1,000 pregnancies in the United States (CDC, 2009). Anencephalic infants are often stillborn, but may survive a few hours to days, but the prognosis is death in these children born without formed brains or cranial coverings. Research has shown a genetic component to neural tube defects, but exact cause is unknown. Increasing folic acid intake by women who could become pregnant has been identified as a possible mechanism for reducing overall risk.

Ventricular System and Cerebrospinal Fluid

Within the brain are four communicating cavities, or ventricles, filled with CSF. In the lower medial portion of each cerebral hemisphere lies a large lateral ventricle that resembles a wishbone and is separated anteriorly from its counterpart by a thin septum (see Figure 12-12). Each lateral ventricle has a body and three horns: frontal, occipital, and temporal. Below the bodies of the lateral ventricles is a central cleft, or third ventricle. It communicates anteriorly with the lateral ventricles through the foramen of Monro and posteriorly with the fourth ventricle through the aqueduct of Sylvius—a long, narrow channel passing through the midbrain. The fourth ventricle is a cavity in the posterior fossa, between the cerebellum and the brainstem. In the roof of the fourth ventricle is the foramen of Magendie, an opening into the cisterna magna; at the lateral margins are the two foramina of Luschka, which open into the cisterna pontis. These cisterns are cavities that serve as reservoirs for CSF.

Much of the CSF originates in the choroid plexuses of the ventricles. These are tufted, vascular structures that allow certain fluid elements of the blood to pass through their ependymal linings. The choroid plexus is found along the floor in each lateral ventricle, on the roof of the third ventricle, and in the posterior portion of the fourth ventricle. Most of the fluid is formed in the lateral ventricles and flows through the interventricular foramen of Monro to the third ventricle and through the aqueduct of Sylvius to the fourth ventricle, where it escapes into the subarachnoid space of the basal cisterns through the foramina of Magendie and Luschka. From the basal cisterns the fluid flows around the spinal cord, over the cerebellar lobes, around the medulla and the base of the brain, and over the cerebral hemispheres in the subarachnoid space. The fluid is absorbed into the venous circulation through villi of the arachnoid (pacchionian granulations) into the great dural venous sinuses, particularly the superior sagittal sinus, and by diffusion through perivascular, perineural, and periradicular channels (see Figure 12-7).

Spinal fluid bathes the brain and spinal cord, helps support the weight of the brain, and acts as a cushion for the brain and spinal cord by absorbing some of the force of external trauma. By variation in its volume, it aids in keeping ICP relatively constant. If the brain atrophies, the amount of CSF increases to fill the dead space; if the brain swells, the amount of CSF decreases to compensate for the increase in brain mass. The fluid can carry certain drugs to diseased parts of the brain. It does not, however, play a significant role in supplying nutrition to the structures that it bathes. The total amount of circulating CSF averages 150 ml in the adult. The ventricles contain about 25 ml, and the remaining CSF circulates in the cranial and spinal subarachnoid space. CSF is secreted at a rate of between 21 and 24 ml/hr, or approximately 450 ml/24 hr. This means that in an adult, CSF is recirculated about three times each day.

Pathologic Conditions Related to Cerebrospinal Fluid. CSF can be examined by the lab to provide diagnostic information. CSF is most commonly obtained by way of lumbar puncture (LP). Because the subarachnoid space surrounding the brain is freely connected to the subarachnoid space of the spinal cord, any abnormal increase in ICP will be directly reflected as an increase at the lumbar site. Tumors, infection, hydrocephalus, and intracranial bleeding can cause increased intracranial and spinal pressure (Pagana and Pagana, 2009). LP is contraindicated when ICP is increased from a suspected intracranial mass that is causing neurologic symptoms. In this situation, the sudden reduction in pressure from the release of CSF could cause brain herniation. The ventricular fluid normally has a protein content of 5 to 15 mg/dl, whereas the protein content of spinal fluid is 25 to 45 mg/dl. These values may be considerably elevated in pathologic conditions of the CNS. The characteristics of normal spinal fluid are as follows:

♦ Appearance: clear and colorless
♦ Pressure: less than 20 cm H_2O
♦ Glucose: 50 to 75 mg/dl, or two thirds of blood glucose level
♦ Chloride: 700 to 750 mg/dl
♦ Cells: white blood cells (WBCs)—neonate, 0 to 30 cells/μl; 1 to 5 years, 0 to 20 cells/μl; 6 to 18 years, 0 to 10 cells/μl; adult, 0 to 5 cells/μl
♦ Protein: lumbar, 15 to 45 mg/dl
♦ Culture: no growth
♦ Gamma globulin: 3% to 12% of total protein (Pagana and Pagana, 2009)

Elevations in CSF pressure can be caused by an expanding mass within the skull, such as a tumor, hemorrhage, or cerebral edema; an increase in formation or decrease in absorption of fluid, as in meningitis, encephalitis, and other febrile conditions; an increase in venous pressure within the skull from an obstruction to normal venous drainage; a blockage of absorption by inflammatory conditions of the arachnoid and perivascular spaces; any mechanical obstruction of the ventricular or subarachnoidal fluid pathways; or decreased absorption of CSF. These pathologic conditions can cause a dangerous increase in ICP, which ultimately could result in brain herniation and death.

The rate of absorption and production of CSF is related to the osmotic and hydrostatic pressures of the blood. Intravenous (IV) injection of hypertonic mannitol, commonly used with a nonosmotic diuretic, can be employed to pull fluid from tissue to the vascular space for excretion by the kidneys, resulting in systemic diuresis and a decrease in ICP.

Hydrocephalus is a condition marked by an excessive accumulation of CSF, resulting in dilation of the intracerebral ventricles where CSF is synthesized and circulated. Enlargement of cerebral ventricles is the result of CSF blockage and interruption of CSF circulation or CSF reabsorption. The causes of hydrocephalus are many, including congenital conditions, aqueductal stenosis, tumors or cysts of the ventricular system, subarachnoid hemorrhage (SAH), posterior fossa tumors, or trauma with increased ICP. Noncommunicating (obstructive) hydrocephalus involves an obstruction of CSF pathways. In communicating hydrocephalus, the normal CSF pathways are open; however, there is an abnormality in CSF absorption with increased ICP. Normal-pressure hydrocephalus (NPH) is a communicating hydrocephalus that produces a normal pressure on random LP (Greenberg, 2005). NPH most commonly develops in the elderly, probably because of abnormal CSF absorption; however, the cause may not be apparent. Symptoms of dementia, unsteady gait, and urinary incontinence are seen with normal pressure and chronic hydrocephalus. Those with acute hydrocephalus present with headache, nausea, vomiting, drowsiness, and papilledema.

The appropriate surgical procedure depends on the precise type of hydrocephalus. Whenever possible, an obstructing lesion that causes hydrocephalus should be surgically removed. For some cases of obstructive hydrocephalus, endoscopic third ventriculostomy may be possible. With endoscopic third ventriculostomy, CSF can be diverted by surgically creating an opening at the floor of the third ventricle, thus eliminating the need for a shunt. However, treatment of hydrocephalus in both the adult and pediatric populations is generally by placement of a ventriculoperitoneal (VP) shunt (Wang and Avellino, 2005). With acute symptoms, temporary placement of an external ventriculostomy catheter used to measure the ICP and drain CSF may be preferred, thus postponing or eliminating the need for a permanent VP shunt.

Cerebral Blood Supply

The brain requires 20% more oxygen than any other organ to maintain its high level of metabolic activity. The arterial supply to the brain enters the cranium through the two internal carotid arteries anteriorly and the two vertebral arteries posteriorly. These communicate at the base of the brain through the circle of Willis (Figure 12-19), which ensures continuity of the

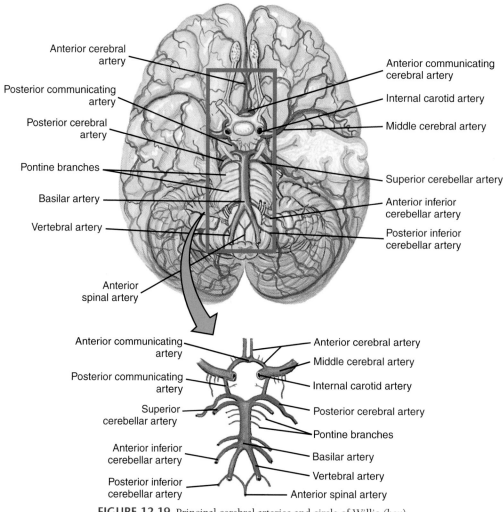

FIGURE 12-19 Principal cerebral arteries and circle of Willis (*box*).

circulation if any one of the four main channels is interrupted. However, these connections are extremely variable and do not always have functional anastomoses. The main branches for distribution of blood to each hemisphere of the brain from the internal carotid arteries are the anterior and middle cerebral arteries. Each artery nourishes a specific area of the brain (Figures 12-19 and 12-20). The anterior cerebral artery supplies the anterior two thirds of the medial surface and adjacent region over the convexity of the hemisphere, thus including about half of the frontal and parietal lobes. The middle cerebral artery supplies most of the lateral surface of the hemisphere, including half of the frontal, parietal, and temporal lobes. The posterior cerebral artery, which originates at the basilar artery, supplies the occipital lobe and the remaining half of the temporal lobe, principally on the inferior and medial surfaces. The brainstem and cerebellum are supplied by branches of the basilar and vertebral arteries.

The cerebral veins do not parallel the arteries as the veins do in most other parts of the body. The external cortical veins anastomose freely in the pia mater, forming larger cerebral veins, and as such they pierce the arachnoid membrane, cross the subdural space, and empty into the great dural venous sinuses. A subdural hemorrhage after head trauma may arise from disruption of these bridging vessels; an epidural hemorrhage often results from lacerations of the middle meningeal artery—a branch of the external carotid artery that supplies the dura mater. The deep cerebral veins, which drain the interior of the hemispheres, empty principally into the great vein of Galen and the inferior sagittal sinus (Figures 12-21 and 12-22).

The blood transports oxygen, nutrients, and other substances necessary for the proper functioning of living tissue. The needs of the brain for oxygen and glucose are critical. The brain can store only small amounts of oxygen and energy-producing nutrients. Constant flow of blood to the brain must be maintained.

The brain uses oxygen in the metabolism of glucose—the chief source of energy. Protein and fat metabolism plays little part in energy production. In the face of an oxygen deficit, the survival time of CNS tissue is very short. In the presence of low levels of blood glucose, CNS function is compromised and unconsciousness results.

Generally, all factors affecting the systemic blood pressure indirectly affect the cerebral circulation. The brain normally receives 20% of the cardiac output. The cerebral blood flow is kept constant by an autoregulation phenomenon such that increases in blood pressure lead to vasoconstriction of cerebral arteries and decreases in blood pressure cause cerebral vasodilation to maintain a relatively constant cerebral blood flow.

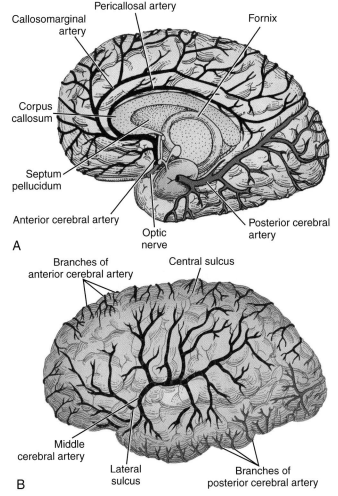

Pericallosal artery

Callosomarginal artery

Fornix

Corpus callosum

Septum pellucidum

Anterior cerebral artery

Optic nerve

Posterior cerebral artery

A

Branches of anterior cerebral artery

Central sulcus

Middle cerebral artery

Lateral sulcus

Branches of posterior cerebral artery

B

FIGURE 12-20 A, Arteries of medial surface of brain. **B,** Arteries of the lateral surface of brain.

When the mean arterial pressure falls below 60 mm Hg, the autoregulation mechanism usually fails.

Vascular Pathologic Conditions of the Brain. Vascular lesions of the brain are most often diagnosed in people who present with acute, spontaneous intracranial hemorrhage.

ANEURYSMS. Aneurysms arise from a complex set of circumstances involving a congenital anatomic predisposition and local or systemic factors that weaken the arterial wall, leading to dilation. The majority of these lesions occur at the branching points of large subarachnoid conducting arteries. The greatest vulnerability to aneurysmal development occurs at points of vessel bifurcation. Acute SAH in this setting can lead to vessel vasospasm (with greatest risk at 4 to 10 days after the SAH), cerebral ischemia, hydrocephalus, increased ICP, diabetes insipidus, syndrome of inappropriate secretion of antidiuretic hormone (SIADH), respiratory failure, brain injury, and risk of rebleeding (Figure 12-23). The vessels of the circle of Willis are most often implicated, including the posterior communicating artery, anterior communicating artery, middle cerebral artery, carotid artery, posterior inferior cerebellar artery, vertebral artery, and basilar artery. Surgical intervention techniques are based on the characteristics of the aneurysm. Small neck aneurysms may be occluded using coils placed by means of interventional radiology techniques. Aneurysmal clipping by way of a craniotomy approach is most often used to treat broad neck aneurysms.

VASCULAR MALFORMATIONS. Vascular malformations of the CNS are characterized by congenital lesions that have the potential to produce symptoms any time during the life of an individual with the malformation. Types of vascular malformations include arteriovenous malformations (AVMs), cavernous malformations, capillary telangiectasias, and venous malformations. AVMs are complex lesions in which direct shunting of arterial blood to the venous system occurs (Figure 12-24). The vascular channels are tightly packed and have a propensity to hemorrhage. Capillary telangiectasias are small vascular malformations commonly seen in the pons. They rarely bleed. Cavernous malformations are cystic vascular spaces, similar to capillary telangiectasias but larger and with a tendency to bleed. Venous malformations are the most common type, comprising anomalous veins, a single tortuous vein, or a number of smaller veins joining at a single point. These are considered benign and rarely bleed. Surgical excision of the cavernous malformation and the AVM is recommended.

HEMATOMAS. Hematomas are collections of blood that coagulate to form space-occupying lesions. An intracerebral hemorrhage, the cause of stroke in many hypertensive patients, results in hematoma formation most often in the basal ganglia, subcortical white matter, cerebellum, and brainstem. These hematomas compress vital structures, depress consciousness, and can be catastrophic. They are often inoperable (Greenberg, 2005).

Intracranial trauma can cause a shearing of arterial and venous vessels that results in hematoma collections in the epidural and subdural spaces. These space-occupying lesions raise ICP and often result in serious neurologic disruption (Figure 12-25). Epidural hematomas are often the result of a blow to the head causing a tear in the middle meningeal artery, which lies on the dura under the skull. These arterial hemorrhages can be life-threatening in that they can cause rapid deterioration in level of consciousness secondary to size of the bleed and brain displacement by the hematoma (Figure 12-26). In contrast to an epidural hematoma, a traumatic subdural hematoma usually results from venous bleeding and collects more slowly. Bridging veins in the subdural space are torn; blood escapes, dissecting a space between the dura and the arachnoid, and collects over one cerebral hemisphere (Figure 12-27). Subdural hematomas may be acute, subacute, or chronic (Figure 12-28). Chronic hematomas can often be evacuated through burr holes, but acute hematomas may require a craniotomy to remove the clot and control bleeding.

CEREBRAL ISCHEMIA. Any area of the brain can become ischemic from an arterial occlusion or embolization. Symptoms may be gradual or sudden. Intracranial plaques most commonly form at the bifurcation of the internal carotid artery, into the middle and anterior cerebral arteries. In select cases, extracranial-intracranial arterial microanastomosis can be performed. Carotid endarterectomy can be performed for extracranial lesions of the carotid artery.

Cranial Nerves

Twelve pairs of cranial nerves arise within the cranial cavity (Figure 12-29). Although they are part of the PNS, from a surgical standpoint they are considered with the head.

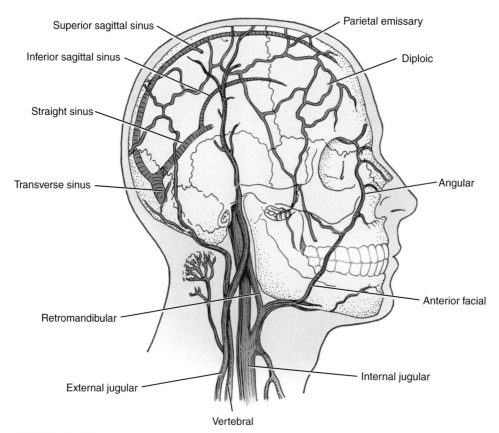

FIGURE 12-21 Semischematic projection of large veins of head. Deep veins and dural sinuses are projected on skull. Note connection (emissary veins) between superficial and deep veins.

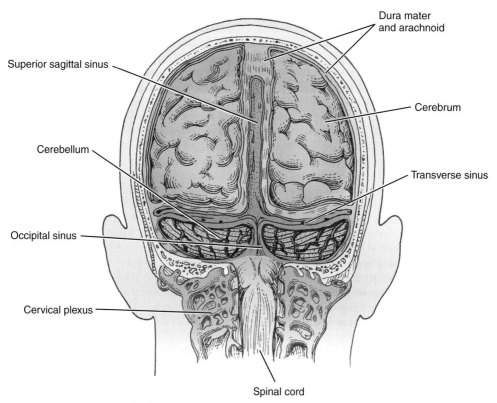

FIGURE 12-22 Venous sinuses shown in relation to brain and skull.

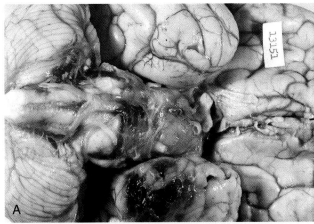

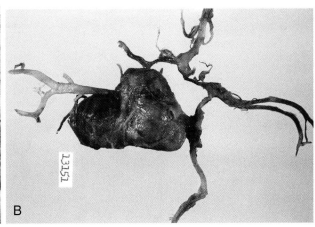

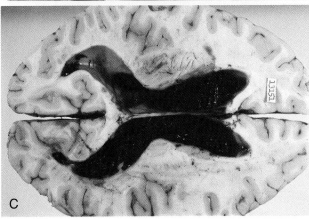

FIGURE 12-23 A, Intracranial aneurysm located at the base of the brain arising from the circle of Willis. **B,** Aneurysm dissected at autopsy. **C,** Intraventricular hemorrhage secondary to ruptured intracranial aneurysm.

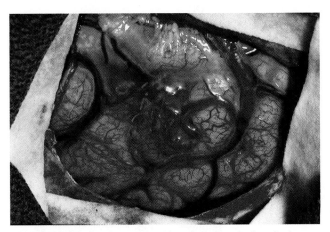

FIGURE 12-24 Arteriovenous malformation (AVM) of cerebral cortex.

First Cranial Nerve. The olfactory nerve, a fiber tract of the brain, is located under the frontal lobe on the cribriform plate of the ethmoid bone. It transmits the sense of smell. Frontal lobe tumors, fractures of the anterior fossa of the skull, and lesions of the nasal cavity may affect the olfactory nerve.

Second Cranial Nerve. The optic nerve is a fiber tract of the brain. It originates in the ganglion cells of the retina and passes through the optic foramen in the apex of the orbit to reach the optic chiasma. A partial crossing of the fibers occurs there; so the fibers from the nasal half of each retina pass to the oppo-

site side. Posterior to the chiasma, the visual pathway is called the *optic tract.* Still farther back, it becomes the optic radiation. Lesions in various parts of this pathway produce characteristic defects in the visual fields. For example, a lesion near the chiasma usually destroys the temporal vision of each eye (bitemporal hemianopia), whereas a lesion of the occipital lobe produces impairment of vision (homonymous hemianopia), affecting the right or left halves of the visual fields of both eyes.

Lesions that affect the optic nerve and are treated by neurosurgery include primary gliomas of the nerve, pituitary tumors that press on the optic chiasma, and occasionally meningiomas of the optic nerve sheath or in the region of the sella turcica and olfactory groove. The optic nerves and chiasma are best exposed through a frontal craniotomy along the floor of the anterior fossa or through a frontotemporal approach along the sphenoid ridge. Cranial base approaches using an orbital osteotomy or orbital-zygomatic osteotomies improve access and exposure of the optic system.

Third, Fourth, and Sixth Cranial Nerves. The third, fourth, and sixth cranial nerves are three pairs of nerves—the oculomotor, the trochlear, and the abducens, respectively. They are conveniently considered together because they are the motor nerves to the muscles of the eyes. They are affected by many toxic, inflammatory, vascular, and neoplastic lesions. The third nerve may be affected by aneurysms of the posterior communicating artery, and pressure against this nerve accounts for pupillary dilation when temporal lobe (uncal) herniation, resulting from increased ICP, is present.

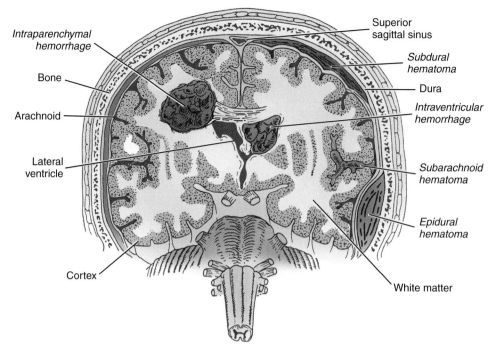

FIGURE 12-25 Types of intracerebral hemorrhage (in italics).

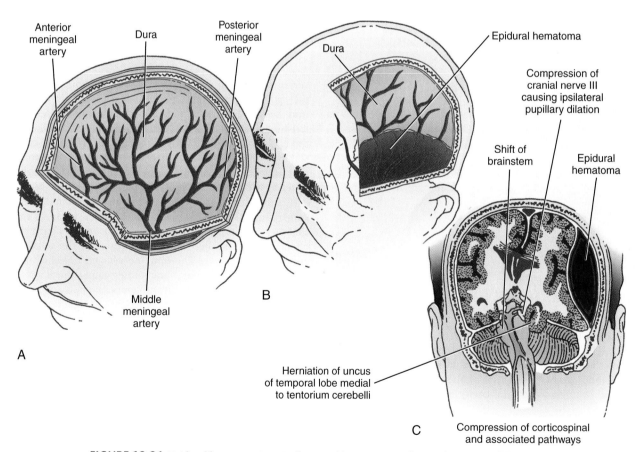

FIGURE 12-26 Epidural hematoma is typically caused by trauma resulting in laceration of the middle meningeal artery. **A,** The middle meningeal artery. The typical traumatic epidural hematoma is caused by a laceration of this vessel. **B** and **C,** A linear fracture of the squamous portion of the temporal bone has torn the middle meningeal artery, which has resulted in an epidural hematoma.

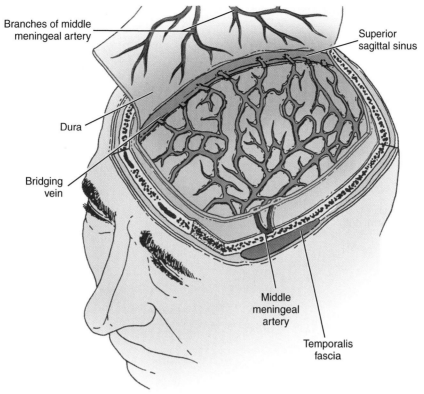

Branches of middle
meningeal artery

Superior
sagittal sinus

Dura

Bridging
vein

Middle
meningeal
artery

Temporalis
fascia

FIGURE 12-27 Veins are shown extending from the surface of the brain to the superior sagittal sinus. Differential movement of the brain within the skull at the time of injury may tear one or more of these veins, leading to the formation of a subdural hematoma.

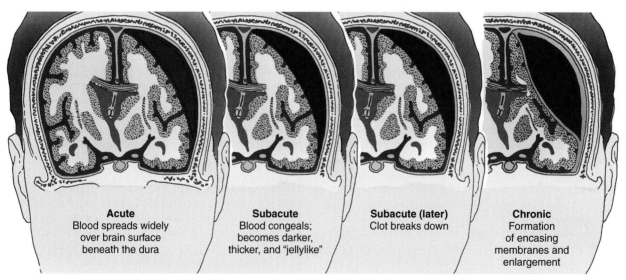

Acute
Blood spreads widely
over brain surface
beneath the dura

Subacute
Blood congeals;
becomes darker,
thicker, and "jellylike"

Subacute (later)
Clot breaks down

Chronic
Formation
of encasing
membranes and
enlargement

FIGURE 12-28 A subdural hematoma is liquid at first and subsequently clots. It is then reabsorbed or develops into a chronic subdural hematoma as a thick, vascular outer membrane. A thin, inner membrane develops around liquefying blood, starting about 2 weeks after injury. The chronic subdural hematoma enlarges as further bleeding occurs within it.

Fifth Cranial Nerve. The trigeminal nerve has two functions: (1) sensory supply to the forehead, eyes, meninges, face, jaw, teeth, hard palate, buccal mucosa, tongue, nose, nasal mucosa, and maxillary sinus; and (2) motor innervation of the muscles of mastication. The sensory fibers that arise from cells in the trigeminal ganglion travel along the medial wall of the middle cranial fossa and then extend peripherally in three divisions: ophthalmic, maxillary, and mandibular. Behind the ganglion the fibers enter the brainstem by way of the sensory root. The motor root, which originates from cells in the brainstem, follows the course of the larger sensory component (Figure 12-30).

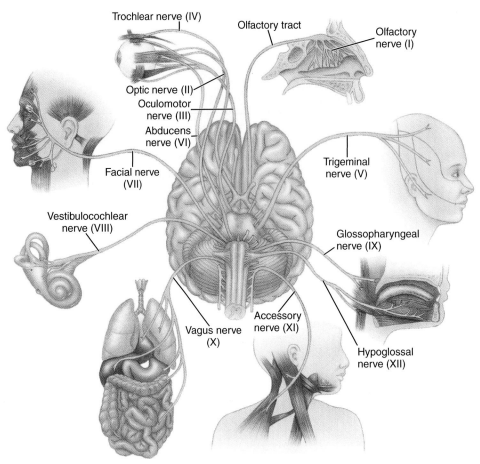

FIGURE 12-29 Ventral surface of brain showing attachment of cranial nerves.

Trigeminal neuralgia (tic douloureux) is characterized by excruciating, piercing paroxysms of pain, affecting one or more of the major peripheral divisions. The recurrent attacks are usually instigated by stimulation of trigger zones present about the face, nares, lips, and teeth. This condition, believed to be caused by a high incidence of vascular compression on the root entry zone of the nerve leading to demyelination, tends to occur unilaterally and in older persons. Medical treatment is frequently unsuccessful in the long term. Types of neurosurgical procedures currently recommended for trigeminal neuralgia include percutaneous rhizotomy using glycerol, radiofrequency, or balloon compression; radiosurgery; and microvascular decompression (Research Highlight). Microvascular decompression requires a suboccipital craniotomy and is the most invasive of the techniques. However, it is the least destructive and probably the most durable treatment.

Seventh Cranial Nerve. The facial nerve supplies the musculature of the face and the sensation of taste for the anterior two thirds of the tongue. It originates in the brainstem, passes through the skull with the eighth nerve by way of the internal acoustic meatus, continues along the facial canal, and exits just posterior to the parotid gland. The nerve may be damaged by vestibular schwannomas (e.g., acoustic neuromas), fractures at the base of the skull, mastoid infections, and surgical procedures in the vicinity of the parotid gland.

Bell's palsy, a facial lower motor neuron paralysis, can affect the seventh nerve. It may last for a few weeks to a few months, but recovery usually takes place. When permanent interruption of the nerve occurs, useful operations for restoration of function include spinal accessory-facial anastomosis and hypoglossal-facial anastomosis. These operations are performed high in the neck behind the parotid gland by use of the operating microscope.

Eighth Cranial Nerve. The acoustic nerve has two parts, both sensory—the cochlear for hearing and the vestibular for balance. The former receives stimuli from the organ of Corti and the latter from the semicircular canals. The major surgical lesion of the eighth nerve is vestibular schwannoma (acoustic neuroma), a histologically benign tumor growing from the nerve sheath at its entrance into the internal auditory meatus. This tumor arises deep in the angle between the cerebellum and pons (cerebellopontine angle). Symptoms may include unilateral deafness, tinnitus, unilateral impairment of cerebellar function, numbness of the face from involvement of the fifth cranial nerve, and, late in the course, papilledema caused by increased ICP. The operative approach is usually through a retrosigmoid craniotomy, exposing the edges of the transverse and sigmoid sinuses. The surgeon must take great care to prevent injury to the pons and to preserve the facial nerve. Attempts are made to preserve the acoustic nerve with smaller tumors when hearing preservation is an option.

Gamma Knife Therapy for Trigeminal Neuralgia

Trigeminal neuralgia is an extremely painful and debilitating condition characterized by unilateral intense pain in the ear, eye, lips, nose, scalp, forehead, teeth, or jaw. A variety of treatments, including microvascular surgical decompression, are offered to patients. These treatments have varying degrees of success and recurrence of the pain is an unfortunate phenomenon. Patients who have persistent or recurrent symptoms despite intervention represent approximately 10% to 30% of patients who undergo microvascular decompression (MVD), 20% to 50% of those who undergo a percutaneous destructive procedure, and 30% to 40% of those who undergo Gamma Knife radiosurgery. The Gamma Knife creates a lesion at the root entry of the trigeminal nerve, resulting in degeneration of the axons and ability to transmit impulses.

Researchers investigated the use of the Gamma Knife as a salvage procedure in patients who had recurrent or persistent pain after surgical treatment and/or failure of medical management. A total of 79 patients underwent salvage Gamma Knife radiosurgery as a treatment for their trigeminal pain. Pain outcome and quality-of-life indicators were measured 1 month after treatment during the patient follow-up visit and periodically after that via surveys and chart analysis.

The median follow-up period measured after the Gamma Knife therapy was 5.3 years. Analysis of the data showed that at 5 years, 20% of patients were pain free and 50% had pain relief; 41% of the group studied required a subsequent procedure.

Researchers concluded that while salvage Gamma Knife therapy for refractive trigeminal neuralgia is an effective and safe treatment, additional research is indicated to gain further understanding about the mechanism of action responsible for recurrent trigeminal dysfunction.

Modified from Little AS et al: Salvage gamma knife stereotactic radiosurgery for surgically refractive trigeminal neuralgia, *Int J Radiat Oncol Biol Phys* 74(2):522-527, 2009.

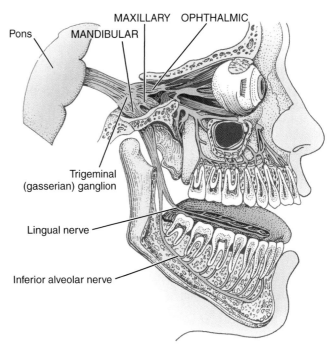

FIGURE 12-30 Trigeminal (fifth cranial) nerve and its three main divisions.

Meniere's disease is an affliction of the eighth nerve characterized by a recurrent and usually progressive group of symptoms including dizziness and a sensation of fullness or pressure in the ears. When medical measures fail to alleviate the problem, sectioning of the eighth nerve may be a surgical option.

Ninth Cranial Nerve. The glossopharyngeal nerve supplies the sense of taste to the posterior third of the tongue, supplies sensation to the tonsils and pharyngeal region, partially innervates the pharyngeal muscles, and primarily innervates the carotid sinus. Stimulation of the baroreceptors of the carotid sinus causes slowing of the heart, vasodilation, and decreased blood pressure. Its sensory component can be sectioned to treat a hypersensitive carotid sinus, or it can be sectioned in conjunction with the fifth nerve to treat painful malignancies of the face, mouth, and pharynx. The ninth nerve lies near the eighth nerve in the posterior fossa and is exposed in a similar way.

Tenth Cranial Nerve. The vagus nerve has many motor and sensory functions, primarily including innervation of pharyngeal and laryngeal musculature, control of heart rate, and regulation of acid secretion of the stomach. In neck surgery, the surgeon carefully avoids injury to the recurrent laryngeal branch because its injury results in vocal cord paralysis. In gastric surgery, the surgeon could sever the vagus nerve at the lower end of the esophagus to treat a peptic ulcer. The neurosurgeon is also concerned with preventing damage to the vagus nerve during posterior fossa surgery.

Eleventh Cranial Nerve. The spinal accessory nerve is a motor nerve to the sternocleidomastoid and trapezius muscles. To restore mobility to the face, it may be anastomosed to the peripheral end of a damaged facial nerve.

Twelfth Cranial Nerve. The hypoglossal nerve innervates the musculature of the tongue. Its neurosurgical interest is similar to that of the spinal accessory nerve.

Table 12-2 gives the function, origin, structures innervated, and assessment of the cranial nerves.

SPINE, SPINAL CORD, AND ADJACENT STRUCTURES

Vertebral Column

The primary roles of the spine are maintaining stability, protecting the neural elements, and allowing range of motion. The vertebral column has four distinct curves: cervical lordosis (a backward bend), thoracic kyphosis (a forward bend), lumbar lordosis, and sacral kyphosis. The spinal column consists of 33 vertebrae: 7 cervical, 12 thoracic, 5 lumbar, 5 sacral (fused as 1 section), and 1 coccygeal, which may have 1 to 3 fused sections (Figure 12-31).

The first cervical vertebra, or atlas, supports the skull. The second cervical vertebra, or axis, can be identified by its odontoid process, a vertical projection extending into the foramen of the atlas like a stick in a hoop. It rests against the anterior tubercle of the first cervical vertebra. Ligaments hold the two together but allow considerable rotational movement. The other cervical, thoracic, and lumbar vertebrae are more alike in structure.

TABLE 12-2

Understanding Cranial Nerves

Cranial Nerve	Function	Origin	Structures Innervated	Assessment
I Olfactory	Sensory	Olfactory bulbs below frontal lobes	Olfactory mucous membranes	Ability to identify familiar odors
II Optic	Sensory	Diencephalon	Retina of eye	Visual acuity Visual fields
III Oculomotor	Motor	Midbrain	Medial, superior, and inferior rectus muscles of eye Inferior oblique eye muscles Sphincter of iris	Extraocular movements Pupillary reaction to light and accommodation
IV Trochlear	Motor	Midbrain	Superior oblique muscle of eye	Extraocular movements
V Trigeminal	Mixed	Pons	*Sensory:* pain, touch, and temperature sensations in cheeks, jaw, and chin; corneal reflex *Motor:* muscles of mastication	Sensation in forehead, cheeks, jaw, and chin Mastication
VI Abducens	Motor	Pons	Lateral rectus muscle of eye	Extraocular movement
VII Facial	Mixed	Pons	*Sensory:* anterior two thirds of tongue *Motor:* muscles of face, forehead, and eye	Taste for anterior two thirds of tongue Movement of facial muscles (smile) Facial symmetry
VIII Acoustic	Sensory	Pons	Cochlear organ of Corti Vestibule and semicircular canals	Hearing acuity Balance
IX Glossopharyngeal	Mixed	Medulla	*Sensory:* posterior third of tongue *Motor:* muscles of pharynx	Taste for posterior third of tongue Movement of pharynx Gag reflex
X Vagus	Mixed	Medulla	*Sensory:* skin of external ear and mucous membranes *Motor:* muscles of larynx, pharynx, and esophagus; thoracic and abdominal viscera	Swallowing Movement of pharynx Gag reflex Cough
XI Spinal accessory	Motor	Medulla	Sternocleidomastoid and trapezius muscles	Shoulder shrug Turn head
XII Hypoglossal	Motor	Medulla	Tongue	Movement and strength of tongue

Each has a body, an oval block of bone situated anteriorly. An intervertebral disk, a fibrocartilaginous elastic cushion, separates one body from another (Figures 12-32 and 12-33). The spinal cord lies in a canal formed by the vertebral bodies, pedicles, and laminae. Articular surfaces or facets project from the pedicles and form joints with the facets of the vertebrae above and below. Transverse processes extend laterally and serve as hitching posts for muscles and ligaments. Spinous processes extend posteriorly and can be palpated in most people. The vertebrae are held together by multiple ligaments and muscles (see Figure 12-33). Motion of the spine occurs at the articular facets and through the elastic intervertebral disks. The intervertebral disks bond the adjacent surfaces of the vertebral bodies. Each disk consists of a fibrous outer annulus that contains the inner nucleus pulposus.

Spinal Cord

The spinal cord is protected by the bony framework of the spinal column. The dura mater is separated from its bony surroundings by a layer of epidural fat. Beneath the dura mater is the arachnoid, a continuation of the same structure in the head. The subarachnoid space contains CSF. A thin layer of pia mater adheres to the cord, and CSF also circulates from the fourth ventricle into the central canal of the cord.

The spinal cord is a downward prolongation of the brainstem, starting at the upper border of the atlas and ending at the upper border of the second lumbar vertebra (Figure 12-34). The cord is oval in cross section. It is slightly flattened in the anteroposterior diameter. A cross section looks like a gray **H** surrounded by a white mantle split in the midline, anteriorly and posteriorly, by sulci (Figure 12-35).

The peripheral white matter carries long, myelinated motor and sensory tracts. The central gray matter consists of nerve cell bodies and short, unmyelinated fibers (see Figures 12-34 and 12-35). The principal long pathways are the laterally placed pyramidal tracts, carrying impulses down from the cerebral cortex to the motor neurons of the cord; the dorsal ascending columns, mediating sensations of touch and proprioception; and the anterolaterally placed spinothalamic tracts, carrying

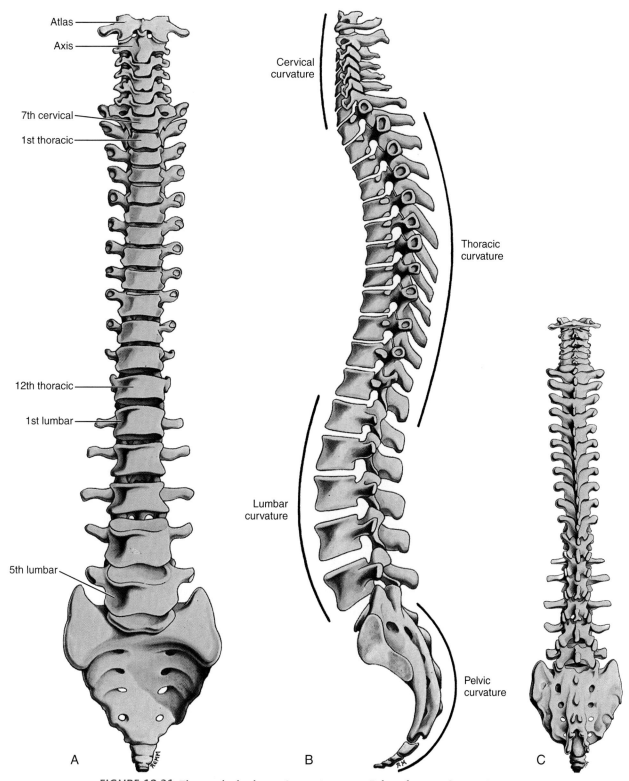

FIGURE 12-31 The vertebral column: A, anterior aspect; B, lateral aspect; C, posterior aspect.

pain and temperature sensations to the thalamus—the sensory receiving station of the brain (Figure 12-36).

Spinal Nerves

At each vertebral level is a pair of spinal nerves, each consisting of an anterior and a posterior root (see Figure 12-35). The anterior, or motor, root contains cell bodies that lie in the anterior horn of the spinal gray matter. The posterior, or sensory, root contains cell bodies that lie in the spinal ganglia located in the intervertebral foramina, the opening through which the nerves exit from the spinal canal and emerge from the cord. The course of the cervical nerves is horizontal, but at each

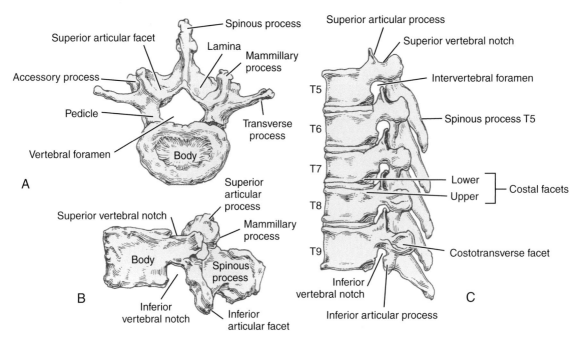

FIGURE 12-32 **A,** Fourth lumbar vertebra from above. **B,** Fourth lumbar vertebra from side. **C,** Fifth to ninth thoracic vertebrae, showing relationships of various parts.

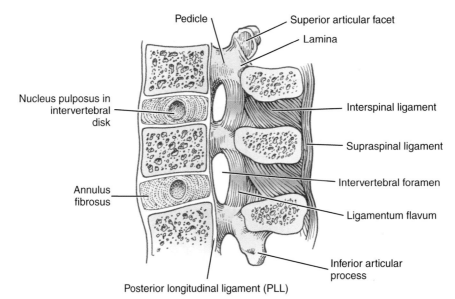

FIGURE 12-33 Median section through three lumbar vertebrae, showing intervertebral disks (nuclei pulposi).

lower level they assume an increasingly oblique and downward direction. In the lumbar region, the course of the nerves is nearly vertical, forming the cauda equina (see Figure 12-34). The normal segmental sensory distribution is valuable in the anatomic localization of sensory disorders (Figure 12-37).

Dermatomes are bands of skin innervated by a sensory root of a single spinal nerve. Knowledge of these dermatomes aids the practitioner in locating neurologic lesions (Figure 12-38).

Spinal Vasculature

The vasculature of the spinal cord and vertebral column is a rich, delicate network. The arterial blood supply to the spi-

nal cord arises from the vertebral arteries as the anterior spinal artery and the posterior spinal arteries. These vessels branch and anastomose on both sides of the cord and within the substance of the cord. They also branch into anterior and posterior radicular arteries that form spinal rami as they accompany the spinal nerve roots through the intervertebral foramina.

A series of venous plexuses surround and innervate the spinal cord at each level in the vertebral canal. They anastomose with each other and form the intervertebral veins as they pass through the intervertebral foramina with the spinal nerves to join the intercostal, lumbar, and sacral veins. The lateral longitudinal veins near the foramen magnum empty into the infe-

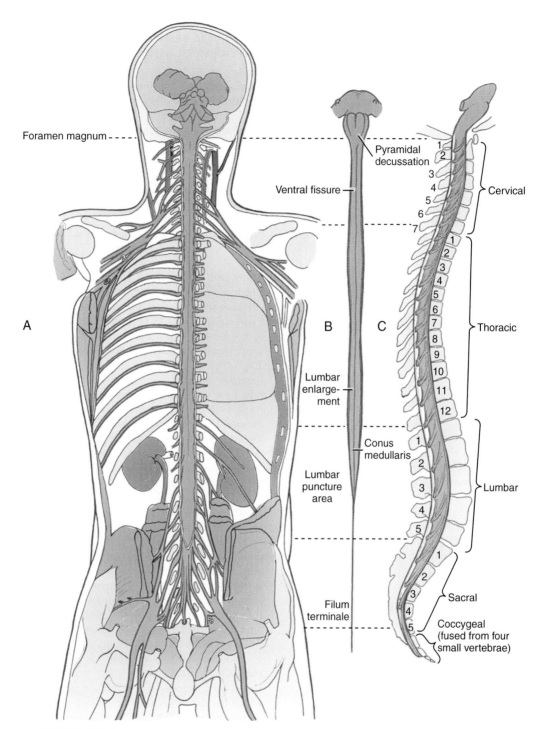

Foramen magnum

Pyramidal decussation

Ventral fissure

1
2
3
4
5
6
7
Cervical

1
2
3
4
5
6
7
8
9
10
11
12
Thoracic

A

B

C

Lumbar enlargement

Conus medullaris

Lumbar puncture area

1
2
3
4
5
Lumbar

1
2
3
4
5
Sacral

Coccygeal (fused from four small vertebrae)

Filum terminale

FIGURE 12-34 Posterior view of brainstem and spinal cord. **A,** Torso dissected from back is shown. Dura mater has been opened and cord exposed. Levels concerned can be easily determined by referring to ribs on left side of thorax. Cord proper terminates opposite body of second lumbar vertebra (**B**) as conus medullaris. **B,** Ventral surface of cord stripped of dura mater and arachnoid. It is symmetric in structure, two halves of which are separated by ventral fissure. This fissure stops at foramen magnum. Caudally, pia mater leaves conus medullaris as glistening thread, or filum terminale. **C,** Cord is exposed from lateral side. Dura mater has been opened. Because cord is shorter than canal and spinal nerves exit through intervertebral foramina, one at a time, lowest portion of canal is occupied only by a bundlelike accumulation of nerve roots—cauda equina. Caudal end of dural sac, enclosing spinal cord and cauda equina, lies somewhere between bodies of first and third sacral vertebrae. Size and position of the three views correspond, and elimination of major vertebral levels is indicated by transverse lines for all three figures.

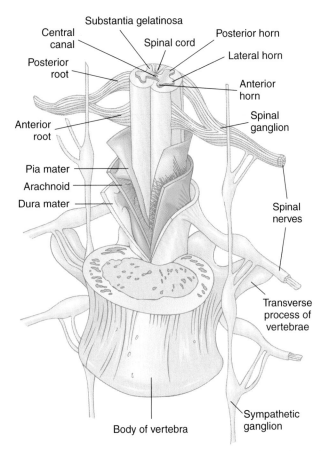

FIGURE 12-35 Spinal cord, showing meninges, formation of spinal nerves, and relationships to vertebra and to sympathetic trunk and ganglia.

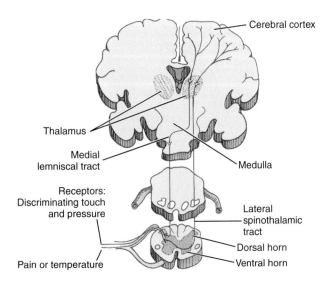

FIGURE 12-36 Lateral spinothalamic and medial lemniscal neural tracts.

rior petrosal sinus and cerebellar veins. The venous network innervates the bony structures and musculature as well as the spinal cord and nerve roots. The surgical technologist considers the possibility of venous bleeding during spinal surgery when planning care.

Pathologic Lesions of the Spinal Cord and Adjacent Structures

Surgery is performed to correct congenital malformations, traumatic injuries, tumors, abscesses, herniated and degenerative intervertebral disks, and intractable pain.

Meningocele. The most common congenital lesion encountered is a lumbar meningocele, or myelomeningocele—a failure of the union of the vertebral arches during fetal development. The fluid-filled, thin-walled sac often contains neural elements. This fetal anomaly is often diagnosed prenatally and is often seen with other CNS abnormalities, which include hydrocephalus, gyral abnormalities, and Chiari's malformation of the hindbrain. Refer to Chapter 17 for a discussion of the surgical treatment of meningocele.

Spine and Spinal Cord Tumors. The most frequently occurring tumors of the spine are metastatic, and the spine is the most common site for skeletal metastasis. Although it is estimated that between 5% and 10% of cancer patients develop *symptomatic* spinal metastasis, it is estimated that as many as 30% to 90% of cancer patients actually develop skeletal metastasis (Donthineni, 2009). Pain is the earliest and most prominent symptom, followed by weakness. Secondary spinal tumors most often originate from carcinomas of the lung, breast, prostate, and blood. Approximately 17% of patients with other primary tumors may experience cord compression as a result of spinal metastases. Metastases to the spine have a predilection toward the thoracic spine, followed by the lumbar and cervical areas (Donthineni, 2009). Treatment goals for metastatic tumors of the spine are pain relief and preservation or restoration of neurologic function. Options include radiation, surgery, or a combination of these. Surgery involves both decompression of the spinal cord and nerve roots and stabilization of the spinal column.

Spinal tumors are classified according to location as *extradural* (outside the dura mater) or *intradural* (inside the dura mater). Intradural tumors may be either *extramedullary* (outside the cord) or *intramedullary* (within the cord). Although metastatic tumors may be found in each category, they are usually extradural. Spinal cord tumors account for approximately 15% of CNS tumors (Greenberg, 2005). Most primary CNS tumors are benign.

Extradural tumors arise outside the spinal cord in vertebral bodies or epidural tissues. They account for 50% to 60% of spinal cord neoplasms and include sarcomas and carcinomas, which may be metastatic from adjacent structures in or around the vertebrae (Harrop, 2005). Other extradural lesions include lymphomas, lipomas, neurofibromas, chondromas, angiomas, abscesses, and granulomas.

Most intradural tumors are extramedullary and benign and, if diagnosed early before severe neurologic deficits occur, offer an excellent prognosis. They manifest their presence by pain of a radicular nature and various motor and sensory disabilities below their segmental locations. Intradural extramedullary tumors represent 35% to 45% of spinal cord tumors (Harrop, 2005). They are usually benign and originate from the dura mater and arachnoid surrounding the cord and from the root sheaths of spinal nerves. Schwannomas (neuromas) are especially common in the thoracocervical area and may be part of generalized neurofibromatosis. Meningiomas also commonly

SURGICAL INTERVENTIONS

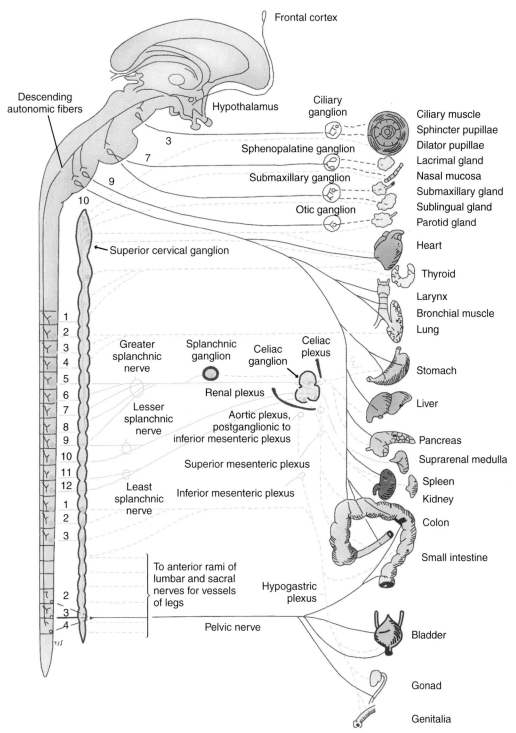

FIGURE 12-37 Sympathetic division of the autonomic nervous system.

occur in intradural extramedullary locations (Figure 12-39). Less frequently, lipomas or other types of tumors are found. Approximately 2% to 7% of spinal cord tumors are intradural intramedullary tumors (Harrop, 2005). These tumors infiltrate the cord tissue and are much more difficult to remove than are

extramedullary tumors. Of the intramedullary tumors, the most common are ependymomas (Figure 12-40) and astrocytomas.

Cord tumors frequently produce spinal fluid blockage and can be pinpointed accurately with MRI. Intraspinal injection of contrast material (myelography) is another option for diag-

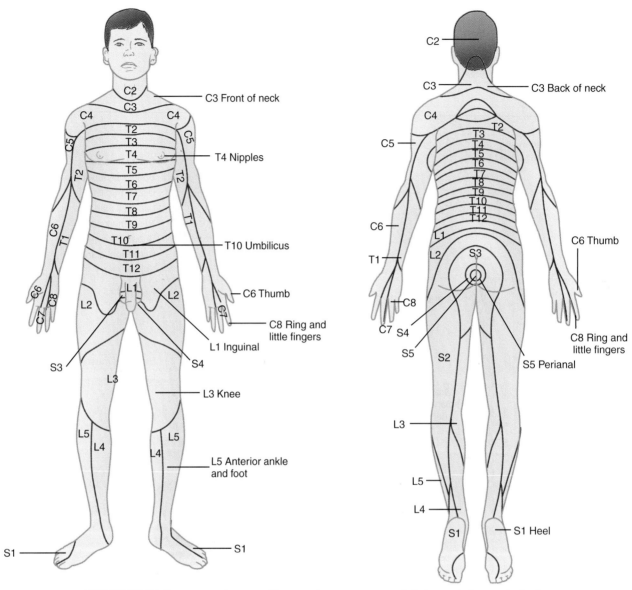

FIGURE 12-38 Dermatomes innervated by posterior nerve roots and their correlation on the body; both anterior and posterior views are shown. *C,* Cervical; *T,* thoracic; *L,* lumbar; *S,* sacral.

nosis. Often, a standard laminectomy is used for exposure and removal.

Spinal Epidural Abscess. Spinal epidural abscess can develop from vertebral osteomyelitis, from infection originating at a distant source and transferred by the blood, or from direct inoculation caused by spinal surgery, LP, or epidural administration of anesthetic. Patients who are immunosuppressed are especially at risk for epidural abscesses. Clinical presentation involves spinal and radicular pain and muscle weakness that can progress to paralysis. Epidural abscess is most easily diagnosed by MRI and typically treated with surgical decompression, culture, and irrigation, along with 4 to 8 weeks of IV antibiotic therapy.

Intervertebral Disk Disease. Intervertebral disk disease is the most frequently encountered neurosurgical problem. The axial skeleton bears both the body's weight and externally applied axial forces while maintaining mobility. Intervertebral disks serve as mechanical buffers that absorb axial loading, bending, and shear forces. Bipedal posture further stresses the intervertebral disks, leading to degenerative disk disorders. Disk rupture occurs with radial fissuring of the annulus. The nucleus pulposus then escapes, extending to the margin of the annulus and posterior longitudinal ligament. Once the nucleus pulposus protrudes beyond the perimeter of the disk space into the epidural space, it results in nerve root compression and radiculopathy (pain produced by pressure or traction on the nerve roots) (Figures 12-41 and 12-42). Most disk protrusions occur at the L4-L5 and L5-S1 interspaces. Interventions include a medical trial of treatment with steroids and analgesics/narcotics, muscle relaxation, rest, epidural steroid injections, and, in failed cases, laminotomy or laminectomy with diskectomy. In far-lateral disk herniations, percutaneous lumbar diskectomy

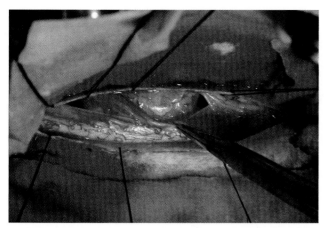

FIGURE 12-39 Intradural spinal cord meningioma. Cord is retracted, exposing tumor between spinal nerve roots.

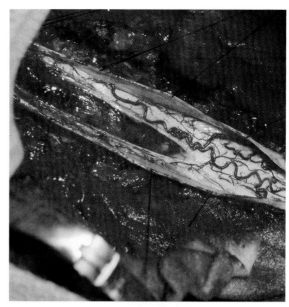

FIGURE 12-40 Intramedullary spinal cord ependymoma.

is often an alternative to laminotomy. This minimally invasive technique gains access to the disk space posterolaterally, using local anesthetic. The disk space is entered by way of a cannula. An aspiration probe may be used to remove the disk matter, or direct removal can be done microscopically or endoscopically.

Intractable Pain. Certain painful spinal lesions, usually of a malignant nature, can be controlled by use of epidural opiates, by use of fentanyl patches, or by temporary or permanent use of a medication pump. Another pain control measure is to divide the pain fibers supplying the affected area. This may be accomplished by sectioning the sensory roots intraspinally (posterior rhizotomy) or by incising the spinothalamic tracts that carry pain and temperature impulses (anterolateral cordotomy). Alternatively, spinal cord stimulation of the affected area can be achieved with the placement of electrodes in the epidural space. A laminectomy for exposure is necessary to perform these surgical procedures.

Peripheral Nerves. The PNS consists of those structures containing nerve fibers or axons that connect the CNS with motor and sensory, somatic and visceral, end-organs. The PNS includes the cranial nerves (III to XII), the spinal nerves, the autonomic nerves, and the ganglia.

The 31 pairs of spinal nerves are each numbered for the level of the spinal column at which they emerge: cervical, C1 through C8; thoracic, T1 through T12; lumbar, L1 through L5; sacral, S1 through S5; and coccygeal, 1. The first pair of cervical spine nerves emerges between C1 and the occipital bone. The eighth cervical nerves emerge from the intervertebral foramina between C7 and T1. The first thoracic nerves emerge between T1 and T2.

In the cervical and lumbosacral regions the spinal nerves regroup in a plexiform manner before they form the peripheral nerves of the upper and lower extremities. Those in the thoracic region form cutaneous and intercostal nerves. The principal nerves of the upper plexus include the musculocutaneous, median, ulnar, and radial. Those of the lumbosacral plexus include the obturator, femoral, and sciatic.

Each spinal nerve divides into anterior, posterior, and white rami. Rami are primary divisions of a nerve. Anterior and posterior rami contain voluntary fibers; white rami contain autonomic fibers. Posterior rami further branch into nerves innervating the muscles, skin, and posterior surfaces of the head, neck, and trunk. Most anterior rami branch to the skeletal muscles and the skin of the extremities and anterior and lateral surfaces. In the process they form plexuses, such as the brachial and sacral plexuses. Spinal nerves contain sensory dendrites and motor axons; some have somatic axons, and some have axons of preganglionic autonomic motor neurons.

The autonomic (involuntary) nervous system consists of all the efferent nerves through which the cardiovascular apparatus, viscera, glands of internal secretion, and peripheral involuntary muscles are innervated (see Figure 12-37). There is a major anatomic difference between the somatic and autonomic nervous systems. In the somatic nervous system an impulse from the brainstem or spinal cord reaches the end-organ through a single neuron. In the autonomic nervous system an impulse passes through two neurons—the first ending in an autonomic ganglion and the second running from the ganglion to the end-organ. Some of the ganglia lie adjacent to the vertebral column to form the sympathetic trunks or chains; others are closely associated with the end-organs.

The preganglionic neurons from the brainstem (which traverse along the cranial nerves) and those from the second, third, and fourth sacral segments to the pelvic viscera end in ganglia in proximity to their end-organs; thus their postganglionic fibers are very short. This is known as the *parasympathetic,* or *craniosacral,* division of the autonomic nervous system. The preganglionic fibers from the thoracic and lumbar spinal cord terminate in the paravertebral ganglia, making up the sympathetic chain, and their postganglionic fibers are relatively long. This is termed the *sympathetic,* or *thoracolumbar,* division of the autonomic nervous system.

The two divisions are distinct anatomically and physiologically. The chemical substance mediating transmission of impulses at most postganglionic sympathetic nerve endings is *norepinephrine,* and the neurotransmitter at all parasympathetic and preganglionic sympathetic neurons is *acetylcholine.*

The majority of organs have dual innervation—part from the craniosacral division and part from the thoracolumbar

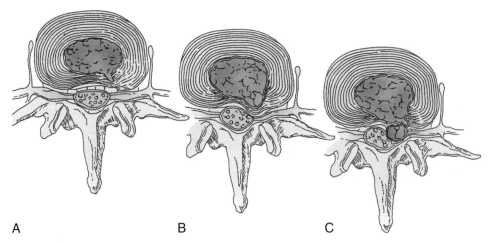

FIGURE 12-41 Stages in the herniation of an intervertebral disk. **A,** Tearing of the rings of the annulus fibrosus. **B,** Protrusion of the disk against the nerve root. **C,** Extrusion of part of the nucleus pulposus, with further nerve root compression.

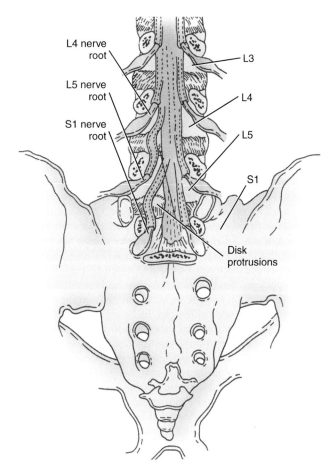

FIGURE 12-42 Posterior view of the lower lumbar spine. A disk protrusion at L4-L5 on the left results in compression of the L5 nerve root where it leaves the dural sac but before it exits from the spinal canal.

division. The functions of these two systems are antagonistic. Together they work to maintain homeostasis. In general, the thoracolumbar division functions as an emergency protection mechanism, always ready to combat physical or psychologic stress. The craniosacral division functions to conserve energy when the body is in a state of relaxation.

Stimuli arising from internal organs or from outside the body traverse visceral and somatic afferent nerve fibers to make reflex connections with preganglionic autonomic neurons in the brainstem and spinal cord. Such stimuli trigger activity of these involuntary systems automatically. When these automatic mechanisms break down or overact, surgery may be indicated. Thoracolumbar sympathectomy was once performed in hypertensive patients as an attempt to decrease blood vessel tone and lower blood pressure. Vagotomy can be performed to decrease acid secretion to the stomach in patients with peptic ulcers. Lumbar sympathectomy is used to relieve vasospastic disorders of the legs. T2 ganglionectomy is done to relieve palmar hyperhydrosis (sweaty palms).

Surgical Technologist Considerations

Assessment

Neurologic Assessment Tools. Basic neurologic assessment tools can be used preoperatively to establish a baseline assessment. Postoperatively, they can be used to establish a return to baseline and to assess postoperative neurologic stability. The postoperative condition of a neurosurgical patient can quickly deteriorate, so an adequate baseline assessment is essential (Rapid Response Team box). The Glasgow Coma Scale is commonly used to assess patients with brain injury (Table 12-3). Three indicators of cerebral function—eye opening, verbal communication, and motor response to verbal and noxious stimuli—are assessed; and the appropriate number of points for each is assigned and totaled. The best possible score is 15, and the worst possible score is 3. The Medical Research Council (MRC) Scale for Muscle Strength Grading can be used to assess muscle strength in the upper and lower extremities of spinal cord injury patients or patients who are having spine surgery (Table 12-4).

Preparation and Planning for Surgery. Communication and organization are essential among the perioperative team

RAPID RESPONSE TEAM

A patient with a neurologic diagnosis may experience irreversible neurologic damage if complications relating to the diagnosis or surgical procedure are not recognized in a timely manner to permit early intervention. In 2008 The Joint Commission established the 16th National Patient Safety Goal; its purpose was to improve the early recognition and response to negative changes in a patient's condition. By January of 2009 all institutions were required to develop and implement a rapid medical response team within their facility (TJC, 2008). Rapid response teams (RRTs) are especially critical for neurosurgical patients because of the rapidity of changes that can occur in the postoperative period. Rapid response teams consist of highly trained personnel that function together to create a pre–code team (Richmond, 2008). The personnel include an ICU nurse, respiratory therapist, medical resident, anesthesia care provider, and sometimes a surgical resident. The RRT can be activated by any bedside clinician, such as surgical technologists, registered nurses, residents, and attending physicians, at the earliest sign of patient deterioration. Most criteria for initiating a RRT call are institution specific, but some examples of the criteria include the following:

- Blood pressure: systolic BP below 90 mm Hg or above 180 mm Hg
- Heart rate: below 45 beats/min or above 125 beats/min
- Respiratory rate: below 8/min or above 24/min
- Oxygen saturation: below 90% or increasing oxygen requirements
- Acute change in mental status
- New onset of chest pain
- Staff member concerned about patient and needs a second opinion
- Patient not responding to treatment already underway for recent change in status (Richmond, 2008)

The RRT arrives at the patient's bedside within minutes to plan and implement interventions to stabilize the patient. While stabilization is occurring, the members of the RRT are communicating to the house staff and bedside clinicians the current and future needs of the patient. The RRT can determine if the patient's needs warrant a transfer to an increased level of monitoring such as an ICU. The main objective of the RRT is to provide early detection and treatment for unstable patients thereby avoiding cardiac or respiratory arrest in non-ICU settings (Winters et al, 2006).

RRT EXAMPLE

Mrs. Jones is post-op day 2 from an L4-S1 decompression and fusion for lumbar spinal stenosis. The previous nurse's report states that there were no complications during the procedure and the patient has been hemodynamically stable and neurologically intact postoperatively. The previous nurse's assessment of Mrs. Jones states that she was alert and oriented times 3, she moved all extremities without difficulty and against resistance, and her speech was clear and appropriate. The report also stated that as the day progressed, Mrs. Jones became increasingly drowsy but it was attributed to the patient-controlled analgesia (PCA) pump filled with morphine. The current nurse's assessment determines that Mrs. Jones is difficult to arouse, uncooperative, and having difficulty speaking; she is also not oriented to place or time. All of the current findings contradict the previous nurse's assessment, and the current nurse knows that the patient's health status is rapidly declining. The nurse immediately pages the facility's rapid response team (RRT), who arrives at the patient's bedside within minutes. The RRT performs an assessment and begins immediate interventions to stabilize Mrs. Jones. She is taken for a stat CT scan of the head, which shows cerebral edema. Mrs. Jones did not return to the nursing unit after the CT scan; she was intubated and transferred to an ICU. It was later determined that Mrs. Jones suffered bilateral symmetric cerebellar hemorrhages from a CSF leak that occurred during the initial spinal surgery.

Modified from The Joint Commission: *National patient safety goals 2008,* available at www.jcrinc.com/common/PDFs/fpdfs/pubs/pdfs/JCReqs/JCP-07-07-S1.pdf. Accessed April 14, 2009; Farag E et al: Cerebellar hemorrhage caused by cerebrospinal fluid leak after spine surgery, *Anesth Analg* 100:545-546, 2005; Richmond R: Rapid response teams, *Health Policy Newslett* 21(2):3, 2008, available at http://jdc.jefferson.edu/hpn/vol21/iss2/3. Accessed April 16, 2009; Winters BD et al: Rapid response teams—walk, don't run, *JAMA* 296:1645-1647, 2006.

members in planning care for the neurosurgical patient in the OR. Preoperative roles and responsibilities include:

1. The perioperative nurse and anesthesia provider will assess the patient and obtain appropriate consents.
2. The surgeon will communicate with the surgical team regarding:
   - Planned and possible surgical procedures
   - Specific approach and position
   - Need for special equipment or instrumentation
   - Need for radiologic support, neuromonitoring, intraoperative blood salvage unit, and image guidance
3. The surgical technologist will prepare the sterile instruments and supplies within the sterile field. Key points in preoperative preparation for neurosurgical procedures include the following:
   - Powered instruments must be assembled, tested prior to use, and kept in safety position when not in use. Nonpowered alternatives (Hudson brace and bits, Gigli saw and handles) should be available in case of drill malfunction.

- Multiple instrument trays may require use of special two-level or additional back tables. Extra Mayo stands or prep trays may also be needed.
- When Mayfield overhead instrument tables are used and the surgical technologist stands on platforms or standing stools, an additional Mayfield table should be positioned within easy reach, draped and prepared with additional instruments and items needed to prevent having to step down and take focus off of the sterile field.
- Draping materials should be organized by order of use to expedite the sometimes complicated process of draping. Additional drapes may be applied around the surgical site to isolate bone dust after creation of bone flap in craniotomy procedures.
- Microscopes should be prepared with appropriate objective lenses, assistant binoculars, camera connections, and so on, and sterilely draped and ready in advance of need. All personnel must take care to prevent inadvertent contamination of draped microscopes.

TABLE 12-3

The Glasgow Coma Scale

	Points
EYE OPENING	
Spontaneous	4
To speech	3
To pain	2
None	1
VERBAL COMMUNICATION	
Oriented	5
Confused conversation	4
Inappropriate words	3
Incomprehensible sounds	2
None	1
MOTOR RESPONSE	
Obeys commands	6
Localizes to pain	5
Withdraws to pain	4
Abnormal flexion	3
Abnormal extension	2
None	1

Modified from Hausman KA: Assessment of the nervous system. In Ignatavicius DD, Workman ML, editors: *Medical-surgical nursing: patient-centered collaborative care,* ed 6, St Louis, 2010, Saunders.

TABLE 12-4

Medical Research Council Scale for Muscle Strength Grading

Grade	Strength
0	No muscle contraction
1	Trace of contraction
2	Active movement with gravity eliminated
3	Active movement against gravity
4	Active movement against gravity and resistance
5	Normal power

From Grant GA, Ellenbogen RG: Clinical evaluation of the nervous system. In Rengachary SS, Ellenbogen RG, editors: *Principles of neurosurgery,* ed 2, St Louis, 2005, Mosby.

- Counts should be performed with the perioperative nurse before the patient enters the OR if possible. Cottonoids should be kept in groups by size. Request that the perioperative nurse prepare an unsterile prep or Mayo stand for discarding and grouping of used cottonoids to facilitate closing count process.
- All medications should be obtained from the perioperative nurse, prepared and labeled. Chemical hemostatic agents such as topical thrombin may require mixing and reconstituting. Absorbable gelatin sponges (Gelfoam) should be cut in sizes that correspond to cottonoid sizes. Clear plastic petri dishes or other containers allow for Gelfoam to be soaked in thrombin and presented to the surgeon for ease of access. Bone wax should be kneaded to soften for use.
- If a sterile cranial fixation device will be used, the appropriate-sized pins (pedi or adult) should be inserted and the device opened for ease of application (Patient Safety box).

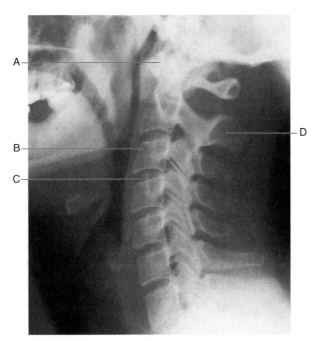

FIGURE 12-43 Lateral x-ray of the cervical spine. **A,** Anterior tubercle of the atlas (C1). **B,** Cervical body. **C,** Intervertebral disk. **D,** Spinous process of the axis (C2).

Diagnostic Procedures. Most patients will have undergone diagnostic procedures before arriving in the OR. Radiologic and other diagnostic studies are of great significance to the surgical team. Any pertinent radiographic images must be available in the OR before the procedure begins. The surgeon can refer to these images to locate the pathologic condition, verify the correct surgical site, and plan the appropriate surgical approach and procedure. Diagnostic studies include the following:

1. *Plain x-rays.* X-rays of the spine can be used initially to identify injury to the spinal column. They are referred to intraoperatively to verify that surgery to the spine is being done at the correct level (Figure 12-43).
2. *CT scan.* A CT scan uses x-ray studies, with or without instilled contrast medium, and computer technology to produce a sequential series of positive images of transverse sections of the brain and spinal cord in which differences in tissue density can be detected and deviations from normal identified. This study remains the criterion standard for evaluation of acute head injury and is considered the first-line screening study.
3. *MRI.* Use of radiofrequency pulses in a powerful magnetic field yields high-resolution images of the human body with no known risk to patients and involves no radiation. Advances in MRI scanning provide enhancement of the scan with the use of gadolinium (contrast medium). A typical MRI study produces views of the brain featured as contiguous slices in three different planes. Axial cuts are from top to bottom. Coronal cuts are from front to back. Sagittal cuts are from side to side. The MRI is the gold standard for the diagnosis of tumors, abscesses, tissue/ligamentous injury, and disk herniation (Figures 12-44 and 12-45).
4. *Stereotactic MRI or CT scan.* Placement of a stereotactic head frame (frame-based system) or fiducials (frameless system) before receiving a CT scan or MRI produces information that

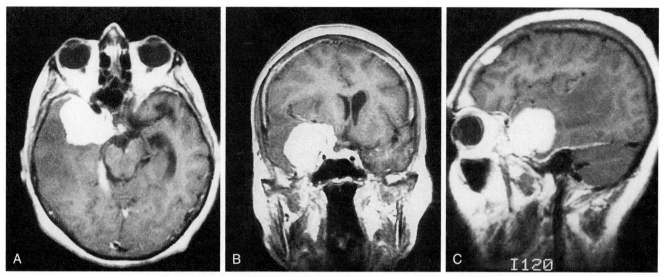

FIGURE 12-44 Gadolinium-enhanced magnetic resonance image (MRI) of a medial sphenoid wing meningioma in (**A**) axial, (**B**) coronal, and (**C**) sagittal planes.

is registered into a computer. The goal of stereotactic surgery is to target a point or volume in space precisely by means of a predefined minimally invasive trajectory (Zonenshayn and Rezai, 2005). The frameless system allows the neurosurgeon to see beyond the actual operative field by using an optical tracking device. This handheld device depicts in three planes on a computer screen where the surgeon is working in the brain relative to deeper structures beyond view.

5. *Magnetic resonance angiography (MRA)*. MRA is a noninvasive means of studying the cerebral vasculature. An MRA study is capable of detecting carotid stenosis, posttraumatic carotid artery dissection, AVMs, and aneurysms.

6. *Angiography (arteriography)*. Injection of contrast medium into the brachial, carotid, vertebral, or femoral arteries is used to study the intracranial blood vessels for size, location, and configuration and to allow diagnosis of space-occupying lesions and vascular abnormalities.

7. *Digital subtraction angiography (DSA)*. DSA is a computerized radiologic procedure. An IV rather than arterial injection is required; a contrast medium injection allows examination of selected arterial circulation. By using computer technology DSA provides an alternative to cerebral angiography for high-risk patients.

8. *Three-dimensional CT angiography*. Contrast-enhanced CT brain scan data are used to generate a three-dimensional image of the intracranial vasculature with minimal risk to the patient.

9. *Stereoscopic display of MRA*. Recent advances in MRI permit high-resolution imaging of blood flow. Projection angiograms can be produced to overcome the tomographic nature of conventional MRI scans. These angiograms are similar to plain x-ray films or digital subtraction angiograms in the demonstration of blood vessels, but the three-dimensional information inherent in them is partially lost in single projections. Stereoscopic image pairs allow the clinician to perceive the relative distance of vessels to one another. MRA permits perception of vascular anatomy in three dimensions.

10. *Myelography*. Contrast medium is injected into the spinal subarachnoid space and fluoroscopy is used to view the

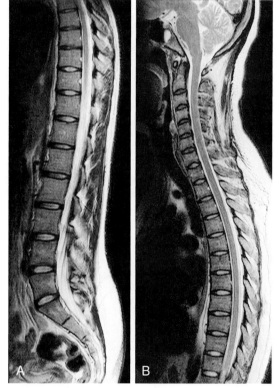

FIGURE 12-45 Sagittal magnetic resonance image (MRI) of (**A**) thoracolumbar spine and (**B**) cervicothoracic spine.

spinal cord, nerve roots, and spinal column and to demonstrate a defect involving these areas.

11. *Ultrasound*. Ultrasound is a noninvasive technique that uses high-frequency sound waves and a computer to create images of blood vessels, tissues, and organs. It is often used to assess the blood flow in the carotid artery. This procedure can be done in or out of the surgical suite. It can be used intraoperatively to localize intradural spinal cord tumors.

12. *Electroencephalogram (EEG).* An EEG is a procedure that records the brain's continuous electrical activity by means of electrodes placed on the scalp or intraoperatively on the brain.

13. *Evoked potentials (EPs).* Evoked potentials are procedures that record the brain's electrical response to visual, auditory, and sensory stimuli.

14. *Wada's test (intracarotid amobarbital [Amytal] test).* Wada's test can be used before brain surgery to lateralize language, memory, and the dominant hemisphere. It can help in lateralization of seizure focus and assess the ability of the hemisphere with the lesion to maintain memory when isolated.

15. *Lumbar puncture.* A spinal needle is used to gain access to CSF in the subarachnoid space. Opening and closing pressures are measured to determine if there is increased pressure surrounding the brain and spinal cord. This can help diagnose hydrocephalus or a spinal tumor. CSF is sent to the lab to evaluate for blood, infection, malignancy, and other neurologic diseases. LP is contraindicated when an intracranial mass is known or suspected because it can cause herniation of the brain in the presence of increased ICP.

Equipment. Neurosurgical procedures require an extensive amount of equipment. The nurse and surgical technologist must analyze the arrangement of the equipment in the OR to ensure that the sterile field is not compromised. Electrical equipment should be placed in proximity to electrical outlets, so that cords are out of high-traffic areas. Monitors should be in comfortable view of the surgeon. A microscope needs a clear path to the surgical field. The surgeon and surgical assistants may require specialized surgical chairs or sitting or standing stools to comfortably perform the surgery.

OR BED AND ATTACHMENTS. A specialized OR bed, such as a Jackson table or Andrews table or frame, may be required for posterior spine surgery. Skull clamps, skull pins, and tongs are commonly used for craniotomies and posterior

cervical spine surgeries to stabilize the head and neck (Figure 12-46). Occasionally, a patient may come to the OR in a halo that was placed for preoperative stabilization of the cervical spine. At least part of the halo will need to be removed so the surgical site can be accessed. Compatible wrenches must be available to accomplish this.

BASIC EQUIPMENT. Neurosurgical procedures typically require one special neurosurgical overhead instrument table, such as the Mayfield table (Figure 12-47), or two large Mayo trays along with one back table. Other basic equipment includes the following: a sequential compression device, a cooling-heating unit, one or two monopolar electrosurgical units (ESUs), a bipolar ESU, and a wall supply or tank of nitrogen with a special pressure gauge for operating air-powered instruments. Usually two suction units are required. Intraoperative blood salvage is used for most spine surgeries, unless infection or malignancy is suspected.

Neurosurgeons usually wear surgical loupes and a fiberoptic headlight, requiring a light source.

OPERATING MICROSCOPE. An operating microscope may be required for surgery on certain areas of the brain, spinal cord, and peripheral nerves. The operating microscope has revolutionized neurosurgery by providing intense light and up to a 12-fold magnification to areas that previously may have been inoperable or inaccessible. Microsurgery allows for greater surgical precision when operating in close proximity to vital structures and has better surgical results.

ENDOSCOPES. Surgeons use endoscopes to perform minimally invasive neurosurgery, such as endoscopic biopsy. The endoscope provides illumination and magnification of structures and an extended viewing angle. Perioperative teams must be prepared to convert from a neuroendovascular procedure to an open procedure if it is determined that the surgery cannot be successfully completed endoscopically. An additional use for endoscopes is in open procedures to see areas that are otherwise visually inaccessible.

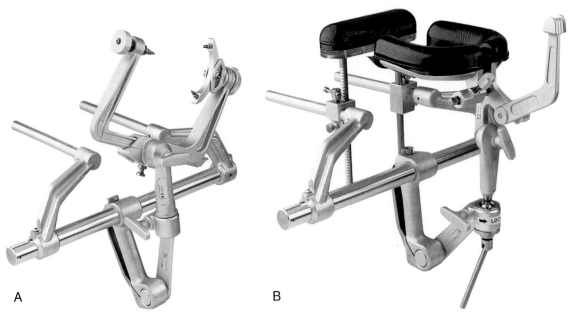

A   B

FIGURE 12-46 **A,** Three-pin fixation skull clamp (Mayfield) for stabilizing head during neurosurgical procedures. **B,** Mayfield horseshoe headrest.

RADIOLOGIC INTERVENTION. Radiology is commonly used intraoperatively for spine surgery. Typically, a radiology technician will operate the equipment. Lead aprons and thyroid shields must be worn or protective shields must be used by all staff in the OR to protect themselves from radiation exposure. X-rays can be taken to check for proper positioning of the spine and to help the surgeon identify a specific level of the spine. This may be done before incision or after partial exposure of the spinous processes and laminae. In both cases an instrument or needle is used to mark a position on the spine, and an x-ray of the spine is taken. The x-ray enables the surgeon to identify the level of the spine that is marked. The surgeon uses that information to identify the correct surgical level. A postoperative x-ray is also taken to verify that the surgery was done to the correct level of the spine.

With fluoroscopy, also called direct image intensification, a C-arm (covered with a sterile drape) is used to take a continuous x-ray that is portrayed on a monitor. This gives the surgeon the ability to view the spine and to directly view screws as they are being placed during an instrumented fusion. This ensures that spinal instrumentation for fusion is properly positioned in the correct levels. Fluoroscopy is also used for placement of nerve-stimulator electrodes in brain or spinal areas and stereotactic procedures.

STEREOTACTIC AND IMAGE-GUIDED EQUIPMENT. Stereotactic and image-guided equipment is commonly employed for neurosurgery. Either a frame-based (requiring a head-frame skull attachment, see Figure 12-48) or a frameless system (using fiducials) can be used. Both systems use a computer to register points, based on information obtained from a stereotactic MRI or CT scan done preoperatively, to determine the least traumatic approach to the target (tumor, lesion, ventricle). Both systems have accompanying attachments and instruments that must be available. The frameless image-guided system requires a monitor to display views of the brain or spine in three different planes: axial, coronal, and sagittal (Figure 12-49).

ULTRASONIC ASPIRATOR. An ultrasonic aspirator (Cavitron Ultrasonic Surgical Aspirator, CUSA) may be used to emulsify and debulk a tumor with high-frequency sound waves. Various settings allow the surgeon to adjust the instrument to remove firm or calcified lesions, or soft masses. The ultrasonic aspirator provides hemostasis and spares adjacent nerves and vessels as it removes the tumor.

AUDIOVISUAL EQUIPMENT. The use of video cameras, recorders, and television monitors is invaluable to teach staff and enhance understanding of the surgical procedure by perioperative personnel who are otherwise unable to visualize the surgeon's actions directly. By viewing the operative field through the monitor, the experienced surgical technologist will be able to anticipate the neurosurgeon's next move and will therefore provide better assistance.

INTRAOPERATIVE MONITORING EQUIPMENT. Equipment for intraoperative monitoring, such as EEG, evoked potentials (EPs), ICP, and Dopplers, may also be required.

Instrumentation, Implants, and Supplies. Typically, instrumentation commonly used in neurosurgery is added to basic surgical instrumentation to make neurosurgical-specific trays, such as a basic craniotomy tray or a laminectomy tray. Specialized trays, instruments, or implants can be added based on the surgical procedure.

Powered surgical instruments are commonly used in neurosurgery. Multiple drills, drill bits, and accessories are available. These tools may be powered by air, battery, or electricity and are operated by a hand control or foot pedal. All drills have a safety control that should be engaged at all times the instrument is not in use. The surgical technologist should monitor the sterile field to ensure that drills and other powered equipment are not left lying on the patient. The use of drills makes bone work easier and reduces operating time. Irrigating the tip of the drill while it is in use prevents overheating of the tissue. By changing drill bits and attachments, different drills can be used to make burr holes, craniotomies, craniectomies, and holes for dural tack-up sutures. They can be used to thin bone for a decompression, to perform decortication for spinal fusion, to harvest hip graft, to shape bone grafts, and to make holes for plating and fixation systems. Examples of specific drills that may be used follow.

The Hall Surgairtome 200 (Figure 12-50) can be used for precision cutting, shaping, and repair of bone. Compressed nitrogen is the power source, as with other air-powered equipment. The Hall Surgairtome 200 can be used to widen the graft area in anterior fusions and to unroof the auditory canal in eighth cranial nerve surgery. For use in less accessible areas, such as the sphenoidal sinus, pituitary fossa, and vertebral bodies, attachments with 12- and 90-degree angles are available. A range of burrs and guards is available.

The craniotome offers a perforator drive for drilling burr holes. Both 12-mm and 7-mm perforators are available in disposable and reusable forms. The perforator driver attachment can be removed and a saw blade and dura guard attached to adapt the instrument for cutting a craniotomy bone flap. A cranioplasty burr and a skull contour burr as well as guards for each type of burr are available.

Another versatile pneumatic tool is the Midas Rex instrument (Figure 12-51). The variety of disposable cutting tools of this foot pedal–controlled instrument and its attachments provides the neurosurgeon with a versatile bone dissector capable of cutting bone by sawing through it or drilling it away. In addition, large craniotomy flaps can be turned with only a

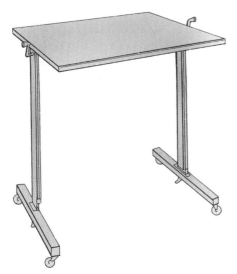

FIGURE 12-47 Mayfield overhead instrument table.

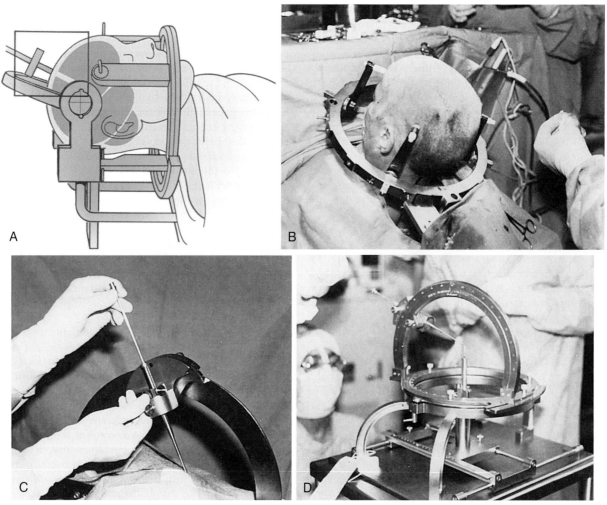

FIGURE 12-48 Stereotactic procedure. Obtaining a biopsy for stereotactic surgery. **A**, Patient fitted with head frame before computed tomography (CT) or magnetic resonance imaging (MRI) scanning. **B**, Awake patient in the sitting position for application of the BRW frame for stereotactic brain biopsy. **C**, Stereotactic surgical procedure with needle insertion for biopsy. **D**, Stereotactic surgical procedure with arc system placed on phantom base to demonstrate and check accuracy of biopsy needle with *xyz* coordinates for precise depth and angle.

single burr hole. Manufacturers' precautions and instructions must be followed for all powered instruments.

A variety of suction tips, retractors, and retractor systems are required for visualization. A transsphenoidal tray and instruments are required for that specialized approach. Microneurosurgical instruments may be needed for delicate brain or spinal cord surgery. Dural grafts and substitutes may be required to repair the dura. Aneurysm instruments, aneurysm clips, or hemostatic clips may be needed for neurovascular surgery. Titanium plates or wire is used to replace a bone plate after a craniotomy. Spinal instrumentation (plating and fixation systems) may be implanted, and bone grafts and substitutes may be used to promote spinal fusion.

Specific surgeries may require shunts or CSF reservoirs, implantable stimulators or pumps, endoscopes and endoscopic instruments, endovascular instruments, catheters, and coils. These supplies must be available if they are to be placed or implanted during surgery.

The surgical technologist needs to assemble instrumentation with consideration for each individual surgery and according to each individual surgeon's preferences. The instrument list for each procedure and neurosurgeon should be documented, referenced, and frequently updated in collaboration with the surgeon. Specific instruments are mentioned in the surgical procedure descriptions that follow.

Preliminary Procedures. A number of procedures or therapeutic measures are performed before the primary surgery begins. It is important that the surgical technologist anticipate these procedures, understand why they are done, and be prepared to facilitate them.

ANESTHESIA CONCERNS. The anesthesia provider collaborates with the surgeon and team to provide appropriate care to the patient. The anesthesia provider must be aware of and plan for situations in which the neurosurgery patient may need to be awake during the surgery for intraoperative assessment. Anesthesia agents must be adjusted if intraoperative monitoring of EPs is to be done. If the cervical spine is unstable or unable to extend, endotracheal intubation may need to be

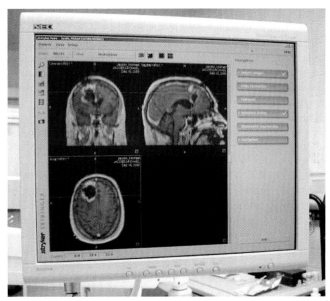

FIGURE 12-49 Frameless stereotactic image-guided navigation monitor showing the brain with tumor in three planes: coronal (*upper left*), sagittal (*upper right*), and axial (*lower left*).

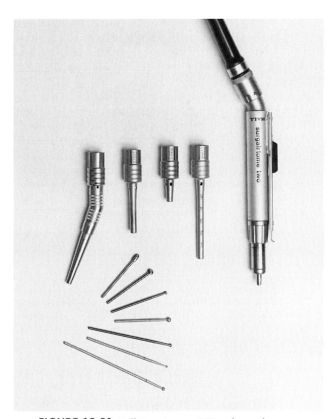

FIGURE 12-50 Hall Surgairtome 200 with attachments.

done while the patient is awake. The position of the bed in the OR should be communicated to the anesthesia provider. For surgery of the head, the bed may be turned 90 or 180 degrees away from the anesthesia machine to provide comfortable access to the surgical site. Anesthesia providers can prepare by having enough length on their tubing to make the turn while maintaining control of the patient's airway.

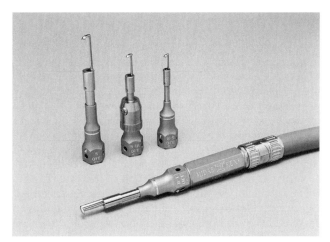

FIGURE 12-51 Midas Rex high-speed drill with attachments.

Anesthesia for neurosurgery requires sufficient IV access. The anesthesia provider may place a central line if peripheral IV lines are insufficient, or if the procedure requires the patient to be positioned in the sitting position. Increased risk of an air embolism during surgery exists when the patient is in a sitting position and when a venous sinus may be breeched. A precordial Doppler ultrasound or a pulmonary artery catheter may be placed to monitor for an air embolus. A catheter in the right atrium can be used to remove an air embolus in the heart. An arterial line may be placed for continuous monitoring of blood pressure and for drawing samples for arterial blood gas (ABG) analysis.

Antibiotic prophylaxis is administered within 30 minutes of incision time and continued at the appropriate dose schedule for at least 24 hours. The preoperative antibiotic dose is the most important dose in the prevention of postoperative infection. Generally, a broad-spectrum cephalosporin is the antibiotic drug of choice, but this depends on the needs of the individual patient. In addition, antibiotics such as bacitracin can be added to the irrigation fluid. Preoperative steroids may be given to minimize inflammation and edema when surgery is done involving the brain or spinal cord. Diuretics may be added for brain relaxation during surgery and to decrease ICP. To prevent seizures antiepileptic drugs are typically given when the cerebral cortex is manipulated. Coagulopathies must be identified and corrected preoperatively.

For all but minor surgeries, a Foley catheter is inserted into the bladder to monitor urinary output during the procedure. It is essential when procedures are expected to be prolonged, when excessive bleeding is anticipated, or when diuretics are to be given intravenously, so that the bladder does not become distended. A Foley catheter is needed by trauma patients for continuous assessment of kidney function.

STEREOTACTIC IMAGE-GUIDED NAVIGATION. To prepare for surgery on the brain, fiducials are placed on bony landmarks or points around the skull before a preoperative MRI or CT scan. Afterward, the fiducials are left in place for entry into the OR. After the patient is anesthetized and positioned, a skull clamp is placed and an image-guided navigation arm is attached to the skull clamp. This provides a fixed point of reference. The arm should be out of the way of the surgical team to ensure that it will not be inadvertently bumped and moved from its fixed point during surgery, thus disrupting the navigation system and potentially making it useless. The location of the fiducials is registered into the computer, allowing the computer to align the preoperative images (of the CT scan or MRI) to the patient's head. The monitor then shows the location of the navigation probe (which is maneuvered by the surgeon) and its trajectory on all three planes (axial, coronal, and sagittal) of the CT or MRI (see Figure 12-49). This enables the neurosurgeon to plan the approach to the target area and to navigate the surgical area using the navigation probe. After the registration process is complete, the fiducials can be removed so that the area can be prepped for surgery. A sterile sleeve is placed over the navigation arm when draping. The navigation system is used to find the target (tumor, lesion, ventricle) using the least traumatic trajectory. It also helps to ensure that the desired amount of tissue is removed. The image-guided navigation system can also be used for spine surgery.

NEUROMONITORING. An EEG can be used intraoperatively to view and record electrical activity by way of electrodes placed on the scalp or directly on the brain. It can be used to identify the location of seizure foci on the brain for possible resection (Research Highlight). Nonconvulsive use of EEG monitors is employed to monitor for burst suppression during carotid endarterectomy. Burst suppression refers to a decrease in brain activity on the EEG monitor and may be related to hypoxemia-related hypoperfusion.

EPs record the brain's electrical response to visual, auditory, and sensory stimuli. They may be used intraoperatively to monitor hearing during resection of acoustic neuromas or to monitor SSEPs (somatosensory evoked potentials) during some spine surgery. SSEPs may also be used to localize the primary sensory cortex in anesthetized patients. SSEPs involve placing needles in significant muscles of the patient and recording a baseline reading before the surgical incision. A significant change in EPs can indicate surgical invasion of the spinal cord, peripheral nerves, brainstem, or midbrain. To avoid permanent injury to the patient, the patient's position may need to be adjusted, or the surgeon may need to adjust retractors or instrumentation, alter a surgical approach, or decide that a subtotal tumor resection is necessary.

Transcranial Doppler (TCD) ultrasound may be used during carotid endarterectomy surgery. TCD provides information relevant to the major causes of perioperative cerebrovascular morbidity, including intraoperative and postoperative emboli, hypoperfusion during cross-clamping, intraoperative or postoperative thrombosis, and postoperative hyperperfusion syndrome. Using information received from TCD, the surgeon can alter the surgical or treatment plan in an attempt to avoid these complications (Whiten and Gunning, 2009).

LUMBAR AND VENTRICULAR DRAINS. The neurosurgeon may place a lumbar drain in the subarachnoid space of the lumbar spine to allow for CSF removal and intraoperative brain relaxation during aneurysm or tumor exposure. It may also be placed to prevent (or postoperatively, to treat) a CSF leak, which is most likely to occur after posterior fossa or transsphenoidal procedures. Alternatively, surgeons may place a ventricular catheter through a burr hole into a ventricle of the brain. In addition to providing the ability to drain CSF, a ventriculostomy provides the most accurate method of monitoring ICP. A transducer-tipped catheter system is a less accurate but less invasive method for monitoring. It does not allow for CSF drainage. With both the lumbar drain and the ventricular catheter, the surgical team must ensure that stopcocks and clamps are properly positioned to avoid overdrainage of CSF, which could result in brain herniation. A separate surgical prep and setup are required for placement of these ICP devices.

Positioning. The perioperative team must collaborate with the surgeon before the procedure to ensure the appropriate OR bed, attachments, and supportive positioning devices are available. Positioning devices that may be needed include a headrest, pillows, blankets, gel pads, a safety belt, tape, a shoulder roll (supine), an axillary roll (lateral), a beanbag (lateral), and chest rolls (prone).

RESEARCH HIGHLIGHT

Results of Surgical Interventions for Epilepsy

This study sought to evaluate the success of epilepsy surgery in patients who required placement of invasive intracranial (IE) electrodes to localize the seizure source. This is a subset of overall patients who might undergo epilepsy surgery, since many patients can have their seizure source localized from surface electroencephalographic monitoring in conjunction with other standard testing (including magnetic resonance imaging and neuropsychologic evaluation).

A retrospective review was undertaken of all patients at one institution who had IE monitoring over a 5-year period. The IE electrodes were placed through skull burr holes. Resective surgery was offered to the patient if a localizable and resectable source for the seizures was clearly identified. Univariate and multivariate analyses were performed to determine those variables that might predispose the patient to being seizure-free and off medication 1 year after the surgery.

In the 172 patients with placement of IE electrodes, 130 elected to have resective surgery. Reasons for not having surgery were multifocal sources for seizures, unlocalizable source, patient decision, and unresectable source. Surgical procedures performed were temporal lobectomy (47%), focal cortical resection (40%), and supplementary motor area (SMA) resection (10%). At 1 year 47% of patients were seizure free, and at 4 years 44% continued to be seizure free. In the univariate analysis, temporal resections were more likely to be seizure free (53%) compared to non–temporal resections (41%). In addition, seizure-free patients were more likely to be younger (21% of patients over 40 years of age were seizure free whereas 58% of patients under 40 were seizure free). The multivariate analysis suggested that temporal lobectomy, SMA resection, and younger age lead to a higher chance of being seizure free.

IE monitoring is not required for all patients with epilepsy being considered for surgical resection. This study suggests that there are certain patient factors and surgical choices that can predict a more successful outcome when IE monitoring is performed.

From MacDougall KW et al: Outcome of epilepsy surgery in patients investigated with subdural electrodes, *Epilepsy Res*, 2009, doi:10.1016/j.eplepsyres.2009.03.014.

Specialized neurosurgical headrests and skull clamps are commonly used for craniotomies and posterior cervical spine surgeries to support and stabilize the head and neck. They can be used with any body position. The basic unit of the neurosurgical headrest attaches to the frame of the OR bed after the standard OR bed headpiece has been removed. An articulated arm allows fine adjustments to the position of the head. A horseshoe-shaped headrest may be used. Alternatively, head clamps, skull pins, and tongs that are attached to the neurosurgical headrest bed attachment and provide maximum stability may be required (see Figure 12-46).

Most skull clamps have three sterile pins that are placed in the skull clamp and covered with antibiotic or povidone-iodine ointment. The surgeon or surgeon's assistant places the skull clamps on the patient's head after anesthetic is administered. The surgeon must place the skull clamp strategically in the skull to provide access to the surgical site and to avoid the frontal sinuses, the superficial temporal arteries, and the eyes. The pins on the clamp partially penetrate the outer table of the skull. If the prone position is used, the surgeon will place the skull clamp while the patient is supine. The surgeon supports the patient's head during the position change and adjusts the final head position after the patient is placed prone (Patient Safety).

After positional adjustments to the patient's body are complete, the skull clamp (and patient's head) is locked into the articulating arm of the headrest by someone other than the person who is supporting the head. The apparatus is tightened from distal to proximal and double-checked for security. Once the patient's head is locked into place, no positional adjustments can be made to the patient's body without first releasing the head. Not doing so could cause injury to the patient's cervical spine. If necessary, an image-guided navigation arm can be attached to certain skull clamps, and the positions of the fiducials are registered into the system before the patient is prepped.

The skull clamp is detached from the basic headrest by loosening the arm from distal to proximal. Finally, while the head is being supported by another person, the skull clamp is loosened, allowing the pins to be released from the skull. Ointment can be applied to the pin sites. Bleeding may occur at the pin sites after the skull clamp is removed. It usually stops with digital pressure, but occasionally a stitch may be required.

The position of the patient's arms must also be considered. For cranial surgery, usually at least one arm is tucked so that the Mayo stand can be positioned over the patient. For cervical spine surgery, both arms are tucked so that the surgical site can be accessed from both sides of the table. When the arms are tucked, the elbows are padded to protect the ulnar nerve,

PATIENT SAFETY

Preventing Injury When Using an Intraoperative Head Fixation System

Specialized bed attachments in conjunction with a skull clamp create a mechanical support system that is often used in head and neck surgery when rigid cranial stabilization is desired. Features of this device include the base unit (which attaches to the OR bed), cross bars, a swivel adaptor (reticulating arm), and the skull clamp. Only properly trained OR staff should be permitted to operate these devices. Mounting instructions for the bed attachment vary by OR bed. The team must verify that the bed attachment is properly secured before the start of patient positioning.

SAFE APPLICATION OF THE SKULL CLAMP

Once the anesthesia provider has determined that the patient is ready for positioning, the designated member of the OR team will pin the patient's head with the skull clamp. The clamp consists of two skull pins in the rocker arm and one skull pin in the extension arm. When properly placed, the pins in the rocker arm are equidistant from the centerline of the patient's head and the single pin in the extension arm is exactly at the centerline. Improper positioning of the skull pins may cause serious injury to the patient. Special attention should be paid to avoiding the areas of the frontal sinus, temporal fossa, blood vessels, and nerves. The person securing the skull clamp must ensure that the pins are at an angle of 90 degrees, the necessary pounds of clamping force are applied, and the rocker arm is in the "CLOSED" position.

SAFE POSITIONING

After the head is safely pinned, the patient can be positioned for surgery. It is important that open communication exists between all members in the OR suite. Every member of the OR team plays a key role in the positioning process, and without good communication critical steps may be missed. Airway management is vital, and the anesthesia provider must have control of the patient's airway at all times. All movements of the patient's head and body must first be cleared by the anesthesia provider. There must be at least three people responsible for positioning the head. One member of the anesthesia team monitors the airway, one member of the surgical team holds the patient's head within the skull clamp, and one member secures the reticulating arm of the bed attachment to the skull clamp. All the components of the bed attachment have a starburst locking mechanism, and it is critical all teeth are engaged and locked securely. It is the responsibility of the team member holding the patient's head to do the final check to ensure all locking mechanisms are engaged properly. There should be no movement detected in any component of the system if secured properly. If even one component of the system is not properly engaged, the patient could possibly be injured.

POSTOPERATIVE MONITORING

Once the procedure is complete and it is time to remove the patient from the fixation system, the same safety measures go into effect. The anesthesia provider maintains control of the patient's airway while one member of the surgical team holds the patient's head within the skull clamp, and a second member of the surgical team releases all the locking mechanisms of the reticulating arm. At this time either the standard headpiece of the OR bed can be reattached or the patient can be moved to the postoperative bed or stretcher. When the skull clamp is released, the surgeon confirms that all three pins are extracted from the patient's head and secured. If bleeding is observed from the pin site, the surgeon may apply pressure to control the oozing, or may use a monofilament suture to close the hole.

Modified from Integra product information, available at www.integra-ls.com/products/. Accessed May 5, 2009; PMI Pro Med Instruments instruction manual, revised September 12, 2008.

the palms face inward, and the wrist is maintained in a neutral position (Denholm, 2009). A drape secures the arms. It should be tucked snugly under the patient, not under the mattress. This prevents the arm from shifting downward intraoperatively and resting against the OR bed rail.

For thoracic and lumbar spine surgery, armboards can usually be placed out of the way of the surgeon and radiology equipment. Armboards are maintained at less than a 90-degree angle to prevent brachial plexus stretch.

As always, the surgical team identifies any potential hazards and takes precautions to prevent them. Sequential compression devices are applied before induction of anesthesia to prevent deep vein thrombosis (DVT) unless they are contraindicated because of a known DVT. Pressure points must be identified and relieved. Joints must be maintained in functional alignment with no pressure or tension on superficial nerves and vessels. A warming/cooling blanket is applied for temperature control. An occlusive dressing applied over the eyes protects them from chemical burns and corneal abrasions that may occur from solutions used to prep the head. Keeping the head positioned above the heart minimizes bleeding when operating on the head.

Supine position or some modification of it can be used for approaches to the frontal, parietal, and temporal lobes; the anterior cervical spine; and the anterior lumbar spine. Lateral position can be used for an approach to the cerebellopontine angle in the posterior fossa, for anterior thoracic and lumbar spine surgery, and for posterior spine surgery. It can be used for lumbar sympathectomies and for placements of nerve stimulators and pumps.

Prone position and modifications of it can be used for access to the posterior spine and for suboccipital and posterior fossa craniotomies. A laminectomy frame or chest rolls are commonly used for prone position. The Jackson table permits access of the C-arm for intraoperative fluoroscopy of the spine. The Andrews table or frame can be used for a modified knee-chest position, which is useful for posterior lumbar spine surgery. The patient's hips and knees are flexed so that the lower body is supported primarily by the knees. The Hicks spinal surgery frame may be used to support this position and allow the abdomen to hang free. The chest is supported on a chest roll. Advantages of this position include decreased bleeding because of the collapse of epidural veins, better exposure resulting from hyperflexion of the spine, absence of pressure on the vena cava, and increased ease of ventilation. Operating time is usually reduced when this position is used. Disadvantages of the knee-chest position include the difficulty of maintaining physical stability on the OR bed, the increased possibility of patient hypotension, and the pooling of blood in the lower extremities.

Fowler's (sitting) position is used for some craniotomies involving a posterior or occipital approach. Advantages of this position include optimum visibility of the operative field and decreased blood loss because of the lowered arterial and venous pressures. Disadvantages are the potential for orthostatic hypotension and air embolism. In the sitting position the venous pressure in the head and neck may be negative, predisposing the patient to air embolism (Risk Reduction Strategies). Other potential problems with this position include neck flexion with airway compromise and difficulty in achieving and maintaining functional alignment.

Skin Preparation. Prevention of infection is a primary concern in neurosurgery. An antiseptic skin prep is performed by the perioperative nurse, surgeon, resident, or surgical assistant. Although studies have shown that shaving the surgical site can contribute to the possibility of infection, usually some hair removal is necessary when operating on the head and posterior cervical spine.

Hair removal from the head causes a disturbance in body image and can be upsetting to patients. A discussion and often a compromise regarding hair removal should take place between the surgeon and patient before the surgery, and an understanding should be reached as to how much hair will be removed. Hair that is removed is the property of the patient. It should be placed in a container, labeled with the patient's name, and kept with the patient after surgery.

Hair removal should be done as close to the time of skin incision as possible to decrease the possibility of surgical site infection. Whenever possible, minimal hair removal is recommended. It is possible to shave a 1- to 2-cm wide area along the length of some craniotomy incisions after the hair is parted at the incision site. After the minimal shave, the hair can be combed away from the incision and held back with prepping solution or antimicrobial ointment. However, other craniotomies require more extensive hair removal. Electric hair clippers are preferred to razors because they are less irritating and less likely to nick the skin, which would predispose the area to infection. After hair removal, the nurse should inspect the patient's skin carefully for any signs of inflammation or infection. If any such signs are noted, they should be reported to the surgeon immediately. The head and hair surrounding the planned incision can be prepped, even though the hair will be draped out of the operative field.

For surgery on the cervical spine it is possible to secure long hair on top of the head and remove neck hair with clippers to a level even with the top of the ears or to the occipital protuberance. Postoperatively, patients with long hair can comb it down over the shaved area until the hair regrows. Patients undergoing thoracic or lumbar spine surgery may not need to be shaved. If a bone graft from the hip will be taken for spinal fusion, that area must be prepped as well as the spinal incision area.

Many neurosurgeons mark the incision line with a marking pen or a marking solution and wooden stick. If a marking solution is used, indigo carmine, gentian violet, or brilliant green is recommended. Methylene blue should never be found in a neurosurgical OR because it produces an inflammatory reaction in CNS tissue. Because the markings tend to wash off during the prep, some surgeons may scratch the scalp along the planned incision with a sharp sterile needle. This increases the risk of infection and should only be done if there is danger of harming the patient by varying from the planned line of incision.

Draping. According to the recommendations of The Joint Commission, the surgical team takes a "time out" during the prepping and draping procedures to be sure that everyone is in agreement that the correct surgery is being done to the correct patient in the correct location. The surgical consent is read aloud by the circulating nurse. In neurosurgical procedures, the right or left side of the head and the level of the spine must be specified. The surgical team should also check that the marking (initials) made to the surgical site in the holding area are in the operative field.

▶▶ RISK REDUCTION STRATEGIES

Preventing and Managing Venous Air Embolism in the Sitting Position

The use of the sitting position is more common in neurosurgical procedures than in other specialties because of its excellent surgical access, improved ventilation, and improved drainage of blood and cerebrospinal fluid from the head and neck, thereby decreasing intracranial pressure. However, patients undergoing posterior fossa, cervical, or supratentorial procedures in the sitting position are at risk for venous air embolism (VAE). VAE is a potentially serious intraoperative condition that may result in significant morbidity and mortality. The incidence of VAE in neurologic procedures performed in the sitting position is 10% to 80% and has a mortality of approximately 1%.

Common sources of VAE are the major cerebral venous sinuses, in particular, the transverse, the sigmoid, and the posterior half of the sagittal sinus, all of which may be noncollapsible because of their dural attachments. Air may also enter through the emissary veins, particularly from the suboccipital musculature, the diploic space of the skull, and the cervical epidural veins. VAE is possible any time there is a negative pressure gradient between the operative site and the right atrial pressure.

PREVENTIVE MEASURES

The nurse and surgical technologist should anticipate assisting the anesthesia provider with the placement of a pulmonary artery pressure (PAP) catheter, precordial Doppler, and a multiorifice central venous line. The pulmonary artery catheter allows the anesthesia care provider to monitor heart pressures. The right atrial central venous catheter is used to measure right arterial pressure, administer vasoactive medication if needed, and provide a route to aspirate air from the right atrium. Depending on availability, transesophageal echocardiography (TEE) may be used to detect VAE. The surgical team should collaborate with the anesthesia provider and neurosurgeon to configure the OR to accommodate the TEE equipment. According to the surgeon's preference, the surgical team should ensure the patient is wearing compression stockings, sequential compression devices, or elastic Ace bandage wraps on the lower extremities to promote venous return and prevent venous stasis. With the help of the anesthesia care provider, the surgical team can place the patient in an antishock suit with separate inflatable chambers for the legs and abdomen, which may not be inflated until a venous air embolism has been detected.

DETECTION OF VENOUS AIR EMBOLISM

The anesthesia provider will monitor the PAP, Doppler, end-tidal CO_2 levels and TEE (if used). Generally, transient decreases in arterial pressure and end-tidal CO_2 levels, which are not otherwise related to anesthetic administration or surgical condition, indicate the presence of VAE. The audible tone of the precordial Doppler changes, and turbulence, or "washing-machine" sounds, may indicate early VAE. If VAE is detected or suspected, the team must be prepared to assist the surgeon and anesthesia provider to rapidly treat the patient.

MANAGING VENOUS AIR EMBOLISM

Once VAE has been diagnosed, a critical component of treatment is to prevent further air entrainment. The surgical technologist should ensure saline-soaked dressings are available on the sterile field so the surgeon can immediately cover the surgical site. The surgeon should then assess and eliminate any entry site to prevent additional air entry. The anesthesia provider is responsible for attempting to aspirate the air by way of the multiorifice right atrial catheter and may administer ephedrine, dobutamine, or norepinephrine to provide inotropic support to the right ventricle. A repositioning to the left lateral decubitus position (right side up) may be indicated to prevent the air in the atrium from moving to the ventricle and causing an air lock. If the patient's position cannot be changed because of the positioning apparatus, the tilt of the OR bed can be adjusted to lower the source of air entry and decrease the negative air pressure gradient. The antishock suit may be inflated, thus increasing right atrial pressure and decreasing the pressure gradient between the right atrium and an entraining vein.

Modified from Goodkin R, Mesiwala A: General principles of operative positioning. In Winn RH, editor: *Youman's neurological surgery*, vol 1, ed 6, Philadelphia, 2009, Saunders; Mirski MA et al: Diagnosis and treatment of vascular air embolism, *Anesthesiology* 106(1):164-177, 2007; Leslie K et al: Venous air embolism and the sitting position: a case series, *J Clin Neurosci* 13(4):419-422, 2006; St-Arnaud D, Paquin MJ: Safe positioning for neurosurgical patients, *AORN J* 87(6):1156-1172, 2008.

Draping for some neurosurgery procedures is complex and requires the cooperation of the surgeon, assistant, and surgical technologist. Four or more towels are placed around the operative site. They may be secured by disposable skin staples, small towel clips, or silk sutures on a cutting needle.

Draping for a craniotomy is challenging. If a minimal shave was done, an adhesive drape with staples placed around the shaved area near the incision can help to keep hair out of the incision. Towels can be contoured to the prepped area of the head and held in place with staples, leaving the operative site exposed. A craniotomy drape can then be placed over the towels. A sterile drainage bag below the incision will help to catch irrigation and blood and drain it into a suction canister. If a stereotactic head frame is used, be sure that the drapes do not interfere with the head frame attachments.

Prepping a hip graft incision site may need to be done with spinal fusion surgery. Two areas may need to be prepped and squared off with towels, which can be held in place with an adhesive drape. A partially unfolded three-fourths drape can be placed between the two planned incision sites before the universal or laparotomy drape is placed. A clamp can be placed over the prepped hip area to positively identify it. The drape can be cut over the prepped area, being sure not to cut an area of the drape that covers a nonsterile area. A second adhesive drape can hold the cut drape in place.

Hemostasis and Visualization. A few minutes before making the incision, the surgeon may inject the incision site with a local anesthetic agent, such as lidocaine or bupivacaine. Lidocaine has a more rapid onset and shorter duration of action than bupivacaine. Along with decreasing the effect of the stimulus of the skin incision, infiltration of the solution will apply pressure within the tissues and decrease bleeding at the time of incision. Using a local anesthetic that also contains epinephrine will constrict blood vessels to further minimize bleeding.

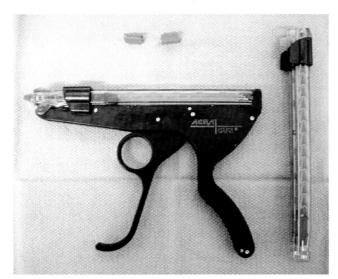

FIGURE 12-52 Automatic clip gun, with disposable scalp clips and cartridge.

Meticulous hemostasis is particularly important in neurosurgery. Many methods are incorporated to limit blood loss. A major consideration is control of hemorrhage from the highly vascular scalp. Skin edges along the wound are compressed with gauze sponges and fingers during the initial incision. Usually, this is followed by application of disposable scalp clips (Figure 12-52). An automatic clip gun may be used to apply clips to include the galea and skin edge. The clips limit bleeding by applying pressure to the scalp edges. They remain in place until closure. Placement of self-retaining retractors also helps to control bleeding of the scalp.

Retraction is required for visualization. Self-retaining retractors such as cerebellar or Gelpi retractors can be used to retract skin, subcutaneous tissue, muscle, or the scalp. Suture can be used to retract the scalp or the dura of the brain or spinal cord. Blunt, malleable retractors are used on brain tissue. Table-mounted self-retaining retractor systems such as the Greenberg help the surgeon to see deep into the brain and may be used with a microscope.

Electrosurgery is routine for neurosurgical procedures. Perioperative personnel must understand the uses and hazards of the ESU and be familiar with the safety measures. Electrocoagulation current seals the blood vessels. To be effective, the electrocoagulating current must contact the vessel in a dry field. For this reason, suctioning is necessary to remove blood as the contact is made between the instrument carrying the current and the bleeding point. A monopolar current is used to cut and coagulate tissue. It can be applied to forceps, a metal suction tip, or another instrument, which acts as a conducting tool. Monopolar electrosurgery is safe to use on the epidermis, dermis, galea, periosteum, muscle, and bone. It is used extensively for exposure of the posterior spine.

Bipolar ESUs provide a completely isolated output with negligible leakage of current between the tips of the forceps, permitting use of electrocoagulating current in proximity to structures where ordinary monopolar electrocoagulation would be hazardous (Figure 12-53). It is safe to use the bipolar ESU to control bleeding on the dura of the brain and spinal cord and near vital

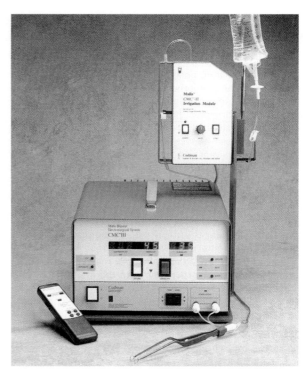

FIGURE 12-53 Malis bipolar coagulator and bipolar cutter, with irrigation module.

nerves and vessels. It can be used to maintain hemostasis and to dissect tissue in the brain. Lactated Ringer's or normal saline solution irrigation is often used during bipolar electrocoagulation to minimize tissue heating, shrinkage, drying, and adherence to the forceps. Some bipolar units have built-in irrigating systems. The use of the bipolar electrocoagulation technique allows hemostasis of almost any size vessel encountered. Vessels as large as the superficial temporal artery, as well as those too small for suture or clip ligation, may be coagulated with bipolar units.

Suction is necessary to evacuate blood, CSF, and irrigation solution from the surgical site. Metal suction tips in multiple sizes, such as the Sachs, Frazier, and Adson, are used not only because they keep the wound dry but also because they can conduct electrocoagulation current from a monopolar unit to the bleeding point. Suction applied directly on normal neural tissue may be harmful and is avoided. Instead, a cottonoid patty may be placed between the suction tip and neural tissue for protection. The intensity of suction can be moderated by placement or removal of a finger over the vent hole on the Frazier and other vented suction tips. Suction can be used to aspirate necrotic or traumatized brain tissue or soft brain tumors after a sample has been obtained for pathologic examination. It is also useful in evacuating abscess cavities, removing fluid from a ventricle or the subarachnoid space, holding a solid tumor during its removal, and applying compression to a bleeding vessel.

Bone wax is a hemostatic material that should be available for all cranial and spinal cord operations. Bone wax may be applied with the surgeon's fingertip or with the tip of an instrument such as a Freer or Penfield elevator. The surgeon firmly rubs or packs the wax into the bleeding surfaces of bone. Bone wax is commonly used in burr holes, along the edges of a craniotomy, and on the cut edges of the spine.

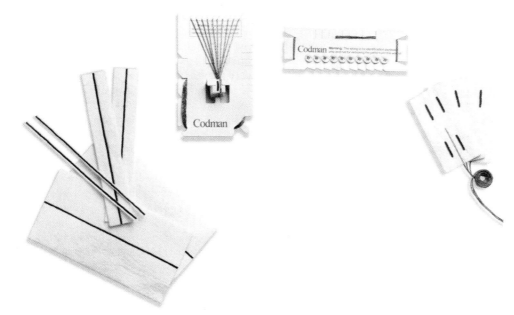

FIGURE 12-54 Cottonoid strips and patties.

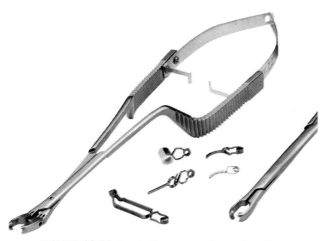

FIGURE 12-55 Standard aneurysm clips and appliers.

Gauze sponges are used to control bleeding before the skull or spinal canal is entered; however, they are coarse and can injure fragile tissues such as the brain and spinal cord. Instead, compressed, absorbent patties made of rayon or cotton (cottonoids) are used to control bleeding beneath the skull and around the spinal cord. Patties are also placed over delicate neural tissue for protection. It is far less traumatic to suction on a patty than directly on the tissue. Patties are available in a variety of sizes, both squares and strips, ranging from ¼ inch to 6 inches long and from ¼ inch to 1 inch wide (Figure 12-54). A supply of various sizes is typically moistened with irrigation solution or thrombin and offered to the surgeon on a waterproof surface. Patties have x-ray–detectable markers and strings attached and are included in the standard sponge count.

Cotton balls moistened with irrigation solution or thrombin may be used as a temporary pack or tamponade in a bleeding tumor bed after a tumor has been removed. The gentle pres-

sure of the cotton balls along with time and patience on the part of the surgeon may stop bleeding not controllable by other means. Cotton balls also have x-ray–detectable strings and are included in the sponge count.

A variety of hemostatic clips are available and used by neurosurgeons to occlude both superficial and deep vessels. Unlike clips that were used in the past, hemoclips and Ligaclips are made of an alloy that is compatible with the MRI scanner. The scrub person removes the clips from a special cartridge with the appropriate applicator and passes them to the surgeon for application to a vessel. Such clips enable the surgeon to occlude vessels in areas difficult to reach by other means and to ligate superficial vessels of the brain before cutting them and without destroying any surrounding tissues. Clips are available in a variety of sizes. Numerous types of special clips are used for permanent or temporary occlusion of vessels or an aneurysm neck in the surgical treatment of an intracranial aneurysm (Figure 12-55).

Neurosurgeons almost routinely use certain hemostatic agents in addition to mechanical hemostasis (Surgical Pharmacology). An absorbable gelatin sponge (Gelfoam) can be applied to an oozing surface, either dry or saturated with irrigation solution or topical thrombin. Larger pieces can be cut into a variety of sizes of strips and squares. Gelfoam is often followed by a patty, which enables the surgeon to maneuver and compress it once it is in the surgical site. Gelfoam is absorbable and can be left in the body.

Oxidized regenerated cellulose is available in two forms: a rayonlike gauze (Surgicel) and a cottonlike form (Fibrillar). These are also absorbable hemostatic agents that are used to control bleeding from oozing surfaces, vessels, and sinuses in the brain. These hemostatic substances are presented in various sizes and shapes and are offered to the surgeon dry. The hemostatic material adheres to the bleeding area with gentle pressure.

Thrombin is a drug that can be topically applied to bleeding surfaces to achieve hemostasis. Typically, Gelfoam or patties are saturated with thrombin and placed on the oozing surface.

Irrigating the wound helps the surgeon identify active bleeding points and may facilitate hemostasis. A syringe with an angiocatheter tip may be used to deliver irrigation for microsurgery. Many neurosurgeons irrigate surgical wounds with an antibiotic solution before wound closure. The antibiotic is mixed with irrigation solution according to the surgeon's preference so that it is ready for use when needed.

Suture. Required suture will vary according to the surgery, the condition of the wound and patient, and the surgeon's preference. Suture can be used for retraction of the scalp for a craniotomy flap. Dura of the brain and spinal cord may be retracted, tacked up, and closed with braided nylon suture. In general, high tensile strength is needed for closure of the galea of the scalp and the fascia and subcutaneous tissue of the back. Braided, absorbable suture can be used in interrupted stitches to close these layers. Skin may be closed with subcuticular absorbable suture, with either a continuous or an interrupted suturing technique using a monofilament, nonabsorbable suture material such as nylon. Use of polypropylene in place of nylon would aid in suture removal post-op due to the blue coloring of the suture material. Alternatively, skin can be closed with staples. Whatever technique is used for skin closure, skin edges should be everted. A drain may be secured to the skin with a nonabsorbable suture such as nylon. In an environment of infection, monofilament, nonabsorbable suture is preferred.

Dressings. Applying dressings to wounds on the head is challenging, especially if a minimal shave was done. For larger incisions in particular, a head wrap can be the best alternative. It keeps a nonadherent dressing in place over the incision site and provides compression to prevent the formation of a postoperative hematoma. A smaller dressing can sometimes be held in place with a transparent dressing or tape. Applying a liquid adhesive, such as Mastisol, to the skin before application of the dressing can help to hold it in place.

SURGICAL PHARMACOLOGY

Hemostatic Agents

Achieving hemostasis in delicate areas can be a challenge for the neurosurgeon. In addition to using meticulous technique to prevent bleeding, topical agents are routinely used as an adjunct to hemostasis. The surgical technologist must be familiar with the agents used in this setting.

Agent	Dosage Form	Mechanism of Action	Side Effects
Topical thrombin	Powder for reconstitution; packaged with diluent and spray pump, or diluent and spray tip syringe, with diluent only	Catalyzes conversion of fibrinogen to fibrin	May cause fever or allergic-type reactions
Gelatin matrix (FloSeal)	Gelatin matrix granules and topical thrombin packaged as a kit with syringes and mixing bowl	Matrix particles form a composite clot that seals bleeding site; thrombin component converts fibrinogen in patient's blood to fibrin	Anemia, atrial fibrillation, infection
Absorbable gelatin sponge (Gelfoam)	Film, powder, and topical forms	Absorbs and holds blood and fluid within its interstices; exerts physical hemostatic effect	Local infection and abscess formation
Collagen hemostat (Avitene, Helistat, Instat)	Pads, powder, sheets, sponges	When in contact with a bleeding surface, attracts platelets that aggregate into thrombi, initiating formation of a physiologic platelet plug	Adhesion formation, allergic reaction, foreign-body reaction, inflammation, potentiation of infection
Oxidized regenerated cellulose (Surgicel)	Fibrous, knitted, or sheer weave fabric	Allows platelets and aggregates of thrombin and particulate blood elements to cling and form a coagulum that can act as a patch	Encapsulation of fluid, foreign-body reactions

Modified from LexiComp Online, available at www.crlonline.com/crlsql/servlet/crlonline. Accessed June 22, 2009; FloSeal package insert product information, available at www.baxter.com/products/biopharmaceuticals/downloads/FloSeal_PI.pdf. Accessed June 22, 2009; Gelfoam package insert product information, available at www.pfizer.com/files/products/uspi_gelfoam_sponge.pdf. Accessed June 22, 2009.

SURGICAL TECHNOLOGY PREFERENCE CARD

Communication and organization are essential among the perioperative team members in planning care for the neurosurgical patient in the OR. Extensive time may be directed toward anesthesia preparation and induction, patient positioning, cranial fixation, neuromonitoring, guided image synchronization, and skin preparation. Elective or scheduled neurosurgical procedures can be long and arduous with complicated steps and setups. The surgical technologist should use this time to organize and prepare everything needed for the procedure so that nothing is left to chance. Neurosurgical trauma procedures, however, take on a special urgency because of the potential for catastrophic damage or death with elapsed time.

Room Prep: Basic operating room furniture in place, thermoregulatory devices, extra blankets, padding, positioning supplies to achieve optimal patient safety. The neurosurgery operating room can become quite crowded with equipment, supplies, and personnel. Care must be taken to prevent contamination of multiple pieces of **sterilely draped** furniture including:

- Microscopes
- Guidance systems
- Fluoroscopic (C-arm) equipment
- Power equipment: drills, craniotomies
- Irrigation warming units

Prep Solution: In room

- Chlorhexidine gluconate (CHG)
- Iodine and iodophors

Catheter: In room and correct size

- Catheter set and tray
  - Latex/rubber
  - Silicone
  - Temperature sensing
- Sizing
  - French
- Retaining
  - Foley
    - 2-way
    - 3-way
- Other urine collection devices

PROCEDURE CHECKLIST

Instruments

- Cranial instruments
- Spinal instruments
  - Powered craniotomes, drills, wire drivers, screwdrivers, saws
  - Bipolar cords, ESU pencils, suction tubing with tips
  - Plates, screws, wires, rods, or other fixation devices
  - Suction aspirators (CUSA or similar)
  - Microinstruments: dissectors, scissors, biopsy forceps, aneurysm clips/appliers, transsphenoidal instruments, etc.
  - Self-retaining retractor systems
  - Cranial fixation braces/head holders
  - Intracranial pressure (ICP) probes

Specialty Suture

- As per surgeon's preference

Hemostasis

- Other hemostatic agents
  - Mechanical
    - Staplers
    - Clip appliers and clips
    - Pressure
    - Ligatures
    - Pledgets
  - Chemical
    - Absorbable gelatin
    - Collagen
    - Oxidized cellulose
    - Silver nitrate
    - Epinephrine
    - Thrombin
  - Thermal
    - Electrosurgical unit
    - Harmonic scalpel
    - Argon beam coagulator
    - Bipolar

Continued

Medications, Irrigation Solutions, and Other:
◆ Warm saline (with or without antibiotics—usually not while dura is open); *never* water
◆ Methylmethacrylate (bone cement, cranioplastic)
◆ Local anesthetic with or without epinephrine
◆ Papaverine—used to reduce vasospasm
◆ Methlyene blue or indigo carmine dye
◆ Fibrin glue—used as sealant for CSF tears/leaks/fistulas
◆ Antibiotic ointments—used over incisional site before placement of dressings

Specimen Types and Care
◆ Specimen care
  • Proper container for each specimen
    • Frozen
    • Fresh
    • Permanent
    • Cultures
  • Labels for each specimen
  • Proper solution for specimen type

Dressings and Drains
Drains are not frequently used in cranial or spinal procedures; however this will be procedure and surgeon specific. Dressings for spinal procedure may be similar to routine abdominal dressings. Cranial dressings will depend on ability to secure the materials: if hair is left in place, a turban-type wrap-around dressing with rolled gauze may be preferred to maintain padding and protection of the incisional site.

Surgical Interventions

MINIMALLY INVASIVE AND SPECIALIZED NEUROSURGERY TECHNIQUES

Microneurosurgery

Adaptation of the operating microscope for neurosurgery has resulted in improvement of many neurosurgical procedures and made new procedures possible. For years, neurosurgeons have worn magnifying loupes to see small structures. Loupes usually have a magnification of 2× or 3.5×. The microscope has a variety of magnifications ranging from 6× to 40×, providing flexibility and precision. The co-axial illumination overcomes the difficulties of lighting neurosurgical wounds (History box).

Use of the microscope restricts the surgeon's field of vision and mobility; therefore the surgical technologist and surgical assistant must be proficient. The operative field, unless video monitoring is available, cannot be seen. Surgical personnel must understand the surgical procedure and the corresponding anatomy, know the names and uses of all microinstruments, and be proficient at passing the instruments to the surgeon without delay that are ready for use. Each time the surgeon must look away and then back to the surgical field, open wound time and anesthesia time are increased while the surgeon becomes reoriented to the field. Therefore the assistance the surgical technologist gives the surgeon saves time and directly benefits the patient.

Microsurgical instruments have been modified and adapted to the requirements of neurosurgery. These instruments often possess the following characteristics: bayonet shape, so that the surgeon's hand remains outside the line of vision and the beam of the microscope light; finely sprung and fluted grip; long length for access to deep structures; and slender and delicate tips that occupy as little space as possible. Microneurosurgical instruments are expensive and delicate. Instructions for handling, cleaning, sterilizing, and storing these instruments should be followed. An instrument that is sprung, bent, dulled,

hooked, or in any way damaged must never be handed to a surgeon for use but must be repaired or replaced. Instruments must be kept free from blood and tissue during use because the microscope also magnifies debris on the instruments, occluding the structure the surgeon is about to approach. Very fine microsutures are available.

Microsurgical techniques have been applied to cranial, spinal, and peripheral nerve operations. Some procedures in which microsurgery is of value are explorations of the posterior fossa, especially for tumors of the fourth ventricle or cerebellopontine angle, and removal of small acoustic neuromas, with resulting preservation of the facial nerve. Small-vessel endarterectomy, cerebral arterial bypass, cerebral aneurysm clipping, and excision of AVMs are performed using the microscope for visualization of the surgical site. Microsurgery also has advantages in the treatment of tumors and AVMs of the spinal cord.

Neuroendoscopy

Neuroendoscopy is a rapidly evolving field of minimally invasive surgery. The endoscope provides illumination and magnification of structures and an extended viewing angle. Brain retraction and manipulation are reduced in endoscopic surgery, resulting in decreased tissue damage (Teo and Mobbs, 2005). The surgical team must be prepared to convert from a neuroendovascular procedure to an open procedure if it is determined that the surgery cannot be successfully completed endoscopically.

Indications for neuroendoscopic surgery are many. Endoscopic tumor removal or CSF diversion through endoscopic fenestration, such as a third ventriculostomy, can be done for the treatment of hydrocephalus and can eliminate the need for a shunt. Interventricular tumors may be removed endoscopically. In addition, the endoscope can be used to assess adequacy of tumor removal and to identify tumor portions left behind or adherent to vital structures. Stereotactic and image-guided surgery is often used with neuroendoscopy successfully. The endoscope is commonly used in the transsphenoidal

HISTORY

Evolution of Surgical Magnification

From 1813 to 1825 English, French, and German opticians attempted to coordinate two monoculars into a single instrument, finally providing the modern binocular, used then as opera glasses. Abbe and Zeiss, circa 1870 to 1880, improved opera glasses with the invention of the binocular roof prism, which enabled greater enlargement of the image without having to deal with the increased length of the optical tube.

In 1886 Westien, a German instrument maker, developed the first surgical loupes for a zoologist interested in performing more accurate dissections. Later, Westien developed binocular loupes for an ophthalmologist. He further adapted magnifying loupes from a stationary device to an instrument to be worn on the head, offering a power of 5× to 6× magnification. These proved impractical because of their weight.

The first teleloupes were developed in 1912. They were the prototype of current surgical loupes, offering a light weight and a magnification of 2×. Their initial popularity was appreciated by ophthalmologists, and in 1948 Riechert, initially an ophthalmologist who later became a neurosurgeon, advocated their use during neurosurgical procedures. It is believed that neurosurgeons' use of surgical loupes was more widespread, but they had not published this fact.

Operating microscopes borrowed the technology of optical systems developed for surgical loupes and underwent further development of their optical and mechanical systems between 1921 and 1952. Monocular scopes, first fixed near the head of the patient, evolved to binocular scopes that attached to the OR bed and later became freestanding floor mounts. The delayed application of the operating microscope in general surgery has been related to the technical deficiencies of the early microscopes, in that they were unstable and immobile and had limited illumination.

In 1952 Littman succeeded in developing a sophisticated, maneuverable microscope for surgical requirements that maintained sharp focus and had a co-axial light system. This prototype was known as the *OPMI 1* and drew the attention of otologic surgeons, ophthalmologic surgeons, and neurosurgeons. The operating microscope has made it possible for neurosurgeons to perform delicate, minimally invasive surgery in anatomic regions requiring magnification and illumination.

Modified from Carl Zeiss: *Technical milestones,* available at www.zeiss.com/C12567A100537AB9/Contents-Frame/63125BAC5434D55DC1256DB900446D61. Accessed June 22, 2009.

approach for pituitary and sellar tumor resection (possibly in collaboration with an otolaryngology surgeon), for microvascular decompression, and for endoscopic biopsy of a lesion. The potential rewards of neuroendoscopy include improved postoperative results, shorter hospitalization times, and fewer postoperative complications (Teo and Mobbs, 2005).

Endovascular Procedures

There are several neurovascular disorders that are amenable to an endovascular procedure. This approach is considered minimally invasive, and is therefore a reasonable option for patients who are not candidates for open surgical procedures because of age, health status, medical condition, or location of the lesion. Interventional neuroradiology uses fluoroscopy to gain access to the intracranial circulation by way of a percutaneous transfemoral catheter.

The endovascular approach to the treatment of both ruptured and unruptured cerebral aneurysms is endosaccular occlusion (Evidence for Practice). This is an excellent technique for aneurysms that are complex, have a neck that is too short for clipping, or are difficult to reach via traditional craniotomy. A flexible platinum coil is fed through the transfemoral catheter and is coiled within the body of the aneurysm, conforming to the aneurysm's shape. The coil is then detached from the catheter. The coil blocks blood flow to the site, thereby preventing rupture or rerupture, both of which can be fatal.

Although surgical excision is still the standard treatment for intracranial arteriovenous malformation (AVM), surgical morbidity may be decreased by utilizing endovascular embolization preoperatively in select cases. A specialized microcatheter is guided directly into the AVM via angiography. The abnormal blood vessels in the AVM are occluded from the inside by means of embolization. There are several materials used to cause embolization, including fibered titanium coils, polyvinyl alcohol particles, and fast-drying biologically inert glues. The AVM may effectively be devascularized and reduced in size through endovascular embolization, and when combined with microsurgery or stereotactic radiosurgery, the AVM may be completely eradicated. Endovascular embolization as the sole treatment of intracranial AVMs is unacceptable, because of unknown long-term occlusion rates and low rates of complete occlusion. In the case of dural arteriovenous fistulas, which comprise 10% to 15% of all intracranial AVMs, endovascular techniques may be curative without the need for further intervention.

Endovascular embolization is also advantageous when employed as a preoperative treatment for select intracranial tumor resections. Highly vascular tumors, as well as tumors that are inopportunely positioned, can be devascularized using techniques similar to those used in the treatment of AVMs, thus decreasing blood loss and risk of hemorrhage during resection.

Carotid artery angioplasty and stenting are the endovascular procedures used to treat carotid artery stenosis. A balloon-tipped catheter is advanced to the location of the offending plaque within the carotid artery and is inflated to press against the plaque. Consequently, the plaque is flattened against the vessel lumen and blood flow is reestablished. A metal-mesh tube is then advanced to the same location to act as a scaffold to prevent reocclusion. Stents may be bare metal, or they may be coated with thrombolytic agents.

Intracranial stenosis has been deemed a high-risk disease in need of alternative therapies. Endovascular intracranial angioplasty and stenting are options, although neither has yet to be evaluated in a controlled clinical trial. Successful use of balloon angioplasty has been documented in mostly academic, high-volume centers, performed by highly skilled and experienced physicians. While the results are encouraging, the technically demanding nature of the procedures carries substantial risk. The Wingspan stent has been approved by the U.S. Food and Drug Administration (FDA) to treat symptomatic patients with

EVIDENCE FOR PRACTICE

Surgical/Endovascular Treatment of Ruptured Aneurysms

The Stroke Council of the American Heart Association (AMA) has formulated recommendations for the surgical/endovascular treatment of ruptured aneurysms. These guidelines are intended to serve as a framework for the treatment of ruptured aneurysms.

♦ Endovascular coil occlusion of the aneurysm is appropriate if the aneurysm is deemed treatable by either endovascular coiling or surgical clipping.

♦ Reasonable consideration of the individual characteristics of the patient and aneurysm must be used in deciding the best means of repair.

♦ The patient should be managed in a surgery center offering both techniques.

♦ Either procedure should be performed to reduce the risk of rebleeding after the initial aneurysmal subarachnoid hemorrhage (SAH).

CLIPPING

The surgeon performs a craniotomy (opening of a portion of the skull) and separates the aneurysm from the surrounding tissue. A small titanium clip, whose features are similar to those of a clothespin, is then placed across the base of the aneurysm. Once the clip is secured, blood can no longer enter or exit the aneurysm sac. By using a needle to drain the remaining blood out of the aneurysm, the sac should empty and eventually collapse. The procedure is ideally performed within 72 hours of diagnosis. It is important to note that following rupture, there is a 40% chance of death and 80% chance of disability. Early detection and treatment offer the best chances of survival.

COILING

Also known as endovascular therapy, coiling is a less invasive treatment option. Especially for those patients who are in poor health, surgical intervention may pose a greater threat than the aneurysm itself. Coiling has proven to be a safe alternative to the traditional treatment of a craniotomy. This procedure does not involve opening of the skull, and is performed from inside the blood vessel. A catheter is inserted into the patient's groin, and is guided up toward the brain under fluoroscopy. A wire is then threaded into the catheter and directed into the aneurysm. Once inside the aneurysm, the wire twists into small coils and continues filling the aneurysm sac until eventually the aneurysm is occluded (Zuccarello and Ringer, 2009).

Previous studies, such as the International Subarachnoid Aneurysm Trial (ISAT) in 2002, found that patients who were initial candidates for both types of procedures had better outcomes 1 year after endovascular coiling as opposed to surgical clipping. Since that time, few studies have emerged to either support these findings or challenge them. It is essential that research continues to determine which course of treatment is the most beneficial.

Modified from Bederson BJ et al: Guidelines for the management of aneurysmal subarachnoid hemorrhage: a statement for healthcare professionals from a special writing group of the Stroke Council, *Stroke* 40:994-1025, 2009; Zuccarello M, Ringer A: Aneurysm clipping, *Mayfield Neuro,* 2009, available at http://mayfieldneuro.com/PE-Clipping.htm. Accessed May 31, 2009.

intracranial stenosis greater than 50% that is refractory to medical therapies. The stent is implanted using the Wingspan technique. Following balloon angioplasty, a self-expanding nitinol stent is placed across the atherosclerotic lesion in the brain. While the Wingspan system appears to be a viable treatment option, a high rate of restenosis has been reported, and its value is not yet firmly established (American Association of Neurological Surgeons [AANS], 2009).

Intraarterial thrombolysis for the treatment of acute ischemic stroke is a consideration for patients who have missed the 3-hour window for therapeutic intravenous thrombolysis. The endovascular route is used to deliver a high concentration of a thrombolytic agent directly to the site of the offending thrombus in combination with mechanical clot extraction. Intraarterial thrombolysis is still being studied for its long-term value. It is currently recommended for selected patients with major ischemic stroke of less than 6 hours' duration caused by occlusion to the middle cerebral artery, and who have contraindications to intravenous thrombolysis, such as recent surgery (Doherty and Way, 2006).

Mechanical clot extraction is an endovascular technique that may be used alone or in conjunction with intraarterial thrombolysis. Success rates are improved when both modalities are used. There are several retrieval devices approved by the FDA for extraction of thrombi from occluded intracranial arteries. A typical retrieval device consists of a coil that is delivered to the thrombus site via endovascular microcatheter and screwed into the clot like a corkscrew to extract the clot. The coils are available in different shapes and configurations to accommodate the specific thrombus. Mechanical clot extraction shows its best utility for cerebral arteries demonstrating large or irregularly shaped clot burdens (Meyers et al, 2009).

Stereotactic Radiosurgery

In stereotactic radiosurgery, stereotactic localization is coupled with delivery of ionizing radiation to destroy a lesion in the brain. Radiosurgery is technically noninvasive and has a low associated morbidity. The use of radiosurgery has increased, and success of treatment has improved with advancements in neuroimaging (CT and MRI) and computer technology. The goal of radiosurgery is to obliterate a relatively small intracranial target with a high irradiation dose while sparing adjacent and distant tissues. Stereotactic imaging and target localization using CT, MRI, or angiography must be fully integrated with the radiation delivery device to achieve pinpoint localization of the target (Pollock and Brown, 2005). Radiosurgical instruments include the Gamma Knife, the Novalis, and the CyberKnife.

Radiosurgery can be used to treat AVMs, tumors, and trigeminal neuralgia. Best results are achieved for lesions smaller than 35 mm. Larger lesions or lesions involving or near cranial nerves can be successfully treated with a fractionated approach where the radiation is precisely delivered in small daily fractions. This technique, called fractionated stereotactic radiotherapy (FSR), has been particularly useful for preserving vision and hearing. Patients with larger lesions often have symptoms of mass effect that are generally not improved with radiosurgery. Radiosurgery and FSR techniques have successfully sterilized a variety of intracranial lesions often with far less morbidity than a surgical approach.

Stereotactic Procedures

The goal of stereotactic surgery is to target a point or volume in space by way of a predefined minimally invasive trajectory (Zonenshayn and Rezai, 2005). This is accomplished with coordinate systems that provide a constant frame of reference. Radiographic modalities (CT, MRI) are used to navigate three dimensionally and locate and destroy target structures. Predetermined anatomic landmarks are used as guides.

Originally, special head-fixation devices were developed for stereotactic brain surgery (see Figure 12-48). Over the past decade frameless systems have surpassed frame-based techniques in popularity and versatility. These systems employ fiducial markers that either affix temporarily to the skin or are implanted into the outer table of the skull, thereby eliminating the need to mount a frame on the patient's head. These markers are visible on the imaging modality being used. By registering the physical location of the fiducials on the patient's skull, the corresponding points on the image can be aligned with the operating space (Zonenshayn and Rezai, 2005).

Both frame-based and frameless stereotactic systems use radiography, fluoroscopy, CT scans, or MRI to permit accurate placement of a probe directed at the target area. The preoperative images are aligned to the patient's head during surgery so that the surgeon has a better idea of the target area.

The many common applications for cranial stereotactic surgery include craniotomies, transsphenoidal approaches, endoscopic surgery, needle biopsies, and therapeutic aspiration. It is also used for catheter placement and third ventriculostomy surgery. Spinal stereotactic surgery is used for screw placement and spinal cord lesions. Common target areas for the stereotactic approach include tumors, infectious lesions, vascular malformations, the basal ganglia, the thalamus, and anterolateral spinal tracts. Target areas can undergo biopsy, be destroyed by chemical or mechanical means, or be electrically stimulated. Stereotactic procedures are also done to place electrodes in various regions of the brain to determine the site of origin of seizures.

Procedural Considerations. As in most image-guided surgery (IGS), carts with a monitor and the computer, along with accessory equipment and supplies, are required. A variety of stereotactic frame systems are available. The surgical technologist must be familiar with the system in place at his or her institution. Frameless stereotactic surgery triggered a new era in surgical navigation and information delivery. This technology provides three-dimensional visualization of anatomic features with real-time localization information (see Figure 12-49).

Operative Procedure

1. The patient's head is placed into a halo head frame with a stereotactic cage before the surgery (framed stereotaxy). Alternatively, fiducials are placed on the patient's skull (frameless stereotaxy).
2. The patient is then taken for a CT or MRI scan of the brain. The target is identified, and computer coordinates are determined and recorded.
3. The nurse brings the patient to the OR with the frame or fiducials left in place. The stereotactic coordinates are registered or entered into the computer, and the procedure is performed through a burr hole. The stereotactic probe is guided by the computer, directing the surgical approach and trajectory (see Figure 12-48).
4. Hollow cannulae, coagulating electrodes, cryosurgical probes, wire loops, and other lesion-producing or biopsy instruments may be introduced for the destruction of areas in the brain. Temporary and permanent nerve-stimulator electrodes are also introduced to augment the pain-control function of the CNS. These instruments are introduced through a burr hole in the skull.

SURGICAL APPROACHES TO THE BRAIN

Burr Holes

A burr hole is the minimum exposure that can be made to gain access to the brain. A small incision is made in the scalp down to the skull. A small self-retaining retractor is placed. The periosteum is retracted using a periosteal elevator. A drill is used to make the appropriate-size burr hole (usually 1 to 2 cm). If necessary, the burr hole can be enlarged using Kerrison rongeurs. The dura is incised, exposing the brain.

Burr holes are necessary for many neurosurgical procedures. They are placed in the skull to remove a localized fluid collection secondary to head trauma that results in an epidural or subdural hematoma. A burr hole can be used to access the intracerebral ventricles for the following reasons: placement of a ventricular catheter to drain obstructed CSF; measurement of ICP; or establishment of a ventricular shunting system. Burr holes are placed for many stereotactic procedures, such as stereotactic biopsy or placement of electrodes. Burr holes are also made before turning the bone flap in preparation for a craniotomy procedure.

Craniotomy

A craniotomy is the removal of a section of the cranium referred to as a bone flap. One or more burr holes are placed, and the dura is dissected away from the cranium. A craniotome with a dura guard attachment is used to excise a section of the cranium, exposing an area of the brain. The surgeon replaces the bone flap to its original location and secures it with wire or titanium plates and screws.

Multiple types of craniotomy incisions are used to expose different parts of the brain. Depending on the location of the pathologic condition, a craniotomy may be frontal, parietal, occipital, temporal, or a combination of two or more of these approaches. The pterional craniotomy is an extremely versatile approach to the anterior and middle fossae. It is useful to access lesions of the frontal or temporal lobes near the sylvian fissure or skull base. A craniotomy may be performed to evacuate intracranial hematomas not accessible through a burr hole, to control bleeding, to debulk or resect tumors, to excise or clip vascular lesions, to aspirate abscess formation, and to decompress cranial nerves.

When turning a scalp flap for a craniotomy, the surgeon may peel the scalp back off the pericranium. The surgeon elevates the bone flap with the overlying muscles still attached (osteoplastic) or strips the periosteum off the skull before the bone flap (free flap) is turned. The bone plate may be separated from the soft tissues, removed from the skull, and set aside for replacement at the end of the procedure. It is placed in an antibiotic solution and remains on the sterile field. The surgical technologist ensures that the bone flap stays separate from other items on the sterile field and alerts the perioperative nurse and any relief surgical technologists of its location to prevent it from being inadvertently discarded. If the bone is not separated from the soft tissues, it is reflected with the temporal muscle and soft tissues. If intracranial swelling is a major concern or the purpose for the craniotomy, the bone plate may not be replaced. If it is not replaced, it may be frozen in a sterile container according to hospital protocol to be used at a future date.

Craniectomy

Craniectomy is the permanent removal of a section of the cranium using burrs and rongeurs to enlarge one or more burr holes. The surgeon performs a craniectomy to gain access to the underlying structures. This procedure may be required to remove tumors, hematomas, and infection of the bone. A suboccipital craniectomy, done with the patient in prone or lateral position, allows access to the posterior fossa. Titanium mesh may be used to repair the cranial defect. Craniectomy is also indicated as treatment for craniosynostosis in infants and young children. Severe head injury with increased ICP can be treated with a craniectomy to give the brain room to swell.

Transsphenoidal Approach

The transsphenoidal route to the pituitary fossa is a less invasive means of removing tumors than the transcranial route. This can be done with a small incision through the nose or through the gingiva under the upper lip. More recently, an endoscope has been used to assist with access through the sphenoid sinus into the pituitary fossa. Tumors of the parasellar region may also be approached using this technique.

Intraoperative Techniques for Cranial Procedures

Extensive time may be directed toward anesthesia preparation and induction, patient positioning, cranial fixation, neuromonitoring, guided image synchronization, and skin preparation. The surgical technologist should use this time to organize and prepare everything needed for the procedure so that nothing is left to chance. Points to consider regarding the intraoperative phase include the following.

- When a Mayfield table is used over the patient, it may be draped in conjunction with the head and rest of patient. It is helpful to use a sterile metal Mayo stand tray filled with instruments for opening so that they can be brought up and placed over the draped overhead table in one step.
- Secondary suction, monopolar ESU, and bipolar may be used on some cranial procedures for ease of access and to ensure visualization and hemostasis. These cords should be attached to the drape and instrument pockets affixed to drapes to prevent tangling or dropping of cords.
- After the scalp is incised, have monopolar ESU, radiopaque sponges, suction, and scalp clips immediately available for hemostasis. Scalps are extremely vascular. The surgical technologist may have to provide additional digital pressure over scalp edges until clips are applied.
- Have self-retaining retractors, suture, spring-loaded clips, or other devices in readiness for each layer of flap opening (scalp, skull if pedicle left, and dura). Have lap sponges or oxidized cellulose (Surgicel) ready for the scalp flap. Be sure

that the opened, folded-over scalp flap is padded and not kinked, causing ischemia of the flap during surgery.

- During burr hole placement, irrigate the cranial perforator to prevent bone burning and to cool the drill; however ask whether bone dust will be saved for placement in the defects before the replacement of the flap. If so, irrigate sparingly and have a specimen cup and periosteal elevator ready to scrape up the built-up bone dust for each hole made. After collection, cover the specimen cup and place on back table until closing.
- When cranial blade is being used to connect burr holes for creation of bone flap, irrigate liberally to keep bone from burning and to remove debris for visualization of exit burr hole.
- It may be necessary to place a metal brain retractor or periosteal elevator to protect soft tissues in case of slipping of cranial cutter when exiting a burr hole.
- The surgical technologist or first assistant should be on guard to prevent bone plate from "popping off" when last cut between burr holes is completed. If brain is under pressure, the free flap can fall off the field. Once off, place flap in covered container on back table and keep it moist.
- Upon removal of a bone flap, be ready with irrigation, bipolar forceps, Gelfoam with thrombin, cottonoids, and bone wax. Dural veins may be severed during removal of the bone flap and hemostasis must be achieved quickly.
- Drill should be changed to hole drilling bit so that reattachment hole can be drilled before opening the dura. These holes will also be used to tent up the opened dural edges to the underside of the skull to prevent dead space and hematoma formation. The first assistant may take this time to prepare the bone flap with plates for closing.
- Before opening the dura, the surgical field is irrigated and bone dust removed or covered with additional draping materials.
- Prepare dural sutures for traction and tacking up.
- *Never* hand instruments over the exposed brain.
- Have all sizes of cottonoids available within easy reach of surgeon and assistant.
- Prepare any necessary retractor systems, microsurgical instrumentation, aneurysm clips, CUSA, biopsy forceps, and so on and have in readiness and within easy reach.
- Irrigating fluids must be maintained at body temperature to prevent vascular spasm. This may require changing the irrigation fluids out periodically on long cases. Sterile solution warmers are helpful for this.
- Verify with surgeon whether antibiotic irrigation will be used. Often they will prefer to not use antibiotics intradurally.
- If microscope is used, the surgical technologist will place instruments in the surgeon's hand and may have to guide the surgeon's hand into the operative field to prevent puncturing the microscope drape or having to divert eyes from the scope.
- Keep eyes on field and monitor if available to anticipate next steps and observe for bleeding.
- All personnel must take care not to move or jar the microscope when in use.
- Following the indicated procedure performed, prepare for closing procedures. If methylmethacrylate is used, check when to start mixing because there is a short window of time that it will remain pliable for use before it sets up. Care must also be taken to prevent fumes from being inhaled.

◆ Allow for lengthy counting of sponges and cottonoids by individual sizes.
◆ Following closure of scalp, instruments, drapes, and overhead table may be removed before application of dressings.
◆ The surgical technologist may have to break scrub to assist in stabilizing the patient's head during removal of the cranial fixation device.

SURGERY OF THE BRAIN AND CRANIUM

Evacuation of Epidural or Subdural Hematoma

After trauma, decompression of the brain, as well as removal and drainage of blood clots and collections of liquefied blood from above or beneath the dura mater, may be required. The need for hematoma evacuation is primarily determined by a declining neurologic status in the patient. Depending on the severity of the injury, evacuation can be accomplished through burr holes or a craniotomy. If elevated ICP is a major concern, the craniotomy plate may be temporarily removed from the skull. This gives the brain more room to swell and may prevent brain herniation and death.

Operative Procedure—Burr Hole Placement for Evacuation of Hematoma

1. A preoperative CT scan is very useful in planning optimal placement of burr holes. The surgeon makes at least two linear or small horseshoe incisions over the site of the lesion. Two or more burr holes are made.
2. If a blood clot or collection of bloody fluid is found outside or beneath the dura mater, the surgeon enlarges the burr hole with a Kerrison rongeur until adequate exposure is obtained.
3. If the hematoma is subdural, the dura is incised.
4. Clot and fluid are evacuated, and hemostasis is accomplished with the ESU or the use of hemostatic clips.
5. The surgeon irrigates through the holes using catheters or bulb syringes. Large amounts of irrigating solution are used until the return appears clear.
6. A drain or catheter may be inserted in the subdural or epidural space for postoperative drainage. Additional burr holes can be made as necessary during the course of the procedure to ensure complete evacuation.

Cranioplasty

Cranioplasty is performed for repair of a skull defect resulting from trauma, malformation, or a surgical procedure. The purpose of cranioplasty is to relieve headache and local tenderness or throbbing, to prevent secondary injury to the underlying brain, and for cosmetic effect.

Procedural Considerations. Repair of a skull defect may be performed acutely in clean procedures. In contaminated procedures, 6 months should pass before repair is attempted (Connolly et al, 2009). When a bone plate is removed for control of elevated ICP, it can be repaired following resolution of ICP issues. If the patient's bone plate was frozen under sterile conditions, it could be replaced with microplates and screws.

The most common materials used for cranioplasty include titanium mesh and/or methylmethacrylate. Commercially prepared cranioplastic synthetics that supply the needed chemicals and mixing containers have simplified the procedures of shaping and molding the prosthesis. Sometimes heavy wire mesh is cut to the shape of the defect, and the methylmethacrylate is molded over the mesh.

Recent technologic advancements use CT scans to produce a computer-generated duplication of the defect. A properly sized prosthesis can be produced and sterilized before the surgery. After the defect is exposed, minor adjustments in the shape of the prosthesis can be made with a burr to achieve an optimal fit.

Operative Procedure—Cranioplasty Using Computer-Generated Prosthesis

1. Typically, the old incision is reopened.
2. Keeping in mind that there is no bony protection between the scalp and the brain, the surgeon carefully elevates the scalp flap from the underlying scar, dura, and brain.
3. Bone edges are exposed with a curette, and the prosthesis is fitted to the defect using a burr. Debris is irrigated out of the wound.
4. Microplates and screws secure the prosthesis in place.
5. The incision is closed as usual for craniotomy.

Operative Procedure—Cranioplasty Using Cranioplastic Material

1. A scalp flap is turned, and the bony defect is exposed.
2. The edges of the defect are trimmed, and a ledge is formed to seat the prosthesis.
3. After the bone defect has been prepared so that it is slightly saucerized, the methylmethacrylate is mixed by combining one volume of liquid monomer with one volume of the powdered polymer. When this has formed a doughy mass, it is dropped into a sterile polyethylene bag. The soft plastic is then rolled on a flat surface into the desired shape, leaving the thickness to the approximate depth of the skull edges. A sterile test tube, syringe barrel, or other round object can be used, although a stainless-steel roller is preferred because of its weight and ease of use.
4. The soft cranioplastic material in the bag is placed over the skull defect and, through light pressing with the ends of the fingers, is fitted into the missing skull area. Assistants stretch the plastic bag as the surgeon molds the plate into the defect and forms an overlapping bevel edge. This overlapping fringe keeps the plate from falling inside the skull, in the same manner as the skull saucerization.
5. When the heat of the chemical reactions is evident, the surgeon lifts the plate out of the bony wound and removes it from the polyethylene bag. Cool saline should be used on the flap while the exothermic reaction takes place.
6. When the plate is cool enough to handle, the surgeon trims excess material and bone using rongeurs or a saw and places the plate in the cranial defect to check for fit.
7. A craniotome is used to smooth the rough spots and bevel the edges so that the plate will blend gradually with the skull.
8. Mixing and fitting the plate take about 7 minutes, the same time needed for the cranioplastic material to harden. Sutures may be used to hold the plate in place, generally at three or more points.

Ventricular Catheter and Shunt Placement for Hydrocephalus

Hydrocephalus is a condition marked by an excessive accumulation of CSF resulting in dilation of the ventricular system (where CSF is manufactured and circulated) and increased ICP. Conditions that result in the development of hydrocephalus and CSF obstruction in both children and adults include congenital hydrocephalus, spina bifida, tumors, intracranial/intraventricular hemorrhage, aqueductal stenosis, and Chiari's malformations. Hydrocephalus is treated by accessing the lateral ventricles for the insertion of a ventricle shunting system. The most commonly used methods to divert CSF from the ventricles are the externalized ventriculostomy catheter and the internalized VP shunt.

Placement of an externalized ventriculostomy catheter requires that a burr hole be made to access either the right or the left lateral ventricle. The ventricular catheter is passed into the ventricle. Flow of CSF is verified. The distal end of the catheter is tunneled beneath the scalp, posterior to the burr hole, externalized, and secured to the scalp with suture. The externalized end of the catheter is connected to an external drainage system, which allows for controlled CSF drainage and for ICP measurement. This system has allowed for temporary shunting in patients with elevated ICP and hydrocephalus from any cause. It is an invaluable adjunct in the clinical assessment and management of head trauma with increased ICP.

For more permanent control of hydrocephalus, an internalized ventricular shunt is placed. The type of shunt and the site of insertion are determined by the neurosurgeon. Three approaches for ventricular insertion are frontal, parietal, and occipital. Although the most common drainage site for an internalized shunting system is the peritoneum by way of open dissection or percutaneous trocar, there are other options. If drainage in the peritoneum is inappropriate because of infection or adhesions, other possible distal insertion sites include the right atrium, the pleural cavity, and the gallbladder (Wang and Avellino, 2005).

The VP shunt system comprises a ventricular (proximal) catheter, a reservoir, a valve, and a peritoneal (distal) catheter. A unitized shunt has fewer separations and connections. The reservoir, if used, is inserted between the catheter and the valve. Access to the system through the reservoir enables the practitioner to assess the patency of the shunt, to obtain CSF for laboratory analysis, to introduce contrast medium for radiologic studies, and in some specific cases to inject medication into the shunt. The one-way valve system directs flow of CSF out of the ventricular system. Valves are available in a variety of different pressure and flow settings. Nonprogrammable valves and shunts are pressure controlled and open to release flow whenever the actual pressure exceeds the pressure that the valve is designed to open (the opening pressure). Some valves are flow controlled and attempt to maintain a constant flow despite pressure changes. A more recent advance is the programmable valve. Programmable valves and shunts allow adjustments to the opening pressure after the shunt is implanted, avoiding surgical procedures to change valves.

Procedural Considerations—Ventriculoperitoneal Shunt Placement. The patient is placed in a modified supine position with a shoulder roll. The head is turned to the opposite side and supported on a donut. Hair is removed from the site where the burr hole will be made to behind the ear and down to the neck. The burr hole site must be prepped, along with the neck, chest, and abdomen on the side of the shunt insertion.

The shunt unit should be handled with extreme care. As with all implantable devices, each manufacturer's specific instructions must be followed and care taken to keep the assembly free of lint, powder, or other foreign bodies that could cause a reaction in the patient's tissues. Lubricants are never used. Blood should be kept clear from the lumen of the catheter to prevent clotting and obstruction. The unit is soaked in normal saline and antibiotic solution and primed before implantation. Air trapping in the valve assembly should be avoided. The valve must be properly oriented to facilitate CSF flow from the ventricles to the peritoneum.

The surgeon may use an endoscope or stereotactic image-guided navigation system to locate small ventricles or to fenestrate the septum between ventricles, thus avoiding the necessity to place multiple ventricular catheters. Surgical technique for VP shunt placement is basically the same for adults and children (Figure 12-56).

Operative Procedure—Ventriculoperitoneal Shunt Placement

1. The surgeon makes a horseshoe-shaped incision to the right or left of midline, along the papillary line. Skin and periosteum are elevated.
2. Scalp bleeding is controlled, and the skin flap is retracted.
3. A burr hole is placed, and the dura is coagulated and incised. The surgeon uses the bipolar ESU to electrocoagulate the pia at the catheter insertion site.
4. The ventricular catheter with an introducer is inserted perpendicularly into the lateral ventricle approximately 4.5 cm in the infant and 6.5 cm in the adult. When the ventricle is penetrated, the surgeon removes the introducer, verifies the CSF flow, and attaches and secures the reservoir and valve with 2-0 silk ties.
5. A subcutaneous tunnel is created from the burr hole to a neck incision, where the peritoneal catheter is then connected.
6. The surgeon makes a subxiphoid or lateral abdominal incision and exposes the peritoneum.
7. Further tunneling is performed from the neck to the chest and abdomen, avoiding the nipples and umbilicus. The surgeon passes the catheter through the tunneling device to the abdominal incision. After spontaneous distal flow of CSF is verified, the distal end of the peritoneal catheter is passed into the peritoneal cavity, leaving enough length to allow for growth in the child and movement in the adult.
8. The catheter is secured to the peritoneum with a purse-string suture. All incisions are closed, being careful not to puncture the shunt system with a suture needle.

Shunt failure can occur at any time, requiring any single portion of the shunt system or the entire system to be replaced. Obstruction, disconnection, malfunction, and infection are routine causes of shunt failure. Revising a shunt typically involves a troubleshooting process. Therefore it is best to prep and drape the patient to provide access to any and all portions of the shunt system. An infected shunt may be externalized until the infection is treated.

Craniotomy

Procedural Considerations. Craniotomy is a technique for exposure of the brain to surgically treat intracranial disease. There are multiple types of craniotomy incisions. A key element

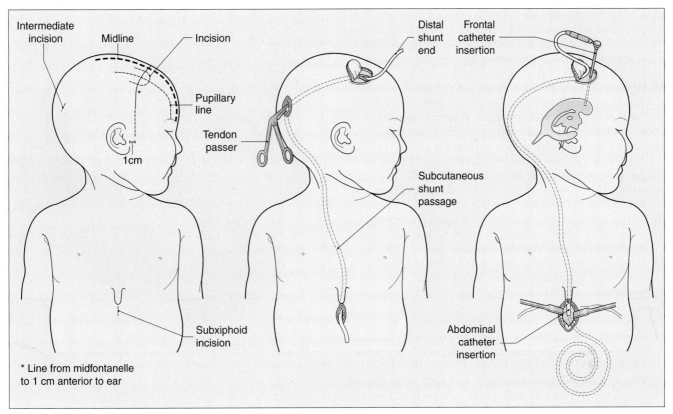

FIGURE 12-56 Placement of a frontal ventriculoperitoneal (VP) shunt. The technique is similar for adult and pediatric patients. The patient is positioned, and coordinates are marked. The shunt is passed subcutaneously. The ventricular catheter and then the peritoneal catheter are inserted.

of these operative approaches is patient positioning, which facilitates exposure, allowing complex procedures to be done through small bony windows with limited dural opening and a minimum of cortex exposure. A skull fixation device provides head stability and allows for rotation, flexion, and extension in the final positioning of the head. If frameless stereotactic image-guided navigation is to be used, registration of fiducials must be done. Careful planning of the incision is imperative for adequate exposure. As a rule, flaps that create a vascular pedicle should be avoided and linear or sigmoid (S-shaped) flaps should be used. This is particularly true for patients with malignant brain tumors who will be treated with radiation, steroids, and chemotherapy. A pedicle flap compromises the blood supply to the incision and, with these other treatments, increases the likelihood of wound infection.

Operative Procedure—Craniotomy for Tumor Resection

1. The surgeon infiltrates the incision site using a local anesthetic with epinephrine.
2. The surgeon and the assistant apply digital pressure along the skin edges as the surgeon incises the skin through the galea.
3. Raney scalp clips are applied to skin edges, and/or self-retaining retractors are placed. The ESU is used on the major scalp vessels for hemostasis.
4. The scalp flap is reflected in the subperiosteal plane with periosteal elevators or with the monopolar device to divide muscle attachments. It is retracted up using devices that

may include retractors, towel clips, suture, or rubber bands and supported with a scalp roll.

5. Burr holes are placed that expose the dura and are widened using curettes and Kerrison rongeurs. The dura is dissected from the cranium using Woodson, Penfield, or Adson dissectors.
6. The craniotomy is accomplished using a craniotome with footplate attachment as the assistant irrigates to cool the bone. The bone flap is carefully elevated from the dura and placed in irrigating solution on the back table.
7. Bone dust is irrigated away from the wound, and hemostasis is established. Bleeding edges of bone are waxed, and bleeding vessels in the dura are electrocoagulated with the bipolar ESU or occluded with thrombin-soaked Gelfoam and patties. The surgeon places hemostatic agents and patties around the craniotomy edges, and then places dural tacking sutures that will remain permanently to prevent postoperative epidural hematoma formation.
8. After hemostasis is achieved, the surgeon opens the dura with a #11 or #15 blade. A dural suture may be placed in the dura before incising it. This tents the dura, ensuring that the surface of the brain is not inadvertently nicked. A Woodson dissector and blade or Metzenbaum scissors are used to extend the dural incision. Bleeding from transected dural vessels can be prevented by coagulating them with the bipolar ESU before cutting them, or to avoid shrinking of the dura, hemoclips can be placed or vessels can be compressed with a hemostat.

9. A self-retaining retractor system is placed if necessary. Cortical dissection is achieved using the bipolar ESU, microscissors, and suction, and the specific surgical procedure is completed. Samples of tumor are sent for pathologic study if applicable.

10. Hemostasis is established. Irrigation can be used to find bleeding sites in the brain. A resection cavity is lined with Surgicel and filled with irrigation. Valsalva's maneuver can be produced with the ventilator to verify hemostasis.

11. The surgeon closes the dura with a 4-0 suture (braided nylon or silk). Gaps in the dura can be repaired using muscle, pericranium, dural substitute, or pericardium. A central dural tacking suture may be placed, and Gelfoam may be placed over the dura.

12. The bone plate is fitted with titanium plates and screws and reconnected to the cranium, or it may be wired into place depending on the surgeon's preference.

13. Muscle/fascia is reapproximated and galea is closed with interrupted absorbable sutures. Skin is closed with suture or staples.

Operative Procedure—Pterional Craniotomy

1. The skin incision for the pterional craniotomy extends from the zygoma to the midline, curving gently just posterior to the hairline (Figure 12-57).

2. The surgeon and the assistant apply digital pressure over folded sponges on both sides of the incision line. The skin and galea are incised in segments, with the length of each segment being equal to that over which the finger pressure is applied. The tissue edges are held with 6-inch toothed forceps as scalp clips are placed on the flap edges. Any remaining active arterial bleeding is controlled by electrocoagulation. If the incision extends into the temporal area, bleeding in the temporal muscle is managed by electrocoagulation, hemostats, tamponade, or suture ligature. Mayo scissors can be used to incise temporal muscle and fascia.

3. The soft tissue is peeled off the periosteum by sharp or blunt dissection or by electrodissection. The scalp flap is reflected over folded sponges and retracted by use of small towel clips and rubber bands or by muscle hooks on rubber bands. In either case, the traction is maintained by securing the rubber band to the drapes with heavy forceps. The flap may be covered with a moist sponge or Telfa strips and a sterile towel. Bleeding is controlled by electrocoagulation (Figure 12-58).

4. When a free bone flap is planned, the muscle and periosteum are incised. Muscle and periosteum are elevated with the skin-galea flap, reflected, and retracted as a unit, as described previously.

5. The periosteum and muscle are incised with a scalpel or ESU knife except at the inferior margins, which are left intact to preserve the blood supply to the bone flap. The periosteum is stripped from the bone at the incision line with a periosteal elevator. Bone wax is used to control bleeding.

6. The scalp edges and muscle are retracted from the bone incision line by a Sachs or Cushing retractor. Two or more burr holes are made (Figure 12-59). A great deal of heat is generated by the friction of the perforator or burr against the bone. The assistant must irrigate the drilling site to counteract the heat and remove bone dust, which collects as the holes are made. A large-gauge suction tip is used to remove both irrigating solution and debris from the field. As the

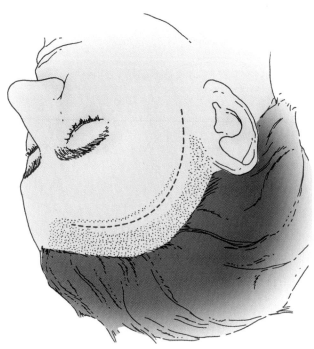

FIGURE 12-57 The skin incision for a pterional craniotomy.

inner table is perforated and the dura exposed, tamponade of the burr hole may be done temporarily with bone wax or a cottonoid strip or patty. Each hole is eventually debrided by a #0 or #00 bone curette or small periosteal elevator. The dura mater is freed at the margins with a #3 Adson elevator, #3 Penfield dissector, or right-angle Frazier elevator or similar instrument. The hole is irrigated and suction applied simultaneously. Active bleeding points in the bone are identified, and bone wax is applied.

7. When all burr holes have been made, the surgeon separates the dura mater from the bone with a dural separator, such as a #3 Penfield dissector or Gigli saw guide. Dural separation is done to prevent tearing of the dura mater, especially over venous sinuses. An air craniotome or Midas Rex drill can be used for cutting the bone flap. Irrigation and suction are required as the bone flap is cut. Soft tissue edges are retracted with Sachs or Cushing retractors.

8. The bone flap with muscle attached is lifted off the dura mater by two periosteal elevators. Bleeding from the bone is controlled with bone wax. The bone flap is covered with a moist sponge, cottonoid material, and then a clean sterile towel and is retracted in the same manner as the scalp flap.

9. The dura mater is irrigated. Moist patties may be inserted between the dura mater and bone and folded back to cover the exposed bone edges. Epidural tack-up sutures are usually placed around the edge of the craniotomy defect to close the epidural dead space. Sterile towels may be placed around the operative site.

10. The surgeon opens the dura (Figure 12-60). A dura hook or a dural stitch may be used to elevate the dura mater from the brain, and a small nick is made in the dura mater with a #15 blade. Alternatively, a small opening may be made in the dura mater without elevating it, after which the dural edges are grasped with two forceps with teeth and are elevated. A narrow, moist cottonoid

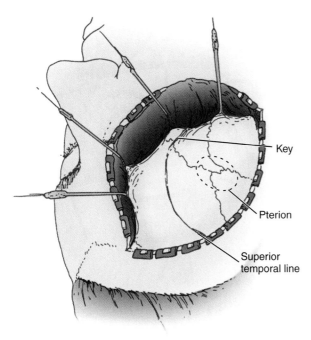

FIGURE 12-58 A commonly employed means of opening the scalp involves incision of the skin, galea, temporalis fascia, and muscle with reflection of the resultant flap in a single layer.

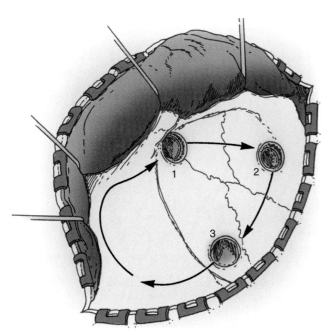

FIGURE 12-59 The pterion craniotomy is performed with power instruments so that three burr holes are placed. The bone is cut as shown, exposing the frontal and temporal dura and the sphenoid ridge.

strip is inserted with smooth forceps (bayonet or Cushing) into the opening to protect the brain as the dura mater is incised and elevated. The dural incision can be made with Metzenbaum scissors, special dura scissors, or a Rayport dura knife. Usually traction sutures are placed at the outer edge of the dura mater and are tagged with small bulldog clamps or mosquito hemostats. Sometimes the tag instruments are attached to the drapes to increase

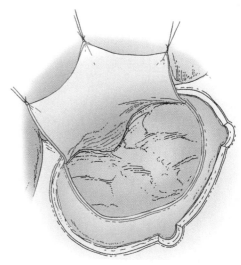

FIGURE 12-60 The dura is opened and reflected back with stay sutures.

traction and keep tension on them. As the dural veins are approached during dural opening, the surgeon ligates or coagulates them before cutting. Ligation is done with hemostatic clips such as Weck hemoclips, McKenzie clips, or Ligaclips. The brain surface is protected by moist cottonoid strips.

11. The surgeon appropriately places cottonoid strips and brain retractors, both self-retaining (Figure 12-61) and manual, while working toward visualizing the particular pathologic entity (Figure 12-62).

12. Pituitary rongeurs as well as the CUSA (Cavitron Ultrasonic Surgical Aspirator) may be needed for tumor removal. Also, a selection of dissectors, bayonet and Gerald forceps, and a bipolar ESU are used. Completely filled irrigating syringes and a full range of moist cottonoid patties and strips must be within easy reach of the surgeon and the assistant. After correction of the pathologic condition and control of bleeding, the brain may be irrigated with an antibiotic solution of the surgeon's choice.

13. The dura mater is usually closed by running or interrupted sutures of absorbable suture or black braided nylon. Dural grafts may be used.

14. The bone flap is replaced and fixated with titanium plates and screws.

15. Periosteum and muscle are approximated with 2-0 or 3-0 absorbable suture. The galea is closed with the same sutures. Skin closure can be interrupted or continuous suture or skin staples.

Surgery for Intracranial Aneurysm

An aneurysm is a vascular dilation usually caused by a local defect in the arterial vascular wall, particularly at points of bifurcation. Vessels at risk within the brain involve those of the major circulation within and around the circle of Willis. Aneurysms are believed to arise from a complex set of circumstances involving a congenital anatomic predisposition enhanced by local and systemic factors. Aneurysmal rupture and hemorrhage into the subarachnoid space are frequently the first sign of an aneurysm, resulting in a sudden, severe headache described as "the worst headache ever." Current neu-

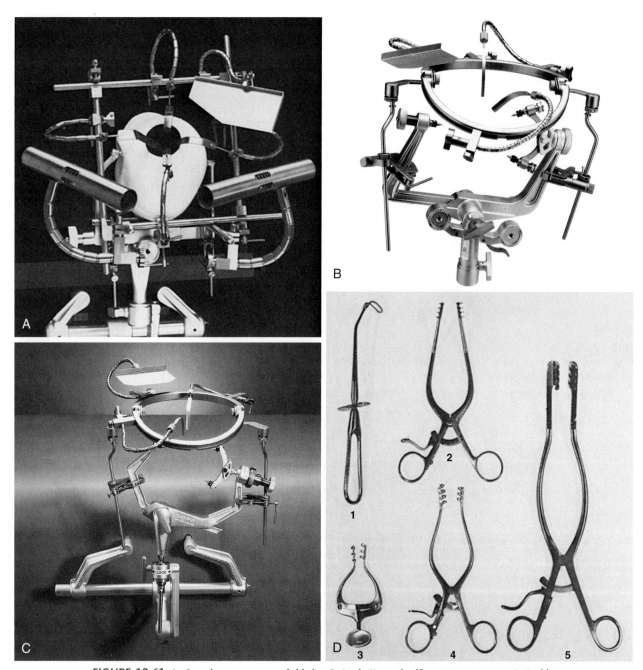

FIGURE 12-61 **A,** Greenberg retractor with blades. **B,** Leyla-Yasargil self-retaining retractor. **C,** Budde halo retractor with attachments. **D,** Retractors: *1,* Cushing subtemporal decompression retractor; *2,* Adson cerebellar retractor; *3,* Jansen mastoid retractor; *4,* Weitlaner retractor; *5,* Beckman laminectomy retractor.

rosurgical techniques have made operations on intracranial aneurysms more feasible; however, fewer than 40% of patients with ruptured aneurysm will return to functional life and 30% die before reaching the hospital (Batjer et al, 2005). Hemorrhage and the cascade of ensuing cerebral trauma are the greatest hazard of the condition and of the operation. To minimize this, control of blood pressure as well as vascular supply to the region beyond the limits of the lesion may be required. Occasionally, control of the cerebral circulation at the level of the cervical carotid artery is desired. The artery may be exposed and controlled by means of preplaced ligatures or clamps that

can be tightened to occlude the vessel if bleeding occurs at the aneurysm site during the operation. This is a separate preliminary surgical procedure.

Procedural Considerations. Aneurysm clips and appliers of the surgeon's choice must be included with the instrumentation. A variety of aneurysm clips are available, and most are spring loaded. Figure 12-55 illustrates a few of the clips and appliers available. Clips may be classified as temporary or permanent, and both must be available with a minimum of two appliers for each type of clip. Temporary clips are commonly used to con-

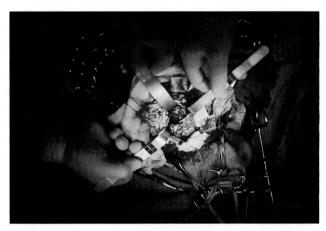

FIGURE 12-62 Craniotomy for choroid plexus papilloma. Tumor is exposed using hand-held malleable brain retractors.

trol giant aneurysms where it may be necessary to evacuate clot and debris before permanent occlusion can be accomplished (Figure 12-63). Temporary clips may also be used to establish the best position for the permanent clip. Temporary clips should be discarded after use. Permanent clips are used to occlude the neck of the aneurysm. Aneurysm clips should not be compressed between the fingers. Clips should be compressed only by the surgeon when seated in their appliers. Once a clip has been compressed, it should be discarded. Clips that have been compressed may be sprung and may slip, causing complications such as bleeding or compression of another vessel or a nerve.

The full armamentarium of aneurysm-occlusion tools should be available for the surgeon. Besides clips, fast-setting aneuroplastic resinous material, a piece of temporal muscle, ligature carriers, or any other material requested by the surgeon should be in the room and ready to use. Fine silk ligatures and hemostatic clips, with or without bipolar electrocoagulation of the neck of the aneurysm, have also been used successfully.

A basic craniotomy setup is required in addition to the special items mentioned. Supplementary suction must be immediately available on the field to prevent hemorrhage from obscuring the surgeon's vision if the aneurysm dome ruptures during the operation. A blood salvage unit should be available for reprocessing of blood for replacement when significant blood loss is expected.

Interventional radiology now plays an important role in the management of intracranial aneurysms. Intravascular balloon occlusion and coiling of aneurysms by interventional radiologists are now considerations in the treatment of aneurysms that meet the criteria for endoscopic therapy. The coils, composed of a soft platinum alloy, allow conformability to the dome of the aneurysm. A guide catheter is introduced into the femoral artery under fluoroscopy and advanced from the aorta into the vessel specific to the aneurysm. Coils are first introduced to outline the border of the aneurysm, and then smaller coils are added to fill the center of the aneurysm. Gradually, blood flow will be reduced, allowing the aneurysm to thrombose (Khatri et al, 2008). Both the neurosurgeon and the radiologist work closely to diagnose and treat these life-threatening anomalies.

Operative Procedure—Craniotomy for Aneurysm Clipping

1. A frontal, pterional, or bifrontal craniotomy may be done to approach an aneurysm in the area of the circle of Wil-

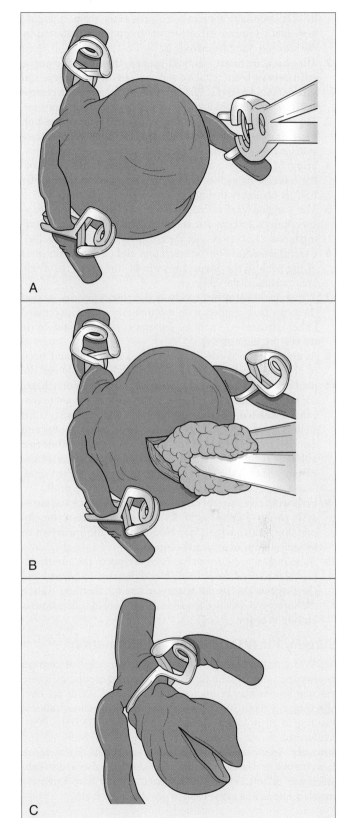

FIGURE 12-63 Temporary arterial occlusion is often necessary in repairing complex large or giant aneurysms. **A,** Temporary clips are placed on the feeder vessels. **B,** The aneurysm sac is opened to allow evacuation of debris and thrombus. **C,** Permanent clip in place.

lis. The bifrontal approach requires extra scalp clips and hemostatic forceps. All aneurysm instruments preferred by the surgeon must be included.

2. After the dura mater has been opened, the surgeon places a self-retaining brain retractor and exposes the optic nerve and subarachnoid cisterns. The olfactory nerve may be electrocoagulated and divided with a long scissors for better exposure.

3. The surgical technologist and perioperative nurse position the operating microscope as directed by the surgeon. Microinstruments, including a micropolar bayonet, are used.

4. Bridging veins are coagulated with bipolar electrocoagulating forceps. Irrigation, which may be a part of the bipolar ESU, is necessary during bipolar electrocoagulation.

5. The surgeon uses microdissectors, hooks, elevators, scissors, knives, forceps, a diamond microknife, and an irrigating bipolar ESU to dissect the covering arachnoidal webs.

6. Careful dissection of the arachnoid and clear visualization of the neck of the aneurysm without rupture of the dome are the aims of the surgeon.

7. The surgeon identifies and frees the parent arteries so that they can be occluded with a temporary clip if necessary. Other structures, such as the optic chiasma and optic nerves, are identified.

8. As the surgeon works slowly toward the dome and neck of the aneurysm, the anesthesia provider may lower the patient's blood pressure for easier control of hemorrhage, should the aneurysm rupture. If the neck of the aneurysm can be isolated, the surgeon places a clip across it. Clips such as the Sundt-Kees and Heifetz have Teflon linings and can be used to approach the aneurysm from a 180-degree angle to avoid excessive manipulation and traction of the parent vessel, if the neck is on the underside of the vessel. These clips support the vessel and serve as a clip graft.

9. Following clip placement, the surgeon may check the aneurysm sac by puncturing it with a needle to see if the clip pressure is adequate to stop blood flow to the aneurysm or to aspirate the aneurysmal contents.

10. As soon as the aneurysm has been occluded, the anesthesia provider returns the patient's blood pressure to normal and the surgeon checks the aneurysm site for bleeding. When the surgeon is satisfied that the operative field is dry, wound closure is begun.

Surgery for Arteriovenous Malformation

An AVM consists of thin-walled vascular channels that connect arteries and veins without the usual intervening capillaries. These vascular lesions may be microscopic or massive. AVMs are rare, affecting only about 300,000 people in the United States (National Institute of Neurological Disorders and Stroke [NINDS], 2009). Malformations vary widely in size, area of involvement, and structure. Arteriovenous fistulas may be congenital or may result from trauma or disease. Vascular anomalies may also lead to subarachnoid or intracerebral hemorrhage or may have extensive irritative effects and cause focal or generalized seizures.

Procedural Considerations. AVMs are difficult to treat successfully. Feeding vessels can be clipped with or without partial removal of the lesion. Total removal, when possible, gives best results. Microsurgical techniques have made total removal without devastating injury to surrounding brain tissue and vessels possible in many cases.

Other methods of treating these malformations include stereotactic radiosurgery with the Gamma Knife. Another method is preoperative embolization, which makes dissection much easier. Surgical glue, such as *N*-butyl cyanoacrylate and tantalum powder, is delivered by means of a catheter into the blood vessels before surgery. During the surgery, the glue is removed along with the AVM. Serial embolization may be performed to reduce the size of the AVM and provide symptom relief when the goal of treatment is not complete obliteration (Schumacher and Marshall, 2006).

Operative Procedure—Craniotomy for Arteriovenous Malformation

1. A supratentorial or infratentorial craniotomy is done, depending on the location of the lesion.

2. The surgeon exposes the feeding arteries distant from the malformation, traces toward it, and then occludes the feeders by clipping, electrocoagulation, ligation, or laser beam coagulation.

3. The malformation is dissected out with suction and bayonet forceps. Additional vessels are clipped or coagulated along the way. Usually one or more draining veins are left to be ligated as the last step in the removal. Closure and dressing are as described for craniotomy.

Craniotomy for Suprasellar and Parasellar Tumors (Pituitary Tumor, Craniopharyngioma, Meningioma, Optic Glioma)

Procedural Considerations. The preferred approach for pituitary tumors and some parasellar tumors is the less invasive transsphenoidal approach. However, for large and complex pituitary and parasellar tumors, a craniotomy may be indicated. A craniotomy setup is used with these additional pituitary instruments: Ray curettes (ring, sharp); angulated suction tips, right and left; large and small spinal needles, #22 or #24; curettes, small, #0 through #4-0; and a Luer-Lok syringe, 10 ml.

Operative Procedure—Craniotomy for Pituitary Tumor Resection

1. The surgeon makes either a bifrontal or a unilateral incision into the frontal or frontotemporal region. Most unilateral approaches are carried out from the right side.

2. Wet brain retractors over moist cottonoids are inserted for exposure of the optic chiasma and the pituitary gland. The frontal and often the temporal lobes are retracted. The olfactory nerve may be coagulated and divided with scissors.

3. A DeMartel, Yasargil, or Greenberg self-retaining retractor is placed to maintain exposure. Aneurysm clips and applicators should be available to control unexpected bleeding from major vessels. The microscope may be moved into place.

4. The surgeon uses the bipolar ESU for hemostasis around the tumor capsule and incises it with a #11 blade on a long knife handle; the tumor is removed with a pituitary rongeur or cup forceps.

5. Small stainless-steel, copper, or Ray curettes, as well as suction, may be used during tumor removal.

6. A wide clip may be applied to the stalk of the pituitary, which may then be cut distally. A long angulated scissors is especially helpful for this.

7. If the tumor capsule is to be removed, bayonet forceps, cup forceps, nerve hooks, and suction aid in the dissection.
8. Closure and dressing are as described for craniotomy.

Extreme caution must be used in removing fluid from the capsule of a craniopharyngioma because the fluid is extremely irritating and may cause chemical leptomeningitis. Calcified pieces of tumor are dissected and removed in the same manner as the capsule of a pituitary adenoma. This is an extremely difficult procedure because of deposits on the carotid arteries, optic nerves, and optic chiasma. The tumor capsule is often left behind on the hypothalamus to avoid stripping off blood vessels supplying this structure. Many moist cottonoid strips are used to protect the surrounding areas from the cystic contents.

Suprasellar meningiomas usually arise from the tuberculum sellae just anterior to the optic nerves and chiasma. Tumor removal is similar to that of a pituitary adenoma except that the electrosurgical cutting loop may be used to excavate the interior of the tumor. After the tumor has been removed, the site of its attachment to the dura is thoroughly electrocoagulated to prevent recurrence. Other meningiomas arising at the base of the skull are treated by similar techniques.

Suboccipital Craniectomy for Posterior Fossa Exploration

The posterior occipital bone is perforated and removed using a drill and rongeurs, and the foramen magnum and arch of the atlas are exposed to remove a lesion in the posterior fossa (Figure 12-64). Posterior fossa lesions include lesions in the cerebellum, the fourth ventricle, and the brainstem; posterior fossa meningiomas; and nerve sheath tumors.

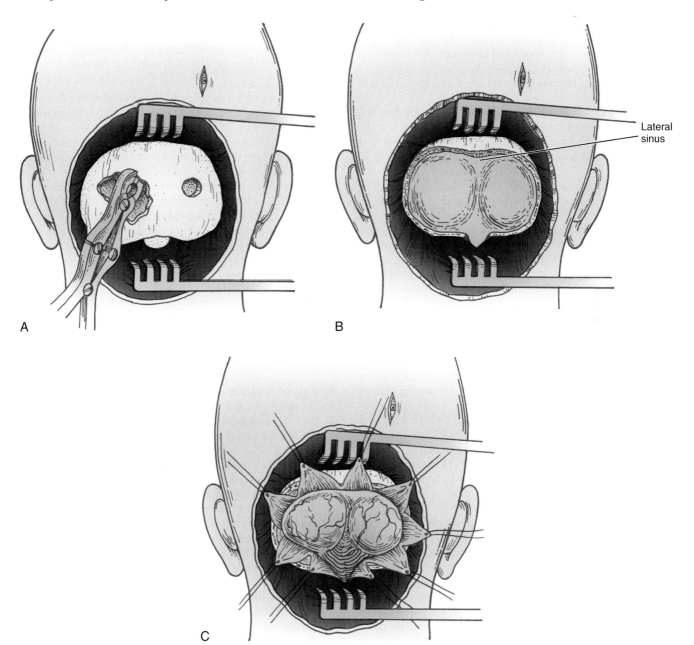

FIGURE 12-64 Suboccipital craniectomy. **A,** Craniectomy being performed. **B,** Dura exposed. **C,** Dura incised and cerebellum exposed.

Procedural Considerations. Depending on the type and size of the lesion, the exposure may be unilateral or bilateral. The operation may include the removal of the arch of the atlas. This approach gives the surgeon access to the fourth ventricle, the cerebellum, the brainstem, and the cranial nerves.

The prone position with the head of the OR bed elevated is the preferred position, but other positions may also be used. An extra-high instrument table or two Mayo stands and standing stool are necessary for the surgical technologist.

Operative Procedure

1. Before the initial surgical incision, the surgeon may make an occipital burr hole for placement of a ventricular catheter. This can be done as a separate procedure or concurrently with the procedure.
2. The incision may be made from mastoid tip to mastoid tip, in an arch curving upward 2 cm above the external occipital protuberance. Alternatively, a posterior midline incision can be used.
3. Scalp bleeding is controlled, and the skin flap is retracted with Weitlaner retractors.
4. The surgeon uses a periosteal elevator to free the muscles, and then divides them with an electrosurgical blade. The incision is deepened. A self-retaining retractor is used. The laminae of the first two or three cervical vertebrae may be exposed.
5. One or more holes are drilled in the occipital bone. The Midas Rex or Anspach drill is used to perform the craniectomy.
6. The dura mater is stripped from the bone. A double-action rongeur, Raney punch, Kerrison punch, or Leksell rongeur is used to enlarge the hole and smooth the edges.
7. Osseous and cerebellar venous bleeding is controlled at each step with bone wax, Gelfoam, and electrocoagulation to prevent air embolism.
8. The dura mater is opened. A small brain spoon or cottonoid strip is used to protect the brain as the initial nick is extended with scalpel or scissors. The dural incision is continued until the cerebellar hemispheres, the vermis, and the cerebellar tonsils can be visualized. Hemostatic clips are used on the dura mater as necessary. Dural traction sutures are placed.
9. The cisterna magna is opened, emptied of spinal fluid, and protected with a cottonoid strip.
10. The cerebellar hemispheres are inspected. Bleeding is controlled with the bipolar coagulator. A needle may be introduced through a small, coagulated incision into the cerebellar hemisphere in an attempt to palpate or tap a deep lesion.
11. Brain retractors over cottonoid strips are placed for exposure. The handle of the retractor must be kept dry to avoid slippage in the surgeon's hand. However, the inserted edge should be wet to prevent damage or tears in the brain surface. These retractors may be positioned in areas that control respiration or other vital functions, so every effort must be made to avoid jarring these instruments in the operative field. When the pathologic entity is identified, a self-retaining retractor may be placed.
12. Long bayonet forceps, bayonet cup forceps, pituitary forceps, suction, and the electrosurgical loop tips may be used

to remove the lesion. Clips may be used to aid in hemostasis. A nerve stimulator may be used to identify cranial nerves; EPs for brainstem monitoring are becoming routine practice.

13. After the lesion has been removed and bleeding controlled, further checking for adequate hemostasis is required. Venous pressure in the patient's head is increased by the anesthesia provider by generating Valsalva's maneuver.
14. The dura mater may be partially or completely closed. The cranial defect may be repaired with titanium mesh. The muscle, fascia, and skin are closed. A dressing is applied.
15. The patient must remain anesthetized until the supine position is achieved and the prongs of the headrest are removed. Particular attention must be given to the patient's head when these prongs are removed to prevent tearing the scalp or damaging the eyes.

Retromastoid Craniectomy for Microvascular Decompression of the Trigeminal Nerve

Trigeminal neuralgia (tic douloureux, fifth cranial nerve pain) is a condition characterized by brief, repeated attacks of excruciating, lancinating pain in the face. The etiology of this facial pain is believed to be the compression of the trigeminal nerve at its exit from the pons by an adjacent artery that has elongated over time to become wedged against the nerve, resulting in demyelination. Pain distribution follows one or all of the trigeminal nerve branches. It is characteristically severe, with sudden onset, short duration, and paroxysmal nature. Triggers often precipitate the pain, such as touching the face, chewing, and talking. When pharmacologic measures fail, surgery to decompress the nerve is undertaken. Frequently more than one treatment is necessary during the course of the disease. Newer options include Gamma Knife radiosurgery.

Procedural Considerations. The patient is in the supine, lateral, or sitting position, depending on the surgeon's preference. An endoscope can be used along with the microscope to improve visualization.

Operative Procedure

1. The surgeon makes a vertical retromastoid incision.
2. The soft tissue is freed from the bone with a periosteal elevator. The bone exposure is maintained with a self-retaining retractor.
3. A burr hole is made, and the dura mater is freed.
4. The surgeon uses a drill and rongeurs to enlarge the burr hole to a diameter of about 2½ inches.
5. With a moist brain retractor, the dura mater overlying the pons and cerebellum is retracted.
6. A self-retaining brain retractor is placed deeper into the wound to retract the cerebellum. The microscope is used to provide light as well as magnification.
7. The surgeon identifies the pons, the superior cerebellar artery, and the trigeminal nerve.
8. Additional blunt dissection frees the vessel from the nerve. A synthetic microsponge is inserted between the vessel and nerve to maintain the separation.
9. The dura and cranial defect are repaired, the incision is closed, and dressings are applied.

Transsphenoidal Hypophysectomy

Endocrine pituitary disorders (such as Cushing's syndrome, acromegaly, malignant exophthalmos, and hypopituitarism resulting from intrasellar tumors) as well as nonpituitary disorders (such as advanced metastatic carcinoma of the breast and prostate, diabetic retinopathy, and uncontrollable severe diabetes) have been successfully treated by transsphenoidal hypophysectomy (TSH). A transnasal or a sublabial incision can be used for rapid access to the sella turcica.

More recently, an endoscope has been used to assist with access through the sphenoid sinus into the pituitary fossa. Otorhinolaryngologic surgeons can be consulted to assist the neurosurgeon with this approach. The endoscope and instrumentation access the sphenoid sinus by the transnasal route. Endoscopic transsphenoidal surgery eliminates the need for an incision and the need for a microscope. When the sphenoid sinus is reached, instruments and technique are similar to the microsurgical technique. Stereotactic image-guided navigation can also be used with the transsphenoidal technique.

All these approaches produce similar results. Complete extracapsular enucleation of the pituitary in cases of hypophysectomy and possible complete removal of small pituitary tumors, with the remaining normal portion of the gland left intact, can be achieved. Patients are relatively free from pain after surgery. No visible scar remains.

Procedural Considerations—Microsurgical Approach for Transsphenoidal Hypophysectomy. General endotracheal anesthetic, combined with a local anesthetic is used. The surgical team places the patient in a semisitting position, with the head against the headrest. The surgeon may use a subnasal midline rhinoseptal approach or a transnasal route, both exposing the sphenoid bone, the sphenoid sinus behind the bone, and the sella containing the tumor. Frequently, an otorhinolaryngologist assists the neurosurgeon in gaining access to the surgical site.

The face, mouth, and nasal cavity are prepped with an antiseptic solution. The surgeon infiltrates the patient's nasal mucosa and gingiva with a local anesthetic agent containing 1:2000 epinephrine to initiate submucosal elevation and diminish oozing from the mucosa. A sterile adhesive plastic drape is applied to the entire face, with additional sterile drapes to ensure a relatively sterile operative field. Sterile sponges (or cotton) are placed in the patient's mouth so that only the upper gum margin is exposed.

Although sterile technique is used, this approach through the nose or mouth is technically not a sterile procedure. Therefore a separate sterile field and instruments must be maintained for adjunct procedures. The thigh or abdomen is prepped if a muscle or fat graft is to be taken. A lumbar drain may be placed preoperatively or postoperatively.

Specialized transsphenoidal instruments are required. The operating microscope is used for the cranial portion of the procedure. A fluoroscopy unit with C-arm may be used to verify the anatomic location of the sella.

Operative Procedure—Microsurgical Approach for a Transsphenoidal Hypophysectomy

1. Using the biopsy setup on a separate small Mayo table, the surgeon may take a small piece of muscle from the previously prepared thigh or a fat graft from the abdomen to be used later in the procedure. This is kept in a moist sponge or soaked in antibiotic solution.

2. An incision is made in the middle of the upper gum margin. The soft tissues of the upper lip and nose are elevated from the bone with an elevator, and the nasal septum is exposed. The nasal mucosa is elevated from either side of the nasal septum, which is flanked by the blades of a Cushing bivalved speculum. The transnasal approach avoids the sublabial incision, instead operating through a bivalve speculum inserted directly through the nares. The inferior third of the anterior cartilaginous septum and osseous vomer are resected, as is the floor of the sphenoidal sinus, exposing the sinus cavity. The floor of the sella turcica can then be identified.

3. The surgeon opens the floor with a sphenoidal punch, and incises the dura mater. The hypophyseal cavity should be opened only in patients undergoing surgery for pituitary adenoma. In these patients, the gland is explored and the tumor is identified and removed.

4. The extracapsular cleavage plane is identified, and the superior surface of the pituitary is dissected until the stalk and the diaphragmatic orifice are found. Cotton pledgets are applied for exposure, hemostasis, and protection of structures.

5. Using a sickle knife, the surgeon sections the pituitary stalk and uses an enucleator to dissect the lateral posterior and inferior surfaces of the gland.

6. The gland is removed, and the sellar cavity may be packed to prevent CSF leakage. The packing is accomplished with muscle obtained previously from the thigh or with the fat graft previously obtained from the abdomen or thigh. The floor is reconstructed with cartilage from the nasal septum.

7. Antibiotic powder may be used and nasal packing introduced for 2 days. If a gingival incision is used, it is closed with suture of the surgeon's preference.

8. Some surgeons prefer to perform this operation by means of a lateral rhinotomy with a transantral-transsphenoidal approach.

NEUROSURGICAL TRAUMA SURGERY

The surgical technologist working in neurosurgery must be prepared for challenges not found in other surgical specialties. Elective or scheduled neurosurgical procedures can be long and arduous with complicated steps and setups. Neurosurgical trauma procedures, however, take on a special urgency because of the potential for catastrophic damage or death with elapsed time. For that reason, a surgical technologist on call must respond as quickly and efficiently as possible.

Traumatic brain injury (TBI) can be caused by seemingly mild bumps, blows, or jolts to the head or severe impact events. Intracranial hemorrhages may be either traumatic (see Figures 12-27 and 12-28) or due to metabolic disorders. They are discussed in previous sections of this chapter. Compound injuries are those where objects penetrate the craniofacial structures and impact the brain (Figure 12-65). Examples include projectiles (Figures 12-66 and 12-67), sharp and blunt objects, and even pieces of the patient's own skull following impact (Figure 12-68).

In the United States from 2002 to 2006, an estimated 1.7 million people sustained a TBI annually (Centers for Disease Control and Prevention [CDC], 2010). Of these people:

- 52,000 die
- 275,000 are hospitalized
- 1,365,000 are treated and released from emergency departments
- Unknown number of patients receive other or no medical care

Further statistics showed that annually:

- TBI contributes to 30.5% of all injury-related deaths in the United States
- About 75% of TBIs are concussions or other mild traumatic brain injuries

- Direct and indirect costs of treatment and lost productivity totaled an estimated $60 billion in 2000 in the United States
- Falls are the leading cause of TBI, with children age 4 and younger and adults over age 75 at highest risk
- Motor vehicle traffic injury is the leading cause of TBI-related deaths with adults between ages of 20 to 24 at the highest rate
- In every age group, males are more likely to sustain TBI than females
- Adults aged 75 or older had the highest rates of TBI-related hospitalization and subsequent death

Traumatic spinal injuries also require urgent medical and sometimes surgical treatment. The most common types of vertebral column injuries are fractures, subluxation (dislocation)

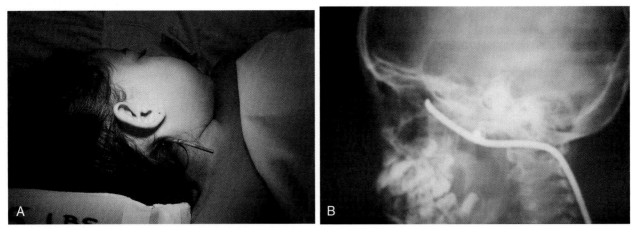

FIGURE 12-65 **A,** Penetrating brain injury. Patient's head is turned to the side with sandbag bracing head. Wire thrown from a lawnmower is seen protruding from the base of the skull on right side. **B,** Skull x-ray showing wire penetrating the base of the skull and lodged in the brain.

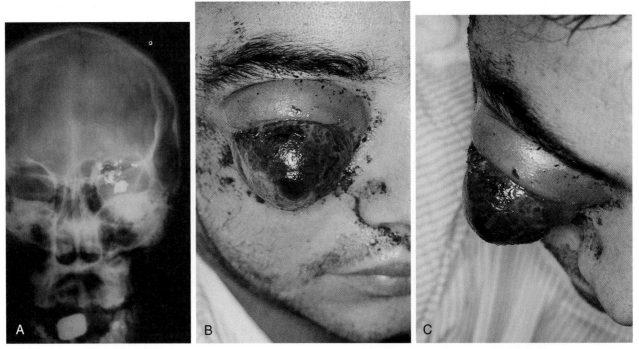

FIGURE 12-66 **A,** Skull x-ray showing bullet fragments in the brain from a gunshot wound of the right orbit. **B,** Proptosis of right eye secondary to gunshot wound of right orbit. **C,** Top view.

injuries, and disk herniation, resulting in neurologic injury in 15% of trauma patients (Mendel et al, 2005). The cervical spine is the most vulnerable to injury. Treatment of a spinal cord injury is initiated at the scene of the accident with efforts to immobilize the spine and keep it in neutral alignment. This may involve use of a rigid neck collar or full carrying board for transport to a hospital. First responders err on the side of caution and presume that spinal cord injury is a possibility that could be exacerbated by movement. The patient may complain of back or neck pain or pressure, respiratory difficulty, weakness, spasms, numbness, tingling, or paralysis. Once the patient arrives in an acute care facility, attention is focused on:

- Maintain ability to breathe
- Preventing shock
- Immobilizing the area to prevent further spinal cord damage
- Avoiding possible complications of urinary retention, respiratory or cardiovascular difficulty, and formation of deep vein thrombosis (DVT) in the extremities
- Sedation if necessary for pain control and diagnostic imaging
- Possible administration of methylprednisolone (Medrol) if injury is identified and fewer than 8 hours have elapsed since time of injury; some patients experience mild improvement of spinal cord injury by decreasing inflammation near the site of the injury

Spinal cord injuries can be classified as either:

- Complete—all sensory and motor function is lost below the level of the injury
- Incomplete—some motor and/or sensory function is present below level of injury

Signs and symptoms of spinal cord injury include:

- Loss of movement

   Tetraplegia or quadriplegia—arms, trunk, legs, and pelvic organs affected

   Paraplegia—all or part of the trunk, legs, and pelvic organs affected

   The Mayo Clinic lists the most common causes of spinal cord injuries in the United States as:

- Motor vehicle accidents—the leading cause at 40% of new injuries per year

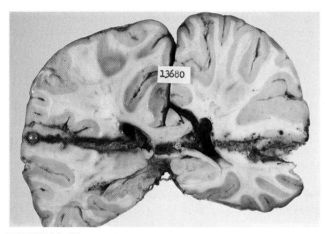

FIGURE 12-67 Air gun pellet track through the brain. Note the large entrance wound defect and pellet lodged in contralateral side.

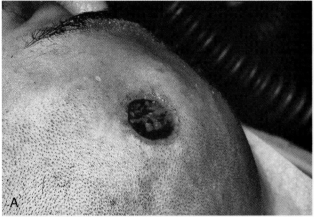

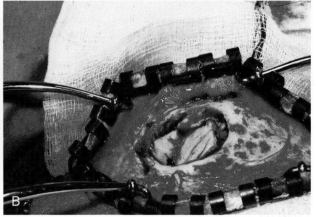

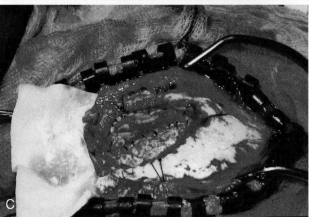

FIGURE 12-68 A, Compound depressed frontal skull fracture secondary to hammer blow. **B,** Depressed skull fragments exposed. **C,** Dural repair following removal of skull fragments.

◆ Acts of violence—up to 15% of injuries result from knife and gunshot wounds as well as other violent acts

◆ Falls—approximately 25% of injuries are caused by falls and are the most common cause of spinal cord injury in patients over the age of 65

◆ Sports and recreation activities—athletics, most commonly impact sports, and diving in shallow water account for approximately 8% of injuries per year

◆ Alcohol—alcohol use is a factor in about 1 out of every 4 spinal cord injuries

Surgical treatment for spinal cord injuries involves surgical decompression and stabilization techniques. These may require use of plates, screws, grafts, prostheses, rods, or external immobilizers. Special care must be taken during positioning and transfer of these patients in the operating room.

SURGERY OF THE SPINE

Surgery of the spinal column is also discussed in Chapter 11, Orthopedic Surgery.

Planning for Spinal Procedures

In times past, the spine was considered the domain of neurosurgeons, but no longer. Some orthopedic surgeons are choosing to specialize in spinal surgery. Regardless of which specialist is operating, the surgical technologist must be familiar with the anatomy, instrumentation, and procedures to provide optimal patient care. The potential hazards with regard to transfer and positioning must be addressed by every member of the surgical team and injury prevented by coordinated routines. General points for the surgical technologist to consider for spinal surgery include:

◆ Prepare for use of imaging equipment, whether x-ray or fluoroscopy, by donning appropriate shielding attire before scrubbing.

◆ Prepare and test all powered instruments before use and lock or place them on safety when not in use.

◆ Remove all bone and disk material from Kerrisons and pituitary rongeurs before returning to surgeon. It may be helpful to carefully use a perforating towel clip to dislodge bone in Kerrison channels if a moistened radiopaque sponge is insufficient.

◆ Always verify which tissues will be saved for possible autograft use or specimen. Some surgeons send all tissues to pathology for examination (e.g., bone, disk fragments, and ligamentum flavum on diskectomies).

◆ In the event of a major intraoperative complication (bleeding from perforated aorta or vena cava or loss of airway) when the patient is in the prone position, the surgical technologist should provide moistened sterile lap sponges and towels to pack the wound, push back Mayo stands and equipment to keep sterile, and assist team members in obtaining the patient transport device for immediate repositioning to supine. If a major vessel is perforated, an immediate laparotomy may be performed. If airway is lost, anesthesia provider will have to reintubate. Following resolution of the emergency, the patient will be repositioned to prone and the wound will require irrigation with antibiotic solutions and the procedure will continue.

◆ As with cranial procedures, the microscope should be prepared with all attachments and settings appropriate for the procedure and surgeon, draped, and left in readiness. Take care to prevent inadvertent contamination.

Anterior Cervical Decompression and Fusion

Anterior cervical decompression and fusion (ACDF) is performed to treat cervical disk herniation or cervical spondylosis (degeneration in the spine) with myelopathy (disorder of the spinal cord) or radiculopathy (disorder of the nerve roots). Symptoms include pain in the neck, shoulders, arms, and hands; and weakness of the upper extremity. An ACDF entails a corpectomy (removal of a vertebral body), diskectomy, and fusion of the vertebral bodies. Bone grafts for the fusion are obtained from the patient's iliac crest (autograft) or from a bone bank (allograft).

Procedural Considerations. Awake endoscopic intubation may be required if the patient's neck is unstable or unable to extend. Neurologic monitoring is commonly employed to prevent further injury during surgery. The patient is placed in the supine position, with a small shoulder roll placed horizontally for mild neck extension. The perioperative nurse ensures the patient's arms are tucked, and the hip is elevated for exposure if bone graft is to be taken from the iliac crest (Figure 12-69). Intraoperative x-ray may be employed to confirm the correct surgical site and verify placement of the graft and related hardware.

Operative Procedure

1. The surgeon may harvest the iliac crest bone graft before the neck procedure begins, or it may be completed after exposure of the anterior cervical spine. An incision is made over the iliac crest, at least 3 cm posterior to the anterior superior iliac spine. The skin and subcutaneous tissues are retracted with a Weitlaner retractor.

2. Soft tissue is dissected until the crest is reached and exposed.

3. The surgeon uses an osteotome or oscillating saw to remove the bone graft. The graft is soaked in antibiotic solution and set aside. The perioperative nurse and surgical technologist perform a sponge and sharp count for this portion of the procedure. Following verification of a correct count, the surgeon irrigates and closes the wound and covers it with a sterile towel.

4. A transverse or horizontal skin incision is made on one side of the neck, directly over the involved cervical level.

5. A Weitlaner retractor is placed, and the surgeon uses sharp dissection to divide the platysma.

6. The medial edge of the sternocleidomastoid muscle is defined with the scissors by blunt and sharp dissection.

7. Using blunt finger dissection, the surgeon creates a vertical plane of dissection between the carotid artery laterally and the trachea and esophagus medially. This plane is held open with retractors.

8. The anterior surface of the spine is identified, and the long muscles of the neck are peeled off the anterior surface of the spine with periosteal elevators or peanut dissectors. The bipolar ESU is used for hemostasis.

9. A 20-gauge spinal needle is inserted a short distance into the disk space, and the location is confirmed radiographically.

10. Self-retaining retractors are inserted into the neck incision. Care is used to protect the carotid artery and the esophagus.

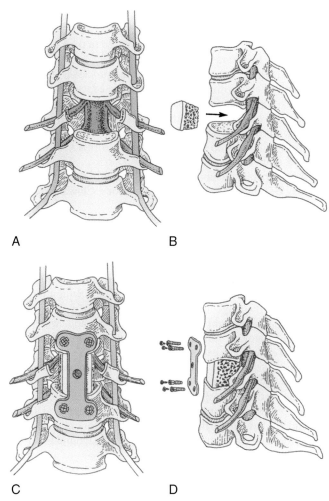

A   B

C   D

FIGURE 12-69 Anterior cervical decompression and fusion. **A** and **B**, A bone graft from the iliac crest or fashioned from bank bone is tailored to fit the site of corpectomy, resting on the vertebral endplates. **C** and **D**, An anterior spinal plate and screws are secured to the vertebral bodies above and below the spanned segment to stabilize and promote a stable fusion.

A combination of sharp and dull blades is used to acquire the best retraction. If a toothed blade is used, the teeth are carefully hooked beneath the long muscle of the neck.

11. The surgeon uses a #15 or #11 blade on a #7 knife handle to incise the disk space; a pituitary rongeur is used to remove the disk material, which may be saved as a specimen. A vertebral spreader may be inserted into the vertebral space to widen the area. Residual disk material is removed with the rongeur or small curettes (angled or straight, #0 to #4-0) until the entire surface of both vertebrae is clean. A small burr may also be used until complete anterior decompression of the nerve root or dural sac is obtained. Nerve hooks may be used for demonstration of adequate decompression.

12. A depth gauge and caliper measure the size of the interbody defect. The bone graft is cut to the appropriate size and placed into the defect with a tamp and a mallet.

13. The anterior cervical plate and screws are secured to the vertebral bodies above and below the bone graft.

14. Lateral x-ray or fluoroscopy is done to confirm location, degree of distraction, and alignment.

15. Hemostasis is obtained, and the wound is irrigated. A drain may be placed. The platysma is closed with absorbable suture. A subcuticular closure of the skin is done, and wound closure strips are applied.

16. A cervical collar is placed before the patient awakens.

Posterior Cervical Approach

The posterior cervical approach is used for laminectomy for decompression, intradural tumor removal, cordotomy, diskectomy, and fusion (Connolly et al, 2009).

Procedural Considerations. A patient with severe spondylosis may require fiberoptic intubation. Intraoperative neurologic monitoring should be used to detect a change in neurologic status. The patient is positioned prone with a three-pin skull clamp (Mayfield). The OR bed is positioned in mild reverse Trendelenburg's position to encourage venous drainage. The patient's arms are tucked. If allograft bone graft is desired for fusion, the posterior iliac spine will be prepped. A cervical collar may be required postoperatively.

Operative Procedure

1. The cervical spinous processes are palpated to plan the incision, and a midline incision is made.
2. Soft tissue dissection is done, and a clamp is placed on the spinous process to verify the correct level with x-ray.
3. Self-retaining retractors help to gain exposure. A subperiosteal dissection is made to the lateral margins of the involved facets using the Bovie, suction, and a cervical Cobb elevator.
4. Hemostasis is maintained with the bipolar ESU, Gelfoam, and patties.
5. A laminectomy is performed using a drill, Leksell rongeurs, curettes, a nerve hook, and Kerrison punch rongeurs.
6. Disk is removed with pituitary rongeurs and curettes.
7. If a fusion is required, instrumentation and allograft or autograft may be needed.
8. The wound is irrigated. A drain may be placed.
9. Bupivacaine may be injected into the paraspinal muscles and subcutaneous tissue for postoperative pain.
10. Absorbable sutures are used to close the fascia and subcutaneous layers. Suture or staples are used for the skin.

Anterior Thoracic Approach

A transthoracic thalamotomy is done to access the spine for a thoracic diskectomy, burst fracture, osteomyelitis, and metastatic disease (Connolly et al, 2009). Usually a thoracic surgeon assists the neurosurgeon in obtaining adequate exposure.

Procedural Considerations. The anesthesia provider may need to place a double-lumen endotracheal tube to allow for deflation of the lung for exposure of the higher thoracic levels. Lateral position with a bean bag is preferred. If intraoperative fluoroscopy is necessary, a Jackson table is needed. A bean bag interferes with fluoroscopy. For T1 to T4, a right-sided approach is preferred to avoid the aortic arch and heart. For T5 to T12, a left-sided approach is preferred because the aorta is safer to manipulate than the vena cava (Connolly et al, 2009). If allograft is desired for fusion, prep the iliac spine.

At times, an anterior thoracic surgery is performed in combination with a posterior thoracic surgery. In this case, the patient is repositioned prone after the completion of the anterior portion of the surgery. The posterior surgical site is prepped and draped, and the posterior portion of the surgery is completed.

Operative Procedure

1. A thoracotomy incision is made, and the latissimus dorsi and other muscles are transected. A rib may be resected with a rib cutter to gain exposure.
2. The parietal pleura is opened, and a thoracotomy retractor is placed. If necessary, the lung is deflated manually.
3. A localization x-ray is done to verify the correct level. The parietal pleura is incised further onto the vertebral body and cleared with blunt dissection. Segmental vessels are ligated as necessary with hemoclips and transected to mobilize the aorta.
4. For diskectomy or decompression, a drill, rongeurs, and curettes may be needed. For spinal fusion, instrumentation and autograft or allograft may be used.
5. The wound is irrigated, and a chest tube is placed. The ribs are reapproximated with a rib approximator and sutured with heavy absorbable suture.
6. The fascia and subcuticular layers are closed.

Laminectomy

Laminectomy is removal of one or more of the vertebral laminae to expose the spinal canal. Laminectomy, hemilaminectomy, and the interlaminar approach are performed to reach the spinal canal and its adjacent structures to treat compression fracture, dislocation, herniated nucleus pulposus, and cord tumor, as well as for spinal cord stimulation. Section of the spinal nerves, including cordotomy and rhizotomy, requires similar surgical exposure.

Procedural Considerations. Laminectomy is done with the patient in the prone or lateral position. It is performed on the cervical, thoracic, or lumbar spine. Laminectomy instruments include the basic neurosurgical set, the retractor of the surgeon's choice, and an assortment of specialty rongeurs.

Operative Procedure—Laminectomy for Spinal Stenosis

1. The surgeon makes a midline vertical incision at the operative site.
2. Two self-retaining retractors (Cone, Weitlaner, or Beckman-Adson) are inserted for exposure.
3. The fascia is incised in the midline with Mayo scissors, electrosurgical cutting tip, or a scalpel.
4. The surgeon uses sharp dissection to expose both sides of the spinous processes.
5. Correct surgical level is verified by lateral spine x-ray film.
6. The paraspinous muscles and periosteum are stripped off the laminae with sharp periosteal elevators. Dissection with the ESU may be used.
7. As each area is stripped, the surgeon packs a radiopaque sponge around the bony structures with a periosteal elevator to aid in further blunt dissection of muscles from the laminae and to tamponade bleeding.
8. A laminectomy retractor is then placed. A Scoville (with a blade on the tissue side and a slightly shorter hook on the bone side), Tower, Crank, or Adson-Beckman retractor can be used.
9. Cottonoid strips or patties may be placed in the extremes of the field for hemostasis.
10. The surgeon removes the spinous processes over the involved area with a rongeur. The bone edges are waxed.
11. The ligamentum flavum is cut with a scalpel, Metzenbaum scissors, or a rongeur. Cottonoid strips or patties are passed through this incision to protect the underlying dura, and a window is cut into the flaval ligament with a #15 blade on a #7 knife handle.
12. Additional ligaments in the lateral gutter of the spinal canal may be removed with a large curette or a Cloward rongeur after first protecting the dural sac.
13. Bleeding from the epidural veins is controlled by packing with narrow cottonoid strips and if necessary by careful coagulation with a bipolar bayonet forceps.
14. Various rongeurs are used to remove the laminae after edges are defined with a curette. Bone drills are commonly used to reduce bone down to epidural fat, saving time and wear on the surgeon's hands.
15. Rongeurs—straight and angled, narrow and wide—are used to remove further bony areas until the cord with its dural covering is exposed and decompressed.
16. The surgeon uses a blunt nerve hook to explore the nerve roots and extradural space.
17. If no further stenosis is felt, hemostasis is secured.
18. The cottonoid strips are removed from the epidural space, and the area is further irrigated. All cottonoid strips and patties and retractors are removed, and the wound is closed.

Operative Procedure—Laminectomy for Intradural Spinal Cord Tumor

1. The fascial incision is made in the midline, both sides of the spinous processes are dissected out, and the paraspinous muscles are reflected bilaterally, one side at a time. The level is confirmed with x-ray.
2. One or more Gelpi or Adson-Beckman self-retaining retractors are placed to maintain the bony exposure.
3. The surgeon performs a midline laminectomy and excises the spinous processes. Various rongeurs (e.g., Leksell, double-action, Cloward) are used to remove the laminae after the edges are defined with a curette. The Midas Rex drill may also be used. The bone edges are waxed for bleeding.
4. The remaining flaval ligament is removed with scissors, scalpel, and Kerrison or Cloward rongeurs. Epidural fat is removed so that the dura mater is fully exposed.
5. A wide, moist cottonoid strip is placed over the superficial soft tissues and muscle down to the bone bordering the exposed dura mater. This provides additional hemostasis.
6. Intraoperative ultrasound may be employed to verify the exact location of the tumor beneath the dura.
7. The surgeon elevates the dura mater with a small hook and nicks it with a #15 blade. A grooved director is inserted beneath the dura mater, and the dural incision is extended over it using long forceps and fine scissors. Alternatively, the surgeon may lengthen the incision with Metzenbaum scissors. Traction sutures of 4-0 silk or braided nylon on dura needles are placed in the dural edges, and the cord is exposed (Figure 12-70). The operating microscope may be used.

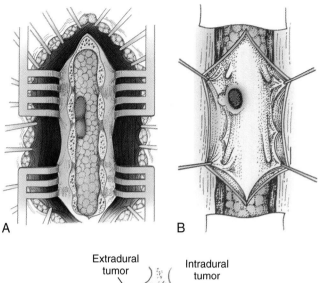

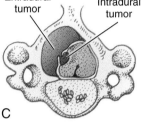

FIGURE 12-70 **A,** Laminectomy completed: dura mater and tumor exposed. **B,** Dura mater incised and retracted, revealing pia arachnoid over spinal cord and part of tumor. **C,** Diagram of cross section of tumor site and location of extradural and intradural pathologic areas.

8. The cord is explored for the pathologic area. Aspiration through a #22 needle on a plain-tipped syringe may be carried out. Whenever possible, the tumor mass is dissected free and removed using suction, the dissecting scissors, the bipolar forceps, small (pituitary) scoops, curettes, pituitary rongeurs, or an ultrasonic aspirator. Bleeding is controlled with moist cottonoids, hemostatic clips, gelatin gauze, and topical hemostatics. Bipolar electrocoagulation is used around the nerves and spinal cord.

9. The wound is irrigated and hemostasis is obtained, being careful to protect the spinal cord.

10. The dura mater is closed with a braided nylon or polytetrafluoroethylene (PTFE) suture.

11. The incision is checked for further bleeding, and the paraspinous muscles are approximated with absorbable suture. The remainder of the wound is closed.

In the case of extradural tumors, invasion of the dura is avoided. Once the dura is opened from a tear or an incision, the neurosurgeon may require that the patient remain flat for 24 hours or longer to allow healing of the dura.

Laminotomy

Laminotomy is the traditional approach to posterior microdiskectomy at the cervical, thoracic, and lumbar levels. Laminotomy is performed on the symptomatic side with resection of a small portion of the medial facet. The goal of this surgery is the resolution of leg pain with little to no residual back pain and a return to preinjury activity and lifestyle. In the twenty-first century, patients with herniated lumbar disks will continue

AMBULATORY SURGERY CONSIDERATIONS

Microdiskectomies

Microdiskectomies are one of several spinal surgeries performed to relieve pain caused by disk herniations. Patients selected for this specific procedure typically complain of leg pain longer than 6 weeks in duration, and receive minimal relief from prescribed pain medications. An MRI confirming the level of nerve root compression as well as a detailed history and physical will determine if the patient is a candidate for surgery.

Ambulatory surgeries are designed for patients who have a nominal health history and pose minimal risk for operative complications. Microdiskectomies have the flexibility of being performed either in a same-day surgery center or in a hospital OR suite. The procedure is typically performed using a general or spinal anesthetic, depending on the needs of the patient. Once the anesthesia provider has control of the airway, the patient is positioned prone for maximum operative accessibility. Positioning may take time, and it is essential that every precaution is taken to prevent patient injury. If the patient is awake, talking should be kept to a minimum, and OR traffic should be closely monitored by the perioperative nurse. Before making the incision the surgeon may inject a local anesthetic containing epinephrine into the lumbar spine to minimize bleeding intraoperatively.

The procedure is approximately 2 hours in duration, and many patients are able to return home the same day. Postoperative pain relief is maximized by the use of intraoperative topical steroids on the nerve root, local anesthetics, and prescribed oral pain medications.

Possible complications include bleeding, infection, and, on rare occasions, nerve damage. Upon discharge the patient is instructed to keep the surgical site clean, restrict activity, and notify the surgeon immediately if he or she experiences excessive pain, swelling, or discharge from the incision site. Follow-up appointments are generally scheduled 2 weeks following the procedure, and most patients can return to work after 4 to 6 weeks.

to have a range of minimally invasive surgical options, many of which will be performed on an outpatient basis. Some of these newer procedures include nucleoplasty (decompression of a contained herniated disk by ablating and coagulating part of the nucleus), intradiskal electrothermal therapy (IDET), and selective endoscopic diskectomy (Singh et al, 2005). Disk replacement is discussed in Chapter 11.

Procedural Considerations. The operating microscope has improved this surgical approach by offering magnification and illumination, which allows for smaller incisions and less tissue dissection. This surgical procedure is associated with less postoperative discomfort and shorter hospital stays. The majority of patients who undergo this procedure can be discharged home on the same day (Figure 12-71) (Ambulatory Surgery Considerations).

Operative Procedure—Lumbar Laminotomy and Microdiskectomy

1. With the patient in prone position or modified knee-chest position, a midline skin incision is made, extending from the spinous process above the involved level to the spinous process below. The correct surgical level is confirmed radiographically.

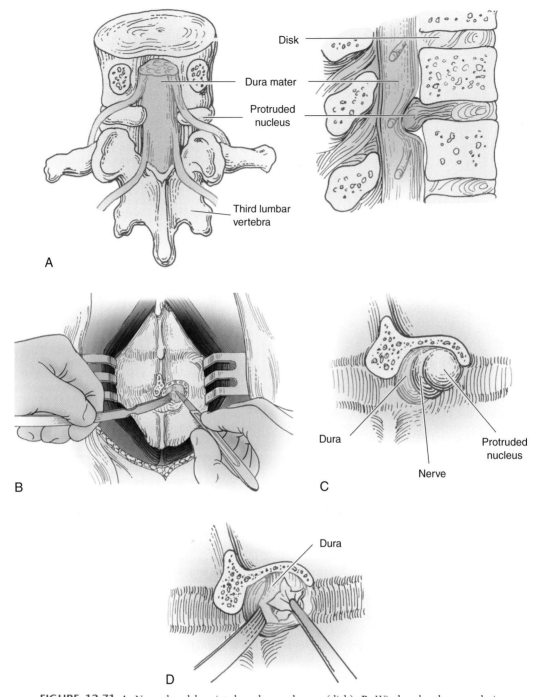

A

B

C

D

FIGURE 12-71 **A,** Normal and herniated nucleus pulposus (disk). **B,** Window has been made in lamina, and ligament has been incised to expose underlying dura mater and nerve root. **C,** Relationship of dura mater, nerve root, and protruded nucleus pulposus (disk). **D,** Retraction of nerve root over dura mater and removal of disk.

2. Dissection is carried down through the subcutaneous tissue to fascia, which is incised through a paramedian incision on the symptomatic side.
3. Paravertebral muscles are then dissected off the spinous processes and laminae.
4. A self-retaining retractor is placed to provide a visual field.
5. The hemilaminotomy, with a small portion of the medial facet removed, is performed.
6. The ligamentum flavum is incised longitudinally and removed with curettes or rongeurs, exposing the thecal sac.
7. A foraminotomy is then performed to expose and decompress the nerve root.
8. The epidural space is explored with a blunt dissector, nerve hook, dental tool, or Penfield #4 dissector.
9. The root is then gently retracted medially, exposing the disk bulge or herniation.

10. A window is made in the disk annulus with a #15 blade, and the disk space is entered.
11. Curettes and disk rongeurs are used to remove loose fragments of disk.
12. After diskectomy, the epidural space and the intervertebral foramen are explored with a blunt nerve hook to confirm patency and resolve nerve root pressure.
13. Hemostasis is achieved, and the wound is irrigated generously with saline/antibiotic solution.
14. The wound is then closed in layers.

For cervical or thoracic disks, only the protruding fragment is removed. Limited, if any, exploration of the interspace is performed because attempts at adequate interspace exploration require retraction of the dural sac, which contains the spinal cord at these levels. Such retraction would result in cord injury and paralysis. For a thoracic disk, a costotransversectomy or transthoracic approach is used.

Endoscopic diskectomy for far lateral disk herniations and annular tears has become an applied surgical approach in this subgroup of patients. Endoscopic spine systems have been developed, and further development and evolution of endoscopic equipment will continue to make minimally invasive procedures attractive to both the patient and the neurosurgeon.

Spinal Cord Stimulators

A spinal cord stimulator (SCS) is an implantable, nondestructive, medical device used to treat chronic intractable pain of the trunk and limbs. The device generates an electrical impulse to the epidural space which produces a tingling sensation that masks the perception of pain.

The goal of the stimulation is to lower the perception of pain, reduce medication use, increase function, and improve quality of life. Patients who are considered good candidates for a spinal cord stimulator placement undergo a trial to check for efficacy prior to permanent implantation. During the trial, a temporary percutaneous lead is placed and connected to an external pulse generator for approximately 3 to 7 days. The patient must experience at least 50% improvement in pain to be considered a candidate for permanent lead placement. The trial is generally performed in the OR using monitored anesthesia care (MAC) or general anesthesia.

The permanent spinal cord stimulator lead is implanted into the epidural space, and the impulse generator (IPG), which is the device battery, is implanted in the abdomen or buttocks. The lead is positioned at a specific level of the spinal cord. The targeted level is determined by the individual patient's symptoms, and by information obtained from the trial. A thoracic spinal cord stimulator is placed for lower back and leg pain. A cervical spinal cord stimulator is placed for upper extremity pain. Peripheral nerve stimulators are an alternative or conjunctive neuromodulation technique that targets peripheral nerves.

Procedural Considerations. Lead placement must be assessed during the surgery. This can be done by waking the patient during the surgery and asking them where they feel the stimulation. To secure the airway, lateral position is used with this method. Alternatively, electromyogram (EMG) monitoring may be used while the patient is under general anesthesia to verify motor responses in the targeted muscle groups. Fluoroscopy is also employed to verify lead placement.

The surgeon determines the battery site and directs the patient's position accordingly. The prone position is used if the battery will be inserted into the subcutaneous tissue of the buttocks. The lateral position is used if the battery is placed in the subcutaneous tissue of the abdomen, or if the patient will be awakened during surgery. The surgical team ensures that the spinal cord stimulator system, the product representative, and the fluoroscopy unit are available, and that the OR bed is compatible with fluoroscopy. The surgeon marks the operative site before the patient is prepped. The surgical prep includes the entire area from the lead placement site to the IPG site.

Operative Procedure
1. The surgeon makes a midline incision at the proper level over the spine and uses sharp and dull dissection through the subcutaneous tissues to reach the fascia.
2. Paravertebral muscles are then dissected off the spinous process and lamina. A self-retaining retractor is placed to provide a visual field.
3. Instruments such as Kerrisons, pituitaries, and rongeurs are then used to perform a surgical laminectomy. The stimulator lead is placed in the epidural space. Proper placement is confirmed by testing with the stimulator programmer while waking and assessing the patient's perception of the stimulation, or while using EMG monitoring. Lead placement is also verified with fluoroscopy or x-ray. Once testing is complete, the surgeon anchors the lead with a 4-0 nonabsorbable suture.
4. The surgeon creates a pocket in the subcutaneous tissue of the buttocks or the abdomen for IPG placement.
5. Using a tunneling device the lead is tunneled from the lead site to the battery location. The IPG is attached. Excess wire is protected by placing it beneath the IPG.
6. The IPG is anchored with 2-0 nonabsorbable suture to prevent migration.
7. Both incisions are irrigated and closed.
8. An abdominal binder is applied to compress the battery site.
9. A postoperative x-ray is obtained to confirm lead placement.

Intrathecal Pump Therapy

An intrathecal pump (ITP) is a specialized device that offers precise, targeted, and adjustable medication treatment for patients with spasticity and/or chronic pain. It delivers medication directly into the CSF via a small catheter attached to a pump.

The pump is controlled via a radio-telemetry link from an external programmer. This controls the rate and mode of infusion. The pump reservoirs are refilled with medication in the physician's office. Baclofen for spasticity or morphine sulfate for pain are most commonly used.

All patients are carefully screened for specific criteria, such as ineffective results or intolerable side effects with oral medication, limited functional abilities, no significant addiction history, and a diagnosed pathology. Contraindications for ITP therapy include active or frequent infections, medication allergy, failed screenings, and lack of patient reliability, resources, or support. ITP complications can include:

◆ Infection
◆ Mechanical failure
◆ CSF leak
◆ Overdose or adverse drug reactions

Each patient undergoes a trial injection that lasts 6 to 8 hours. Positive results must be noted before final implantation. Trials are performed in the physician's office, while final implantation is performed in the OR using MAC or general anesthesia.

Procedural Considerations. The nurse ensures the availability of the intrathecal pump system and the prescribed intrathecal medication before the procedure. A representative from the manufacturer should be present to assist with pump programming. Intraoperative fluoroscopy is used to verify proper placement of the catheter, so a compatible OR bed is necessary. The surgeon will determine the patient's preference for pump placement (right or left abdomen) and mark the abdomen and back incisions. The back incision is typically marked at the area of L3-4. The abdominal incision is marked strategically to avoid the belt line, umbilicus, and the iliac crest. The patient is placed in the lateral position, using pillows and side braces as positioning aids. The surgical prep extends from the posterior incision site to the abdominal pump site.

Operative Procedure

1. The surgeon makes an incision in the patient's back and extends it through the subcutaneous tissue to the fascia. Hemostasis is obtained with the ESU.
2. A Tuohy needle is inserted paraspinally and at a 30-degree angle through the fascia into the intrathecal space, usually at L3-4. The surgeon confirms proper needle placement by removing the inner stylet of the Tuohy needle and visualizing a flow of CSF through the outer cannula.
3. The surgeon threads the catheter through the needle and feeds it to the proper level of the spine. This is determined by the patient's symptoms and the type of medication that will be administered. The catheter placement is verified under fluoroscopic visualization and is secured with anchors and a 4-0 nonabsorbable suture.
4. The abdominal incision is made to create a pocket approximately 2.5 cm deep subcutaneously for pump placement.
5. Using a tunneling device the surgeon tunnels the catheter from the back to the abdominal pocket. The flow of CSF is once again verified through the catheter before it is connected to the pump. The pump is placed in the abdominal pocket and secured with 2-0 nonabsorbable suture to prevent migration.
6. Both the back and abdominal incisions are irrigated and closed.
7. Dressings are applied to both incisions, and an abdominal binder is secured. In the recovery room, the pump is set with the external programmer.

Additional spine techniques are covered in Chapter 11.

PERIPHERAL NERVE SURGERY

Sympathectomy

Sympathectomy is excision of a portion of the sympathetic division of the autonomic nervous system. Most sympathectomies are performed on the paravertebral chain and are named for the region resected, such as cervical, thoracolumbar, and lumbar. The periarterial sympathectomy, vagotomy, and presacral neurectomy are other procedures that are occasionally performed on the autonomic system. The principal diseases treated by sympathectomy are vascular disorders of the extremities, intractable pain from certain nerve injuries, chronic abdominal conditions, and hyperhidrosis (overactivity of sweat glands).

The position of the patient depends on the region to be resected. Basic dissecting instruments and the microscope are used. For retropleural and transthoracic approaches, rib-resecting instruments are added. For the thoracic approach, Beckman or Scoville laminectomy retractors and an assortment of handheld retractors, including malleables, Deavers, and Richardsons, are added. For the abdominal approach, Balfour self-retaining retractors are added.

Cervicothoracic Sympathectomy—Dorsal. Dorsal sympathectomy entails removal of the cervicothoracic chain, often from the fourth cervical to the third thoracic ganglion. Sympathetic denervation of the upper extremities and heart may be accomplished by cervicothoracic sympathectomy. The vasospastic phenomenon of Raynaud's disease is relieved by this procedure. It also may be beneficial in relieving intractable angina pectoris.

PROCEDURAL CONSIDERATIONS. For the anterior approach, both the laminectomy set and rib instruments are used, plus deep retractors and a nerve stimulator. The setup for the posterior approach is the same as that for the anterior approach, plus rib-resecting instruments, periosteal elevators, small rib retractors, a firm rubber pad, and OR bed attachments for the posterolateral position.

OPERATIVE PROCEDURE—ANTERIOR APPROACH

1. The patient is placed in a supine position with the head rotated to the opposite side. General endotracheal anesthesia is necessary because puncturing the pleura is a possibility.
2. A transverse incision is made one fingerbreadth above the clavicle, the clavicular head of the sternocleidomastoid muscle is severed, and the deep cervical fascia is divided.
3. The phrenic nerve and the jugular vein are protected, and the anterior scalene muscle is divided to expose and isolate the underlying subclavian artery. One of its branches, the thyroid axis, is ligated and divided.
4. The stellate ganglion, deep against the vertebral body, is brought into view and lifted on a nerve hook. The sympathetic chain is traced upward to the middle cervical ganglion and divided. Deep dissection behind the pleura exposes the upper thoracic ganglia, which are removed to below the third thoracic ganglion. Clips may be placed on the sympathetic nerves before their division.
5. The wound is closed, and dressings are applied.

OPERATIVE PROCEDURE—POSTERIOR APPROACH

1. The patient is placed in the lateral position, and a paravertebral incision is centered over the third rib. The trapezius muscle is divided, and the rhomboid is split in line with its fibers. The third and fourth ribs are isolated extrapleurally, and the posterior 4 to 5 cm is resected. The transverse processes may be removed to provide better exposure.
2. The sympathetic trunk, which lies on the anterolateral aspect of the vertebral body, is reached by carefully reflecting the pleura. The trunk is picked up on a nerve hook, traced up and down, and removed, usually from the stellate ganglion to the fourth thoracic ganglion. Clips may be applied to the nerve before the fibers are severed.

3. A firm rubber tube may be left in the wound during closure. Suctioning apparatus is applied to this tube as the last deep fascial suture is drawn tight; all air is aspirated, and the tube is quickly withdrawn.

4. The subcutaneous tissue and skin edges are closed.

Nerve Repairs

Peripheral nerve injuries are the most common indication for nerve repair. Nerve tumors are rare in comparison. When the continuity of a nerve is destroyed, function distal to the site of injury is lost. Recovery will occur only if regeneration of nerve axons takes place from the healthy proximal segments. These axons must grow down the axis cylinders of the nerve beyond the injury if they are to reinnervate their end-organs and allow function to return.

When a nerve is divided, the cut ends retract, become scarred, and form neuromas. Regenerating axons from the proximal segment cannot bridge such a gap or penetrate the scar tissue. An unobstructed path down the axis cylinder must be made available if nerves are ever again to move muscles or transmit sensation. All procedures are directed toward obtaining the best possible conditions for regeneration.

Procedural Considerations. A basic dissecting instrument set, microinstruments, a microscope, and a nerve stimulator are used. For lesser procedures such as spinal accessory–facial anastomosis in the neck, division of the volar carpal liga-ment for median nerve compression at the wrist, or repair of a small digital nerve, suitable modification may be made. The positioning, skin prep, and draping of the patient depend on the site of the injury. A large area is prepped.

General anesthesia is usually preferred, with the patient positioned for maximum accessibility to the injured nerve. Exposure must be adequate because considerable mobilization of the nerve is often necessary. A dry field may be achieved using a tourniquet on the involved extremity.

Operative Procedure

1. The site of injury is explored, with careful attention to hemostasis. Nerve ends are dissected from surrounding scar tissue, and neuromas are excised. Moist umbilical tapes, vessel loops, or Penrose tubing may be passed around the nerve to handle it more easily and with less trauma.

2. The nerve repair anastomosis is made with multiple fine sutures placed only through the nerve sheath or epineurium (Figure 12-72). Tension at the suture line is eliminated by maneuvers such as freeing a long length of nerve on either side of the point of injury, transposing the nerve to shorten its course, appropriately positioning the extremity with plaster splinting during the postoperative period, and, rarely, using a nerve graft. Some surgeons apply a cuff of inert material, such as silicone, around the anastomosis.

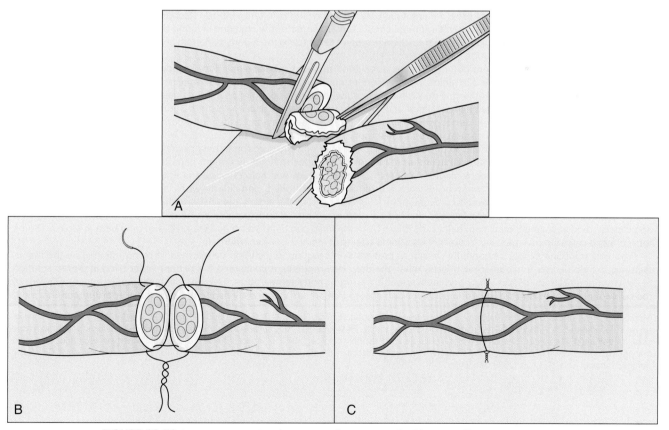

FIGURE 12-72 Nerve repair. **A**, Serial resection of neuroma to healthy nerve fibers. **B**, Placement of sutures in epineurium. **C**, Approximation and tying of sutures.

NEUROSURGERY SUMMARY

Neurosurgery is a complicated and demanding specialty. Surgical technologists who have a desire to challenge themselves to hone their skills to the sharpest possible may find that, once they have put the effort into researching the fine points provided in this chapter, the secret is simply to apply the foundations of quality surgical patient care learned in school to practice. Organization and meticulous attention to detail are qualities that best serve the surgical technologist working in neurosurgery. The efforts spent in researching procedures in advance, reviewing anatomy, keeping abreast of the most current techniques, and daring to enter the room where craniotomies, laminectomies, shunts, and nerve repairs are being done will pay off with the sense of accomplishment and satisfaction of contributing to the success of the entire surgical team.

GERIATRIC CONSIDERATIONS

The Elderly Patient—Neurosurgery

Neurosurgical procedures can be lengthy, requiring special considerations in positioning, preparing the surgical site (prepping) and keeping the aging patient warm. Protection of skin integrity is of utmost importance in all surgical patients. Elderly patients undergo a loss of subcutaneous fat, poor skin turgor, and tissue fragility. They should be lifted into position, rather than slid or dragged, to prevent shearing injuries. Aging changes in the musculoskeletal system accentuate bony prominences and decrease the range of motion. These skeletal changes coupled with limitations imposed by chronic pain make positioning one of the most important considerations of care. The provision of appropriate positioning devices is pivotal to the protection from injury for this population of surgical patients. Arms are placed on padded armboards with the palms up and fingers extended. Armboards are maintained at less than a 90-degree angle to prevent brachial plexus stretch. If there are surgical reasons to tuck the arms at the side, the elbows are padded to protect the ulnar nerve, the palms face inward, and the wrist is maintained in a neutral position (Denholm, 2009). A drape secures the arms. It should be tucked snuggly under the patient, not under the mattress. This prevents the arm from shifting downward intraoperatively and resting against the OR bed rail.

Often, because of musculoskeletal deformity and chronic pain, elderly patients cannot fully extend the spine, neck, or upper and lower extremities. Using padding devices to compensate for these limitations not only makes the patient more comfortable during the procedure but also prevents residual pain or injury postoperatively. Depending on the situation, positioning the patient before anesthesia induction may be best so that the patient can assist their own positioning efforts in regard to comfort.

Aging skin is more susceptible to rashes, infection, and inflammation. A common complaint of the elderly is dry skin that may be part of the natural aging process or can be related to diseases such as anemia, malignancy, kidney disease, or diabetes. Medications, such as corticosteroids, may cause skin to become more fragile. Changes in the dermal receptor cells can alter the ability of the elderly to perceive sensations of pressure and touch, as well as changes in temperature. Decreased muscle tissue and activity, reduced subcutaneous fat, and diminished peripheral circulation are some of the changes in aging that can have a negative impact on thermoregulation (Wold, 2008). The perioperative environment can expose the elderly patient to cool temperatures and hazardous chemicals, thus requiring extra caution.

Temperature fluctuations are common in elders as a result of impaired thermoregulation. Response to cold, including vasoconstriction and shivering, is diminished in elders, and the core temperature must be lower to trigger a response than that required in younger adults. Intraoperative hypothermia may be associated with altered coagulation and increased surgical site bleeding (Rutherford et al, 2008). Other complications associated with hypothermia include vasoconstriction, poor tissue perfusion, and reduced oxygen tension, predisposing the patient to wound infection (Kulaylat and Dayton, 2008). For elderly patients with coronary artery disease, hypothermia may cause increased oxygen consumption, which could lead to myocardial ischemia (Sherwood et al, 2008).

The perioperative team collaborates with the anesthesia provider and the surgeon to ensure measures are in place to minimize the effects of hypothermia. Prevention of hypothermia is critical because the elderly patient generally lacks reserves to withstand prolonged shifts in temperature. Increasing the ambient OR temperature will help stabilize the effects of heat loss. Devices such as warmed blankets or forced-air warming devices are highly recommended, particularly when a lengthy surgical procedure is expected. Special care should be taken to prevent injury, such as burns, to the elderly patient with the use of such devices. When the body is exposed to cold temperatures, blood is shunted away from peripheral body parts to the head. Because the head lacks fat storage capacity and vasoconstriction capabilities, heat loss from the head can be as much as 25% to 60% of total body heat loss. Some form of head covering may be used to prevent additional effects of inadvertent hypothermia.

Prepping solutions should be carefully chosen to prevent skin irritation and should be warmed (if recommended by the manufacturer) to help decrease hypothermic effects. When the prep is completed, it is ensured the patient is not lying in a prep solution or on wet linens to reduce skin injury and inadvertent lowering of body temperature. The surgical technologist must be aware of the consequences of using cold irrigation solutions and ensure that any irrigation provided to the surgeon is appropriately warmed.

Modified from Denholm B: Tucking patient's arms and general positioning, *AORN J* 89(4):755–757, 2009; Kulaylat MN, Dayton MT: Surgical complications. In Townsend CM, editor: *Sabiston textbook of surgery*, ed 18, Philadelphia, 2008, Saunders; Rutherford EJ et al: Hematologic principles in surgery. In Townsend CM, editor: *Sabiston textbook of surgery*, ed 18, Philadelphia, 2008, Saunders; Sherwood ER et al: Anesthesiology principles, pain management, and conscious sedation. In Townsend CM, editor: *Sabiston textbook of surgery*, ed 18, Philadelphia, 2008, Saunders; Wold GH: *Basic geriatric nursing*, ed 4, St Louis, 2008, Mosby.

REVIEW QUESTIONS

1. What is the name of the neurosurgical dissectors numbered 1 through 5?
   a. Hudson
   b. Penfield
   c. Cushing
   d. Kittner

2. Which of the following is a commonly used three-pin cranial fixation device?
   a. Cloward
   b. Greenberg
   c. Layla
   d. Mayfield

3. Which of the following instruments has a pistol-grip–type shape and is used to dissect bone for access in laminectomy procedures?
   a. Bayonet
   b. Kerrison
   c. Myerding
   d. Taylor

4. Which of the following terms describes the removal of the large anterior portion of a vertebra during spinal decompression and fusion?
   a. corpectomy
   b. hypophysectomy
   c. diskectomy
   d. sympathectomy

5. Which of the following congenital anomalies is characterized by protrusion of meninges, spinal nerves, and CSF due to failure of neural tube closure?
   a. anencephaly
   b. hydrocephalus
   c. myelomeningocele
   d. spina bifida occulta

6. Which of the following are frequently used for mechanical hemostasis on incised scalp edges during cranial procedures?
   a. Filshie clips
   b. hemoclips
   c. ligaclips
   d. Raney clips

7. Which of the following surgical approaches is used for access to the structures of the sella turcica and may be combined with assistance from an otorhinolaryngologist?
   a. frontoparietal
   b. suboccipital
   c. bifrontal
   d. transsphenoidal

8. Which of the following is/are being assessed intracranially with use of an ICP monitor?
   a. pressure
   b. patterns
   c. pulsations
   d. placement

9. Expanding intracranial lesions such as epidural hematomas may cause brain herniation through which of the following structures?
   a. corpus callosum
   b. foramen magnum
   c. sella turcica
   d. superior sagittal sinus

10. Which of the following diagnostic studies does *not* require use of ionizing radiation?
    a. CT scan
    b. myelogram
    c. MRI
    d. arteriogram

11. Which of the following intracranial structures produces cerebrospinal fluid (CSF)?
    a. circle of Willis
    b. basal ganglia
    c. sylvian fissure
    d. choroid plexus

12. Giantism and dwarfism are conditions related to disorders of which of the following?
    a. cranial nerves
    b. pituitary gland
    c. medulla oblongata
    d. sylvian fissure

13. Which of the following is a *noninvasive* treatment for some intracranial lesions?
    a. gamma knife
    b. stereotactic biopsy
    c. endovascular coiling
    d. transsphenoidal endoscopy

14. Into which two structures is a VP shunt system placed?
    a. lateral ventricle and pleural cavity
    b. third ventricle and pulmonary vein
    c. lateral ventricle and peritoneal cavity
    d. third ventricle and posterior fossa

15. Which of the following thermal methods of hemostasis is most commonly used for intracranial surgical procedures?
    a. CO_2 laser
    b. bipolar ESU
    c. monopolar ESU
    d. ultrasonic scalpel

16. Which of the following positions may require placement of a catheter in the right atrium of the heart to remove an air embolism during craniectomy?
    a. lateral
    b. prone
    c. supine
    d. sitting

17. Which of the following is a bone replacement material created by mixing powder and liquid, creating an exothermic response?
    a. bone wax
    b. methylmethacrylate
    c. topical thrombin
    d. microfibrillar collagen

18. How would a subdural hematoma most likely be caused?
    a. tearing of bridging dural veins
    b. laceration of the middle meningeal artery
    c. rupture of the posterior communicating artery
    d. penetration of the superior sagittal sinus

19. Carpal tunnel syndrome involves compression of which of the following peripheral nerves?
    a. thoracodorsal
    b. peroneal
    c. median
    d. ulnar

20. Which of the following is a fatal congenital anomaly characterized by lack of cranial formation and neural tube closure?
    a. hydrocephalus
    b. craniosynostosis
    c. anencephaly
    d. myelomeningocele

21. Define and briefly describe the following surgical procedures:
    Craniotomy
    Cranioplasty
    Laminectomy

Critical Thinking Question

A 41-year-old female patient is scheduled for a craniotomy for clipping of aneurysm. The approach will be right peritoneal for access to the right middle cerebral artery where the aneurysm is located. The patient has been anesthetized in the supine position and the surgeon has requested cranial stabilization. For cranial fixation and stabilization, which devices would likely be used? What is done with the hair that has been clipped and collected from the patient's head? The surgeon and assistant use digital pressure to help reduce blood loss during the initial incision. What might the surgical technologist anticipate providing during digital pressure? What else might the surgical technologist anticipate as the skin incision is extended into the temporal area?

REFERENCES

Al-Mefty O, Heth J: Meningiomas. In Rengachary SS, Ellenbogen RG, editors: *Principles of neurosurgery*, ed 2, St Louis, 2005, Mosby.

American Association of Neurological Surgeons (AANS): Endovascular surgery, available at www.neurosurgerytoday.org/what/fact/endo_vascular.pdf. Accessed May 1, 2009.

American Association of Neurological Surgeons (AANS): Traumatic brain injury, available at www.aans.org/Patient%20Information/Conditions%20and%20Treatments/Traumatic%20Brain%20Injury.aspx. Accessed August 28, 2010.

American Cancer Society (ACS): *Cancer facts and figures 2009*, Atlanta, 2009, American Cancer Society.

Batjer HH et al: Intracranial aneurysm. In Rengachary SS, Ellenbogen RG, editors: *Principles of neurosurgery*, ed 2, St Louis, 2005, Mosby.

Centers for Disease Control and Prevention: Get the stats on traumatic brain injury in the United States, available at www.cdc.gov/traumaticbraininjury/pdf/BlueBook_factsheet-a.pdf. Accessed August 29, 2010.

Centers for Disease Control and Prevention—National Center on Birth Defects and Developmental Disabilities (CDC-NCBDDD): Anencephaly, available at www.cdc.gov/ncbddd/birthdefects/anencephaly.htm. Accessed August 29, 2010.

Centers for Disease Control and Prevention—National Center on Birth Defects and Developmental Disabilities (CDC-NCBDDD): Encephalocele, available at www.cdc.gov/ncbddd/birthdefects/Encephalocele.htm. Accessed August 28, 2010.

Centers for Disease Control and Prevention—National Center on Birth Defects and Developmental Disabilities (CDC-NCBDDD): Medical progress in the Prevention of Neural Tube Defects, available at www.cdc.gov/ncbddd/bd/mp.htm. Accessed August 28, 2010.

Central Brain Tumor Registry of the United States (CBTRUS): Statistical report: primary brain tumors in the United States, 2007-2008, available at www.cbtrus.org/reports//2007-2008/2007report.pdf. Accessed June 20, 2009.

Connolly ES et al: *Fundamentals of operative techniques in neurosurgery*, ed 2, New York, 2009, Thieme.

Denholm B: Tucking patient's arms and general positioning, *AORN J* 89(4):755–757, 2009.

Doherty GM, Way LW: *Current surgical diagnosis and treatment*, ed 12, Columbus, 2006, McGraw-Hill.

Donthineni R: Diagnosis and staging of spine tumors, *Orthop Clin North Am* 40:1–7, 2009.

Greenberg MS: *Handbook of neurosurgery*, ed 6, New York, 2005, Thieme.

Harrop JS: Intradural spinal neoplasms. In Vaccaro AR, editor: *Spine core knowledge in orthopaedics*, St Louis, 2005, Mosby.

Khatri R et al: Interventional neuroimaging, *Neurol Clin* 27:109–137, 2008.

MayoClinic.com: Spinal cord injury—causes, available at www.mayoclinic.com/health/spinal-cord-injury/DS00460/DSECTION=causes. Accessed August 29, 2010.

MayoClinic.com: Spinal cord injury—symptoms, available at www.mayoclinic.com/health/spinal-cord-injury/DS00460/DSECTION=symptoms. Accessed August 29, 2010.

MayoClinic.com: Spinal cord injury—treatment and drugs, available at www.mayoclinic.com/health/spinal-cord-injury/DS00460/DSECTION=treatments-and-drugs. Accessed August 29, 2010.

McCutcheon IE: Metastatic brain tumors. In Rengachary SS, Ellenbogen RG, editors: *Principles of neurosurgery*, ed 2, St Louis, 2005, Mosby.

MedlinePlus: U.S. National Library of Medicine and the National Institutes of Health: Kernicterus, available at www.nlm.nih.gov/medlineplus/ency/article/007309.htm. Accessed August 27, 2010.

Mendel E et al: Injuries to the cervical spine. In Vaccaro AR, editor: *Spine core knowledge in orthopaedics*, St Louis, 2005, Mosby.

Meyers PM et al: Indications for the performance of intracranial endovascular neurointerventional procedures, a scientific statement, *Circulation* 119:2235–2239, 2009, available at http://circ.ahajournals.org/cgi/reprint/CIRCULATIONAHA.109.192217. Accessed May 1, 2009.

National Cancer Institute (NCI): Adult brain tumors treatment, available at www.cancer.gov/cancertopics/pdq/treatment/adultbrain/HealthProfessional/page3. Accessed June 20, 2009.

National Institute of Neurological Disorders and Stroke (NINDS): NINDS Anencephaly, 2010, available at www.ninds.nih.gov/disorders/anencephaly/anencephaly.htm. Accessed August 28, 2010.

National Institute of Neurological Disorders and Stroke (NINDS): NINDS arteriovenous malformation information page, 2009, available at www.ninds.nih.gov/disorders/avms/avms.htm. Accessed April 14, 2009.

Oyesiku NM: Nonfunctioning pituitary adenomas. In Rengachary SS, Ellenbogen RG, editors: *Principles of neurosurgery*, ed 2, St Louis, 2005, Mosby.

Pagana KD, Pagana TJ: *Mosby's diagnostic and laboratory test reference*, ed 9, St Louis, 2009, Mosby.

Pollock BE, Brown PD: Stereotactic radiosurgery. In Rengachary SS, Ellenbogen RG, editors: *Principles of neurosurgery*, ed 2, St Louis, 2005, Mosby.

Rajshekhar V: Surgical management of neurocysticercosis, *Int J Surg*; 8(2):100–104, 2010. Epub 2010 Jan 4, available at www.ncbi.nlm.nih.gov/pubmed/20045747. Accessed August 27, 2010.

Schumacher HC, Marshall RS: Arteriovenous malformations: treatment & medication, emedicine, 2006, available at http://emedicine.medscape.com/article/1160167-treatment. Accessed April 14, 2009.

Singh K et al: Intradiscal therapy: a review of current treatment modalities, *Spine* 30(17s):s20–s26, 2005.

Sloan AE et al: Gliomas. In Rengachary SS, Ellenbogen RG, editors: *Principles of neurosurgery*, ed 2, St Louis, 2005, Mosby.

Teo C, Mobbs R: Neuroendoscopy. In Rengachary SS, Ellenbogen RG, editors: *Principles of neurosurgery*, ed 2, St Louis, 2005, Mosby.

Wang P, Avellino AM: Hydrocephalus in children. In Rengachary SS, Ellenbogen RG, editors: *Principles of neurosurgery*, ed 2, St Louis, 2005, Mosby.

Whiten C, Gunning P: Carotid endarterectomy: intraoperative monitoring of cerebral perfusion, *Curr Anaesth Crit Care* 20:42–45, 2009.

Zonenshayn M, Rezai A: Stereotactic surgery. In Rengachary SS, Ellenbogen RG, editors: *Principles of neurosurgery*, ed 2, St Louis, 2005, Mosby.

Plastic and Reconstructive Surgery

Overview

Derived from the Greek word *plastikos*, which means to mold or give form, plastic surgery is a medical specialty that restores or gives shape to the body. There are two different subspecialties of plastic surgery. *Cosmetic surgery* restores or reshapes normal structures of the body, to improve appearance and self-esteem. *Reconstructive surgery* treats abnormal structures of the body caused by birth defects, developmental problems, disease,

tumors, infection, or injury to restore function and correct disfigurement or scarring (American Society of Plastic Surgeons [ASPS], 2009a.) As a surgical specialty, plastic surgery owes much of its heritage to knowledge gained from the wars of the twentieth century (History box).

Despite the economic downturn, 12.1 million cosmetic surgical procedures were performed [by surgeons certified by the American Society of Plastic Surgeons (ASPS)] in 2008, an increase of 3%; the majority were minimally invasive procedures. Females constituted 91% of all patients undergoing cosmetic procedures. Hispanic, Asian, and African American patients showed an increase in cosmetic procedures; the number of Caucasians undergoing cosmetic procedures decreased by 2%. Office-based cosmetic procedures increased by 13%, with a total of $10.3 billion dollars spent on the cosmetic procedures in the United States (Ambulatory Surgery Considerations). The 4.9 million reconstructive procedures also showed a 3% increase, although breast reductions decreased by 16% (ASPS Stats, 2009).

This chapter was originally written by Victoria Dreger, MSN, RN, MA, CNOR, for the 14th edition of Alexander's Care of the Patient in Surgery and has been revised by Jeff Feix, LVN, CST/CSFA, FAST, for this text.

Surgical Anatomy

Plastic and reconstructive surgery is not limited to a single anatomic or biologic system. It is based on thorough understanding of the anatomy and biology of tissue. Operative techniques are complex and staged to achieve the expected results. The surgery also involves removing, reducing, enlarging, and recontouring, as well as camouflaging scars into existing skin lines (Figure 13-1). The tissues of the body can be transferred to use as various types of flaps. Free flaps are the transfer of tissue along with its vascular pedicle. When nerve is anastomosed with these flaps, they are called neurovascular free flaps. Flaps are used to cover defects or create new structures such as breasts, digits, or facial structures. Body parts can also be transplanted. By improving the patient's deformity, the patient's self-esteem will improve and the patient will feel more comfortable in public and social activities. The body changes as we age. The patient's concern with aesthetics, the variety of acquired defects, the diversity of operative techniques, and the psychologic responses of patients offer unique learning experiences and challenges for perioperative patient care.

Surgical Technologist Considerations

Preparation of the OR Suite. Assemble all necessary medical and surgical supplies, equipment, suture material, positioning aids, implantable devices, and medications. Ensure that lights and video equipment are in working order, that emergency supplies are present, and that compressed gases are adequate. Depending on the procedure to be performed, the OR bed may need to be configured differently from the standard room setup. Plastic and reconstructive surgeons frequently use preoperative photographs of the patient when attempting to restore or modify appearance. These photographs help the surgeon maintain perspective since features may change because of surgical positioning. Preoperative and postoperative photos, in order to be accurate, should be taken with the same lighting, angle, and distance (Hagan, 2008).

Equipment and Special Mechanical Devices. Essential equipment for any OR includes a fully functional bed that may be positioned for any number of special needs and also has accessory attachments, such as headrests and aids for extremity positioning. The room must also have well-positioned and numerous electrical outlets, good overhead lighting, suction equipment, mounted x-ray view boxes, and computer terminals for those facilities using electronic medical records. Step stools, tables, chairs, hand tables, tourniquets, microscopes, and intravenous (IV) poles should be in appropriate supply and accessible. Surgeons often provide their own digital cameras although facilities may have them available for use.

INSTRUMENTATION. Basic instrument trays are available for the plastic surgery OR. A "local" tray may include Bishop Harmon and Adson tissue forceps (with and without teeth); straight and curved iris, Stevens, and Metzenbaum scissors; fine mosquito forceps; and skin hooks. Minor and major trays for plastic surgery may contain a range of tissue forceps, scissors, hemostats, and retractors. With the addition of instruments for specific surgeries, these trays usually suffice for all plastic surgery operations. Adequate instrumentation should be available to avoid flash sterilization (Risk Reduction Strategies).

HISTORY

Origins and Growth of Plastic Surgery

Historically, battlefield combat has been an impetus for the development of new medical and surgical techniques based on the injuries sustained. As battlefield technology and the weapons of war became more sophisticated throughout history, the degree of injury and tissue devastation became more horrific. The trench warfare of World Wars I and II gave rise to a whole new category of facial injuries. Helmets protected combatant's skulls and the trenches offered some protection to the chest, but the face was exposed, and as a result, devastating burns and fractures of the face occurred. Special hospitals were created to address these problems, and even before the United States joined the first World War, the Harvard unit sent 35 physicians and surgeons, 3 dentists, and 75 nurses from various medical centers to assist in caring for the wounded. These visionaries were soon developing new techniques and procedures to correct the disfiguring injuries. They were credited as being the first generation of modern plastic surgeons, and helped give much needed respect to the specialty.

While World War I helped reinvent plastic surgery, the specialty has been identified as long ago as 600 BC, when a Hindu surgeon described using a cheek flap to reconstruct a nose. Another flap technique, this time using the forehead to reconstruct a severed nose, was performed around 1000 AD in India. The Italian surgeon Gaspare Tagliacozzi, also known as the "father of plastic surgery," developed still another flap surgery using the upper arm to reconstruct a nose. History tells us that the condition of the nose, whether from war, punishment, or social disease (syphilis), presented a story that often was undesirable. This resulted in impetus in the different societies to camouflage the injuries, thus propelling advances in plastic surgery.

Following the end of the first World War, plastic surgery turned its attention to the rest of society, and concentrated on deformities caused by birth or trauma. Soon, some surgeons began using their talents to improve less than desirable facial features. For example, Fanny Brice underwent a rhinoplasty in her apartment in 1923 to change the appearance of her nose from "prominent to decorative." In 1924 a New York newspaper had a contest to transform the city's homeliest woman into a beauty. Dr. John Howard Crum performed the first facelift on record in the Grand Ballroom of the Pennsylvania Hotel in New York City in 1931, during which "a pianist accompanied him with appropriate popular tunes, flashbulbs popped, and men and women fainted."

Modified from Feldman E: Before & after: cosmetic surgery was born 2,500 years ago and came of age in the inferno of the western front, *Am Herit* 55(1):60-70, 2004; *The history of plastic surgery: the early years,* available at www.plasticsurgery.org/About_ASPS/History_of_Plastic_Surgery. html. Accessed July 6, 2009.

AMBULATORY SURGERY CONSIDERATIONS

Patient Choices in Facility

There has been a dramatic shift toward encouraging patients to be more involved and informed in all of their healthcare decisions. Many organizations are focusing on active participation of patients in their own care. One aspect of this is choosing the outpatient facility for their plastic surgery. In keeping with this trend, the American Society of Plastic Surgeons (ASPS) has developed a brochure, with an excerpt available on-line, to help patients choose a facility. The brochure includes the following information:

◆ *Types of facilities*: For ambulatory (discharge same day as surgery) procedures, the facility may be part of the surgeon's office, a surgical suite adjacent to the office, a free-standing facility, or part of a hospital.

◆ *Choice and benefits*: Some patients prefer no overnight stay at a hospital. Cost savings and convenience along with added privacy and personalized care may all be factors.

◆ *Accreditation*: As a result of the strict guidelines for equipment, staff, anesthesia services, and hospital access, patients are encouraged to determine if a facility is accredited, as it could indicate the quality of the facility. (All ASPS member surgeons are required to operate in an accredited medical facility.)

◆ *Insurance*: The accreditation mentioned above also impacts financial aspects. Although facility fees are typically not covered by insurance providers for elective procedures, facility fees for reconstructive procedures may be covered. Reimbursement may be expedited for facilities that carry accreditation because the accreditation ensures that certain quality standards are met at that facility. Also, similar services at a hospital generally cost more than in an ambulatory facility.

◆ *Individual considerations*: Each patient must discuss the options with his/her surgeon. Depending on medical history and condition requiring surgery, ambulatory surgery may not be appropriate for everyone.

Modified from American Society of Plastic Surgeons: *Ambulatory facilities: same day facilities: choosing same day surgery facilities*, Arlington Heights, Ill, 2008, available at www.plasticsurgery.org/Patients_and_Consumers/Planning_Your_Surgery/Same_Day_Surgery_Facilities.html. Accessed June 17, 2009.

DERMATOMES. Dermatomes are used for removing split-thickness skin grafts (STSGs) from donor sites; they are of three basic types: knife, drum, and motor-driven (Figures 13-2 through 13-5). Sterile mineral oil and a tongue blade should be available when STSGs are being obtained.

SKIN MESHERS. Several types of skin meshers are available. Each is designed to produce multiple uniform slits in a skin graft, approximately 0.05 inch apart. These multiple apertures in the graft can then expand, permitting the skin graft to stretch and cover a larger area. Meshing also facilitates drainage through the graft, preventing fluid accumulation under a graft. The graft is placed on the carrier and passed through the mesher (Figures 13-6 and 13-7). The manufacturer supplies sterile carriers for meshers. They are usually available in several sizes, which determine the expansion ratio of the skin graft.

PNEUMATIC-POWERED INSTRUMENTS. Pneumatic-powered instruments use an inert, nonflammable, and explosion-free compressed gas as their power source. The motor may be activated by a foot pedal or hand control. The various

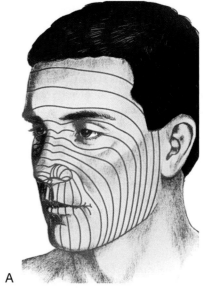

A

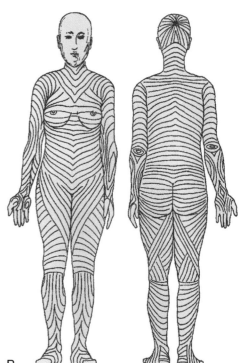

B

FIGURE 13-1 The surgeon adheres to several principles when planning skin incisions, one of which is to reduce the amount of tension across the wound, thus minimizing scarring. Elective incisions should preferably parallel relaxed skin tension lines (RSTLs) in the face (**A**) and the body (**B**).

attachments should be sterilized as recommended by the manufacturer to prolong instrument life and ensure effective sterilization. The following attachments may be used in plastic surgery:

◆ Wire driver and bone drill
◆ Oscillating saw
◆ Derma-Tattoo (used with reciprocating-saw handpiece)
◆ Reciprocating saw
◆ Dermabrader
◆ Sagittal saw

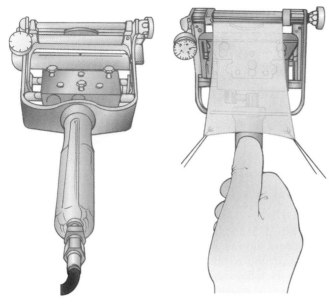

FIGURE 13-2 Powered Brown dermatome.

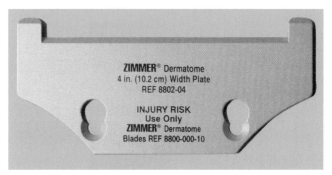

FIGURE 13-4 Blade of Zimmer electric air dermatome.

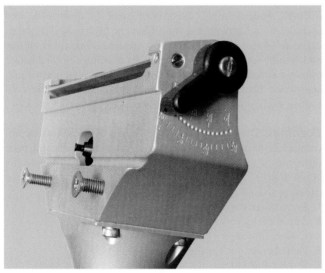

FIGURE 13-3 Head of Zimmer electric air dermatome.

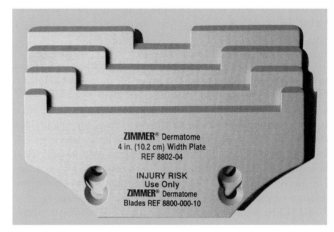

FIGURE 13-5 Four sizes of blades of Zimmer electric air dermatome.

A pneumatic tourniquet with an inflatable cuff is used in most hand surgery procedures as well as in other upper and lower extremity surgical interventions. The tourniquet is described in Chapter 10.

ELECTROSURGICAL UNIT. The electrosurgical unit (ESU) is employed and safety precautions should be followed. Monopolar ESU will require the use of a grounding pad (return electrode/dispersive electrode). Specialized tips will be used with the ESU pencil including needle point and guarded along with the standard tip. The use of specialized tips allows the use of higher coagulation settings to obtain hemostasis with little or no effect on adjacent tissue or structures. Inspect ESU tip and cord on handpiece for damage before use, be sure tip is securely seated into the place handpiece in nonconductive holster when not in use, keep tip free of eschar or tissue build-up. Methods to do so include moistened sponge, instrument wipe, and abrasive electrode cleaner, but *not* a scalpel blade.

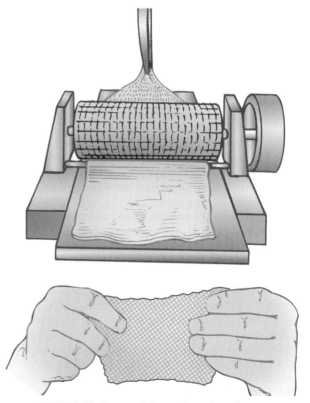

FIGURE 13-6 Manual skin graft meshing device.

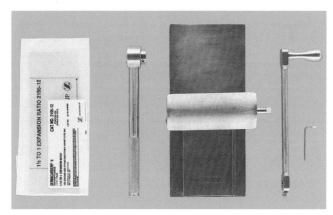

FIGURE 13-7 Mesh graft dermatome (skin expander) with derma-carrier (*left,* in package).

BIPOLAR COAGULATION UNIT. Bipolar electrosurgery is the use of electrical current in which the circuit is completed by means of two parallel poles located close to one another. One pole is positive; the other is negative. The flow of current is restricted between these two poles, which are usually the tines of the bipolar forceps. Because the poles are so close, low voltages are used to achieve the tissue effect. Because electrical current does not flow through the patient, a return electrode (dispersive pad) is not necessary. This makes bipolar electrosurgery very safe and permits precise electrocoagulation.

LASERS. A variety of lasers are employed for plastic surgical procedures. The perioperative team must ensure that the laser safety accessories specific to the type of laser being used are available. Types of lasers and their common uses are presented in Box 13-3, pp. 637-639.

FIBEROPTIC INSTRUMENTS. Examples of fiberoptic instrument attachments used in plastic surgery are a headlight for rhinoplasties, augmentation mammoplasties, and other procedures; a mammary retractor for augmentation mammoplasties; a rhytidectomy retractor; abdominoplasty retractors; and endoscopic face and forehead fiberoptic instrumentation.

LOUPES. Loupes (Figure 13-8) are magnifying lenses used by many plastic surgeons for microvascular surgery and nerve repairs and for numerous other instances in which cosmetic results are improved by the magnification effect. The nurse should inquire about the use of loupes before the surgeon dons a headlight because adjustments will need to be made to the headlight alignment if the loupes are required in midprocedure. Adjusting or removing the headlight in midprocedure has the potential to contaminate the sterile field.

MICROSCOPE. The microscope is frequently used in nerve repairs and microsurgical anastomoses; the nerves or vessels to be repaired, such as in hand surgery, and the suture used to do so (sometimes 9-0, 10-0, or even 11-0 size) can be finer than human hair and thus requires magnification. While each microscope has different features, an important matter to avoid confusion is whether the surgeon control overrides the assistant view, or if each can separately adjust the field of view.

WOOD'S LAMP. The Wood's lamp is an ultraviolet lamp used in a darkened room to determine the viability of skin flaps. After IV injection of fluorescein, the blood vessels appear bright purple (the skin appears yellow). Sodium fluorescein is excreted in the urine, and patients should be informed of this.

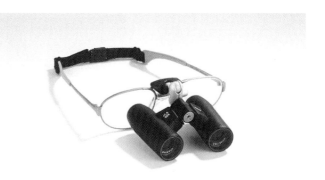

FIGURE 13-8 Loupes from Carl Zeiss, used for magnification.

SPECIAL SUPPLIES. Surgeon-specific and procedure-specific special supplies are frequently added to instrument setups for plastic and reconstructive procedures. These commonly include the following: sterile marking pen or methylene blue; ruler; local anesthetic of choice for injection, with syringes and needles; and ESU, with active electrode (pencil) and tip of choice, with tip cleaner.

Sutures. Sutures range from permanent to absorbable and include monofilament and multifilament materials. The surgical technologist should be a good steward of costly resources and should verify the type and number of sutures needed before opening suture packages, as well as needle preference, to prevent waste. Many plastic surgical procedures have multiple techniques, each of which necessitates very specific suture choices.

Dressings. Dressings are an essential part of the operative procedure in plastic surgery and may contribute to the ultimate outcome of the surgical intervention. Dressings are usually applied while the patient is still anesthetized. In general, the dressing should accomplish the following five goals:
1. Immobilize the surgical part.
2. Apply even pressure over the wound.
3. Collect drainage.
4. Provide comfort for the patient.
5. Protect the wound.

Pressure dressings may be used to eliminate dead space, to prevent seroma and hematoma formation, and to prevent third spacing associated with liposuction and reconstructive procedures involving transfer of large muscle or tissue flaps. In some cases pressure can be achieved by the use of catheters or drains placed within the operative site and connected to closed-wound suction devices, such as a Hemovac or Jackson-Pratt. In smaller wounds a butterfly cannula may be inserted into the operative site, with the needle end placed into a red-top tube, such as a blood collection tube, that has a vacuum (evacuated tube).

Common general dressings and supplies available in sterile form and various sizes:
◆ Nonadherent gauze (e.g., Betadine gauze, Adaptic, Nu Gauze, Xeroform, Biobrane, Scarlet Red)
◆ Petrolatum gauze, ½ inch (or other packing material, such as Merocel sponge for nasal packing)
◆ Telfa
◆ Fine mesh gauze
◆ Interface
◆ Gauze dressing sponges, 4 × 4 inches, 2 × 2 inches

- Kling, Kerlix fluff, and Kerlix gauze rolls (2, 4, and 6 inches wide)
- Abdominal pads (most commonly used are 5 × 8 inches)
- Cotton sheets and balls
- Webril
- Tape (paper; silk; and foam; skin tapes, flesh-colored and regular [⅛, ¼, ½, and 1 inch wide])
- Benzoin spray or swab or Mastoplast
- Ace bandages
- Coban
- Casting supplies and splints (as required for postoperative immobilization)
- Abdominal binders and other postoperative garments
- Slings

In some instances, such as a free flap, transparent dressings are used so that the flap can be monitored and observed for vascular flow. Compression garments and support devices are also frequently used by plastic surgeons. Proper fit is essential to minimize vascular compromise. Compression garments are typically applied over a light dressing. A proper garment is selected based on its characteristics (e.g., fabric, stretch, softness, antimicrobial properties) and proper sizing according to measurement instructions. Educating patients of the needs and benefits of compression garment use as well as providing hints for their proper application (avoid ripping with long nails, instructions on how to don the garment) promotes comfort and compliance (Gladfelter, 2007).

Implant Materials. The range of materials available for implantation and augmentation in the specialty of plastic and reconstructive surgery has benefited from ongoing research. The perioperative team is responsible for complying with tracking regulations for implantable materials and devices (Patient Safety).

Biologic materials (autogenous grafts) are preferred when available. Autologous human tissue successfully utilized includes fat, solid dermis, and collagen. Human cadavers are used as a source for acellular collagen (AlloDerm) (Figure 13-9). This product is available in various sizes of sheeting and must be rehydrated in several steps. AlloDerm integrates with the body's tissue and helps to prevent rejection over the long term.

Implant failure may be directly linked to bacterial contamination; therefore meticulous aseptic technique with minimal handling is essential when using implants of any sort. Most alloplastic implants are presterilized from the manufacturer.

Anesthesia. A variety of anesthesia techniques are employed with plastic surgery procedures. Local, regional, tumescent, conscious sedation, deep sedation, and general anesthesia may be used, depending on the type of procedure, the patient's anesthetic history, the American Society of Anesthesiologists (ASA) physical status classification, and the surgeon's preference.

PATIENT SAFETY

Tracking Medical Devices

A variety of implantable devices are used in aesthetic and reconstructive plastic surgery procedures. Tracking of these devices is critical to patient safety. The manufacturer of the device must have a mechanism to locate implantables after they have been distributed. Devices may be recalled for sterility issues, malfunction, or any event that is found to pose a serious health risk.

The U.S. Food and Drug Administration (FDA) regulates the process of tracking medical devices and directs the tracking of devices whose failure would result in serious, adverse health consequences; devices that are intended to be implanted in the human body for more than 1 year; and devices that are life-sustaining and life-supporting and are used outside of a facility such as a hospital, nursing home, or ambulatory surgery center.

The perioperative team plays an important role in the accurate documentation of implantable devices for tracking purposes. Information that is typically gathered for tracking purposes includes:

- Device identification (i.e., lot, batch, model number, serial number)
- Date of device manufacture and shipping
- Name, address, telephone number, and social security number of the patient who received the device
- Location the device was implanted
- Name, address, and telephone number of the physician who is caring for the patient, if different from the prescribing physician

If an implantable device is sterilized within the sterile processing department of the facility, monitoring requirements include the use of a process challenge device containing a biologic indicator. The load should be quarantined until the result of the biologic indicator is determined. Documentation should include a record of the sterilizer load identification number on the patient's medical record, or the patient's name on the load record. Lot identification provides a method for tracing problems in the event of a recall. Flash sterilization of implantable devices is not recommended.

Patients have the right to refuse tracking of their devices and may refuse to have their social security number used for tracking. The patient's consent for tracking should be obtained before the procedure. If the patient refuses to have the device tracked, the nurse will document the refusal along with the required product information and report these data to the manufacturer.

Under the Safe Medical Device Act, institutions must also report any incident of death or serious injury relating to the use of a medical device. The FDA has classified and identified more than 1700 different devices that must be reported if the device is suspected of causing serious injury or death to an individual. Surgical technologists and nurses should work within their institutional policies to report these incidents.

Modified from Association for the Advancement of Medical Instrumentation: *Comprehensive guide to steam sterilization and sterility assurance in health care facilities*, Arlington, Va, 2006, AAMI; Chard R: Clinical issues, *AORN J* 90(1):117, 2009; Denholm B, Downing D: Clinical issues, *AORN J* 87(2):432-434, 2008; U.S. Food and Drug Administration: *Medical device tracking, guidance for industry and FDA staff*, available at www.fda.gov/cdrh/comp/guidance/169.html. Accessed July 6, 2009; U.S. Food and Drug Administration: *Medical device reporting*, available at www.fda.gov/cdrh/devadvice/351.html. Accessed July 6, 2009.

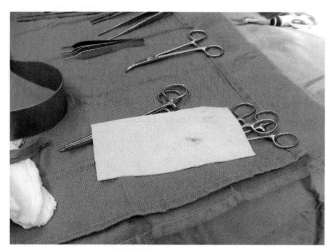

FIGURE 13-9 AlloDerm.

Preoperative Skin Preparation. Most surgical interventions require that the operative site and adjacent areas be cleansed before surgery. The physician may prescribe that the patient carry out this treatment before surgery. Special attention is given to the fingernails for patients undergoing hand surgery; to hair for surgery of the head, face, or neck; and to oral hygiene for surgery in or near the mouth. Shaving is avoided and clippers, not a razor, are used if needed, because shaving creates an access for the entry of bacteria into the operative site (Health Stream, 2007). The eyebrows and eyelashes, in particular, are left intact to preserve facial appearance and expression. The surgical site is marked before surgery by the surgeon to designate the correct site and to define landmark areas. Either a povidone-iodine solution, an iodine-alcohol mixture, chlorhexidine gluconate (CHG), or another broad-spectrum agent may be selected for the antimicrobial skin prep. The use of CHG should be avoided around the ears and eyes. It is important to place shields on the eyes if prepping the periorbital site or performing an extensive head and neck prep, place plugs in the ear canals, and prevent pooling of the prep agent. When prepping for a skin graft procedure, separate skin prep setups are needed for the graft and donor sites.

Positioning and Draping. The OR bed must be positioned so that the remaining space in the room can comfortably accommodate anesthetic equipment, members of the surgical team, instrument tables, and any adjunct equipment (hand table, drills, microscope, laser) to be used. The patient is carefully positioned on the OR bed so that all operative sites may

SURGICAL TECHNOLOGY PREFERENCE CARD

Plastic and reconstructive surgery patients will range from infant to adult and include corrections for birth defects, trauma, burns, cancers, and cosmetic reasons.

Planning with the perioperative team is essential in plastic and reconstructive surgery with a wide variety of surgical procedures and patient populations. Specialty supplies, instruments, and prostheses will be used, frequently requiring strict sterile technique and efficient room layout. Allowing additional time preoperatively to organize the room and check the availability of supplies and prostheses provide for efficient communication between the circulator and scrub during the procedure. Additional setups for some procedures may be needed, so additional furniture and equipment should be organized to ensure sterility and no mixing of instruments.

Room Prep: Basic operating room furniture in place, thermoregulatory devices, padding, positioning supplies, ESU, and in some cases laser or a microscope

Prep Solution: In room and may require more than one site prepped

◆ Chlorhexidine gluconate (CHG)
◆ Povidone-iodine solution
◆ Iodine alcohol solution

Catheter: In the room and correct size for patient

◆ Catheter set and tray
  • Latex/rubber
  • Silicone
  • PVC
◆ Sizing
  • French
◆ Nonretaining
  • Red rubber
◆ Retaining
  • Foley
    • 2-way

PROCEDURE CHECKLIST

Instruments

◆ Standard plastic instruments
◆ Skin grafting instrumentation
◆ Orthopedic and debridement instrumentation
◆ Microscopic instrumentation
◆ Anticipated additional instruments

Specialty Suture

◆ As per surgeon's preference

SURGICAL TECHNOLOGY PREFERENCE CARD—cont'd

Hemostatic Agents
- Mechanical
  - Staplers
  - Clip appliers and clips
  - Pressure
  - Ligatures
- Chemical
  - Epinephrine
  - Thrombin
- Thermal
  - Electrosurgical unit
    - Monopolar
    - Bipolar
  - Laser

Specialty Supplies
- Prostheses
- Vessel loops
- Microscopic sponges
- Irrigation/aspiration unit
- Skin grafting supplies

Additional Supplies: both sterile and nonsterile
- If the physician is requesting supplies, instruments, or equipment not normally used, check to be sure all have arrived to the room before opening any sterile supplies
- Sponges
- Drapes
- Gowns and gloves for team members
- "Have available" supplies

Medications and Irrigation Solutions
- Syringes, hypodermic needles, labels, and a marking pen
- Warm solutions for pediatric patients
- Marcaine with epinephrine
- Antibiotic of choice for irrigations to soak prostheses or for debridement

Drains and Dressings
- Correct size and type for planned surgery
  - Open—not attached to a drainage system
    - Penrose
    - Cigarette
  - Closed—attached to a drainage system
    - Hemovac
    - Jackson-Pratt
- Specialty dressings
  - Dressing bras
  - Telfa and medicated nonadherent dressings
  - Cotton balls for skin grafts

Specimen Care
- Proper container for each specimen
- Labels for each specimen
- Proper solution for specimen type
- Be prepared for multiple frozen sections

Before opening for the procedure, the surgical technologist should:
- Arrange furniture
- Gather positioning devices
- Damp dust lights, furniture, and surfaces
- Verify functionality of equipment
- Place items to be opened in their appropriate places
- Ensure all prosthesis sizes are on hand if one is to be used

When opening sterile supplies:
- Verify exposure to sterilization
- Use strict sterile technique
- Open bundles in appropriate location
- Open additional supplies onto sterile field
- Open the sterile field as close to the surgical start as possible

be appropriately exposed and the airway easily observed and accessed.

Correct draping procedures depend on the location of the operative site or sites. Disposable drapes are often used because of their barrier qualities, ease of handling and storage, and versatility in adapting to a variety of plastic surgery procedures. Two of the most frequently used draping techniques in plastic surgery are the head drape and the hand drape. Both of these draping techniques have the goal of providing maximum mobility of the operative part. The head drape includes a fluid-resistant drape that encircles the head and the addition of a drape to cover the remainder of the body. The following techniques represent methods of obtaining maximum accessibility and sterile coverage for facial surgery:

1. A barrier sheet, folded in half, and two towels are placed beneath the patient's head with the towels uppermost. The folded barrier sheet covers the headrest or head portion of the OR bed. One towel is brought around the patient's head on each side to cover all hair, leaving the entire face (and ears, as necessary) exposed; the towel is then secured with nonpenetrating towel clamps. For craniofacial procedures a towel folded lengthwise in quarters may be placed under the head to assist with moving the head from side to side. Two additional towels are then placed diagonally across the neck, just under the chin; they are secured to each other (with nonpenetrating towel clamps) in the middle over the neck and are secured on each side to the towel around the head. A full sheet is then added to cover the patient from neck to feet.
2. After the head portion of the drape is placed, a split, or U, drape is added to cover the patient from neck to feet.

Surgical Interventions

Reconstructive Plastic Surgery

Reconstructive plastic surgery seeks to restore or improve function after trauma, disease, infection, congenital anomalies, or acquired defects while trying to approximate an aesthetic appearance.

REMOVAL OF SKIN CANCERS

The estimated number of new skin cancer cases diagnosed in 2009 is 1 million (National Cancer Institute [NCI], 2009). The three most common skin cancers are basal cell, squamous cell, and melanoma (Gutierrez and Peterson, 2007). Basal cells account for approximately 70% of all skin cancers (Figure 13-10, *A*). If basal cell cancer is left untreated, it will grow locally, but rarely metastasizes (Box 13-1). Treated early, it may be cured by simple excision and closure (with pathologic diagnosis to ensure disease-free margins). Squamous cell skin cancers are considered more aggressive (Figure 13-10, *B*). Surgical treatment is the same as that for basal cell carcinomas. Melanoma accounts for the smallest percentage of skin cancers (5%), but it is treated much more aggressively because of its high mortality rate, comprising 75% of skin cancer deaths (Sladden et al, 2009) (Figure 13-10, *C*). Excision of melanoma may involve sentinel node mapping and excision. Early diagnosis of melanoma is imperative to successful treatment (Evidence for Practice). A Cochrane Database Systematic Review is underway (Sladden et al, 2009) since various international organizations varied in their recommendations regarding optimal excision margins. Excision margins that are too narrow

may result in higher local recurrence rates and/or mortality; wider excisions may increase hospital length of stay and require costlier procedures such as skin grafting and anesthesia.

Procedural Considerations

Consideration must be given to the type of skin cancer to be excised and the anticipated closure technique. Simple excision and closure with adjacent tissue will be the simplest technique, requiring a local plastic tray accompanied by skin markers and the electrosurgical unit (ESU), and usually involving use of a local anesthetic with epinephrine. A simple excision may be performed with the patient administered a local or general anesthetic or after induction of sedation. If additional procedures will be performed (e.g., reconstruction with skin graft, flap, or sentinel node mapping), refer to those sections for additional procedural considerations.

Operative Procedure—Simple Excision

1. The site is prepped and draped.
2. The surgeon infiltrates the site with a local anesthetic.
3. The lesion is curetted or excised and may be sent for frozen section or pathologic diagnosis.
4. Hemostasis is obtained.
5. The surgeon closes the wound if necessary.

Mohs' Surgery

Mohs' surgery is a specialized excision used to treat basal and squamous cell skin cancers. The procedure involves excising the lesion layer by layer and examining each layer under the microscope until all the abnormal tissue is removed.

Procedural Considerations. Mohs' surgery is usually completed on an ambulatory basis with the patient administered a local anesthetic. The procedure can be very time-consuming to accomplish, but it typically results in the preservation of the surrounding healthy tissue. Because the procedure is lengthy, patient preparation and comfort are essential to facilitate cooperation during the procedure. A minor plastic surgery set is required, along with fine (5-0 or 6-0) suture material.

Operative Procedure. Current procedures involve removal of all visible portions of the skin cancer lesion. A horizontal layer of tissue is removed and divided into sections that are color-coded with dyes. A map of the surgical site is then drawn. Frozen sections are immediately prepared and examined microscopically for any remaining tumor. If tumor is found, the location or locations are noted on the map and another layer of tissue is resected. The procedure is repeated as many times as necessary to completely remove the tumor.

BURN SURGERY

A majority of burns result from exposure to high temperatures, which injures the skin. Flame, scalding, or direct contact with a hot object may cause thermal skin injury. Similar destruction of skin can result from contact with chemicals such as acid or alkali or contact with an electrical current. The latter, however, often involves extensive destruction of the underlying tissue and physiologic systems in addition to the skin. A 2007 fact sheet on burn statistics includes the following information: approxi-

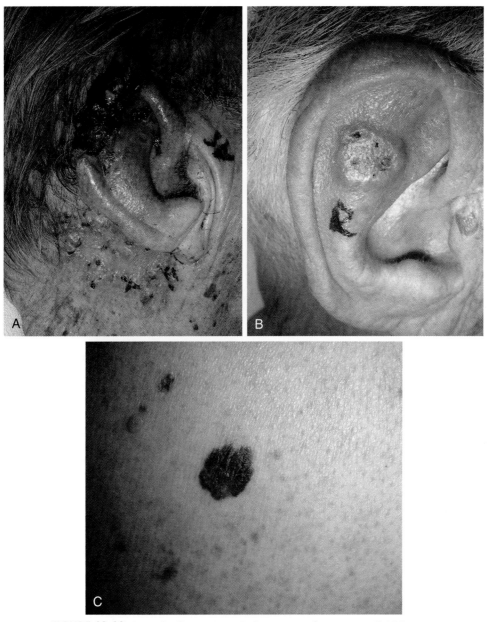

FIGURE 13-10 **A**, Basal cell carcinoma. **B**, Squamous cell carcinoma. **C**, Melanoma.

mately 500,000 burn injuries receive medical treatment yearly; 40,000 patients are hospitalized in the United States for burn injuries, with 25,000 of those admitted to the 125 hospitals with specialized burn centers (American Burn Association [ABA], 2007).

Intact skin provides protection against the environment for all underlying tissues and organs. It aids in heat regulation, prevents water loss, and is the major barrier against bacterial invasion. The tissue injury resulting from a burn disrupts this normal protective function, resulting in local and systemic effects (Box 13-2). Burn patients are therefore some of the most acutely ill patients brought to the OR. The greater the degree of injury to the skin, expressed in percentage of total body surface area (BSA) and depth of burn, the more severe the injury. One method of measuring BSA in adults is by use of the rule of nines (Song et al, 2007) (Figure 13-11).

Partial-thickness (first- and second-degree) burns heal by regeneration of skin from dermal elements that remain intact. First-degree burns involve the epidermis, which appears pink or red; sunburn is usually a first-degree burn. Second-degree burns, also called partial-thickness burns, involve the epidermis and some of the dermis. Full-thickness (third-degree) burns (Figure 13-12) involve the epidermis, the entire dermis, and the subcutaneous tissues; they require skin grafting to heal because no dermal elements remain intact. Both partial- and full-thickness burns may require debridement of necrotic tissue (eschar) before healing can occur by skin regeneration or grafting. An allograft may be used to cover the burned area during the initial healing process. However, the allograft must be carefully tested for immunodeficiency diseases. A xenograft (e.g., pig skin) may also be used for covering the burned area.

Procedural Considerations

The essentials of skin grafting are discussed under Skin and Tissue Grafting. This section therefore deals only with the procedure for debridement of burn wounds.

A basic plastic instrument set is required, plus a knife dermatome, an ESU, topical thrombin solution, a pneumatic tourniquet for isolated extremity burns, and a topical antimicrobial agent of choice.

Because patients who have sustained burns are vulnerable to hypothermia from the loss of body surface area (BSA), the temperature and humidity in the OR are increased and exposure is limited only to the areas related to the planned surgical event. Anesthesia is often induced while the patient is on the burn

---

BOX 13-1

Important Trends for Skin Cancer

INCIDENCE

Approximately 1 million cases per year with the majority being the highly curable basal or squamous cell cancers, accounting for more than 50% of all cancers; not as common is the most serious malignant melanoma, with an estimated 68,720 cases per year.

MORTALITY

Total estimated deaths for 2009 were 8650 from malignant melanoma and 11,590 from other skin cancers.

RISK FACTORS

- Excessive exposure to ultraviolet radiation from the sun
- Fair complexion
- Occupational exposure to coal tar, pitch, creosote, arsenic compounds, and radium
- Exposure to human papillomavirus and human immunodeficiency virus
- Skin cancer negligible in African Americans because of heavy skin pigmentation

WARNING SIGNALS

Any unusual skin conditions, especially a change in the size or color of a mole or other darkly pigmented growth or spot.

PREVENTION AND EARLY DETECTION

Avoid sun when ultraviolet light is strongest (e.g., 10:00 AM to 3:00 PM); use sunscreen preparations, especially those containing ingredients such as *para*-aminobenzoic acid (PABA). Basal and squamous cell cancers often form a pale, waxlike, pearly nodule or a red, scaly, sharply outlined patch; melanomas are usually dark brown or black pigmentation; they start as small molelike growths that increase in size, change color, become ulcerated, and bleed easily from a slight injury.

TREATMENT

The four methods of treatment are surgery, electrodesiccation (tissue destruction by heat), radiation therapy, and cryosurgery (tissue destruction by freezing). For malignant melanomas, wide and often deep excisions and removal of nearby lymph nodes are required.

SURVIVAL

For basal cell and squamous cell cancers, cure is virtually ensured with early detection and treatment. Malignant melanoma, however, metastasizes quickly; this accounts for a lower 5-year survival rate for Caucasian patients with this disease.

Modified from American Cancer Society (ACS): *Cancer facts and figures 2009*, Atlanta, 2009, The Society; Huether SE: Structure, function, and disorders of the integument. In Huether SE, McCance KL: *Understanding pathology*, ed 4, St Louis, 2008, Mosby.

EVIDENCE FOR PRACTICE

Melanoma Awareness, Prevention, and Detection

It is estimated that more than 68,720 men and women will be diagnosed with melanoma in 2009, according to the American Cancer Society. In the most recent time period, rapid increases have occurred among young white women (3.8% annual increase since 1995 in those aged 15 to 34 years) and older white men (8.8% annual increase since 2003 in those 65 and older). Although the exact cause of developing a melanoma is not known, certain risk factors have been identified:

- **Ultraviolet (UV) radiation:** sunlight, tanning beds
- **Moles:** more than 50 = greater risk
- **Fair skin:** fair skin, freckling, red or blond hair
- **Family history:** 10% have a relative with melanoma
- **Immune system compromise:** taking antirejection medications after organ transplantation surgery
- **Age:** increased risk in older adults
- **Gender:** men more than women
- **Previous melanoma:** increased risk for having another melanoma

PREVENTION

Limit UV radiation exposure:

1. Wear protective clothing (tight weave) and a hat with a broad brim.

2. Shade is good—avoid too much sunlight; remember that it reflects off water, sand, concrete, and snow.
3. Use sunscreen—SPF 15 or higher; apply 20 to 30 minutes before sun exposure; reapply every 2 hours; protect your lips.
4. Do not forget your eyes—look for sunglasses with 99% UV absorption.
5. Stay away from tanning beds and lamps—more UV exposure; try using self-tanning lotions.
6. Children need sunscreen—their skin is fragile; most damage to skin is acquired before the age of 18 years.
7. Take an inventory—know your moles and what they normally look like so you can detect changes if and when they occur.

KNOW YOUR A-B-C-Ds

A: Asymmetry—one half of the lesion looks different from the other side.

B: Border irregularity—instead of a smooth edge, the border is ragged or irregular.

C: Color—the color is usually irregular as well; may have a number of different hues and colors.

D: Diameter—lesions larger than 6 mm have a greater chance of being a melanoma.

EVIDENCE FOR PRACTICE

Melanoma Awareness, Prevention, and Detection—cont'd

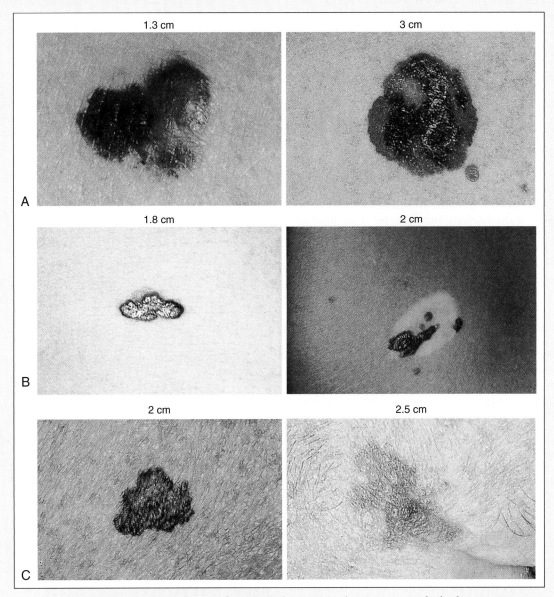

Malignant melanomas. Note presence of "ABCDE" characteristics (*a*symmetry, irregular *b*order, variation in *c*olor, *d*iameter >6 mm, enlargement and *e*levation). **A**, Superficial spreading melanoma. **B**, Nodular melanoma. **C**, Lentigo malignant melanoma.

Modified from American Cancer Society (ACS): *Cancer facts and figures 2009,* Atlanta, 2009, The Society.

unit bed; transfer to the OR bed is done carefully and gently, with attention to maintaining the airway. Most burn patients arrive in the OR with dressings covering their wounds. The dressings are removed after the patient has been anesthetized to minimize pain and loss of body heat through the open burn wounds. Throughout the procedure, the temperature in the OR is constantly monitored to prevent hypothermia. The OR team caring for burn patients coordinates activities to prevent any delays in obtaining required equipment or supplies. A variety of topical agents are used to dress wounds.

Operative Procedure

1. The surgeon excises all nonviable tissue down to underlying muscle fascia.
2. An alternative method is tangential excision of the burn wound, which is performed with a knife dermatome. This type of excision is usually carried down only to the bleeding subcutaneous fat, rather than to fascia.
3. Hemostasis is obtained with the ESU or use of topical thrombin solution.

4. Dressings saturated with the topical antimicrobial agent of choice are applied.

Although skin grafting may be done at the time of wound debridement, it is usually performed several days later, particularly in burns that are extensive.

EXCISIONAL DEBRIDEMENT

Excisional debridement is the act of removing dead or devitalized tissue to promote healing. Plastic surgeons use debridement in conjunction with treatment of injuries, trauma, and infection.

TREATMENT OF PRESSURE ULCERS

Pressure ulcers result from prolonged compression of soft tissues overlying bony prominences (Figure 13-13). However, whether excessive pressure is sufficient to create an ulcer depends on the intensity and duration of the pressure as well as on tissue tolerance. Factors that contribute to pressure ulcer development are immobility, sensory and motor deficits, reduced circulation, anemia, edema, infection, moisture, shearing force, friction, and nutritional debilita-

---

BOX 13-2

Pathophysiology of Burn Injuries

Thermal and chemical injuries disrupt the normal protective function of the skin, causing local and systemic effects. The extent of these effects depends on the type, duration, and intensity of exposure to the causative agent. With electrical burns, heat is generated as the electrical current passes through body tissues, causing thermal burns along the path taken by the current. Local damage is marked by histamine release and severe vasoconstriction, followed in a few hours by vasodilation and increased capillary permeability, which allows plasma to escape into the wound. Damaged cells swell and platelets and leukocytes aggregate, causing thrombotic ischemia and escalating tissue damage. Systemic effects, which are caused by vascular changes and tissue loss, include hypovolemia, hyperventilation, increased blood viscosity, and suppression of the immune system. The severity of the burn determines the extent of local and systemic effects. Severity is judged by the depth of the burn and the quantity of tissue involved. The depth of the burn is classified by degree. First-degree (superficial) burns affect the epidermis only; second-degree burns (split thickness) affect the epidermis and dermis; third-degree burns (full thickness) affect all skin layers and extend to subcutaneous tissue, muscle, and nerves; fourth-degree burns involve all skin layers, plus bone. The percentage of body surface area (BSA) system of the American Burn Association classifies quantity as follows:

◆ Minor burn: full-thickness burns over less than 2% of BSA; partial-thickness burns over less than 15% of BSA

◆ Moderate burns: full-thickness burns over 2% to 10% of BSA; partial-thickness burns over less than 15% to 25% of BSA

◆ Major burns: full-thickness burns over 10% or more of BSA; partial-thickness burns over 25% or more of BSA; any burn to face, head, hands, feet, or perineum; inhalation and electrical burns; burns complicated by trauma or other disease processes

From Langford RW, Thompson JD: *Mosby's handbook of diseases,* ed 3, St Louis, 2005, Mosby.

---

tion (Cuzzell and Workman, 2010). The most common sites of pressure ulcers are the sacrum, the ischium, the trochanter, the malleolus, and the heel; these are called decubitus ulcers. These ulcers are different from chronic ulcers such as vascular, diabetic, and neurogenic ulcers. Surgical interventions for pressure ulcers are usually based on ulcer staging (also referred to as *grading*). In stage I the ulcer involves the epidermis and has soft tissue swelling that is irregular and ill-defined; heat and erythema at the ulcer site are characteristic. A stage II ulcer involves the epidermis and dermis but not the subcutaneous fat. Stage III ulcers show full-thickness skin loss with injury to underlying tissue layers and may contain necrotic material. Thorough excisional debridement is performed, and IV antibiotic therapy is instituted. Although debrided stage III ulcers often heal on their own, surgical excision and closure may be done to

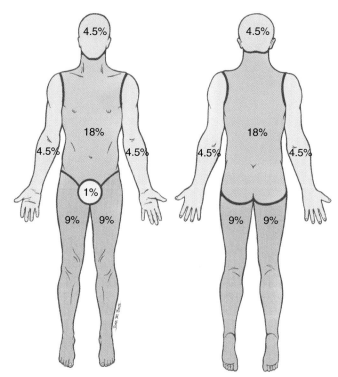

FIGURE 13-11 The "rule of nines." The amount of skin surface burned in an adult can be estimated by dividing the body into 11 areas of 9% each.

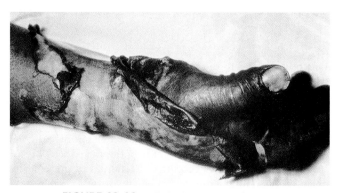

FIGURE 13-12 Full-thickness thermal injury.

prevent a lengthy spontaneous closure, which may result in a weak, unstable scar with resultant recurrence. Stage IV ulcers are the deepest, requiring more radical excisional debridement. Adequate soft tissue cover may be obtained by either split-thickness or full-thickness skin grafting or tissue flaps (Figure 13-14). Tissue expansion may be used when there is not enough tissue adjacent to the ulcer site to provide flap coverage.

The use of a CO_2 laser minimizes blood loss and possibly reduces infection rates in the presence of gross contamination. Although many techniques and flaps are surgical options, basic principles apply to all pressure ulcer closure procedures. The following procedure is for an adjacent flap.

Procedural Considerations

A basic plastic instrument set is required, as well as assorted sizes of osteotomes (straight and curved), a mallet, the Gigli saw and handle, assorted curettes, a Key periosteal elevator, a duckbill rongeur, bone wax, the dermatome of choice, the ESU, a sterile marking pen, and a closed-wound drainage system. The patient is positioned and draped so that the pressure ulcer, adjacent flap donor site, and skin graft donor site are well exposed.

Operative Procedure

1. The area to be excised and the local flap are outlined.
2. The surgeon excises the ulcer along with the underlying bony prominence.
3. Large suction catheters are placed into the defect left by excision of the ulcer and beneath the flap.
4. The flap is sutured in place.
5. A split-thickness skin graft generally is used to resurface the flap donor site.
6. A stent dressing is placed over the skin graft, and gauze dressings or a plastic spray dressing is applied over the suture lines of the flap.

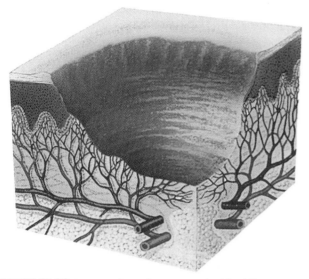

FIGURE 13-13 Pressure ulcers often appear after blood flow to an area slows or is obstructed because of pressure on bony prominences. Infections often follow, since lack of blood flow causes tissue damage or death.

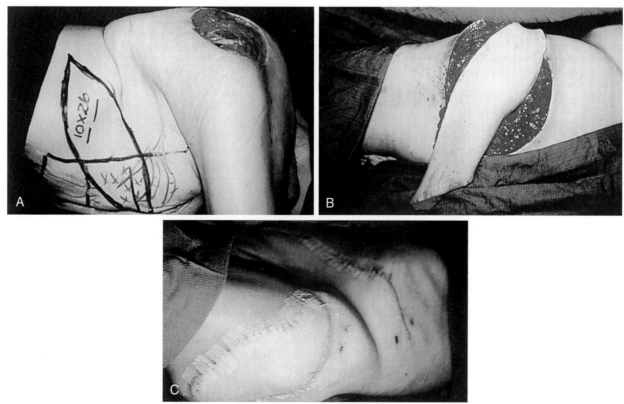

FIGURE 13-14 A, Rotational flap from abdomen for pressure sore coverage. **B,** Placement of flap. **C,** Completed coverage with flap placement.

SURGICAL PHARMACOLOGY

Topical Medications Used in Burn Therapy

Agent	Indication	Implications
Petroleum-based antimicrobials (bacitracin, Neosporin, polymyxin B)	Partial-thickness burns	Provides barrier protection to wound. Has mild antimicrobial activity. Cleaning wound before applying prevents caking. Maintain layer adequate to keep wound from drying.
Silver sulfadiazine (Silvadene)	Deep partial to full-thickness burns Wound infection	Has broad-spectrum antimicrobial action against gram-negative bacteria, gram-positive bacteria, and *Candida* organisms. Penetrates eschar to inhibit bacterial growth at dermis-eschar interface. Soothes pain with ¼-inch layer applied directly to wound or on impregnated gauze applied 2-3 times daily. May cause slimy, grayish appearance with repeated applications. Inhibits epithelial tissue development. Discontinued when eschar no longer present. Side or toxic effects include skin rash on unburned tissues, transient decrease in WBCs for 24-48 hr after application. Contraindicated in patients with sulfa hypersensitivities.
Mafenide acetate (Sulfamylon)	Deep partial to full-thickness burns Wound infection	Is bacteriostatic against gram-negative and gram-positive bacteria. Is applied in ¼-inch layer directly to wound or on impregnated gauze 2-3 times daily. 11.1% cream: penetrates thick eschar and cartilage; inhibits epithelial tissue development. 5% solution: antimicrobial solution used to prevent and treat wound infections. Discontinued when eschar no longer present. Side or toxic effects include pain on application (may necessitate pain management), metabolic acidosis (when applied to more than 40% total body surface area), hypersensitivity rash, pruritus, fungal growth.
Silver nitrate (5% solution)	Deep partial to full-thickness burns Wound infection	Is bacteriostatic against gram-negative and gram-positive bacteria. Has poor penetration of eschar. Side or toxic effects include staining of the wound black (making assessment difficult), pain on application (may necessitate pain management), staining of clothing and linens, decreases in electrolytes (sodium, potassium, calcium, chloride).

Modified from Green-Nigro CJ: Burns. In Monahan F et al, editors: *Phipps medical-surgical nursing*, ed 8, St Louis, 2007, Mosby.

DIABETIC FOOT CONDITIONS

In the past decade, the incidence of diabetes and concomitant severe foot infections has risen significantly. The severity of these infections is conveyed by diagnoses and sequelae (e.g., necrotizing fasciitis, gas gangrene, ascending cellulitis, and infection with systemic toxicity or metabolic instability). Because patients with diabetes mellitus may have peripheral neuropathies, they may not feel and therefore not notice any tenderness or early signs of infection. These foot infections can lead to hospitalization and eventual lower extremity amputation for patients with preexisting ulcerations; surgical management is often required for the severe infections. The experienced surgeon determines when and how to intervene. Main principles for management include stabilization of the patient; adequate debridement along with antibiotic therapy; vascular evaluation and revascularization as necessary; delayed soft tissue reconstruction; and postoperative information and intervention for medical and surgical issues. In addressing all these aspects, the surgeon optimizes the possibility for limb salvage. This overview serves as a reminder to emphasize the importance of overall adherence in managing diabetes mellitus to prevent further complications (Zgonis et al, 2008).

These complex patients are best handled with multidisciplinary consultations to coordinate care and determine optimal timing for soft tissue reconstruction. Primary closure may not be an option and secondary healing is not necessarily reliable. The proactive surgical approach aims to salvage the diabetic limb by improving overall health and to provide a stable, mechanically sound limb that will resist further breakdown once the patient is able to walk again. To prevent complications, patients need ongoing support and validation. Hospital care focuses on dressing changes, wound care, physical therapy, limb position, shower privileges, and laboratory testing. Postoperative nursing care should provide instruction for follow-up and frequency of monitoring of the surgical results, ambulatory status, work and social restrictions, and bathing.

SKIN AND TISSUE GRAFTING

Skin grafting provides an effective way to cover a wound if vascularity is adequate, infection is absent, and hemostasis is

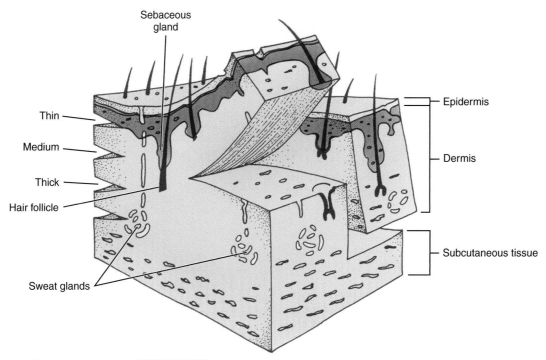

FIGURE 13-15 Split-thickness and full-thickness skin grafts.

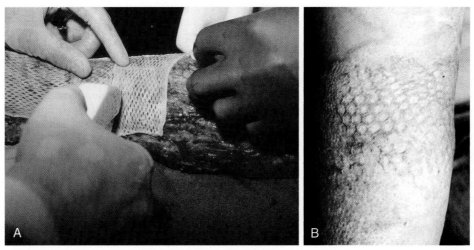

FIGURE 13-16 A, Split-thickness skin is meshed and used to cover a marginal wound. Minimal expansion is used, and the holes provide drainage. **B,** Appearance of the graft after healing.

achieved. Skin from the donor site is detached from its blood supply and placed in the recipient site, where it develops a new blood supply from the base of the wound. Color match, contour, and durability of the graft are all considerations in selection of an appropriate donor area. Other types of grafts that are available for surgical reconstruction include bone, cartilage, nerve, tendon, and autologous fat grafts.

Split-Thickness and Full-Thickness Skin Grafts

Skin grafts can be either split-thickness (STSGs) or full-thickness grafts (FTSGs) (Figure 13-15). A split-thickness (or partial-thickness) skin graft contains epidermis and only a portion of the dermis of the donor site; it varies from a thin graft to a thick graft. Although this type of graft becomes vascular-

ized more rapidly and the donor site heals more rapidly than a full-thickness graft, it may exhibit postgraft contraction, be minimally resistant to surface trauma, and be least like normal skin in texture, suppleness, pore pattern, hair growth, and other characteristics. A split-thickness skin graft may be meshed (Figure 13-16); meshed grafts can expand to many times their original size. Meshing allows the graft to be placed on an irregular recipient area; however, its appearance may be aesthetically undesirable. A full-thickness skin graft contains both epidermis and dermis; any remaining subcutaneous tissue is trimmed before the FTSG is applied to the graft site. The advantages of this type of graft are that it causes minimal contracture, can be used in areas of flexion, has a greater ability to withstand trauma, can add tissue where a loss has occurred or where padding is required, and is aesthetically more acceptable than an STSG. The donor site can be closed primarily, leaving a minimal defect.

The donor site for an STSG heals by regeneration of epithelium from dermal elements that remain intact. Thus only a dressing is placed over this donor site. Because no dermal elements remain when an FTSG is taken, this donor site does not heal spontaneously. It heals either when the wound edges of the donor site are sutured together (primary closure) or when an STSG is applied over it. A scar remains at the donor site of a skin graft; therefore donor sites that are covered by clothing are generally chosen.

For a graft to survive, the vascularity of the recipient area must be adequate, contact between the graft and recipient bed must be maintained, and the graft-bed unit must be adequately immobilized.

Color, temperature, signs of infection, blanching of the skin, excessive pain and discomfort, edema, vasoconstriction, and venous congestion should be noted and any change reported to the surgeon.

Any changes should be documented. If the patient is discharged to home after surgery, patient and family education should include reportable signs and symptoms of potential complications.

A stent or tie-over dressing is often placed over a skin graft (Figure 13-17). This exerts even pressure, ensuring good contact between graft and recipient site. It also eliminates potential shearing forces at the graft and recipient site interface that might disrupt new blood vessels growing into the graft.

Procedural Considerations. A plastic local instrument set is required, with the addition of a dermatome of choice, a skin mesher, and sterile marking pen. The patient is positioned so that both donor and recipient sites are well exposed. Both areas are prepped and draped to maintain adequate exposure and mobility, as required.

Operative Procedure
1. The recipient site is prepared as necessary. This step may involve excision of a benign or malignant skin tumor, debridement of an open wound, or release of a scar contracture.
2. Careful planning and marking before harvesting the graft from the recipient site are essential. Patterns matching intended recipient site and the donor site are outlined with a sterile marking pen.
3. STSGs are harvested with a knife dermatome or powered dermatome of the surgeon's choice (Figure 13-18).
4. Moist sponges soaked in normal saline, an antibiotic solution, or a solution of 20 mg of phenylephrine HCl (Neo-Synephrine) per 1000 ml of normal saline may be applied to the donor sites to aid hemostasis. Medication labels indicating strength are placed on all solutions, including Neo-Synephrine, to further identify all solutions on the sterile field. These sponges are removed, and the donor site is covered with Biobrane or OpSite.
5. If the graft is to be meshed, it is now applied to specifically supplied carriers for use with certain skin meshers.
6. A graft that is not immediately applied to the recipient site dries quickly, particularly a meshed graft. The surgical technologist should ensure that the graft is kept on the carrier and covered with moist gauze sponges to prevent inadvertent loss of the graft. Meshed skin should not be removed from its carrier until it is applied directly to the recipient

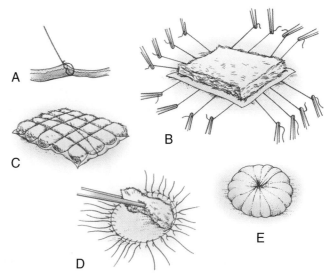

FIGURE 13-17 **A,** Method of fixation of skin graft to edges of wound. **B,** Nonadherent dressing is applied over skin graft, on top of which is placed a generous pad of acrylic fiber. **C,** Long ends of suture are tied over fiber to produce area of pressure between graft and base. **D,** Similar dressing is applied to circular graft. **E,** Long suture ends are tied over circular graft (often called *stent dressing*).

site. Whether applied as a sheet or meshed, the STSG may be sutured or stapled with a skin stapler. Nonadherent gauze is usually applied as the first layer of dressing over a graft. Moist dressings should be applied to all meshed grafts to prevent desiccation and loss of the graft.
7. Fat adherent to the graft is trimmed. The graft is applied to the recipient site and usually sutured at the edges, and these sutures are left long to tie over a stent dressing. Blood clots beneath the graft are removed by saline irrigation before the dressing is applied.

Composite Graft

Composite grafts are composed of skin and underlying tissues that are completely separated from the blood supply of the donor site and transplanted to another area of the body. The survival of a composite graft depends on ingrowth of new blood vessels from the recipient site around the periphery of the graft. Therefore composite grafts are usually small so that no portion of the graft is more than 1 cm from its periphery. An example of compound tissues used as composite grafts is hair transplants, composed of skin, fat, and hair follicles, which are used to treat male pattern baldness. The term *composite* thus indicates a defect that requires a graft be transferred to the area to meet more than one type of tissue deficiency.

Procedural Considerations. A plastic local instrument set is required, plus a sterile marking pen. The patient is positioned, prepped, and draped such that adequate exposure of both donor and recipient sites is achieved.

Operative Procedure
1. The recipient site is prepared by excising tissue, such as a scar or a benign or malignant skin lesion.
2. When feasible, the surgeon makes a pattern of the recipient site and transfers it to the donor site.

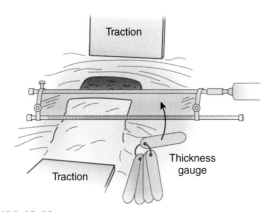

FIGURE 13-18 Harvesting a split-thickness skin graft (STSG) with the Humby knife.

3. The surgeon excises the composite graft. The donor site is either closed by approximating its skin edges or left unsutured (as in hair transplant donor sites).
4. Meanwhile, the composite graft is kept in a moist sponge until it is sutured to the edges of the recipient site.
5. Dressings of choice are applied to the composite graft and donor site.

Replacement of Lost or Absent Tissue

When coverage for a defect cannot be achieved through skin grafting, plastic surgeons rely on other techniques to replace tissue. Just as the flap has evolved, other techniques for tissue restoration through biologic engineering have also evolved. Four principal avenues have been explored to make new tissues for biologic replacement: the injection of isolated cell populations, the placement of polymer scaffolds to guide tissue regeneration, the development of encapsulated systems, and the transplantation of cells in polymer matrices (Marler and Upton, 2006). A discussion of flap techniques follows.

Flaps

The term *flap* refers to tissue that is detached from one area of the body and transferred to the recipient area with either part or all of its original blood supply intact. In a free flap the flap is detached from one part of the body with its vascular pedicle and then reestablished by reanastomosis with the recipient vascular system; thus it has a self-contained vascular system. The base or pedicle of the flap is that portion through which the blood supply enters or exits. Because flaps carry their own blood supply, they generally are used to cover recipient sites that have poor vascularity and full-thickness tissue loss. Flaps are used for reconstruction or wound closure. They are useful for covering exposed bone, tendon, or nerve. They may be used if surgery through the wound may be necessary at a later date to repair underlying structures. Flaps containing skin and subcutaneous tissue retain more properties of normal skin and shrink less than skin grafts. Flaps, however, have some disadvantages, such as bulky appearance, failure to match tissue of the recipient site in texture or color, and the possibility of requiring multiple operations and prolonged hospitalization.

Flaps may be classified according to blood supply. *Random pattern flaps* consist of skin and subcutaneous tissue vascularized by random perforators with limited length/width ratio.

Axial pattern flaps have a well-defined arteriovenous supply along the long axis; they can be comparatively long in relation to width. Flaps may also be classified according to position or how they are rotated after elevation. *Advancement flaps* are cut and advanced to reconstruct a nearby defect. *Transposition flaps* are advanced along an axis that forms an angle to the flap's original position. *Rotation flaps* are similar to transposition flaps but are semicircular and rotate along a greater axis. *Island flaps* of isolated sections of skin and subcutaneous tissue are tunneled beneath the skin to new sites. *Pedicle flaps* were the forerunners of muscle and musculocutaneous flaps. These consist of skin and underlying muscle; they are very mobile and can be rotated into distant defects. *Free flaps* are actually a form of tissue transplantation. Using microvascular techniques, a defined amount of skin, muscle, or bone can be isolated, totally detached, and reattached at the recipient site by microvascular anastomoses between recipient site blood vessels and the major vessels that supply the flap. The vascular pedicle may contain functional nerves, yielding sensory flaps to provide protective sensation or motor flaps to restore function. Bone and joints may be transplanted as free flaps, as in the case of toe-to-thumb site transfers.

Procedural Considerations. The perioperative nurse and surgical technologist should consult with the surgeon in advance of the procedure to determine the donor site, the patient's position(s), and the surgical sequence of the procedure. Generally the surgical site and flap area are marked preoperatively with the patient in a functional position because landmarks and aesthetics are influenced by surgical positioning. If marking is undertaken on the anesthetized and surgically positioned patient, inaccuracies in tissue placement could occur. Flap procedures may involve two teams of surgeons working simultaneously: one raising the flap and closing the resulting defect, and the other preparing the site, repositioning the flap in its new site, and, in the case of a free flap, microscopically reanastomosing the blood vessels. For any lengthy procedure, a Foley catheter, sequential compression devices, warming units, and positioning aids that are safe for the skin will be needed. Skin grafts are sometimes used to achieve closure of the flap donor site; if this is anticipated then the surgical technologist should add appropriate instrumentation for harvesting a skin graft.

A basic plastic instrument set is required, plus the following:
- ESU
- Sterile marking pen
- Extra hemostats
- Dermatome of choice
- Skin mesher
- Microvascular instruments (as appropriate)

Operative Procedure—Advancement, Transpositional, Rotational, Island, and Pedicle Flaps

1. The recipient site is prepared in the same manner as for a skin graft.
2. Patterns matching the recipient and donor sites are drawn/marked.
3. The surgeon incises, elevates, and transfers the flap to the recipient site.
4. The edges of the flap are sutured to the periphery of the recipient site.

5. The flap donor site is repaired by approximating the skin edges directly or by covering the defect with a skin graft or another flap.

6. Drains are usually placed under flaps.

7. Dressings are applied with particular attention given to immobilization of the flap, which may require a stockinette, padding, or plaster of paris.

8. NOTE: Before a pedicle flap is detached from the donor site, the surgeon may want to determine the adequacy of circulation within the flap. One method to check circulation involves placing rubber-shod clamps across the base of the pedicle and injecting sodium fluorescein intravenously. After 10 minutes have elapsed, all lights in the OR are turned off and a Wood's lamp is held over the flap to determine the presence or absence of fluorescence within the flap. Fluorescein may be injected locally for the same purpose.

Operative Procedure—Free Flaps. See Operative Procedure for free TRAM flap described under Reconstructive Breast Surgery.

RECONSTRUCTIVE BREAST SURGERY

The loss of a breast because of cancer may have a devastating effect on a woman. Fortunately, the option of breast reconstruction is available to virtually any woman who loses her breast to cancer (ASPS, 2009c). Reconstruction has the ability to offer hope and a return to wholeness and normalcy. Normal, of course, is subjective, and although breasts may be reconstructed, there is a wide range of outcomes, and it must be stressed that breast reconstruction is not a one-time surgery. Revisions are the rule and not the exception. Techniques and options continue to evolve and improve, and women have many options. Breast reconstruction may be offered at one of many times during this process—initially, at the time of mas-

tectomy; before or after adjunct therapy; or even many years later. The important fact is that each woman and her oncologic status are individual, so the decision for reconstruction must be made according to the woman's wishes coupled with her most favorable circumstances. Reconstruction has no known effect on the recurrence of breast cancer (ACS, 2009). Breast reconstruction options include alloplastic (artificial materials), autogenous (flaps), or a combination of both. Flaps may be pedicle-based or free flaps, requiring microsurgical techniques for their reconstruction.

Breast Reconstruction Using Tissue Expanders

Mastectomy may leave a shortage of skin that prevents creation of a breast mound. For these patients, extra tissue can be created locally with the use of tissue expanders (Figure 13-19). Tissue expansion is a technique used to stretch normal tissue that is adjacent to a defect, mechanically creating redundancy of normal tissue to correct the defect. For breast reconstruction, the expander resembles the shape of a breast prosthesis. The expander has a metal-backed, self-sealing silicone valve at its dome. Another type of expander used less frequently has a small, dome-shaped reservoir with a fill tube that is positioned subcutaneously at a distance from the expander but connected to it. Following surgery, the tissue expander is gradually filled with percutaneous injections of normal saline during routine office visits. The expander may be filled as often as weekly, or it may remain unused until chemotherapy or radiation is completed. Once the tissue expander is filled to the appropriate volume, it may be removed and replaced with a permanent reconstructive mammary prosthesis, either saline or silicone, as an ambulatory surgical procedure. Silicone can be used for breast augmentation for patients older than 21 years. If silicone is chosen, both the surgeon and the patient must participate in an adjunct clinical study at this time; the patient may opt out. Another option is the use of combination tissue expander

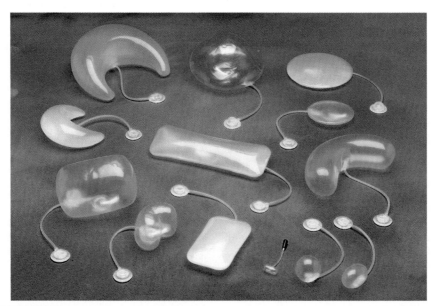

FIGURE 13-19 Tissue expanders are inflatable plastic reservoirs of various shapes and volumes that are implanted under the skin. The skin over the expander is stretched during a period of several weeks as the expander is gradually filled by percutaneous injection of saline into an incorporated part of the remote-fill port. Expanders are useful for breast reconstruction.

and breast prosthesis, which remains in place once the desired amount of saline has been sequentially added. The benefit of this prosthesis is the ability to add or remove saline in case an adjustment proves necessary. The recent introduction of allografts helps to achieve better shape and fast expansion and is less painful.

Procedural Considerations. A basic plastic set may be used with the addition of fiberoptic breast retractors. Positioning is usually supine with both arms extended on armboards. Both inframammary folds are marked preoperatively, and both sides of the chest should be prepped and draped. The breast shape expander is supplied in a sterile package from the manufacturer and is available in a variety of sizes. Meticulous sterile technique is required, and the expander should be handled as little as possible. This procedure may be performed immediately following mastectomy or at a later date. Drains are usually placed to prevent hematoma and seroma formation, the latter of which could cause rotation or malposition of the tissue expander. If a surgical bra is used, care must be taken that it is not too tight and does not compromise circulation to the skin flaps.

Operative Procedure

1. Skin flaps are assessed for adequate blood supply, and then the pectoralis fascia is incised along its lateral border. The surgeon creates a submuscular pocket for the temporary expander by undermining the muscle over the sternal attachments and down over the lower ribs.
2. Recently, allograft material is being used to bridge the gap created from the elevated pectoral and serratus muscles to the inframammary fold.
3. The tissue expander is tested before insertion for watertight integrity.
4. After hemostasis is achieved, the surgeon checks the expander for integrity and then inserts it into the pocket. Muscle coverage is assessed, and if adequate the reservoir is positioned subcutaneously and connected, the wound is closed, and the expander is filled with sterile saline solution until slight blanching of the skin is achieved. The amount is recorded on the patient record.

Second-Stage Tissue Expander Breast Reconstruction

Once the tissue expander has been expanded to the desired size, the patient is taken back to surgery for the next stage of her breast reconstruction. This is a relatively minor procedure in which the tissue expander is deflated and replaced with a permanent mammary prosthesis (Figures 13-20 and 13-21, *A* and *B*). At this time, if there is asymmetry of the contralateral breast, surgery may be performed to create bilateral symmetry. The patient may require correction of breast ptosis through mastopexy, with or without the addition of a breast implant; alternatively, a reduction mammoplasty may be needed on the opposite breast. This procedure is usually performed on an outpatient basis in which the patient is administered a general anesthetic.

Breast Reconstruction Using Myocutaneous Flaps

Flaps are described by the types of tissue they contain, the blood supply of the tissues, and the method by which the flaps are moved from the donor site to the recipient site. The latissimus dorsi myocutaneous flap is used during reconstruction of the breast after mastectomy. This procedure may be staged. Because the flap consists of skin combined with muscle, it is described as *myocutaneous*. This flap is used when significant tissue deficiency occurs after a mastectomy or when abdominal flap (trans-

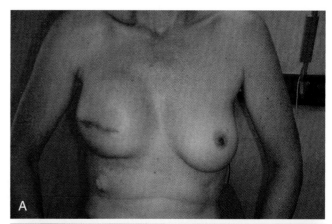
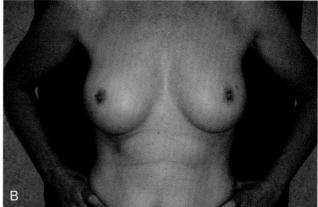

FIGURE 13-21 A, Tissue expander is used to create extra tissue after mastectomy so a breast mound can be created. **B,** Postoperative result after tissue expander replaced with breast prosthesis.

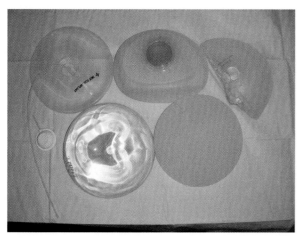

FIGURE 13-20 While discussing options in surgeon's office, samples of tissue expanders, textured and smooth saline and silicone implants, are shown to patients for their selection.

verse rectus abdominis myocutaneous [TRAM]) reconstruction is not an option. The latissimus dorsi muscle is a wide, flat muscle extending over the midthoracic portion of the back and inserting into the humerus. Its blood supply comes from the thoracodorsal artery and from perforators of the upper lumbar arteries and intercostal vessels. This rich vascularity allows the surgeon flexibility in orienting and positioning the flap to the pattern of the deficit on the anterior chest wall. Latissimus dorsi flaps are usually used in conjunction with a reconstructive breast prosthesis, in order to create a more natural breast mound.

According to the U.S. Department of Labor, The Women's Health and Cancer Rights Act of 1998 (WHCRA) mandates financial coverage of all breast reconstruction related procedures. One other option is the superior gluteal artery perforator (SGAP) flap, which is becoming more refined recently. Some women choose to use their own tissue for reconstruction, as they prefer what they consider more realistic, supple breasts that would not need to be replaced or removed as is possible with implants. The SGAP flap does require microsurgical skills and is not offered at all institutions. Factors for choosing reconstructive options include the patient's size and availability of appropriate abdominal or gluteal tissue. Even very thin patients generally have enough skin and fat for the SGAP procedure, and the consistency of the buttock fat (thicker than abdominal) provides the more supple result. Positioning is especially challenging, and some operative efficiency may be achieved by using two OR beds (Edwards et al, 2009).

Procedural Considerations. The surgeon marks the donor site of the latissimus dorsi with its skin island, along with the intended recipient site, before surgery with the patient in a sitting position. In the OR, the patient is placed in a lateral position, donor side up, with the arm extended and safely supported. The perioperative team should assemble extra padding and positioning aids in preparation for the patient's arrival. Once the donor muscle has been mobilized and exteriorized through the area of defect, the back incision is closed and the patient repositioned supine with the arm extended on an armboard. Instrumentation should include a basic plastic instrument set, fiberoptic breast retractor, vascular instruments, sterile marking pens, suction, and long tissue forceps and scissors, and a Doppler probe should be available.

Operative Procedure
1. Initially the island of skin is incised transversely across the back, being careful to ensure that a bra or bathing suit will cover the resulting scar (Figure 13-22, *A*).
2. The surgeon frees the muscle, subcuticular fat, and fascia from the overlying skin by undermining so that part or all of the muscle may be mobilized (Figure 13-22, *B*).
3. The skin island and the muscle are then tunneled under the axilla to the chest wall (Figure 13-22, *C*). The insertion of the muscle on the humerus and accompanying blood vessels are left undisturbed. The latissimus dorsi muscle fills the space left by the missing pectoralis muscle.
4. The island of skin is oriented to the recipient site, and the surgeon sutures both into place (Figure 13-22, *D*).
5. A mammary prosthesis is placed under the muscle before suturing to reconstruct the breast mound.
6. The wound is drained by closed-wound drains.

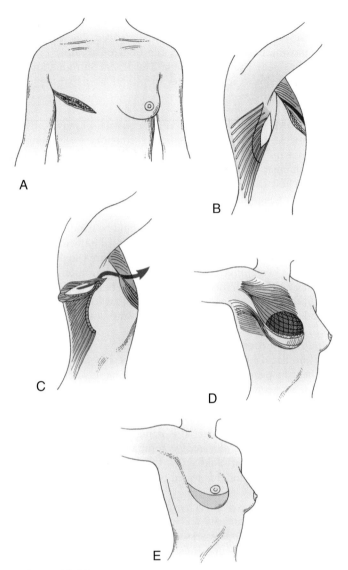

FIGURE 13-22 Latissimus dorsi flap for reconstruction after mastectomy (see text for procedure).

7. The nipple-areola complex may also be reconstructed by sharing the nipple on the unaffected side or by using groin, adjacent tissue, thigh, or auricular tissue. This can be done at the time of reconstruction or at a later date as a minor procedure with the patient administered a local anesthetic (Figure 13-22, *E*).
8. If a surgical bra is used, care must be taken not to compromise blood supply to the flap.

Transverse Rectus Abdominis Myocutaneous Flap

TRAM flaps are the most common pedicle-based flaps used for breast reconstruction. The rectus muscle is the broad, wide abdominal muscle that reaches from under the ribs to the pubis, and either one or both sides of the muscle may be used for reconstruction. The blood supply (superior epigastric artery and vein) is carried within the muscle pedicle. The muscle along with its pedicle is severed at its most distal origins and pulled through a subcutaneous tunnel to the chest to form a breast. Although this procedure has the added benefit of

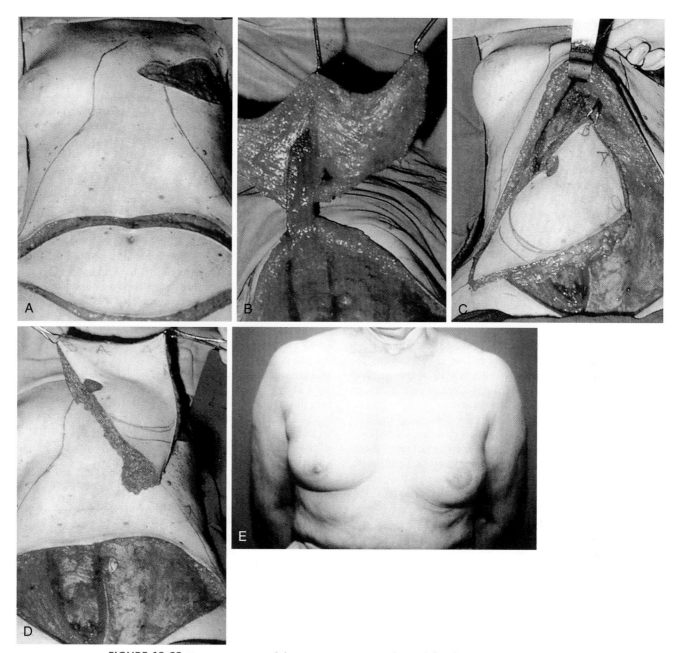

FIGURE 13-23 Transverse rectus abdominis myocutaneous (TRAM) flap for postmastectomy breast reconstruction (see text for procedure).

an abdominoplasty, if there is inadequate abdominal tissue the patient may require a small mammary prosthesis.

The several types of TRAM techniques are based on blood supply, but the procedure still follows a basic format. As with other types of breast reconstruction, TRAM flaps may be performed immediately following mastectomy or planned for a later stage in the patient's recuperative phase.

Procedural Considerations. The surgeon marks the surgical landmarks preoperatively with the patient in a standing position. A basic plastic instrument set is used as for the latissimus dorsi flap. The patient is positioned supine with arms extended on armboards. Positioning the patient for this procedure is particularly difficult because of the need to promote

closure of the abdominal wound, support circulation to the flap, and protect the patient from injury. The OR bed is often flexed; additional padding of the lower extremities may be required. The skin prep should extend from the lower neck to midthigh.

Operative Procedure

1. The surgeon excises the skin from the mastectomy scar and makes the abdominal incision. The abdominal flap is dissected with care being taken not to shear the skin and subcutaneous tissue from its underlying muscle attachments (Figure 13-23, *A*).

2. The transverse rectus abdominis muscle is divided from its inferior-most attachment (Figure 13-23, *B*).

3. The flap is rotated and passed through to its new location on the chest wall (Figure 13-23, *C* and *D*) and sutured medially; the thinnest portion of the flap is superior and medial, and the thickest portion is inferior and lateral.

4. Because of the amount of tissue available, an implant is often unnecessary (Figure 13-23, *E*).

Free Transverse Rectus Abdominis Myocutaneous Flap

The free TRAM flap is indicated when there is concern about the absence of one or both of the rectus muscles following the procedure or when there are concerns about vascularity, either with the pedicle used in the standard TRAM flap with any other factors that may compromise vascularity of the flap. A newer technique of the free TRAM (deep inferior epigastric perforator procedure) has the advantage of not requiring the entire rectus muscle, because only a small portion of the rectus muscle that carries a segment of the deep inferior epigastric perforator vessels is needed to move with the fat and skin to its new location. It is also used when the buttock tissue (superior gluteal perforator flap) is planned to replace the absent breast or breasts.

Procedural Considerations. Care of the patient undergoing a free TRAM procedure is identical to that of patients undergoing pedicle TRAM flaps with the addition of the surgical microscope. Refer to the Procedural Considerations under Transverse Rectus Abdominis Myocutaneous Flaps (TRAM). Two surgical teams may be used, one for harvesting and one for site preparation. Meticulous attention must be paid to positioning and protection from pressure injuries because of the length of the procedure. During the preoperative verification process, the perioperative team should determine if the patient has made preoperative autologous blood donations and if the appropriate blood work has been performed.

Operative Procedure
1. The site is prepped, and the recipient site blood vessels are identified for anastomosis.
2. The surgeon dissects and isolates the recipient vessels.
3. Donor vessels are selected based on pedicle length, and the flap is prepared.
4. The anesthesia provider administers heparin to prevent clotting and vasospasm.
5. Once recipient vessels are ready, the surgeon severs the flap.
6. The microscope is positioned in place and draped with a sterile drape.
7. The free flap is transferred to the recipient site, and the surgeon anastomoses the blood vessels.
8. The breast mound is shaped and sutured in place.
9. The donor site is closed, covering with a skin graft if necessary.

Nipple Reconstruction

Although nipple reconstruction can be performed at the time of breast reconstruction or replacement of the tissue expander with a mammary prosthesis, some surgeons prefer to wait and let the new breast tissues "settle" and mature in order to reconstruct the new nipple in the most accurate anatomic position. Generally this may take a minimum of 6 to 8 weeks. Tissue for the new nipple can be recruited locally by raising a flap or be grafted from the opposite nipple. The areola is reconstructed with skin grafting from the groin, buttock crease, or auricle (Figure 13-24). The areolar skin may be tattooed to create a very pleasing nipple-areolar complex (Figure 13-25, *A* and *B*).

MICROSURGERY

Microsurgery is a fundamental tool in reconstructive plastic surgery. It allows an almost unlimited choice of reconstructive methods, replacement of lost tissue with similar components, and optimal selection of donor sites with minimal morbidity (Wei and Suominen, 2006). Reconstructive microsurgical procedures include, but are not limited to, replantation of amputated body parts, repair of facial nerves, repair of lacerated nerves and blood vessels, treatment of extensive trauma to extremities and hands, reconstruction following removal of extensive cancers, and female to male transsexual reassignment. Today's physicians skilled in microsurgery can successfully anastomose the ends of a vessel measuring less than 1 mm in diameter. The surgeon's use of an operating microscope or loupes for microsurgical procedures depends on the procedure to be performed, condition of the tissue, and personal preference. Endoscopic harvesting of tissues for microsurgical grafting is possible in some circumstances. The success of microsurgery depends on several factors besides patient factors: (1) the individual and collective experiences of the surgical team and the members' ability to work together, relieving each other as necessary during long operations; (2) the surgeon's knowledge of the physiology of the microcirculation; (3) many hours of practice in the laboratory by the surgical team; and (4) the availability of proper microscopes, microvascular instruments, and microvascular suture.

Replantation of Amputated Body Part

Replantation is an attempt to reattach a completely amputated digit or other body part. Revascularization is the procedure performed on incomplete amputations, when the part remains attached to the body by skin, artery, vein, or nerve. Good candidates for replantation are those with the following amputations: (1) thumb, (2) multiple digits, (3) distal portion of hand at palm level, (4) wrist or forearm, (5) elbow and above the elbow, and (6) almost any body part of a child.

The success of digital replantation depends primarily on the microsurgical repair of one digital artery and two digital veins. Replantation of an amputated part is ideally performed within 4 to 6 hours after injury, but success has been reported up to 24 hours after injury if the amputated part has been cooled. Proper care of the amputated body part or parts before surgery is vital to successful replantation. The ultimate aim of replantation is the restitution of function beyond that provided by a prosthesis.

Procedural Considerations. A regional anesthetic is usually given to replantation patients if the anticipated length of surgery permits. Because of the length of these surgeries (12 to 16 hours), positioning is important. The OR bed and armboards should be carefully padded with pressure-reducing materials to support the supine patient. The surgeon may request the room temperature increased before the patient arrives because the warm room will reduce vasoconstriction in the extremities. A warming device, such as a forced-air warming blanket, is usually applied to maintain the patient's core body tempera-

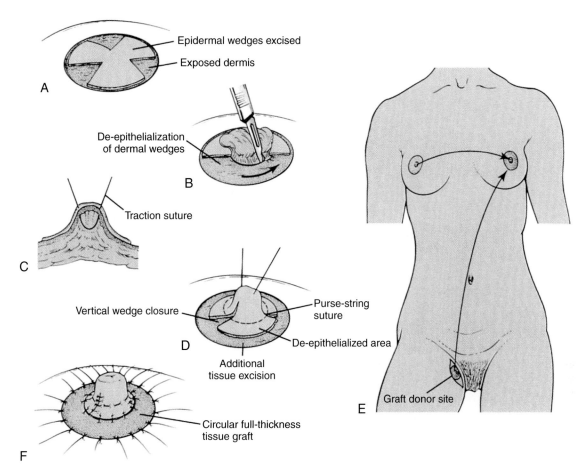

FIGURE 13-24 **A,** Circumferential demarcation of the nipple periphery with removal of dermal wedges. **B,** Dermal wedges are deepithelialized from the rim toward the center. **C,** A traction suture is used to elevate the central future nipple tip. **D,** Traction is applied to the future nipple tip as the wedges are approximated to create a permanent projected surface. A purse-string suture is placed, and excess tissue is excised. **E,** Possible full-thickness donor site areolar color match may be found in the labial folds. **F,** The donor graft is measured, cut, and secured to the dermal ring of the neonipple-areolar complex.

ture. The surgeon usually brings the amputated part to the OR before the patient arrives to ensure ample time for preparation of the amputated part for replantation. The amputated body part should be maintained by wrapping it in saline-soaked gauze sponges, placing it in an occlusive bag, and immersing it in a container of iced saline. If radiographs of the amputated body part and amputation site have not been taken before the patient's arrival in the OR the perioperative team should arrange for these to be taken. Radiographic films are crucial to determine bone trauma and loss.

The hand drape (described later in this paragraph) can be applied to either upper or lower extremities, as required by the surgical procedure. Before a hand drape is placed, a pneumatic tourniquet cuff is often applied to the upper arm over padding. The patient is supine on the OR bed, with the affected arm extended and supported on a hand table. While an assistant holds the patient's arm with both hands around the tourniquet cuff, the skin prep solution is applied from fingertips to tourniquet cuff. Care is taken to keep the cuff dry and free of solution. Then two folded barrier sheets are used to cover the hand table. The first sheet is placed with the folded edge nearest the patient (thus forming a cuff). A double-

thickness, 4-inch stockinette is used to cover the extremity, and the edge is rolled over the tourniquet. The upper arm and upper half of the body are covered by a folded sheet, with the folded edge placed across the part of the stockinette that covers the tourniquet cuff. A small, nonperforating towel clamp that grasps the edge of the folded top sheet, the stockinette, and the edge of the cuff of the bottom sheet is placed on each side of the arm. This excludes the tourniquet cuff from the sterile field. The remainder of the body is covered with one or two additional sheets. A commercially prepared extremity drape that has an aperture incorporated into the drape may also be used.

Instrumentation includes a plastic hand instrument set, microvascular instruments, a Kirschner wire driver, Kirschner wires, an operating microscope, and a bipolar ESU.

Operative Procedure
1. The surgeon shortens the bone ends to eliminate tension on vascular anastomoses to be done later; the bone is stabilized by means of internal fixation with Kirschner wires.
2. Flexor and extensor tendon repairs are usually performed next.

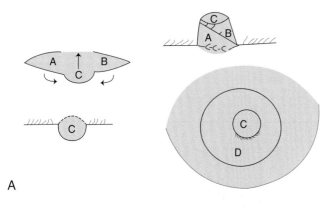

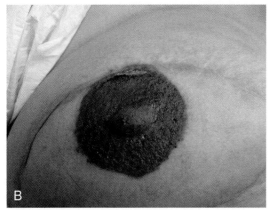

A

B

FIGURE 13-25 *A,* Breast nipple reconstruction. *A* and *B* represent wing flaps raised from side and wrapped around *C;* the central flap was raised superiorly. *D* represents areolar skin created with skin grafted either from pigmented groin skin or from opposite areolar skin by tattooing. *B,* Areolar tattoo.

3. The digital nerves are repaired with the aid of loupes or the operating microscope.
4. With microsurgical instruments and techniques, two digital veins are repaired, followed by repair of one digital artery. If ischemic time has been prolonged, digital vessel repair may precede repair of tendons and nerves.
5. The skin is sutured.
6. A bulky supportive hand dressing is applied.

Toe-to-Hand Transfer

The reconstructive procedure of toe-to-hand transfer involves surgical removal of a single toe or multiple toes and anastomosis of the vessels of the toes to those on the hand to restore finger and thumb functions. It is lengthy surgery (12 to 16 hours) and entails a two-team approach; one team is at the foot for toe removal, and one team is at the recipient site—the hand.

Procedural Considerations. The patient is placed in the supine position on the OR bed. The patient is administered an anticoagulation regimen during the anastomosis procedure. Two tourniquets are needed—one on the thigh of the operative foot and one on the operative arm. Both extremities are separately prepped and draped. Instrumentation includes a plastic hand set, microvascular instruments, power Kirschner wire driver, and Kirschner wires. Additional equipment includes the operating microscope, two tourniquet power

sources, two bipolar ESUs, a sterile marking pen, and an Esmarch bandage.

Operative Procedure

1. The surgeon preparing the hand determines adequate blood flow and vessel location on the thumb site (Figure 13-26, *A*). This may prevent a needless amputation of the toe.
2. Appropriate skin flaps are incised to expose the veins on the dorsum of the hand and clamped with vessel microclips.
3. The radial artery or its branches are dissected out and prepared for anastomosis.
4. The flexor and extensor pollicis longus tendons are located and transfixed.
5. The bone at the base of the thumb is prepared for the toe.
6. The nerves to the thumb are dissected out with adequate length for suturing without tension.
7. The toe is circumscribed with a racket-shaped incision (Figure 13-26, *B*), and the veins are isolated through the dorsal aspect and clamped with vessel microclips.
8. The extensor tendon is dissected proximally and transected over the base of the metatarsal.
9. The dorsalis pedis artery is dissected to the digital vessels with ligation of all branches of that vessel to prepare for the anastomosis.
10. On the plantar surface, the digital nerves and flexor tendons are transected at levels of adequate length for anastomosis (Figure 13-26, *C*).
11. The toe is transected at the level previously determined for adequate length of the thumb.
12. The toe vessels are anastomosed microsurgically to the thumb vessels. The toe is attached to the thumb area by Kirschner wires (Figure 13-26, *D*).

An aesthetic and functionally effective hand can be achieved through this procedure (Figure 13-26, *E*).

RECONSTRUCTIVE MAXILLOFACIAL SURGERY

The need for maxillofacial surgery results from blunt or penetrating trauma, disease, or congenital anomaly. Regardless of the cause, the principles are the same: establishment of preinjury/predisease/normal anatomic dental occlusion, anatomic reduction, stabilization of the fracture, and healing for functional results (Pfiedler Enterprises, 2007). The technique and approach must be individualized to optimize the visual reduction (or reconstruction) of the procedure as well as minimize facial scarring and nerve injury, whether it be a mandibular free flap tissue and bone reconstruction or open reduction and internal fixation of any number and combination of facial fractures. In addition to midface fractures, other common facial fractures include nasal, orbital (blow-out) floor, zygomatic, and mandibular fractures.

Procedural Considerations for Maxillofacial Surgery

The perioperative nurse and surgical technologist should consult with the surgeon about the precise injuries and the expected surgical treatment plan: open or closed reduction; intraoral or extraoral approach; the order of multiple procedures; need for intraoperative x-rays; and type, number, and

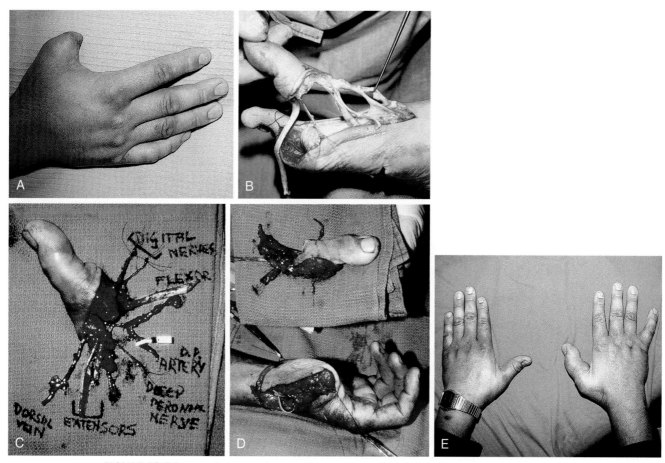

FIGURE 13-26 Toe-to-hand transfer. **A,** Preoperative appearance of hand. **B,** Harvest of toe. **C,** Identification of vessels and nerves. **D,** Transfer of toe to thumb site. **E,** Postoperative view of toe-to-thumb site transfer.

sizes of screws and compression plates to be placed if rigid fixation is to be employed. Orbital fractures may require alloplastic implant material. Wire is used less frequently for immobilization because of the greater degree of stability afforded by plating systems. The head should be immobilized and stabilized in a gel-type head ring; the position is almost always supine. Both eyes should be protected, and care must be taken not to displace endotracheal tubes. Instrumentation needs include a plastic surgery set, periosteal elevators, power drill for plating systems, bone hooks, Rowe disimpaction forceps (for maxillary fractures), the ESU, sterile marking pens, and suction. For application of arch bars, the surgical technologist should assemble arch bars, wires, elastics, wire cutters, wire twisters, and dull retractors for good exposure of the teeth.

Reduction of Nasal Fracture

Usually a closed reduction of the bony nasal fragments is performed by digital and instrumental manipulation. Occasionally an open reduction with interosseous wire fixation of nasal bone fragments is necessary. A nasal fracture may involve a fracture of the nasal bones or cartilage (including the septum). Closed reduction of a nasal fracture is most often performed with the patient administered topical and local anesthetics. Procedural considerations and the surgical intervention are described in Chapter 10.

Reduction of Orbital Floor Fractures

The orbital floor is the eggshell-thin bone on which the eye and periorbital tissues rest. It separates the orbit from the maxillary antrum. Orbital floor fractures usually occur in combination with fractures of the infraorbital rim (maxillary and zygomatic fractures). An isolated depressed orbital floor fracture with an intact infraorbital rim is called a *blow-out* fracture.

Fractures of the walls of the orbit may be caused by direct blows or by extension of a fracture line from adjacent bones. Isolated orbital floor, or blow-out, fractures usually occur after injury to the region of the eye by an object the size of an apple or an adult's fist (Figure 13-27). Orbital contents herniated into the maxillary sinus, and the inferior rectus or inferior oblique muscle, may become incarcerated at the fracture site. A Caldwell-Luc antrostomy may be done with reduction of the fracture from below, or the fracture site may be approached directly through the lower lid along the orbital floor; the prolapsed tissue is reduced, the orbital floor is reduced, and the orbital floor defect is bridged with bone grafts, molded metal implants, or plastic material.

Procedural Considerations. A graft set may be used for implantation of autogenous graft or synthetic graft materials of various sizes and thicknesses, along with a flexible

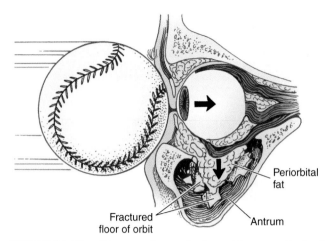

FIGURE 13-27 Ball has struck rim of orbit and has pressed orbital contents backward, displacing fragments of bone into maxillary sinus. Inferior rectus muscle is incarcerated in fracture. Inferior oblique muscle may also be involved.

narrow-width retractor. Interosseous wiring may be required for fractures of the frontozygomatic junction. Microplates and screws to stabilize fractures involving the fragile facial and orbital bones may also be used. A general anesthetic is usually administered.

Operative Procedure

1. The surgeon tests the maximum ocular rotation by exerting traction with a forceps on the tendon of the inferior rectus muscle to determine if the inferior muscle sling is trapped in the fracture.
2. To distribute tension over the lower lid and stretch the orbicularis muscle, the surgeon inserts a traction suture through the lower lid margin.
3. With a #3 knife handle and a #15 blade, the surgeon incises the lower lid in the lid fold above the orbital rim.
4. The skin is separated from the orbicularis muscle, and the orbital septum is identified by blunt dissection. Dissection is continued down to the periosteum of the orbital rim by means of scissors, loop retractors, elevators, and forceps.
5. The periosteum of the orbital rim is incised with a #15 blade. With periosteal elevators, the floor of the orbit is exposed and explored. When the fracture site is identified, bone spicules (needle-shaped bone fragments) are removed and the herniated contents are freed from the maxillary antrum. The contents of the orbit are elevated by means of narrow-width, flexible retractors. A 4-0 traction suture is placed around the tendon of the inferior rectus muscle.
6. An autogenous graft is taken from the iliac crest, or an alloplastic material of proper size is used to repair the bony defect. The material may or may not be anchored to the orbital rim by wire sutures.
7. The periosteum is carefully closed with 4-0 absorbable sutures.
8. The skin is closed with 6-0 nonabsorbable sutures, and a pressure dressing is applied.

Reduction of Zygomatic Fractures

Fractures of the zygoma (the cheek or malar bone) are corrected by either closed or open reduction. The two most com-

mon types of zygomatic fractures are depressed fractures of the arch and separation at or near the zygomaticofrontal, zygomaticomaxillary, and zygomaticotemporal suture lines, which constitutes a trimalar fracture. Although fractures of the zygoma can interfere with the ability to open and close the mouth properly, their chief consequence is a flattening of the cheek on the involved side, which results from a depressed trimalar or zygomatic arch fracture. Treatment is directed toward elevating the depressed fracture and maintaining the reduction. Closed reduction is the procedure used for treatment of zygomatic arch fractures, whereas most trimalar fractures are reduced by means of open reduction with internal fixation.

Procedural Considerations. A plastic instrument set, a Suraci zygoma hook-elevator, and a jaw hook are required for a closed reduction. A basic plastic instrument set, along with the following instruments and supplies, is required for an open reduction: a Hall II air drill; stainless-steel wires (#26, #28, and #30); the Suraci zygoma hook-elevator; a jaw hook; a Kerrison rongeur; two Blair retractors; the bipolar ESU; a sterile marking pen; epinephrine 1:200,000 for injection; and a miniplating rigid fixation set. The patient is placed in the supine position on the OR bed. The head drape is used.

Operative Procedure. Closed reduction is performed by elevating the depressed fracture with a percutaneous bone hook. Stabilization of a trimalar fracture may then be achieved by inserting a transantral Kirschner wire from the fractured side to the normal side.

The technique of open reduction of a trimalar fracture is as follows:
1. Incisions are marked along the lateral area of the eyebrow and lower eyelid over the zygomaticofrontal suture line and zygomaticomaxillary suture line (infraorbital rim) fractures, respectively.
2. After injection with epinephrine 1:200,000 for hemostasis, the surgeon incises along the premarked lines down to bone, and suture lines are identified and exposed.
3. The depressed zygoma is elevated with a Kelly hemostat or periosteal elevator placed behind the body of the zygoma through the lateral eyebrow incision. Bone hooks placed percutaneously or at the fracture sites may be used instead.
4. The surgeon drills holes into bone on each side of the fracture lines. Stainless-steel wires are passed through the hole and twisted down tightly to maintain the reduction. (Reduction and stabilization of two of the three fractures are sufficient.) Alternative methods of stabilization of the fractures are interosseous wiring of the zygomaticofrontal fracture and placement of a transmural Kirschner wire or stabilization with micro/mini plates and screws.
5. Using a subcuticular technique, the surgeon closes the incisions.
6. An eye-patch dressing may be applied.

Reduction of Maxillary Fractures

Midface fractures are usually classified according to a system developed in the early 1900s by Dr. Rene Le Fort: (1) Le Fort I, or transverse maxillary, fracture—this horizontal fracture includes the nasal floor, septum, and teeth; (2) Le Fort II, or pyramidal maxillary, fracture (unilateral or bilateral)—this type often involves the nasal cavity, hard palate, and the orbital rim;

and (3) Le Fort III, or craniofacial dysjunction, fracture—this type includes fractures of both zygomas and the nose (Pfiedler Enterprises, 2007) (Figure 13-28). Like a mandibular fracture, a maxillary fracture also produces malocclusion. In addition, depending on the severity of the fracture, it may produce considerable deformity of the middle of the face, usually perceived as a flattening or smashed-in appearance.

Closed reduction with intermaxillary fixation suffices for treatment of Le Fort I and some Le Fort II fractures. The more severe Le Fort II and all Le Fort III fractures require open reduction in addition to intermaxillary fixation.

Procedural Considerations. The basic plastic instrument set is required as well as an air drill; stainless-steel wires (#25, #26, and #28); Rowe maxillary forceps, right and left; a Brown fascia needle; polyethylene buttons (for suspension wire pull-through for Le Fort III repair); a small, foam-rubber pad; a sterile marking pen or methylene blue; the ESU; epinephrine 1:200,000 for injection; periosteal elevators; and a rigid fixation system. A separate Mayo setup for the application of arch bars is required, as described for reduction of mandibular fractures. The patient is placed in the supine position on the OR bed. The head drape is used.

Operative Procedure. Arch bars are applied before or after the open reduction, or they may be the only mode of treatment in closed reduction. In addition to ligating the maxillary arch bar to the teeth, it must also be suspended from stable bones superior to the fractured maxilla (which is unstable). In Le Fort I fractures, suspension may be around both zygomatic arches by passage of percutaneous wires. In Le Fort II and Le Fort III fractures, suspension wires are placed through holes drilled bilaterally into the zygomatic process of the frontal bone. This requires incisions into both lateral eyebrow areas. The following description pertains to open reduction of Le Fort II and Le Fort III fractures:

1. After injection of epinephrine 1:200,000 for hemostasis, the surgeon makes bilateral incisions to expose the infraorbital rims and zygomaticofrontal suture lines.
2. The surgeon applies Rowe maxillary forceps intranasally and intraorally to disimpact and reduce the maxilla. Holes are drilled into bone on each side of fracture lines along the infraorbital rim (and zygomaticofrontal area for Le Fort III fractures, after reducing the zygomatic fractures).
3. Stainless-steel wires are passed through these holes and twisted down tightly to maintain the reduction.
4. Suspension wires are passed from the eyebrow incisions, behind the zygomatic arches, and into the mouth with the Brown fascia needle. A pullout wire is looped through each suspension wire within the eyebrow incision, brought out through the skin near the hairline, and tied down over a polyethylene button and foam-rubber padding. Self-tapping screws, mini compression plates, and bone grafts may also be used, based on the surgeon's preference. Incisions are closed.
5. When indicated, reduction of a nasal fracture is then performed.

Reduction of Mandibular Fractures

The purpose of treatment for a mandibular fracture is to restore the patient's preinjury dental occlusion. With some types of fractures, a closed reduction with immobilization by means of intermaxillary fixation is sufficient for treatment. With a

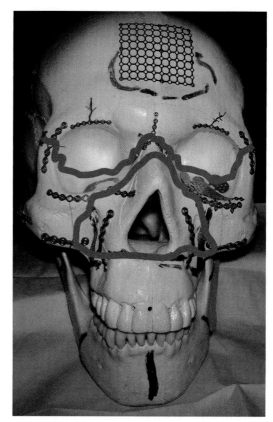

FIGURE 13-28 Practice skulls are provided in seminars to practice fixation techniques. See text for Le Fort classification of fractures.

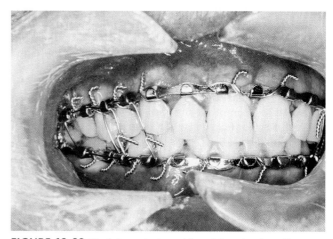

FIGURE 13-29 Teeth in occlusion with arch bars in place. Tongs on arch bars will accept latex bands, which maintain occlusion for several weeks (wires around tongs are shown).

majority of mandibular fractures, however, an open reduction with wire fixation is necessary, plus supplemental intermaxillary fixation to achieve adequate immobilization for healing.

Intermaxillary fixation is most often accomplished when arch bars are applied to the maxillary and mandibular teeth. Stainless-steel wires (#24 or #25) are placed around the necks of the teeth and are ligated around the arch bars to hold the latter in place. Latex bands are attached to the tongs on the maxillary and mandibular arch bars to fix the teeth in occlusion (Figure 13-29). If the patient is edentulous, arch bars are attached to dentures or specially fabricated dental splints. The dentures or splints are held in place by means of wires placed around the mandible (for the mandibular arch bar) and through the nasal spine and around the zygomatic arches (for the maxillary arch bar). Scissors or wire cutters must be sent with the patient to the PACU and the postoperative patient care unit to prevent aspiration if the patient vomits or chokes.

Procedural Considerations—Open Reduction.
In addition to a basic plastic instrument set, the following instruments and supplies are needed for an open reduction of a fractured mandible: a Hall II air drill, two Dingman bone-holding forceps, a nerve stimulator, a sterile marking pen, stainless-steel wires (#24, #26, and #28), the ESU, epinephrine 1:200,000 for injection, and a rigid fixation system.

For the application of arch bars or other types of interdental wiring techniques, a separate Mayo setup with the following instruments and supplies is required: a set of coil arch bars and latex bands; stainless-steel wire (#25 or #26); two Mayo-Hegar needle holders, 8 inch; a wire suture scissors, 4¾ inch; a wire twister; a Yankauer suction tube; two Wieder tongue depressors, large and small; six mosquito hemostats, curved, 5¼ inch; a Brown fascia needle (if dentures or splints are used); a Freer septal elevator; and a small drain.

If arch bars are applied before the open reduction is performed, this former setup must be kept completely separate from the instruments used for the open reduction. Because the mouth is a contaminated area, a complete change of gowns, gloves, and drapes is necessary after the intraoral procedure.

Operative Procedure
1. Arch bars may be applied before or after the open reduction.
2. A line inferior and parallel to the lower border of the mandible at the fracture site is marked, and the area is infiltrated with epinephrine 1:200,000 for hemostasis.
3. The surgeon places the incision to expose the inferior border of the mandible. The nerve stimulator may be used to aid in identification of the marginal mandibular branch of the facial nerve in fractures of the posterior body and angle of the mandible.
4. The fracture is reduced by manipulation. Holes are drilled into the mandible on each side of the fracture line with the Hall II air drill while an assistant holds the reduced fracture with the aid of Dingman bone-holding forceps.
5. Stainless-steel wire is inserted through the holes and twisted tightly to secure the fracture fragments in anatomic alignment.
6. In the event that rigid fixation is desired with the use of plates and screws, the appropriate drill bit, tap, and depth gauge are chosen. With these items, the proper-size prosthesis is placed and the fracture is approximated, aligned, and placed in anatomic position.
7. A small drain is sometimes placed into the wound, and the wound is closed in layers (periosteum, platysma muscle, and skin).
8. The latex bands may be applied to the arch bars at this time but more frequently are applied later, after the patient is fully awake and reactive.
9. A moderate compression dressing is applied to cover the submandibular wound and drain.

Elective Orthognathic Surgery

A large number of patients have either acquired or congenital facial defects that affect the maxilla, the mandible, or both. The condition of many of these patients can be improved dramatically with orthodontic care; however, many also require surgical rearrangement of the maxilla or mandible.

Procedural Considerations.
Psychosocial and functional deficits are related to abnormalities of the maxilla and mandible. Surgical correction of these defects can improve patients' quality of life. Surgery is usually delayed until an adequate number of permanent teeth are in place for postoperative immobilization. Coordinated preoperative planning is of great importance to the success of these procedures.

Operative Procedure
1. Arch bars are applied for postoperative immobilization.
2. Intraoral incisions provide exposure.
3. The maxilla or mandible is cut as indicated by the preoperative workup.
4. Bone is advanced or set back to a predetermined position.
5. Bones are wired in place, with grafts placed in defects as needed.

GENDER REASSIGNMENT

Transsexualism is defined as the condition in which an individual with chromosomes and internal and external organs normal to one gender identifies psychologically and socially with attributes of the opposite gender. Reassignment of gender by means of surgery is the last step to be taken in treatment of transsexuals. It is performed only after the patient has been treated with hormones of the opposite gender, has experienced a period of cross-gender living, and has had intensive psychiatric evaluation. Most institutions performing this type of surgery have gender-identity teams who evaluate and treat transsexuals. These teams usually include a variety of professionals: psychiatrist, psychologist, endocrinologist, plastic surgeon, urologist, gynecologist, and social worker.

The surgical techniques for assignment of male to female are technically easier. A breast augmentation may be performed if hormone therapy has not sufficiently changed breast size. Construction of the neovagina includes radical penectomy, bilateral orchiectomy, urethroplasty, perineal dissection, creation of a neovaginal vault, vaginoplasty, and vulvoplasty.

The surgical technique for female to male is technically more difficult and requires multiple surgical procedures. Considerations that must be addressed are twofold: the neophallus must be constructed to (1) allow the patient to stand to void and (2) permit stimulation of a sexual partner during intercourse. This may require a radial artery forearm free flap with a later-stage surgical insertion of a penile prosthesis for attaining an erection.

AESTHETIC SURGERY

Aesthetic surgery may be performed after induction of general anesthesia, monitored anesthesia care, or local anesthesia with moderate sedation.

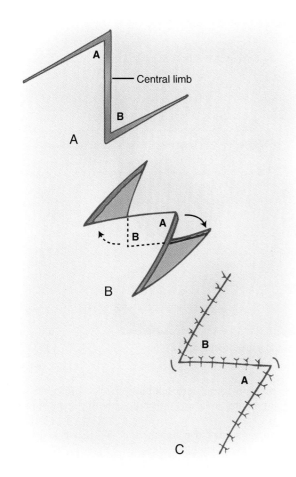

FIGURE 13-30 Z-plasty for scar revision. **A,** The central limb of the Z-plasty is over the scar that needs to be revised. **B,** Two other limbs are incised—each equal in length to the central limb and diverging from it at an equal angle. The flaps are then transposed. **C,** Flaps transposed, and original Z rotated 90 degrees and reversed.

Scar Revision

Scar revision involves the rearranging or reshaping of an existing scar so that the scar is less noticeable. The simplest form of scar revision is excision of an existing scar and simple resuturing of the wound. This may improve scars that are wide.

The Z-plasty is the most widely used method of scar revision (Figure 13-30). It breaks up linear scars, rearranging them so that the central limb of the Z lies in the same direction as a natural skin line. Scars that are parallel to skin lines are less noticeable than scars that are perpendicular to skin lines. A contracted scar line can also be lengthened with a Z-plasty.

Procedural Considerations. A plastic local instrument set and a sterile marking pen are required. The procedure may be performed with the patient administered a local or general anesthetic. The patient is positioned, prepped, and draped so that the scar that is to be revised is well exposed.

Operative Procedure
1. The surgeon marks the pattern for the planned revision.
2. The scar is excised.

3. The surrounding tissue is undermined, and the wound edges are approximated according to the surgeon's markings.
4. Dressings may or may not be applied.

Endoscopic Brow Lift

The aging process affects the area above the eyes and brows in several ways. Loss of skin elasticity can cause the appearance of a heavy brow and emphasize hooding of the upper eyelids. Repetitive muscle action results in horizontal forehead lines and furrows as well as creases between the brows. The goal of endoscopic brow/forehead surgery is to minimize the heaviness of the brow and improve the frown lines of aging, reduce upper eyelid hooding, reposition the eyebrows if necessary, and create a more youthful, refreshed appearance of the forehead and brow area, all through multiple, short incisions in the scalp.

Procedural Considerations. Positioning the patient at the very top of the OR bed is necessary for good utilization and mobility of the endoscopic instruments. For patients with medium to long hair, the hair may be sectioned and tied with sterilized rubber bands to minimize interference with the planned incision. The surgeon marks the patient's incision lines and anatomic landmarks before the surgery. The entire head (scalp, face, ears, and neck) should be prepped and draped with impervious drape material. The patient's eyes may be protected with ointment and shields for the duration of the procedure; ear canals may also be protected from pooling of prep solution by using sterile cotton balls. During preparation of the room, the perioperative nurse and surgical technologist perform a check of all endoscopic equipment to ensure it is functioning properly. Endoscopic instrumentation includes elevators, scissors, clamps, needle holders, camera, and light sources. Depending on the method of fixation, screws and accompanying instrumentation may be necessary.

Operative Procedure
1. The surgeon injects a local anesthetic and places three to five small scalp incisions (one midline and one or two paramedian).
2. Using blunt dissection, the surgeon elevates the forehead skin.
3. The endoscope is placed to allow visualization of muscles, vessels, nerves, and tissues.
4. Using endoscopic instruments the surgeon dissects the corrugator and procerus muscles and soft tissues. The area is redraped to produce a smoother appearance and desired repositioning of brows.
5. Screws are placed in the outer table of the cranium at designated points, and sutures are placed through the galea and tied around screws to facilitate elevation of the brow and forehead.
6. The surgeon staples or sutures the scalp incisions for closure.

Rhytidectomy (Facelift)

As the aging process progresses, the skin of the face and neck becomes loose and redundant. This is particularly noticeable in the "jowl" areas and just beneath the chin. A facelift is performed to correct the sagging skin. A common misconception is that a facelift involves only the face. Actually, one of the most common complaints of aging is the appearance of the neck and submental skin. The typical facelift treats the face and neck and involves removal and redraping of excess skin of the face and neck once repositioning of the underlying muscle and

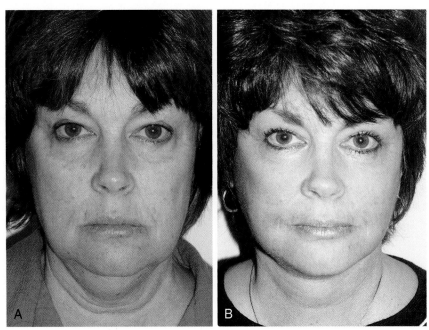

FIGURE 13-31 A, Preoperative and **B,** postoperative rhytidectomy.

platysma has been performed. The result is a smooth, rested appearance, without unnatural tightness or distortion of facial features (Figure 13-31). Rather than excising the redundant skin directly, incisions adjacent to or within hairlines are used so that the scars are virtually indiscernible.

Procedural Considerations. The patient is positioned supine with the head and shoulders slightly elevated. Attention should be given to safety by using proper positioning to prevent pressure injuries, using sequential compression devices (SCDs), maintaining normothermia, and preventing eye injuries by using shields. Depending on the complexity of the procedure and planned surgical time, the urinary catheter may be inserted.

Specialized scissors of varying lengths should be available, along with smooth and toothed tissue forceps and various sizes of needle holders. A fiberoptic lighted retractor is standard for facelifts. To avoid flash sterilization, contact with the surgeon or office staff should be initiated before the day of surgery to discuss special requests.

There are numerous techniques for rhytidectomy, and a well-prepared surgical technologist will ask the surgeon about the specific technique in order to have the appropriate suture material and special needles available. The underlying superficial muscular aponeurotic system (SMAS) may be repositioned, the cheek may be elevated independently, the midface may be lifted, and there may or may not be accompanying liposuction. Facelift procedures are customized specific to the anatomic needs of the individual patient. The entire head, neck, ears, and scalp are prepped and draped.

Operative Procedure
1. The surgeon marks bilateral incision lines from the temporal scalp, around the earlobe, around the posterior margin of the auricula, and into the occipital scalp (Figures 13-32 and 13-33).

2. The incision lines, both temples, cheeks, upper neck, and the submental area are injected with the local anesthetic agent.
3. The surgeon may use liposuction on the neck, jowls, or cheeks before placing the incisions.
4. After the incisions are made, the surgeon elevates the temporal and cheek skin. The SMAS is plicated cephalad and caudally, elevating and tightening the SMAS and platysma.
5. The surgeon elevates and repositions the malar pad; it is then anchored with suture.
6. The facial skin flap is then elevated in a superior and slightly posterior direction and tacked, and excess skin is trimmed at the flap edges.
7. Through a submental incision, the surgeon undermines the neck, and identifies and plicates the plastysmal bands. Excess tissue is trimmed and tacked postauricularly. Small drains are placed beneath the skin flaps and secured.
8. Incisions are closed in one or two layers.
9. A moderate pressure dressing is applied.

Blepharoplasty

The aging process causes a sagging or relaxation of eyelid skin and the orbital septum. As the latter becomes weaker, it allows periorbital fat to bulge. These changes are perceived as baggy eyelids, which give the patient a chronically tired appearance. The goal of blepharoplasty is to improve the patient's appearance by removing excess eyelid skin, removing or repositioning bulging periorbital fat, and tightening and smoothing the muscles under the eye (Figure 13-34). The upper eyelid skin can be so redundant that it encroaches on the patient's field of vision, and removal of excessive hooding of the upper eyelid skin may even improve peripheral vision. The upper eyelid crease may also be enhanced. Not all patients need removal of skin; for selected individuals, CO_2 skin resurfacing may be the procedure of choice to achieve

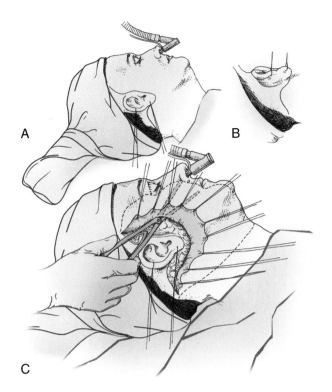

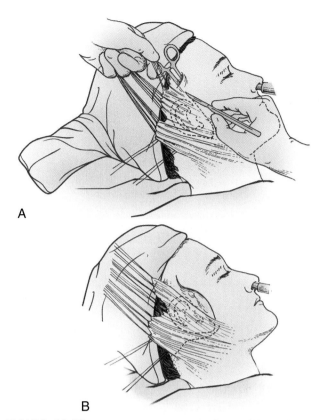

FIGURE 13-32 Rhytidectomy: line of incision and undermining. **A,** Traction sutures of 4-0 silk placed into auricle; temporal incision curved posteriorly for better support of upward pull. **B,** Incision carried under earlobe and then curved posteriorly upward and then caudad toward midline. **C,** Skin undermined almost to nasolabial fold, to area of mental foramen, and to midline of neck as far down as thyroid cartilage. Care is taken to avoid injury to submandibular branches of facial nerve and facial artery.

FIGURE 13-33 Rhytidectomy: removal of superfluous skin. **A,** Skin drawn upward to proper degree of tension, and incision made along posterior margin of clamp. **B,** Incision continued upward around posterior margin of auricle and then backward to excise skin specimen.

a smoother appearance of the lower eyelid skin. Incisions in the subconjunctival mucosa of the lower lids are sometimes used for this group of patients if resection or repositioning of the periorbital fat is also indicated. Blepharoplasty is often performed with rhytidectomy. Blepharoplasty may be performed on both the upper and lower lids, upper lids only, or lower lids only.

Procedural Considerations. A plastic local instrument set is required. Delicate, short instruments are used, with special attention to scissors (curved Kaye blepharoplasty); fine Adson forceps with teeth; calipers; and fixation forceps. Webster needle holders are frequently desired. A bipolar ESU unit may be used. A needle tip for the active electrode may be requested if the monopolar ESU is used. (With the monopolar ESU, a lower setting is used. The perioperative nurse should verbally repeat back the settings requested by the surgeon.) Blepharoplasty is usually performed using a local anesthetic with monitored anesthesia care. The patient is in the supine position on the OR bed. The face is prepped, and the head drape is used. Corneal shields may be used to protect the cornea.

Operative Procedure—Upper Lids
1. The surgeon marks the lines of incision and injects local anesthetic.

2. The incision is placed, and excess skin is removed. Hemostasis is obtained (Figure 13-35, *A* to *C*).
3. The surgeon trims the orbicularis oculi muscle and identifies and excises the septum orbitale. Excess periorbital fat is trimmed and coagulated.
4. Upper lid incisions are closed; and the procedure is repeated for the opposite upper lid.
5. Finely crushed ice on moist gauze 4 × 4 pads may be applied to the periorbital region; other means of reducing swelling, such as cold compresses or a mechanical cold mask, may be similarly applied. Compresses are changed as often as they become warm.

Operative Procedure—Lower Lids
1. The surgeon marks the lines of incision and injects local anesthetic.
2. A subciliary incision (1 mm below eyelashes) is made and brought out in a natural line in the outer canthal skin.
3. The skin-muscle flap is raised, leaving a 3-mm strip of muscle attached to the tarsus (Figure 13-35, *D*).
4. The skin-muscle flap is dissected down below the level of the orbital rim.
5. The surgeon incises the arcus marginalis, and redundant fat with the overlying septum orbitale is draped over the orbital rim (Figure 13-35, *E*) and sutured.

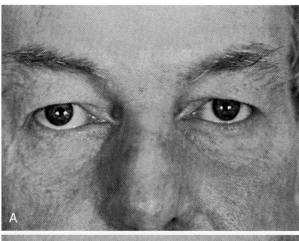

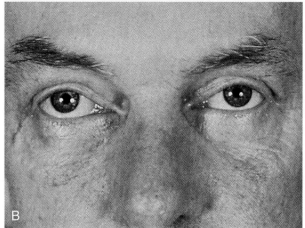

FIGURE 13-34 **A**, Preoperative and **B**, postoperative blepharoplasty.

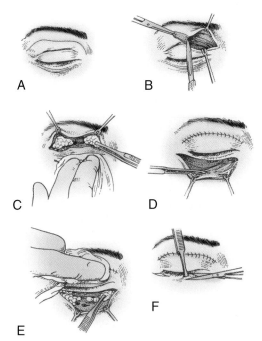

FIGURE 13-35 Blepharoplasty for baggy eyelids. **A**, Areas of proposed skin excision marked with methylene blue or a sterile marking pen. **B**, Strip of skin excised from upper lid; fat pad shining through orbital fascia and orbicular muscle of eye. **C**, Orbital fascia opened in two places (medially and laterally). Pressure on eyeball causes fat pads to bulge. They are eased out meticulously. **D**, Upper lid incision sutured with continuous 6-0 suture material of choice. Orbital muscle fibers of lower lid are separated from skin. **E**, Orbital fascia opened; fat pads bulge because of digital pressure and are teased out meticulously. **F**, Skin tailored to fit and sutured.

6. Hemostasis is obtained. Skin is redraped in an upward and outward fashion with attention to prevention of ectropion.
7. Excess skin is trimmed (Figure 13-35, *F*).
8. Lateral muscle is sutured to periosteum.
9. The surgeon closes the lower lid incision, and repeats the procedure for the opposite lower lid.
10. Compresses are applied as described in the upper lid procedure.

Rhinoplasty

Deformities of the external nose and nasal septum may be congenital or secondary to previous trauma. The goal of rhinoplasty is to improve the appearance of the external nose. This is accomplished by reshaping the underlying framework of the nose, which allows the overlying skin and subcutaneous tissue to redrape over the new framework. Reshaping the nasal skeleton usually includes use of a rasp for dorsal hump reduction, partial excision of lateral and alar cartilages, shortening of the septum, and osteotomy of nasal bones. A procedure to alter the nasal septum—septoplasty, or submucous resection (SMR)—often accompanies rhinoplasty. The goal of SMR is to improve the nasal airway by resecting a segment of septal cartilage. Septoplasty reshapes the existing septal cartilage; it may aid in altering the appearance of the nose or in improving the airway. Rhinoplasty may be performed as an open procedure by making an external incision across the base of the columella, or it may be performed entirely through the nostrils by

using internal incisions. Small external incisions at the alar bases are used to narrow the nostrils, and internal incisions placed alongside the base of the nasal bones are used to narrow the entire nose once the hump is removed or dorsum is incised. A full description of rhinologic procedures may be found in Chapter 10.

Laser Surgery

Several different types of lasers are commonly used in plastic and reconstructive surgery (Box 13-3). One of the most popular types of laser is the skin resurfacing, or CO_2, laser. The laser is attracted to the water in the skin cells and ablates the cells at a predetermined depth. The collagen material is also heated, resulting in smoother and slightly tighter skin. This treatment has virtually replaced dermabrasion, because it is much more consistent in terms of depth of penetration and less dependent on user technique or skill.

Tattoo removal and destruction of vascular lesions, such as facial telangiectasias, spider veins, and hemangiomas, may be achieved with the use of other types of lasers. Whether using lasers for skin resurfacing or tattoo removal procedures, the areas must first be numbed with a local anesthetic. Use of sedation depends on the anxiety level of the patient as well as the total surface area to be treated. Vascular lesions may be treated without local anesthesia, although there is some temporary discomfort with each pulse of the laser.

Liposuction

Liposuction is a surgical technique designed to remove excess deposits of fat and improve the contour of the body (Figure 13-36). It is not a treatment for obesity or simply a weight reduction procedure; rather, the ideal candidate is of normal weight and desires to remove localized fat that has proved resistant despite diet and exercise. By extension, liposuction patients must adhere to lifestyle changes (e.g., proper nutrition, adequate exercise) to maintain optimal results (Logan and Broughton, 2008). Although most often associated with contour correction, liposuction may also be used for treatment of gynecomastia or to remove lipomas. Areas that may be suctioned include face, neck, back, breasts (not a replacement for reduction mammoplasty, only contour correction), waist, abdomen, midriff, flanks, upper arms, hips, medial and lateral thighs, knees, and ankles (Figures 13-37 and 13-38).

Multiple techniques have been developed to enhance the final results as well as ease the removal of the fat. These techniques are not always used in isolation of each other; rather, some may be combined both to achieve the best possible outcome and to address the surgeon's preferences. Each procedure has specific equipment needed for that technique and often has highly specific cannulae and other instrumentation. Since multiple areas are usually treated, the surgical technologist should determine the sequence of liposuction the surgeon prefers to be prepared for positioning.

Procedural Considerations. Immediate preoperative preparation includes asking the patient to stand while the area of deformity is outlined. The surgeon usually draws two lines on the skin surface—one delineating the major area of defect and the other placed a short distance outside the first area. These lines make it easier for the surgeon to make a smooth transition toward the normal tissue by adjusting the amount of fat removed from the center to the periphery of the deformity. The patient may remain standing and be prepped circumferentially with a spray bottle of antimicrobial skin solution.

Preoperative patient education should include a discussion of the compression garment, which is typically worn for 2 to 4 weeks postoperatively. Patients should also be informed about the likelihood of the puncture sites leaking tumescent solution during the first 24 hours of the postoperative period. Absorbent dressings are required to minimize soiling of clothing and bedding during this period as well as to maintain the cleanliness of the compression garment.

Depending on the areas targeted for liposuction, draping may require a good deal of innovation. Minimal instrumentation is necessary—knife handle, towel clips, tissue forceps, scissors, clamps, and needle holder are used along with the suction cannulae specific to the proposed liposuction technique. A general anesthetic, moderate sedation, or epidural anesthetic may or may not be used. However, the surgeon typically injects a medicated solution into the fatty areas before removal because of concerns about large fluid volume shift and blood loss after lipectomy. The solution contains IV solution (e.g., lactated Ringer's), lidocaine, and epinephrine. Using more than 70 ml/kg of wetting solution for infiltration can lead to fluid overload; this may present as increased blood pressure, jugular vein distention, bounding pulses, cough, dyspnea, lung crackles, and pulmonary edema. For safety issues, the nurse and surgical technologist need to communicate and verify with the surgeon the total lipoaspirate and volume of wetting solution used. Additionally, it is imperative that warmed wetting solution be used for suction-assisted lipectomy (Logan and Broughton, 2008).

In the tumescent technique, large volumes of this solution are administered. The "super-wet" technique uses less solution; usually the amount of fluid injected approximates the amount of fat to be removed—thus the name, which refers to the swollen and firm ("tumesced") state of the tissues when they are filled with solution. The perioperative nurse and surgical technologist should inquire if the surgeon will be infiltrating tumescent solution and, if so, what ingredients are used for his or her technique. Also, they should ask whether the surgeon uses internal or external ultrasound (sound waves that liquefy fat) or power-assisted liposuction. One of the newer techniques is the use of

---

BOX 13-3

Lasers in Plastic Surgery

Common uses for lasers in plastic surgery include exfoliation, treatment of vascular malformations, removal of hair and tattoos, and tightening of collagen fibers in aging skin. A variety of lasers are available; selection of the appropriate laser is dependent on the patient's diagnosis because the effect of the laser on the skin tissue is dependent on its wavelength. The types of lasers and their common uses are described below.

Laser	Use
CO_2	Desiccation of benign lesions of skin, skin resurfacing, cutting tissue
Excimer	Eye surgery, psoriasis
Argon	Hemangiomas, telangiectasias
Nd:YAG	Benign pigmented lesions and red tattoos
Candela dye	Tattoos, pigmented benign lesions, hemangiomas
Helium-neon	Biostimulation, wound healing alleviation, acupuncture
Diode	Hair removal, tattoo removal
Ruby	Nevi removal, dark tattoos
Erbium:YAG	Rhytides
Q-Switch	Benign pigmented lesions and dark tattoos

Continued

BOX 13-3

Lasers in Plastic Surgery—cont'd

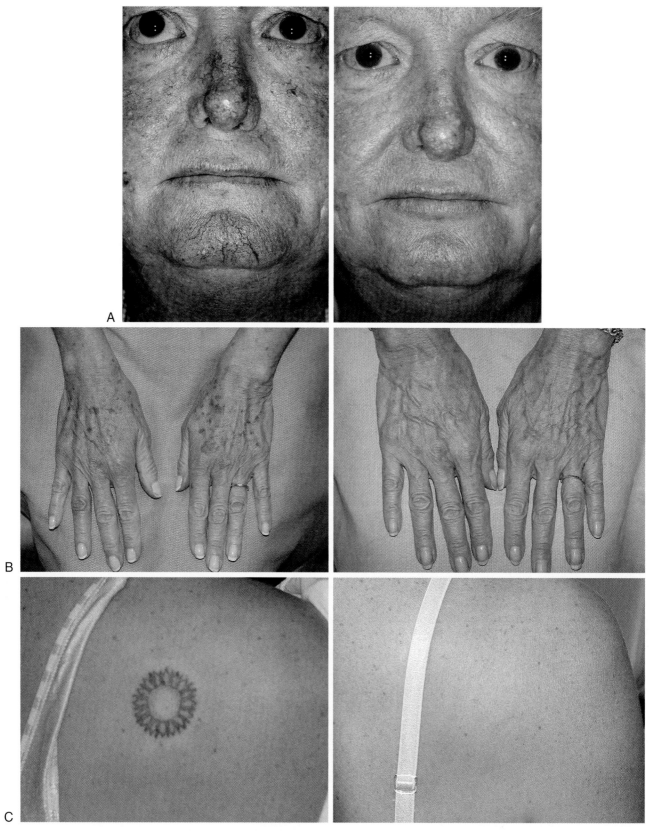

A, Laser removal of large facial telangiectasia. B, Laser removal of photoaging and lentigines on hands of woman in her sixties. C, Laser removal of multicolored tattoo on the posterior shoulder.

BOX 13-3

Lasers in Plastic Surgery—cont'd

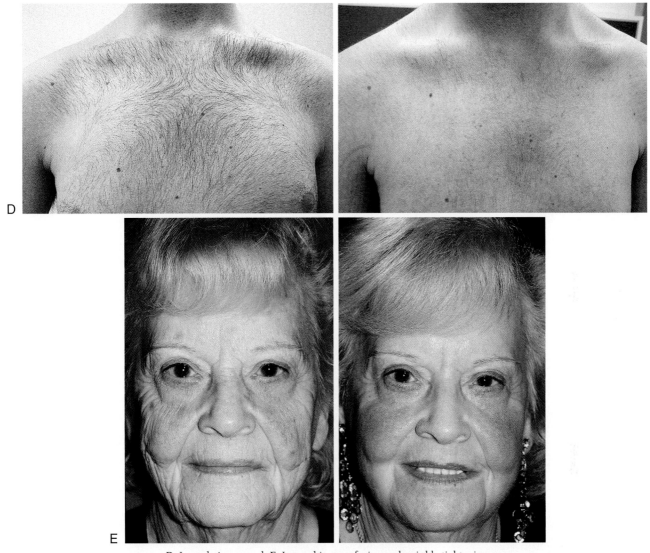

D, Laser hair removal. **E,** Laser skin resurfacing and wrinkle tightening.

Modified from Choi JE et al: Treatment of Becker's nevi with a long-pulse alexandrite laser, *Dermatol Surg*, April 27 [Epub ahead of print], 2009; Kono T et al: Long-pulsed neodymium:yttrium-aluminum-garnet laser treatment for hypertrophic port-wine stains on the lips, *J Cosmet Laser Ther* 11(1):11-13, 2009; Krupashankar DS: Standard guidelines of care: CO_2 laser for removal of benign skin lesions and resurfacing, IADVL Dermatosurgery Task Force, *Indian J Dermatol Venereol Leprol* 74(suppl):S61-S67, 2008; Mendonca DA et al: Venous malformations of the limbs: the Birmingham experience, comparisons and classification in children, *J Plast Reconstr Aesthet Surg*, Dec 27 [Epub ahead of print], 2008; Onesti MG: Surgical and laser treatment of Sturge-Weber syndrome, *Aesthet Plast Surg*, Mar 19 [Epub ahead of print], 2009.

VASER (vibration amplification of sound energy at resonance) liposelection or VASER-assisted liposuction, which incorporates thermal energy to liquefy the fat, thus aiding greatly in its removal.

Operative Procedure

1. The surgeon places stablike incisions in concealed areas to access sites to be liposuctioned.
2. Tumescent solution is infused.
3. Depending on technique, at this point either internal or external ultrasound or the VASER technique is performed at predetermined settings and length of time.
4. Liposuction is performed with the use of various sizes and lengths of cannulae. The cannula is attached to large-bore, firm suction tubing and connected to an aspirating unit. The high vacuum pressure caused by the unit causes the fat cells to emulsify so that they can be suctioned through the vacuum opening near the rounded tip of the cannula. Areas are usually cross-suctioned to achieve the best outcomes. Stab wounds may be closed with absorbable suture or left open to drain.
5. The patient's skin is cleaned, and bulky dressings and compression garments are applied.

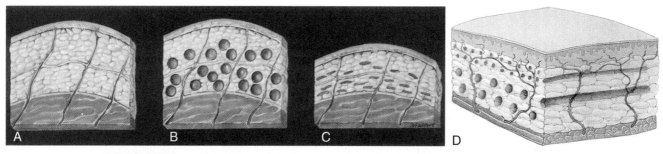

FIGURE 13-36 A, Normal appearance of excess fat. **B,** Removal of deep fat by larger-diameter cannulae. **C,** Corrected contour following removal of excess fat by liposuction. **D,** Removal of superficial fat involves using narrower-gauge cannulae.

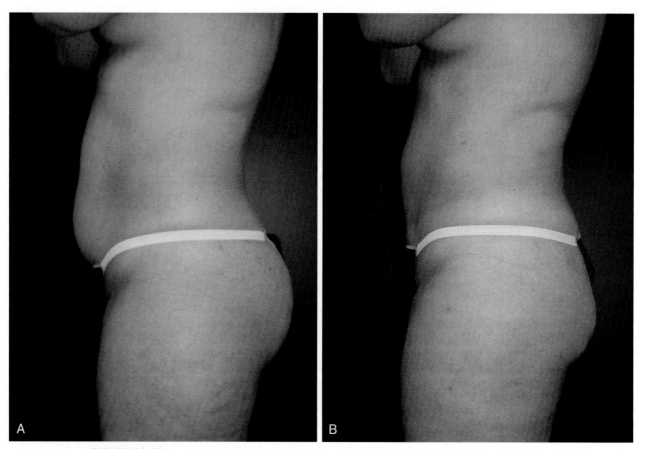

FIGURE 13-37 Female 43-year-old patient. **A,** Before and **B,** 6 months after liposuction of the abdomen and buttocks.

Abdominoplasty

Abdominoplasty is particularly useful in improving the appearance (and to a certain extent, function) of persons who have lost a great deal of weight or who suffer from laxity of abdominal skin following pregnancy. Obesity produces distention and stretching of the skin of the abdomen. Weight loss reduces the volume of the underlying fat; however, it does not produce concomitant reduction in the excess surface area of the overlying skin, which results from destruction or insufficiency of elastic fibers in the skin. The rectus abdominis fascia is also stretched in obese patients, and weight loss does not restore its integrity.

There are several versions of the abdominoplasty procedure and the choice of which technique to use depends upon the degree of deformity of the abdominal skin and muscle. All techniques are designed to improve the appearance of the abdomen by tightening the abdominal area (abdominal wall/rectus muscles) and removing excess skin or fullness.

If there is minimal to no laxity of the skin and mostly fullness of the lower abdomen, then a "mini-abdominoplasty" may be indicated. With this technique it is not necessary to relocate or incise the umbilicus and a short incision, resembling a Pfannenstiel, may be effectively utilized. However, if there is laxity of the periumbilical and upper and lower abdominal skin accompanied by protrusion of the abdomi-

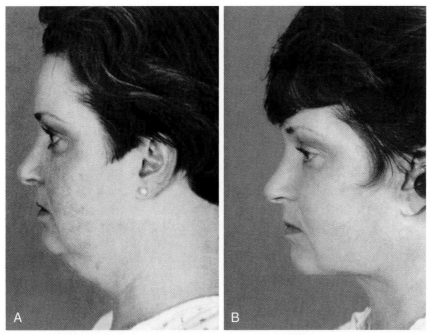

FIGURE 13-38 Submental liposuction. **A,** Preoperative. **B,** Postoperative.

nal wall with diastasis (separation) of the rectus muscle, then full abdominoplasty is the procedure of choice. This version requires relocation of the umbilicus and an incision that stretches from hip to hip. Endoscopic abdominoplasty is another option if only muscle repair (correction of the diastasis deformity or shortening of the rectus muscles) is needed.

Procedural Considerations. A basic plastic instrument set is required, as well as extra retractors and clamping instruments, an ESU, and a sterile marking pen. Frequently tumescent anesthetic solution will be added to minimize bleeding, reduce postoperative discomfort, and aid in dissection. The perioperative nurse and surgical technologist should ask the surgeon about the use of tumescent as well as preference for ingredients. A lighted fiberoptic retractor should be available. Sequential compression devices or antiembolism hose are usually in place or applied in the OR. The patient is in the supine position with slight flexion at the hips. Draping is such that the entire abdomen, lower costal margins, upper thighs, and both anterior iliac spines are exposed.

Operative Procedure
1. The surgeon makes a low transverse abdominal incision across both inguinal areas laterally and the superior border of the mons pubis in the midline down to fascia.
2. A large flap of skin and subcutaneous tissue is elevated away from the fascia of the anterior abdominal wall.
3. The umbilicus is circumscribed and left in its normal position.
4. The surgeon elevates the abdominal flap until the xiphoid process of the sternum and the lower costal margins are reached.
5. If diastasis of the rectus abdominis fascia is present, the surgeon plicates it with suture from the xiphoid process to the mons pubis.

6. The flap of abdominal skin and subcutaneous tissue is pulled inferiorly, and excess tissue is excised.
7. A small incision is made in the midline of the flap to accommodate the umbilicus, which is then sutured peripherally to the flap.
8. Drains are inserted, followed by closure of the lower abdominal incision in layers.
9. Postoperatively the patient is placed in the hospital bed in high-Fowler position.

Post–Bariatric Surgery Body Contouring

Successful bariatric surgery produces significant weight loss. The weight loss may result in a trunk that lacks waist and hip definition; ptosis of the mons pubis; and various degrees of skin, fat, and abdominal wall laxity. Upper and lower back rolls accompany the anterior truncal deformities; the buttocks are lower and lack fullness. Upper arms and thighs exhibit similar deformities.

Treatment is aimed at removing the excessive skin and creating a desirable body contour. Most patients are candidates for some form of circumferential recontouring (belt lipectomy) (Figure 13-39) in combination with any number of other recontouring procedures: brachioplasty (Figure 13-40), thigh lifts (Figure 13-41), and mastopexy. For the perioperative nurse, these surgeries offer a logistical challenge because of the combination of procedures and positioning required. The malabsorptive effects of the original bariatric surgery may compromise postoperative wound healing after body contouring procedures.

Procedural Considerations. Any form of body contouring will begin in the preoperative area, where extensive measuring and marking are performed by the plastic surgeon. The perioperative nurse and surgical technologist should inquire about the ordering of the procedures and positioning if more than one is planned. Sequential compression devices and a Foley catheter should be used once the patient arrives in the

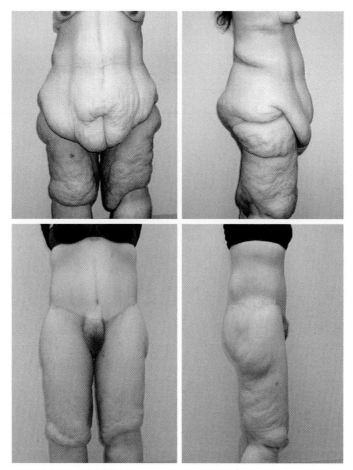

FIGURE 13-39 Belt lipectomy and thigh liposuction. The patient was a 40-year-old woman 40 months after gastric bypass surgery with a weight loss of 269 pounds.

OR. During prepping and draping, attempts should be made to preserve the patient's body temperature. Repositioning is a standard part of these procedures. Pressure points should be well padded with appropriate positioning aids to maintain functional alignment and stable positioning. With each repositioning activity, the patient must be reassessed for safety in terms of skin and nerve compression and competence of the grounding pad, Foley catheter, and all monitoring devices (Ide et al, 2008). A basic plastic surgery instrument set with additional towel clamps is used. Other supplies include a stapler for skin approximation, multiple drains, and the ESU. The surgeon may choose to use tissue adhesive products in combination with suture material to reduce the incidence of seroma. Compression garments may be applied, but care must be taken not to compromise the vascularity of the skin flaps.

Operative Procedure—Belt Lipectomy

Sites addressed are the abdomen, including mons pubis, upper and lower back, lateral trunk skin, buttocks, and lateral upper thighs.

1. The surgeon infuses dilute tumescent solution to aid in hemostasis and facilitate undermining of flaps.
2. Incisions are made and taken down to the level of the fascia, and flaps are elevated to previously marked margins. Liposuction cannulae without vacuum attachments may be used for undermining.

3. Liposuction is used if indicated for contouring only.
4. Muscle plication is performed when indicated.
5. The surgeon approximates and sutures the superficial fascia with permanent sutures.
6. Skin flaps are approximated, and excess skin is excised.
7. Closed-wound suction drains are inserted and secured with suture.
8. The patient is repositioned; depending on position at the start of the procedure, this could be lateral decubitus or supine.
9. Similar techniques are used for defects in areas presented by the new position and repeated until all areas are addressed, including relocation of the umbilicus.
10. The patient is cleaned, incisions are dressed, and a garment is applied at the surgeon's preference.
11. The patient is transferred to a stretcher or bed and placed in the flexed position.

Breast Surgeries

A variety of surgical procedures are available to enhance the aesthetic appearance of the breasts. Patients may choose to enlarge, reduce, and change the position of their breasts.

Augmentation Mammoplasty. Breast augmentation is performed for correction of hypomastia, to correct breast asymmetry, and to recreate the breast after mastectomy. A prosthesis is inserted to enlarge or form the breast mound.

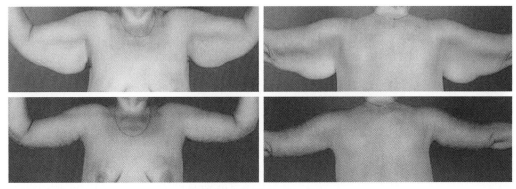

FIGURE 13-40 Brachioplasty.

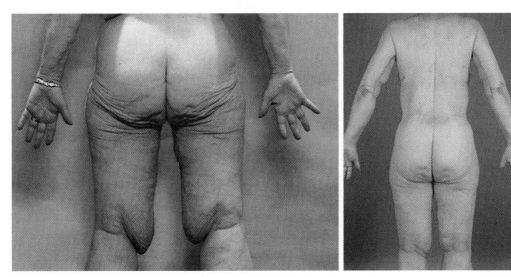

FIGURE 13-41 Thigh lift.

Breast Implants. The two basic types of breast implants are saline filled and silicone gel filled. Both are now approved by the FDA for elective breast augmentation; in November 2006 the FDA approved the use of silicone gel filled breast implants for breast augmentation and breast reconstruction and revision surgeries (Gladfelter and Murphy, 2008). Of the total breast implants performed in 2008, 53% used saline and 47% used silicone (ASPS Stats, 2009).

Implants are configured into round or teardrop (also known as anatomic) shapes and may have a smooth or textured surface. The surfaces are designed to minimize capsular contracture and migration. The choice to use a round or an anatomic implant is based on the shape and form of the existing breast.

PROCEDURAL CONSIDERATIONS. The perioperative nurse and surgical technologist verify style and size of implant and handle the implant according to the manufacturer's recommendations. Handling implants as little as possible assists in efforts to reduce the potential for implant contamination. A basic plastic instrument set is used, plus lighted fiberoptic retractors. The breast implants are packaged in sterile containers from the manufacturer and given to the scrub person when breast size is determined. Breast implants should only be filled with sterile injectable saline using a closed system designed for that purpose. The patient is supine. The arms may be extended on armboards to approximately 60 degrees. Prepping and draping are carried out in the routine manner to expose the operative site.

OPERATIVE PROCEDURE. The surgeon may perform augmentation mammoplasty through circumareolar, inframammary, axillary, or transumbilical incisions using an open or endoscopic approach. Depending on the anatomy of the patient and the surgeon's preference, breast implants may be placed subglandularly, subpectorally (Figure 13-42), or biplanar (partial muscle coverage).

OPERATIVE PROCEDURE—UNFILLED SALINE IMPLANTS

1. The surgeon may inject local anesthetic to decrease bleeding and provide analgesia.
2. An incision is made, the pocket is dissected, and hemostasis is achieved.
3. The surgeon may utilize breast implant sizers (gel or saline) to evaluate the size of the pocket and determine the size of the final implant.
4. With the sizers in place, the anesthesia provider elevates the patient to the 90-degree position so the surgeon can evaluate the appearance from various angles and plan for any adjustments or revisions to the pocket.
5. The sizers are removed, and the surgeon finalizes the pocket.

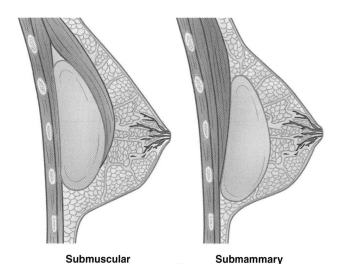

A **Submuscular**
with more fullness above

B **Submammary**
with more superior slope

FIGURE 13-42 **A**, Augmentation mammoplasty implant under muscle. **B**, Implant under breast tissue.

6. The perioperative nurse verifies the implant type and size again with the surgeon and dispenses it to the sterile field.
7. The surgeon rolls the implant into a cylindric shape in preparation for insertion.
8. The pocket is irrigated with saline or antibiotic solution.
9. The surgeon inserts the implant and unrolls it, and once it is properly positioned, the surgeon inflates the implant with an appropriate amount of saline.
10. The procedure is repeated for the opposite breast.
11. The incision is closed in two layers.
12. The patient is cleaned, and bandages and a surgical bra are applied.

Capsulotomy. Capsule contracture results from an exaggerated scar response to a foreign prosthetic material. All surgical implants undergo some degree of encapsulation, but clinical problems arise when this scar formation becomes excessive (Maxwell and Hartley, 2006). Depending on the extent of the contracture, an open capsulotomy may be used to release the constrictive tissue, or a capsulectomy may be indicated to actually remove the tissue (A Board Certified Plastic Surgeon Resource [ABCPSR], 2009).

PROCEDURAL CONSIDERATIONS. The patient is prepared and positioned in the same manner as for breast augmentation. Although patients receive education about capsule contracture as part of the informed consent process for breast augmentation, the actuality of the event may cause emotional distress for the patient. The patient may verbalize disappointment over the results and express fear related to additional postoperative changes in the appearance and functioning of the breast. In addition, the patient now faces the surgical and anesthetic risks associated with a second surgical procedure and may also be struggling with a possible financial burden because these procedures may not be covered by the patient's health plan. An empathetic and understanding approach is paramount to easing the patient's anxiety.

OPERATIVE PROCEDURE
1. The surgeon incises the skin and exposes the capsule.

2. The capsule is scored in multiple areas to achieve the desired release. Depending on the degree of contracture, circumferential incisions may be necessary to release the contracture.
3. If capsulotomy is not effective in releasing the capsule, a partial or full capsulectomy may be required to physically remove all or a portion of the capsule.
   a. The capsule is excised, and the breast implant is removed.
   b. The breast implant may be replaced in the same area, exchanged and replaced, or placed in a new pocket.
4. The site is irrigated with antibiotic solution. Drains are placed if a capsulectomy was performed.
5. The surgeon closes the incision in two layers.
6. The patient's skin is cleaned, and dressings are applied.

Reduction Mammoplasty. Reduction mammoplasty is indicated for the patient with macromastia with resulting back pain, intertrigo (chronic skin infection), or deep grooving in the shoulders from the bra straps because of the weight of the breasts (Box 13-4) (Research Highlight) (Figure 13-43, *A*). The procedure may also be performed to achieve symmetry after a mastectomy on the contralateral side. Excessive breast tissue and its overlying skin are excised, with reconstruction of the breast contour, size, shape, and symmetry (Figure 13-43, *B*).

PROCEDURAL CONSIDERATIONS. A basic plastic instrument set is used with the addition of a "cookie cutter" areola marker or a "keyhole" pattern marker, a sterile marking pen, skin stapler, tape measure, baby Deaver retractors, and two closed-wound suction systems. The ESU and a scale for weighing specimens should also be available, and tissue from each side should be carefully weighed and marked appropriately. The perioperative nurse should ensure the scale is calibrated correctly before weighing any tissue. Numerous blades will be used if deepithelializing breast skin. If the nipple is removed and placed as a free nipple graft, extra suture will be necessary for tie-over bolsters. There are numerous choices in the reduction mammoplasty technique; therefore before opening suture or other supplies, the surgical technologist should ask the surgeon which technique will be employed. The surgeon will mark the skin to be excised and the new site for the nipple preoperatively with the patient in a sitting position.

The patient is supine with arms slightly extended on padded armboards. The hips should be positioned at the break in the OR bed so that the patient may be raised to a sitting position if necessary. Standard prepping and draping are done. Care should be taken not to remove the preoperative markings.

OPERATIVE PROCEDURE. The standard reduction mammoplasty procedure is described below. If the surgeon is using the "short scar" technique, the breast tissue is incised and removed according to the technique chosen. The nipple pedicle technique, wherein the nipple is mobilized and secured in a new position, may be chosen, or a free nipple graft may be utilized.

1. The surgeon incises and removes the skin between the new and the old nipple sites, with the nipple remaining attached to the underlying breast tissue. On patients with very large breasts, the nipples are removed and then reapplied as free grafts when the reduction is complete.
2. The redundant segment of breast tissue inferior to the nipple is excised through an inverted-T incision. Tissue from each breast is weighed and kept separate.

BOX 13-4

BREAST REDUCTION OVERVIEW

Patient Education for Breast Reduction

GENERAL INFORMATION

Women with very large, pendulous breasts (a condition known as macromastia) can experience a number of physical and emotional problems. Macromastia is generally defined as excessive breast size, usually a bra cup size of D or larger. This condition is seen in young girls to middle-aged women. The condition probably is caused by hormonal factors but is also associated with obesity. Often there is a family pattern of large breasts.

COMMON SIGNS AND SYMPTOMS

- Breast size that is out of proportion to the torso and larger than the accepted norm
- Upper back and neck pain
- Shoulder pain
- Arm pain
- Breast pain
- Rashes and sometimes infections of the skin under the breasts
- Shoulder grooving from bra straps
- Hyperpigmentation (dark marks) in the bra strap lines
- Difficulty in finding bras or clothing that fits
- Possibly shyness or other personality changes because of appearance and the effects of excessively large breasts

DIAGNOSIS

The surgeon will confirm the diagnosis of macromastia by examining the breasts carefully and relating the findings of the patient's history.

TREATMENT

- Women with large breasts have often tried custom bras and weight loss as a way of reducing breast size or adding support. Physical therapy and pain medications may also be used in an effort to relieve symptoms. After trying these methods without success, many women seek surgical help in the form of breast reduction surgery. Technically, breast reduction surgery is known as reduction mammoplasty.
- The best candidates for breast reduction usually have at least two of the symptoms listed in the aforementioned Common Signs and Symptoms category.
- Breast reduction surgery should be delayed if the breasts are still growing; also, if the patient is gaining or losing weight, they should consider delaying breast reduction until their weight has stabilized.
- The aims of the operation are the following:
  - To remove enough breast tissue to be able to construct a normal-appearing breast mound
  - To reposition the nipple-areola complex in a suitable position in the "new" breast

There are many operations to reduce large breasts. A common technique is shown in the figures.

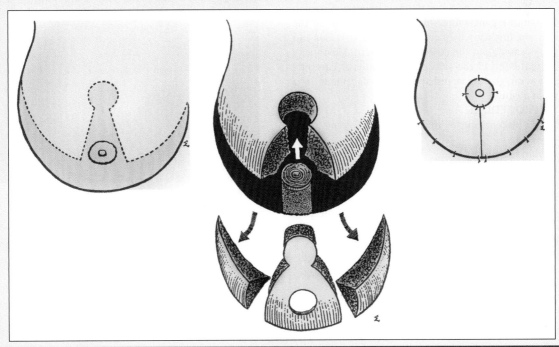

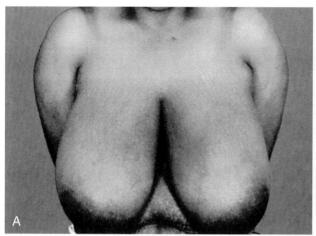
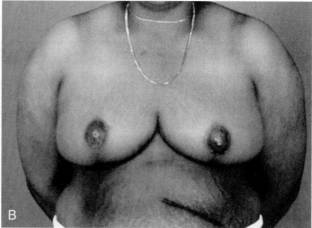

FIGURE 13-43 **A,** Preoperative view of reduction mammoplasty. **B,** Postoperative view.

3. The surgeon mobilizes the nipple and adjacent tissue and sutures them in place.
4. The medial and lateral skin edges are approximated in a vertical suture line inferior to the nipple.
5. The inframammary elliptic incision is trimmed and closed transversely. Closed-wound suction catheters may be placed. The wound is dressed.

Mastopexy. Breast ptosis is corrected by moving the nipple to a more normal position and removing excess breast skin (Figure 13-44). With mastopexy surgery there is usually minimal to no removal of breast tissue, although it may be necessary to add a breast implant to achieve the desired result.

PROCEDURAL CONSIDERATIONS. The surgeon will mark the patient before surgery. Positioning is similar to that used for breast augmentation. Skin incision choices are periareolar only; periareolar combined with a vertical (known as a short scar or vertical mastopexy); the classic inverted T, which adds an inframammary incision to the previous incision; or the horizontal inframammary, which combines the periareolar and inframammary, leaving out the vertical component. Mastopexy may involve reduction of the skin envelope only or combine skin removal with glandular reshaping and placement in a more desirable position.

OPERATIVE PROCEDURE
1. Incisions are placed; one or more of the following techniques are used:
   a. Excess skin is removed.
   b. The breast cone is reshaped by invagination of lower midbreast tissue.
   c. The lower submammary breast tissue pedicle is advanced below the breast tissue and tacked superiorly to the pectoral muscle.
   d. Lower midbreast tissue is incised and overlapped.
   e. A superiorly based (on the nipple-areolar complex pedicle) wedge tissue flap is created, turned under, and superiorly attached.
   f. The upper pole of breast tissue is mobilized and advanced superiorly and tacked to the pectoral muscle fascia.
2. The breast may be sutured entirely at this time or approximated, and the same procedure is applied to the opposite breast, closing both at the end of the procedure.

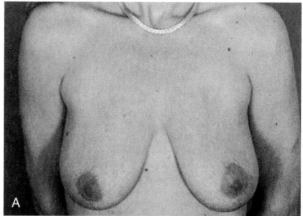
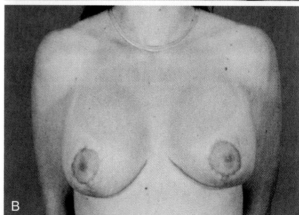

FIGURE 13-44 Mastopexy. **A,** Preoperative view. **B,** Postoperative view; ptosis corrected.

3. The operative area is cleaned, dressings of choice are applied, and a surgical bra is applied.

Excision of Gynecomastia. Gynecomastia is a relatively common pathologic condition that consists of bilateral or unilateral enlargement of the male breast. It occurs primarily during puberty or after the age of 40 years. Although it may be produced by a variety of diseases or be the result of side effects related to certain medications, it is usually related to excessive hormone

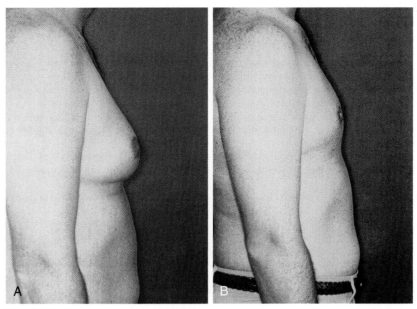

FIGURE 13-45 A, Preoperative view of gynecomastia. B, Postoperative view after excision of gynecomastia.

RESEARCH HIGHLIGHT

A Phenomenologic Study in Breast Reduction Patients

Researchers explored women's perception of life after breast reduction surgery in an effort to understand subjective issues for these patients. A limitation of this study was the use of a small convenience sample of nine patients interviewed at follow-up visits; in addition, one of the researchers was a novice in this field. However, the data collected gave a qualitative aspect to an event that had been studied for surgical technique or physical symptoms. The study intended to gather detailed, descriptive information to reflect women's experiences after this surgery.

After obtaining informed consent data were collected in a private exam room in the office. Open-ended questions were asked, such as "What is life like following your breast reduction?" Prompts (e.g., "tell me more") were also used in an unstructured interview. Field notes were taken and interviews audiotaped for later analysis.

Findings revealed the following themes; explanations through patient quotes were listed in the article:

◆ Enhanced physical health
◆ Improved body image
◆ Increased self-esteem
◆ Increased self-confidence
◆ Dissatisfaction with the postoperative recovery period/though pleased overall with above aspects (this may be due to method, in that patients requiring follow-up care 5 months to 3 years after surgery may have more issues than a typical patient)

Implications for future research emphasize the need for adequate patient education for realistic expectations. Future research includes determining whether patients are receiving adequate information prospectively to have realistic expectations following surgery. Understanding the rationale for postoperative difficulties or for the extended time in making the decision to have breast reduction surgery could lead to new patient care interventions. Finally, this research should be replicated in patients who did not need to return to the plastic surgeon's office following the routine 90-day postoperative period.

Modified from Woodman R, Radzyminski S: Women's perception of life following breast reduction: a phenomenological study, *Plast Surg Nurs* 27(2): 85-95, 2007.

production or alterations in hormonal balance. It may also be seen in elderly men and in men after excessive use of marijuana. All subareolar fibroglandular tissue is removed, and the resultant defect is surgically closed (Figure 13-45). The patient may be positioned in a supine position or semi-Fowler position, according to the surgeon's preference. Supplies and equipment needed are the same as those for a simple mastectomy, plus a basic plastic instrument set. Because suction-assisted lipectomy (SAL) may be used for contouring, suction cannulae, associated supplies, and an aspirator should also be available. All breast tissue removed should be weighed and then sent for pathologic examination. Although infrequent, men are not immune from breast cancer.

OPERATIVE PROCEDURE
1. The surgeon instills local anesthetic and makes a stab wound incision for introduction of the liposuction cannula.
2. Liposuction is performed. If satisfactory removal of breast tissue is accomplished, the incision is closed and a compression garment applied.
3. If additional surgery is required, the surgeon makes a periareolar incision. Through this incision, the fibrous and ductal attachments of the underlying glandular tissue to the nipple are divided.
4. A cuff of fatty tissue is left attached to the underlying nipple surface to protect the blood supply.

GERIATRIC CONSIDERATIONS

The Elderly Patient—Plastic and Reconstructive Surgery

Some aesthetic surgical procedures are accomplished using local anesthesia. Medication safety practices recommend the following:

◆ Follow the seven rights (7 R's) of medication delivery: right patient, medication, dose, route, time, technique, and documentation.

◆ Use at least two patient identifiers when administering medications. Identifiers include the patient's name, assigned identification number, or bar coding in a patient ID bracelet that includes two or more specific patient identifiers.

◆ Identify/verify any patient allergies and sensitivities (e.g., medications, latex, foods, adhesives, chemicals).

◆ Review patient's medication history (including herbal remedies, over-the-counter [OTC] drugs); identify possible medication interactions or contraindications.

◆ When receiving information from the surgeon, physician assistant, or assistant-in-surgery regarding desired local anesthetic medication, "repeat back" the medication name and strength, receiving confirmation from the person who gave the information that it is correct.

◆ Comply with the institution's "Do not use" list and list of look-alike/sound-alike drugs. Look-alike and sound-alike drugs should be stored separately.

◆ The circulating nurse and scrub person should audibly review and confirm the medication ordered before transfer to the sterile field. Medication verification should include drug/solution/agent name, strength, dosage, and expiration date. The medication order is sometimes part of a standing protocol on the preference card/pick list.

◆ Label all medications and containers with solutions (e.g., syringes, medicine cups, basins) on and off the sterile field, even if there is only one medication being used.

◆ Verify any medication listed on the physician's preference card/pick list with the physician before delivery to the field, labeling, or administration.

◆ Label any medication or solution when it is transferred from its original package to another container.

◆ Label each medication or solution one at a time. Verify name and concentration, complete preparation for administration, deliver to the sterile field, and label on the field before another medication/solution is prepared.

◆ Use medication vial transfer devices to dispense medications onto the sterile field without contaminating the medication during dispensing.

◆ Keep original packages from medications or solutions available for reference in the OR/procedure room until the surgery/procedure ends.

◆ Labels should contain the drug name, strength, amount (if not apparent from the container), expiration date when not used within 24 hours, and expiration time when expiration occurs in less than 24 hours.

◆ Differentiate look-alike and sound-alike products by using "tall man" lettering on products or highlighting/circling the distinguishing information to prevent errors.

◆ Verify all labels verbally and visually by two qualified individuals.

◆ Discard any unlabeled medication or solution immediately.

◆ The scrub person should actively communicate medication/solution name, amount, and dose when transferring it to the surgeon.

◆ At shift change or when personnel are relieved ("hand-off"), all medications and solutions on and off the sterile field and their labels should be reviewed by entering and exiting staff.

◆ Discard all labeled containers used during the surgical procedure at the procedure's end.

◆ Follow procedures for reporting and responding to medication errors (adverse drug events [ADEs]), including near-misses.

Modified from AORN Guidance Statement: Safe medication practices in perioperative practice settings, *AORN Standards and Recommended Practices*, Denver, 2009, The Association; Beyea SC: *Perioperative nursing data set*, ed 2, Denver, 2007, The Association; Cole LM: Documentation to reduce medication errors, *OR Nurse* 2(7):17–19, 2008; Giarrizzo-Wilson S: Clinical issues—medication practices, *AORN J* 81(6):1326–1329, 2005; Improving the OR's medication safety, *OR Manager* 23(1):17–18, 2007; ISMP Medication Safety Alert: *NurseAdvise-ERR: positive identification—not just for patients, but for drugs and solutions*, 3(8), 2005; JCAHO: *What every health care organization should know about sentinel events*, Chicago, 2005, The Association.

5. The breast tissue mass is dissected. Carrying the dissection to the pectoralis fascia is usually necessary to remove the entire mass.

6. Hemostasis is achieved.

7. Closure is performed, the area cleaned, and a compression garment applied.

PLASTIC AND RECONSTRUCTIVE SURGERY SUMMARY

The plastic/reconstructive surgical patient population is varied from young to old, and interventions are performed for cosmetic and reconstructive purposes. Burns, congenital and acquired defects, trauma, and self-esteem issues bring the patient into the operating room for repair.

The anatomy involved is the integumentary system, which includes the skin, hair, and nails. This system is the largest organ within the human body, and underlying structures of bone and nerve are also frequently involved.

Special equipment and supplies include prosthetic devices, dermatomes, skin meshers, specialized plastic instrumentation sets, bone saws, drills, loupes, microscope, local anesthetic of choice, marking pens, scales, dye of choice, and dressing material from simple 4 × 4s to dressing bras to casting material.

Surgical interventions for skin cancer, burns, debridement, and pressure ulcers are frequently performed with skin grafting employed. The type of skin grafting will depend upon the area requiring the graft and what structures need to be replaced. Skin grafting requires the use of special equipment to procure and prepare the graft for successful implantation. Dressings with surgeon-specific special supplies are essential as well. Tissue or muscle flaps may be required in major reconstructive interventions.

Breast reconstruction offers several options to the surgical patient and surgeon. Tissue expanders, flaps, prostheses, and microsurgery can be employed for specific patient outcomes. Replantation of body structures is seen in trauma patients and success depends upon the part amputated and what is required to replant the structure.

Maxillofacial reconstructive surgery can be performed for nasal, orbital, zygomatic, maxillary, and mandibular fractures. Patients will also seek maxillofacial interventions for cosmetic reasons due to acquired or congenital defects.

Aesthetic or cosmetic surgical interventions are frequently performed and can be done under local to general anesthesia.

Scar revisions, brow lifts, face lifts, blepharoplasty, rhinoplasty, and liposuction are common facial interventions. Use of the laser has improved patient outcomes in this area.

Liposuction is used in various parts of the body, depending upon the patient and their surgical goals. Abdominoplasty is another common intervention, and the increase in bariatric surgery has produced more patients seeking this correction after weight loss.

Mammoplasty for breast augmentation or reduction is another common intervention. The use of implants is seen in augmentation procedures and the type of prosthesis selected depends both on surgeon preference and the patient's surgical goals.

REVIEW QUESTIONS

1. Once the dermatome is used to remove a skin graft, what is needed next to prepare the graft for implantation?

2. What surgical intervention is indicated for removal of malignant melanoma?

3. What is essential for a skin graft to survive?

4. What is the most common pedicle-based flap used for breast reconstruction?

5. Define and briefly describe the following surgical procedures:
   Breast reconstruction using a myocutaneous flap
   Reduction of maxillary fractures
   Blepharoplasty of upper and lower lids

Critical Thinking Question

1. When performing excision of malignant melanoma, what should the surgical technologist consider when preparing the instrumentation and supplies?

2. What is the most important factor to consider when the surgical intervention involves breast implants?

REFERENCES

A Board Certified Plastic Surgeon Resource (ABCPSR) (2009): Capsular contracture, available at www.aboardcertifiedplasticsurgeonresource.com/breast_augmentation/capsular_contracture/index.html. Accessed June 28, 2009.

American Burn Association (ABA): Burn incidence and treatment in the US: 2007, available at www.ameriburn.org/resources_factsheet.php. Accessed June 27, 2009.

American Cancer Society (ACS): Breast reconstruction after mastectomy, 2009, available at www.cancer.org/docroot/CRI/content/CRI_2_6X_Breast_Reconstruction_After_Mastectomy_5.asp?sitearea=. Accessed Nov. 21, 2009.

American Society of Plastic Surgeons (ASPS): Quick facts: percentage change 2008 vs. 2007, available at www.plasticsurgery.org/media/stats/2008-quick-facts-cosmetic-surgery-minimally-invasive-statistics.pdf. Accessed June 11, 2009.

American Society of Plastic Surgeons (ASPS) Stats, 2000/2007/2008 National plastic surgery statistics: Cosmetic and reconstructive procedure trends 2009, available at www.plasticsurgery.org/media/stats/2008-cosmetic-reconstructive-plastic-surgery-minimally-invasive-statistics.pdf. Accessed June 20, 2009.

American Society of Plastic Surgeons (ASPS) 2009a: Patients and consumers: planning your surgery: plastic surgery and total patient care, available at www.plasticsurgery.org/Patients_and_Consumers/Planning_Your_Surgery/Plastic_Surgery_and_Total_Patient_Care.html. Accessed June 19, 2009.

American Society of Plastic Surgeons (ASPS) 2009b: Patients and consumers: planning your surgery: psychological aspects: your self-image and plastic surgery, available at www.plasticsurgery.org/Patients_and_Consumers/Planning_Your_Surgery/Psychological_Aspects_Your_Self-Image_and_Plastic_Surgery.html. Accessed June 26, 2009.

American Society of Plastic Surgeons (ASPS) 2009c: Breast reconstruction, available at www.plasticsurgery.org/public_education/procedures/Breast-Reconstruction.cfm. Accessed July 8, 2009.

Association of periOperative Registered Nurses (AORN): Recommended practices for managing the patient receiving local anesthesia. In *Perioperative standards and recommended practices*, Denver, 2009, The Association.

Cuzzell J, Workman ML: Interventions for clients with skin problems. In Ignatavicius DD, Workman ML, editors: *Medical-surgical nursing: patient-centered collaborative care*, ed 6, St. Louis, 2010, Saunders.

Edwards C et al: The SGAP flap for the postmastectomy patient, *OR Nurse* 3(3):28–34, 2009.

Gladfelter J: Compression garments 101, *Plast Surg Nurs* 27(2):73–77, 2007.

Gladfelter J, Murphy D: Breast augmentation motivations and satisfaction: a prospective study of more than 3,000 silicone implantations, *Plast Surg Nurs* 28(4):170–174, 2008.

Gutierrez KJ, Peterson PG: Alterations in integumentary function. In *Saunders nursing survival guide, Pathophysiology*, St Louis, 2007, Saunders.

Hagan KF: Clinical photography for the plastic surgery practice—the basics, *Plast Surg Nurs* 28(4):188–192, 2008.

Health Stream: *Infection prevention for surgical site care, (study guide).* (Grant funds provided by Enturia). (Health Stream is accredited as provider of continuing nursing education by the American Nurses Credentialing Center's Commission on Accreditation), Denver, 2007, Health Stream, p. 13.

Ide P et al: Perioperative nursing care of the bariatric surgical patient, *AORN J* 88(1):30–54, 2008.

Logan JM, Broughton G: Plastic surgery: understanding abdominoplasty and liposuction, *AORN J* 88(4):587–600, 2008.

Marler JJ, Upton JJ: Tissue engineering. In Mathes SJ, editor: *Plastic surgery*, vol 1, ed 2, Philadelphia, 2006, Saunders.

Maxwell GP, Hartley RW: Breast augmentation. In Mathes SJ, editor: *Plastic surgery*, vol 1, ed 2, Philadelphia, 2006, Saunders.

National Cancer Institute, U.S. National Institutes of Health (NCI): Skin cancer, available at www.cancer.gov/cancertopics/types/skin. Accessed June 27, 2009.

Pfiedler Enterprises: Maxillofacial injuries: Perioperative patient care, 2007, CECredit booklet [Pfiedler Enterprises is approved as an Authorized Provider by the International Association for Continuing Education and Training (IACET), Washington, DC] and was offered through AORN for ANCC credit (grant funds provided by Stryker Craniomaxillofacial).

Sladden MJ et al: Surgical excision margins for localised cutaneous melanoma (Protocol). Cochrane Database of Systematic Reviews 2004, Issue 3. Art. No.: CD004835. DOI: 10.1002/14651858.CD004835, available at http://mrw.interscience.wiley.com/cochrane/clsysrev/articles/CD004835/frame.html. Accessed May 13, 2009.

Song DH et al: Plastic and reconstructive surgery essentials for students, 2007, available at www.plasticsurgery.org/d.xml?comp=x1504. Accessed June 27, 2009.

Wei F, Suominen S: Principles and techniques of microvascular surgery. In Mathes SJ, editor: *Plastic surgery*, vol 1, ed 2, Philadelphia, 2006, Saunders.

Zgonis T et al: Surgical management of diabetic foot infections and amputations, *AORN J* 87(5):935–946, 2008.

Thoracic Surgery

Overview

Thoracic surgery, like other specialties, has evolved with the development of surgical techniques and treatments, such as blood transfusion, anesthetic delivery, and screening procedures. During the past 50 years the understanding of pathophysiology and improved techniques have expanded the field of thoracic surgery. The thoracic specialty extends beyond the surgical arena into infectious disease, trauma, and oncology. Improved technology and the determination to treat diseases previously considered untreatable with operative and other invasive procedures continue to improve the recovery rate for patients experiencing thoracic diseases. As the ability to treat thoracic disease has improved, the responsibilities of the surgical team have expanded, resulting in accomplishments throughout the years that have provided an extensive knowledge base and specialized perioperative practitioners.

This chapter was originally written by Brian Blanchard, MSN, CRNP, for the 14th edition of Alexander's Care of the Patient in Surgery *and has been revised by Betsy Boatwright, CST, for this text.*

Surgical Anatomy

The skeletal framework of the thorax is formed anteriorly by the sternum and costal cartilages, laterally by the 12 pairs of ribs, and posteriorly by the 12 thoracic vertebrae (Figure 14-1). This airtight compartment is enclosed in the root of the neck by Sibson's fascia and is separated from the abdomen by the diaphragm.

The sternum forms the anterior thoracic wall in the midline. It consists of three parts: (1) the upper part, or manubrium; (2) the body, or gladiolus; and (3) the lower cartilage, or xiphoid process. The manubrium articulates with the clavicles and the first two ribs on each side; the gladiolus articulates with the remaining true ribs by separate costal cartilages; and the xiphoid fuses with the gladiolus in early development and is attached to the diaphragm by the substernal ligament.

Normally the lateral walls of the thorax are formed by the 12 pairs of ribs. Posteriorly, each pair of ribs articulates with its corresponding thoracic vertebrae. Anteriorly, the first seven ribs articulate with the sternum. The eighth, ninth, and tenth ribs articulate with the costal cartilages of the rib above; however, the eleventh and twelfth ribs are not fixed to the costal arch (see Figure 14-1).

The muscles of each hemithorax (Figures 14-2 and 14-3) include the 11 external and 11 internal intercostal muscles,

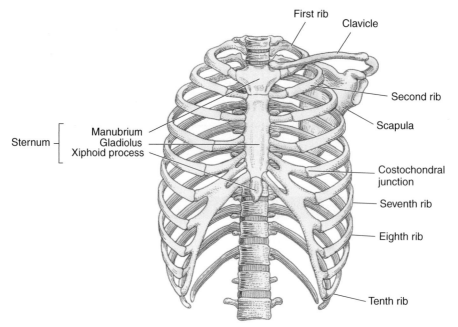

FIGURE 14-1 Bony thorax.

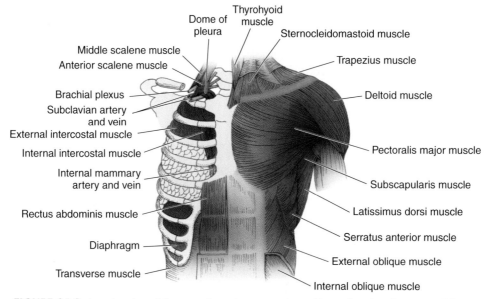

FIGURE 14-2 Anterior view of thorax and contiguous portions of base of neck and anterior abdominal wall. *Right half,* Superficial layer of muscles and fascia; *left half,* relations of deep muscles of neck and abdomen to rib cage, intercostal muscles, diaphragm, and internal mammary vessels; relations of muscles, nerves, and vessels with first rib; and anterior relations of lung.

which fill the spaces between the ribs. An intercostal artery, vein, and nerve accompany each intercostal muscle. The arteries communicate with the internal thoracic artery anteriorly and arise from the aorta posteriorly. The intercostal veins follow the course of the arteries and communicate with the mammary veins anteriorly and with the azygos and hemiazygos veins posteriorly.

During surgery, great care is taken to prevent injury to the intercostal nerve, which passes forward and alongside the posterior intercostal artery and shares with the superior branch of the artery the intercostal groove on the inferior edge of the corresponding rib. When the nerve must be disturbed, an anesthetic agent may be injected to prevent postoperative pain.

The thoracic outlet is a junction bound anteriorly by the manubrium, anterolaterally by the first ribs, and posteriorly by the first thoracic vertebrae and posterior angles of the first ribs of the space. The great vessels of the head, neck, and arm pass through this space. Compression of these structures causes thoracic outlet syndrome.

The mediastinum is divided into anterior, middle, and posterior compartments. The anterior mediastinum is bound anteriorly by the sternum and posteriorly by the pericardium and

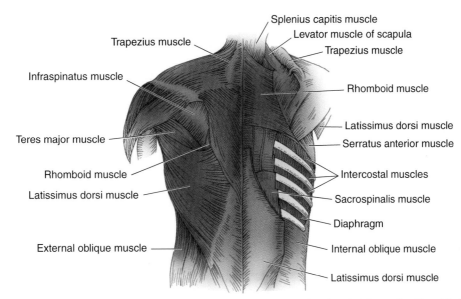

FIGURE 14-3 Posterior view of thorax and contiguous portions of neck and abdominal wall. *Left half,* Superficial muscles; *right half,* deeper muscles.

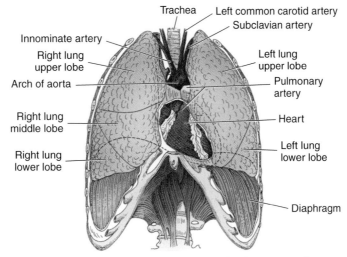

FIGURE 14-4 Organs of thoracic cavity. Part of pericardium has been removed to expose heart.

great vessels. It contains the thymus gland, lymph nodes, and pericardial fat. The middle mediastinum is bound anteriorly by the pericardium and great vessels and posteriorly by the anterior border of the vertebral bodies. The posterior mediastinum is bound anteriorly by the vertebral bodies and extends posteriorly to the chest wall.

The chest cavity is subdivided into the right and the left pleural cavities, which contain the lungs separated by the mediastinum, which lies medially between the two pleural membranes. The parietal pleura, the membrane that lines the inner surface of each hemithorax, is adjacent to the inner surfaces of the ribs posteriorly and the mediastinum medially and covers the surface of the diaphragm except at the central portion. Part of the parietal membrane is reflected back at the root of each lung to form a sac around it. This reflection is called the *visceral pleura*. The pleural space holds about 50 ml of pleural fluid, a serous secretion that provides lubrication between these two membranes to minimize friction

during inspiration and expiration (Coughlin and Parchinsky, 2006).

The lungs are the essential organs of respiration. The base of each lung rests on the diaphragm, whereas its apex (upper end) projects into the base of the neck at a level above the first rib. The bronchus, the nerves, the lymphatics, and the pulmonary and bronchial vessels enter and leave the lung on the mediastinal surface in a structure known as the *hilum,* or *root,* of the lung. Deep fissures divide the spongy, porous lung into lobes. The primary bronchi divide and then subdivide into each lobe and eventually become bronchioles. The right lung has an upper, a middle, and a lower lobe; the left lung has only an upper and a lower lobe (Figure 14-4). However, the lungs are similar in that each is composed of 10 major segments (Figure 14-5). Each segment extends to the pleural surface, expanding in volume from its center to its peripheral edges. Each segment also has its own bronchus and branches of the pulmonary artery and vein.

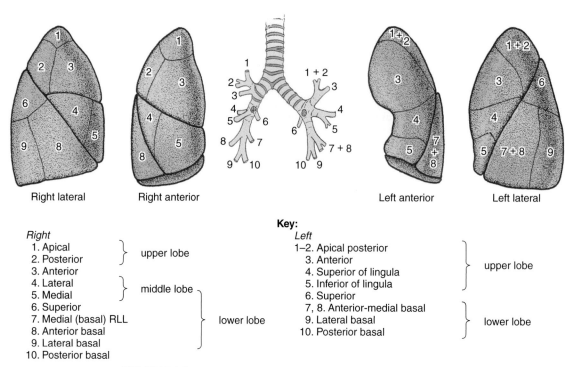

Right lateral   Right anterior   Left anterior   Left lateral

Key:

Right
1. Apical   ⎫
2. Posterior   ⎬ upper lobe
3. Anterior   ⎭
4. Lateral   ⎫ middle lobe
5. Medial   ⎭
6. Superior
7. Medial (basal) RLL
8. Anterior basal   lower lobe
9. Lateral basal
10. Posterior basal

Left
1–2. Apical posterior   ⎫
3. Anterior   ⎬ upper lobe
4. Superior of lingula ⎪
5. Inferior of lingula ⎭
6. Superior
7, 8. Anterior-medial basal   ⎫
9. Lateral basal   ⎬ lower lobe
10. Posterior basal   ⎭

FIGURE 14-5 Segments of the pulmonary lobes. *RLL,* Right lower lobe.

The bronchial arteries, arising from the aorta, supply nourishment to the lungs. They vary in their number and course. The arrangement may include two branches to the left lung and one branch to the right lung, which later branches into two, or there may be one or two branches for each lung. The pulmonary arteries carry the blood to the pulmonary parenchyma, and the pulmonary veins transport the oxygenated blood to the left atrium.

The nerves of the lungs are a part of the autonomic nervous system. They regulate constriction and relaxation of the bronchi and of the blood vessels within the lungs.

Although the thoracic cavity is an airtight space, the lungs receive outside air through the nasal passages, trachea, and bronchi. The main function of the lungs is to exchange carbon dioxide for oxygen. Normally, as the thorax expands, the lungs also expand as air is drawn in; during expiration, the thorax relaxes and the lungs passively contract as air is forced out. Inspiration normally takes place when the intrathoracic pressure is slightly below atmospheric pressure (76 cm Hg, or 760 mm Hg) and when a partial vacuum exists between the parietal and visceral pleural (intrathoracic) surfaces. As the muscles of inspiration contract to enlarge the chest cage, the lungs passively follow the diaphragm and chest wall because of decreased intrathoracic pressure. The acts of inspiration and expiration are the result of air moving in and out of the lung, causing pressure to equalize with that of the atmosphere at the end of expiration.

The normal intrapleural pressure varies from –9 to –12 cm H_2O during inspiration and from about –3 to –6 cm H_2O during expiration. The greatest amount of air that can be expired after a maximum inspiration is termed the *vital capacity,* and the volume of gas remaining in the lungs after maximal expiration is *residual volume.* Size, age, gender, and pulmonary disease of the patient influence vital capacity. Any condition that interferes with the normally negative intrapleural pressure affects respiratory function.

Surgical Technologist Considerations

The surgical technologist must be prepared for the demands of thoracic surgery. From bronchoscopy to mediastinoscopy and resection to lobectomy, surgical technologists' responsibilities include prepping, draping, special equipment knowledge, instrumentation, suture, and supplies. It is important to note that thoracic surgery also usually entails special care and labeling of specimens, including frozen section, cytology, and cultures.

Medications on the sterile field may include a local injectable, as well as a warm antibiotic irrigation. Depending on the procedure, the surgeon and the anesthesia provider may decide to do a block or epidural for additional pain control. Many sizes and types of chest tubes will be needed, as well as stapling devices. There are many types of anastomotic devices on the market. It is important to familiarize yourself with what your facility has available for use by the surgeon.

Additional Considerations

During thoracic surgery, the surgical technologist is concerned with both preparatory patient considerations (e.g., verification of the patient, surgical procedure, and site; positioning; draping) and the requirements of the surgical intervention (e.g., medication delivery; instrument, equipment, and supply availability).

Positioning. The type of position used in thoracic surgery is determined by the operative procedure planned. Bronchoscopy is performed in the supine position with a shoulder roll. Tho-

SURGICAL TECHNOLOGY PREFERENCE CARD

In thoracic surgery, positioning of the patient is one of the most important parts of the procedure. From a mediastinoscopy to a segmental resection, it is vital for the surgeon to have good visualization. It is also important to get familiar with the surgeons' preferences. Taking time to bring in special equipment and supplies will be efficient for the entire perioperative team. Keep in mind the possibility of multiple specimens, labeling, and how the specimen will be processed. Use safe specimen handling practices. Knowledge of the scopes, including how to care for and handle them, is an additional responsibility of the surgical technologist.

Room Prep: Basic operating room furniture is in place, along with a video system, light source, camera, insufflation device, positioning supplies—pillows, axillary roll, lateral arm holder, egg crate padding, and vac pac

Prep Solution
◆ Chlorhexidine gluconate (CHG); make sure the prep is dry before draping occurs

Catheters
◆ Foley catheter—should have a urine meter and is typically a 16 French in size
◆ Latex allergy patients—accommodations are made before the patient with a latex allergy enters the room; all latex allergy precautions are instituted

PROCEDURE CHECKLIST

Instruments
◆ Standard—thoracotomy/thoracoscopy set, self retaining thoracic retractor
◆ Laparoscopic—scope, camera, light cord, electrosurgical instruments and cords (monopolar and bipolar)
◆ Have available aspirating needle, biopsy clamps, minimally invasive set, and long instruments

Suture
◆ 3-0 monofilament suture, long and double armed for ligature
◆ 0 silk suture for chest tubes
◆ 2-0 and 0 silk ties—long and can be passed on a clamp or free hand
◆ Pericostal sutures to appose the ribs—braided and absorbable suture with a large swaged-on needle
◆ Fascia—0 or 1 braided absorbable suture
◆ Subcutaneous—2-0 braided absorbable
◆ Skin—3-0 monofilament or staples

Other Hemostatic Agents
◆ Staplers—have a variety available with reloads
◆ Clip appliers—have a variety of sizes, long in length, and clips
◆ Platelet gel—derived from the patient's own blood and mixed with thrombin
◆ Electrosurgical unit (ESU) and harmonic scalpel

Additional Supplies
◆ Physician's special requests—including suture, clamps, and staplers
◆ Sponges—laps, raytec, and kitners
◆ Suction canisters—multiple, possibly a spider setup
◆ Specimen containers—variety of culture tubes, specimen cups, and formalin containers
◆ Chest tubes and drainage systems—have a variety available
◆ Smoke evacuation system

Medications and Irrigations
◆ Warm antibiotic irrigation
◆ Epidural or spinal block kit
◆ Injectable local anesthetic

Drains
◆ Correct size and type for procedure and surgeon preference
◆ Autologous blood retrieval system
◆ Jackson-Pratt to a closed reservoir for fluid collection

Specimen Care
◆ Multiple specimens are common—label correctly and use the correct container and solution

Before opening for the procedure, the surgical technologist should:
◆ Check procedure against a surgeon's preference card
◆ Arrange OR furniture—depending on surgical site and surgeon preference
◆ Gather positioning devices and specialty carts in the OR
◆ Gather and arrange needed equipment—verify function of equipment

racotomy can be performed with the patient in one of three common positions: (1) lateral for the posterolateral approach, (2) semilateral for the anterolateral approach (Figure 14-6), and (3) supine for the median sternotomy approach. Arms are placed on padded armboards with the palms up and fingers extended. Armboards are maintained at less than a 90-degree angle to prevent brachial plexus stretch. If there are surgical reasons to tuck the arms at the side, the elbows are padded to protect the ulnar nerve, the palms face inward, and the wrist is maintained in a neutral position (Denholm, 2009). A drape secures the arms. It should be tucked snuggly under the patient, not under the mattress. This prevents the arm from shifting downward intraoperatively and resting against the OR bed rail.

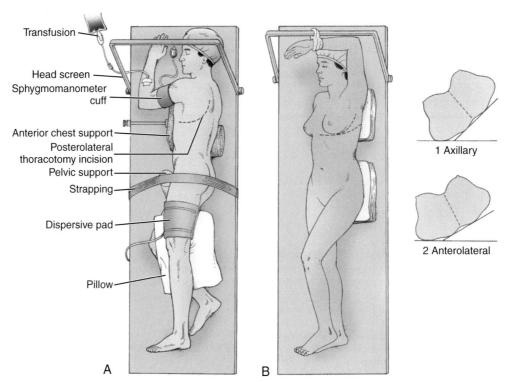

FIGURE 14-6 Positions for thoracotomy incisions. **A,** Lateral position for posterolateral incision. **B,** Semilateral position for axillary or anterolateral position.

Draping. Draping may be minimal for bronchoscopic procedures. The principles of draping for other procedures are followed in thoracic procedures. Drapes may consist of a fenestrated sheet or single sheets surrounding the incision site. To prevent instruments from falling from the field, the surgical technologist may place a magnetic pad on the drapes below the incision site when the patient is placed in lateral position. A forced-air warming blanket is placed on the patient before draping to maintain normothermia. Sequential compression devices are often applied also to prevent the development of deep vein thrombosis (DVT).

Instrumentation. Bronchoscopy instruments are designed to directly inspect and observe the larynx, trachea, bronchi, or mediastinum; to remove secretions; to obtain washings or tissue for bacterial and cytologic studies; or to remove tissue. They are also designed to remove foreign bodies. Instrumentation for thoracic surgery includes the laparotomy instrument set (see Chapter 2) and specialty items. Instruments used for a thoracotomy or chest procedure include a combination of delicate and heavy instruments. Stapling equipment commonly is used as suturing devices and requires staplers and reload staples of appropriate sizes. The delicate instruments are used to cut tissue and vessels or to clamp tissue in an atraumatic manner. The heavier instruments are used for bone cutting, dissecting, or retracting. Instrumentation must also be available for hemostasis and suturing of all types of tissue.

The surgical technologist should determine the arrangement of items on the instrument table and Mayo stand; this arrangement should be an effective standard method that applies principles of work simplification and thorough knowledge of

procedures. Lengthy incisions are often required for thoracic procedures; therefore it is critical that an instrument count be performed before closure.

The back table will include instruments required for the type of thoracic surgery being performed. Common setup includes a basin set, thoracotomy/thoracoscopy set, and a self-retainer retractor, such as a Karlin or Beuford. Although surgeons may have a preference for the type of scope and camera used in endoscopic procedures, either monopolar or bipolar electrosurgery is commonly employed. Preferences will also include an aspirating needle, endo graspers, endo forceps, punches, or biting biopsy clamps, as well as minimally invasive needle holders and scissors. Extra long instruments should also be available.

The Mayo stand includes long and standard Metzenbaum and Mayo scissors and long DeBakey, Russian, and Gerald forceps. Blades needed include 20, 10, 15, and 11 on both long and standard handles. Long hemoclip appliers in medium and large sizes, as well as an extended electrosurgical pencil (active electrode), and long silk ties on a pass are common. Clamps include Duvals, long Allises tonsils, and hemostats. The Allison lung retractor is the most common handheld thoracic retractor. Figures 14-7 through 14-9 show examples of instruments used in thoracic procedures.

A long double-armed monofilament suture is needed for any unexpected bleeding. Closing suture on an open procedure includes pericostal sutures. These are placed to appose the ribs and are commonly a braided absorbable suture material on a rather large needle.

Equipment. In thoracic surgery, a variety of equipment is used, including a forced-air warming unit, fiberoptic head-

PATIENT SAFETY

Patient Identification

Like the hospital gown, the wrist identification band is a traditional part of the "patient" persona and is linked to the routine of verification before administering medications, treatments, or procedures. When the wristband is present and has correct information, it can be a reliable identifier.

Patients undergoing thoracic procedures are at risk for identification errors because their wristbands are often removed to provide access for starting intravenous (IV) and other invasive monitoring lines or may be inaccessible because of positioning or draping. Correctly identifying the patient is an important Joint Commission National Patient Safety Goal. Research from The Joint Commission found that incorrect patient identification was involved in 13% of surgical errors and 67% of transfusion errors. The OR team must be familiar with the institutional policy regarding patient identification and the methods and procedures used to accomplish it. If a band is removed it should never be retaped in a new location or taped or pinned to the patient's gown. The band that is retaped or repaired may not maintain its integrity. A band pinned to a gown is easily lost if the gown is removed or replaced. The OR team should anticipate that identification bands may need to be removed for access purposes and ensure replacement bands are available. If the patient's arms are not accessible, the OR team should consider placing the new band on the patient's ankle.

Some organizations use color-coded identification bands to indicate allergies, blood type, or do-not-resuscitate (DNR) orders. The OR team must be familiar with the color coding used by the institution to avoid misidentification.

Technology is available to support the patient identification process. Many identification bands include bar codes that can be read with handheld bar code readers. Bar codes allow the surgical team to verify identity and capture other important data. A bar code identification band meets the American Hospital Association's guidelines for a tamperproof, nontransferable identification band.

Newer technology uses radiofrequency identification (RFID) systems for accurate patient verification. RFID remotely collects information and stores it on a system consisting of tags (transponders) and readers (interrogators). Microchips inside the tags contain more than 100 times the information of bar codes. The chip can contain patient information such as name, blood type, allergies, and medications.

The Joint Commission recommends using a two-patient identifier system, a preprocedural identification process, and a time-out procedure. First, the two-patient identifier simply means that the surgical team must use more than one method of identification to identify the patient. Using the wristband alone is not enough. Second, the preprocedural identification is performed by the surgeon and the OR team. This is used to correctly identify each patient just before going into the operating suite. Lastly, the time-out procedure is performed in the operating suite by the surgeon and the perioperative team—time is taken to properly identify the patient, procedure, and site of surgery. This is the final identifier before the actual operation is performed.

Modified from The Joint Commission International Center for Patient Safety: *Using identification bands to reduce patient identification errors,* available at www. jcipatientsafety.org/show.asp?durki=12346. Accessed April 11, 2009; The Joint Commission: *2009 National Patient Safety Goals (NPSGs),* available at www. jointcommission/NR/rdonlyres/31666E86-E7F4-423E-9BE8-F05BD1CB0AA8/0/HAP_NPSG.pdf. Accessed May 7, 2009; Inglesby JM, Inglesby T: Automatic identification barcoding and RFID, *Patient Safety Quality HealthCare,* available at www.psqh.com/sepoct05/barcodingrfid2.html. Accessed May 7, 2009.

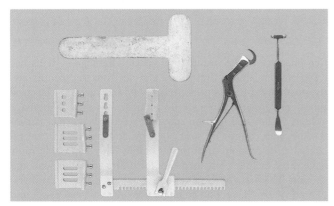

FIGURE 14-7 *Top, left to right:* 1 malleable T retractor; 1 Giertz (first rib) (rib guillotine) rongeur; 1 Matson rib stripper and elevator. *Bottom left:* Burford rib spreader with shallow blade attached; 1 shallow blade; 2 deep blades.

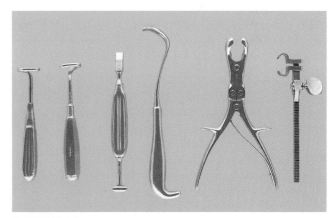

FIGURE 14-8 *Left to right:* 2 Doyen rib elevators and raspatories, *left and right:* 1 Alexander rib raspatory (periosteotome), double-ended; 1 Semb lung retractor; 1 Semb gouging rongeur, double-action; 1 Bailey rib contractor.

lights, fiberoptic light sources, video equipment, sequential compression devices, and anesthesia supplies. Double-lumen endotracheal tubes are commonly used for thoracotomies.

The neodymium:yttrium-aluminum-garnet (Nd:YAG) or CO_2 laser can be used for treating tracheobronchial lesions with use of a bronchoscope. Obstruction of the mainstem bronchus and trachea caused by benign and malignant lesions can also

be effectively treated with laser therapy. Use of laser equipment requires a thorough understanding of the equipment, the safety issues, the responsibilities, and the planned surgical procedure.

One or more chest catheters (tubes) may be inserted for postoperative closed-chest drainage. The chest tubes provide a conduit for drainage of air, blood, and other fluid from the intrapleural or mediastinal space and reestablishment of nega-

Laboratory Studies and Tests for Assessment of Patients Undergoing Thoracic Procedures

Laboratory Study	Normal Results	Significance of Abnormal Findings
PERFUSION STUDIES—ARTERIAL BLOOD GASES (ABGs)		
pH	7.35-7.45	Changes indicate metabolic or respiratory acidosis.
$Paco_2$	35-45 mm Hg	Elevations indicate possible COPD, asthma, pneumonia, anesthetic effects, or use of opioids (respiratory acidosis). Decreased levels indicate hyperventilation/respiratory alkalosis.
HCO_3^-	21-28 mEq/L	Elevations indicate possible respiratory acidosis as compensation for primary metabolic alkalosis. Decreased levels indicate possible respiratory alkalosis as compensation for primary metabolic acidosis.
Pao_2	80-100 mm Hg	Elevations may indicate possible excessive oxygen administration. Decreased levels indicate possible COPD, asthma, chronic bronchitis, cancer of bronchi and lungs, respiratory distress syndrome, or any other cause of hypoxia.
O_2 saturation	95%-100%	Decreased levels indicate possible impaired ability of hemoglobin to release oxygen to tissues.
COMPLETE BLOOD COUNT		
RBCs	*Male:* 4.7-6.1 million/mm³ *Female:* 4.2-5.4 million/mm³	Elevated levels may be due to excessive production of erythropoietin, which occurs in response to a hypoxic stimulus, such as COPD. Decreased levels may indicate anemia, hemorrhage, or hemolysis.
Hemoglobin	*Male:* 14.8 g/dl *Female:* 12-16 g/dl	Same as for RBCs.
Hematocrit	*Male:* 42%-52% *Female:* 37%-47%	Same as for RBCs.
WBCs	5000-10,000/mm³	Elevations indicate possible acute bacterial infections or inflammatory conditions (smoking). Decreased levels may indicate overwhelming infection or immunosuppression.

COPD, Chronic obstructive pulmonary disease; *HCO₃⁻,* bicarbonate ion; *Paco₂,* partial pressure of arterial carbon dioxide; *Pao₂,* partial pressure of arterial oxygen; *RBC,* red blood cell; *WBC,* white blood cell.
From Pagana KD, Pagana TJ: *Mosby's diagnostic and laboratory test references,* ed 9, St Louis, 2009, Mosby; Rees HC: Assessment of the respiratory system. In Ignatavicius DD, Workman ML, editors: *Medical-surgical nursing: patient-centered collaborative care,* ed 6, Philadelphia, 2010, Saunders.

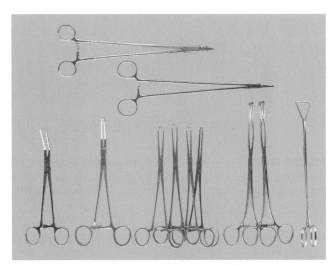

FIGURE 14-9 *Top:* 2 Crile-Wood needle holders, 11 inch. *Bottom, left to right:* 1 Sarot bronchus clamp, angled; 1 Lee bronchus clamp, angular; 4 Allis tissue forceps, long; 3 Duval lung forceps, 2 front views and 1 side view.

tive pressure in the intrapleural space. Drainage systems use three mechanisms to drain fluid and air from the pleural cavity: positive expiratory pressure, gravity, and suction. The chest tubes are connected to a sterile water-seal or gravity drainage system. Water-seal suction may be necessary when a persistent air leak cannot be controlled by drainage alone. Several compact, disposable units are available. The disposable units have three or four compartments for drainage, water seal, and suction. The first chamber collects the drainage from the intrapleural space, the second chamber provides the water seal, and the third provides the suction control determined by the level of water (Figure 14-10). If two chest tubes are inserted, they may be attached by a Y connector to a single drainage unit or may be attached individually to two separate units. Chest tubes are generally removed within 5 to 7 days.

Surgical Interventions

ENDOSCOPY (DIAGNOSTIC OR THERAPEUTIC)

Endoscopy refers to examination of hollow body organs or cavities with instruments that permit visual inspection of their con-

▶▶ RISK REDUCTION STRATEGIES

Chest Tube Safety

The use of chest tubes is almost synonymous with thoracic surgery. Effective strategies for the management of chest tubes and chest tube drainage systems promote reduction of risk to patients for this aspect of thoracic surgery.

According to the U.S. Agency for Healthcare Research and Quality (AHRQ), major sources of adverse outcomes include breaks in sterile technique, inadequate anesthesia, incorrect insertion techniques, and inadequate self-protection by clinicians. The agency issued the following findings:

◆ Trying to perform multiple procedures concurrently is a major source of error.
◆ Equipment trays should be positioned near the surgeon's dominant hand.
◆ A patient's discomfort can make it difficult to perform a sterile procedure. While adequate anesthesia is important, the patient may also need verbal and physical comforting. If a patient's movements cannot be controlled, the anesthesia team should be called.
◆ Correct techniques can prevent damage to the lung and surrounding tissue, contamination of the wound, and leakage of fluid.
◆ Universal Precautions against bloodborne infections are crucial to protect clinicians and their patients. In U.S. urban trauma centers, HIV rates among trauma patients are as high as 10%, and hepatitis C rates are as high as 15%; therefore Universal Precautions should be practiced for all chest tube insertions.

Additional management strategies include the following:

◆ Ensure that the dressing on the chest around the tube is tight and intact. Palpate the area for puffiness or crackling that may indicate subcutaneous emphysema.
◆ Assess for difficulty breathing.
◆ Assess breathing effectiveness by pulse oximetry.
◆ Check alignment of the patient's trachea.
◆ Keep the drainage system lower than the patient's chest.
◆ Keep the chest tube as straight as possible, avoiding kinks and dependent loops; do not "strip" the chest tube.
◆ Ensure the chest tube is securely taped to the connector and the connector is taped to the tubing that enters the collection chamber.
◆ Assess bubbling in the water-seal chamber; should be gentle bubbling on patient's exhalation, forceful cough, position changes.

The physician or rapid response team should be notified when the following are observed:

◆ Tracheal deviation
◆ Sudden onset or increased intensity of dyspnea
◆ Oxygen saturation less than 90%
◆ Drainage greater than 70 ml/hr
◆ Visible eyelets on the chest tube
◆ Chest tube falls out of the patient's chest or disconnects from the drainage system

Modified from Problems and Prevention: *Chest tube insertion. Patient safety: findings in action,* AHRQ Publ No. 06-P024, Sept 2006, Agency for Healthcare Research and Quality, Rockville, Md, available at www.ahrq.gov/qual/chesttubes.htm. Accessed May 12, 2009; Workman ML: Care of patients with noninfectious lower respiratory problems. In Ignatavicius DD, Workman ML, editors: *Medical-surgical nursing: patient-centered collaborative care,* ed 6, Philadelphia, 2010, Saunders.

tents and walls. The endoscopic procedures pertinent to thoracic surgery are bronchoscopy, mediastinoscopy, and thoracoscopy. Each endoscopist has preferences regarding the type of endoscope, positioning of the patient, type of anesthetic, and equipment. Invasive diagnostic or therapeutic measures enhance the decision to pursue surgical intervention by providing information related to the disease process, including histologic characteristics, location of the lesion, and lesion extent. Therapeutic endoscopy provides treatment by removal of the lesion or foreign body.

Standard Bronchoscopy Using Rigid Bronchoscope

Standard bronchoscopy is the direct visualization of the mucosa of the trachea, the main bronchi and their openings, and most of the segmental bronchi. It also includes removal of material for microscopic study if necessary.

Bronchoscopy is an integral part of the examination of patients with pulmonary symptoms such as persistent cough or wheezing, hemoptysis, obstruction, and abnormal roentgenographic changes. Common causes of bleeding (hemoptysis) are bronchiectasis, carcinoma, and tuberculosis. Congenital anomalies and suspected presence of a foreign body, especially in infants and children, are responsible for emergency examination of the respiratory tract.

The surgeon performs bronchoscopy to determine the presence of a lesion in the tracheobronchial passages, to identify and localize that lesion accurately, and to observe periodically the effects of therapy. It can be completed for dilating struc-

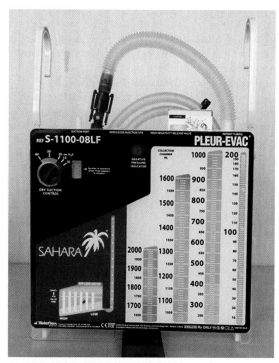

FIGURE 14-10 Commercial chest drainage system.

AMBULATORY SURGERY CONSIDERATIONS

Ambulatory Thoracic Surgery

The concept of ambulatory surgical procedures is not new to the thoracic specialty; patients undergoing bronchoscopy or endoscopic sympathectomy have often completed their procedures on an outpatient basis. With the increased trend toward more minimally invasive procedures and improved technology to accomplish those procedures, the indications for ambulatory thoracic surgery are growing. Proper patient selection is key to the success of an ambulatory thoracic program. The surgeon must weigh the risks and benefits of performing surgery on a patient and allowing a discharge to home within several hours of the procedure. Anesthesia risk can be assessed according to the individual patient's American Society of Anesthesiologists (ASA) physical status classification. The surgeon considers the complexity of the surgery, the patient's medical and surgical history, and other factors on a case-by-case basis before surgery to ensure the most appropriate patients are selected for outpatient procedures. Because the majority of thoracic procedures entail entry into the chest, the patient's level of pain, amount of chest tube output, presence or absence of an air leak, and pneumothorax status must be closely monitored before the final determination for discharge that same day.

There are many ambulatory surgical centers in the United States that offer an array of thoracic services. Mediastinoscopies, endoscopic and minimally invasive procedures on the lungs and nerves of the mediastinum, are the most frequently performed thoracic surgeries on an outpatient basis. Through proper patient selection, excellent surgical technique, and exceptional postoperative care the majority of patients treated at these centers can safely be discharged to home the day of surgery. Essential teaching points to cover with the patient and caregiver include pain control, respiratory treatments (to include deep breathing and coughing as ordered by the surgeon), and activity. Because the chest wall has been entered, the importance of seeking emergency care if the patient experiences difficulty breathing, sudden chest pain, palpitations, uncontrollable cough, or bloody sputum is emphasized.

Though they do not meet the standard definition of outpatient surgery, there is a movement toward programs to fast-track thoracic patients to earlier discharge to reduce inpatient stays. These fast-track programs usually operate, recover, and discharge a patient within a few days of being admitted. The postoperative recovery periods at these centers focus on pain relief and advances in chest tube management. Patients are often able to be discharged home safely with chest tubes in place using either a Heimlich valve or a portable drainage collection system. As more fast-track programs evolve and are able to demonstrate successful outcomes, new indications for outpatient care are likely to evolve.

Modified from Cerolio R, Brant AS: Does minimally invasive thoracic surgery warrant fast tracking of thoracic surgical patients? *Thorac Surg Clin* 18:301-304, 2008; Molins L et al: Outpatient thoracic surgery, *Thorac Surg Clin* 18:321-327, 2008.

---

tures, debriding tumors, or evacuating clots. In suspected carcinoma, the aspirated secretions obtained by bronchoscopy may contain malignant cells.

Procedural Considerations. Flexible bronchoscopy on an adult patient may be completed after induction of local (topical) anesthesia or monitored anesthesia care; a child usually receives a general anesthetic. Patients undergoing rigid bronchoscopy should be paralyzed and ventilation continued to minimize trauma. The adult patient administered a local anesthetic may experience discomfort and anxiety. To reduce anxiety, the perioperative nurse should introduce members of the surgical team, explain intraoperative activities, and provide reassurance to the patient. The oral structures, including the teeth and lips, should be assessed for integrity. Loose teeth may require removal before or during the procedure.

The anesthesia provider or nurse providing moderate sedation may administer IV sedatives or analgesics during the procedure. The topical (or local) anesthetic setup should include a headlight for visualization, laryngeal mirrors of various sizes, a lingual spatula, sprays with straight and curved cannulae, and anesthetic drugs, as ordered. Other items include the laryngeal syringe with straight and curved cannulae, Jackson cross-action forceps, and the Schindler pharyngeal anesthetizer, if desired. Luer-Lok 10-ml syringes and 20- and 22-gauge needles are needed for transtracheal injection. The surgical technologist ensures that all requested instrumentation is available to avoid delays and ensure the procedure is performed efficiently for the patient.

Anesthetic drugs frequently used for local or topical anesthesia are lidocaine (Xylocaine), procaine (Novocain), and tetracaine (Pontocaine, Cetacaine) with or without epinephrine. Pauses of 3 to 4 minutes are taken between applications of the anesthetic agent to the tongue, palate, and pharynx and then to the larynx and to the trachea. The surgeon or anesthesia provider applies the anesthetic agent by means of a spray or laryngeal syringe with a straight or curved cannula.

Some physicians prefer to have the patient sit upright and gargle with the topical anesthetic mixture, rinse it around in the mouth, and then expectorate it, thereby producing a partial anesthesia of the buccal mucosa and pharynx.

For direct bronchoscopy, the surgeon or anesthesia provider uses a long metal cannula attached to a syringe to apply the anesthetic agent to the surface of the vocal cords; then the agent is injected through the anesthetized glottis into the trachea. This act causes the patient to produce a sharp, sudden cough. For intrabronchial anesthesia, a portion of the anesthetic agent is introduced through the bronchoscope.

The patient may be positioned either in the supine position—with the shoulders elevated on a small roll, gel pad, or a sandbag to gently extend the head and neck—or in the sitting position.

The setup includes the bronchoscope, telescopes of desired types, fiberoptic light cords, and the fiberoptic light source. Each standard scope requires a fiberoptic light carrier, cord, and light source. The surgical technologist ensures that duplicates of each, along with the appropriate replacement lightbulbs for the light source, are available for immediate use. The light source should be tested periodically and immediately before use. To test the fiberoptic light carrier and telescope, the instrument should be held vertically by the ocular end. The endoscope should always be tested immediately before passage into the patient. The light-intensity dial should be set at the proper level, as specified by the manufacturer. The light source should be switched on and off to test its function. During a procedure, the perioperative nurse switches the light source to standby mode whenever it is not in active use to conserve the life of the bulb and promote cooling.

Other supplies that will be needed are suction tubing, aspirating tubes, specimen collectors, sponge carriers, and the desired type of forceps. The metal sponge carrier consists of two parts: an inner rod, which has two jaws protruding from its distal end; and an outer band, which is screwed down on the inner rod so that a sponge can be held securely within the jaws. Small gauze sponges are used to keep the field dry, remove secretions, and apply a topical anesthetic agent. Cytologic specimen collectors, such as the Clerf or Lukens, are used to hold secretions as they are obtained. Aspirating tubes of different lengths and designs are used to remove secretions and collect material for microscopic examination and culture(s). The straight aspirating tube with one or two openings at the distal end is used to remove material from the pharynx, larynx, and esophagus. The curved aspirating tube with a flexible tip is used to remove secretions from the upper and dorsal orifices of the bronchi.

The surgeon uses various types of forceps to remove foreign bodies or tissues for histologic study. Biting-tip forceps may be used to secure tissue for pathologic study. Forceps with jaws that veer laterally at about a 45-degree angle from the instrument's axis permit visualization during the biopsy maneuver. Bronchoesophageal forceps consist of a stylet, a cannula with a handle, a screw, a locknut, and a setscrew. Forceps for laryngeal and bronchial regions are designed to remove tissue specimens. The circulating nurse will prepare several specimen containers with the identifying patient information label, along with laboratory slips for specific requests. If brush specimens are collected, slides and alcohol are required. Specimen safety practices are followed, and the surgical technologist and circulating nurse should "repeat back" the type and location of each specimen collected.

The standard bronchoscope is a rigid speculum used for visualizing the tracheobronchial tree. The rigid bronchoscope might be selected for biopsy of a large central mass, for removal of a foreign object, or to control hemorrhage during biopsy of a vascular mass. The rigid bronchoscope remains the instrument of choice for removal of foreign bodies in infants and children. A fiberoptic light carrier is inserted into the bronchoscope to illuminate the distal opening. A side channel is incorporated into the bronchoscope to permit aeration of the lungs with oxygen or anesthetic gases. An additional device, the Sanders Venturi system, which is available to the anesthesia provider, provides adequate patient ventilation during bronchoscopies and laryngoscopies.

The endoscopist risks contamination in the presence of communicable diseases. For this reason, the endoscopist and assistants should wear facemasks and eye protection or wear a transparent shield attached to a headband. With increasing numbers of patients with tuberculosis, particulate respirators are recommended as protective devices. Aseptic technique is used to prevent cross-contamination.

Operative Procedure

1. The patient's head is placed in position for visualization of the bronchus—to the left when the right main bronchi are inspected and to the right when the left bronchi are inspected. The head is lowered for inspection of the middle lobe.
2. The endoscopist places a tooth guard to protect the patient's teeth. The bronchoscope is inserted over the surface of the tongue, usually through the right corner of the mouth. The patient's lip is retracted from the upper teeth with a finger of the endoscopist's left hand. The epiglottis is identified and elevated with the tip of the bronchoscope.
3. The endoscopist passes the distal end of the scope through the true vocal cords of the larynx, and views the upper tracheal rings. A small amount of anesthetic solution may be sprayed through the tube on the carina of the trachea and into the bronchus with the bronchial atomizer or spray. The patient's head is moved to the left to obtain a view of the right bronchi. The right-angle telescope is inserted with the light adjusted into the bronchoscope.
4. The segmental bronchial orifices of the upper right lobe bronchi are viewed, and the telescope is removed. The endoscopist uses suction and aspirating tubes to clear the field of vision and remove accumulated secretions.
5. The endoscopist inserts an oblique 45-degree–angle telescope or right-angle telescope and advances it to inspect the middle lobe branches. The patient's head is lowered to view the right middle lobe or turned to the right to view the left main bronchus.
6. Secretions are aspirated by the endoscopist for study. Biopsy forceps are used if indicated; foreign bodies are removed with forceps.
7. The bronchoscope is removed, and the patient's face is cleansed.

Bronchoscopy Using the Flexible Bronchoscope

Flexible bronchoscopy is performed to view structures that cannot be observed with a rigid scope. Flexible bronchoscopy may be performed in addition to a standard rigid bronchoscopy or as an independent procedure. If performed independently, the patient may remain on the transporting stretcher during the procedure. Flexible bronchoscopy is completed for the same reasons as rigid bronchoscopy. Flexible fiberoptic telescopes permit visualization of the upper, middle, and lower lobe bronchi. They can be passed in patients with a jaw deformity or cervical bone rigidity with less difficulty than the rigid scope. Flexible fiberoptic bronchoscopes are more frequently used, as is video endoscopy.

Procedural Considerations. Patient considerations are as described for rigid bronchoscopy. Instruments and equipment used include the flexible bronchoscope, fiberoptic light source, flexible biopsy forceps, flexible brush (optional; if used, slides and alcohol are necessary to collect specimen), labeled specimen collectors, pathology requests, syringe for wash, and suction tubing with collection tube attached to collect the wash specimen.

Operative Procedure

1. The lubricated bronchoscope is passed through the adapter on the endotracheal tube, which is held secure by the anesthesia provider. If local or monitored anesthesia care is used

for the procedure, the lubricated bronchoscope may be passed nasally.

2. The suction tube is positioned with the specimen collector attached for collection of bronchial washings. When indicated, the suction tubing is connected to the bronchoscope; the container for collection is held securely in an upright position to prevent loss of the specimen through the suction.

3. The endoscopist or surgical technologist injects approximately 5 ml of saline solution into the channel. Suction is quickly reapplied. This procedure may be repeated as necessary.

After completion of the procedure, the perioperative nurse sends the specimens to the laboratory for analysis.

Mediastinoscopy

Mediastinoscopy is the direct visualization and possible biopsy of lymph nodes or tumors at the tracheobronchial junction, under the carina of the trachea, or on the upper lobe bronchi or subdivisions. Mediastinoscopy may precede an exploratory thoracotomy in known cases of lung carcinoma or may be completed to assist in accurately staging the patient's lymph node status. Patients with positive findings may be treated with radiation or chemotherapy, as indicated. The mediastinoscope is a hollow tube with a fiberoptic light carrier. A fiberoptic light source with a light-intensity dial provides power and control of illumination.

Procedural Considerations. The setup for mediastinoscopy includes a set of instruments for incising, cutting, retracting, and suturing similar to those needed for a minor procedure. In addition, the desired type of mediastinoscope, fiberoptic light cords, fiberoptic light source, suction tubing, aspirating tubes, biopsy forceps, electrosurgical unit (ESU), and an 8-inch, 20-gauge endocardiac needle are required. Depending on institutional policy, a thoracotomy tray may be in the OR on standby in the event of uncontrolled bleeding after biopsy.

The anesthesia provider administers a general anesthetic agent and assists with positioning the patient as described for a tracheostomy (see Chapter 10).

Operative Procedure

1. The surgeon makes a short (approximately 2-cm) transverse incision above the suprasternal notch, and exposes and incises the pretracheal fascia.

2. Using blunt (digital) dissection, the surgeon tunnels alongside the trachea into the mediastinum.

3. The surgeon introduces the mediastinoscope under direct vision deep to the fascial plane and advances it along the side of the trachea toward the mediastinum.

4. The scope is manipulated to visualize the tracheal bifurcation, bronchi, aortic arch, and associated lymph nodes.

5. Lymph node tissue is located for biopsy and aspirated with a small-gauge needle and syringe to verify that it is a nonvascular structure.

6. The surgeon inserts a biopsy forceps through the scope, and obtains a tissue specimen. Pressure can be applied to the excision site with a bronchus sponge on a holder. The mediastinum is reinspected for bleeding.

7. The mediastinoscope is withdrawn.

8. Subcutaneous tissue is sutured with absorbable sutures. The surgeon closes the skin with nonabsorbable material on a small cutting needle.

9. A small dressing is applied.

Video-Assisted Thoracic Surgery

Video-assisted thoracic surgery (VATS) is a minimally invasive operative technique that has evolved over the past decade. It uses an endoscopic approach to visualization of the thoracic cavity for diagnosis of pleural disease or treatment of pleural conditions, such as cysts, blebs, and effusions; for biopsy of mediastinal masses; to perform wedge resections, lobectomy, pericardectomy, lung volume reduction surgery, and cervical sympathectomy; to obtain hemostasis; and to evacuate blood clots or divide adhesions (Khraim, 2007). Pleurodesis with instillation of talc, tetracycline, or other sclerosing treatment can be accomplished through the thoracoscope (Surgical Pharmacology). VATS has many benefits, including the elimination of a thoracotomy incision, decreased pain, shortened hospital stay, and reduced morbidity. VATS may also be used in conjunction with robotically assisted thoracic procedures such as robotic lobectomy.

Procedural Considerations. Endoscopic instrumentation and equipment used for a thoracoscopy include 5- and 10-mm telescopes, light cord, camera, graspers, dissectors, scissors, ligators, and endoscopic soft tissue instruments (scissors, hemostats, suction tips, retractors) and stapling devices. Accessory equipment for video (television monitors, videocassette recorder, printer, light source for camera and scope, slave television monitor) and insufflation is also used. The perioperative nurse will assist in positioning the patient supine, semilaterally or laterally, depending on the anatomic structures involved.

Operative Procedure

1. The surgeon creates a 2- to 3-cm incision between the fifth and seventh intercostal spaces for insertion of the 10- or 12-mm trocar. The zero-degree telescope is inserted to view the site so that the approach can be determined.

2. If the procedure can be completed by thoracoscopy, the surgeon creates additional puncture sites for insertion of additional trocars to allow instrument manipulation. The size of trocars and types of instruments vary for the diagnosis.

3. After the selected procedure, the surgeon inserts a chest tube through one of the surgical puncture sites and secures it to the skin. Trocar sites are closed, and small dressings or adhesive skin tapes are applied.

Endoscopic Thoracic Sympathectomy

Hyperhidrosis is defined as excessive sweating, usually affecting the palms, axillae, and soles of the feet. It may also affect the face, groin, or legs. Patients with severe hyperhidrosis may produce 40 times the normal amount of sweat (Solish et al, 2008). Hyperhidrosis affects approximately 2.8% of the general population, with 1.4% of these individuals projected to have axillary hyperhidrosis and 0.5% to have sweating that is intolerable or interferes with daily activities (Weksler et al, 2008). Familial history of hyperhidrosis is implicated in 30% to 65% of cases (Solish et al, 2008). Endoscopic thoracic sympathectomy (ETS) is a thoracoscopic intervention used to surgically treat hyperhidrosis (Research Highlight). To treat

SURGICAL PHARMACOLOGY

Agents for Chemical Pleurodesis

Pleurodesis is undertaken as a treatment for malignant pleural effusion and for unresolved spontaneous pneumothorax. A variety of chemical agents are used to cause adherence of the pleural layers. Adherence of the pleural layers is thought to prevent the accumulation of pleural fluid in the case of pleural effusion and to prevent subsequent pneumothoraces. Commonly used agents for chemical pleurodesis are listed. Other agents may be used according to the surgeon's preference, surgical region, and agent availability. Surgical technologists should consult with the surgeon before the procedure to determine the agent used.

Agent	Mechanism of Action	Dosage	Side Effects
Talc	Stimulates mesothelial cells to coordinate an inflammatory response	5-10 g in 250 ml of sodium chloride	Pain, infection, ARDS, pulmonary edema
Antineoplastics	Chemical pleural irritation and fibrosis of pleural surfaces	Bleomycin: 60 units mixed with 100-200 mg of lidocaine	Pain, fever, neutropenia
Cyclines	Indirectly stimulate pleural macrophages, activating pleural mesothelial cells; low pH initiates an inflammatory reaction, causing fibrosis	Minocycline: 7 mg/kg Doxycycline: 500 mg in 30-50 ml of sodium chloride	Pain, fever, hemothorax, neutropenia
Silver nitrate	Coagulates cellular protein to form pleural eschar	20 ml of 0.5% silver nitrate	Pain, fever
Quinacrine	Causes systemic inflammatory response	500 mg in 200 ml of saline	Pain, fever
Iodopovidone	Mechanism of action unknown	20 ml of 10% iodopovidone in 80 ml of saline	Severe pain, hypotension

ARDS, Acute respiratory distress syndrome.
Modified from Colt HG, Davoudi M: The ideal pleurodesis agent: still searching after all these years, *Lancet Oncol* 9(10):912-913, 2008; Demmy TL, Nwogu C: Malignant pleural and pericardial effusion. In Selke FW et al, editors: *Sabiston and Spencer surgery of the chest,* ed 7, Philadelphia, 2005, Saunders; Dikensoy O, Light RW: Alternative widely available, inexpensive agents for pleurodesis, *Curr Opin Pulmonary Med* 11:340-344, 2005; Khaleeq G, Musani AI: Emerging paradigms in the management of malignant pleural effusions, *Respir Med* 102:939-948, 2008; Kilic D et al: Management of recurrent malignant pleural effusion with chemical pleurodesis, *Surg Today* 35:634-638, 2005.

RESEARCH HIGHLIGHT

Thoracoscopic Sympathectomy versus Medical Management for Severe Hyperhidrosis

Hyperhidrosis can be an extremely disabling condition for which medical management is the first-line treatment. While many patients are able to control their hyperhidrosis through medical management (e.g., topical aluminum chloride, anticoagulants, botulinum toxin A injections, use of iontophoresis [a treatment that uses water to conduct an electrical current through the skin's surface that results in microscopic thickening of the outer layer of the skin, which blocks the flow of sweat to the skin surface]), these treatments are temporary, require a high degree of patient commitment, and are associated with side effects. The researchers in this study sought to compare the outcomes of medical versus surgical management for palmoplantar hyperhidrosis (e.g., excessive sweating of the hands and feet) and evaluate the efficacy and side effects of both treatments.

Researchers conducted a prospective and retrospective study of 192 patients who met the criteria of (1) massive palmar sweating to the point of dripping or near-dripping, (2) plantar sweating approximating the palmar sweating, (3) simultaneous onset either in early childhood or at puberty, and (4) exacerbation with the use of ordinary hand lotion. The vast majority of patients met all four criteria, and no patient had fewer than three of the criteria. A total of 46 patients in the prospective group used the medical treatments for at least 2 weeks, and their responses and side effects were noted. If the medical treatment was unsatisfactory because of intolerable side effects or lack of response, the group was offered endoscopic thoracic sympathectomy (ETS). Only 1 patient from the prospective group and 1 patient from the retrospective group were satisfied enough with the results of medical management to forgo ETS surgery; 89 patients in the retrospective group underwent ETS.

Data analysis revealed that six (3.2%) patients who underwent ETS experienced severe compensatory sweating that resulted in significant discomfort. One patient experienced a pneumothorax, but no other significant complications were reported from ETS. Complications reported from medical management included palmar reactions (from topical solutions), with cracking and continued sweating through the cracks, and mouth dryness/discomfort, blurred vision, mental changes, and headaches. All of the patients who used botulinum toxin A experienced palmar pain, and one third of patients in the iontophoresis group developed pain and irritation from the treatments. Researchers concluded that ETS can "safely and confidently" be recommended as a first-line treatment of severe palmoplantar hyperhidrosis.

Modified from Baumgartner FJ et al: Superiority of thoracoscopic sympathectomy over medical management for the palmoplantar subset of severe hyperhidrosis, *Ann Vasc Surg* 23:1-7, 2009.

palmar hyperhidrosis, the surgeon interrupts the sympathetic chain at the T2 level. Compensatory sweating, defined as increased sweating in other areas following the procedure, is the most common side effect of this procedure. The incidence of mild compensatory sweating varies from 14% to 90% and the incidence of severe compensatory sweating ranges from 1.2% to 30.9% (Dumont, 2008). Many patients who undergo ETS do so on an ambulatory basis or require only an overnight stay. The procedure produces dramatic and immediate results and is associated with a positive outcome for the patient. ETS may also be used to surgically treat pain syndromes (e.g., complex regional pain syndrome), facial blushing, and Raynaud's syndrome.

Procedural Considerations. The patient is positioned supine, and the anesthesia provider inserts a double-lumen endotracheal tube. Video monitors are placed on each side of the patient to allow the surgeon an unobstructed view from either side, because the procedure is performed bilaterally.

Operative Procedure

1. The anesthesia care provider deflates the patient's lung as directed by the surgeon.
2. The surgeon uses the scalpel to make a small (2 mm or less) incision between the patient's second and third ribs in the axillary plane.

3. A disposable thoracic port is inserted through the incision, and the surgeon inserts a small (2- or 5-mm) telescope through the port.
4. The surgeon identifies the sympathetic chain at the T2 level (Figure 14-11, *A* and *B*), and uses endoscopic scissors to open the pleura.
5. The nerve is grasped with a bipolar forceps and divided with bipolar electrocoagulation (Figure 14-11, *C*). Alternatively, clips may be applied to the nerve.
6. The port is removed, and a small thoracic catheter is inserted through the incision.
7. The surgeon closes the incision, and the lung is reexpanded. As the air is forced out of the pleural cavity, the catheter is removed and wound closure is completed.
8. The procedure is repeated for the opposite side.
9. Adhesive skin tapes are placed over the incision sites.
10. A postoperative chest x-ray film is obtained in the PACU to rule out any residual pneumothorax.

Robotic-Assisted Surgery

Robotic-assisted thoracic procedures have evolved since the introduction of robotic technology in the 1990s; they enhance the speed, accuracy, and safety of VATs (Kernstine et al, 2008). During traditional thoracotomy the surgeon's view is hampered by the size of the incision and rigidity of the chest wall. An advantage to the robotic-assisted approach is the superior three-dimensional view of the operative field and thoracic cavity,

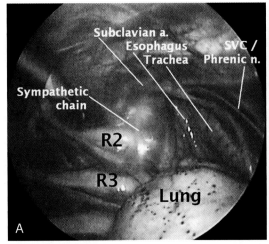
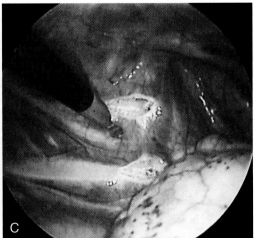
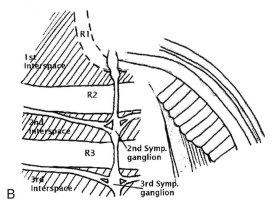

FIGURE 14-11 A, Thoracoscopic view of right superior posterior mediastinum. The sympathetic chain runs over the anterior surface of the posterior rib heads. The first rib is not visualized but can be palpated. **B,** Schematic diagram. The first rib is outlined. The sympathetic ganglion and its rami are seen just below the respective rib level. **C,** Sympathectomy over the right second and third ribs. The ganglia themselves are spared. *a,* Artery; *n,* nerve; *R1,* first rib; *R2,* second rib; *R3,* third rib; *SVC,* superior vena cava; *Symp,* sympathetic.

allowing the surgeon superior visualization, increased magnification, and better maneuverability. Smaller incisions are used for robotic surgery, so patients experience less postoperative pain and morbidity (Figure 14-12). A variety of robotic-assisted procedures are performed by specially trained surgeons, including mediastinal tumor resection, lobectomy, and sympathectomy. Continued advances in technology will allow for the development of additional applications and procedures within the thoracic specialty. The procedure for robotic-assisted lobectomy is described below.

Procedural Considerations. In addition to preparing for the robotic procedure, the perioperative nurse and surgical technologist ensure that they have also gathered instrumentation and supplies to convert to an open procedure in the event an emergency arises or the surgeon is unable to complete the procedure through the minimally invasive approach. The nurse assists the anesthesia provider with inserting a double-lumen endotracheal tube and helps to position the patient in the lateral position with the operative side up. After the patient is prepped and draped, the anesthesia provider places the patient in reverse Trendelenburg's position. The nurse assists with positioning the robot, video monitors, and three-dimensional vision console equipment.

Operative Procedure

1. The surgeon consults the patient's preoperative CT scans to determine the placement of the thoracoports based on the location of the lesion.
2. The surgeon incises the skin at the seventh to eighth intercostal space along the midposterior axillary line and inserts the 12-mm thoracoport.
3. The robotic system is positioned, and the surgeon inserts a 30-degree scope through the thoracoport and connects the scope to the camera arm.
4. The surgeon incises the skin at the sixth to seventh, fourth to fifth, and fifth to sixth intercostal spaces, inserts the remaining thoracoports, and passes the dissecting instruments through the ports and connects them to the instrument arms.
5. A combination of blunt and sharp dissection is used by the surgeon around the hilar structures to gain exposure to the pulmonary vessels.
6. The surgeon ligates the pulmonary vein and artery using suture and/or robotic clips.
7. The surgeon dissects the lobar bronchus and nodes.
8. A 3.5-mm endostapler is passed through the appropriate thoracoport, clamped, and fired to complete the bronchial transection.
9. The specimen is placed in a sterile removal bag and removed via the port site.
10. The surgeon tests the bronchial stump for leaks under water.
11. The pleural space is vented and the surgeon places a closed suction drain before closing the incisions.
12. Dressings are applied.

LUNG SURGERY

Thoracotomy

Thoracotomy involves an incision in the chest wall through a median sternotomy or a lateral or posterolateral incision for the

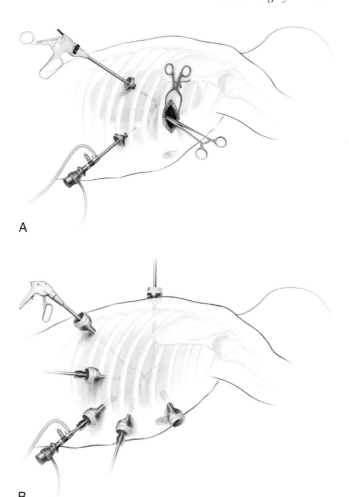

A

B

FIGURE 14-12 Comparison of VATS lobectomy to robotic lobectomy: The two patients shown are undergoing hilar dissection. **A,** VATS resection. There are three incisions shown, one for the videoscope and the other two for the right-angle clamp and stapler. The manipulation of the instrumentation and the arcs of rotation occur outside of the chest. The fulcrum of the instrumentation occurs at the chest wall, compressing and distending the intercostal nerves. **B,** Robotic resection. The arcs of rotation and management of the instrumentation for dissection are within the chest, allowing surgical dissection to occur in small spaces.

purpose of operating on the lungs (History box). Thoracotomy may be performed for a variety of benign and malignant conditions. Lung cancer (Figure 14-13) is a common diagnosis associated with thoracotomy. Patients with lung cancer may have specific treatment based on their tumor, node, and metastasis (TNM) characteristics. The TNM system defines tumor (T) as the size, location, and spread (pulmonary or extrapulmonary). The designation of nodes (N) refers to spread to a lymph node or group of lymph nodes. Metastasis (M) relates to metastatic tumor activity in distant organs (e.g., brain, liver). Staging is based on TNM findings (Figure 14-14). Intraoperative patient care is similar for various thoracotomy procedures, with consideration of the patient's history and disease process, planned procedure, and individualized patient needs. Basic thoracic instrumentation is used and may include a sternal saw and stapling devices. Preparation by the anesthesia care provider with careful monitoring of the patient is a priority. Insertion of a

Important Events in Thoracic Surgery

As early as 3000 BC, treatments related to the lungs and chest were undertaken as a result of injuries and wounds. It was not until the eighteenth century, however, that physiologic studies and animal experiments included the respiratory system. Several early reports discussed trauma, noting that wound closure helped the patient breathe easier. Thus the relationship between respiration and lung function was first established. During World War I there was increased awareness of the value of immediate closure of chest wounds.

The first thoracic procedure, recorded in 1499, was an unsuccessful excision of a herniation of the lung. From that time, the physiologic effect on the lungs and perceived difficulty entering the chest resulted in hesitancy to perform thoracic procedures. Until the 1880s the only thoracic procedures performed were to drain empyema and lung abscess or to treat traumatic chest injury. In 1823 the first purposeful resection of a part of the lung for accidental injury was reported by Milton Antony, and in 1861 the French surgeon Péan removed part of a lung for tumor.

Treatment of tuberculosis (TB) also provided an impetus for new developments in thoracic procedures. Thoracoplasty became widely used as a means of collapsing the lungs for treatment of TB, followed by other forms of treatment. In 1907 an article was published describing surgical techniques for access to the thoracic cavity. In 1913 Jacobeus is credited with dividing adhesions with an electrosurgical unit (ESU) passed through one cannula while through another he passed a cystoscope-like instrument he called a *thoracoscope*. Student textbooks in the 1920s contained only a short paragraph on cancer of the lung. From that time until the first successful pneumonectomy in 1933, many attempts were made to remove carcinomas, with limited success.

In 1899 the first important article on tumors of the chest wall was written. It summarized case reports of 46 other cases and classified the various tumor types. The first accounts of pulmonary resection were published in 1896, and one of the first cases of cancer of the lung to be reported in the United States was in 1851. Equipment and instrument development also improved the ability to study lung function. Although the bronchoscope was introduced in 1937, it was not used to study chest diseases until later. Using the bronchoscope became more important to remove secretions when Papanicolaou identified the advantages of applying cytologic technique to diagnosis of cancer.

The nursing care of patients with thoracic conditions evolved over time as medical and surgical treatments advanced and technology made new treatments available. Modern-day thoracentesis is generally accomplished using a presterilized disposable kit from a manufacturer. In the 1920s nurses who assisted with thoracentesis were responsible for acquiring a rubber sheet to protect the bed, sterile sheets to create a sterile field, sterile cotton, a hypodermic syringe and needle, sterile gloves and powder for the physician, and the aspirating set. The aspirating set consisted of a graduated 5- to 8-pint glass bottle with a rubber stopper fitted with a bifurcated metal tube and stopcocks. Rubber tubing with metal connectors was attached to the metal tube, and the sterile aspirating needle was connected to one branch of the tubing. The other branch of the tubing was connected to an exhaust pump. The nurse was responsible for testing the apparatus before the physician arrived, because the apparatus was used instead of a syringe for aspiration. Postprocedure treatment for the patient was described as "the patient must remain quietly in bed, in the recumbent position and no exertion or sudden movements should be allowed. The greatest precautions should be taken to prevent the entrance of infection."

Modified from Meade RH: *History of thoracic surgery,* Springfield, Ill, 1961, Charles C Thomas; Scott RJE: *Pocket cyclopedia of nursing,* New York, 1923, The Macmillan Co.

---

double-lumen endotracheal tube, an arterial line for monitoring ABG samples, and a central venous line to ensure patent access for fluids are procedures performed by the anesthesia provider. An epidural catheter may be inserted for intraoperative and postoperative pain management. Patient preparation by the surgical team includes positioning, placement of devices for prevention of complications (e.g., sequential compression devices, thermal-regulating blanket, electrosurgical dispersive pad), insertion of a urinary catheter, and ongoing evaluation and communication of the patient's status to the family throughout the procedure.

Pneumonectomy

Pneumonectomy is the removal of an entire lung, usually to treat malignant neoplasms. Other reasons for this procedure include removal of an extensive unilateral bronchiectasis (e.g., irreversible dilation of the bronchi) involving the greater part of one lung, drainage of an extensive chronic pulmonary abscess involving portions of one or more lobes, removal of selected benign tumors, and treatment of any extensive unilateral lesion. Other resections are often combined with pneumonectomy, such as resection of mediastinal lymph nodes, resections of portions of the chest wall or diaphragm, and removal of parietal pleura.

Procedural Considerations. The basic thoracic instrumentation is used. The perioperative nurse facilitates positioning the patient in the lateral position for a posterolateral incision.

Operative Procedure

1. The surgeon incises the skin, subcutaneous tissue, and muscle with a scalpel and the ESU. Hemostasis is attained. If a rib is to be excised, bone instruments are required.
2. The ribs and tissue are protected with moist sponges; the rib retractor is placed (Figure 14-15) and opened slowly and gently.
3. The surgeon frees any peripheral adhesions to mobilize the lung and divides the pulmonary ligament. Dissection to the hilum of the involved lobe is carried out.
4. The superior pulmonary vein is gently retracted, and the pulmonary artery is dissected.
5. The surgeon clamps the branches of the pulmonary artery and vein of the involved lobe, places double ligatures, and divides them with fine right-angled vascular clamps, scissors, and nonabsorbable suture.
6. The inferior pulmonary vein is exposed by incising the hilar pleura and retracting the lung anteriorly. The inferior pulmonary vein is clamped, doubly ligated, and divided.

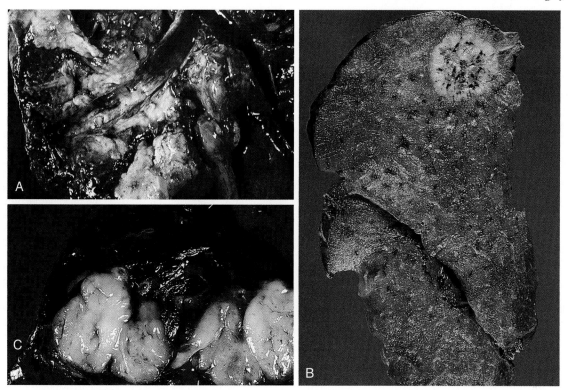

FIGURE 14-13 Lung cancer. **A**, Squamous cell carcinoma originating from the main bronchus. **B**, Peripheral adenoma. **C**, Small cell carcinoma.

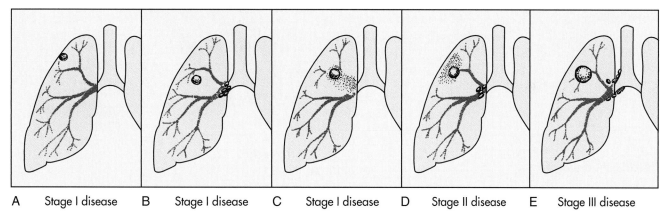

| A | Stage I disease | B | Stage I disease | C | Stage I disease | D | Stage II disease | E | Stage III disease |

FIGURE 14-14 Staging of lung cancer by TNM system. **A** and **B**, Stage I disease includes tumors classified as T_1 with or without metastasis to the lymph node in the ipsilateral hilar region. **C**, Also included in stage I are tumors classified as T_2 but having no nodal or distant metastases. **D**, Stage II disease includes those tumors classified as T_2, with metastasis only to the ipsilateral hilar lymph nodes. **E**, Stage III includes all tumors more extensive than T_2 or any tumor with metastasis to the lymph nodes in the mediastinum with distant metastasis.

7. The surgeon applies a bronchus clamp and divides the bronchus near the tracheal bifurcation. The stump is closed with atraumatic nonabsorbable mattress sutures or bronchus staples. If staples are applied, the scalpel is used to complete division of the bronchus. The lung is removed from the chest.

8. The surgical technologist supplies normal saline to irrigate the pleural space and check for hemostasis and air leaks during positive-pressure inspiration.

9. A pleural flap is created and sutured over the bronchial stump (other methods of securing the bronchus might be used).

10. Hemostasis is ensured in the pleural space.

11. Chest tubes (28-French to 30-French) are inserted into the pleural space and exteriorized through a stab wound at the eighth or ninth interspace near the anterior axillary line (Figure 14-16). An upper tube is inserted through a second stab wound if indicated to evaluate leaking air. The tubes are secured with heavy sutures and connected to water-seal drainage after closure of the pleural space.

12. The surgeon places the rib approximator (Figure 14-17) and begins closure with interrupted sutures.

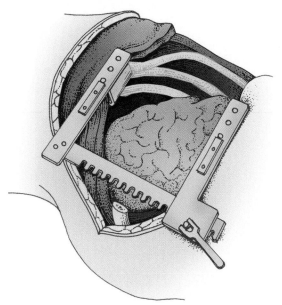

FIGURE 14-15 Rib retractor placed for thoracotomy.

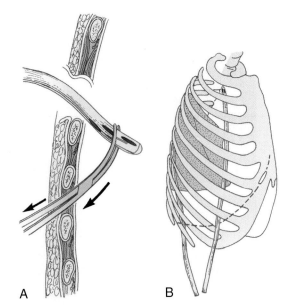

FIGURE 14-16 A, Introduction of chest drainage tube through a stab wound. **B,** Placement of apical and basal drainage tubes after upper and middle lobectomy.

13. The muscle, subcutaneous tissue, and skin are closed. Drains are anchored to the chest wall with suture.
14. The dressing is applied.
15. Chest tube connections are secured with Parnham bands or tape and labeled (anterior or posterior).

Lobectomy

Lobectomy is excision of one or more lobes of the lung. It is performed when the primary tumor is located in a particular lobe or to remove metastatic lesions when the tumor is peripherally located and hilar nodes are not involved. Other conditions affecting the lung and treated by lobectomy might be bronchiectasis; giant emphysematous blebs or bullae; large, centrally located benign tumors; fungal infections; and congenital anomalies.

Procedural Considerations. Basic thoracic instrumentation is used. The patient is placed in a lateral position for a posterolateral approach; the supine position may be used for upper- and middle-lobe resections. The procedure varies with the specific lobe to be removed depending on the anatomic structure.

Operative Procedure

1. The surgeon incises the skin, subcutaneous tissue, and muscle using a blade and the ESU. Hemostasis is attained. If a rib is to be excised, bone instruments are required.
2. The ribs and tissue are protected with sponges. The rib retractor is placed and opened slowly and gently.
3. The surgeon enters the pleura and frees the peripheral adhesions with scissors, blunt dissection, or a sponge on a sponge-holding forceps.
4. The hilar pleura is incised and separated.
5. The branches of the pulmonary arteries and veins are isolated, clamped, doubly ligated, and divided with fine, right-angled vascular clamps, scissors, and nonabsorbable suture.
6. The surgeon identifies the main trunk of the pulmonary artery and the fissure between the lobes.

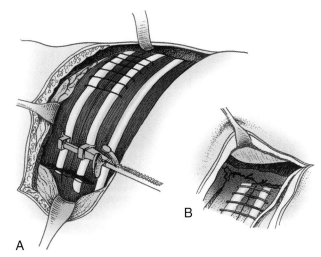

FIGURE 14-17 A, Rib approximator placed for closure of incision. **B,** Heavy-gauge suture used for closure of ribs.

7. The bronchus clamp is applied. The remaining lung is inflated to identify the line of demarcation. The bronchus is divided with a scalpel or heavy scissors.
8. Bronchial secretions are suctioned.
9. The surgeon closes the bronchus with atraumatic nonabsorbable mattress sutures or bronchus staples. If staples are applied, a blade is used to complete division of the bronchus.
10. Incomplete fissures are divided between hemostats with fine Metzenbaum scissors. Edges may be sutured closed.
11. A pleural flap is created and sutured over the bronchial stump (other methods of securing the bronchus might be used).
12. The pleural cavity is thoroughly irrigated with normal saline, and hemostasis is ensured. The remaining lobes are inflated to check for air leaks, and the degree of expansion of the remaining lobes is assessed.

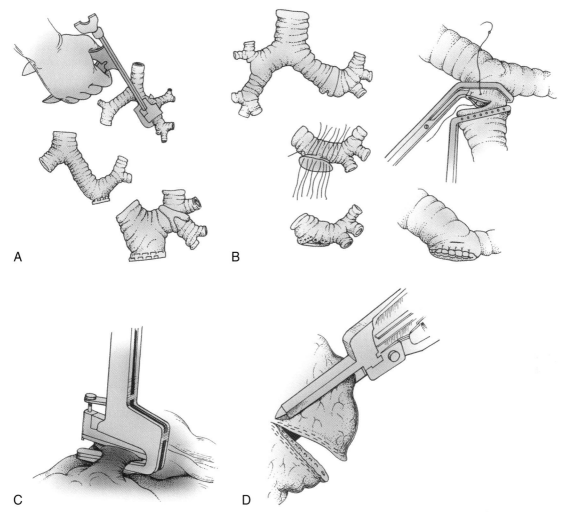

FIGURE 14-18 **A,** Staple suturing of bronchus. **B,** Conventional suturing of bronchus; application of bronchus clamp and incision; closure of stump. **C,** Staple suturing of pulmonary vessels. **D,** Staple suturing of lung tissue (wedge resection or lung biopsy).

13. The pleural space is irrigated, and the procedure is completed as described for a pneumonectomy.

Segmental Resection

Segmental resection is removal of one or more anatomic subdivisions of the pulmonary lobe. It conserves healthy, functioning pulmonary tissue by sparing remaining segments. Segmental resection is indicated for any benign lesion with segmental distribution or diseased tissue affecting only one segment of the lung with compromised cardiorespiratory reserve. The most common cause for removal is bronchiectasis. Other conditions requiring removal include chronic, localized inflammation and congenital cysts or blebs.

Procedural Considerations. Basic thoracotomy instrumentation is used. The patient is placed in lateral position.

Operative Procedure

1. The surgeon incises the skin, subcutaneous tissue, and muscle using a blade and the ESU.
2. The parietal pleura is incised with a scalpel and scissors. Adhesions are divided with sharp or blunt dissection.

3. The segmental artery is identified to provide accurate identification of the bronchus of the diseased segment.
4. The surgeon ligates the segmental pulmonary vein and branches.
5. The surgeon clamps the bronchus with the bronchus clamp, and the remaining lung is inflated. The intersegmental boundary is confirmed, and proper placement of the clamp is ensured.
6. The visceral pleura is incised around the diseased segment, beginning anterior to the hilum and progressing toward the periphery. Exposure is facilitated with a malleable or other type of retractor. The intersegmental vessels are clamped with thoracic hemostats and ligated.
7. The surgeon transects the segmental bronchus and closes the stump with atraumatic nonabsorbable mattress sutures or bronchus staples (Figure 14-18).
8. Dissection is continued to separate segmental surfaces, and vessels are ligated as needed. The segment of the lung is removed.
9. The surgeon creates a pleural flap and sutures it over the bronchial stump (other methods of securing the bronchus may be used).

10. The anesthesia provider reinflates the lung and the surgeon irrigates with normal saline. Bleeding is controlled with ligatures or hemoclips.
11. The procedure is completed as described for pneumonectomy.

Wedge Resection

Wedge resection is removal of a wedge-shaped section of parenchyma that includes the identified lesion, without regard for intersegmental planes. The resection is also used for removal of small, peripherally located benign primary tumors and peripherally located inflammatory disease, as well as for biopsy in patients with chronic, diffuse lung disease.

Procedural Considerations. Thoracic instrumentation is used. The team positions the patient to allow access to the operative site with consideration of the area of lung to be resected.

Operative Procedure
1. The surgeon incises the skin, subcutaneous tissue, and muscle using a blade and the ESU.
2. The rib retractor is placed.
3. The surgeon controls bleeding and secures the small bronchi with clamps and ligature. Large bronchi are ligated or sutured to prevent persistent air leak.
4. The wedge is outlined for excision, with a margin of normal tissue left, using one of the following techniques:
   a. Long hemostatic clamps are applied in three rows to outline the wedge. Excision is accomplished with a scalpel. The tissue is sutured with a running absorbable suture behind the clamps before removal. The edges of the tissue are oversewn with a continuous or interrupted suture (Figure 14-19).
   b. The lobe is grasped with a lung clamp, and the thoracic stapling instrument is applied to the parenchymal portion of the lung. Staples are applied, and the wedge is excised with the scalpel. Staples are reapplied to the opposite side of the lesion adjoining the staple lines.
5. The specimen is removed. The surgeon checks for air leaks by irrigation and inspection. Bleeding is controlled with ligation or hemoclips. The procedure is completed as described for pneumonectomy.

Lung Volume Reduction Surgery

Lung volume reduction surgery (LVRS) is an alternative surgical treatment for patients with chronic pulmonary emphysema (Figure 14-20). The surgery is intended to increase expiratory airflow, maximal exercise capacity, and respiratory muscle strength, thereby relieving dyspnea. The procedure may also be referred to as *lung volume reduction,* or *pneumoplasty.* Candidates for the procedure are those who have progressive, severe dyspnea secondary to pulmonary dysfunction; those whose medical management is ineffective; and those in whom disease distribution is limited to target areas of severity. The two operative approaches for LVRS are median sternotomy and video-assisted thoracic surgery (VATS). Median sternotomy provides excellent bilateral exposure and flexibility, whereas the VATS approach has the advantage of a shorter hospitalization, fewer days of postoperative air leaks, and fewer days on the ventilator (McKenna, 2007). Patients undergoing LVRS participate in vigorous pulmonary rehabilitation as a standard practice in preparation for surgery. Pulmonary rehabilitation programs not only improve airway clearance and diaphragmatic function but also ensure that optimal conditioning is achieved, which improves surgical outcomes, improves tolerance for surgery, and decreases postoperative complications. An alternative procedure, bronchoscopic lung volume reduction (BLVR), using either an implanted valve system or a distributed sclerosant, is currently being evaluated in clinical trials in the United States (Mamary and Criner, 2008).

Procedural Considerations. The basic thoracotomy setup and instrumentation are used, along with stapling devices, chest tubes, and a water-seal drainage system. A laser may be required, as may other materials for sealing the resected edges (e.g., bovine pericardium, collagen). Positioning is a particular concern for this patient population, who are often malnourished and are at increased risk for positioning injury.

Operative Procedure
1. The surgeon exposes the patient's lungs through a transverse anterior thoracotomy incision using the sternal saw to separate the sternum. Adhesiotomies are performed, and the inferior pulmonary ligaments are incised.
2. The anesthesia provider deflates the patient's lungs to allow for visualization of the portions of the lung where air is trapped in emphysematous lung tissue.
3. A lung-grasping forceps is used to hold the portion of the lung to be excised. A surgical stapling device is lined with bovine pericardium and positioned on either side of the lung. The stapling of emphysematous lung tissue continues, and staple lines are overlapped to prevent air leaks. Alternative means of sealing the resection line include the use of a pleural flap or the application of collagen.
4. The anesthesia provider reinflates the lung to identify air leaks. If air leaks are found, the lung is deflated and the stapling procedure continues.
5. One or two chest tubes are placed into each pleural space. The chest tubes are connected to water-seal drainage systems without suction.
6. The surgeon reapproximates the ribs and sternum using stainless-steel surgical wire. The muscle layer, subcutaneous tissue, and skin are closed, and dressings are applied.

Lung Biopsy

Lung biopsy is the resection of a small portion of the lung for diagnosis. The biopsy allows removal of relatively large specimens for microscopic examination of the lung tissue. Indications include (1) failure of closed methods (needle biopsy) for diagnosis and (2) the presence of small, localized lesions that can be removed by biopsy.

Procedural Considerations. In addition to the basic instrument setup, a rib retractor, a lung-grasping forceps, dissecting scissors, a chest tube and water-seal system, and an endostapling device are required. More than one specimen container may be needed. The patient is positioned in a semilateral position for an anterolateral incision.

Operative Procedure
1. A short incision (approximately 5 cm) is made at the fifth intercostal space. The surgeon incises the pleura and retracts the ribs.

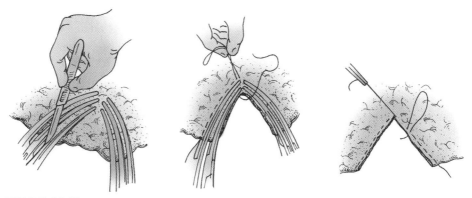

FIGURE 14-19 Wedge resection. Clamps applied to edge of lung tissue to be excised with blade and sutured with a running suture and oversewn.

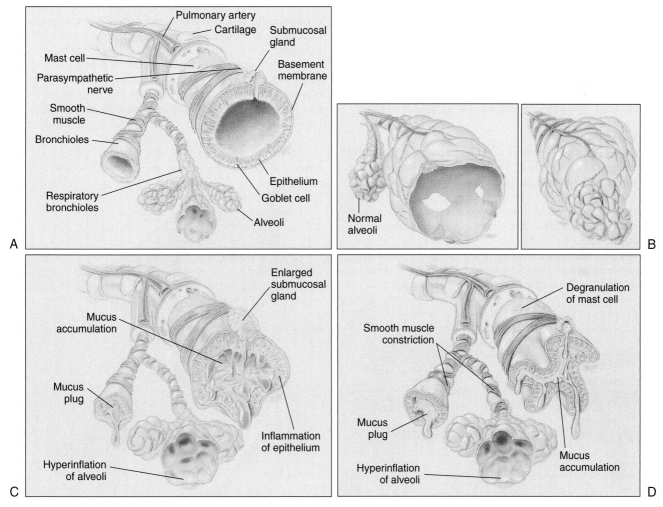

FIGURE 14-20 Airway obstruction caused by emphysema, chronic bronchitis, and asthma. **A,** The normal lung. **B,** Emphysema enlargement and destruction of alveolar walls with loss of elasticity and trapping of air; *(left)* panlobular emphysema showing abnormal weakening and enlargement of all air spaces distal to the terminal bronchioles (normal alveoli shown for comparison only); *(right)* centri-lobular emphysema showing abnormal weakening and enlargement of the respiratory bronchioles in the proximal portion of the acinus. **C,** Chronic bronchitis: inflammation and thickening of mucous membrane with accumulation of mucus and pus leading to obstruction; characterized by cough. **D,** Bronchial asthma: thick mucus, mucosal edema, and smooth muscle spasm causing obstruction of small airways; breathing becomes labored, and expiration is difficult.

2. The lung is secured and exteriorized using a Duval lung clamp.

3. Using a Satinsky clamp or a stapling device, the surgeon segments the tissue to be biopsied. The tissue to be removed is excised with a scalpel. After application of the clamp, tissue edges are approximated with absorbable suture.

4. Bleeding is controlled by the application of a moist sponge at the incision site. The area is irrigated and inspected for air leaks.

5. The chest tube (28F to 30F) is inserted and connected to suction.

6. The incision is closed, the chest tube is anchored to the chest wall, and a dressing is applied.

Decortication

Decortication of the lung is removal of any fibrinous deposit, cancer, or restrictive membrane on the visceral and parietal pleura that interferes with pulmonary ventilatory function. It may also be done in conjunction with a pleurectomy for patients with pleural-based tumors, such as mesothelioma. The procedure results in blood loss and trauma and should be used only if the underlying lung is healthy. The objective is to return the lung to near-normal function.

Procedural Considerations. The basic thoracic instrumentation is used. The patient is placed in a lateral position.

Operative Procedure

1. The surgeon incises the skin, subcutaneous tissue, and muscle using a blade and the ESU.

2. A rib, usually the fifth or sixth, is stripped (Figure 14-21) and resected.

3. The surgical technologist provides moist sponges to protect the ribs and tissue. The rib retractor is placed and slowly and gently opened.

4. Parietal adhesions are divided to the margins of the lung, mediastinal surface, and pericardium with thoracic scissors, forceps, and a moist sponge on sponge-holding forceps.

5. The fibrous membrane is incised and separated from the visceral pleura using blunt and sharp dissection, handling the tissues gently (Figure 14-22). The procedure is completed as described for pneumonectomy.

Drainage of Empyema

The accumulation of pus in the pleural space might be associated with acute or chronic infection. Acute empyema may result from a lung abscess, pneumonia, or infection after thoracotomy. Parapneumonic effusions occur in 20% to 60% of patients hospitalized for bacterial pneumonia; 5% to 10% of these parapneumonic effusions progress to empyema. The mortality of empyema in the elderly and debilitated is 25% to 75% (Lee, 2005). Empyema (other than a pure tuberculous type) must be drained to prevent fibrothorax, and patients with empyema may require further treatment with decortication. When the infection is not extensive the procedure can be performed with the patient administered a local anesthetic. Prolonged intrapleural infection results in chronic empyema, which can create additional complications such as mediastinal shift, swallowing difficulties, respiratory limitations, bronchus erosion, and chest deformity. Talc poudrage may be the treatment of choice for patients able to tolerate additional procedures and who experience relief of pleural effusion by thoracentesis. Postoperative empyema or empyema occurring in immunosuppressed patients is effectively treated with a rib resection and drainage.

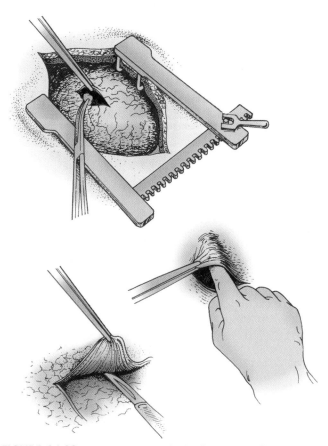

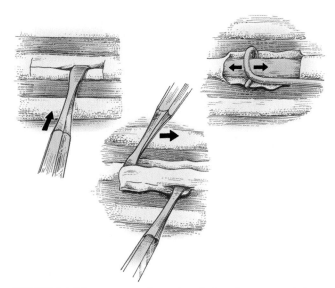

FIGURE 14-21 Separation of muscles of rib with a periosteal elevator and rib stripper.

FIGURE 14-22 Decortication. Methods of separating fibrous membrane from visceral pleura.

Procedural Considerations. If the patient is administered a general anesthetic, the basic thoracic instrumentation is used. The team positions the patient in a lateral position for an anterolateral incision. A catheter for instillation of the sclerosing agent is required. The chest cavity is irrigated profusely during and on completion of the procedure.

Operative Procedure

1. The surgeon incises the skin and tissues with a scalpel to expose the affected area of the lung. Suction is used to prevent spillage of drainage from the chest.
2. The adjacent rib is resected, and the intercostal neurovascular bundle is divided.
3. The underlying thickened pleura is incised, and gross pus is evacuated. An inflammatory response might be created by stripping the parietal pleura from the visceral pleura by sharp or blunt dissection.
4. A large-bore catheter (46F) is inserted, and the sclerosing agent is instilled when indicated.
5. The surgeon closes the incision site as described for other thoracotomy procedures.
6. A dressing is applied.

Open Thoracostomy—Partial Rib Resection

Partial rib resection is removal of a portion of selected rib or ribs through an open thoracostomy incision to allow healing and reinflation of an infected lung. The procedure is performed for treatment of chronic empyemic lesions to establish a mechanism for continuous drainage.

Procedural Considerations. The basic thoracic instrument set and bone-cutting instruments are used. An ESU, chest tube, and water-seal drainage system are required, as are culture tubes for aerobic and anaerobic laboratory analysis. The patient is placed in a lateral position for a posterolateral incision. The surgical procedure can be completed with the patient administered a local anesthetic.

Operative Procedure

1. The surgeon incises the skin, subcutaneous tissue, and muscle using a blade and the ESU.
2. The rib is resected, and the pleura is incised. Suction is used to control anticipated drainage.
3. Aerobic and anaerobic swabs for culture and sensitivity are obtained. The chest cavity is irrigated.
4. A large chest tube is inserted through the pleural opening. The incision is closed or packed open (depending on the extent of the disease process).
5. The chest tube is secured with a suture of heavy-gauge material on a cutting needle.
6. The chest tube is connected to a water-seal drainage system, and connections are secured.
7. A dressing is applied. A number of layers of dressing may be necessary to absorb drainage.

Closed Thoracostomy—Intercostal Drainage

Closed thoracostomy is insertion of a chest catheter through an intercostal space for establishment of closed drainage. The procedure provides continuous aspiration of air, blood, or infectious fluid from the pleural cavity. It is indicated for treatment of spontaneous pneumothorax, traumatic hemothorax, pleural effusion, and acute empyema. Malignant pleural effusions (Figure 14-23) may be managed by drainage and chemical pleurodesis by way of the thoracostomy tube.

Procedural Considerations. The thoracostomy may not take place in an OR setting. The procedure is usually done with monitored anesthesia care and local anesthesia. A local anesthesia set, including syringes, needles, and an anesthetic agent of choice for local injection, will be needed. The minor instrument set is used, in addition to disposable chest catheters, water-seal drainage system, two aspirating needles, and culture tubes. The patient is placed in a lateral or sitting position. Despite the administration of local anesthetic, thoracostomy can be uncomfortable for the patient. The surgical team should provide explanations and emotional support to the patient during the procedure.

Operative Procedure

1. The surgeon estimates the correct depth of insertion and marks the catheter. The operative site is anesthetized.
2. An aspirating needle attached to a syringe is introduced into the chest cavity to verify the presence of purulent drainage, air, or blood.
3. The surgeon incises the skin and introduces a clamp through the incision into the intercostal space and pleural cavity.
4. Next, the surgeon inserts a catheter through the incision site and clamps it to prevent egress of air as it is inserted into the cavity.
5. The incision site is sutured, and the catheter is secured.
6. The catheter is attached to water-seal drainage, and the tubing is secured. The clamp is removed, and a dressing is applied.

Decompression for Thoracic Outlet Syndrome

Thoracic outlet syndrome is a compression of the subclavian vessels and brachial plexus at the superior aperture of the thorax (Figure 14-24). The first rib is the usual cause of the com-

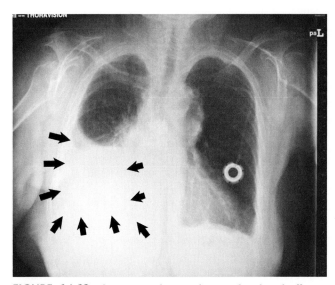

FIGURE 14-23 Chest x-ray showing large right pleural effusion outlined by arrows.

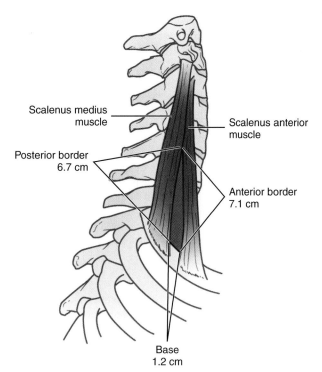

Scalenus medius muscle

Scalenus anterior muscle

Posterior border 6.7 cm

Anterior border 7.1 cm

Base 1.2 cm

FIGURE 14-24 The scalene (anterior) triangle showing its measurements and the narrow space through which the neurovascular bundle passes.

pression, because of either a congenital deformity or a traumatic injury that results in anatomic changes. Fibromuscular bands may also form between the cervical rib and other structures (i.e., scalenus tubercle) and cause compression. Symptoms depend on whether nerves, blood vessels, or both are compressed at the thoracic outlet. Decompression is accomplished through partial or entire removal of the rib using an open technique or video-assisted endoscopic techniques.

Procedural Considerations. Soft tissue and bone instrumentation is used. An ESU is required. The patient is positioned in a lateral decubitus position.

Operative Procedure—Open Technique

1. The surgeon incises the skin, subcutaneous tissue, and muscle using a blade and the ESU. Soft tissue dissection continues to identify the neurovascular bundle.
2. The first rib is meticulously dissected subperiosteally using the periosteal elevator. The rib elevator, stripper, and rib raspatories may be required. Undue traction on the brachial plexus and damage to the subclavian artery or vein are avoided during the dissection.
3. A wedge is taken from the midportion, or the rib is removed in its entirety using rib shears.
4. A drain is placed, and the incision is closed. A dressing is applied.

Excision of Mediastinal Lesion

Excision of a mediastinal lesion involves removal of a lesion from the anterior, middle, and posterior sections of the mediastinum. Identifying the compartment is important for planning a surgical approach to the resection, for optimal exposure and access. A mediastinoscopy should be performed to determine the diagnosis of an anterior mediastinal lesion. Indications for excision of a mediastinal lesion include miscellaneous cysts and tumors, thymoma, lymphoma, and neurogenic tumor.

Procedural Considerations. The thoracic instrumentation set is used. A procedure on the superior mediastinum might require use of thyroid instruments (see Chapter 7). The ESU and bone wax are needed. The patient is placed in a supine position for a median sternotomy incision (alternatively, lateral position may be used).

Operative Procedure—Thymectomy

1. The surgeon incises the skin, subcutaneous tissue, and muscle using a blade and the ESU.
2. The sternum is transected with a power saw or sternal knife. Bleeding is controlled at the bone edges with bone wax.
3. The thymus gland is dissected; vessels are clamped, ligated, and divided. The gland is removed.
4. The incision is closed. The sternum is reapproximated and closed with heavy wire. The skin is sutured closed. A dressing is applied.

Lung Transplantation

Since 1988 more than 17,000 lung transplants have been performed (Organ Procurement and Transplantation Network, 2009). Indications for single-lung transplantation (SLT) include restrictive lung disease, emphysema, pulmonary hypertension, and other nonseptic end-stage pulmonary diseases. Double-lung transplantation (DLT) is indicated for patients with cystic fibrosis or patients with a chronic infection in end-stage pulmonary failure. The procedure involves the allografting of one or both lungs from a cadaver or donor who has met clinical criteria for brain death. Developments in SLT include donor contribution from living relatives for patients who have chronic disease and a high risk for death while waiting on the donor transplantation list. Contraindications for transplantation include multisystem disease other than the lung, history of carcinoma or sarcoma, current infection, significant renal or hepatic dysfunction, cigarette smoking within 3 or 4 months, drug or alcohol abuse, psychologic instability, or poor medication compliance. Although the surgical technique is increasingly successful, it is anticipated that future application of lung transplantation techniques may be limited by donor supply. As the field of lung transplantation continues to evolve, questions will need to be answered regarding quality of life after transplantation and whether the single or double procedure is ultimately best for patients with chronic obstructive lung disease and primary pulmonary hypertension. Issues include the shortage of suitable donors, improved methods for early detection of chronic rejection, and improved immunosuppressive agents and regimens.

Procedural Considerations. Selection of the donor and recipients, preservation of the lung, and administration of anesthetic agents are considerations in this procedure. Recipient patients will have been started preoperatively on immunosuppressive therapy and infection prophylaxis. The patient's positioning will vary for the techniques being employed. The instrumentation is similar to that used for a thoracotomy. Cardiopulmonary bypass (CPB) may be required, as described in Chapter 16, along with the ESU, cold perfusion solution, and surgical stapling devices. Continuous hemodynamic monitoring, oximetry, and ventricular function assessment by transesophageal echocardiography (TEE) are all performed intraoperatively.

Operative Procedure—Single-Lung Transplantation
DONOR HARVESTING

1. The patient's skin is prepped from chin to knees and laterally to the midaxillary line. A median sternotomy incision or thoracotomy incision may be used.
2. The surgeon opens the pleura longitudinally posterior to the sternum, and divides the pericardium back to the hilum on both sides. The inferior pulmonary ligament is dissected, pleural adhesions are incised, and the proximal pulmonary arteries are dissected at their origin.
3. After heparinization and hypotensive anesthesia, the superior vena cava is ligated and divided and heavy silk ties are placed around each vessel.
4. The surgeon dissects the aortic arch free, and divides the ligamentum arteriosum. The anterior and inferior margins of the pulmonary artery are separated from the main artery and ascending aorta. Umbilical tapes are placed around the pulmonary artery and aorta. A purse-string suture is placed for infusion of the cardioplegia solution in the heart.
5. Once cardioplegia and pulmoplegia are accomplished, the heart is prepared for removal; veins and arteries are separated, and the heart is removed and placed in cold Collins solution.
6. Using blunt and sharp dissection the surgeon dissects the pulmonary arteries free from the mediastinum to the hilum anteriorly and then posteriorly to the anterior aorta and hilum. The trachea is dissected free. The lungs are inflated before stapling and dissection. The lungs are removed and immersed in cold Collins solution.

RECIPIENT PREPARATION AND TRANSPLANTATION

1. The patient is positioned laterally, and a wide skin prep is performed for exposure of the chest and abdomen (nipple line to knees).
2. An incision is made for a thoracotomy. The procedure depends on which lung is to be removed. If the right lung is being removed, the pulmonary vein is isolated extrapericardially; the pulmonary artery is isolated as close to the lung as possible. The surgeon ligates and divides the azygos vein; the pulmonary artery is dissected.
3. If the left lung is being removed, the ligamentum arteriosum is divided.
4. The anesthesia provider collapses the lung to be removed, and the proximal pulmonary artery is occluded. If instability occurs after occlusion, partial femoral arteriovenous bypass is initiated. If the patient remains stable, the pneumonectomy is performed.
5. Pulmonary veins are divided extrapericardially. The first branch of the pulmonary artery and descending branch are separated. The blood supply to the bronchus is preserved by not dissecting tissue around the bronchus.
6. The surgeon divides the bronchus and removes the lung. The pericardium is opened around the pulmonary veins to allow room for the atrial clamp.
7. Inferior and superior pulmonary veins are incised and joined.
8. Three anastomoses are completed for a single-lung transplant: bronchus to bronchus, pulmonary artery to pulmonary artery, and recipient pulmonary veins to donor atrial cuff. Techniques used to minimize bronchial anastomotic complications include shortening the donor bronchial stump, reinforcing the anastomosis with a vascularized tissue pedicle such as omentum or intercostal muscle pedicle flap, or using an intussuscepting bronchial anastomosis technique.

GERIATRIC CONSIDERATIONS

The Elderly Patient—Thoracic Surgery

Pulmonary complications in the elderly account for nearly 50% of postoperative complications in the total population of surgical patients (Wold, 2008). Lungs lose elasticity, which contributes to a decrease in functional residual capacity, residual volume, and dead space. Lungs increase in size and are lighter in weight with aging. A rigid chest wall is the result of calcification of costal cartilages, osteoporosis, and dorsal kyphosis. Muscles responsible for inhalation and exhalation may be weakened, resulting in a diminished ability to increase and decrease the size of the thoracic cavity. All these changes contribute to a minimal tidal exchange, which makes the elderly patient more susceptible to pulmonary complications, such as adult respiratory distress syndrome (ARDS), pneumonia, and aspiration. Lung changes are not usually obvious at rest. However, when the person becomes active, breathing may be more difficult. The ability to cough and clear the upper airway is lessened, and such reduction may increase the chance of respiratory tract infections and diseases, some of which can be severe enough to threaten the elderly person's life.

Meiner (2011) notes the following implications of anesthesia and surgery on the respiratory system:

◆ The elderly surgical patient has an increased risk of aspiration resulting from diminished laryngeal reflexes.
◆ If the surgery is an emergency, aspiration risk increases because of delayed gastric emptying in aging patients and the potential for a full stomach.
◆ The risks of postoperative atelectasis are increased because of decreased muscle strength, decreased cough reflex, and the normal pain associated with surgery.
◆ Airway clearance problems increase due in part to postoperative immobility.
◆ The sensation of thirst is decreased in older patients, increasing risks of hypovolemia and thickened secretions that are more difficult to clear from the airway.

Preventing these anesthetic and postoperative problems is facilitated by encouraging deep breathing, use of incentive spirometry, early ambulation, adequate hydration, and frequent position changes.

Modified from Meiner SE: *Gerontologic nursing*, ed 4, St Louis, 2011, Elsevier; and Wold GH: *Basic geriatric nursing*, ed 4, St Louis, 2008, Mosby.

9. After anastomoses and restoration of circulation, the lung is fully inflated and observed.
10. After closure of the chest, the surgeon performs a bronchoscopy to remove secretions and to ensure that the anastomosis is intact.

THORACIC SURGERY SUMMARY

Generally, thoracic surgery covers procedures and disease associated with the lungs. The surgical technologist needs to be familiar with anatomy, related diseases, procedures, surgical interventions, and potential complications that can arise during thoracic surgery.

A surgical procedure varies according to the preference of the surgeon. However, the surgical care of the thoracic patient is the same, no matter what region of the country you practice in. In every thoracic procedure, you should know the surgeon's preferences; the importance of prepping, positioning, and draping; and the required equipment and instrumentation. The surgical technologist needs to be able to think several steps ahead in the thoracic procedure; this facilitates the ability of the team to anticipate the needs of the surgeon.

REVIEW QUESTIONS

1. The three most common positions for a thoracotomy are:
   a. supine, lateral, and semilateral
   b. Trendelenburg's, supine, and semilateral
   c. reverse Trendelenburg, supine, and semilateral
   d. lithotomy, lateral, and semilateral

2. The three mechanisms a drainage system will use to drain fluid and air from the plural cavity include:
   a. positive pressure, hemovac, and gravity
   b. Jackson-Pratt, suction, and gravity
   c. positive pressure, suction, and Penrose
   d. positive pressure, suction, and gravity

3. The _____ forms the anterior thoracic wall in the midline.
   a. ribs
   b. sternum
   c. aorta
   d. inferior vena cava

4. In a mediastinoscopy, the surgeon makes a _____ incision above the suprasternal notch.
   a. thoracoabdominal
   b. lateral
   c. transverse
   d. anterolateral

5. _____ is a treatment for malignant pleural effusion and for spontaneous pneumothorax.
   a. wedge resection
   b. segmental resection
   c. decortication
   d. pleurodesis

6. Endoscopic procedures commonly used in thoracic surgery include the following:
   a. bronchoscopy, thoracoscopy, and mediastinoscopy
   b. bronchoscopy, thoracoscopy, and pelviscopy
   c. laparoscopy, thoracoscopy, and mediastinoscopy
   d. bronchoscopy, thoracoscopy, and EGD

7. A bronchoscopy procedure allows visualization of the:
   a. pericardium
   b. bronchi
   c. diaphragm
   d. lungs

8. The nerves of the lungs regulate constriction and relaxation of the bronchi and _____.

9. The main function of the lungs is to exchange _____ for oxygen.

10. A chest tube is used to _____.

11. Define and briefly describe the following procedures:
    Pneumonectomy
    Lobectomy
    Lung transplantation

Critical Thinking Question

In surgery involving the bronchus, describe the appropriate care for the surgical instruments used.

REFERENCES

Amdo T: Imaging bronchoscopic correlations for interventional pulmonology, *Radiol Clin North Am* 47:271–287, 2009.

Coughlin AM, Parchinsky C: Go with the flow of chest tube therapy, *Nursing* 36(3):36–41, 2006.

Denholm B: Tucking patient's arms and general positioning, *AORN J* 89(4):755–757, 2009.

Dumont P: Side effects and complications of surgery for hyperhidrosis, *Thorac Surg Clin* 18:193–207, 2008.

Fox J et al: Bloodless surgery and patient safety issues, *Perioperative Nursing Clinics* 3:345–354, 2008.

Kernstine KH et al: Robotic lobectomy, *Operative Techniques in Thoracic and Cardiovascular Surgery* 13(3):204.e1–204.e23, 2008.

Khraim FM: The wider scope of video-assisted thoracoscopic surgery, *AORN J* 85:1199–1208, 2007.

Lee RB: Benign pleural disease: empyema thoracis. In Selke FW et al: *Sabiston and Spencer surgery of the chest*, ed 7, Philadelphia, 2005, Saunders.

Mamary AJ, Criner GJ: Lung volume reduction surgery and bronchoscopic lung volume reduction in severe emphysema, *Respir Med* 4:44–59, 2008.

McKenna RJ: Thoracoscopic lung volume reduction surgery, *Operative Techniques in Thoracic and Cardiovascular Surgery* 12(2):141–149, 2007.

Organ Procurement and Transplantation Network (OPTN): Transplants by donor type 1988-2009, available at: http://optn.transplant.hrsa.gov/latestData/rptData.asp. Accessed May 6, 2009.

Rees HC: Assessment of the respiratory system. In Ignatavicius DD, Workman ML, editors: *Medical-surgical nursing: patient-centered collaborative care*, ed 6, St Louis, 2010, Saunders.

Solish N et al: Evaluating the patient presenting with hyperhidrosis, *Thorac Surg Clin* 18:133–140, 2008.

Weksler B et al: Thoracic sympathectomy: at what level should you perform surgery? *Thorac Surg Clin* 18:183–191, 2008.

CHAPTER 15

Vascular Surgery

LEARNING OBJECTIVES

After studying this chapter the reader will be able to:
- Identify relevant anatomy
- Correlate surgical anatomy with physiological conditions of the vascular system
- Contrast the unique characteristic of the veins and arteries with regard to function and blood flow
- Discuss the properties, purposes, and problems associated with the peripheral vascular system
- Discuss diagnostic methods for determination of surgical interventions and approaches
- Identify tissue layers involved in opening and closing vascular incisions
- Identify specialized instruments, equipment, and supplies used in open and endoscopic vascular procedures
- List the pharmacologic and hemostatic agents used during vascular surgery
- Apply broad vascular surgical concepts and knowledge to clinical practice for enhanced surgical patient care

Overview

Atherosclerosis continues to be one of the leading causes of death and disability in the Western world. It is estimated that peripheral atherosclerosis, including carotid, mesenteric, renal, and peripheral arterial disease (PAD) (also referred to as peripheral arterial occlusive disease [PAOD]), affects about 5% of Americans older than 60 years and up to 15% who are older than 70 years (Linsky et al, 2008). This is particularly striking, given that by the year 2030 the percentage of the U.S. population older than 65 years will increase to 20% (Federal Interagency Forum on Aging-Related Statistics, 2008). Many of these people will require interventions for the syndromes of peripheral ischemia, aneurysm, and venous disease.

Interventional therapy for peripheral atherosclerosis has become common. Aortic procedures are now routinely performed with minimal mortality. Carotid endarterectomy has also proven to be safe and effective. Peripheral angioplasty and bypass have a high initial success rate, but restenosis, graft failure, and progression of distal disease still lead to limb loss in certain patients after several years. Thus emphasis has been placed on decreasing morbidity and hospital stay associated with revascularization. Minimally invasive methods and strategies, including endovascular aortic aneurysm repair (Pearce, 2005), carotid artery stenting (Liu et al,

This chapter was originally written by Patricia Wieczorek, MSN, RN, CNOR, for the 14th edition of Alexander's Care of the Patient in Surgery and has been revised by Betsy Boatwright, CST, for this text.

2009) (Research Highlight), stenting for lower-limb ischemia (Rosen and Karmy-Jones, 2009), and percutaneous transluminal angioplasty (Zeller et al, 2009), have been developed, and their application and popularity continue to increase. New technologies, such as miniature shavers and laser arthrectomy devices for arterial plaque, continue to be developed (Nguyen and Garcia, 2008). The surgical technologist must be prepared for the demands of vascular surgery. This chapter reviews surgical anatomy, perioperative team considerations, and surgical interventions for a variety of vascular procedures.

Surgical Anatomy

Basic knowledge of anatomy is essential when caring for perioperative patients with a vascular disorder. Figure 15-1 depicts the principal arteries and veins of the body. Arteries and veins have three layers:

◆ Tunica intima (innermost layer)
◆ Tunica media (muscular middle layer)
◆ Tunica adventitia (fibrous outer layer)

   Arteries differ from veins in function and slightly in structure (Figure 15-2). Structurally, arteries have a thicker muscle layer and more elastic fibers than veins. The properties of elasticity and distensibility enable arteries to compensate for changes in blood pressure and volume. Because of the thicker muscle layer, severed arteries are capable of contracting and constricting enough to stop hemorrhage. In contrast, veins are more fragile than arteries, and whether its cause is traumatic or iatrogenic, venous bleeding may be difficult to control. Another difference is the presence of semilunar intimal folds, or valves, in veins that prevent backflow. Veins and arteries are nourished by a tiny network of vessels (the vasa vasorum), as well as from

RESEARCH HIGHLIGHT

Long-Term Results of Carotid Stenting versus Endarterectomy in High-Risk Patients

With the continued evolution of endovascular techniques, carotid stenting has become an option in high-risk patients. The authors previously reported that carotid stenting did not produce inferior results to carotid endarterectomy for the treatment of carotid artery disease at 30-days and at 1-year postprocedure. This study now reports the results of those same patients at 3 years. The prespecified major endpoint at 3 years was a composite of death, stroke, or myocardial infarction within 30 days after the procedure or death or ipsilateral stroke between 31 days and 1080 days. Data were available for 260 patients (77.8% of the initial group). The prespecified endpoint occurred in 41 patients in the stenting group (cumulative incidence, 24.6%) and 45 patients in the endarterectomy group (cumulative incidence, 26.9%); 15 patients in each group had a stroke. The authors concluded that in their trial of patients with severe carotid artery stenosis and increased surgical risk, no significant difference was seen in the long-term outcomes between the two groups. Further studies focusing on preprocedural variables are recommended as well as longer-term outcome results.

Modified from Gurm H et al: Long-term results of carotid stenting versus endarterectomy in high risk patients, *N Engl J Med* 358(15):1572-1581, 2008.

the intraluminal blood flow. Both are regulated by the autonomic nervous system, with veins having fewer nerve fibers than arteries. The two systems are connected (except for the pulmonary artery and pulmonary venous system): major arteries carry oxygenated blood, they branch into smaller arteries and arterioles, and then blood moves into capillaries to venules and to veins. The work of exchanging nutrients and metabolic waste is done at the capillary level.

   Blood flow is a complex process that depends on many factors. Blood flows through arteries such that the blood in the center of the vessel moves faster than the blood at the periphery. Because the movement of the blood is in parallel lines, it is referred to as *laminar*. When flow is disrupted by an obstruction, stenosis, curve, or bifurcation, the particle motion is referred to as *turbulent*. Turbulence may be evidenced by the presence of a bruit (e.g., turbulent noise), detected by auscultation, or detected by a characteristic Doppler signal. Flow depends on blood viscosity, vessel wall resistance, and the peripheral resistance of the arterioles. There must be a difference in pressures, or a pressure gradient, to allow blood to flow. The gradient is provided by the contraction of the left ventricle. The negative pressure created by the relaxed right ventricle assists in venous return by creating a suctioning effect and the skeletal and visceral muscles help propel venous return toward the heart.

ARTERIAL DISEASE

Aneurysmal Disease

The most common cause of an arterial aneurysm is atherosclerotic degeneration of the arterial wall (Gloviczki and Ricotta, 2008). The pathogenesis is a multifactorial process, involving atherosclerosis along with genetic predisposition, aging, inflammation, and localized activation of proteolytic enzymes (Gloviczki and Ricotta, 2008). A true aneurysm is a dilation of all layers of the artery wall. A dissecting aneurysm results from a tear in the artery wall, allowing blood to dissect between the layers of the vessel wall. A false aneurysm, or pseudoaneurysm, is not an aneurysm but a disruption through all the layers of a vessel wall with the escaping blood being contained by the perivascular tissues. False aneurysms may result from trauma, infection, or disruption of an arterial suture line after surgery. True aneurysms are most frequently found in the abdominal aorta but are also found in the thoracic aorta and iliac, femoral, and popliteal arteries. More men than women are affected, and aneurysmal disease tends to be a disease of older persons. As early as 1977, a familial tendency was observed that subsequent research verified; as many as 18% of patients with abdominal aortic aneurysms have a first-degree relative with a similar diagnosis (Gloviczki and Ricotta, 2008).

   Abdominal aortic aneurysms (AAAs), which account for most aneurysms, occur primarily between the renal arteries and the aortic bifurcation (Ignatavicius and Walicek, 2010). An aneurysm involves intimal damage of the aorta and weakening of the tunica media (Alberto et al, 2008) or elastic portion (collagen and elastin defects) of the arterial wall. Gradually the vessel wall in the damaged area expands and atheroma develops within the aneurysm sac (Figure 15-3). An AAA has minimal symptoms and is generally discovered on routine history and physical examination. In men, the diameter of the

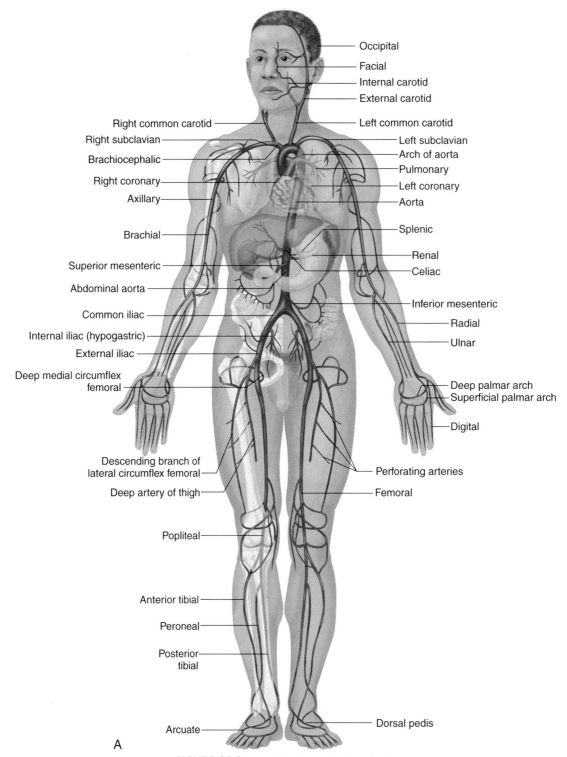

Occipital
Facial
Internal carotid
External carotid
Right common carotid
Left common carotid
Right subclavian
Left subclavian
Brachiocephalic
Arch of aorta
Right coronary
Pulmonary
Left coronary
Axillary
Aorta
Brachial
Splenic
Superior mesenteric
Renal
Celiac
Abdominal aorta
Inferior mesenteric
Common iliac
Radial
Internal iliac (hypogastric)
Ulnar
External iliac
Deep medial circumflex femoral
Deep palmar arch
Superficial palmar arch
Digital
Descending branch of lateral circumflex femoral
Perforating arteries
Deep artery of thigh
Femoral
Popliteal
Anterior tibial
Peroneal
Posterior tibial
Arcuate
Dorsal pedis

A

FIGURE 15-1 A, Principal arteries of the body.

infrarenal aorta normally measures between 14 and 24 mm and in women it measures between 12 and 21 mm. An AAA is diagnosed if the diameter is 3 cm or larger for men or 2.6 cm or larger for females (Gloviczki and Ricotta, 2008). Mortality is low with elective resection of the aneurysm. Dissection and rupture of the aneurysm (aortic dissection) dramatically increase operative mortality because of the abrupt and mas-sive hemorrhagic shock that accompanies the rupture. Aortic dissection is believed to arise from a sudden tear in the aortic intima, opening the way for blood to enter the aortic wall.

Acute Arterial Insufficiency

Arterial insufficiency may result from an acute occlusion, as in embolic disease, or from the rupture of an unstable ath-

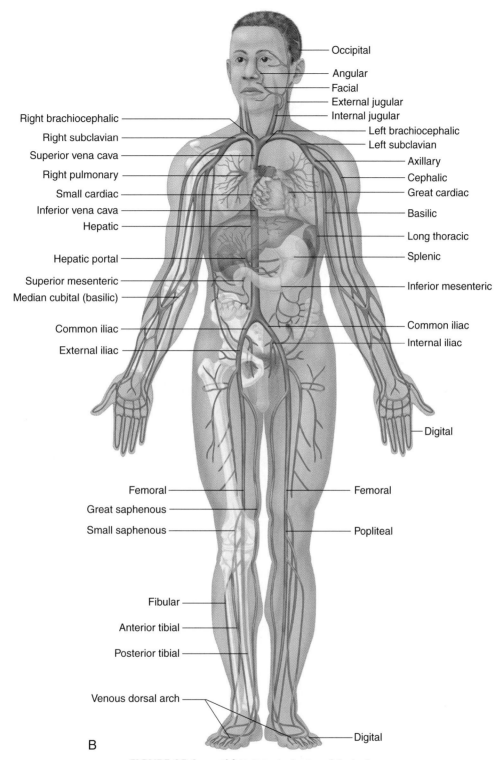

Occipital
Angular
Facial
External jugular
Internal jugular
Left brachiocephalic
Left subclavian
Axillary
Cephalic
Great cardiac
Basilic
Long thoracic
Splenic
Inferior mesenteric
Common iliac
Internal iliac
Digital
Femoral
Popliteal
Digital

Right brachiocephalic
Right subclavian
Superior vena cava
Right pulmonary
Small cardiac
Inferior vena cava
Hepatic
Hepatic portal
Superior mesenteric
Median cubital (basilic)
Common iliac
External iliac
Femoral
Great saphenous
Small saphenous
Fibular
Anterior tibial
Posterior tibial
Venous dorsal arch

B

FIGURE 15-1 cont'd B, Principal veins of the body.

erosclerotic plaque, causing acute thrombosis of the vessel. Emboli usually arise from the heart as a result of atrial fibrillation but may occasionally result from a myocardial infarction (MI), where a clot forms on the endocardium (the lining of the heart) in an area of muscle damage. Atherosclerotic plaque can also break loose from other areas and result in an acute arterial blockage. Patients with acute arterial occlusion usually present with the onset of the six *P*'s: sudden severe *p*ain, *p*ulselessness, *p*aresthesia, *p*aralysis, *p*allor, and *p*oikilothermia (coolness) of an extremity (Ignatavicius and Walicek, 2010). Heparin is the mainstay to prevent the enlargement of emboli while allowing time for collateral blood flow to develop. However, in the threatened limb there are basically two options: surgical removal of the clot (embolectomy) or

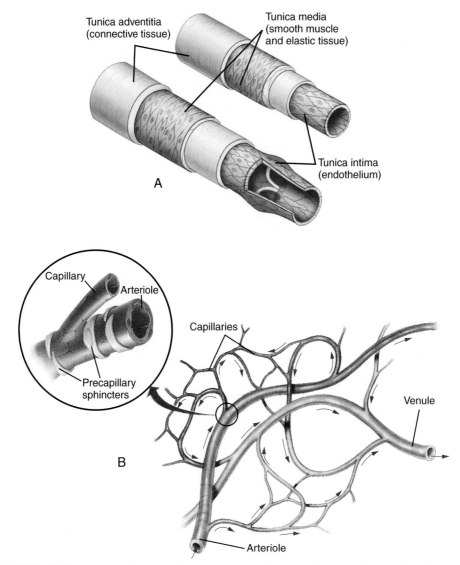

FIGURE 15-2 A, Layers of artery and vein. Drawings of a sectioned artery and vein show the three layers of large vessel walls. **B,** Microcirculation. The smaller blood vessels—arterioles, capillaries, and venules—cannot be observed without magnification. Note that the control of blood flow through any particular region of a capillary network can be regulated by the relative contraction of precapillary sphincters in the walls of the arterioles *(inset)*. Note also that capillaries have a wall composed of only a single layer of flattened cells, whereas the walls of the larger vessels also have a smooth layer.

chemical removal of the clot with the use of a thrombolytic medication. If the limb reaches the point where the muscle is rigid, the limb is not salvageable and amputation is a lifesaving procedure.

Chronic Arterial Insufficiency

Chronic arterial insufficiency occurs because of the deposition of calcium and cholesterol within the wall of the artery. Arteriosclerosis is a natural part of the aging process and occurs when the walls of the arterial vasculature undergo changes such as increased thickness and hardening, reducing the elasticity of the arteries. The decrease in elasticity should not be confused with atherosclerosis obliterans, which is a pathologic process that affects the intimal layer of the artery with the buildup of a fibrous plaque of lipids that can calcify and

necrose. Atherosclerosis is the most common cause of PAOD, the probable mechanism being initial damage to the intima and subsequent activation and aggregation of the body's platelets. Inflammation follows, with the deposition of lipoproteins forming an atheroma. Calcification of this lesion leads to the development of an atherosclerotic plaque, resulting in inadequate muscle perfusion and ischemia (Rosen and Karmy-Jones, 2009). The process is a gradual one, and a localized lesion usually indicates systemic disease. The body develops a network of collateral vessels as an adaptive mechanism to supply the tissues with oxygenated blood. Many theories have been postulated to explain the process of atherogenesis. The inflammatory process of intimal injury, as just described, seems to be the current and most widely accepted hypothesis. Box 15-1 presents risk factors for atherosclerosis. A large number of vascular sur-

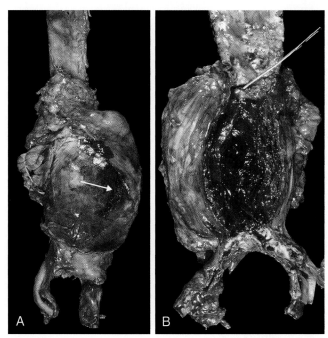

FIGURE 15-3 Abdominal aortic aneurysm. **A,** External view, gross photograph of a large aortic aneurysm that ruptured (*arrow*). **B,** Opened view. The wall of the aneurysm is thin and the lumen is filled with a large quantity of thrombus. The probe indicates the track of the rupture.

gical procedures revolve around the results of chronic arterial insufficiency.

Arterial Insufficiency: Cerebrovascular Disease and Stroke

Cerebrovascular accident (CVA or stroke) is a leading cause of death in the United States and most industrialized countries. In the United States, approximately 795,000 persons experience a stroke each year (Lloyd-Jones et al, 2009). Cerebrovascular disease may manifest itself as a transient ischemic attack (TIA) or as a major or minor stroke. A TIA is an episode of neurologic dysfunction that resolves in 24 hours. It may be caused by atheromatous debris or a thromboembolism from a carotid artery or the vertebral basilar system. Vascular lesions in the carotid artery occur primarily at the bifurcation of the common carotid artery into the internal and the external carotid arteries. The internal carotid artery supplies the brain with needed oxygenated blood. Obstruction in this arterial vessel leads to cerebrovascular insufficiency.

The right and the left carotid and vertebral arteries supply the brain (Figure 15-4). The first major branch of the internal carotid artery is the ophthalmic artery. Thromboembolic events that affect this artery may result in visual disturbances, ocular TIAs, or "amaurosis fugax" (complete or partial loss of vision). Patients will often describe amaurosis fugax as a curtain over a partial field of vision, usually the top. Clinical conditions that generally indicate the need for a carotid endarterectomy (CEA) are transient cerebral ischemia, asymptomatic severe stenosis, and stable strokes. Carotid disease may recur after a CEA. Redo surgery for restenosis poses the same complication risks as the original procedure.

Arterial Insufficiency: Peripheral Vascular Disease

The initial and most important symptom of vascular disease in the aortoiliac vessels and distal arteries is intermittent claudication. The term *claudication* is derived from the Latin word "claudicare," which means "to limp" (History box). This is the most common symptom of lower-extremity PAD and occurs distal to the arterial obstruction while the patient is exercising. Many patients are asymptomatic and do not experience pain. When this symptom does occur, it is typically located in the working muscle, occurs with the same amount of exercise each time, and is relieved with rest. This is referred to as functional ischemia; blood flow is adequate at rest but inadequate to sustain exercise. The increased muscle demand for oxygen with exercise cannot be met distal to the arterial obstruction. Anaerobic metabolism occurs, and muscle cramping develops. Surgery is not usually performed for claudication unless it is unusually disabling.

The second symptom—rest pain, which is located in the foot—develops as the vascular disease progresses (Faisal and Cooper, 2008). At this stage the ischemia is termed *critical*. Rest pain occurs without exercise and is a constant discomfort, often aggravated at night. The body is now unable to meet the oxygen needs of distal tissues even at rest. Rest pain may be somewhat relieved by analgesics or by lowering the legs off the bed. Gravity assists in increasing the tissue perfusion and oxygen supply to decrease the pain. Unless the vascular disease is corrected, nonhealing ulcers and gangrene can develop. Gangrene occurs when the arterial vessels are unable to meet the oxygen needs of distal tissues even at complete rest.

VENOUS DISEASE

Acute Venous Insufficiency

Acute venous insufficiency is caused by a clot in the deep venous system, or deep vein thrombosis (DVT). Such venous insufficiency can be a diagnosis of DVT, phlebitis, thrombophlebitis, or phlebothrombosis, which merely indicates that

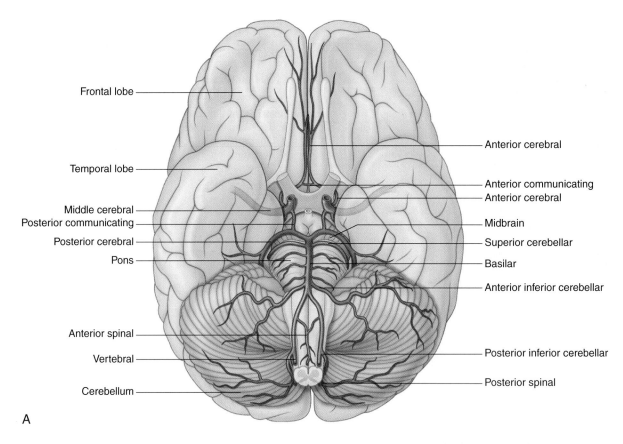

Frontal lobe

Temporal lobe

Middle cerebral
Posterior communicating
Posterior cerebral
Pons

Anterior spinal

Vertebral

Cerebellum

Anterior cerebral

Anterior communicating
Anterior cerebral

Midbrain
Superior cerebellar
Basilar
Anterior inferior cerebellar

Posterior inferior cerebellar

Posterior spinal

A

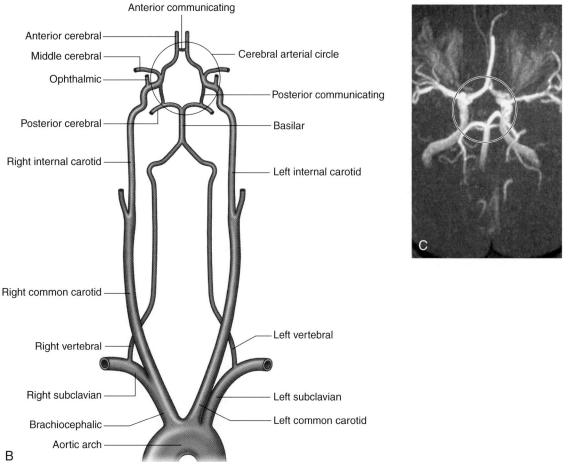

Anterior communicating

Anterior cerebral

Middle cerebral

Ophthalmic

Posterior cerebral

Right internal carotid

Right common carotid

Right vertebral

Right subclavian

Brachiocephalic

Aortic arch

Cerebral arterial circle

Posterior communicating

Basilar

Left internal carotid

Left vertebral

Left subclavian

Left common carotid

B

C

FIGURE 15-4 Arteries at the base of the brain. **A,** Diagram shows the cerebral arterial circle (of Willis) and related structures on the base of the brain. Note the arterial anastomoses. **B,** Origins of blood vessels that form the cerebral arterial circle. **C,** Magnetic resonance image of the cerebral arterial circle.

there is a clot, usually in the lower extremity. Virchow, a pathologist, identified the three elements that trigger venous thrombosis. Referred to as Virchow's triad, these elements, or risk factors, are endothelial injury, venostasis, and hypercoagulability (Ignatavicius and Walicek, 2010). The cause of hypercoagulability is sometimes unknown but is seen in patients with tissue trauma (e.g., surgery, burns, or stroke), malignancy, sepsis, pregnancy or estrogen use, and diabetes mellitus. The patient may be asymptomatic or present with limb swelling, pain, and a skin color change. The danger lies in the potential emboli migrating to the right ventricle and proceeding to the lungs. Pulmonary emboli (PEs) can be fatal. The majority of pulmonary emboli cases are caused by DVT. The majority of these originate in the lower extremities. The use of heparin and bed rest is the usual medical treatment. In cases that preclude the use of systemic heparin or in which heparin is ineffective, surgical insertion of a vena cava filter may be indicated.

Chronic Venous Insufficiency

Patients with chronic venous insufficiency (CVI) have not been treated surgically as often as patients with arterial disease for several reasons. CVI is generally not life-threatening or limb-threatening. Improved imaging techniques (e.g., duplex ultrasonography) allow better diagnoses of the precise problem. The treatment of the majority of venous disorders is nonsurgical and aimed at increasing venous return and decreasing edema. CVI, which presents with stasis ulcers from postphlebitic syndrome, usually occurs in one leg. The leg is usually very swollen with a cyclic edema, which does not change visibly after overnight leg elevation. Stasis ulcers and hyperpigmentation usually are found in the "gaiter" area and above the medial malleolus on the leg. The condition is caused by incompetent perforator valves. The perforating veins connect the superficial and deep venous systems. The usual management is to apply 20 to 30 mm Hg of external pressure by means of special pressure stockings. Surgical interventions such as valvuloplasty (direct repair of the valve), valve transposition or transplantation (moving a valve from the arm to the leg), or perforator interruptions are occasionally performed but have had limited success. Patient selection is critical, and long-term results are mixed.

Surgical Technologist Considerations

A surgical technologist's direct responsibilities, from carotid to arteriovenous (AV) fistula, and from abdominal aortic aneurysm (AAA) to femoral bypass, include prepping, draping, equipment required, and, of course, instrumentation, suture, and supplies. The back table should be set up in a standardized fashion for vascular surgical procedures. Standardized setups allow the surgical technologist to be more efficient and reduce the potential for errors when the surgical technologist is relieved by another scrub person. The back table might have a large vascular set, a peripheral vascular (PV) fine set, small and medium clip appliers, the surgeon's specials, and a basin set. A variety of Weitlaners, Henley retractors, and the possibility of endoscopic vein harvest, graph preparation, or a tunneling device are special considerations. In every PV procedure, the use of an electrosurgical unit, suction, Doppler, and headlights are expected. Special supplies for a PV procedure include vessel loops, bulldogs for hemostasis, umbilical tapes, drains, kitner sponges for dissection, and grafting materials including patches. It is the job of the surgical technologist to prepare and keep sterile any grafting devices.

Preoperative Tests. A variety of tests may be required to plan for surgical interventions. Segmental pressure measurements give partial anatomic information in that they assist in locating lesions. Hemodynamic tests provide information on the flow of blood, such as that to the brain or an extremity, and the effects on flow caused by a vascular lesion.

ANGIOGRAPHY. Invasive diagnostic tests may be performed preoperatively to identify the extent and location of the patient's peripheral vascular disease (Faisal and Cooper, 2008). The introduction of a contrast medium through a catheter into the arterial or venous system of the patient facilitates this visualization. Angiography also involves injecting a contrast medium into the patient's arterial system and taking serial radiographs of the movement of the dye through the arteries. Digital subtraction angiography (DSA) is one such technique that uses a computer along with contrast medium injection to make the image (Figure 15-5). Usually one side of the film shows the bone for orientation, and the other side subtracts the density of the bone and soft tissue to allow a clearer view of the vessels. Arteriography provides information on arterial anatomy and the location of stenotic or occluded vessels and assists the surgeon in planning bypass procedures. A veno-

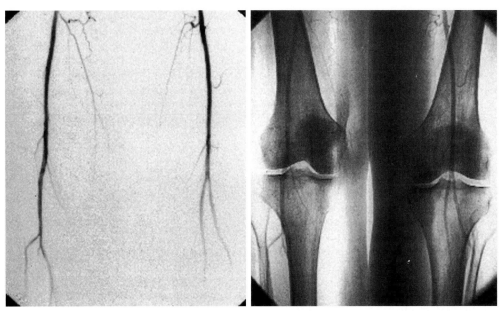

FIGURE 15-5 Digital subtraction angiography.

gram (contrast venography) is performed to show venous abnormalities in extremities, the vena cava, and the hepatic and renal systems. Ascending venography can differentiate between acute and chronic thrombosis and can define anatomy. Descending venography assesses valve competence of the lower extremities.

DOPPLER SCANNING. The Doppler effect is the change in the frequency of echo signals that occurs whenever there is a change in the distance between the sources of a sound and the receiving object. The probe, or transducer, is aimed toward the blood vessel at an angle of 45 to 60 degrees. This directs an ultrasound beam that is reflected back to the probe by moving red blood cells (RBCs). The velocity of the flow of cells is converted into an audible signal heard through a speaker. The signal is described as a swishing sound. The sound is called a signal, not a pulse. The tip of the probe is made of an element called a ceramic piezoelectric crystal, which can send, receive, and convert signals when an electric current is applied. The element becomes thicker and thinner, thus resulting in a pressure wave converted to an audible signal. The simplest form is the continuous wave (CW) Doppler probe. It has two elements: one sends a high-frequency wave, and the other receives it. In a pulsed Doppler probe, the same element sends and receives signals. The pulsed Doppler probe has the advantage of being able to differentiate among vessels of different depths. A normal arterial Doppler signal is either biphasic or triphasic. The first sound corresponds to systolic flow and is forward-moving and of high velocity. The second sound is related to early diastole and has a lesser reversal of flow. The third sound is later diastole and is smaller, forward-flowing, and of a lower velocity. The pitch is described as rising quickly in systole and dropping quickly in early diastole. An abnormal signal, indicating stenosis or occlusion, is heard as low-pitched and monophasic. These abnormal arterial signals may sound like venous signals.

The Doppler probe can provide information in three forms: the audible signal, a visible graph printout similar to an elec-

trocardiogram (ECG) tracing, and a spectral analysis that appears on a screen and may be recorded on paper as well. The Doppler transducer is the most widely used instrument for vascular study. It has the advantages of being readily available, inexpensive, and easy to use. A small, portable battery unit is durable and can be transported and stored easily. When the probe is used on intact skin, a water-soluble gel is needed to conduct a signal. Probes can be used directly on a vessel intraoperatively. The probes are heat-sensitive and must either be sterilized according to manufacturer's instructions or be inserted into a sterile sleeve or probe cover. If they are handled gently, the probes have a reasonable life span. Care must be taken to protect the sensitive tip from being dropped or crushed. The biggest drawback of the Doppler probe is a negative finding in the presence of a stenotic lesion pronounced enough to produce a flow disturbance that results in an altered signal.

A bruit is a sound disturbance that is sometimes described as a low-pitched, blowing sound. It can be heard through a stethoscope over an area of blood flow turbulence that occurs at points of vessel stenoses. Bruits do not provide information on the extent of a lesion—only that an abnormal flow may exist. They occur at points of significant stenosis and are not heard when severe flow restriction or total flow occlusion occurs. The Doppler probe is noninvasive and painless for patients.

ULTRASONOGRAPHY. Ultrasonography is done to obtain information about structures through the emission of high-frequency sound waves. These sound waves are reflected, or bounced back, to the probe or transducer that emits them and are electronically transformed into an image.

B-Mode Ultrasonography. B-mode is brightness modulation, a technique in ultrasound imaging that projects a two-dimensional image on an oscilloscope screen. The image appears as dots from the echoes of the signal. The strength of the echo is shown by the intensity and brightness of the dots on the screen.

Duplex Ultrasonography. A duplex ultrasound machine is a combination of the pulsed Doppler image and the so-called real-time B-mode image ultrasonogram. "Real time" simply refers to the image projecting current, undelayed information. B-mode image is best when the probe is perpendicular to the vessel, but the Doppler probe does not pick up signals at a perpendicular angle. Some manipulation of the probe angle is required to obtain the best results. Color duplex imaging converts the detected signals caused by blood flow into a color, depending on the direction of flow. Flow toward the probe may be displayed as red, away from the probe as blue, and turbulence as multiple colors. This imaging provides both hemodynamic and anatomic information. The technology is also used in transesophageal echocardiography (TEE) and is the diagnostic method of choice for venous insufficiency.

Pulse Volume Recording (PVR), or Sequential Volume Plethysmography. A plethysmograph measures and records the changes in the sizes and volumes in extremities by measuring the blood volumes at blood pressure cuffs placed at

---

SURGICAL TECHNOLOGY PREFERENCE CARD

In peripheral vascular surgery, whether the procedure is a femoropopliteal (fem-pop) bypass or an abdominal aortic aneurysm, there are special considerations for the vascular patient. In each vascular procedure your back table will look similar, as will your preoperative routine. It is important to have the patient films in the room and available for viewing throughout the entire procedure. A surgeon will have the patient get special diagnostic testing, preoperatively, specifically for the intent on viewing them during the procedure. If grafts are going to be used, you should check with the surgeon regarding type and size of graft and its preparation. Also, you should check with blood bank that all blood and blood products are available as ordered. Throughout the procedure, it is important to note the amount of irrigation used.

Room Prep: Basic OR furniture, warmer for irrigation, video assist system for endoscopic vein harvest, and headlight

Prep Solution
- Chlorhexidine gluconate (CHG) is commonly used
- Make sure the prep is completely dry before draping the patient

Catheter
- Check with the surgeon and anesthesia provider
- Insertion is common for longer procedures and when using a lot of irrigation
- Accommodate appropriately for any allergy to latex

PROCEDURE CHECKLIST

Instruments
- Standard—peripheral vascular (PV) set, PV fine set, special instruments, hemoclip appliers
- Endovein harvest—scope, camera, light cord, bipolar cord
- "Have available" blunt and sharp Weitlaners, Henley retractors, long hemoclip appliers

Suture
- Anastomosis—double-armed monofilament ranging from 7-0 to 3-0
- Ligature—silk ties ranging from 4-0 to 0
- 2-0 silk to sew in the drains
- Closing suture—0 monofilament for fascia, 2-0 braided absorbable for subcutaneous and staples

Other Hemostatic Agents
- Gelfoam and thrombin, surgicel, fibrillar
- Clip appliers—have a variety of sizes, long in length
- Platelet gel—derived from the patient's own blood and mixed with thrombin
- ESU and harmonic scalpel

Additional Supplies
- Graft cart, Endovascular cart, and PV suture and supplies cart
- Physician's special requests—including suture, clamps, and staplers
- Sponges—laps, raytec, and kitners

Medications and Irrigations
- Warm antibiotic irrigation
- Epidural or spinal block kit
- Injectable local anesthetic
- Heparinized irrigation

Drains
- Correct size and type for procedure and surgeon preference
- Jackson-Pratt to a closed reservoir for fluid collection

Specimen Care
- Label correctly, using the "Repeat and Verify" when passing off the field
- Follow all other specimen safety measures

Before opening for the procedure, the surgical technologist should:
- Check procedure against a surgeon's preference card
- Arrange OR furniture—depending on surgical site and surgeon preference
- Gather appropriate carts needed in the room for the procedure
- Gather and arrange needed equipment—verify function of equipment

intervals along the extremity. The methods include electrical impedance, mercury in Silastic strain gauges, and air or fluid displacement. This test, which is used to determine the location of an arterial lesion and estimate the severity of the disease, requires careful limb positioning and a cooperative patient. A negative study is a good predictor of low risk for pulmonary embolus (PE).

This test is inexpensive, has good predictive value, and is accurate in detecting thrombosis. It has the disadvantage of a high rate of false-positive results in the presence of old DVT, congestive heart failure (CHF), and external compression.

Magnetic Resonance Imaging. Magnetic resonance imaging (MRI) measures the behavior of atoms in a strong magnetic field. This test provides detailed and three-dimensional images of anatomy for evaluation of carotid, aortic, and lower-extremity disease (Faisal and Cooper, 2008). An MRI provides more detail than ultrasonography or computed tomography (CT) scan and avoids the complications of contrast medium injection and exposure to x-rays. MRI is contraindicated for patients with preexisting implantable devices.

Implementation

Site Verification: "Time Out." Patient safety is of utmost importance. It is the entire surgical team's responsibility to verify that the correct patient is receiving the correct procedure on the correct site immediately before the start of any surgical procedure. The surgical site needs to be marked and visible after draping if laterality is involved. The "time out" is a requirement of The Joint Commission. During the time-out, the patient's name, procedure, site verification, and laterality are reviewed. Other items that may be discussed include the consent, anesthesia plan/concerns, the patient's allergies, antibiotics ordered, the patient's position, required instruments and special equipment, availability of blood, and anticipated length of the procedure. Such briefings improve team communication and intraoperative patient care (Makary et al, 2007).

Intraoperative Monitoring. Intraoperative monitoring for patients with vascular disorders includes the use of the basic ECG, pulse oximeter, and blood pressure cuff. For patients undergoing saphenous vein stripping or amputation, these are usually adequate. For lengthy procedures, such as arterial bypass or reconstruction, an arterial line is usually placed percutaneously into the radial artery. This is kept open by a pressurized heparin drip line attached to a transducer, and a waveform monitor reads the systolic and diastolic pressures. The monitor calculates the mean arterial pressure (MAP), which aids in the evaluation of the perfusion of systemic and cardiac circulation. This arterial line also allows easy access for collecting specimens for arterial blood gas (ABG) analysis. Continuous assessment of the patient's arterial pressure is a critical part of the surgical procedure. Pulmonary capillary wedge pressure, as an index of left atrial pressure (LAP), may be monitored depending on the patient's physiologic status. A general anesthetic may be administered and the patient intubated; local or regional anesthesia may also be used, depending on the surgical intervention. Epidural catheters may be placed to provide intraoperative anesthesia that can be augmented to accommodate increased surgical time, as opposed to a spinal anesthetic, which provides a finite period of anesthesia. Epi-

dural catheters may be left in place postoperatively for pain management as well. Because many patients undergoing vascular surgery have generalized atherosclerotic disease, the surgical team should be constantly alert for cardiac dysrhythmias and blood pressure changes. Acid-base balance and pulmonary gas exchange are assessed from the ABG analysis.

A central venous pressure (CVP) catheter or pulmonary artery (PA) catheter may be inserted, usually by way of the right internal jugular vein. The CVP line allows assessment of blood volume and vascular tone. The PA catheter monitors cardiac output, fluid balance, and the cardiac response to medications. PA catheters are commonly used for patients undergoing aortic surgery or for patients with cardiac disease.

TEE may be used to monitor the heart noninvasively during aortic surgery. The device looks similar to a bronchoscope and can be passed down the esophagus to provide an ultrasonic image. The cardiac structures, blood flow, wall motion, and great vessels can be observed. Use of TEE requires highly skilled personnel and may not be available in all surgical settings.

Electroencephalographic (EEG) monitoring is used for patients undergoing a carotid endarterectomy and allows for immediate observation of the slowing of brain waves caused by cerebral ischemia or reduced perfusion. The surgeon may elect to place a temporary shunt in the artery if this occurs during clamping, potentially reducing the chances of perioperative stroke.

A urinary catheter is inserted for many procedures, including the following: if the proposed procedure involves the renal arteries or clamping of the aorta above the renal arteries; if considerable blood loss is anticipated; if the planned procedure time is lengthy; or whenever spinal or epidural anesthesia is used, because they delay the patient's ability to void voluntarily. Urinary catheterization facilitates accurate hourly measurements of urine during and after the surgical procedure and assists in the assessment of renal perfusion and fluid status.

Positioning. Positioning of the patient undergoing vascular surgery is of particular importance because of restricted circulation distal to the area of arterial obstruction and a generalized state of poor circulation. Particular care must be exercised in positioning elderly patients. Awareness of joint range-of-motion limitations attributable to immobility or joint surgery is critical even for a procedure as routine as urinary catheter insertion. A footboard may be applied to the OR bed to prevent the weight of drapes resting on the patient's lower extremities. A head support may be used to position the head. A roll may be placed between the scapulae. For surgical procedures involving a lower extremity, the patient's thigh may be externally rotated and abducted with the knee flexed. A small bolster may be used under the knee to support the patient's leg. Proper skeletal alignment during surgery prevents injury to the neuromuscular system. The surgical team pays close attention to the skin overlying bony prominences, especially the heels, sacrum, and elbows, and uses the proper supports and pads to prevent pressure and potential positioning injury to the patient. If the procedure will be lengthy, a pressure-reducing mattress or pad can be placed on the OR bed to help prevent patient injury. Arms are placed on padded armboards with the palms up and fingers extended. Armboards are maintained at less than a 90-degree angle to prevent brachial plexus stretch. If there are surgical reasons to tuck the arms at the side, the elbows are padded to protect the ulnar nerve, the palms face inward, and the wrist is maintained in a neutral position (Denholm, 2009). A drape secures the arms. It should be tucked snuggly under the patient, not under the mattress. This prevents the arm from shifting downward intraoperatively and resting against the OR bed rail. During the procedure the perioperative nurse and surgical technologist continually monitor the sterile field to ensure heavy instruments and drapes do not rest on the patient's body and cause pressure injuries.

Skin Preparation and Draping. Skin preparation for vascular surgery may be extensive. Hair should be removed preoperatively only if it interferes with the procedure; if hair removal is necessary, it should be done immediately before the surgical procedure using clippers (Evidence for Practice), not a razor (Association of periOperative Registered Nurses [AORN], 2009). For abdominal aortic surgery, the patient's skin is prepped from the nipple line to the midthigh area. For peripheral vascular surgery on the lower extremities, the patient is prepped from the umbilicus to the feet. The patient's legs are prepped circumferentially. For carotid surgery, the patient is prepped from the ear and chin on the affected side to below the clavicle. It is important that alcohol-based prep solutions are allowed to dry completely before applying the surgical drapes and starting the surgical procedure.

Draping should permit the surgeon free access to involved areas. For example, abdominal surgery may also require exposure of the groin region for possible exploration of the femoral arteries. A femoral-popliteal bypass on one leg may require access to the other leg for saphenous vein harvesting. Impervious drapes should be used to prevent contamination of the surgical field from blood and irrigation fluids.

Medications and Solutions. In vascular surgery, several medications may be present on the sterile field at any given time. These may include heparin, heparinized saline, and papaverine, as well as local anesthetic medications and contrast dye. All medications and solutions on and off the sterile field must be labeled (Crum, 2006) (Risk Reduction Strategies). Heparin is the most common medication used in vascular surgery (Surgical Pharmacology) and may be given as an intravenous (IV) bolus by the anesthesia provider for systemic anticoagulation. When administered parenterally, heparin has a rapid onset of action, peaks in minutes, and has a 2- to 6-hour duration. Because it is metabolized in the liver and excreted by the kidneys, the effects of heparin may be prolonged in patients with liver and renal disease. The anticoagulant effects may be monitored by measurement of the activated partial thromboplastin time (APTT) or partial thromboplastin time (PTT). Patients are given anticoagulants just before the placement of a vascular clamp to prevent a thromboembolic event. The effects of systemic heparin may or may not need to be reversed at the end of the surgical procedure. Monitoring the activated clotting time (ACT) intraoperatively provides useful data for judging the need for reversal or additional medication. The effects of heparin can be reversed by the administration of protamine sulfate.

Since protamine sulfate is derived from fish sperm and testes, caution is advised when administering it to patients who are allergic to fish or who have received protamine-containing

insulin. One milligram of protamine neutralizes 100 mg of heparin. The dose should be calculated to offset half of the last dose of heparin. Protamine must be given slowly, at a maximum rate of 50 mg in 10 minutes, or dyspnea, flushing, bradycardia, and severe hypotension may occur. Another reason for monitoring heparin dose is that protamine, given in the absence of circulating heparin, acts as an anticoagulant and could delay hemostasis intraoperatively.

Heparinized saline solution is often used during vascular surgery for irrigation. It may be used to irrigate a blood vessel lumen during surgery, usually after the patient has been systemically heparinized. It is also commonly used to flush the lumen of tubes used to shunt blood. The strength of the heparin solution will vary according to the manufacturer's recommendations for certain implant devices or by the surgeon's preference. A reasonable range is 250 to 1000 units in 250 ml of normal saline.

Surgeon preferences differ regarding solutions with which to distend, irrigate, or store vein grafts. Some surgeons prefer a cold solution to decrease the metabolic demands of the vessel, whereas others believe this may lead to spasm. Spasm may be of particular concern when working with the small vessels of the distal leg or foot. Papaverine hydrochloride (HCl) may be added to a heparinized saline solution for its direct antispasmodic effect on the smooth muscle of the vessel wall and for its vasodilating properties. A reasonable dose is 120 mg in 250 ml of saline. The pressure of a handheld syringe to distend vein grafts has been viewed as a potential cause of graft failure or graft stenosis because this causes endothelial damage. Papaverine HCl, as a smooth muscle relaxant, allows distention at a lower pressure and may decrease the risk of injury. Concentrations for infiltration range from 0.05 to 0.6 mg/ml, or 12.5 to 150 mg per 250 ml of solution.

Topical hemostatic agents may be needed. Absorbable hemostatics are effective by creating an environment that promotes the adhesion of platelets. For example, an absorbable gelatin sponge may be applied to a bleeding surface to provide

EVIDENCE FOR PRACTICE

Reducing the Risks of Surgical Site Infections: Preoperative Hair Removal

Surgical site infections (SSIs) can be devastating to patients. An infection may mean a prolonged hospital stay, additional surgical procedures, or even death in an extreme case. A systematic literature review by Tanner (2007) showed that clinical studies done 20 years ago indicated that shaving with a razor increased the frequency of SSIs and that using clippers is the preferred method for hair removal when hair removal is deemed necessary. The increased SSI risk associated with shaving versus clipping is attributed to microscopic cuts in the skin that later serve as foci for bacterial multiplication. The Centers for Disease Control and Prevention (CDC) developed guidelines to reduce the risks of surgical site infections using this evidence of best practice from the literature. Following the CDC's recommended guidelines for hair removal to reduce the risks of SSIs equates to providing optimal patient care.

Modified from Tanner J: Preoperative hair removal: a systemic review, *J Periop Pract* 17(3):118-121, 2007; Mangram A et al: Guidelines for prevention of surgical site infection, *Infect Control Hosp Epidemiol* 20(4): 247-278, 1999, available at www.cdc.gov/ncidod/dhqp/pdf/guidelines/SSI. pdf. Accessed April 28, 2009.

a matrix into which clots form. It may be applied dry, moistened with saline, or soaked in a topical thrombin-saline solution; 100 to 2000 NIH units of thrombin per 1 ml of saline or blood may be applied to control bleeding.

Infections of prosthetic vascular grafts are rare but are extremely serious. Infection may be life-threatening for patients with aortic grafts or may be limb-threatening in lower-extremity procedures. Protecting the prosthetic graft from contact with the skin is essential to prevent bacterial contamination. Prophylactic IV antibiotics that provide coverage for any likely organisms to be encountered in the procedure should be administered within 1 hour before the surgical incision (Hawn et al, 2006). In some institutions, medical staff–approved protocols are available for selection of the appropriate antibiotic.

Vascular Prostheses. Vascular grafting materials and techniques are of major importance to the field of vascular surgery for bypass procedures and reconstruction. The understanding, study, and comparison of new prosthetic grafts; utilization and preparation of autogenous grafts; and knowledge of long-term patency rates are critical to improving patient outcomes. Grafts are made in various sizes and configurations; they may be straight, tapered, or Y-shaped (i.e., bifurcated); or they may be pieces of material cut for use as a patch. The arteriotomy from a carotid endarterectomy may be closed primarily or with a patch of either vein or synthetic fabric. In aortic surgery, a straight tube or a bifurcated synthetic graft is used. Dacron (polyester) grafts are the usual choice and have been used successfully for many years. Large vessels, such as the aorta, have high flow rates and thus have a low incidence of thrombus formation and excellent graft-patency rate. Desirable characteristics for vascular grafts are that they are reasonably priced, readily available in a variety of sizes, suitable for use anywhere in the body,

biocompatible and hypoallergenic, and able to survive repeated sterilizations. Grafts should be easy to handle and last a lifetime while permitting blood passage without clotting or infection.

Prosthetic grafts are nonantigenic; tissue incorporates well, which helps prevent infection, and such grafts generally resist thrombosis. For years, knitted polyester grafts were preferred over woven polyester because they were easier to handle, although they had to be preclotted because of their high porosity. Woven grafts are somewhat stronger and bleed less through the fabric interstices but can be less flexible. Newer grafts have been developed to incorporate the best of both by using velour polyester. They are often impregnated with albumin, collagen, or gelatin to provide ease in handling without the need to preclot. The surgical technologist ensures the graft is preclotted by submerging it into a basin containing a small quantity of the patient's own blood collected before systemic heparinization. This makes the graft impervious by allowing fibrin to fill in the fabric spaces.

The other popular prosthetic material is polytetrafluoroethylene (PTFE), which is available in straight, tapered, and bifurcated styles of varying lengths and may have external support rings to prevent compression. These grafts do not stretch, and needle-hole bleeding may be troublesome.

Cryo-preserved saphenous vein grafts are commercially available for patients who have no veins available because of previous bypass procedures, saphenous vein stripping, or poor quality or size of available veins. The nurse and surgical technologist must follow the manufacturers' instructions for rinsing these grafts to remove all traces of preservative.

Volumes have been written about vascular grafts, and the reader should consider this chapter an introduction only. The American National Standards Institute (ANSI), the U.S. Food and Drug Administration (FDA), and the Association for the

SURGICAL PHARMACOLOGY

Heparin—A High-Alert Medication

Heparin sodium is an anticoagulant that interferes with blood coagulation by blocking conversion of prothrombin to thrombin and fibrinogen to fibrin. It has no effect on a blood clot that has already formed or on ischemic tissue injured as a result of inadequate blood supply caused by a clot.

It is considered a high-alert drug, so designated by The Joint Commission and the Institute for Safe Medication Practices (ISMP) because it may cause life-threatening or permanent harm to the patient if administered incorrectly.

It is used for prophylaxis and/or treatment of vascular thromboembolic disorders, such as venous thrombosis and peripheral arterial embolism, and for prevention of thromboembolus during vascular surgical procedures. The number of units per milliliter varies in available dosage forms (supplied in vials). The most often used form is 5000 units/ml. One milligram of heparin is the equivalent of 100 units. Heparin may be administered by the anesthesia provider as an intravenous medication, administered by the surgeon as a full-strength injection during certain vascular procedures, or prepared as an irrigating solution by the scrub person. Standardized practices in the OR should be used to reduce the risk of an adverse drug event from the administration of anticoagulants such as heparin.

Sound-alike caution: Hespan. Institutions should identify and at a minimum annually review look-alike/sound-alike drugs to prevent errors involving the interchange of such drugs.

Labeling requirements: Any medication container, such as a syringe, medicine cup, or basin, containing heparin or a heparin solution must be labeled whether it is on or off the sterile field in perioperative or other procedural settings. Labels should be verified by two qualified individuals if the person preparing the medication is not the person administering it; this may be the case during relief of OR personnel (Crum, 2006).

Modified from *Drug information handbook for perioperative nursing*, Hudson, Ohio, 2006, Lexi-Comp; The Joint Commission: Preventing errors relating to commonly used anticoagulants, *Sentinel Event Alert*, September 24, 2008, available at www.jointcommission.org/SentinelEvents/SentinelEventAlert/sea_41.htm. Accessed April 15, 2009; ISMP Medication Safety Alert! ISMP Quarterly Action Agenda—January-March 2008, *The Institute for Safe Medication Practices*, available at www.ismp.org/Newsletters/acutecare/articles/A2Q08Action.asp. Accessed April 15, 2009; Crum BG: Revised national patient safety goal on medication handling, *AORN J* 83(4):955-957, 2006.

Advancement of Medical Instrumentation (AAMI) are a few of the organizations active in setting standards and regulating usage and development of grafts.

Autogenous vein grafting for infrainguinal bypass is considered the criterion standard. Undamaged endothelial cells inhibit the clotting mechanism by the natural release of fibrinolytic substances and plasminogen factors. Two methods of grafting veins have been extensively studied, and the results are not totally conclusive that one method is better than the other. These are the in situ graft and the reversed vein graft. The in situ method leaves the vein in its place, side branches are ligated to prevent arteriovenous fistulas, and the valves that would impede arterial flow are disrupted with instruments specifically designed to cut valves, called *valvulotomes* (Figure 15-6). Reoperation is more frequent with the in situ method because of missed valves and residual arteriovenous fistulas. Reversal of a vein graft is performed per the surgeon's preference or when it must be harvested from the contralateral limb. Vein grafts are used in below-knee (BK) bypass procedures. Above-knee (AK) bypasses may use PTFE or other synthetic grafts for vein sparing, or they may be used in high-risk patients who may not tolerate the longer vein harvesting or have a life expectancy of less than 3 years. *Atraumatic* clamps with rubber, plastic, or hydrostatic jaw clamps are used to protect vein grafts from injury. Distal bypasses, particularly those in persons with diabetes, are more successful today as a result of improved tissue handling. The surgeon may also use the pneumatic tourniquet as an alternative to clamping the vessels.

Sutures. Most vascular sutures are made of synthetic nonabsorbable materials, such as Dacron, polyester, PTFE, and polypropylene. Vascular sutures have swaged-on needles of various sizes and are available in sizes 0 to 10-0. The suture may be single-armed or double-armed (i.e., a needle on one or both ends). The size and curve of the needle depend on the vessel and its location. Teflon felt or leftover pieces of graft material (synthetic or vein) may be used as pledgets or buttresses under a suture. They are used when tissue is friable to keep the suture from tearing through or when an anastomosis leaks and needs a better seal. The pledget may be loaded onto the vascular suture or added by the surgeon to a suture already in use. The pledget remains on the suture line (Figure 15-7).

Vascular Monitoring Equipment. Assessing blood flow through diseased vessels by palpation is often difficult. Physical assessment of the patient's hemodynamic status during surgery can be further complicated by spasm of the vessel walls, the cool environment of the OR, and alterations in blood pressure caused by hemorrhage. Therefore the surgeon often uses vascular monitoring equipment to evaluate tissue perfusion and flow. The Doppler device is critical when pulses cannot be palpated. With a coupling gel, the unsterile Doppler probe can be placed on the patient's skin distal to the surgical site. Some probes can be sterilized and used within the sterile field to assess the flow in an arterial graft or determine whether the blood supply to the intestines or other structures is intact after aortic surgery. Besides providing an audible signal, the Doppler probe can provide a permanent record of the sound if a recorder is attached.

An EEG accurately determines reduced cerebral perfusion during a CEA. This enables the surgeon to decide whether to use a temporary shunt in the carotid artery or if the patient can tolerate clamping. Sterile IV tubing connected to an arterial transducer can also be used to check pressure gradients intraoperatively. The stump pressure of unclamped carotid arteries before thromboendarterectomy can also determine the need for intraoperative shunting. Trained personnel are necessary to operate this equipment.

Instrumentation. Most vascular procedures begin with a basic laparotomy set (for scissors, clamps, and retractors) and a vascular set. Items specific to each surgical procedure are then

---

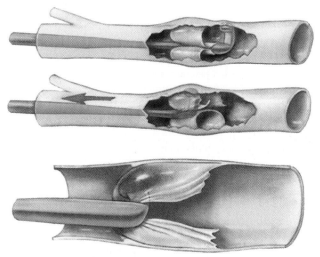

FIGURE 15-6 Valve incision with valvulotome.

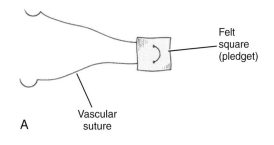

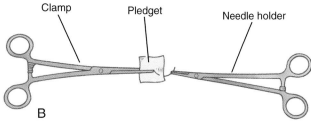

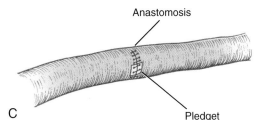

FIGURE 15-7 Pledgetted suture. **A,** Double-armed vascular suture prepared with pledget. **B,** Technique for surgeon to add pledget to suture already in use. **C,** Appearance of suture line with pledget in place.

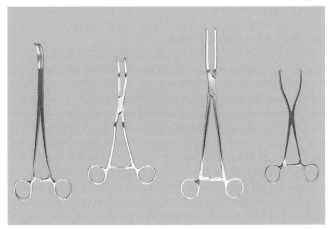

FIGURE 15-8 *Left to right:* 1 Semb ligature-carrying forceps, 9 inch; 1 Lambert-Kay aortic clamp; 1 Fogarty clamp-applying forceps, angled; 1 bulldog clamp applier.

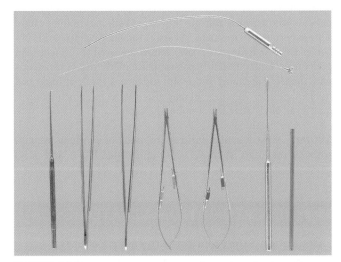

FIGURE 15-9 *Top:* 1 Frazier suction tube with stylet, long. *Bottom, left to right:* 1 blunt hook, 2-mm round tip; 2 Reul coronary tissue forceps, delicate, 8 inch; 2 Jarit microsurgical needle holders with locks; Carb-Bite jaws, smooth, 7 inch; 1 Penfield dissector, single-ended, #4; 1 Beaver knife handle, knurled, 6 inch, without insert.

added. For abdominal surgery, a large self-retaining retractor should be added. Additional individually wrapped, sterile aortic clamps; some long clamps (cystic duct and right angle); and long forceps for larger patients should be available in the OR. Smaller vascular clamps and vascular bulldog clamps should also be kept sterile in the OR. For peripheral procedures, a variety of Weitlaner self-retaining retractors should be available. Carotid surgery requires carotid shunt clamps, shunts, microforceps, and dissectors for peeling plaque from the artery. The surgeon may use the saphenous vein as a graft conduit by removing and reversing it or by using it in situ. A variety of instruments are available for disrupting the valves to permit arterial flow in the in situ procedure. Amputations do not require vascular instrumentation. A minor basic set and appropriately sized bone instruments are needed.

A Mayo stand will include DeBakey forceps, and ring Gerald forceps. Metzenbaum and straight Mayo scissors, as well as tenotomy and Potts scissors are needed. Retractors will include a small Richardson, appendicle, vein retractors, and a variety of Weitlaners both sharp and blunt, both small and medium. Also needed are rubber shods to hold suture, and micro and standard vein hooks to detangle suture if necessary. Typically, a Castroviejo needle holder is used in vascular procedures. The suture used is typically a monofilament such as prolene, and it is most commonly double armed.

Figures 15-8 through 15-11 show commonly used instruments in vascular surgery.

Surgical Interventions

ABDOMINAL AORTIC ANEURYSM RESECTION

Abdominal aortic aneurysmectomy is surgical obliteration of the aneurysm, which may or may not include the iliac arteries, with insertion of a synthetic prosthesis to reestablish functional continuity. The majority of AAAs begin below the renal arteries (infrarenal), and many extend to involve the bifurcation and common iliac arteries. Severe back pain, along with symptoms of hypotension, shock, and distal vascular insufficiency, usually indicates rupture and represents a true emergency condition. The prime surgical consideration when a rupture occurs is the control of hemorrhage by occlusion of the aorta proximal to the point of rupture. AAAs are usually asymptomatic and are found on routine physical examination. They occur more frequently in men than in women. Aneurysmal disease is caused by a disruption of the tunica media, which structurally weakens

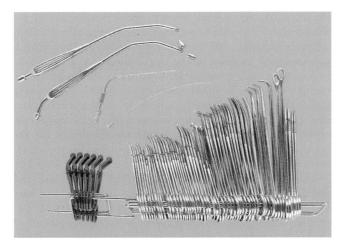

FIGURE 15-10 *Top to bottom:* 2 Yankauer suction tubes with tips; 1 Frazier suction tube with stylet. *Bottom, left to right:* 6 paper drape clips; 10 Halsted mosquito hemostatic forceps, curved; 6 Crile hemostatic forceps, curved, 5½ inch; 6 Providence Hospital hemostatic forceps (delicate tip), curved 5½ inch; 4 Crile hemostatic forceps, curved 6½ inch; 4 Allis tissue forceps; 4 Westphal hemostatic forceps; 6 tonsil hemostatic forceps; 2 Mayo-Péan hemostatic forceps, long, curved; 2 Carmalt hemostatic forceps, long; 2 Adson hemostatic forceps, long; 2 Mixter hemostatic forceps, long, fine, and heavy tips; 2 Foerster sponge forceps; 2 Crile-Wood needle holders, 7 inch; 2 Ayers needle holders, 7 inch, fine tips.

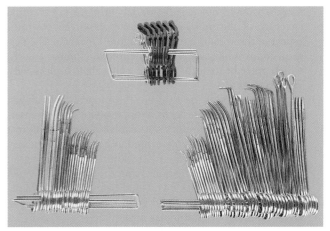

FIGURE 15-11 *Top, left to right:* 2 Backhaus towel forceps; 6 paper drape clips. *Bottom, left to right:* 2 Ochsner hemostatic forceps, straight, long; 2 Mayo-Péan hemostatic forceps, long: 4 tonsil hemostatic forceps; 1 Westphal hemostatic forceps; 4 Providence Hospital hemostatic forceps (delicate tip), 5½ inch, curved; 4 Crile hemostatic forceps, 5½ inch, curved; 4 Halsted mosquito hemostatic forceps, curved. *Second stringer:* 4 Halsted mosquito hemostatic forceps, curved; 6 Crile hemostatic forceps, 5½ inch, curved; 1 Westphal hemostatic forceps; 4 tonsil hemostatic forceps; 4 Carmalt hemostatic forceps, long; 2 Adson hemostatic forceps, long; 2 Allis tissue forceps, long; 4 Ochsner hemostatic forceps, long, straight; 3 Mixter hemostatic forceps, long, heavy tip; 2 Mixter hemostatic forceps, long, fine tip; 4 Foerster sponge forceps; 2 Ayers needle holders, 8 inch; 2 Crile-Wood needle holders, 8 inch.

the aortic wall. Aneurysmal aortas are found to have a significantly decreased amount of collagen and elastin in the vessel wall. Rupture carries less than a 50% death rate for patients in stable condition with a contained rupture. Risks from AAA surgery include massive hemorrhage and hypotension, injury to the ureters, renal failure, spinal cord ischemia, and death. Because peripheral vascular disease is a manifestation of a systemic disorder, it is not surprising that patients with aneurysms often have concomitant coronary artery disease. Patients are at risk of myocardial ischemia, myocardial infarction, hypotension, and hypertension. Myocardial infarction is the leading cause of death after AAA repair; therefore it is imperative that a patient with cardiac symptoms or ECG abnormalities have a thorough preoperative cardiac assessment.

The perioperative team must be alert to the fact that at the time the aortic clamp is released to permit distal flow, "declamping shock" or severe hypotension may occur. This may be attributable to the presence of inadequate volume replacement, the sudden reestablishment of flow to dilated distal vessels, or the release of acidic metabolites. Declamping shock and hemorrhage have been proposed as causes of renal failure from acute tubular necrosis.

Procedural Considerations

The patient is placed in the supine position. General endotracheal anesthesia is used. The anesthesia provider inserts a central venous catheter and arterial line. A urinary catheter is then inserted, the surgical site is prepped for a midline abdominal incision, and the surgical technologist assists with draping to permit access to the groin region for possible exploration of femoral arteries. The nurse ensures the patient's pedal pulses are marked before the beginning of the procedure so that they may be located easily when the surgeon requests a check of the

pulses. This assessment of pulses can be done manually or with a Doppler probe.

Operative Procedure—Transperitoneal Approach

1. The surgeon opens the patient's abdomen through a long midline incision (Figure 15-12, *A*) from the xiphoid process to the symphysis pubis and achieves hemostasis.
2. An abdominal self-retaining retractor is inserted into the wound. The surgeon and assistant retract the patient's small bowel, including the duodenum, to the right; they may place it outside the abdomen and cover it with moist laparotomy packs for better exposure.
3. The retroperitoneum overlying the aneurysm is incised and extended superiorly to expose the aneurysm and also inferiorly over the bifurcation and beyond the iliac arteries. Metzenbaum scissors, smooth forceps, and hemostats are used.
4. Careful blunt and sharp dissection is used to expose the aorta above the aneurysm to permit placement of an aortic clamp while avoiding the renal artery and ureters. The surgeon inspects the iliac vessels and bifurcation for evidence of small aneurysms, thrombosis, and calcification.
5. The anesthesia provider administers a dose of heparin intravenously, and the surgeon applies and closes an aortic clamp such as a DeBakey, Fogarty, or Satinsky around the aorta. Distal runoff vessels are also clamped. Opening of the aneurysm is undertaken with a scalpel or electrosurgical blade and heavy scissors (Figure 15-12, *B*).
6. The aneurysm is completely opened, and all atheromatous and thrombotic material is removed. The aneurysm walls

may be excised but usually are left in place for eventual coverage of the prosthesis. In either case, the posterior aspect of the aorta is left intact (Figure 15-12, *C*). The surgeon controls bleeding, especially from the lumbar vessels, which enter posteriorly, by oversewing their orifices with vascular suture.

7. At the direction of the surgeon, the surgical technologist prepares the prosthetic graft of appropriate size for insertion. If the aneurysm does not involve the aortic bifurcation, a straight tubular graft is used; otherwise, a bifurcated or Y-shaped graft is necessary. Preclotting of a knitted graft may be accomplished by immersing the graft into a small quantity of the patient's own blood before systemic heparinization, or a manufactured graft impregnated with collagen, albumin, or gelatin may be used.

8. The aortic cuff is prepared for anastomosis by irrigating it with heparinized saline solution and by removing all fibrotic plaques. One or two vascular sutures (double-armed) are used to accomplish the anastomosis by a through-and-through continuous suture (Figure 15-12, *D*). Additional interrupted sutures may be needed if the anastomosis leaks on completion. A strip of Teflon felt may be used along the suture line for reinforcement.

9. The surgeon opens and inspects the distal vessels for back-bleeding, and may inject heparinized saline solution to prevent clotting.

10. Each limb of the graft is anastomosed to the iliac artery, using a smaller vascular suture and similar technique (Figure 15-12, *E*). After the first side of the anastomosis has been completed, blood is permitted to circulate and the remaining limb of the graft is clamped to prevent leaking during the last part of the anastomosis.

11. The aneurysm may be closed over the graft.

12. The peritoneum is closed to exclude contact of the intestine with the graft, and the abdominal wound is closed.

ENDOVASCULAR ABDOMINAL AORTIC ANEURYSM REPAIR

Endovascular aneurysm repair (EVAR) differs from open surgical repair in that the surgeon introduces the prosthetic endograft or stent-graft into the aneurysm through a surgically exposed femoral artery and fixes it in place to the nonaneurysmal infrarenal neck and iliac arteries with self-expanding or balloon-expandable stents rather than sutures (Figure 15-13). A major abdominal incision is thus avoided, and patient morbidity related to the procedure is much reduced. The benefits of this procedure are a hospital stay of 1 to 2 days, a rapid return to normal physical activity, and a reduction in the mortality and complication rates compared with those of the conventional surgical procedure (Egorova et al, 2008). The procedure may also be applicable to high-risk patients.

A number of commercially manufactured stent-grafts have been developed since the first endovascular aneurysm repair was carried out in 1991, using a Dacron graft sutured onto balloon-expandable Palmaz stents. Early tubular grafts have largely been replaced by modular bifurcated grafts that have expanded the applicability of this therapy. Different graft configurations, depending on the anatomic problem, are available. For patients with an AAA that is limited to the aorta and in whom there is both a neck between the renal arteries and

the aneurysm and a neck between the lower portion of the aneurysm and the iliac bifurcation, a graft of tubular configuration is available. For those patients in whom the abdominal aneurysm extends to the iliac bifurcation, a bifurcated or Y-shaped graft is available. For those patients who have both an AAA and an aneurysm of one or both iliac arteries, a tapered tube graft that excludes both the aortic aneurysm and one iliac aneurysm is usually selected. The technical details of endovascular repair vary with each specific device, but the general principles are similar. Candidates for this procedure include patients with a proximal infrarenal neck at least 1 to 2 cm in length and common iliac arteries for proximal and distal fixation of an endograft, without excessive tortuosity and with appropriate iliofemoral access. Long-term follow-up data are ongoing, and patients undergoing this procedure should understand that prolonged follow-up with periodic imaging will be required and that reintervention may become necessary. Nonetheless, the future of endoluminal grafting continues to evolve and has the potential of significant rewards (Schermerhorn et al, 2008).

Procedural Considerations

The team positions the patient supine on a radiolucent OR bed with a special marker board. The board has remotely controlled radiopaque cursors that are used to fluoroscopically detect proximal and distal positions for graft deployment. An ample supply of lead gowns needs to be available. The anesthesia provider may administer a general anesthetic or an epidural anesthetic. If an epidural anesthetic is used, mechanical ventilation is available in case conversion to the traditional surgical procedure is required. The anesthesia provider inserts a central venous catheter and an arterial catheter for hemodynamic monitoring. A urinary catheter is inserted, and the patient's abdomen and groin areas are prepped and draped to allow conversion to the traditional surgical technique if necessary.

Operative Procedure

1. The surgeon performs bilateral groin cutdowns and dissects both common femoral arteries.

2. After the anesthesia provider administers IV heparin, the surgeon clamps the right common femoral artery, performs an arteriotomy, and introduces an 8-French (8F) sheath into the right external iliac artery.

3. The left femoral artery is punctured, and the surgeon places a 12F sheath into the left external iliac artery. An angiocath is inserted, and an arteriogram is obtained to clearly mark the renal arteries and aortic bifurcation. The final length of the device to cover the aorta from the renal arteries to a suitable section of the common iliac arteries is chosen.

4. A snare is introduced into the aorta through the left femoral artery, and a pull wire is introduced into the aorta by way of the right femoral artery. The pull wire is snared above the aortic bifurcation and retracted into the left iliac artery. This step is done to help position the limbs of the graft into the iliac arteries.

5. The surgeon inserts the grafting device into the right femoral artery, advances it into the proximal part of the aorta, and positions it above the aortic bifurcation. Fluoroscopy is used to determine proper position of the stent.

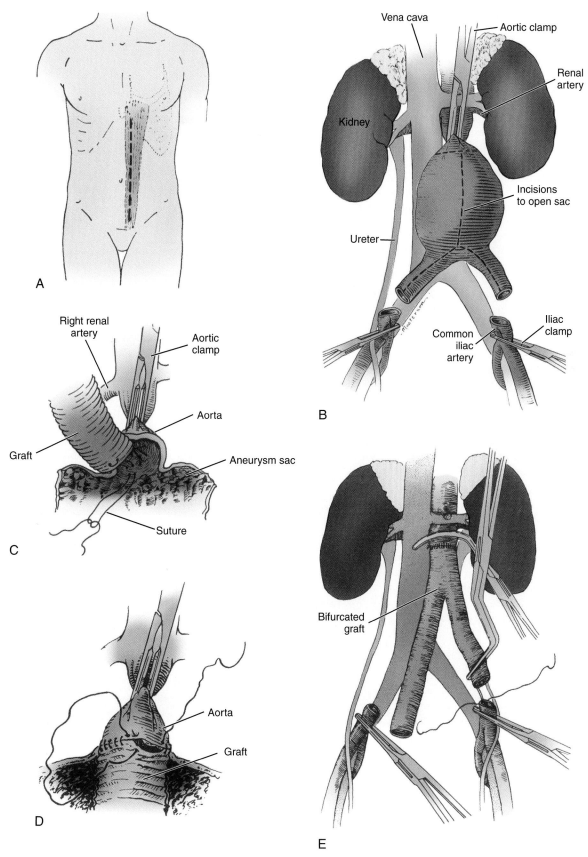

FIGURE 15-12 Resection of abdominal aortic aneurysm. **A,** Midline abdominal incision. **B,** Aneurysm sac is opened. **C,** Prosthetic graft is sewn to back wall of aorta, creating a cuff. **D,** Completion of aortic graft anastomosis. **E,** Iliac artery anastomosis.

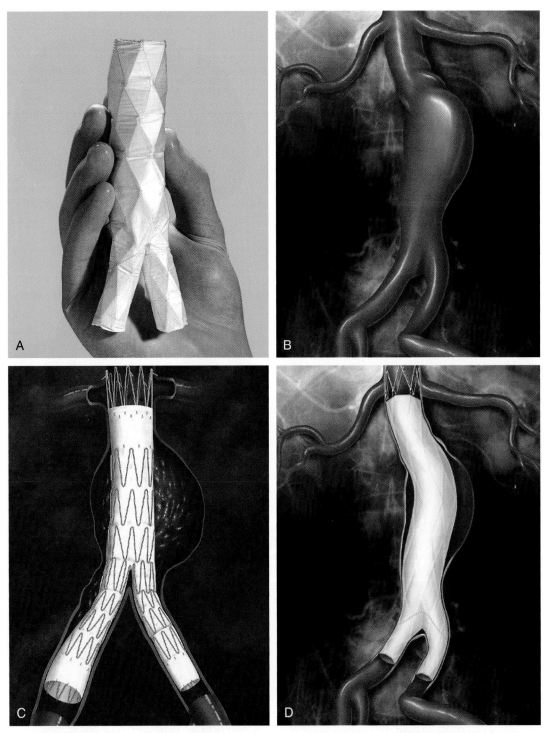

FIGURE 15-13 **A,** Endoluminal graft: demonstrating size compared to an adult hand. **B,** Graphic diagram of a descending aortic aneurysm. **C,** Graphic diagram of an endoluminal graft in place: descending aorta and iliac arteries. **D,** Graphic diagram of an endoluminal graft postoperatively. (Courtesy VAS Communications, Phoenix, Arizona.)

6. The device is exposed by retracting a covering jacket, and the graft limbs are positioned in the iliac arteries. The hooks of the graft become attached to the walls of the aorta and the iliac arteries as the attachment systems are deployed.

7. The balloon on the device is inflated to secure the proximal attachment system to the aorta and the contralateral and ipsilateral systems to the iliac arteries.

8. An arteriogram is obtained to confirm proper positioning and complete exclusion of the AAA. Ideally, the graft is positioned to occlude the inferior mesenteric artery to prevent persistent blood flow within the aneurysmal sac.

9. After all the sheaths are removed, the surgeon closes the wounds with subcuticular sutures.

PERCUTANEOUS TRANSLUMINAL ANGIOPLASTY

Percutaneous transluminal angioplasty (PTA) is performed with a local anesthetic and minimal sedation, as a same-day surgery admission. Although initially performed only in the common iliac artery for stenosis, PTA is routinely used to treat short-segment occlusions as well as external iliac lesions. Iliac artery PTA may be particularly useful to help improve inflow before a more distal surgical reconstruction.

The use of iliac artery stents has also begun to play an increasing role in the management of patients with aortoiliac occlusive disease. Iliac artery stents are most useful after initial suboptimal results from PTA. However, they are used primarily in the treatment of complex lesions. When PTA is not an option, a number of surgical alternatives are available. Depending on the condition of the patient and the patient's pathologic anatomy, the options include aortobifemoral bypass, aortoiliac thromboendarterectomy, axillofemoral bypass, iliofemoral bypass, and femorofemoral bypass.

FEMORAL-POPLITEAL AND FEMORAL-TIBIAL BYPASS

Femoral-popliteal bypass is the restoration of blood flow to the leg with a graft bypassing the occluded section of the femoral artery. The bypass may be a saphenous vein or straight synthetic graft. The patient must have a patent outflow artery for a successful bypass procedure. If popliteal patency is doubtful, artery exploration is necessary as the first procedure. Involvement of the popliteal artery may necessitate the exposure and use of the tibial vessels for the lower anastomosis. If this occurs, the procedure could require the use of microvascular instruments and technique.

Procedural Considerations

The patient is placed in a supine position. The hip is externally rotated and abducted with the knee flexed. Prepping and draping include the entire groin and leg. The instrument setup includes the basic minor and vascular sets, plus the following: Gelpi retractors, Garrett or Weitlaner retractors, a device to tunnel, and supplies and equipment for operative arteriograms.

Operative Procedures

Exploration of Common Femoral Artery

1. A vertical incision, extending downward about 3 to 5 inches along the medial aspect of the thigh, is made by the surgeon over the femoral artery below the inguinal area, and the field is exposed with a self-retaining retractor.
2. The surgeon locates the common femoral artery and dissects it in both directions for complete exposure.
3. The surgical technologist supplies moist umbilical tapes or vessel loops, which the surgeon passes around the common femoral, the superficial femoral, and the deep femoral arteries.

Exploration of Above-Knee Popliteal Artery

1. The surgeon makes a vertical incision along the medial aspect of the lower area of the thigh. If the popliteal artery is diseased, an additional incision below the knee is made to expose the distal popliteal artery.

2. A Weitlaner retractor is used to retract the muscles and expose the artery.
3. The surgeon flexes the patient's knee, dissects the popliteal artery, and passes a moist umbilical tape around the popliteal artery. Arteriograms may be performed at this time if doubt exists about the patency of the popliteal artery or distal arterial tree.
4. The saphenous vein is exposed via joined femoral and popliteal incisions the length of the thigh or through multiple short incisions along the medial area of the thigh. If the vein is suitable, the surgeon resects the necessary length or prepares it for in situ grafting. If a prosthesis will be used, the surgeon determines the length and size and the surgical technologist preclots the graft as previously described.
5. The surgeon ligates the side branches of the saphenous vein with fine silk. Finally, because of venous valves, the vein is reversed so that the end originally in the groin is anastomosed to the popliteal artery.
6. If a synthetic graft is used, the surgeon passes a tunneling device beneath the sartorius muscle from the popliteal fossa to the groin.
7. The graft is carefully pulled through the tunnel and positioned to prevent kinks or twists.
8. The anesthesia provider administers IV heparin to the patient before the surgeon applies a vascular clamp to the femoral artery. An incision is made into the femoral artery with a #11 knife blade and extended with a Potts angulated scissors.
9. The graft is anastomosed to the artery with fine vascular sutures.
10. The patient's knee is flexed, and the surgeon places vascular clamps on the popliteal artery at the site of the distal anastomosis.
11. An incision is made into the popliteal artery as explained for femoral arteriotomy.
12. The graft is sutured to the popliteal (or tibial) artery, and before completion the femoral occluding clamp is momentarily opened to eliminate air and debris.
13. All occluding clamps are removed, and the graft is assessed for anastomotic leaks.
14. The incision is closed as described previously.

FEMORAL-POPLITEAL BYPASS IN SITU

In situ femoral-popliteal bypass is the restoration of blood flow to the leg, bypassing an occluded portion of the femoral artery with the patient's saphenous vein, which remains in place. The procedure includes incising the venous valves and interrupting the venous tributaries. The adequacy of the patient's saphenous vein may be validated before the surgical procedure by an ultrasound duplex scan. Varicose veins or a previous saphenous vein ligation and stripping are contraindications to the procedure. The advantages of a vein-bypass procedure include increased graft availability and improved patency. A disadvantage is the time-consuming aspect of this technique.

Procedural Considerations

The surgeon uses microvascular scissors, a valvulotome, or a leather in situ valve cutter kit to incise the valves within the vein. An angioscope may be used to monitor the lysis of valve leaflets.

Operative Procedure

1. The procedure is similar to that for a femoral-popliteal bypass. The surgeon extends the groin incision downward over the course of the saphenous vein. A skin bridge may be left between the groin and the popliteal incisions.
2. The saphenous vein is exposed and divided at its proximal and distal ends. Venous tributaries are occluded with vessel clips, such as hemoclips, or fine nonabsorbable sutures.
3. The surgeon passes a valvulotome from below to the top, usually through side branches. The valvulotome is used to incise the internal valve (see Figure 15-6). In angioscopically assisted bypass, valve lysis is done under direct vision.
4. The saphenous vein is distended with heparinized saline, papaverine, or heparinized blood to identify any valvular obstruction or open venous tributary. Another pass of the valve cutter alleviates the obstruction. Open branches of the saphenous vein can also be ligated with vessel clips or fine nonabsorbable sutures.
5. The incompetent saphenous vein is used to bypass the occluded segment of the femoral artery (see steps 8 through 14 of the femoral-popliteal bypass procedure described under Exploration of Above-Knee Popliteal Artery).

FEMOROFEMORAL BYPASS

Femorofemoral bypass is an extraanatomic (a route that is outside the normal path) bypass that is performed to restore blood flow to one leg when an inflow procedure is necessary but a major aortic procedure is not desired. This type of bypass procedure is also used when the surgical risks for the patient are high because of a complicated medical condition or there are technical problems with the procedure (Figure 15-14). Studies continue to examine the long-term patency rate and outcomes for this patient population. Severe cardiac or pulmonary disease may prevent the patient from undergoing a more extensive procedure. Subcutaneous vascular grafting is an option in these conditions because the procedure bypasses normal vascular anatomy and can be performed using a local anesthetic with adjunct moderate sedation and analgesia. The patient must have one good iliac artery for inflow for a femorofemoral bypass to be considered. Another extraanatomic procedure that can be done in these instances is an axillofemoral bypass involving the subcutaneous placement of a prosthesis from the axillary artery to the femoral artery on the same side (Figure 15-15).

Procedural Considerations

The patient is positioned supine on the OR bed with a small pad placed under each knee. The area prepped for surgery extends from the umbilicus to midthigh area. The genitalia are covered with a sterile towel.

Operative Procedure

1. A longitudinal incision is made by the surgeon over each femoral artery from the inguinal ligament to just below the femoral bifurcation.
2. Each common femoral artery, superficial femoral artery, and deep femoral artery are dissected free, mobilized, and secured with umbilical tapes or vessel loops.
3. The surgeon creates a graft tunnel between the two femoral arteries across the symphysis pubis in the subcutaneous tis-

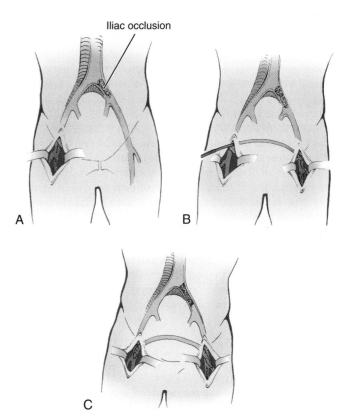

FIGURE 15-14 Femorofemoral bypass to restore blood flow to left leg. **A,** Left iliac artery occlusion and right femoral artery exposure. **B,** Exposure of the right and left femoral arteries: tunneling device creating a path for the graft in the subcutaneous tissue. **C,** Femorofemoral bypass graft in place.

sue with digital dissection, scissors dissection, or the passage of a clamp or tunneling device across the preperitoneal space.
4. A Dacron or PTFE vascular graft is passed through the subcutaneous tunnel with care to prevent kinking of the graft.
5. The anesthesia provider administers IV heparin, and the surgeon places vascular clamps on the common femoral, superficial femoral, and deep femoral arteries. A longitudinal arteriotomy is made in the common femoral artery.
6. The surgeon performs an end-to-side anastomosis using nonabsorbable vascular sutures to join the graft with the common femoral artery. A similar anastomosis is done on the other side.
7. After the clamps are released and flow is restored, the patient's pulses are checked with a sterile Doppler; the perioperative nurse may be asked to assess the patient's feet for warmth and color.
8. The femoral incisions are closed.

ARTERIAL EMBOLECTOMY

Arterial embolectomy entails an incision made in the affected artery to remove thromboembolic material and restore blood flow. Emboli may be clot particles, a foreign body, air, fat, or a tumor that circulates through the bloodstream and becomes lodged as the vessel decreases in size. More often the direct source is a cardiac mural thrombus, associated with cardiac or vascular disease. Pain or numbness distal to the obstruction is

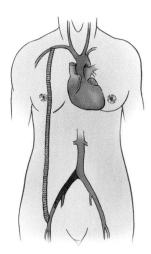

FIGURE 15-15 Axillofemoral bypass graft for right iliac artery occlusion.

the initial symptom, accompanied by other signs of vascular occlusion, such as pallor and absence of pulses.

Procedural Considerations

The patient is placed in the supine position, the skin area is prepped, and draping is completed to permit access to the affected area. The instrument setup includes the basic instrument and vascular sets, including embolectomy catheters and irrigation catheters. Heparinized saline is required.

Operative Procedure—Femoral Embolectomy

1. After making a groin incision the surgeon exposes the femoral artery to permit the application of vascular clamps (Figure 15-16, *A* and *B*).
2. An incision is made into the artery with a #11 blade and a Potts scissors. An embolectomy catheter is carefully inserted beyond the point of clot proximally and distally. The balloon is inflated, and the catheter is withdrawn along with the detached clot (Figure 15-16, *C* and *D*).
3. As backflow is obtained, the surgeon applies a vascular clamp below the arteriotomy (Figure 15-16, *E*).
4. The artery may be flushed by injection of heparinized saline solution through a small irrigating catheter. Angioscopy or an arteriogram may or may not be requested at this time.
5. The arterial closure is completed with vascular sutures (Figure 15-16, *F*). The wound is closed, and dressings are applied.

AMPUTATION

Amputations involving the lower extremity are performed to eliminate ischemic, gangrenous, necrotic, or infected tissue; relieve pain; and promote maximum independence. Amputations may be necessary because of trauma or malignancy or when the lower limb cannot be salvaged by arterial reconstruction. In the immediate postoperative period, patients may experience phantom limb pain, described as shooting, burning, throbbing, stabbing, or squeezing. Phantom limb pain may recur, but less frequently, in the months following surgery (Hanley et al, 2006).

Procedural Considerations

It is critical to verify the correct limb for this procedure. Because amputations are often performed with the patient administered a regional anesthetic, the surgical team must be sure that the patient does not witness the wrapping or transport of the amputated limb. Toes or partial foot amputations may be done in certain instances, but often a below-knee (BK) or above-knee (AK) amputation is indicated. Syme's amputation, through the ankle, is seldom performed because of improved prosthetics and rehabilitation that favor mid-calf amputation. The level is based on the health of the patient, level of vascularity, and potential for healing and rehabilitation. Severe infection or toxemia may require amputation as a lifesaving procedure. Operative risks for amputation are higher than those for reconstruction, possibly because of more extensive vascular disease. BK amputations are best done at the junction of the upper and middle thirds of the lower leg. This allows for an immediate postoperative prosthesis, aids in better healing, and may reduce phantom limb pain. AK amputations may be at the middle or lower third of the thigh. Flaps are tailored to provide fascial and skin coverage to cushion the smoothed end of the bone. Meticulous hemostasis and drainage are needed to decrease hematoma formation, since healing is both problematic and critical in these patients. Persons with diabetes are at highest risk for amputation because of their neuropathy, altered response to infection, and vascular insufficiency.

Operative Procedure

1. The surgeon determines the level of amputation, and marks the incision line to create a long posterior flap for a BK amputation. For an AK amputation, the anterior and posterior flaps are fairly equal in size (Figure 15-17).
2. Blood loss may be reduced by using a sterile tourniquet after the leg is raised to drain venous blood. The tourniquet is inflated and the surgeon makes the incision and divides the muscle and soft tissue. The periosteum is raised with an elevator.
3. The surgeon cuts the bones—the tibia with a Gigli or oscillating saw and the fibula with a bone cutter—and bevels their anterior aspect and smoothes them with a rongeur and rasp. The specimen is handed off the field.
4. The stump is gently irrigated, and hemostasis is achieved.
5. A closed-wound drainage system may be inserted.
6. Fascia is closed with interrupted sutures.
7. Skin is approximated and closed with interrupted suture or staples.
8. An immediate postoperative stump dressing may be applied to prevent flexion contracture.

CAROTID ENDARTERECTOMY (CEA)

CEA is the removal of an atheroma (plaque) at the carotid artery bifurcation to increase cerebral perfusion and decrease the risk of embolization and consequent stroke (Liu et al, 2009). In most settings, the patient is discharged on the first postoperative day. Lessening the likelihood of any transient or permanent neurologic deficit is a major concern during a CEA. The use of a temporary carotid artery shunt (Figure 15-18), such as an Argyle or Javid shunt, allows for continuous blood flow through the carotid artery and to the brain.

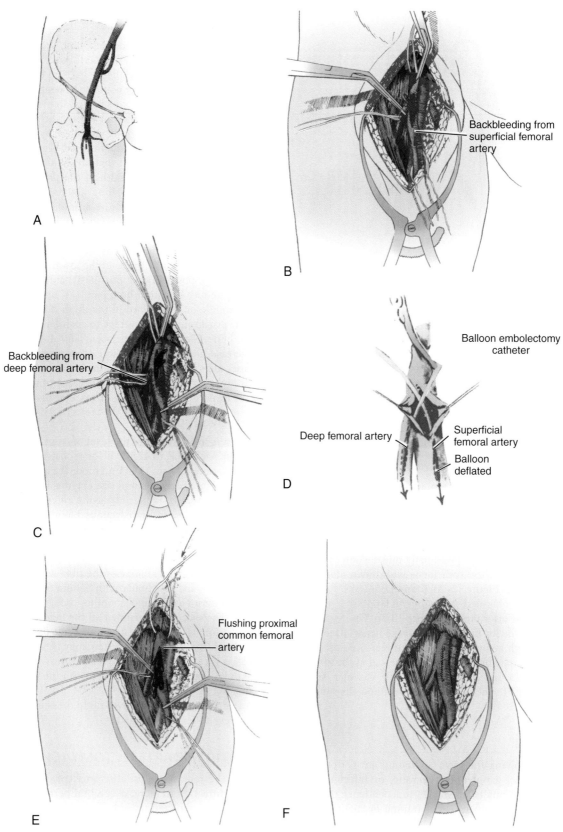

FIGURE 15-16 Femoral embolectomy. **A,** Femoral arteriotomy. **B,** Clamp on common femoral and deep femoral (profunda femoris) arteries. Backflow of blood from superficial femoral artery (SFA) is checked. **C,** Clamp on common femoral artery and SFA. Backflow of blood from deep femoral artery is checked. **D,** Balloon embolectomy catheters are passed into SFA and profunda. **E,** Proximal (common femoral) artery is unclamped and flushed. **F,** Arteriotomy is closed.

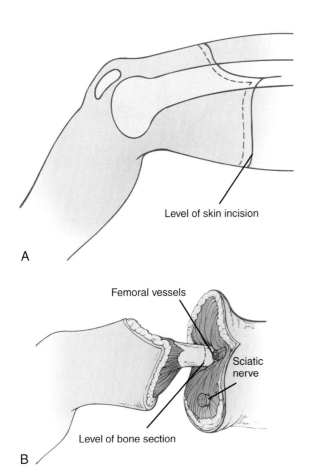

Level of skin incision

A

Femoral vessels

Sciatic nerve

Level of bone section

B

FIGURE 15-17 Leg amputation, above knee, through the middle third of the thigh. **A,** Level of skin incision. **B,** Level of bone resection.

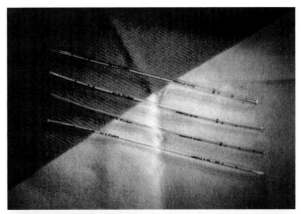

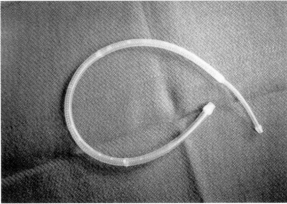

FIGURE 15-18 Example of temporary carotid artery shunts that are used to permit blood flow during carotid endarterectomy procedures.

Some disadvantages in using this temporary device are that additional dissection is necessary for its placement and that there is a possibility of dislodging debris when the shunt is inserted. Also, it is difficult to view the endarterectomy endpoint and suturing a patch is more difficult.

Two techniques that facilitate continual assessment of cerebral perfusion are the use of a cervical plexus block for anesthesia and the use of electroencephalography. A conscious patient with a cervical plexus block can be observed for neurologic deficits encountered during the procedure. The patient who is administered a general anesthetic can be monitored with an EEG. If either method demonstrates reduced cerebral perfusion, the surgeon may decide to use a temporary carotid artery shunt. The shunting device should always be available and sterile at the beginning of the procedure.

Procedural Considerations

The patient is positioned supine on the OR bed with the head supported on a head support. The head is turned away from the operative side, and the neck may be slightly hyperextended. A roll may be placed between the scapulae.

Operative Procedure

1. The surgeon makes a longitudinal incision over the area of the carotid bifurcation (Figure 15-19, *A*) and places a Weitlaner self-retaining retractor for exposure.

2. With Metzenbaum scissors, the surgeon dissects the soft tissue to expose the carotid artery and its bifurcation (Figure 15-19, *B*).

3. A moistened umbilical tape or vessel loop is passed around the vessel for ease of handling. Systemic heparin is given to the patient by the anesthesia provider.

4. The surgeon clamps the external, common, and internal carotid arteries.

5. The surgeon uses a #11 knife blade to create an arteriotomy over the stenotic area and lengthens the incision with a Potts angulated scissors to expose the full extent of the occluding plaque.

6. Using a blunt dissector, the surgeon dissects the plaque or plaques free from the arterial wall. Heparin solution is used as an irrigant to clean the intima.

7. The surgeon closes the arteriotomy with fine vascular sutures. A synthetic (polyester or PTFE) or autogenous (vein) patch graft may be used to restore the arterial lumen if it is small (Figure 15-20). Before complete closure, blood flow is temporarily restored through the arteries to wash away any free plaques, air, or thrombi. For this to be done, the occluding clamps are opened and closed individually, with flushing of any debris away from the internal carotid artery. The closure of the arteriotomy is completed (Figure 15-21).

8. The occluding clamps are removed from the external and common carotid arteries; the internal carotid artery clamp is removed last. This sequence ensures that any minor

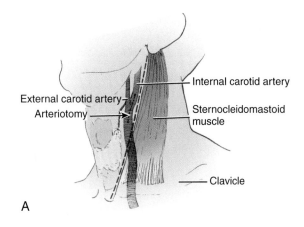

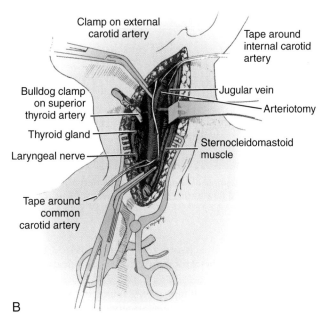

FIGURE 15-19 Left carotid endarterectomy. **A,** Incision and anatomy. **B,** Exposure of carotid bifurcation.

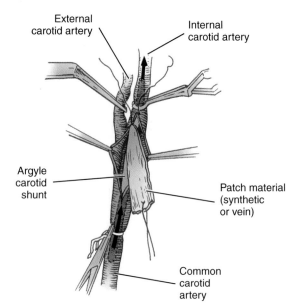

FIGURE 15-20 Left carotid endarterectomy illustrating initial placement and suturing of a patch (a shunt is in place).

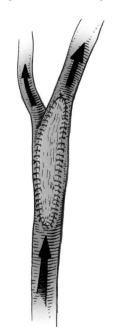

FIGURE 15-21 Left carotid endarterectomy (patch angioplasty) with patch sewn in place.

debris missed will be flushed harmlessly into the external rather than the internal carotid artery.

9. Additional interrupted sutures may be needed to control leakage.

10. A closed drainage system is inserted by way of a separate stab incision.

11. The wound is closed, and dressings are applied.

CAROTID ENDARTERECTOMY WITH SHUNT

Operative Procedure

1-5. The first five steps as described for carotid endarterectomy are followed.

6. To maintain cerebral blood flow the surgeon inserts either a piece of tubing (polyethylene or Silastic) with a suture tied around its center or a commercially prepared shunt device into the common carotid artery and the internal carotid artery. The surgeon then stabilizes the tube or shunt with vessel loops or shunt clamps (Figure 15-22).

7. The surgeon removes the plaque as described for carotid endarterectomy and the arteriotomy is closed with or without a patch.

8. Before the arteriotomy closure is completed, the surgeon releases the shunt clamp or vessel loop on the internal carotid artery and removes the shunt. The external carotid occluding clamp is removed, followed by the common carotid artery clamp, and, last, the internal carotid artery occluding clamp.

9. The wound is closed, and dressings are applied.

ARTERIOVENOUS FISTULA

Arteriovenous fistulas—direct connections between an artery and a vein—are the standard means of vascular access for long-

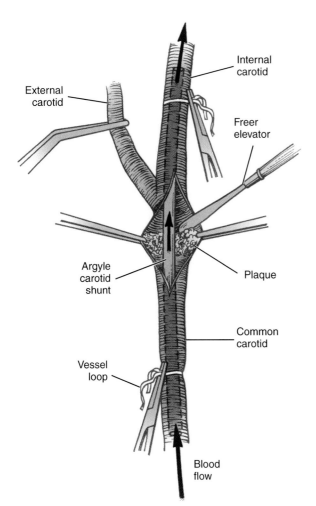

FIGURE 15-22 Left carotid endarterectomy. Argyle carotid shunt in place to allow blood flow to the brain. Stenotic plaque being removed with Freer elevator.

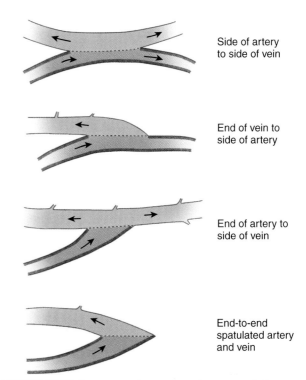

FIGURE 15-23 Four types of anastomoses between radial artery and cephalic vein.

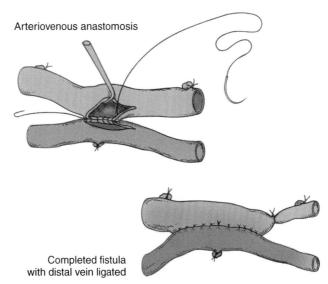

FIGURE 15-24 Arteriovenous anastomosis. The artery is anastomosed to the vein.

term renal dialysis. The dilated vein can then be used for direct cannulation with large-bore needles for hemodialysis. This method is preferable to an external shunt, which carries a high risk of thrombosis and infection. The best access is achieved using the patient's own vessels and creating a subcutaneous connection between the artery and vein, referred to as an arteriovenous shunt, or bridge fistula. Other choices include using a bovine carotid artery, a human umbilical vein graft, or a synthetic vascular graft, usually PTFE. Four anastomoses that can be created between the artery and vein are side of artery to side of vein, end of artery to side of vein, end of vein to side of artery, and end of vein to end of artery (Parker et al, 2008) (Figure 15-23). The Brescia-Cimino fistula is a connection between the radial artery and cephalic vein at the wrist (Figure 15-24). A basic principle of creating a fistula is to start in the distal arm and move proximally with subsequent fistulas. These include ulnar artery to basilic vein and brachial artery to brachial or cephalic vein (Figure 15-25).

Arteriovenous shunts are indicated for long-term renal dialysis access. Patients with end-stage renal disease have their creatinine clearance levels observed. When the creatinine clearance level falls to 10 ml/min, a Cimino fistula may be created in anticipation of the need for dialysis. A Cimino (or Brescia-

Cimino) type of fistula has proved to have the longest patency and lowest infection rate. It is created to connect the patient's artery to a vein that will dilate and become thick-walled (its muscle layer hypertrophies). This occurs from the high rate of blood flow delivered by the connection to the artery. The arterialization, or maturation process, necessary to allow the fistula to withstand the repeated needle punctures of dialysis takes about 3 weeks.

Bridge fistulas do not need to mature and therefore are available for immediate dialysis use. For connections between an artery and a vein that are in proximity, a U-shaped graft is

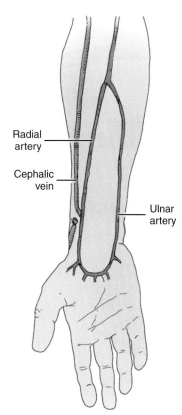

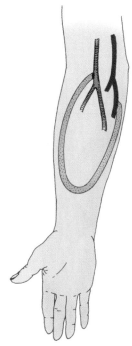

FIGURE 15-26 An example of a loop fistula. A synthetic graft has been used to create a loop brachiocephalic fistula.

FIGURE 15-25 End of the cephalic vein anastomosed to the side of the radial artery at a site superior to the usual location of the radiocephalic fistula. This technique can be useful if the distal radial artery is small or the cephalic vein at the wrist is thrombosed.

placed. Grafts that are far apart require a straight or slightly curved graft. Although the saphenous vein, an umbilical vein graft, and the bovine carotid artery are used, the PTFE grafts work the best and are most commonly used for bridge fistulas. Some surgeons prefer to use a specially designed PTFE step-graft, or tapered graft. These have a short segment of 4 mm in diameter at one end and the majority of the graft with a 7-mm diameter. This graft may avoid an output or flow rate that is so high it causes cardiac overload. Primary sites for bridge fistulas include the upper arm between the brachial artery and axillary vein and the forearm between the brachial artery and antecubital vein or between the brachial artery and basilic vein (Figure 15-26). The axillofemoral graft for dialysis is reserved for those patients who have exhausted other fistula sites. A regular-walled (versus a thin-walled) graft is placed from the axillary artery to the common femoral vein. PTFE grafts can be used immediately, but it may be better to wait 2 weeks for anastomotic healing to occur.

The side-to-side fistula was the original subcutaneous method introduced by Brescia in 1966. The side-to-side fistula is technically the easiest to perform and creates the highest flow rate. The arterial end-to-vein side fistula has a lower flow rate. The arterial side-to-vein end fistula is technically more difficult to create but has a lower incidence of venous hypertension. The end-to-end construction has the lowest rate of venous hypertension but also has the lowest flow rate. There is a trend toward performing fewer side-to-side fistulas and more artery side-to-vein end fistulas.

Since the patency of fistulas is limited, dialysis patients return for revision or embolectomy in attempts to salvage their function. Unfortunately, the success rate for salvage is low and access may be better managed by the creation of another site or a bridge fistula. Risk factors for complications include female gender, African American race, older than 65 years, and presence of diabetes. Treatment for the most common complication, stenosis, is surgery. Stenosis usually results in thrombosis. Stenosis most often involves the venous anastomosis, and a patch angioplasty is usually performed to revise a thrombosed fistula. Other complications include aneurysm and pseudoaneurysm formation, infection, subclavian steal syndrome, and high-output CHF.

VARICOSE VEIN EXCISION AND STRIPPING

Varicose veins are enlarged and distended veins that are visible and palpable beneath the skin. Varicose veins are described as primary or secondary. Primary varicose veins are more prevalent and are not associated with a pathologic condition of the deeper venous system, that is, post-thrombotic syndrome or a history of DVT. Secondary varicose veins are believed to be a result of insufficiency of the deep venous system. Disease may prevent the normal functioning of these valves, resulting in distention; as the vein wall weakens and dilates, venous pressure increases and the valves become incompetent. The veins gradually become dilated. Veins in the lower extremities are most frequently affected, particularly the long saphenous vein. Risk factors include female gender, increased age, pregnancy, geographic location, and race (more prevalent in Caucasians).

Dilation of the saphenous vein produces venous stasis, which may be followed by secondary complications, such as stasis ulcers. Venous obstruction causes an increase in venous pressure, which leads to an increase in capillary pressure. This

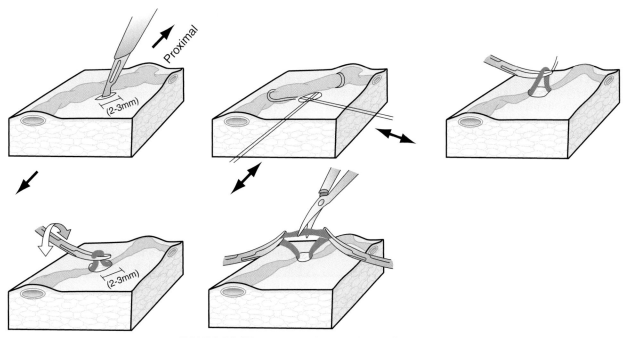

FIGURE 15-27 Technique of stab avulsions of varicosities.

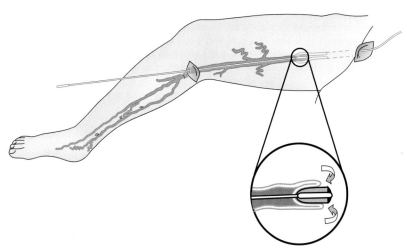

FIGURE 15-28 Inversion stripping of the saphenous vein for superficial venous reflux caused by an incompetent saphenofemoral junction.

causes fluid to leak from the capillaries and produce edema. The objective of surgical intervention is to remove the diseased veins, thus preventing ulceration, secondary edema, pain, and fatigue in the extremity.

Procedural Considerations

Before sedation or entrance into the OR, the patient should stand and the varicose veins should be marked with an indelible marker. This ensures adequate visualization for complete removal of the varicosities, since the patient is often placed in the Trendelenburg's position intraoperatively to decrease venous congestion, which could interfere with visualization of the varicosities. The patient is positioned supine on the OR bed with the legs slightly abducted. Ligation or stripping of the lesser saphenous veins and branches may require placing the patient in the prone position. In the stab avulsion technique, multiple small (2 to 3 mm) incisions are made over the identified varicosities, and the affected vein segments are removed (Figure 15-27). Stripping indicates removal of a long segment of vein by means of a special device (Figure 15-28). Drapes are placed to enable flexing and lifting at the knee. Instruments include a basic minor instrument setup, plus the following: Weitlaner self-retaining retractors, #11 blades, skin hooks, mosquito hemostats, vein strippers with various tips available, and elastic bandages. Endovenous laser ablation (EVLA) is an innovative nonsurgical procedure for varicose veins and offers patients an alternative treatment to surgical vein stripping (Ambulatory Surgical Considerations).

Operative Procedure

1. The surgeon makes an incision in the upper area of the thigh, parallel to the crease in the groin, and clamps and ligates any bleeding vessels.

AMBULATORY SURGERY CONSIDERATIONS

Post-Discharge Follow-Up: Endovenous Laser Ablation for Varicose Veins

Endovenous laser ablation (EVLA) is an innovative nonsurgical procedure for varicose veins that offers an alternative treatment to the often painful surgical ligation (or stripping) of veins, which is performed with the patient administered a general anesthetic and often has a long recovery time. During EVLA, by delivering laser energy through a fiberoptic catheter a particular vein is sealed to prevent blood flow. The catheter is inserted into the vein with ultrasound guidance. The entire procedure can be done in 1 hour as an ambulatory surgery procedure with the patient administered a local anesthetic. Once the procedure is completed, the skin puncture site is approximated with an adhesive strip. A graduated compression stocking or wrap is applied to the affected extremity from the base of the toes to the groin; it is constantly kept in place for 2 weeks and thereafter for 6 weeks when ambulatory to help maintain occlusion of the vein. Immediate and frequent ambulation is encouraged to decrease the incidence of DVT formation.

An important consideration for vascular procedure patients in the ambulatory setting is postoperative and discharge education. Patients need detailed instructions regarding recovery and convalescence since this phase is not complete upon discharge. Those instructions should include possible complications, activity level, wound care, pain management, and the plan for follow-up. Postoperative phone calls, 24 to 48 hours after discharge, have proven beneficial to identify any adverse events and answer patient questions. In a study by Forster and colleagues (2008), an automated system was developed for follow-up. Several patients requested to speak to a nurse directly for worsening postoperative symptoms and for additional clarification of the discharge instructions. Although all patients received detailed education, new questions arose. The post-discharge phone call can stress the importance of wearing the compression stocking or wrap to prevent complications.

Modified from Orenstein BW: Replacing vein stripping, *Radiol Today* 6(12):22-27, 2005; Forster AJ et al: Automated patient assessments after outpatient surgery using an interactive voice response system, *Am J Manag Care* 14(7):429-436, 2008.

GERIATRIC CONSIDERATIONS

The Elderly Patient—Vascular Surgery

The most frequent vascular conditions treated surgically in the older population are abdominal aortic aneurysms, carotid artery disease, and peripheral vascular disease. In patients 65 years and older the mortality from elective aneurysm repair is less than 5% in spite of existing co-morbidities. Emergency repair for ruptured aneurysm carries an operative mortality of more than 50% (Berger et al, 2008). Peripheral vascular surgery for limb salvage can be safely performed in patients older than 80 years and may be indicated for ischemic rest pain and nonhealing ulcers.

The following factors are important considerations in older adults with peripheral vascular disease (Meiner, 2011):

- Subjective—does the patient report:
    Pain in an extremity (what is the location, intensity, duration and onset of the pain?)
    Knowledge of precipitating factors (does the pain occur at activity or at rest?)
    Can the patient describe relieving factors (does rest, changing position, or activity relieve the pain?)
    Presence of intermittent claudication (what is the frequency and how far can the patient walk before the pain occurs?)
    A family history of peripheral vascular disease
    Anxiety or depression
- Objective—observe:
    Skin changes (color, temperature, appearance, or sensation)
    Condition of the nails
    Circulation in the extremities (pulses and capillary filling)
    Muscle tone

The older adult who undergoes vascular surgery procedures is expected to develop improved tissue perfusion and viability. This patient and family members need to be educated about controlling risk factors. They should stop smoking, lose weight, control their blood pressure, and diabetes if these are health issues for them, eat a low fat and low cholesterol diet, and exercise to tolerance on a daily basis. They need to be reminded not to cross their legs while sitting and not to wear constricting garments, like a girdle. Foot care is important, as is proper-fitting footwear. All older adults should be taught to note and report to their healthcare provider changes in the color, temperature, or sensation in the affected area of surgery or any damage to their skin integrity.

Modified from Berger DH et al: Surgery in the elderly. In Townsend CM et al: *Sabiston textbook of surgery*, ed 18, Philadelphia, 2008, Saunders; Meiner SE: *Gerontologic nursing*, ed 4, St Louis, 2011, Elsevier.

2. The saphenous vein is identified and isolated. Margins of the wound are separated with a Weitlaner self-retaining retractor.

3. The surgeon double ligates the saphenous vein branches with black silk ties, or they are transfixed, clamped, and divided. The proximal stump is dissected upward to the point at which it enters the femoral vein, where it is carefully ligated.

4. If the saphenous vein is to be excised, the surgeon makes an incision at its distal portion at the ankle, and the vein is identified, ligated, and divided.

5. A vein stripper is inserted and advanced to the proximal end of the vein in the groin, where it is secured with a heavy suture, and the tip is attached.

6. As the surgeon pulls the stripper up the leg, external compression is applied by the assistant or surgical technologist.

7. Tributaries may be excised through numerous small incisions along the course of the vein.
8. The surgeon closes the groin wound in layers, and other small incisions are closed with skin sutures or staples. Dressings and circular compression bandages are applied.

VASCULAR SURGERY SUMMARY

As with any surgical service, in vascular surgery it is imperative to know the anatomy and physiology of the surgical area. The ability to differentiate between an embolus and an aneurysm will help the surgical technologist be prepared for the procedure. In every vascular procedure, you should comprehend the surgeon's preferences, the importance of prepping, positioning, and draping; and the required equipment and instrumentation. If the use of specialized equipment such as fluoroscopy is anticipated, having the necessary drape open and prepared will keep the procedure moving smoothly.

Understanding that vascular surgery can result in substantial blood loss, surgical technologists should be prepared with sponges, suture, vascular clamps, and specific retractors to gain the necessary exposure. If a graft is required, having the appropriate graft material along with the correct size and the clotting solutions will streamline insertion of the graft and result in better surgical patient care.

The surgical technologist should be prepared with a drain, should it be necessary, and the appropriate dressing for the procedure.

REVIEW QUESTIONS

1. The most common cause of arterial aneurysm is atherosclerotic degeneration of the:
   a. artery walls
   b. venous walls
   c. venous valves
   d. none of these

2. A false aneurysm is also called a(n):
   a. embolus
   b. stroke
   c. chronic arterial insufficiency
   d. pseudoaneurysm

3. Surgical removal of a clot is referred to as a(n):
   a. stroke
   b. embolectomy
   c. pseudoaneurysm
   d. chronic arterial insufficiency

4. A true aneurysm is a dilation of all _____ layers of the arterial wall:
   a. two
   b. four
   c. three
   d. one

5. Abdominal aortic aneurysm occurs primarily between the _____ arteries and the aortic bifurcation.
   a. femoral
   b. renal
   c. iliac
   d. pulmonary

6. The introduction of a contrast medium through a catheter into the arterial or venous system to facilitate visualization is:
   a. angioplasty
   b. emboloectomy
   c. ultrasonography
   d. angiography

7. The fem-pop bypass graft involves the:
   a. femoral artery and the iliac artery
   b. femoral artery and the renal artery
   c. femoral artery and the popliteal artery
   d. popliteal artery and the iliac artery

8. An arteriovenous fistula is a direct connection between a(n):
   a. artery and an artery
   b. vein and an artery
   c. vein and a vein
   d. none of the above

9. A carotid endarterectomy is the removal of _____ at the carotid bifurcation.
   a. fat
   b. air
   c. clot
   d. plaque

10. A unique characteristic of vascular suture materials is that it is often:
    a. composed of polypropylene
    b. double-armed
    c. packaged with swaged-on needles
    d. used with a pledget to keep the suture from tearing when it is tied

11. Define and briefly describe the following procedures:
    Endovascular abdominal aortic aneurysm repair
    Femorofemoral bypass
    Carotid endarterectomy

Critical Thinking Question

Because the need for intraoperative arteriography or fluoroscopy for endovascular procedures is a possibility, what should the surgical technologist consider when preparing for these procedures?

REFERENCES

Alberto P et al: Prevalence of risk factors, coronary and systemic atherosclerosis in abdominal aortic aneurysm: comparison with high cardiovascular risk population, *Vasc Health Risk Manag* 4:877–883, 2008.

Association of periOperative Registered Nurses (AORN): Recommended practices skin antisepsis; preoperative patients. In *Perioperative standards and recommended practices*, Denver, 2009, The Association.

Crum BG: Revised national patient safety goal on medication handling, *AORN J* 83(4):955–957, 2006.

Denholm B: Tucking patient's arms and general positioning, *AORN J* 89(4):755–757, 2009.

Egorova N et al: National outcomes for the treatment of ruptured abdominal aortic aneurysm: comparison of open versus endovascular repairs, *J Vasc Surg* 48:1092–1100, 2008.

Faisal A, Cooper L: Peripheral arterial disease: diagnosis and management, *Mayo Clin Proc* 83(8):944–949, 2008.

Federal Interagency Forum on Aging-Related Statistics: *Older Americans 2004: key indicators of well-being.* Federal Interagency Forum on Aging-Related Statistics, Washington, DC, March 2008, U.S. Government Printing Office.

Gloviczki P, Ricotta JJ: Aneurysmal vascular disease. In Townsend CM et al, editors: *Sabiston textbook of surgery*, ed 18, Philadelphia, 2008, Saunders.

Hanley MA et al: Self-reported treatments used for lower-limb phantom pain: descriptive findings, *Arch Phys Med Rehabil* 87:270–277, 2006.

Hawn MT et al: Timely administration of prophylactic antibiotics for major surgical procedures, *J Am Coll Surg* 203:803–811, 2006.

Ignatavicius DD, Walicek SH: Interventions for clients with vascular problems. In Ignatavicius DD, Workman ML, editors: *Medical-surgical nursing: patient-centered collaborative care*, ed 6, St Louis, 2010, Saunders.

Linsky RA et al: Contemporary management of peripheral arterial disease: a review, *Med Health R I* 91(10):305–308, 2008.

Liu Z et al: Carotid artery stenting versus carotid endarterectomy: systematic review and meta-analysis, *World J Surg* 33:586–596, 2009.

Lloyd-Jones D et al: Heart disease and stroke statistics—2009 update: a report from the American Heart Association Statistic Committee and Stroke Statistics Committee, *Circulation* 119:e21–e181, 2009.

Makary MA et al: Operating room briefings and wrong site surgery, *J Am Coll Surg* 204:236–243, 2007.

Nguyen MC, Garcia LA: Recent advances in atherectomy and devices for treatment of infra-inguinal occlusive disease, *J Cardiovasc Surg* 49:167–177, 2008.

Parker FM et al: Access and ports. In Townsend CM et al, editors: *Sabiston textbook of surgery*, ed 18, Philadelphia, 2008, Saunders.

Pearce WH: The endovascular repair of abdominal aortic aneurysms: what's new in ACS surgery, available at www.medscape.com. Accessed February 5, 2005.

Rosen P, Karmy-Jones RC: Endovascular interventions on the superficial femoral and popliteal arteries, The Cardiothoracic Surgery Network, available at www.ctsnet.org/potals/endovascular/procedures101/article-3.html. Accessed March 20, 2009.

Schermerhorn ML et al: Endovascular vs. open repair of abdominal aortic aneurysms in the Medicare population, *N Engl J Med* 358:464, 2008.

Wu HW et al: Improving patient safety through informed consent for patients with limited health literacy, NQF Project Brief, 2005, available at www.qualityforum.org/projects/completed/informed_consent.asp. Accessed April 14, 2009.

Zeller T et al: New techniques for endovascular treatment of peripheral artery disease with focus on chronic critical limb ischemia, *VASA* 38(1):3–12, 2009.

CHAPTER 16

Cardiac Surgery

After studying this chapter the reader will be able to:
- Correlate cardiac surgical anatomy with correction of select cardiac defects
- Contrast the unique characteristic of the veins and arteries with regard to function and blood flow
- Discuss the properties, purposes, and problems associated with cardiac surgery
- Discuss diagnostic methods for determination of surgical interventions and approaches
- Identify tissue layers involved in opening and closing incisions used in cardiac surgery
- Identify specialized instruments, equipment, and supplies used in open and minimally invasive cardiac surgery
- List the pharmacologic and hemostatic agents used during cardiac surgery
- Apply broad cardiac surgical concepts and knowledge to clinical practice for enhanced surgical patient care

CHAPTER OUTLINE

Overview

Cardiac surgery (History box) reflects individual and collaborative innovation, risk-taking, and problem-solving. Anastomotic techniques to join blood vessels, advances in the development of atraumatic vascular instruments, endovascular approaches in the repair of great vessels, and improvements in myocardial protection strategies represent a few of the many advances that have led to remarkable achieve-

ments in the surgical repair of congenital and acquired cardiovascular diseases (Stoney, 2008). Cardiac surgeries continue to evolve and reflect societal mandates for personal safety, enhanced functional outcomes, institutional efficiency, staff competence, and operational cost-effectiveness (Lytle, 2008). Evidence of these achievements can be seen in the rapid growth of endoscopic and robotic technology, minimally invasive procedures, off-pump techniques, combined (hybrid) surgical and percutaneous interventions, and molecular-level treatments for cardiovascular disease. Many newer procedures require smaller incisions, promote faster healing, and enable patients to achieve their desired functional outcomes more quickly.

These trends have not replaced the need for traditional techniques; rather, they have expanded treatment options for coronary artery disease (CAD), valvular dysfunction, thoracic aneurysms, conduction disturbances, congenital abnormalities (Sommer et al, 2008a, b, c), heart failure, intracardiac masses (Kuchukarian et al, 2007), and end-stage cardiac disease. Therapeutic options may employ laser, radiofrequency, and cryo energies. Stem cell therapy, used to induce cardiac neorevascularization at the cellular level (Menasche, 2009), and mechanical assist devices are effective alternatives to allograft transplant organs, which are in scarce supply. Great strides have been made to reduce mortality from coronary artery disease (Gardner, 2009; American Heart Association, 2009a), but significant challenges associated with the aging population, obesity, diabetes, and other risk factors continue to affect the cardiovascular system and the need for surgical treatment.

Surgical Anatomy

The heart (Figure 16-1) is a four-chamber muscular pump that propels blood into the systemic and pulmonary circulatory systems. It is enclosed in a pericardial sac within the mediastinum, which lies between the lungs, posterior to the sternum, and anterior to the vertebrae, esophagus, and descending portion of the aorta. The diaphragm is positioned below the heart (Figure 16-2). The cardiac wall is composed of three layers: the epicardium, the outer lining; the myocardium, or muscular layer, which is the important functional layer; and the endocardium, the inner lining (Figure 16-3).

HISTORY

History of Cardiac Surgery

Although the notion of the heart as the seat of the soul is an ancient concept, cardiac surgery is one of the youngest clinical specialties, partly because of religious restrictions and partly because of physiologic constraints. Rehn's suture repair of a right ventricular stab wound in 1896 opened the door to the specialty of cardiac surgery. The introduction of positive-pressure endotracheal anesthesia allowed surgeons to access the heart and enter the pleural cavities without causing the lungs to collapse; the introduction of electrical defibrillation and chemical arresting solutions made it possible to stop, and then restart, the heart with predictability. Diagnostic techniques to visualize anatomy and physiology of the heart, record electrical activity, measure blood pressure and flow, and assess ventricular function expanded opportunities to precisely identify the cardiac pathologic condition and to tailor the surgical intervention to the needs of the patient. The ability to isolate the heart and lungs from the circulation without producing irreversible cerebral anoxia was first demonstrated in 1953 when Gibbon repaired an atrial septal defect using extracorporeal circulation with a pump oxygenator that he and his wife had designed. Anastomotic techniques devised by Carrel in the early twentieth century made it possible for numerous advances, including innovations in the repair of aortic aneurysms developed by DeBakey and Cooley in the 1950s, direct myocardial revascularization with the internal mammary artery and saphenous vein introduced by Favaloro and others in the mid-1960s, and cardiac transplantations presented by Barnard and Shumway in the late 1960s. The development of plastics, polyesters, and new metal compounds fostered the creation of prosthetic implants for cardiac valve replacement, first performed in 1960 by Harkin and Starr for the aortic and the mitral valves, respectively. Implantation of a long-term total artificial heart by DeVries in 1988 was possible in no small part because of developments in the chemical industry and laid the foundation for subsequent devices now widely employed to provide mechanical support—or replacement—for one or both failing ventricles.

Adapted from Lytle BW: Who we are—who we will be, *J Thorac Cardiovasc Surg* 135(5):965-975, 2008; Stoney WS: *Pioneers of cardiac surgery*, Nashville, Tenn, 2008, Vanderbilt University Press; Westaby S: *Landmarks in cardiac surgery*, Oxford, England, 1997, Isis Medical Media.

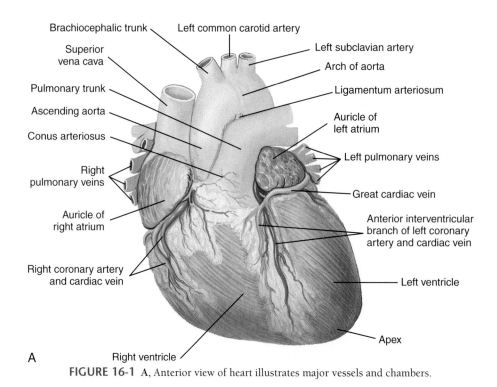

FIGURE 16-1 A, Anterior view of heart illustrates major vessels and chambers.

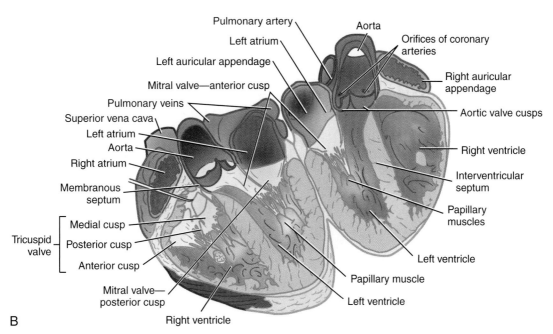

B

FIGURE 16-1, cont'd B, Drawing of a heart split perpendicular to the interventricular septum illustrates the anatomic relationships of the leaflets of the atrioventricular and aortic valve, and the receiving chambers (atria) and the pumping chambers (ventricles). Systemic venous blood returns to the heart by way of the inferior and superior venae cavae. It enters the right atrium, flows through the tricuspid valve into the right ventricle, and is ejected through the pulmonic valve (not shown) into the pulmonary circulation. The blood is oxygenated in the lungs and returns to the left atrium through the pulmonary veins. From the left atrium, it flows through the mitral valve into the left ventricle, where it is ejected through the aortic valve into the aorta and the systemic circulation.

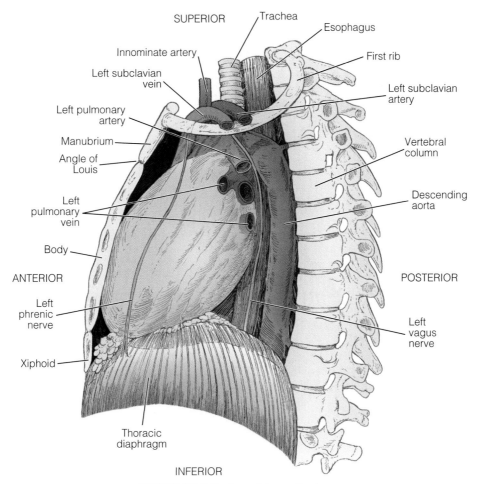

FIGURE 16-2 Regions of the mediastinum.

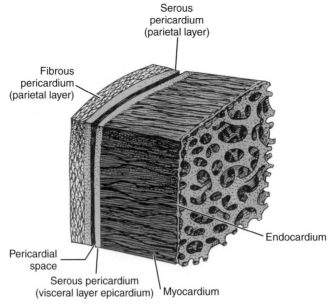

FIGURE 16-3 Cross section of cardiac muscle showing its three layers (endocardium, myocardium, epicardium) and pericardium.

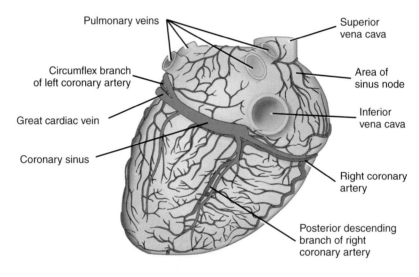

POSTERIOR VIEW

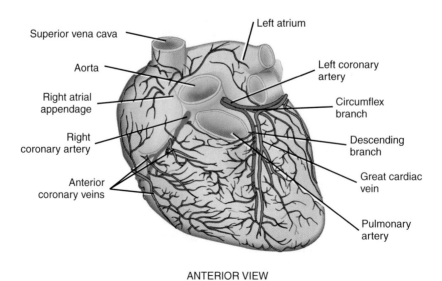

ANTERIOR VIEW

FIGURE 16-4 Anterior and posterior surfaces of the heart, illustrating the location and distribution of the principal coronary arteries and veins.

Two thirds of the heart is located to the left of the midline, and the remaining one third is to the right. Although functionally divided into right and left halves, the heart is rotated to the left, with the right side located anteriorly and the left side situated relatively posteriorly. Each half of the heart contains an upper and a lower communicating chamber: the atrium and the ventricle, respectively. The right atrium (RA) receives desaturated blood from the inferior and superior venae cavae and from the coronary circulation by way of the coronary sinus. The left atrium (LA) receives oxygenated blood from the lungs by way of the pulmonary veins. From the atria, blood flows through the atrioventricular (AV) valves into the ventricles.

The left ventricle (LV) pumps blood into the major vessels of the *systemic circulatory system* by way of the aorta and its main branches to the head, upper extremities, abdominal organs, and lower extremities. The right and left internal (thoracic) mammary arteries, used as grafts during coronary bypass surgery, branch off the subclavian arteries and course behind and parallel to the edges of the sternum. The arteries of the circulatory system subdivide into arterioles and eventually into capillaries, where internal respiration and metabolic exchange occur. From the capillary beds, desaturated blood flows into the venules and veins and finally returns to the RA.

In the *pulmonary circulatory system,* blood is pumped from the right ventricle (RV) through the pulmonary valve into the main pulmonary artery (PA). The PA divides into the right and left pulmonary arteries, which further subdivide into the arterioles and capillaries of the lungs. External respiration occurs in the capillary beds and the alveoli, where carbon dioxide is exchanged for oxygen. Freshly oxygenated blood from the lungs flows through the pulmonary veins into the left atrium.

Coronary circulation (Figure 16-4) supplies oxygen and nutrients to, and removes metabolic waste from, the myocardium; internal respiration occurs in the *myocytes.* The heart receives its blood supply from the left and right coronary arteries, which originate in the sinuses of Valsalva behind the cusps of the aortic valve in the ascending aorta. The left main coronary artery divides into the left anterior descending (LAD) coronary artery and the circumflex coronary artery; along with the right coronary artery (RCA), these arteries represent the three main vessels of the coronary arterial system. In coronary arteries affected by coronary artery disease (CAD), focal or diffuse atherosclerotic plaques develop and progressively enlarge, jeopardizing myocardial blood flow and oxygenation, producing ischemic pain (in many, but not all, cases). Occlusion of an artery by expanding atherosclerotic lesions causes myocardial infarction (MI) and irreversible damage to the region of the myocardium perfused by the obstructed artery. Coronary artery bypass procedures increase blood flow to the affected ischemic areas by attaching a bypass graft conduit to the artery distal to the narrowed portion of the artery. A totally occluded (infarcted) artery does not benefit from bypass surgery because the myocardial injury is irreversible.

The main coronary arteries are situated in the epicardium, which facilitates accessibility during coronary bypass procedures. From these arteries arise the septal perforators and other branches that penetrate the entire myocardium. The cardiac veins empty into the right atrium by way of the coronary sinus; the thebesian veins, prominent in the walls of the right atrium and the right ventricle, open directly into these chambers.

Nerve impulses to the heart travel from the medulla oblongata along the middle cervical nerve, composed of sympathetic fibers, and the vagus nerve, composed of parasympathetic fibers. Sympathetic fibers increase the force and rate of contraction, while parasympathetic fibers control heart rate. Running vertically along the right and left sides of the pericardium are major branches of the phrenic nerve, which innervate the diaphragm and stimulate it to contract. Identifying this nerve is important to protect the diaphragm in procedures in which the lateral pericardium is incised or excised. Within the myocardium itself, certain areas of tissue are modified to form a *conduction system* (Figure 16-5). The process of excitation and contraction originates in the sinoatrial (SA) node, located in the area where the superior vena cava (SVC) meets the right atrium. The impulse spreads to the atria through internodal pathways and travels to the AV junction (which contains the AV node) located medial to the entrance of the coronary sinus in the right atrium, close to the tricuspid valve. From the AV junction, the impulse spreads to the bundle of His, which extends down the right side of the interventricular septum. The bundle of His divides into the right and left bundle branches, which terminate in a network of fibers called the *Purkinje system.* Purkinje fibers are spread throughout the inner surface of both ventricles and the papillary muscles, which when stimulated produce contraction of the heart muscle. The location of conduction tissue is clinically significant during surgical repair of atrial or ventricular septal defects.

During myocardial contraction and relaxation, spiral fibers of the heart contract and relax (Figure 16-6, *A*). To prevent regurgitation of blood, the four cardiac valves (Figure 16-6, *B* and *C*, and Figure 16-7) open and close to maintain unidirectional blood flow. The AV valves are located between the atria and the ventricles. The right AV valve is called the *tricuspid valve* and contains three leaflets. The left AV valve, called the *mitral valve,* consists of two leaflets (see Figure 16-6). Each AV valve is a complex system consisting of a fibrous annulus surrounding the valve orifice, the valve leaflets (or cusps), the chordae tendineae, the atrium, and the papillary muscles, which anchor the valve to the inner ventricular wall (see Figure 16-1). The mitral valve annulus is a dynamic structure with a three-dimensional "saddle" shape, which has stimulated the design of newer prosthetic annuloplasty rings (Fedak et al, 2008). When the ventricle contracts, these muscles and the chordae tendineae, connected to the valve leaflets, prevent the leaflets from everting into the atrium. All parts of the system must function for the valve to work properly. If the shape of the ventricle has been changed by dilatation or hypertrophy, for example, the altered geometry of the ventricle impairs ventricular function. Conditions such as hypertension, myocardial injury, and aortic stenosis promote a pathologic *remodeling* of the heart that can lead not only to valvular dysfunction but also to heart failure and malignant dysrhythmias (Hill and Olson, 2008).

The semilunar valves are at the outlets of the left and right ventricles. These valves are known as the *aortic* and *pulmonic* valves, respectively. They are less complex than the AV valves, and they open and close passively with cyclic fluctuations in the blood pressure and volume that occur during systole and diastole.

Abnormalities such as stenosis, insufficiency, or a combination of both impair the mechanical function of the valves.

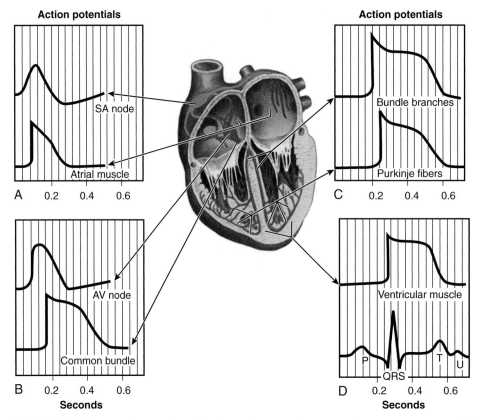

FIGURE 16-5 Heart with normal conduction pathways and transmembrane action potential of sinoatrial (*SA*) node, **A**; atrioventricular (*AV*) node (AV junction), **B**; bundle branches, **C**; and ventricular muscle, **D**.

Stenosed valves have leaflets that are fibrous and stiff, with uneven and adherent margins. Regurgitant, insufficient, or incompetent valves, such as those with leaflet degeneration or perforations, dilated annuli, or ruptured chordae tendineae, produce regurgitation of blood into the originating chamber. These conditions, or a combination of stenosis and insufficiency, strain the myocardium by increasing intracardiac pressure, volume, and workload. The sound of blood flowing through a narrowed or incompetent valve produces an abnormal sound called a *murmur.*

Any of the four valves may be congenitally deformed. Acquired valvular heart disease most commonly affects the mitral and aortic valves and is believed to be exacerbated by increased stress associated with the higher pressures within the left chambers of the heart.

Surgical Technologist Considerations

The history obtained by the surgical team includes information about the patient's health status as well as the response to the disease and the recommended intervention or interventions. Patients with cardiac disease may display symptoms including ischemic chest pain (angina pectoris), fatigue, dyspnea, and syncope. Depending on their severity, these *subjective* symptoms affect the patient's functional status and ability to engage in activities of daily living.

Atypical ischemic chest pain is more likely in women than in men, and angina may be attributed to vasospastic angina, mitral valve prolapse, or psychologic factors. CAD is unusual in premenopausal women, but after cessation of menses the risk is similar to that of men (McSweeney and Lefler, 2008; Mosca et al, 2007). Estrogen hormone replacement therapy is not recommended in postmenopausal women, according to the *Evidence-Based Guidelines for Cardiovascular Disease Prevention in Women: 2007 Update* (Mosca et al, 2007) (Evidence for Practice).

A cardiovascular disease risk factor profile (Box 16-1) is helpful to the surgical team when planning for both hospitalization and discharge. For example, the presence of diabetes is notable because diabetes affects the vascular system and may retard healing and predispose the patient to infection. Of special concern are the epidemic growth of type 2 diabetes in particular and the role of hyperglycemia in general. Although type 2 diabetes was formerly considered an adult-onset disease, children are increasingly vulnerable because of a greater incidence of increased body weight, sedentary lifestyle, and accelerated insulin resistance in this population (Warziski et al, 2008). Altered glucose metabolism (in the absence of diagnosed diabetes mellitus) has shown a significant correlation to atherosclerosis (Lamendola, 2008), and control of hyperglycemia during coronary bypass surgery is an important strategy to reduce the risk of adverse clinical outcomes (Lorenz et al, 2005). This information becomes an integral component of assessment by the surgical team, especially in patients at risk.

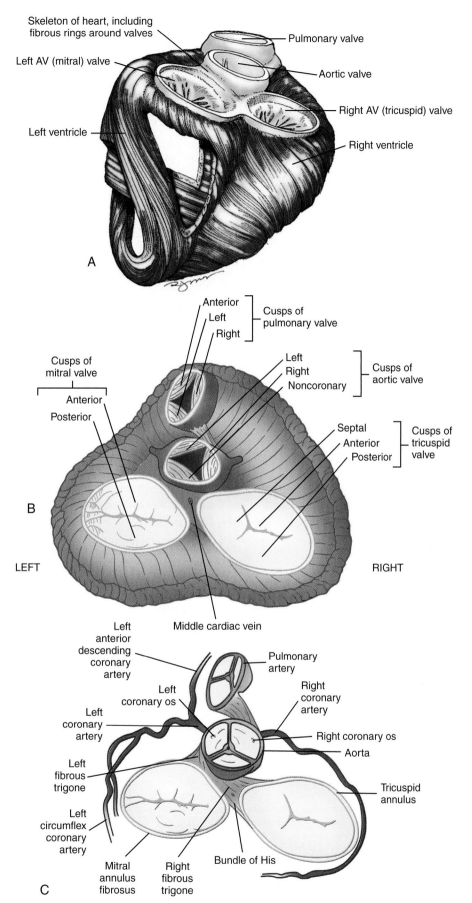

FIGURE 16-6 A, Location of the heart valves in relation to the spiral fibers of the myocardium. *AV,* Atrioventricular. **B,** Superior view of cardiac valves: pulmonary *(top);* aortic *(middle);* mitral *(bottom left);* and tricuspid *(bottom right).* **C,** Superior view of valves in relation to coronary arteries and conduction tissue.

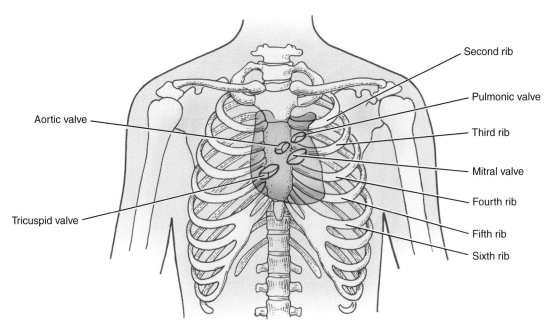

FIGURE 16-7 Anatomic position of cardiac valves. Note relationship of left ventricular apex to fourth and fifth ribs—a frequent site for minimally invasive incisions.

EVIDENCE FOR PRACTICE

Practice Guidelines for Females Undergoing Coronary Artery Bypass Surgery

Numerous inconsistencies surround the issue of gender-based differences between the outcomes of women and men undergoing coronary artery bypass grafts (CABGs). The Society of Thoracic Surgeons (STS) Workforce on Evidence-Based Surgery reviewed published information and proposed the following guidelines that focus specifically on *perioperative* management and are based on available evidence. Additional recommendations, not reviewed here, are incorporated in the guidelines.

1. Use of the internal mammary artery (IMA)
   a. IMA underused in women
   b. Use of IMA associated with significant reduction in mortality (compared with CABG using venous conduits alone)
   c. At least one IMA used to bypass stenotic coronary artery
2. Management of hyperglycemia
   a. Diabetes more common in women than in men undergoing CABG
   b. Adverse effects of diabetes more pronounced in women
   c. Hyperglycemia produced incremental risk in CABG
   d. Maintain blood glucose levels below 180 mg/dl
3. Intraoperative management of anemia
   a. Hematocrits below 22% associated with operative mortality
   b. Strategies to increase red blood cell concentration: hemoconcentration, ultrafiltration, minimizing pump prime volume, rapid autologous priming
   c. Maintain adequate hematocrit level at or greater than 22%

4. Use of off-pump CABG
   a. Improved outcomes after off-pump CABG versus on-pump CABG may be related to increased use of IMA with off-pump CAB
   b. No major differences in outcomes associated with *valve* surgeries
   c. Absent of firm evidence that off-pump CABG is superior, the guidelines suggest that the indications for off-pump CABG are the same for women as for men
5. Optimization of thyroxine treatment for women with hypothyroidism
   a. Hypothyroidism associated with impaired contractility and increased risk of myocardial infarction
   b. Greater incidence of women with hypothyroidism (compared with men) undergoing CABG
   c. Maintain in a euthyroid state during surgery
6. Consideration of preoperative hormone replacement therapy (HRT)
   a. HRT not a significant predictor of mortality in multivariate analyses
   b. HRT associated with complications such as thromboembolism
   c. HRT not used for postmenopausal women undergoing CABG

Modified from Edwards FH et al: Gender-specific practice guidelines for coronary artery bypass surgery: perioperative management, *Ann Thorac Surg* 79:2189-2194, 2005; Puskas JD et al: Off-pump techniques benefit men and women and narrow the disparity in mortality after coronary bypass grafting, *Ann Thorac Surg* 84:1447-1456, 2007; Toumpoulis IK et al: Assessment of independent predictors for long-term mortality between women and men after coronary artery bypass grafting: are women different from men? *J Thorac Cardiovasc Surg* 131:343-351, 2006, available at http://jtcs.ctsnetjournals.org/cgi/content/full/jtcs;131/2/343. Accessed July 4, 2009.

Inflammation has been increasingly implicated in the development of coronary artery disease; in particular, elevated homocysteine levels (which increase platelet aggregation) and high C-reactive protein (CRP) levels (CRP is a biologic marker for inflammation and is associated with increased risk for CAD) have been implicated (Ruz and Lennie, 2008; Seymour et al, 2009). Targeting low-density lipoprotein ("bad" cholesterol) levels of less than 100 mg/dl is often recommended (Grundy, 2008); some authors also stress the importance of increasing the levels of high-density lipoproteins ("good" cholesterol) (Superko and King, 2008).

Additional recognized risk factors include metabolic syndrome (central obesity, hypertension, insulin resistance, and dyslipidemia) and obesity (Lamendola, 2008). Hypertension and obesity increase the workload of the heart; obesity may also increase the risk for postoperative infection because adipose tissue is poorly vascularized. Patients who are obese and those who are underweight (compared with patients in the high-normal and overweight categories) have a higher risk of death after coronary artery bypass surgery (Jin et al, 2005).

BOX 16-1

Risk Factors for Coronary Artery Disease

NONMODIFIABLE

- Age
- Male gender (but postmenopausal women have risk similar to that of men)
- Heredity, genetic makeup, family history
- Race
- Menstrual status (estrogen levels may be modifiable; postmenopausal women have risk similar to that of men)

MODIFIABLE

- Elevated levels of serum cholesterol and other lipids
- Hypertension
- Cigarette smoking
- Obesity, metabolic syndrome
- Diabetes mellitus
- Psychologic stress
- Personality type
- Physical inactivity

NEWER, NOVEL CONTRIBUTING FACTORS

- Elevated homocysteine levels (increase platelet aggregation)
- Inflammation (the atherosclerotic process is inflammatory)
- High C-reactive protein level (CRP is a marker for inflammation associated with atherogenesis)
- Periodontal disease (a marker for inflammation and possible infection)
- Atrial and ventricular natriuretic peptides (hormones secreted by the atria and ventricles in response to volume expansion and fluid retention; predictive of a variety of cardiac problems)

Modified from Libby P et al, editors: *Braunwald's heart disease*, ed 8, Philadelphia, 2008, Saunders; Moser DK, Riegel B, editors: *Cardiac nursing: a companion to Braunwald's heart disease*, St Louis, 2008, Saunders; Hlatky MA et al: Criteria for evaluation of novel markers of cardiovascular risk: a scientific statement from the American Heart Association, *Circulation* 119:2408-2416, 2009; Seymour GJ et al: Infection or inflammation: the link between periodontal and cardiovascular diseases, *Future Cardiol* 5(1):5-9, 2009, available at www.medscape.com/viewarticle/587591. Accessed April 3, 2009; American Heart Association, 2009; Daniels LB, Maisel AS: Natriuretic peptides, *J Am Coll Cardiol* 50 (25), 2007, available at www.medscape.com/viewarticle/567064. Accessed January 17, 2008.

Among the newer biomarkers denoting cardiovascular diseases are the *natriuretic peptides*—cardiac hormones synthesized and secreted by the atrium (atrial natriuretic peptide [ANP]) and the ventricle (B-type natriuretic peptide [BNP]). Discovered in 1981, the natriuretic peptides have a regulatory effect that causes myocardial relaxation in response to acute increases in ventricular volume. Measurement of circulating peptides is increasingly used to identify heart failure and sudden cardiac death (Korngold et al, 2009; Hlatky et al, 2009). Another biomarker under intensive study as a risk factor is lipoprotein(a) (Lp[a]), which has been identified from genetic studies as a causal link to myocardial infarction. According to the researchers (Kamstrupp et al, 2009), Lp(a) levels need to be tested only once in a lifetime as the levels do not change over time. Optimal therapy has not been established, but niacin has been shown to reduce the level of Lp(a) in some individuals.

The risk for complications and major adverse cardiac events (MACE) after cardiac surgery has also shown some gender differences (Puskas et al, 2007; Edwards et al, 2005). Investigations of risk factors in men and women for sternal wound infection showed that three significant risk factors were identified and occurred at significantly different rates in men and women: smoking, use of a single internal mammary artery (IMA), and age more than 70 years. Smoking and the use of a single IMA for bypass grafting were more common risk factors in men compared with women; women tended to be older than men at the time of surgery (Hussey et al, 2001). Fewer MACE were seen in women undergoing coronary bypass surgery without the use of cardiopulmonary bypass (CPB) compared to surgery with CPB (Puskas et al, 2007); however, malignant ventricular dysrhythmias (e.g., ventricular tachycardia), a calcified aorta, or preoperative renal failure were poor prognostic signs in women (Gray and Sethna, 2008). These findings can be incorporated into patient/family teaching plans with recommendations for lifestyle changes as indicated.

Other risk factors associated with postoperative infection include previous cardiac surgery, extensive length of surgery, use of cardiopulmonary bypass (CPB) and/or blood transfusion, amount of postoperative blood loss, and length of preoperative hospitalization. Female gender, obesity, and arterial occlusive disease of the legs are related to impaired wound healing at the saphenous venectomy site after coronary bypass surgery; bilateral IMA grafts in patients with diabetes, obesity, and postoperative inotropic support have also been implicated (Newby and Douglas, 2008; Pradhan et al, 2008).

A history of rheumatic fever or frequent tonsillitis as a child is significant because the sequelae of rheumatic fever and streptococcal infections can lead to damage of the cardiac valves. Although the incidence of rheumatic fever has declined significantly in wealthy countries, rheumatic heart disease is a significant problem in less industrialized countries (Carapetis, 2007). Given the increasing number of immigrants to the United States, it is expected that treatment for rheumatic heart disease will continue to grow.

Diagnostic Studies. Most patients referred for surgery have had clinical evaluations including both invasive and noninvasive studies (Box 16-2). After the history and physical assessment, a resting electrocardiogram (ECG) is ordered. An exercise ECG (stress test) is often performed because ST-segment changes indicating myocardial ischemia may be apparent only

Diagnostic Tests Commonly Performed for Cardiovascular Disorders

NONINVASIVE*
- Resting ECG
- Exercise ECG (stress test)
- Chest radiography
- Echocardiogram (TTE, TEE)
- Carotid Doppler echocardiogram
- Resting MUGA
- Exercise thallium
- Exercise MUGA
- CT scan
- PET scan with stress
- CMRI, MRA

INVASIVE
- Aortography
- Arteriography
- Digital subtraction angiography
- Electrophysiology
- Cardiac catheterization
- Ventriculography
- Endomyocardial biopsy

*When dye is injected into the vascular system, the test is considered semiinvasive.
CT, Computerized tomography; *CMRI*, cardiovascular magnetic resonance imaging; *ECG*, electrocardiogram; *MRA*, magnetic resonance angiogram; *MUGA*, multiple uptake gated acquisition; *PET*, positron emission tomography; *TEE*, transesophageal echocardiogram; *TTE*, transthoracic echocardiogram.
Modified from Libby P et al, editors: *Braunwald's heart disease*, ed 8, Philadelphia, 2008, Saunders; Pagana KD, Pagana TJ: *Mosby's diagnostic and laboratory test reference*, ed 9, St Louis, 2009, Mosby.

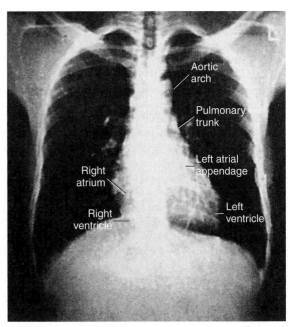

FIGURE 16-8 Anteroposterior chest radiograph (normal).

during or after exercise. In patients with intractable dysrhythmias, electrophysiology (EP) studies may be performed to locate the site of irritable atrial or ventricular foci that can be surgically ablated, excised, or controlled with pharmacologic therapy. EP studies are also performed to determine the need for internal defibrillators or antitachycardia devices. Bradycardia may be an indication for pacemaker insertion.

Chest radiography provides information about the size of the cardiac chambers, thoracic aorta, and pulmonary vasculature as well as the presence of calcium in valves, pericardium, coronary arteries, and aorta (Figure 16-8). Lateral chest radiographs of patients with prior sternal operations show the chest wires and extent of pericardial adhesions. Magnetic resonance imaging (MRI) is used to assess myocardial viability and can also be employed to image vascular structures with MRI angiograms that provide great clarity (Figure 16-9, *A*). In patients with suspected aortic or other vascular abnormalities, a computerized tomography (CT) scan of the chest with intravenous injection of a contrast medium is used to create x-ray serial "slices" of the body area under study (Figure 16-9, *B*), and CT angiography is especially useful for imaging the aorta and great vessels. CT scans may be contraindicated in very unstable patients because the patient's position in the tubelike scanner makes patient access difficult. Less frequently performed is arteriography with radiographic contrast material (dye) to determine the size and location of the lesion and the site of the intimal tear in aortic dissections (Figure 16-10); digital sub-

traction angiography (DSA) provides clear images and requires less contrast material (Libby et al, 2008).

Echocardiography is a noninvasive test that evaluates both the structure and the function of the heart by transmitting sound waves to the heart and measuring those sound waves reflected back to the transducer (Figure 16-11). The sound waves are processed by the transducer, which creates visual images of the structure's movements. This test is commonly used to assess ventricular and valvular function before, during, and after surgery and to determine the degree of valvular stenosis or regurgitation. It can also demonstrate a tumor, thrombus, or air in the ventricular or atrial cavities. Two-dimensional and color-flow Doppler techniques have greatly enhanced the functional assessment of valvular performance and carotid artery stenoses. Echocardiography is the gold standard for diagnosing mitral stenosis, and it is widely used to assess other valvular disorders and congenital heart disease. Transesophageal echocardiography (TEE) is also employed to evaluate the effectiveness of valve repairs and other surgical procedures.

Radionuclide imaging is employed to illustrate wall motion and blood flow through the heart and to quantify cardiac function. These noninvasive techniques are generally well tolerated by patients, especially when patients may be too unstable to withstand a cardiac catheterization. These techniques may also be used as a complement to catheterization.

Cardiac catheterization provides definitive information about the extent and location of ischemic heart disease and is an adjunct to echocardiography for diagnosing valvular heart disease (Todd and Phippen, 2009). A radiopaque plastic catheter is inserted retrograde through the aortic valve into the left side of the heart by a percutaneous puncture or a cutdown to the vessels of the brachial artery (Sones technique) or the femoral artery (Judkins technique). The right side of the heart is approached percutaneously by the superior or inferior vena caval route. To perform coronary angiography that demonstrates intracoronary anatomy, a contrast medium is injected into the coronary

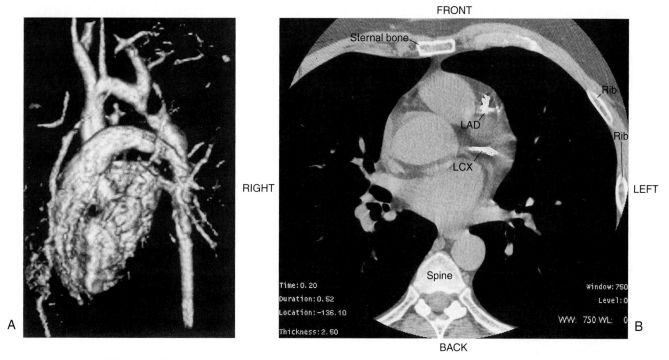

FIGURE 16-9 **A,** Three-dimensional reconstruction of a contrast medium–enhanced magnetic resonance angiogram of the thoracic aorta, illustrating a severe coarctation (narrowing) of the aorta. **B,** High-resolution cross-sectional computed tomography (CT) scan of the heart, illustrating calcification within the left anterior descending (*LAD*) coronary artery and left circumflex (*LCX*) coronary artery.

ostia. Obstructions (Figure 16-12), flow, and distal perfusion can be assessed. Ventriculography illustrates contractile weaknesses of the ventricles as well as shunting and regurgitation of blood. These studies are used to assess the degree of myocardial dysfunction and to plan interventions such as coronary artery bypass grafting, valve repair or replacement, repair of congenital anomalies, and cardiac transplantation. The cardiologist can compute the orifice of a stenosed valve or determine the degree of regurgitation of an incompetent valve.

Ventricular, atrial, and pulmonary pressures are recorded, and cardiac output and ejection fraction are estimated (Box 16-3). Oxygen saturation of cardiac chambers and the ratio of pulmonary to systemic blood flow (Q_p/Q_s) are calculated for patients with shunts and congenital or acquired defects. Cinearteriograms record the movement of the heart, and cut films or digitized versions of the cines may be displayed during surgery.

The cardiac catheterization laboratory also performs percutaneous coronary interventional (PCI) therapies for evolving and acute myocardial infarctions (Leeson et al, 2008). Coronary thrombolysis with fibrinolytic drugs can dissolve fresh blood clots and reopen, or recanalize, the artery; antiplatelet agents such as aspirin, dipyridamole, and clopidogrel are often prescribed to block platelet aggregation that can lead to restenosis. Percutaneous transluminal coronary angioplasty (PTCA) followed by insertion of intracoronary (bare metal or drug-eluting) stents is often performed to dilate and maintain the patency of the recanalized artery. Laser angioplasty and atherectomy to excise intraluminal plaque may also be employed (Todd and Phippen, 2009). In many instances these interventions may obviate the need for surgical bypass graft-

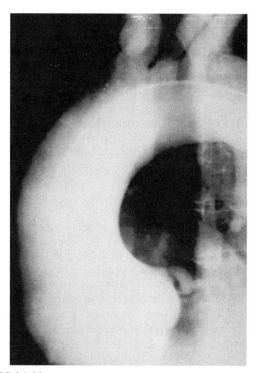

FIGURE 16-10 Aortogram of ascending aortic dissection, with aortic valve insufficiency. Note regurgitation of dye into left ventricle.

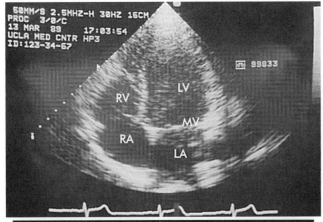

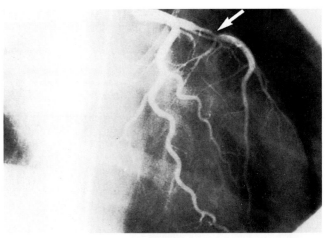

FIGURE 16-12 Right anterior oblique (RAO) view of left coronary artery injection demonstrating high-grade stenosis of the left anterior descending coronary artery (*arrow*) at the lead of the first septal perforator.

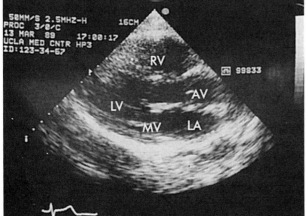

FIGURE 16-11 Two-dimensional echocardiography showing two views of the cardiac chambers. *LA,* Left atrium; *LV,* left ventricle; *MV,* mitral valve; *RA,* right atrium; *RV,* right ventricle.

BOX 16-3

Hemodynamic Concepts

Cardiac output	Amount of blood (in liters) ejected by left ventricle per minute; product of heart rate times stroke volume.
Cardiac index	Cardiac output corrected for differences in body size.
Preload	Volume and pressure of blood in the ventricle at the end of diastole. Central venous pressure (CVP) measures right-sided heart preload; pulmonary artery wedge pressure (PAWP) indirectly measures left-sided heart preload.
Afterload	Impedance, or resistance, the heart must overcome to pump blood into the systemic circulation; left ventricular wall tension during systole; systemic vascular resistance.
Contractility	Inotropic state of the heart; ability of the ventricle to pump.
Ejection fraction	Percentage of end-diastolic volume ejected into systemic circulation; indicator of ventricular function.

ing, although the progressive nature of CAD may eventually lead to patients requiring surgical revascularization. OR availability may be recommended for unstable patients undergoing stent insertion and atherectomy, but the need for on-site cardiac surgical availability has been questioned. One study demonstrated that patients undergoing PCI at facilities without surgical backup had rates of morbidity, emergency cardiac surgery, and mortality related to emergency surgery that were similar to those in facilities with surgical backup (Kutcher et al, 2009).

EP studies are performed to diagnose conduction disturbances and to provide therapeutic interventions, such as radiofrequency or cryologic ablation of foci producing atrial fibrillation or accessory pathways seen in Wolff-Parkinson-White syndrome. Insertion of a pacemaker for bradydysrhythmias or an internal cardioverter defibrillator for ventricular tachydysrhythmias is commonly performed in EP laboratories. However, insertion of these devices may require an OR when percutaneous access is unfeasible or when concomitant cardiac surgery is being performed.

Safety Considerations. The safety of the patient is a primary responsibility of the entire perioperative team. Equipment should be functioning properly and undergo routine testing by the biomedical engineering department. Supplies should be used according to manufacturers' instructions, and instru-

ments should be regularly scrutinized to ensure that there are no burrs that could injure tissue, that the jaws of vascular and other clamps align properly, and that small items are accounted for at the end of surgery. Toxic material, such as the glutaraldehyde storage solution of bioprosthetic valves, should be thoroughly rinsed before implantation. Monitoring the aseptic practices of team members as well as visitors is an important safety consideration.

Staff safety is also important. Protective personal equipment should be consistently and properly worn. Gloves should be used by the OR staff whenever there is contact with a patient. The effects of electrical, chemical, and other potentially hazardous materials within the OR can be minimized by reinforcing safe practices to decrease the risks of injury.

Special Facilities. The OR must be large enough to accommodate bulky, highly specialized equipment while maintaining aseptic technique. Multiple electrical outlets, auxiliary lighting, and additional suction outlets should be available. Ceiling-mounted, mobile booms for housing electrosurgical units (ESUs), headlight sources, suction, medical gases, electrical outlets, and other items can reduce floor clutter and enhance the safety of the environment for patients and staff.

A growing number of hybrid suites have been designed that combine the traditional surgical controlled environment and the fluoroscopic imaging capabilities of interventional cardiologic laboratories. A typical hybrid procedure may consist of a surgical coronary anastomosis under direct vision or with a robot that is combined with percutaneously inserted coronary artery stents under fluoroscopy (Jansens et al, 2009).

Instrumentation and Equipment. A basic back table for CABG will include a basin set with large pitchers, an open heart instrument set, a mammary retractor, a self-retaining sternal retractor, and the camera, light cord, and scope for the endovein harvest. A sternal saw and internal defibrillator paddles are also required. The surgical technologist will also have the cardiovascular fine set that will include tenotomy scissors, Gerald forceps, suture tags, and coronary epicardial retractors for the finer parts of the procedure. Most vascular surgeons have a set of doctor specials that include the forward and backward Potts scissors, their favorite forceps for taking down the mammary, titanium bulldogs, fine rummells, or vascular clamp.

Vascular clamps, which are designed to occlude blood flow partially or completely, must be maintained in good condition if they are to prevent fracture of the delicate tunica intima of the blood vessels and still retain their specific holding qualities. There are many variations in construction of vascular instruments. The jaws may consist of single or double rows of fine, sharp, or blunt teeth or special crosshatching or longitudinal serrations. The working angles of the clamps also vary. All clamps are designed to hold the vessels securely and without trauma (Figure 16-13).

Minimally invasive procedures require special instrumentation to access the heart by way of smaller incisions in the anterior and/or lateral aspects of the chest wall (Figure 16-14). Retractors, dissecting instruments, suturing devices, coronary artery stabilizers, and vascular clamps are available.

Sternal and rib retractors are available to meet specific needs. IMA retractors expose the retrosternal artery bed by elevating the sternal border (Figure 16-15). Some sternal retractors have attachments that provide improved exposure of the left atrium during mitral valve replacement (MVR) (Figure 16-16). Exposure of the left or right atrium or the aortic root may also be accomplished with handheld retractors. Special rib spreaders provide exposure for mini-thoracotomy procedures. Coronary artery stabilizer systems with left ventricular apical suction retractors (Figure 16-17) are widely employed for beating heart coronary bypass surgery.

Other equipment commonly used (or available) for cardiac surgery may include the following:
- Sternal saw and motor
- Irrigation fluid cooling/warming machine
- Autotransfusion/cell saver system
- Electrical fibrillator

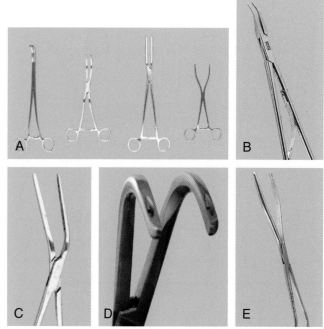

FIGURE 16-13 **A,** *Left to right,* 1 Semb ligature-carrying forceps, 9 inch; 1 Lambert-Kay aorta clamp; 1 Fogarty clamp-applying forceps, angled; 1 bulldog clamp applier. **B,** Close-up of Weck hemoclip applier. **C,** Fogarty clamp-applying forceps, angled. **D,** Semb ligature-carrying forceps, close-up of tip. **E,** Bulldog clamp applier. (From Tighe SM: *Instrumentation for the operating room,* ed 6, St Louis, 2003, Mosby.)

- Direct current (DC) defibrillator with internal paddles (Figure 16-18) and adhesive external pads
- Thermia unit (mattress or forced-air warming)
- External and internal pulse pacemaker generator (single and dual chamber)
- Pump oxygenator/CPB machine
- Epicardial pacemaker leads (temporary and permanent)
- Fiberoptic headlight and light source
- Intra-aortic balloon pump (IABP)
- Mechanical ventricular assist devices (VADs)
- Cryoablation energy ablation source (for atrial fibrillation surgery)
- Radiofrequency energy ablation source (for atrial fibrillation surgery)
- Ultrasonic cutting/coagulation device (harmonic scalpel)
- TEE probe and monitor
- Minimally invasive, video-assisted vein-harvesting system
- Thoracoscopic equipment
- Video equipment

Lasers (for transmyocardial laser revascularization) and robots (for valve repair; retraction during port-access, video-assisted procedures) increasingly are also part of the equipment found in a cardiac OR.

The Mayo stand for a CABG includes a needle box; heavy silk ties; knife handles for a 20, 10, 11, 15; and Beaver blades. Forceps include DeBakey, Gerald, and fine coronary anastomosis forceps. Scissors include Metzenbaum and Mayos of varying lengths, the forward and backward Potts, and the tenotomy scissors. Mosquitos, hemostats, tonsil clamps, large and small

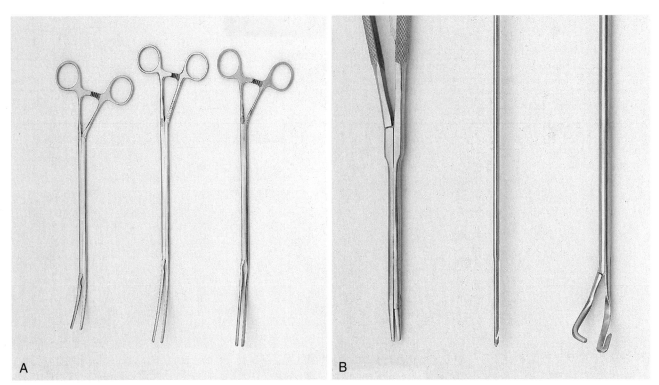

A

B

FIGURE 16-14 A, Transthoracic DeBakey vascular clamps are designed to pass through the chest wall by way of smaller incisions for minimally invasive procedures. **B,** Close-up views of minimally invasive needle holder, trocar/suture puller, and knot slider.

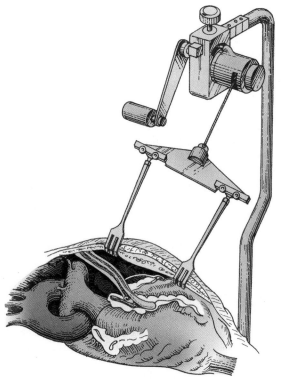

FIGURE 16-15 Retractor used to elevate sternal border for exposure of the internal mammary artery.

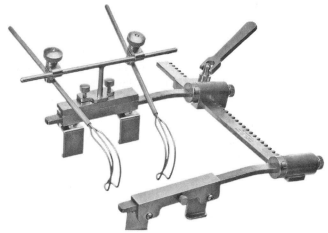

FIGURE 16-16 Sternal self-retaining retractor with attachments for left atrial retraction during mitral valve replacement.

tubing clamps, and hemoclip appliers all have their place on the Mayo stand. An experienced surgical technologist will have the cross clamp and partial occluding clamps' inserts loaded and ready to go before the patient comes in the room.

If the procedure includes a valve repair or replacement, additional instruments will be needed. Valve sets include a suture ring, extra hemostats, long serrated scissors, ronguers, and handheld valve retractors. If the procedure is minimally invasive, or endothoracic, a minimally invasive set of instruments that includes scissors, forceps, and graspers, will be needed in addition to the standard open instrument sets available in the operating room.

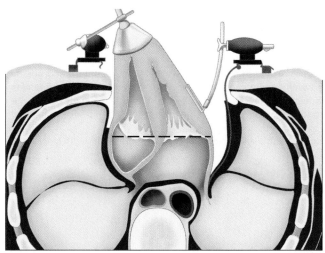

FIGURE 16-17 Cross section of chest showing (*top left*) left ventricular apical suction cup to expose lateral and posterior coronary arteries for bypass grafting during off-pump surgery. The platform stabilizer (*top right*) isolates and immobilizes the section of the coronary artery to be anastomosed.

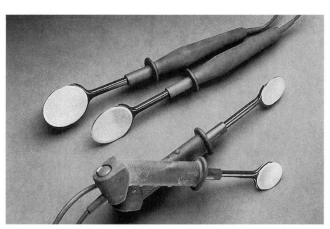

FIGURE 16-18 Internal defibrillator paddles are available in an array of sizes and designs: the paddles may be activated through the handles or by pressing the button on the defibrillator. Smaller internal paddles are used for infants and children.

Suture Materials. A variety of nonabsorbable cardiovascular sutures with atraumatic needles are available from most suture manufacturers. Synthetic sutures of Teflon, Dacron, polyester, or polypropylene are usually selected for insertion of prostheses and for vascular anastomoses. Most sutures are double armed with a needle on each end. Because of the number of stitches required for prosthetic valve repair and replacement, alternately colored suture and slotted, numbered suture holders may be helpful to avoid confusion. Polytetrafluoroethylene (PTFE) sutures can be used for replacement of mitral valve chordae. Vessel loops and umbilical tapes are commonly used to identify and to retract blood vessels and other structures. Wire (monofilament or twisted cable) commonly is used to approximate the sternum (Figure 16-19), with plastic, metal, or nylon bands occasionally added to reinforce fragile bone. Skin staplers may be used to close skin incisions; a staple remover must accompany the patient to the postanesthesia area if staples have been used to close the chest.

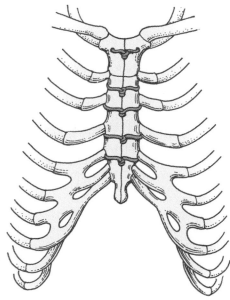

FIGURE 16-19 Technique for wire closure of the sternum. A variety of closing mechanisms have become available. These may consist of monofilament wire (shown), twisted wire cables, or (in some instances) plates and screws. In selected patients in whom disruption may be anticipated, such as elderly, obese, or malnourished patients, two or more heavy bands of nylon may be passed around the sternum and secured by a twisted stainless-steel wire in addition to the wire sutures. A figure-of-eight technique may also be employed.

Supplies

The following supplies are generally used in most cardiac procedures. Depending on the surgeon's preference, other items may be added or substituted.

- Rubber shods (placed on the tips of hemostats to protect suture clamped by the hemostat)
- Pill sponges (gauze dissectors)
- Various-sized Silastic or polyvinyl chloride tubing
- Tourniquet catheters
- Disposable drapes
- Foot-control and hand-control ESU pencils, ultrasonic scalpel
- Adapters, connectors, stopcocks
- Extra syringes and needles for injections, infusions, and blood samples
- Sterile marking pen to identify anastomotic sites and mark grafts
- Irrigation cannulae
- Disposable vascular (bulldog) clamps
- Coronary occluders and stabilizers
- Autotransfusion supplies
- Chest tubes, chest drainage system
- Topical hemostatic agents
- Femoral arterial blood pressure supplies (hypodermic needle, guidewire, stopcocks, pressure tubing)
- Intra-aortic balloon pump (IABP) insertion supplies (hypodermic needle, guidewire, vascular dilators, stopcocks, pressure tubing, IABP catheter)
- CPB and myocardial protection cannulae, tubing, connectors, stopcocks

SURGICAL TECHNOLOGY PREFERENCE CARD

Coronary artery bypass graft (CABG) is known as "open heart surgery." In cardiac surgery, it is imperative that the surgical technologist be thoroughly familiar with the routine of the surgeon and the entire perioperative team.

Cannulation of the heart for cardiopulmonary bypass (CPB) can be performed in a variety of ways. Although suture and needle size are the surgeon's preference, cardiac surgeons that employ CPB will usually cannulate the aorta (blood in) and venae cavae (blood out), protect the heart by cooling it, use antegrade or retrograde cardioplegia to arrest the heart, and place a left ventricular (LV) sump for decompression of the heart. After cannulation, the surgeon institutes CPB with the assistance of the perfusionist, and then the cross clamp is applied.

Room Prep: Basic OR furniture, warmer for irrigation, video assist system for endoscopic vein harvest, surgeon's headlight and loops, cell saver suction, and CO_2 blower

Prep Solution: In room and warmed according to manufacturer's instructions
- Chlorhexidine gluconate (CHG) is commonly used
- Make sure the prep is completely dry before draping the patient.

Catheter
- Insertion is routine for cardiac procedures
- Accommodate appropriately for any allergy to latex

PROCEDURE CHECKLIST

Instruments
- Standard—basin set, defibrillator paddles, sternal saw
- Endovein harvest—scope, camera, light cord, bipolar cord
- Open heart tray, CV fine set, sternal retractor, and mammary retractor

Suture
- Heavy silk ties—ranging in size from 2 silk to 0 silk
- Cannulation suture—of the surgeon's preference
- Vein graft suture—of the surgeon's preference
- Valve suture
- Sternal closing sutures including steel wires

Additional Supplies: both sterile and nonsterile
- Graft cart, Endovascular cart, and CV suture and supplies cart
- Physician's special requests—including suture, clamps, staplers, or new devices
- Disposable bulldogs and Fogarty inserts, vessel tips, and cannulae
- Suture boots, pledgets, and assorted hypodermic needles and syringes

Medications and Irrigation Solutions
- Warm antibiotic irrigation
- Heparin and papaverine
- Normosol irrigation, starting with room temp, moving to warm when patient comes off pump

Other Hemostatic Agents
- Surgicel, Fibrillar, HemoStase, bone wax
- Clip appliers—have a variety of sizes and long in length
- Platelet gel—derived from the patient's own blood and mixed with thrombin
- Electrosurgical unit (ESU) supplies and harmonic scalpel

Drains and Dressings
- Chest tubes—correct size and type for procedure and surgeon preference
- Jackson-Pratt to a closed reservoir for fluid collection on smaller procedures
- Autologous blood retrieval system

Specimen Care
- Label correctly, using the "Repeat and Verify" when receiving and passing the specimen off the field
- Implement all other specimen safety measures
- Valves should be sent for cultures to pathology

Before opening for the procedure, the surgical technologist should:
- Check procedure against the surgeon's preference card
- Arrange OR furniture—including perfusion, anesthesia, and the endo harvesting system
- Gather appropriate carts needed in the room for the procedure
- Gather and arrange needed equipment—verifying function of equipment
- Take time to make sure the prosthetic valve is in the room

Prosthetic Material. In addition to these general supplies, special supplies are needed for repair or replacement of cardiovascular structures. Intracardiac patches, heart valves, and synthetic grafts should be handled with care to prevent damage or the introduction of foreign materials. Teflon, a fluorocarbon fiber, and Dacron, a polyester fiber, are available in a variety of meshes, fabrics, felts, tapes, and sutures and are also combined with other materials in prosthetic heart valves (Figure 16-20).

Teflon patches are made in a variety of forms for intracardiac and outflow tract use. Varying degrees of firmness, thickness, and porosity are available for specific uses. Low reactivity, strength retention, and tissue acceptance are important properties to be considered in the selection of such patches.

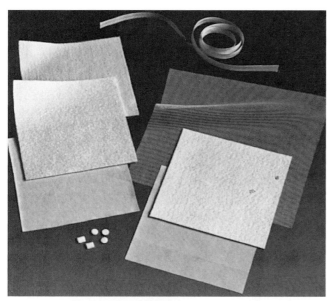

FIGURE 16-20 Assorted prosthetic materials to repair intracardiac and extracardiac defects: tapes, Teflon and Dacron patches, and pledgets.

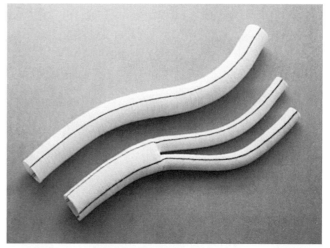

FIGURE 16-21 Straight and bifurcated arterial tube grafts.

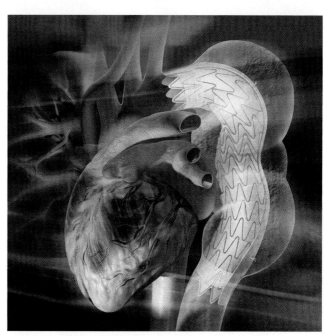

FIGURE 16-22 Thoracic aortic endovascular stented prosthesis made from expanded polytetrafluoroethylene (PTFE). The compressed device is inserted percutaneously through the femoral artery by way of a delivery catheter and guided to the desired position in the thoracic aorta under fluoroscopy. When the correct position has been confirmed, the device expands automatically after it is deployed from the delivery catheter. The delivery catheter is then withdrawn, and hemostasis of the femoral incision site achieved.

Dacron arterial tube grafts are commonly used in cardiac surgery, although reinforced expanded PTFE grafts are also available. There are two types of Dacron grafts: knitted and woven. Woven prosthetic grafts are usually employed when the patient has been fully heparinized because the interstices of woven grafts are tighter than those in knitted grafts and bleeding is usually reduced. Compared to woven grafts, the advantages of knitted grafts are that they do not fray as readily, they are easier to handle, and they reendothelialize more quickly. Grafts are available in a variety of sizes and may be straight or bifurcated (Figure 16-21). Knitted and woven grafts impregnated with collagen to reduce interstitial bleeding are useful in the thoracic aorta and do not have to be preclotted, even when the patient is fully heparinized for cardiopulmonary bypass. Graft sizers are available for determining the correct size.

Specially designed tube grafts for the aortic arch incorporate prosthetic branches for the head vessels (brachiocephalic, left common carotid, and subclavian arteries); and tube grafts for replacement of the aortic root and ascending aorta are available with preformed sinuses of Valsalva incorporated into the prosthesis (Cameron et al, 2009).

Endovascular, expandable stented tube grafts are available for both the abdominal aorta and the descending portion of the thoracic aorta (Figure 16-22). The endovascular graft is inserted percutaneously into the femoral artery and advanced to the desired position in the abdominal or descending thoracic aorta, where the prosthesis is opened, implanted, and secured (Tinkham, 2009; Thompson and Bertling, 2009).

Valve Prostheses. Valve prostheses are selected according to their hemodynamics, thromboresistance, durability, ease of insertion, anatomic suitability, and patient acceptability; cost, patient outcome, and value are also important considerations (Rahimtoola, 2003, 2004). Most mechanical prostheses employ a tilting disk design. The ball-and-cage prosthesis was the first implanted mechanical valve (Starr and Edwards, 1961) but currently is implanted infrequently. Prosthetic valves allow complete closure with slight regurgitation to prevent stasis of blood (Figures 16-23 to 16-26).

Bioprostheses are derived from porcine, bovine, or equine tissue (Figures 16-27 to 16-29). Porcine valves consist of an aortic valve from a pig that can be sutured to a Dacron-covered stent (Figure 16-27, *A*), or the porcine aortic valve may be "stentless" (without a sewing ring) to enhance the hemodynamics, especially in patients with a small aortic root (i.e., orifice less than 21 mm) (see Figure 16-27, *B*) (Pepper et al, 2009). The bovine (calf) (see Figure 16-28) pericardial bio-

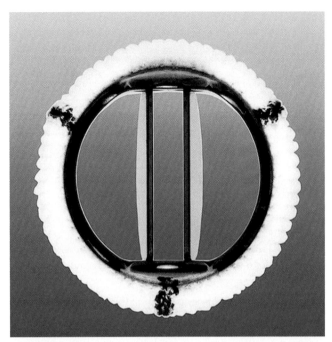

FIGURE 16-23 St. Jude Medical bileaflet tilting disk valve prosthesis.

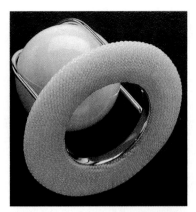

FIGURE 16-25 Starr-Edwards ball-and-cage aortic valve prosthesis.

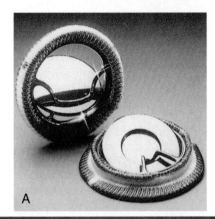

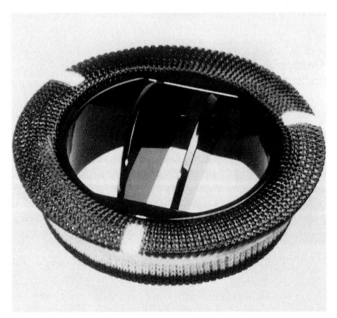

FIGURE 16-24 CarboMedics supraannular aortic prosthesis designed for the small aortic root.

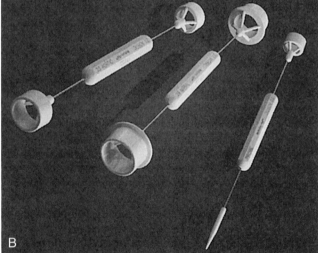

FIGURE 16-26 A, Medtronic-Hall tilting disk valve prosthesis. **B,** Double-ended sizing obturators for the Medtronic-Hall prosthesis *(left and center)* and probe *(right)* to test leaflet movement. All valve prostheses have sizing obturators specific to the prosthesis itself.

prosthesis is created by cutting leaflet-shaped pieces from the pericardium and sewing them onto a Dacron ring; the equine (horse) pericardial prosthesis is created by cutting pieces of the pericardium, shaping the pieces into a tube, and attaching the prosthesis to a ring of Dacron material. The advantage of these biologic valves is that administration of long-term anticoagulants is not necessary in most patients. Obturators for sizing prosthetic valves as well as valve holders are specific to the prostheses (see Figure 16-26, *B*). Tables 16-1 and 16-2 compare mechanical and biologic prosthetic heart valves. Tissue-

engineered heart valves may offer a future potential cure for valvular heart disease (Hjortnaes et al, 2009).

Aortic valve allografts (homografts) have little or no risk of thromboembolism, optimal hemodynamic function, no need for anticoagulation drugs, and no risk of sudden catastrophic failure. Moreover, they demonstrate a lower incidence of infective endocarditis than that found in mechanical or bio-

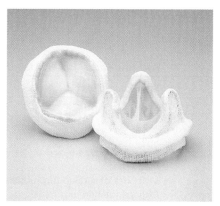

FIGURE 16-28 Carpentier-Edwards bovine pericardial aortic bioprosthesis.

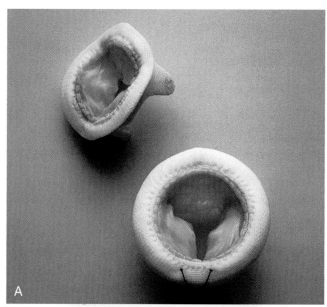

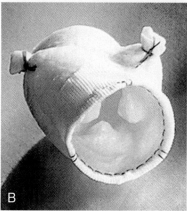

FIGURE 16-27 A, Medtronic Mosaic porcine aortic (*top*) and mitral (*bottom*) bioprostheses. **B,** Stentless porcine aortic valve. The absence of a stent and sewing ring provides a greater orifice area through which blood can flow.

logic valves and their long-term durability is comparable with that of bioprostheses. Allograft root replacement is also a valuable technique in the setting of prosthetic valve endocarditis. The entire ascending aorta and valve (see Figure 16-29) or the valve alone (Figure 16-30) may be inserted. Allografts are cryopreserved and must be thawed in saline according to the vendor's protocol before implantation. Because stentless aortic valves (see Figure 16-27, *B*) are more easily available than allografts, they are increasingly preferred for aortic root replacement.

Conduits consisting of mechanical or biologic aortic valves attached to a tube graft (Figure 16-31) are used in procedures such as repair of aortic dissections requiring replacement of the aortic valve and ascending aorta. If vein grafts must be inserted into the conduit or if a direct coronary ostial anastomosis is required, an eye electrocoagulator is used to make the opening into the graft and at the same time heat-seal the cut edges of the prosthesis. Conduits with *biologic* valves interposed between tube graft materials may be used when patients are at increased risk for bleeding complications associated with the need for

chronic anticoagulation therapy. Allograft conduits may be used for these procedures as well.

Although allografts and stentless bioprostheses avoid the complications associated with prosthetic mechanical valve replacement, valve repair rather than replacement is preferred, particularly with mitral and tricuspid valves. Fedak and colleagues (2008) listed more than 30 mitral valve rings and bands commercially available in 2007; the authors also described additional newer prostheses in development for both surgical and interventional percutaneous reparative procedures. When repairing the native valve with an annuloplasty ring, obturators specific to various kinds of annuloplasty rings are used to size the annulus (Figure 16-32, *A* and *B*).

Safety considerations include storing prosthetic materials in a clean, protected environment and using them according to manufacturers' instructions. Before implantation, biologic valves must be rinsed in three saline baths to remove the glutaraldehyde (or other) storage solution (Mirzaie et al, 2007). The prescribed amount of physiologic fluid in each rinsing bath and the recommended rinsing time for each bath vary among bioprosthetic manufacturers. Surgical technologists should adhere to the specific instructions for each prosthesis (Risk Reduction Strategies). It should be noted that some bioprostheses do not require rinsing because they are stored in a physiologically neutral solution (i.e., not glutaraldehyde). However, before and during insertion, all bioprostheses should be kept moist with saline. Mechanical valves should be protected from scratching and other injury.

Preinduction Care. The patient is transferred to the OR suite, where a focused preoperative assessment is performed and the chart is reviewed for completion and documentation of informed consent, advance directives, laboratory results, diagnostic data, and other pertinent information. The identity of the patient and the intended operation, including identification and confirmation of the site and side, and the required position as applicable, is verified. Verification of which leg (i.e., right or left) will be used for vein harvest in bypass patients may not be necessary if this decision depends on the operator's preference rather than a specific clinical indication. However, some institutions may require site marking of bypass harvesting sites, and the nurse should follow institutional policy for guidance.

Preoperatively, cardiac surgical patients may exhibit more stress and anxiety than other types of patients. The periop-

TABLE 16-1

Mechanical Valve Prostheses*

	Ball-and-Cage (Rarely Used)	Tilting Disk	
	Starr-Edwards	Medtronic-Hall, Omniscience	St. Jude Medical, CarboMedics
Model/description	6120 Mitral 1260 Aortic	Spherical (single) tilting disk	Bileaflet tilting disk
Advantages	Long-term durability Good hemodynamics Inaudible Least risk of sudden thrombosis	Long-term durability Good hemodynamics in all sizes Low profile	Long-term durability Good hemodynamics in all sizes Low profile Low TE rate for mechanical valve
Disadvantages	Anticoagulation required	Anticoagulation required	Anticoagulation strongly recommended
	Higher incidence of TE than disk valves Large profile Suboptimal hemodynamics in small aortic sizes (less than 23 mm) High profile not optimal in small LV or aortic root Higher risk of TE in mitral position	Potential for sudden thrombosis Noisy Higher risk of TE in mitral position If Coumadin must be discontinued, there is increased risk of catastrophic thrombosis	Potential for sudden thrombosis Some noise Higher risk of TE in mitral position If Coumadin must be discontinued, there is increased risk of catastrophic thrombosis
Special considerations	Sizers and handles specific to prosthesis; must be sterilized Poppet of aortic valve removable to facilitate tying sutures; replaced before aorta closed; mitral poppet not removable Aortic model has three struts; mitral has four	Sizers and handles specific to prosthesis; must be sterilized	Sizers and handles specific to prosthesis; must be sterilized Frequently used in children needing prosthetic valve
Resterilization	Not recommended	Not recommended	Not recommended

*All prostheses should be stored in a cool, dry, contamination-free area.
LV, Left ventricle; *TE,* thromboembolism.
Adapted from Ascione R et al: Mechanical heart valves in septuagenarians, *J Cardiac Surg* 23:8-16, 2007.

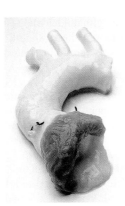

FIGURE 16-29 Aortic allograft with aortic valve and arch vessels attached.

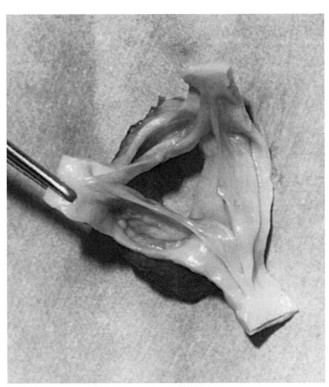

FIGURE 16-30 Aortic valve allograft.

TABLE 16-2

Biologic Valve Prostheses

	Heterograft (Xenograft)		Allograft (Homograft)
	Stentless Porcine Bioprostheses	**Stented Porcine Heterograft; Bovine and Equine Pericardial Valve Prostheses**	**Allograft (Homograft)**
Model/description	For use in aortic position Stentless (aortic): no sewing ring; includes porcine aortic root with coronary ostial branches	Pericardial valve used in aortic position Porcine heterograft used in aortic, mitral, and tricuspid positions Porcine heterograft (from excised pig aortic valves; leaflets attached to sewing ring) Aortic bovine and equine pericardium (cut and shaped into trileaflet valve)	Aortic valve allograft (cadaver, organ donor, excised cardiomyopathic heart from transplant recipient; mitral valve allograft also available)
Advantages	Incidence of TE very low; anticoagulation rare after AVR Stentless has excellent flow, especially in small aortic annulus (≤21 mm) No hemolysis Good hemodynamics Use may avoid need for aortic root enlargement Central flow Gradual failure allows elective reoperation Little residual gradient Durability good after age 60 yr Stentless graft has many advantages of allograft valves	Incidence of TE very low; anticoagulation rare after AVR No hemolysis Good hemodynamics in all sizes Central flow Gradual failure allows elective reoperation Residual gradient minimal	Incidence of TE very low; anticoagulation rare; used for AVR and MVR No hemolysis Excellent hemodynamics (especially with stentless technique) Central flow Gradual failure allows elective reoperation No residual gradient
Disadvantages	Durability may be less than 15 yr Accelerated fibrocalcific degeneration in children, patients with hypertension, or patients needing chronic renal dialysis Cross-clamp time and CPB longer than those for insertion of stented valve because of greater complexity of subcoronary insertion	Durability not yet established In small aortic root of large body, may produce prosthesis-patient mismatch Accelerated calcification may be a problem in children, renal patients, or those with hypertension	Limited availability Insertion technique more complex than stented valve Possible immunologic reaction (newer decellularization process strips cells from graft and reduces immune response)
Special considerations	Sizers and handles specific to prosthesis; must be sterilized before insertion; must be rinsed in saline to remove storage solution before insertion; follow manufacturer's instructions for rinsing; frequent irrigation recommended to prevent drying Diets low in calcium recommended for children, renal patients	Sizers and handles specific to prosthesis; must be sterilized before insertion; must be rinsed in saline to remove storage solution before insertion; follow manufacturer's instructions for rinsing; frequent irrigation recommended to prevent drying Diets low in calcium recommended for children, renal patients	No specific sizers; may use sizers for heterografts; cryopreserved allograft must be thawed per protocol; used for aortic or mitral valve replacement; stent can be attached if indicated for use in other positions
Resterilization	Not recommended	Not recommended	Not recommended

AVR, Aortic valve replacement; *CPB*, cardiopulmonary bypass; *MVR*, mitral valve replacement; *TE*, thromboembolism.

Modified from Oakley RE et al: Choice of prosthetic heart valve in today's practice, *Circulation* 117:253-256, 2008; Kumar AS: *Techniques in valvular heart surgery*, New Delhi, India, 2008, CBS Publishers and Distributors; Pepper J et al: Stentless versus stented bioprosthetic aortic valves. A Consensus Statement of the International Society of Minimally Invasive Cardiothoracic Surgery (ISMICS) 2008, *Innovations* 4(2):49-60, 2009; Cheng D: Stentless versus stented bioprosthetic aortic valves: a systematic review and meta-analysis of controlled trials, *Innovations* 4(2):61-73, 2009.

▶▶ RISK REDUCTION STRATEGIES

Varying Rinsing Procedures for Biologic Heart Valves

Glutaraldehyde storage solution is used for many bioprostheses, and rinsing procedures for its removal vary among bioprosthetic heart valve manufacturers. Both the amount of rinsing solution in each rinsing basin and the time for each rinse (total of three rinsing baths) should be followed according to each manufacturer's instructions. Some manufacturers (see ATS Medical) recommend a *fourth* basin for storing the bioprosthesis until implantation. The following sampling of rinsing processes reflects the differences among manufacturers' recommended rinsing procedures. The person rinsing the valve should collaborate with the circulating nurse when following the instructions for that particular valve.

PERICARDIAL (EQUINE) AORTIC VALVE (ATS MEDICAL 3F)

Prepare *four* rinse basins with a minimum of *500 ml of saline* solution in each basin. Gently agitate the valve for *30 seconds in each of the first three basins* for a total of *1.5 minutes (90 seconds)*. Allow the bioprosthesis to remain in the *fourth basin* until required by the surgeon.

ATS Medical 3f rinse procedure, ATS 3f Aortic Bioprosthesis (Model 1000), Implant Procedure, ATS Medical, Minneapolis, Minn, available at www.atsmedical.com/uploadedFiles/Public_Site/Physicians_International/Biological_Valves/st_broc_3f.pdf. Accessed July 9, 2009.

PERICARDIAL (BOVINE) VALVE (CARBOMEDICS)

Prepare three rinse basins with a minimum of *300 ml of saline* solution in each basin. Gently agitate the valve for *2 minutes in each basin for a total of 6 minutes*. Allow the bioprosthesis to remain in the third basin until required by the surgeon.

CarboMedics rinse procedure, available at www.carbomedics.com/professional_faq.asp?faq=HPBio#27. Accessed July 3, 2009.

PERICARDIAL (BOVINE) VALVE (EDWARDS LIFE SCIENCES PERIMOUNT MAGNA 3000TFX)

Prepare two rinse basins with a minimum of *500 ml of saline solution in each basin*. Gently agitate the valve (keeping it submerged) *for a minimum of 1 minute in each basin for a total of at least 2 minutes*. Allow the bioprosthesis to remain in the third basin until required by the surgeon.

From Edwards Life Sciences: *Instructions for use*, available at http://www.edwards.com/products/heartvalves/mmimplantprep.htm?MagnaMitral=1. Accessed November 25, 2009.

PORCINE VALVE (MEDTRONIC MOSAIC 305)

Prepare three rinse basins with a minimum of *500 ml of saline solution in each basin*. Gently agitate the valve (keeping it submerged) *for 2 minutes in each basin for a total of 6 minutes*. Allow the bioprosthesis to remain in the third basin until required by the surgeon.

Medtronic rinse procedure, available at www.medtronic.ch/cardsurgery/products/pdf/200102908b%20EN.pdf. Accessed July 3, 2009.

PORCINE STENTLESS VALVE (MEDTRONIC STENTLESS FREESTYLE 995)

Prepare three rinse basins with a minimum of *500 ml of saline solution in each basin*. Gently agitate the valve (keeping it submerged) *for 2 minutes in each basin for a total of 6 minutes*. Allow the bioprosthesis to remain in the third basin until required by the surgeon.

From Medtronic: *Instructions for use*. Package insert. Medtronic, Inc., Minneapolis, MN, 2007.

PERICARDIAL VALVE (SORIN *FREEDOM SOLO*)

This is a newer valve detoxified by, but not stored in, glutaraldehyde (other bioprostheses are stored in glutaraldehyde); *eliminates the need for rinsing* (although the prosthesis should be kept moist with saline to prevent drying of the tissue).

Mirzaie M et al: A new storage solution for porcine aortic valves, *Ann Thorac Cardiovasc Surg* 13:102-109, 2007, available at www.atcs.jp/pdf/2007_13_2/102.pdf. Accessed July 3, 2009; see also the review at www.ces.clemson.edu/bio/documents/Publications/Simionescu%20-%20Expert%20Opinion%202004.pdf.

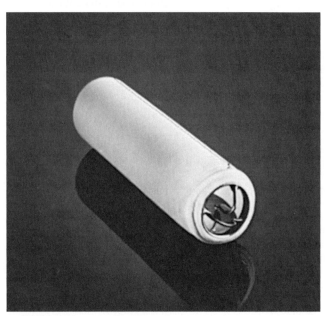

FIGURE 16-31 Valved conduit with Medtronic-Hall tilting disk valve prosthesis.

erative team should anticipate and prepare for this reaction because anxiety increases myocardial oxygen consumption. Efforts to reduce the family's anxiety level are also important and result in less emotional stress being transmitted to the patient.

A peripheral arterial pressure line and venous infusion lines are inserted. A local anesthetic may be used at the insertion sites, and a sedative may be injected intravenously. Occasionally, a patient's response to sedation results in impaired respiration as evidenced by shallow respirations, decreased oxygen saturation, and a respiratory rate of 8 breaths (or less) per minute (Mancini and Bubien, 2008).

Admission to the OR. Depending on the patient's response to sedative medications received preoperatively, the patient may require assistance onto the OR bed. Warm blankets should be provided for comfort and to reduce shivering; the nurse should ensure that the blanket temperature does not produce thermal injury (Bujdoso, 2009).

After application of the ECG leads and the pulse oximeter finger cot, the hands, elbows, and feet can be padded. The perioperative team confirms that the peripheral arterial pressure line is functioning properly and may reposition the arm as necessary in collaboration with the anesthesia provider. Pulse

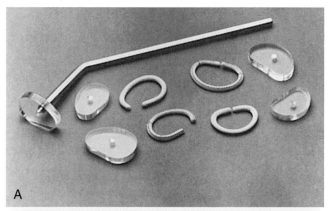

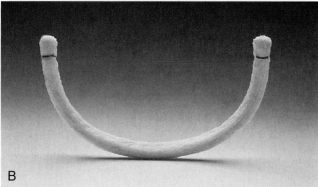

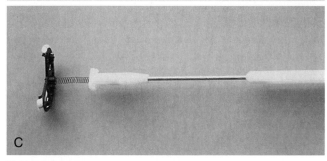

FIGURE 16-32 **A,** Carpentier-Edwards "classic" tricuspid and mitral annuloplasty rings, sizers, and sizer handle. The tricuspid rings are notched in the area corresponding to conduction tissue in the tricuspid annulus to avoid suture injury. **B,** Cosgrove annuloplasty ring. **C,** Ring attached to ring holder and handle.

oximetry function is confirmed. Additional monitoring devices are listed in Table 16-3. A "time out" is performed to comply with The Joint Commission's *Universal Protocol.*

Anesthesia Induction. The choice of anesthetic agent or agents depends on the cardiovascular effects of the anesthetic, the patient's hemodynamic status and general health, and the anticipated length of stay in the surgical intensive care unit (SICU). Newer, fast-acting anesthetic agents are used to "fast-track" patients postoperatively, whereby the patient is extubated in the OR, or very shortly after admission to the SICU, to speed the recuperation process (Camp et al, 2009).

Because the period of induction is one of the most critical during the procedure, close monitoring of the patient is required, especially for patients with ventricular ischemia from congenital or acquired disease (Moss and Moss, 2009). Anesthetic management focuses on maintaining an adequate car-

diac output by keeping myocardial oxygen demand low and the oxygen supply high (DiNardo and Zvara, 2008).

Medication Safety. In addition to anesthetic medications, multiple other drugs are employed to cause vasodilation or vasoconstriction, enhance heart rate and contractility, promote anticoagulation, result in diuresis, and provide antibiotic prophylaxis (Surgical Pharmacology). Antibiotic prophylaxis for infection prevention in the cardiac patient is an important consideration and the perioperative team should confirm that the antibiotic has been infused before the surgical incision is made (Simmonds et al, 2008). According to Engelman and colleagues (2007), *Staphylococcus aureus* is the most frequently cultured organism in cardiac surgical site infection (SSI). The recommended primary prophylactic antibiotic for adult cardiac surgery is a first-generation cephalosporin (usually cefazolin); vancomycin (one preoperative dose and an additional dose) may be a reasonable adjunct to cephalosporin. In patients allergic to penicillin, vancomycin may be considered the primary prophylactic antibiotic with additional gram-negative coverage.

Additional safety precautions include labeling all medications on the field (including irrigating fluids and H_2O). Of particular importance are heparinized solutions, papaverine (to reduce spasm in IMA and radial artery conduits), and saphenous vein infusions. Containers and syringes are labeled and the circulating nurse and the scrub person visually and verbally confirm drug name, dose, route, strength, and outdate of every medication passed onto the field.

Monitoring. Extensive monitoring of hemodynamic and other variables is indicated during cardiac surgery (see Table 16-3). After intubation (or before, depending on the anesthesia provider's preference), additional pressure lines may be inserted to measure central venous pressure (CVP) and pulmonary artery pressures (PAPs). Maximal sterile barriers should be used for insertion of central lines (Clancy, 2009; Hu et al, 2004) (Evidence for Practice). Peripheral and central arterial and venous pressures are usually monitored directly by means of a transducer and oscilloscope.

An indwelling urinary catheter is inserted for measuring urine output and monitoring renal function, especially during and after CPB. The urinary catheter may contain a thermistor temperature probe. Other temperature probes may be placed, usually in the esophagus, nasopharynx, or rectum, or on the forehead. Temperatures can also be recorded from the pulmonary artery catheters and the arterial infusion line of the bypass circuit. Ventricular septal temperatures can be recorded by insertion of a needle probe while the patient's heart is arrested. Monitoring of cerebral oxygenation and the level of anesthesia awareness is frequently employed.

The skin is carefully inspected before ECG and ESU dispersive pads are placed. Bony prominences, such as the coccyx and the back of the head, are padded to prevent pressure necrosis resulting from hypoperfusion and hypothermia during bypass. Because elderly patients are especially vulnerable to skin breakdown, additional precautions to avoid pressure injuries are recommended (Walton-Geer, 2009). Monitoring aseptic practice is an important infection control strategy.

Positioning. The supine position provides optimal exposure for the institution of CPB and the surgical repair of the heart

TABLE 16-3

Perioperative Patient Monitoring

Monitoring Device	Location	Measures
Electrocardiogram (ECG)	Lateral, posterior electrode placement	Electrical activity of heart
Arterial line	Peripheral radial artery	Arterial blood pressure (direct)
	Central femoral artery	
	Aorta (with needle attached to pressure tubing, or with sensor in bypass circuit)	
Blood pressure (BP) cuff	Upper arm	Arterial BP (indirect)
Central venous pressure (CVP)	Right atrium (RA)	RA pressure (e.g., CVP)
Pulmonary artery (PA) catheter (Swan-Ganz)	RA (proximal port)	RA pressure (e.g., CVP)
	Right ventricle (RV) (midline port)	RV pressure
	Distal PA (distal port)	PA and pulmonary artery wedge pressure (PAWP)
		Indirect measure of left atrial and left ventricular (LV) pressure
		Cardiac output
Left atrial (LA) line	Left atrium	LA, LV pressure
Pulse oximeter	Finger, earlobe	Oxygen saturation of arterial hemoglobin
Urinary drainage catheter	Urinary bladder	Urine output, renal perfusion/function, temperature
Temperature probes	Esophagus	Temperature (core and peripheral)
	Nasopharyngeal	
	Urinary bladder	
	Rectum	
	Ventricular septum	
	Bypass circuit	
	Tympanic	
	Face/forehead (adhesive patch)	
Neurologic monitoring		
Electroencephalogram (EEG)	Head	Electrical activity of brain; awareness
Transcranial Doppler		Detects cerebral arterial emboli
Bispectral index (BIS)		Detects anesthesia awareness
Cerebral oximetry		Measures cerebral tissue oxygen saturation with sensors placed bilaterally on patient's forehead
Transesophageal echocardiogram (TEE)	Esophagus	Cardiac function, presence of air, integrity of valve repair

Adapted from DiNardo JA, Zvara DA: *Anesthesia for cardiac surgery,* ed 3, Malden, Mass, 2008, Blackwell Publishing; Savino JS, Cheung AT: Cardiac anesthesia. In Cohn LH, editor: *Cardiac surgery in the adult,* ed 3, New York, 2007, McGraw-Hill; Moss CJ, Moss R: Assist the anesthesia provider. In Phippen ML et al, editors: *Competency for safe patient care during operative and invasive procedures,* Denver, 2009, Competency and Credentialing Institute.

and great vessels. In addition, respiratory impairment and discomfort are reduced with this approach (Bishop, 2009). When the supine position is used, the hands and arms are tucked along either side of the body. The legs may be slightly "froglegged" to provide access to the femoral arteries for insertion of pressure lines and IABP lines or to excise the saphenous vein. Measures to avoid pressure injury (especially in the elderly, debilitated, or obese patient) include padding the coccyx and applying heel protectors. Measures to protect the occipital area from pressure ulcers include placing pillows under the head and repositioning the head during surgery. Significant factors associated with the development of pressure ulcers include preexisting diabetes mellitus; lower preoperative hemoglobin, hematocrit, and serum albumin levels (Walton-Geer, 2009); and the presence of intra-aortic balloon pumps.

A semilateral position may be employed for thoracoabdominal aneurysms in order to expose both the descending thoracic aorta and the abdominal aorta. A thoracotomy position may be used for some minimally invasive procedures including surgery on the descending thoracic aorta. For minimally invasive surgery, the right or left side of the chest may be elevated with a roll or other positioning device to provide adequate exposure for one or more small thoracotomy incisions. The presence of severe mediastinal adhesions may also necessitate this approach in some repeat valve operations. Thoracotomy positioning aids should be available to position arms and legs per the surgeon's protocol.

Prepping and Draping. For procedures requiring excision of the saphenous vein, the prep extends from the jaw to the toes and includes the anterior (or lateral) area of the chest, abdomen, groin, and legs. The legs and feet are prepped circumferentially and the chest and abdomen from bedline to bedline.

In procedures not requiring saphenous vein excision, the prep extends to a level below the knees to give the surgeon access to the femoral artery or saphenous vein in the thigh area. (Some surgeons prefer to have both legs prepped circumferentially for all cardiac procedures.) Femoral artery access may be required for arterial pressure monitoring or insertion of an intra-aortic balloon. Saphenous vein exposure facilitates access if a bypass conduit is required. In the lateral position, the

SURGICAL PHARMACOLOGY

Medications Used in Adults During Cardiac Surgery

Medication	Purpose/Description/Delivery
ANALGESICS AND ANESTHETICS	
Thiopental	Induction, ultra–short-acting barbiturate, intravenous bolus
Fentanyl (Sublimaze)	Synthetic narcotic, intravenous bolus and/or infusion
Sufentanil (Sufenta)	Synthetic narcotic, intravenous bolus and/or infusion
Alfentanil (Alfenta)	Synthetic narcotic, intravenous bolus and/or infusion
Remifentanil (Ultiva)	Synthetic narcotic, intravenous bolus and/or infusion
Morphine sulfate	Narcotic, intravenous bolus
Halothane (Fluothane)	Inhalation anesthetic, maintenance
Enflurane (Ethrane)	Inhalation anesthetic, maintenance
Isoflurane (Forane)	Inhalation anesthetic, maintenance
Methohexital (Brevital)	Three times more potent and faster clearance than thiopental
Remifentanil (Ultiva)	Synthetic narcotic, intravenous bolus and/or infusion
Propofol (Diprivan)	Intravenous anesthetic; bolus and/or infusion; very fast acting
Sevoflurane (Ultane)	Inhalation anesthetic, maintenance
Desflurane (Suprane)	Inhalation anesthetic, maintenance
MUSCLE RELAXANTS	
Vecuronium (Norcuron)	Intubation, maintenance of muscle relaxation
Atracurium	Maintenance of muscle relaxation; relatively free of circulatory effects
Doxacurium	Maintenance of muscle relaxation; relatively free of circulatory effects
Pancuronium (Pavulon)	Maintenance of muscle relaxation
Pipecuronium	Maintenance of muscle relaxation; relatively free of circulatory effects
Rocuronium (Zemuron)	Fast-acting muscle relaxant; allows hemodynamic stability
Succinylcholine	Fast-acting muscle relaxant, 0% renal elimination
AMNESIACS	
Midazolam (Versed)	Hypnotic; anxiety-reducing sedative
Scopolamine	Sedative; amnesic
Lorazepam (Ativan)	Hypnotic sedative; premedication
CARDIOVASCULAR AGENTS	
Anticholinergics	
Atropine	Decreases vagal tone; treats sinus bradycardia
Glycopyrrolate (Robinul)	Similar to atropine but has less incidence of dysrhythmias than atropine with slower onset
Vasopressors	
Norepinephrine (Levophed)	Increases force and velocity of contraction; increases systemic and pulmonary vascular resistance
Phenylephrine (Neo-Synephrine)	Arteriolar and venous vasoconstriction; increases blood pressure and systemic vascular resistance
Vasodilators	
Nitroglycerin (Tridil)	Dilates coronary arteries; reduces preload
Phentolamine (Regitine)	Decreases systemic and pulmonary resistance
Prostaglandin E_1 (Prostin VR)	Vascular smooth muscle dilator, potent pulmonary vascular dilator; used to maintain patency of ductus arteriosus in cyanotic neonates, patients with severe pulmonary hypertension
Nitroprusside (Nipride)	Arteriolar and venous vasodilation; reduces preload and afterload
Inotropic Agents	
Amrinone (Inocor)	Increases cardiac output, force and velocity of contraction
Calcium chloride	In iodized form, increases cardiac output, blood pressure (BP), and contractility
Dopamine (Intropin)	In low doses, increases renal and mesenteric perfusion; with moderate doses, increases heart rate, contractility, and cardiac output; in higher doses, increases systemic and pulmonary vascular resistance
Dobutamine (Dobutrex)	Increases contractility with less increase in heart rate than occurs with dopamine; has vasodilation effect on vascular bed
Ephedrine	Increases contractility, cardiac output, BP
Epinephrine (Adrenalin)	Increases rate and strength of contraction, BP (effective bronchodilator)
Isoproterenol (Isuprel)	Increases heart rate, contractility, cardiac output; decreases systemic vascular resistance
Milrinone (Primacor)	Increases cardiac output, force and velocity of contraction

Continued

SURGICAL PHARMACOLOGY

Medications Used in Adults During Cardiac Surgery—cont'd

Medication	Purpose/Description/Delivery
Antidysrhythmics	
Lidocaine (Xylocaine)	Acts on ventricles; decreases automaticity of ischemic ventricular tissue
Bretylium (Bretylol)	Prolongs duration of action potential and refractory period; useful for ventricular dysrhythmias refractory to therapy
Digoxin (Lanoxin)	Decreases ventricular rate in atrial fibrillation or flutter and other supraventricular dysrhythmias; avoid in patients with Wolff-Parkinson-White syndrome and other accessory atrioventricular pathways
Nifedipine (Procardia)	Calcium channel blocker; reduces coronary artery spasm; produces coronary vasodilation; extremely light-sensitive; must be given orally or by way of nasal or oral mucosa; antihypertensive
Procainamide (Pronestyl)	Decreases automaticity and conduction in all cardiac tissue (normal and ischemic); stabilizes cellular membranes
Quinidine	Similar to procainamide; atrial and ventricular dysrhythmias
Verapamil (Calan, Isoptin)	Calcium channel blocker; used to treat atrial dysrhythmias; slows ventricular rate in atrial fibrillation or flutter; can be given intravenously
Adenosine	Supraventricular dysrhythmias
DIURETICS	
Furosemide (Lasix)	Decreases renal absorption of sodium and chloride; increases excretion of water and electrolytes, especially potassium, sodium, chloride, magnesium, and calcium
Mannitol	Osmotic diuretic; pulls free water out of organs (reducing cerebral edema); protects kidneys
ANTICOAGULANTS/COAGULANTS	
Heparin	Systemic anticoagulation during CPB; blocks activation of thrombin (and intrinsic clotting cascade)
Protamine sulfate	Heparin antagonist
Bivalirudin	Short-acting direct thrombin inhibitor
ANTIBIOTICS	
Cephalosporins (Mandol, Ancef, Keflex, Keflin, Cefadyl)	Broad-spectrum prophylaxis
Tobramycin (Nebcin)	Aerobic gram-negative and gram-positive bacteria
Vancomycin	Severe endocarditis
Bacitracin	Topical irrigation
MISCELLANEOUS	
Diazepam (Valium)	Sedative, induction of anesthesia
Nitric oxide (NO)	Vascular (especially pulmonary) relaxation; inhaled; reduces pulmonary hypertension
Lidocaine 1% (plain)	Local anesthetic for insertion of invasive monitoring
Naloxone	Opioid antagonist; reverses narcotic-induced respiratory depression
Papaverine	Reduces arterial spasm (e.g., mammary artery)
Potassium	Replaces electrolyte loss
Sodium bicarbonate	Corrects acidosis
Insulin (e.g., NPH)	Corrects hyperglycemia in diabetic patients
Topical hemostatic agents	Intraoperative control of bleeding
Desmopressin (DDAVP)	Pharmacologic hemostatic agent

Adapted from Savino JS, Cheung AT: Cardiac anesthesia. In Cohn LH, editor: *Cardiac surgery in the adult,* ed 3, New York, 2007, McGraw-Hill Medical; Simmonds PK et al: Cardiovascular pharmacologic agents. In Conte JV et al, editors: *The Johns Hopkins manual of cardiac surgical care,* ed 2, St Louis, 2008, Mosby; Seifert PC, Collins J: Cardiac surgery. In Phippen ML et al, editors: *Competency for safe patient care during operative and invasive procedures,* Denver, 2009, Competency and Credentialing Institute.

patient is prepped bedline to bedline anteriorly and posteriorly at least to the knees.

After the prep, the patient is draped so that the anterior areas of the chest, abdomen, and inguinal area are accessible. The perineum is covered, and a towel folded lengthwise (to create a "belt") may be placed across the umbilicus to connect the side drapes. When the saphenous vein is to be excised, both legs remain exposed, with only the feet covered. When draping, the surgical technologist should consider the placement of bypass lines so that they remain securely attached and do not become contaminated. A small drape or towel may be placed over the groin area when access to it is not immediately necessary. If the femoral artery needs to be accessed, the drape can be discarded. Similarly, towels may be placed over the legs after saphenous vein excision to reduce inadvertent cooling.

Optimal Draping for Central Venous Catheters

Central venous catheters are associated with bacterial colonization of the catheter, local infection at the site of insertion, and bloodstream infection. According to Clancy (2009), 250,000 central line–associated bloodstream infections (CLABSIs) occur in U.S. hospitals each year, and add $36,000 in additional cost per patient. In addition to the use of maximal barriers, infection prevention measures include handwashing, skin cleansing with chlorhexidine gluconate, avoiding the femoral site, and removing catheters as soon as possible.

The use of maximal barriers—although time-consuming, more expensive, and more cumbersome than other techniques employing minimal draping—has been shown to reduce the number of CLABSIs. Hu and colleagues (2004) calculated the total direct medical costs and the incidence of CLABSIs, bacterial colonization of the catheter, and death. When compared to minimal barriers, the researchers determined that the use of maximal barriers resulted in the following: lower costs (from $621 to $369 per patient), decreased bloodstream infections (from 5.3% to 2.8%), decreased catheter colonization with local infection (from 5.5% to 2.9%), and decreased death rates (from 0.8% to 0.4%). The authors calculated that $68,000 would be saved with maximal barrier application for every 270 catheter placements, 7 episodes of catheter-related infections would be avoided, and 1 death would be prevented. The results of this study support routine maximal draping for the insertion of central lines.

Modified from Clancy CM: Reducing central line-related bloodstream infections, *AORN J* 89(6):1123-1125, 2009; Hu KK et al: Use of maximal sterile barriers during central venous catheter insertion: clinical and economic outcomes, *Clin Infect Dis* 39, November 15, 2004.

Incisions. A variety of incisions can be used. The standard median sternotomy is most common but mini-sternotomy, mini-thoracotomy, or full thoracotomy incisions are used according to the surgeon's preference and type of procedure (Figure 16-33).

MEDIAN STERNOTOMY. The skin incision for full sternotomy extends from the sternal notch to the linea alba below the xiphoid process (Figure 16-34). For mini-sternotomy, the sternum is partially divided starting from either the sternal notch or the xiphoid process (depending on the cardiac structures to be exposed). The sternum is divided with a saw, and a sternal retractor is inserted. If the IMA or the saphenous vein will be used, it is made available at this time. The pericardium is incised and the pericardial edges are retracted with (six to eight) sutures sewn to the subcutaneous tissue; this technique enhances exposure by elevating the heart and creates a well to contain irrigation solutions.

In repeat sternotomy, adhesions from a previous cardiac operation must be dissected. The sternum may be divided with an oscillating saw and the retrosternal tissue dissected free. Increased risk of fibrillation from manipulation of the heart and bleeding and laceration of the right ventricle should alert the perioperative nurse and surgical technologist to the possibility of instituting femoral vein–femoral artery bypass (discussed later). In addition, disposable defibrillation patches are applied preoperatively to the left lateral chest and the right upper posterior chest; these patches can be activated for defibrillation if the heart has not been exposed. Sterile external paddles may also be available.

Anteroposterior and lateral chest radiographs are useful to determine the extent of retrosternal adhesions and to count the number of chest wires for removal. On occasion, a patient presents for repeat mitral valve surgery. If the initial operation was performed through a thoracotomy incision, sternal adhesions may be minimal or nonexistent and the special precautions associated with repeat sternotomy may not be necessary. Conversely, if the primary chest incision was a sternotomy, a right or left lateral thoracic incision may provide better exposure because of the presence of fewer adhesions.

MINI-THORACOTOMY. For minimally invasive cardiac procedures, a variety of smaller (up to approximately 4 to 8 cm) incisions and/or ports can be used. These include anterolateral chest incisions small enough for the insertion of specially designed instruments (see Figure 16-14), including video cameras and robotic arms. Minimally invasive cardiac procedures using smaller incisions may be performed under direct visualization or, increasingly, by means of video assistance.

CARDIOPULMONARY BYPASS. The temporary substitution of a pump oxygenator for the heart and lungs allows the surgeon to stop the heart to perform cardiac procedures under direct vision in a relatively dry, motionless field. It also allows the surgeon to manipulate the heart without the attendant risk of producing ventricular fibrillation and reduced cardiac output that jeopardize perfusion to the myocardial, peripheral, and cerebral tissues.

Under some circumstances, access to the anteroapical portion of the heart can be achieved without excess manipulation of the heart. Special retraction/stabilization devices (see Figure 16-17) allow the surgeon to create coronary artery bypass grafts (CABGs) to the anterolateral coronary arteries without the use of CPB and induced cardiac arrest. This enables surgery to be performed on a beating heart (discussed later).

In traditional CPB circuits, systemic venous return to the heart flows by gravity drainage through cannulae (Figure 16-35) placed in the superior and inferior venae cavae (Figure 16-36) or through a single two-stage cannula in the right atrium (Figure 16-37) into tubing connected to the bypass machine. Blood is oxygenated, filtered, warmed or cooled, and pumped back into the systemic circulation through a cannula placed in the ascending aorta or occasionally in the femoral artery (Figure 16-38) or the axillary artery (Khonsari et al, 2008). Because the CPB machine (Figure 16-39) oxygenates blood, the lungs do not need to function and can be deflated to provide better exposure of the mediastinal structures.

A percutaneous method of instituting femoral vein–femoral artery CPB can be used for minimally invasive (or conventional open) procedures (Figure 16-40) and in emergency situations where the environment is not conducive to traditional CPB methods (e.g., in the cardiac catheterization laboratory, the intensive care unit, and the emergency department). The system employs thin-walled, wire-reinforced catheters inserted into the femoral vein or artery, or both. The resistance of the small-bore cannula used in the femoral vein can impede gravity drainage; to overcome this, a centrifugal pump may be used to actively siphon blood to the pump oxygenator. Other advances include the use of heparin-bonded bypass circuits and tubing; this reduces (but does not obviate altogether) the amount of heparin required to achieve systemic anticoagulation and can reduce bleeding and the associated need for blood products. Efforts to reduce platelet destruction and the inflammatory

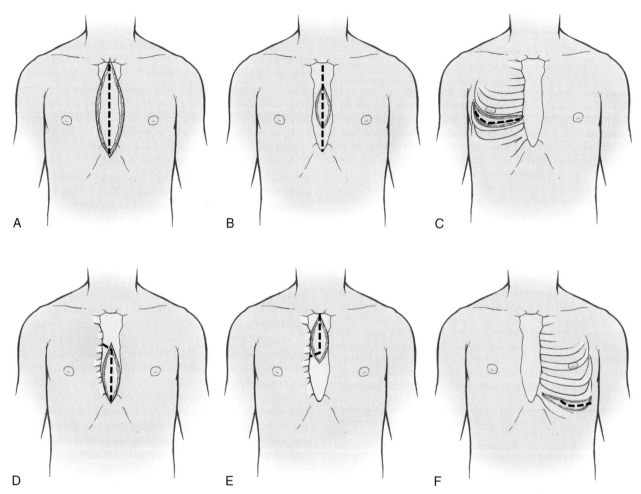

FIGURE 16-33 Schematic representation of traditional incision and sternotomy, **A**, compared with a variety of less-invasive incisions (*dotted lines* represent chest wall incisions). Limited skin incision/full sternotomy, **B**, is gaining popularity because of improved cosmesis and reduced trauma from the limited chest wall retraction. The parasternal approach, **C**, is used less frequently because of the residual chest wall defect. Partial lower or upper sternotomy, **D** and **E**, respectively, has been used predominantly in valve procedures. Right anterior thoracotomy, **F**, is a useful approach, particularly in mitral valve reoperations.

response by coating components of the CPB circuits with phosphorylcholine and other newer materials have shown some encouraging results (Schulze et al, 2009).

By diverting blood away from the heart, CPB also decompresses the ventricles, thereby reducing myocardial wall tension, which is a significant determinant of myocardial oxygen demand. This principle is evident when CPB or other means of ventricular support are employed to "rest" the heart. Further decompression is achieved by venting the left ventricle to remove air and accumulated thebesian and bronchial venous return as well as systemic return flowing around the venous cannulae (Figure 16-41). The venting catheter is inserted into the left ventricle by way of the right superior pulmonary vein or, less commonly, through the left ventricular apex. The venting line is connected to the suction lines of the bypass machine. A small venting catheter may also be inserted into the ascending aorta to remove air. Occasionally a vent is inserted into the pulmonary artery. Venting can reduce the incidence of gaseous microemboli. Ambient air removal can also be accomplished in

cases when the heart is opened (e.g., valve surgery) with the insertion of a CO_2 gas diffuser; the gas is insufflated into the pericardial well. The CO_2 gas dissolves in blood approximately 25 times faster than room air; CO_2 retained within the cardiac chambers is better tolerated than ambient air and less harmful to tissue (Svenarud et al, 2004).

Improved bypass technology has also reduced the incidence of bypass-related microemboli and cellular injury with the use of finer filters for air and particulate emboli and moderation of the strength of siphoning pressures (Groom et al, 2009). Membrane oxygenators incorporated into the bypass circuit (see Figure 16-38) perform gas exchange (removing CO_2 and adding oxygen to the blood) more efficiently and less traumatically. Gases diffuse through a semipermeable membrane that separates the oxygenating gas and the venous blood. Although membrane oxygenators preserve platelet and red blood cell function better than the older "bubble" oxygenators, there does remain considerable morbidity associated with the use of CPB.

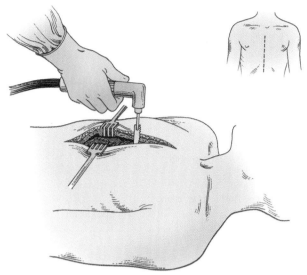

FIGURE 16-34 Median sternotomy with sternal saw.

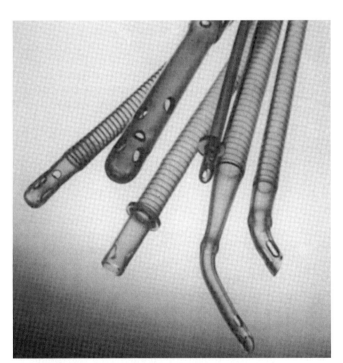

FIGURE 16-35 Arterial and venous perfusion cannulae.

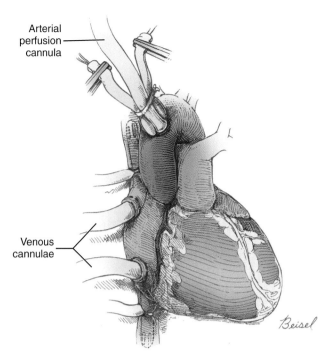

FIGURE 16-36 Bicaval cannulation of the superior and inferior venae cavae; aortic cannulation.

Extracorporeal circulation causes fluid retention and inter-compartmental fluid shifts, multiple organ dysfunction, showers of microemboli, inflammatory responses, and unique bleeding complications (Gourlay and Qureshi, 2008; Groom et al, 2009; Seifert, 2009). The mechanism of injury is believed to be related to the exposure of the blood to the abnormal surfaces of the bypass circuit, hypothermia, shear forces, and altered blood flow. These can initiate a systemic inflammatory response (complement activation), which releases vasoactive substances. Attempts to minimize the inflammatory reaction have focused on modifying the acti-

vation of platelets and blood factors that play a major role in initiating the response (Sniecinski and Levy, 2008). To avoid the complications associated with CPB, clinicians have stimulated greater use of "beating heart" ("off-pump") techniques for myocardial revascularization. It should be noted that "off-pump" techniques are not indicated for procedures requiring the heart to be opened (e.g., mitral valve surgery, left ventricular aneurysm repair) because air within the opened chamber would embolize to the brain. CPB enables the heart to be isolated from the systemic circulation so that after the repair is completed (and before the cross-clamp is removed) residual air can be removed through various venting techniques.

Two types of pumps are available: roller pumps and centrifugal pumps. Roller pumps have roller heads that propel blood forward by compressing blood-filled tubing against a smooth, metal housing. Centrifugal pumps use cones or blades that rotate at high speed to produce forward flow. All pumps produce some hemolysis from turbulence and shear forces, but careful calibration and minimal use of connectors can provide relatively atraumatic flow for short periods (e.g., less than 6 hours). Arterial blood flow on bypass is largely nonpulsatile, although modifications to the pump can simulate phasic (systolic/nonsystolic) flow (Gourlay and Qureshi, 2008); the arterial blood pressure is usually manifested by a mean arterial waveform on the oscilloscope during CPB.

Suction lines are ordinarily used during CPB to return shed blood to the venous reservoir and the oxygenator. These lines may combine conventional handheld suction tubes and ventricular decompression lines or sumps (see Figure 16-42). Before the initiation of CPB, the entire extracorporeal circuit must be primed and rendered free of air to prevent air emboli.

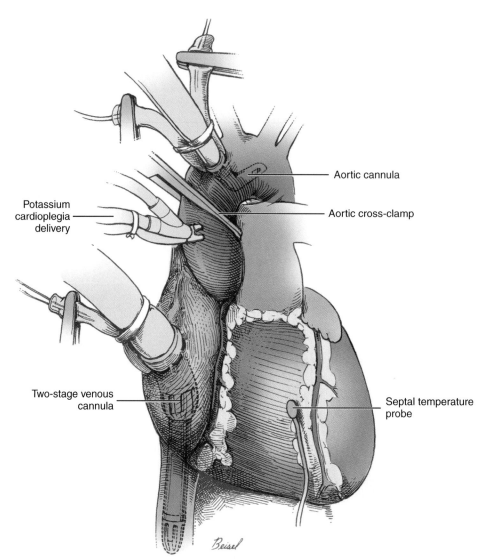

FIGURE 16-37 Diagram showing aortic and venous cannulae during aortic cross-clamping. Also shown is antegrade cardioplegic solution delivery catheter in the aorta proximal to the cross-clamp and a temperature probe. The single (two-stage) venous cannula has openings in the distal end of the cannula to drain the inferior vena cava; the openings in the midportion (right atrial area) of the cannula drain the superior vena cava and the coronary sinus venous return.

The priming solution is usually a combination of colloid and crystalloid fluids with a balanced electrolyte component. Priming volumes (i.e., within the CPB circuit) are generally between 1400 and 2000 ml (Frumento and Bennett-Guerrero, 2008). When the patient's blood volume mixes with the prime, there is some hemodilution and a subsequent reduction of the hematocrit (Hct) level. Advantages of hemodilution include reducing the number of homologous serum reactions and the incidence of hepatitis and human immunodeficiency virus (HIV) as well as providing better perfusion of the capillary beds because of reduced blood viscosity. Hct levels as low as 25% may be adequate during CPB, but once CPB is terminated, transfusion of red blood cells may be required to enhance the blood's oxygen-carrying capacity. In low-weight, low-hematocrit patients, hemodilution may not be tolerated. One method to decrease hemodilution is to employ the technique of

rapid-autologous-prime (RAP). First, the perfusionist shortens the length of bypass tubing (thereby reducing the volume of prime solution in the CPB circuit). After the surgeon inserts the arterial cannula into the aorta and connects it to the arterial tubing leading to the bypass machine (but before initiation of bypass), the perfusionist allows a predetermined amount of the patient's arterial blood to drain from the line and fill part of the bypass circuit; the perfusionist then clamps the circuit. The clamps are removed at the initiation of bypass (Frumento and Bennett-Guerrero, 2008).

The amount and kind of drugs used in the priming solution vary among institutions, but heparin is routinely added to block clot formation in the bypass circuit. Anticoagulation is routinely monitored during bypass, and more heparin is given as needed to maintain an activated clotting time (ACT) exceeding 600 seconds. Other ingredients are added to main-

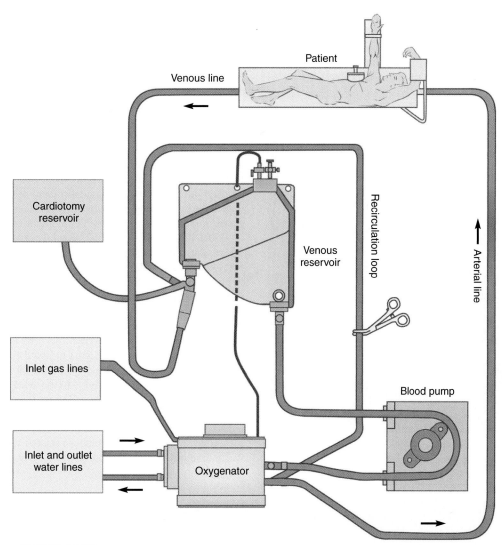

FIGURE 16-38 Cardiopulmonary bypass circuit. Venous blood is drained by gravity from the right atrium or venae cavae into an oxygenator that incorporates a blood reservoir and a heat exchanger, which warms or cools the blood as needed. The ventilating gas flowing into the oxygenator removes carbon dioxide and adds oxygen to the blood. Saturated blood leaves the oxygenator and is pumped from the reservoir into the arterial system by the use of a roller pump. Filters and monitors are incorporated into the circuit. Additional roller pumps are used to suction shed blood from the pericardial well and the intracardiac chambers (cardiotomy suckers); the blood is returned to the cardiotomy reservoir. Another roller pump is used to vent air and blood through a right superior pulmonary venous catheter that is inserted into the left ventricle.

tain normal pH and electrolyte status (Frumento and Bennett-Guerrero, 2008).

Arterial blood flow rates are estimated according to the patient's height, weight, and body surface area. Depending on the arterial and venous pressure values and the results of blood gas determinations, the flow is adjusted.

Myocardial Protection. Improvement in the results of cardiac surgery is attributable in great part to progress made in the protection of the myocardium. Coronary circulatory interruptions, ischemia, and hypoperfusion accompanying induced cardiac arrest are often necessary to permit the surgeon

sufficient time to repair cardiac lesions under direct vision. Unless measures are taken to protect the myocardium during these periods, irreversible damage can result. The main protective strategies are cooling the heart (and the rest of the body) to reduce metabolic demand, rapidly arresting the heart so that myocardial energy resources are preserved, and restoring intracellular homeostasis (e.g., by correcting pH, oxygen, and electrolyte imbalances) to avoid postischemic reperfusion injury (Mentzer et al, 2007).

HYPOTHERMIA. Hypothermia in cardiac surgery is the deliberate reduction of body temperature for therapeutic purposes. A moderate degree of hypothermia, to 28° C (82.4° F), permits reduction of oxygen consumption by 50%. At 20° C (68° F) there is a further reduction of about 25%. Systemic circulatory cooling is achieved with the heat exchanger of the heart-lung machine. When very cold temperatures (less than 20° C [68° F]) are desired for myocardial protection in pro-

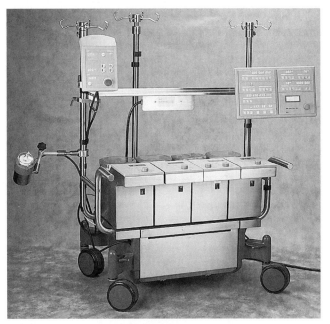

FIGURE 16-39 Cardiopulmonary bypass pump. Modular system with integrated centrifugal pump driver.

longed, complex cases, additional surface cooling of the heart with topical application of cold saline/slush or continuous irrigation of the pericardial wall can be used. Large ice chips in pericardial irrigating fluids should be avoided to prevent injury to the phrenic nerve within the right and left lateral pericardium and other cardiac tissue. Insulation pads placed behind the heart can reduce heat conduction from relatively warmer organs. Transmural cooling of the heart is achieved with cardioplegia (discussed later).

Ventricular fibrillation can occur during the cooling process although it is less likely at temperatures greater than 32° C (89.6° F). Other complications are related to the adverse effects that hypothermia has on coagulation and wound healing; this may delay hemostasis after heparin reversal and have an impact on recuperation (Edmunds, 2004; Mentzer et al, 2007).

CARDIOPLEGIC ARREST. Rapidly arresting the heart during diastole is beneficial because an arrested heart uses less energy than a fibrillating or beating heart. Cardioplegia with hypothermia can reduce energy requirements even further (Mentzer et al, 2007). Both "warm" and "cold" heart surgery proponents concur that infusing a warm initial bolus of cardioplegia acts as a form of active resuscitation in energy-depleted hearts. There is also concurrence that providing a warm terminal bolus of cardioplegia helps to avoid reperfusion injury (caused by oxygen free radicals and lactic acid buildup) by providing oxygen and other nutrients to the heart. The controversy lies in the use of normothermic ("warm") cardioplegia during the period of arrest when the actual surgical repair or bypass construction occurs. Proponents of warm arrest techniques seek to avoid the complications associated with hypothermia; warm cardioplegia is delivered continuously while the surgical

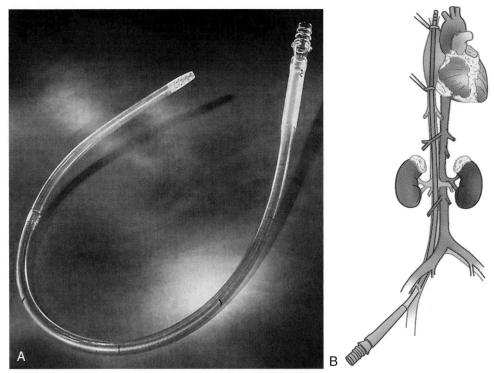

FIGURE 16-40 A, Venous endovascular cannula. **B,** The catheter tip is inserted into the femoral vein and threaded to the right atrium; the distal tip is positioned in the superior vena cava (SVC) to drain the upper body.

repair is performed (Salerno, 2007). Opponents of continuous warm cardioplegia cite the technical difficulty associated with a constant flow of cardioplegia obscuring the surgical site. Some authors favor intermittent cold cardioplegia infusions because if cardioplegia infusions are even momentarily interrupted to enhance visualization, myocardial protection is jeopardized (Mentzer et al, 2007; Khonsari et al, 2008).

CARDIOPLEGIA DELIVERY. Cardioplegic arrest is accomplished by infusing the coronary arteries with a 4° to 10° C (39.2° to 50° F) solution containing potassium (2 to 50 mEq/L) and buffering agents to counteract ischemic acidosis. Potassium acts by depolarizing the myocardial cell membrane and arresting the heart in diastole.

Delivery of the solution may be by the antegrade or the retrograde route (Figure 16-42). With antegrade delivery, a needle is inserted into the aortic root proximal to the aortic cross-clamp; the cardioplegic solution is infused under pressure that closes the aortic valve leaflets. The only remaining route for the solution is into the right and left coronary arteries and the coronary circulation (see Figure 16-37). If the aortic valve does not close properly, the cardioplegic solution will flow preferentially into the left ventricular chamber, causing distention; in these cases direct cannulation of the coronary ostia is performed. Direct infusion into vein grafts protects the myocardium distal to coronary lesions and enhances transmural cooling. Retrograde infusion is achieved with a catheter placed transatrially into the coronary sinus; the perfusate enters the coronary venous system and flows through the myocardial circulation, leaving through the coronary ostia. The retrograde route is especially useful in the presence of coronary artery obstructions and left ventricular hypertrophy.

When the heart is sufficiently arrested, the ECG reflects a straight line; when electrical activity is noted on the monitor (fine fibrillation), the cardioplegic solution is reinfused when continued cooling is desired (approximately every 15 to 20 minutes).

Minimally invasive techniques for myocardial protection have also been developed (described under Cardioplegic Deliv-

ery). Percutaneously inserted catheters can infuse antegrade cardioplegic solution through a catheter threaded into the aortic root; retrograde cardioplegic solution is infused through a catheter inserted into the internal jugular vein and then passed into the SVC, the right atrium, and the coronary sinus.

CIRCULATORY ARREST. In some highly complex procedures, such as those involving the aortic arch, it may be impossible to place an occluding clamp across the aorta. In these cases, circulatory arrest may be used to maintain a dry operative site. Because all blood flow will be interrupted, additional protection is required to protect myocardial, cerebral, and other tissue from ischemia.

The patient is cooled with the heat exchanger to approximately 18° C (65° F), at which point the bypass pump is turned off (Pretre and Turina, 2007). The incision is made, and the repair is performed. The small amount of collateral drainage entering the field can be removed with a suction catheter. When

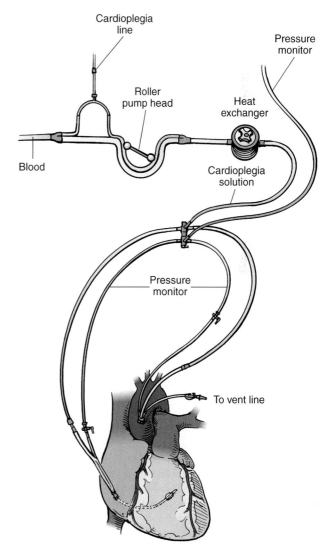

FIGURE 16-42 Antegrade-retrograde cardioplegia system. The antegrade cardioplegia catheter is inserted into the aorta proximally to the cross-clamp; the catheter is Y-ed into a vent line and into the retrograde cardioplegia catheter, which is inserted transatrially into the coronary sinus. The coronary sinus pressure is monitored; its pressure should remain less than 50 mm Hg.

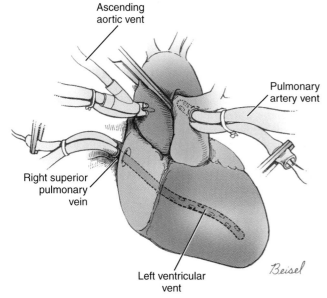

FIGURE 16-41 Types of venting catheters.

the repair is completed, air is removed and CPB is slowly reinstituted. Rewarming is performed at a rate of approximately 1° C every 3 minutes.

CEREBROPLEGIA. Circulatory arrest poses additional risk to the brain. Cerebral protection, cerebroplegia, is provided by the infusion of oxygenated blood to the brain. *Antegrade* cerebral perfusion is achieved with the insertion of cannulae directly into the innominate artery, the right common carotid artery, or another branch of the aortic arch. *Retrograde* cerebral perfusion is accomplished using a cannula that has been Y-ed to the superior vena cava drainage cannula that connects to the arterial infusion line. When blood flow is stopped (during circulatory arrest), the venous line is clamped, the connection to the arterial line is opened, and the retrograde cerebral perfusion line is used to infuse cerebroplegia into the head vessels (Pretre and Turina, 2007). Blood returning from the head (through the carotid or vertebral arteries) is suctioned from the field.

Termination of Cardiopulmonary Bypass. Near the end of the repair, the heart is allowed to rewarm while the perfusionist rewarms the patient systemically with the oxygenator's heat exchanger. Air is evacuated from the left ventricle and the proximal portion of the aorta. The cross-clamp is removed. The heart often converts spontaneously to sinus rhythm, but internal (or external) defibrillation may be necessary. Temporary epicardial pacing wires may be sutured to the right atrial appendage or the right ventricle; these are used postoperatively if the patient has transient bradycardia, supraventricular tachycardia, or other dysrhythmias. Atrial fibrillation (AF) is a common postoperative complication that is associated with a greater risk of embolic events and increases the patient's length of stay (Sethares et al, 2008).

When the heart is contracting, the patient is gradually weaned from CPB. Ventilation of the lungs is restarted. Venous flow is gradually reduced by clamping the venous line or lines, and a commensurate reduction in arterial flow is made by the perfusionist. When heart action is sufficient and systemic and pulmonary blood pressures are stabilized, the bypass is terminated and the cannulae are removed.

Measures to actively promote body heat retention are implemented to enhance clotting mechanisms, immune function, and oxygenation. Maintenance of normothermia after the termination of CPB has also been recommended to reduce the risk of postoperative infection (Savino and Cheung, 2007).

Closing. After hemostasis is achieved, catheters are inserted into the pericardium for mediastinal drainage of shed blood. If either or both pleurae have been entered, chest tubes are inserted to drain shed blood entering from the pericardium and to create negative intrapleural pressure to facilitate lung expansion. The tubes are connected to a water-seal drainage system or an autotransfusion drainage system by using straight or Y connectors. Chest tube drainage of greater than 100 ml/hr requires investigation of possible causes (Sethares et al, 2008). The clinician anticipates possible blood studies to determine

whether clotting factors require replacement, hemostasis of anastomoses is present, or bypass conduits require exploration. Reopening the chest may be necessary to control bleeding.

Chest closure in median sternotomy is achieved with wire sutures (see Figure 16-19). The wire sutures are twisted, excess wire is cut, and the wire ends are buried into the sternal periosteum. Some surgeons use small metal crimpers to approximate and hold the wires (rather than twisting and burying the wire ends). In a frail sternum, a long sternal closing wire may be threaded longitudinally along the right and left lateral margins of the sternum; the crossed sternal wires are inserted through the longitudinal wires and then approximated to close the sternum. This reinforces the sternal closure and reduces the possibility of sternal dehiscence. In some thin patients with little subcutaneous tissue over the sternum, one (or more) of the sternal wires may continue to cause discomfort after the sternum has fully healed. In these patients the surgeon may elect to remove the wire as an ambulatory (outpatient) procedure (Ambulatory Surgery Considerations).

The linea alba is closed with suture. A layer of sutures is placed to approximate the fascia over the sternum; the subcutaneous tissue and skin are closed. If metal staples are used on the skin, a staple remover should accompany the patient to the recovery area. Thoracotomy incisions are closed in standard fashion.

Before transferring the patient, the perioperative nurse telephones a report to the recovery area, usually the cardiovascular SICU.

Perioperative documentation follows the standard protocol and includes a description of the procedure performed and identification of medications and all implanted material (with lot and serial numbers). Hospital policy should be followed to ensure compliance with the Safe Medical Devices Act.

Postoperatively, complications associated with cardiac surgery are outlined in Table 16-4. Excessive or sudden hemorrhage producing cardiac tamponade may initiate the need for a rapid response team to control the hemorrhage and achieve hemostasis.

TABLE 16-4

Complications of Cardiac Surgery

Body System	Complication	Treatment Measures
Cardiovascular	Bleeding	Transfusion Replacement of clotting factors Control of hypertension Maintenance of normothermia Possible return to OR for exploration and hemostasis
	Cardiac tamponade	Release of constricting blood via chest tube insertion or operative exploration
	Myocardial ischemia/infarction	Monitor ECG for ischemic changes Measure serum enzymes Minimize oxygen demand Administer medications to reduce cardiac workload and dysrhythmias Insertion of an IABP
	Dysrhythmias	Administer antidysrhythmic drugs Correct electrolyte imbalances Correct acid-base, hypovolemia Employ pacemaker therapy Cardiovert or defibrillate as necessary Maintain adequate CO
Pulmonary	Hemothorax/pneumothorax	Maintain chest tube patency Check chest tubes for air leaks Insert additional chest tube (pleural or mediastinal)
	Atelectasis/pneumonia	Check ventilator settings and endotracheal tube Suction endotracheal tube Monitor breath sounds Monitor pulse oximetry Obtain chest x-ray film Elevate head of bed Ensure proper function of NG tube After extubation, encourage mobilization and use of incentive spirometry Frequent staff handwashing
	Pulmonary embolus	Frequent patient mouth care Employ compression stockings Assess for acute chest pain and SOB Perform radiologic examination Possible surgical embolectomy
	Failure to wean from ventilator	Maintain aggressive pulmonary toilet Monitor pulse oximetry Frequent mobilization (even while on ventilator) Pain and anxiety management Incentive spirometry once extubated Possible tracheostomy
Kidneys	Renal insufficiency/failure	Promote adequate CO, renal perfusion Monitor urine output Diuretics for oliguria Administer volume (vs. drugs) to increase renal perfusion Possible dialysis
Gastrointestinal (GI)	Ileus	Assess bowel sounds and distention Maintain NG tube function Progress diet slowly
	GI bleeding	Maintain NG tube function to differentiate upper and lower GI bleeding Stress ulcer prophylaxis Monitor complaints of nausea Use extra caution with anticoagulants
Neurologic	Stroke	Avoid hypotension Assess neurologic function Restart preoperative antidepressant drugs
	Neurocognitive dysfunction/postcardiotomy delirium	Avoid hypoperfusion Correct metabolic derangements Avoid hypoxemia Orient frequently to time and place Discontinue medications that may promote delirium Ensure a safe environment

Continued

Complications of Cardiac Surgery—cont'd

Body System	Complication	Treatment Measures
Immune	Nosocomial infection	Frequent staff hand cleansing
		Strict aseptic technique
		Dressing care, urinary catheter care
		Early removal of central lines, urinary catheters, chest tubes
		Administer antibiotics
	Mediastinitis	Strict aseptic technique
		Administration of antibiotics
Metabolic	Hyper/hypoglycemia	Limited blood transfusion
		Glucose (hyperglycemic) control
		Possible return to OR for debridement and muscle flap repair
		Avoid hyperglycemia (maintain glucose at less than 200 mg/dl)
		Avoid hypoglycemia
		Monitor for potential rebound from insulin administered during surgery

CO, Cardiac output; *ECG,* electrocardiogram; *IABP,* intra-aortic balloon pump; *NG,* nasogastric; *OR,* operating room; *SOB,* shortness of breath.
Modified from Sethares K et al: Care of patients undergoing cardiac surgery. In Moser DK, Riegel B, editors: *Cardiac nursing: a companion to Braunwald's heart disease,* St Louis, 2008, Saunders; Gray RJ, Sethna DH: Medical management of the patient undergoing cardiac surgery. In Libby P et al, editors: *Braunwald's heart disease,* ed 8, Philadelphia, 2008, Saunders; Babb M: Clinical risk assessment: identifying patients at high risk for heart failure, *AORN J* 89(2):273-288, 2009.

Surgical Interventions

The following section describes operations for acquired forms of heart disease. Both traditional "open" procedures and minimally invasive techniques are described. Traditional procedures are performed through a median sternotomy incision using aortocaval CPB (see Figures 16-36 and 16-37) and antegrade-retrograde cardioplegia (see Figure 16-42) with routine chest drainage and closure. Minimally invasive procedures are described for CPB, saphenous vein harvesting, coronary artery bypass grafting, atrial fibrillation, and MVR. These procedures may be performed through a median sternotomy or an anterior left or right thoracotomy; some lesions may be approached through a cephalad or caudal mini-sternotomy.

EXTRACORPOREAL CIRCULATION PROCEDURES

Operative Procedures

Aortic-Caval Cannulation by Way of Sternotomy

1. A longitudinal pericardial incision is made, and the pericardial edges are retracted by suture to the chest wall.
2. If the aorta is to be cannulated for arterial blood return to the patient, it is partially dissected from the pulmonary artery.
3. Purse-string sutures are placed in the aorta (twice) and right atrium (or both venae cavae) for the eventual placement of the perfusion cannulae. Tourniquets are placed over the suture ends and held with a hemostat.
4. For ascending aortic cannulation, the aorta is incised inside the purse-string sutures with a knife (the surgeon places a finger over the aortotomy); the cannula is inserted, and the purse-string sutures are firmly secured with the tourniquet. It is important to have the distal end of the cannula clamped before it is inserted into the aorta to prevent backbleeding from the aorta. To prevent air emboli, the arterial connection is made under a saline drip, or by having the perfusionist slowly pump priming solution out of the arterial line. Arterial cannulation is generally performed before caval cannulation so that direct access for blood replacement is available if needed.
5. Venous cannulation is performed in one of the following ways:
   a. Single, two-stage cannulation for venous return to the pump-oxygenator: An incision is made into the right atrial appendage and the two-stage cannula (see Figure 16-37) is inserted into the atrium. The distal end of the cannula is placed into the inferior vena cava (IVC). The purse-string suture is secured with a tourniquet, and the catheter is permitted to fill partially with blood before being connected to the venous line.
   b. Double cannulation: For double cannulation, a second incision is made into the atrial wall within the purse-string suture and the cannulae are placed in the inferior and superior venae cavae (see Figure 16-37). To force all venous return into the cannulae, umbilical tapes with tourniquets may be placed around each cava and then tightened. This forces systemic venous return to enter the cannulae, producing total CPB (see Figure 16-41).
6. In procedures where greater exposure of the right atrium is required (e.g., tricuspid valve surgery, closure of atrial septal defects in adults), a right-angle cannula may be inserted into the SVC (Figure 16-43).

Femoral Vein–Femoral Artery Cannulation

1. A vertical or oblique incision is made into the femoral triangle, and the femoral vein and artery are exposed. Umbilical compression tapes are passed around the vessels above and below the proposed venotomy and arteriotomy. Vascular clamps may be applied above and below the incision into each vessel.
2. A purse-string suture is placed in the femoral artery. A needle is inserted into the artery, followed by a guidewire. The needle is removed, and dilators are threaded over the guidewire to enlarge the artery. The dilators are removed, and the

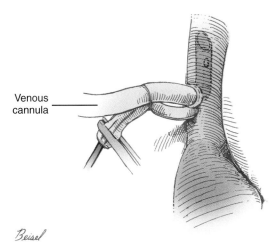

FIGURE 16-43 Right-angle cannula in superior vena cava.

Venous cannula

Beisel

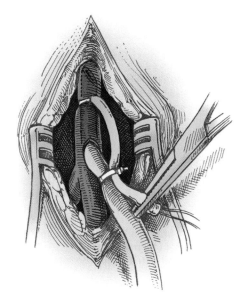

FIGURE 16-44 Cannulation of femoral artery.

perfusion catheter (occluded distally with a tubing clamp) is inserted retrograde into the arteriotomy as the proximal clamp or tourniquet is released. The proximal tourniquet is tightened (Figure 16-44). The cannula is connected to the arterial line.

3. An incision is made into the femoral vein, and the venous catheter is inserted into the vein as the proximal clamp or tourniquet is released. After the cannula is in place, the proximal tourniquet is tightened to prevent bleeding from the venotomy. The cannula is occluded at the distal end with a tubing clamp to prevent bleeding from the cannula. The cannula is connected to the venous line, and the tubing clamp is removed.

MINIMALLY INVASIVE CANNULATION. Femoral cannulation techniques are employed. Femoral arterial cannulation is as just described. Venous drainage is achieved with an extended catheter inserted into the exposed femoral vein, and the distal tip is advanced to the SVC to the inferior portion of the RA (see Figure 16-40). Side ports along the distal portion of the cannula allow drainage of blood from the SVC, the right atrium, and the IVC. Because of the higher resistance to drainage flow compared with right atrial cannulation, a centrifugal pump or vacuum-assisted drainage incorporated in the CPB circuit is used to augment venous drainage.

PUMP-OXYGENATOR PREPARATION. After the arterial and venous connections are completed and the lines secured, bypass is slowly begun and the desired flow rate is gradually achieved. Arterial infusion is calibrated to match venous outflow in order to maintain a consistent cardiac output and blood volume. Perfusion flow is adjusted as necessary during the operation (Mongero and Beck, 2008).

Axillary Artery Cannulation. Although infrequently used for arterial perfusion, the right axillary artery (AA) is a useful cannulation site when circulatory arrest is necessary for surgery on the aorta. Another indication for its use occurs in the presence of acute or chronic aortic dissection when retrograde flow through the femoral artery may produce femoral artery dissection and malperfusion of the central organs (e.g., the kidneys). The AA is usually free of atherosclerosis and has excellent collateral flow from the thyrocervical trunk to the

suprascapular and transverse cervical arteries, which helps to avoid upper extremity ischemia during cross-clamping (Kokotsakis et al, 2005). Use of the AA also facilitates antegrade cerebral perfusion during hypothermic arrest. The artery can be cannulated directly, but the risk of dissection favors indirect cannulation via an 8-mm to 10-mm Dacron tube graft anastomosed to the artery (Khonsari et al, 2008; Kokotsakis et al, 2005).

The patient is positioned supine with a roll under the shoulders to enhance access to the artery; the OR bed may be tilted to the left for better exposure of the artery during cannulation. The right arm may be positioned next to the body with the elbow flexed slightly; the arm may be extended in some procedures, depending on surgeon preference. Additional patient safety considerations are listed in the Patient Safety box.

CANNULATION PROCEDURE

1. The right axillary (or subclavian) artery is exposed via a small incision below and parallel to the midportion of the right clavicle. The tissue is dissected toward the insertion of the pectoralis minor muscle and the deltopectoral groove; the pectoralis major muscle is dissected and divided, and the axillary vein and underlying artery are exposed and gently mobilized for about 2 cm.

2. The brachial plexus is located (cephalad to the vessels); manipulation is avoided to protect the plexus during cannulation and the operative procedure.

3. A partial occlusion clamp is applied to the artery and an 8-mm to 10-mm Dacron tube graft is anastomosed end-to-side to the artery with 4-0 or 5-0 polypropylene suture.

4. A straight arterial cannula is inserted through the graft and a heavy silk tie or umbilical tape is tied around the graft over the cannula to prevent bleeding.

5. Arterial flow is slowly initiated. Blood pressures via both the right and left radial arteries are compared to confirm the absence of a pressure gradient; after confirmation, arterial flow is increased to the initial desired rate of 2.2 to 2.8 $L/min/m^2$.

PATIENT SAFETY

Patient Safety Considerations for Axillary Artery Cannulation

During high-risk, low-volume procedures, such as axillary artery (AA) cannulation, less frequently encountered patient safety factors should be scrutinized with care. These factors include understanding the purpose and plan for the procedure, having the necessary supplies, anticipating possible complications, and preparing for alternate techniques. The considerations listed are pertinent to the use of the axillary artery.

BLOOD PRESSURE (BP) MONITORING
◆ Use bilateral radial artery BP lines to compare right- and left-sided pressures and to confirm the absence of a pressure gradient.
◆ Use a right radial artery line to monitor antegrade cerebral perfusion during hypothermic arrest.
◆ Cerebral perfusion pressure should be kept at 50 mm Hg (or less).

PREVENTION OF INJURY TO BRACHIAL PLEXUS
◆ Traction and manipulation should be avoided.
◆ Do not use electrosurgical energy in area of brachial plexus.

CANNULATION
◆ Ensure absence of preexisting dissection in *axillary* artery when *aortic* dissection is present.
◆ There is increased risk of dissection with *direct* cannulation of axillary artery; attachment of tube graft for *indirect* cannulation is often performed.
◆ During cardiopulmonary bypass (CPB) the BP tends to be higher on the side of the arterial (axillary) cannulation; contralateral BP line should be used for monitoring.
◆ Known, severe atherosclerosis of the axillary artery is a contraindication to its use.

AVOIDANCE OF VASCULAR INJURY
◆ Closing the artery after completion of CPB should avoid narrowing the arterial lumen; the graft can be cut in a way that does not impinge on the vessel lumen and also does not leave residual graft material, which can allow stasis of blood and increase the risk for thromboembolus.

HEMOSTASIS
◆ If metal ligating clips are used to close the graft, ensure proper function of the clip applier.

Adapted from Khonsari S et al: *Cardiac surgery: safeguards and pitfalls in operative technique*, ed 4, Philadelphia, 2008, Lippincott Williams and Wilkins; Kokotsakis J et al: Right axillary artery cannulation: surgical management of the hostile ascending aorta, *Texas Heart Inst J* 32(2):189-193, 2005.

6. Completion of bypass and removal of the AA cannula: After CPB has been discontinued, the arterial cannula is gradually withdrawn and the AA graft is clamped (or ligated with two large metal clips); the graft is cut a few millimeters above the artery and oversewn with polypropylene suture. The surgeon is careful to avoid narrowing the AA or leaving a graft "stump" (which could become a source of emboli) during closure (Khonsari et al, 2008; Kokotsakis et al, 2005).

Cardioplegic Delivery

ANTEGRADE CARDIOPLEGIA. A purse-string suture and tourniquet are placed into the anterior ascending aorta proximal to the aortic cross-clamp, and a needle-tipped catheter is inserted. Both the catheter and the cardioplegic tubing are flushed to remove residual air. The catheter tubing is Y-ed into a vent line so that alternatively the needle can be used to infuse the cardioplegic solution into the aortic root or vent air and blood from the aorta and left ventricle. Individual lines incorporated into the antegrade infusion system can be used to selectively infuse the coronary bypass graft or grafts. Handheld cardioplegic cannulae may be used to infuse cardioplegic solution directly into the coronary ostia, but the risk of injuring ostial tissue usually favors this technique when retrograde delivery cannot be achieved.

RETROGRADE CARDIOPLEGIA. A purse-string suture is placed into the lateral wall of the right atrium, and a tourniquet is applied to the suture. A stab wound is made into the atrium, and the retrograde catheter is inserted and palpated into the coronary sinus. Blood is aspirated from the catheter, and the catheter is connected to the flushed retrograde infusion line and to a pressure line. Infusion pressure should be between 20 and 45 mm Hg (Khonsari et al, 2008). Because a full right atrium facilitates insertion of the catheter, inser-

tion is performed before the initiation of CPB when possible. If the patient is already on CPB, the surgeon can fill the atrium by clamping the venous drainage line momentarily, thereby diverting blood into the heart.

MINIMALLY INVASIVE ENDOVASCULAR ANTEGRADE-RETROGRADE CARDIOPLEGIA. A system of endovascular multilumen catheters designed to infuse solutions, vent air and blood, measure intravascular pressures, and occlude the aorta may be used (Figure 16-45). Fluoroscopy or TEE can be employed to confirm proper catheter placement.

The intravascular aortic catheter has three lumens. The first lumen has an inflatable balloon at the tip that, when inflated inside the vessel, occludes the aorta and serves as an internal "cross-clamp." The second lumen can be used either to infuse antegrade cardioplegic solution or to vent the ventricle. The third lumen is used to measure aortic root pressure. The catheter is introduced into the femoral artery and advanced into the ascending aorta. Either the femoral artery used for arterial inflow or the contralateral femoral artery is used.

A triple-lumen coronary sinus retrograde cardioplegic catheter is inserted percutaneously through the jugular vein into the SVC. The catheter is guided into the coronary sinus under fluoroscopy. One lumen allows manual catheter balloon inflation; another lumen is used to infuse retroplegic solution; and the third lumen measures coronary sinus pressure.

A third catheter is used as a venting-and-decompression device. It is inserted into the jugular vein (through a separate sheath from the retrograde catheter) and advanced into the main pulmonary artery.

These catheter systems allow surgeons to use minimally invasive techniques to treat lesions, such as mitral valve stenosis, that cannot be performed safely with a beating heart.

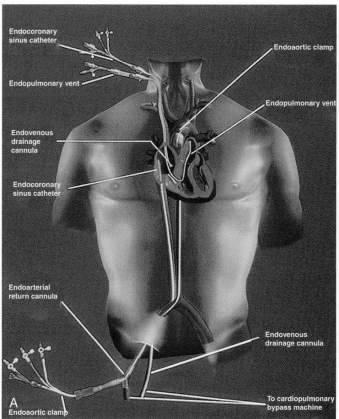
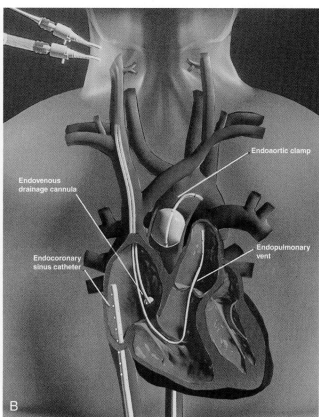

FIGURE 16-45 A, Endovascular cardiopulmonary bypass and myocardial protection system (see text). **B,** Intracardiac placement of catheters.

Termination of Cardiopulmonary Bypass

1. After the intracardiac procedure has been completed, all air is evacuated from the left ventricle. A warm dose of cardioplegic solution may be given, after which the cross-clamp is removed. The warm solution dilates the coronary vascular bed and enhances coronary perfusion once the cross-clamp is removed.

2. Defibrillation is often spontaneous with removal of the aortic cross-clamp and the entry of warm blood into the coronary circulation. If not, internal defibrillation is necessary. Endovascular, minimally invasive procedures will require external defibrillation with sterile external paddles or patches. Temporary epicardial pacing wires attached to the atrium and to the ventricle are used to adjust the heart rate and optimize cardiac output.

3. Venous flow to the pump is reduced. Arterial flow is also reduced to equal the reduced venous return. When heart action is sufficient and systemic arterial blood pressure is stabilized, venous return is further reduced and the patient is taken off bypass by clamping all lines and stopping the pump.

4. As the cannulation catheters are removed, the purse-string sutures are tightened and tied. Additional sutures may be required for hemostasis.

5. Chest tubes are inserted into the pericardium (and the pleural cavity if the pleura has been opened).

6. Protamine sulfate, a heparin antagonist, is administered.

7. The pericardium is usually left open so that accumulating drainage does not produce cardiac tamponade.

Closure of Femoral Incisions

1. The femoral catheters are removed, and the arteriotomies are closed with nonabsorbable cardiovascular suture. Compression tapes and bulldog clamps, if used, are removed.

2. The incision is closed with absorbable sutures, and the skin is closed with interrupted or continuous sutures.

3. Dressings are applied to all incisions.

PERICARDIECTOMY

Pericardiectomy is the partial excision of the adhered, thickened fibrotic pericardium to relieve constriction of compressed heart and large blood vessels. The adhered portions of the scarred, thickened pericardium restrict diastolic filling and myocardial contractility. As the pericardial space is obliterated and calcification of the pericardium occurs, the heart is further compressed. Ascites, elevated venous pressure, decreased arterial pressure, edema, and hepatic enlargement result. In most patients the etiology is unknown although there are documented cases caused by chronic pericarditis, which may be of tubercular, rheumatic, viral, or neoplastic origin. Either the supine position or the left lateral position may be used for a left anterolateral thoracotomy (Lachman et al, 2009; Kouchoukos et al, 2003).

Procedural Considerations

The use of CPB is rare, but it may be requested on a standby basis. The supplies and instruments for bypass should be available.

Operative Procedure

1. The lungs are hypoinflated to enhance exposure of the heart. The right and left phrenic nerves are identified and carefully protected. The pericardium is incised.

2. The outer, thickened pericardium is removed as indicated. Cartilage scissors may be required. The fibrous portions adhering to the atria and ventricles are carefully dissected with dry dissectors and scissors. Caution is exercised to prevent perforation of the atria and right ventricle; thus small islands of adherent pericardium may be retained.

3. Dissection is continued, and the large blood vessels are exposed and freed as indicated.

4. Drainage catheters are placed near the heart or through the pleural spaces, and connections to the water-seal drainage system are established.

SURGERY FOR CORONARY ARTERY DISEASE

The growth of minimally invasive surgical techniques (including off-pump CABGs) and percutaneous coronary interventions (PCIs) is most evident in the treatment of CAD. PCIs with bare metal or drug-eluting stents are performed in more than 2 million patients annually. Although there is some evidence that drug-eluting stents have a higher rate of thrombotic occlusion than bare metal stents, Kirtane and colleagues (2009) found comparable results with either type of stent.

When compared to PCI with stent insertion, CABG remains the standard of care for patients with left main or three-vessel CAD (Serruys et al, 2009; Patel et al, 2009; Li et al, 2009) although there is ongoing controversy about the preference for PCI or CABG among subsets of patients with CAD (Smith, 2009). Hybrid rooms facilitate a combination of both traditional surgical techniques and fluoroscopically guided PCI.

In addition to PCI, revascularization procedures for the ischemic myocardium include an expanding array of options such as port-access, robotic, endoscopic, and video-assisted procedures using smaller thoracic or sternal incisions (Table 16-5). Other forms of revascularization include left ventricular aneurysmectomy and transmyocardial laser revascularization. Endoscopic saphenous vein and radial artery excision is performed frequently.

Off-pump coronary artery bypass (OPCAB) is popular, and procedures employing CPB can be performed with

TABLE 16-5

Thoracic Incisions

Incision	Position	Possible Indications	Special Patient Needs
Median sternotomy: Incision along center of sternum	Supine	Most adult cardiac procedures except those on branch pulmonary arteries, distal transverse aortic arch, and descending thoracic aorta; OPCAB	Padding for hands, elbows, feet/heels, back of head, dependent bony prominences
Mini-sternotomy: Partial upper or lower sternal incision starting either from sternal notch or from xiphoid process and extending to midportion of sternum; lower-end sternal splitting (LESS)	Supine	MAS, or OPCAB procedures	Same as median sternotomy
Parasternotomy: Resection of right or left costal cartilages (from second to fifth cartilage, depending on surgical target)	Supine; small roll may be placed under affected side	Left: MAS CABG Right: MAS CABG, valve procedures	Same as median sternotomy; risk of postoperative chest wall instability
Anterolateral thoracotomy: Curvilinear incision along subpectoral groove to axillary line	Supine with pad or pillow under operative site; arm supported in sling or overarm board; arm on unaffected side may be tucked along side	MAS, MIDCAB, trauma to anterior pericardium and left ventricle; repeat sternotomy	Padding for extremities; pillow or other device to elevate affected side; armboard or sling for arm on affected side
Left anterior mini-thoracotomy; right anterior mini-thoracotomy: One or more small incisions (or ports) on left or right side	Supine with small roll under affected side	Left: MAS, MIDCAB, port-access for robotic surgery Right: MAS valve procedures, surgery for atrial fibrillation ("mini-MAZE"); port-access for robotic surgery	Same as anterolateral thoracotomy
Lateral thoracotomy: Curvilinear incision along costochondral junction anteriorly to posterior border of scapula	Placed on side with arms extended and axilla and head supported; knees and legs protected	Lung biopsies; first-rib resection; lobectomy	Armboard, overarm board, axillary roll, padding for extremities, pillow between legs; sandbags, straps, wide tape, or other devices to support torso

TABLE 16-5

Thoracic Incisions—cont'd

Incision	Position	Possible Indications	Special Patient Needs
Posterolateral thoracotomy: Curvilinear incision from subpectoral crease below nipple, extended laterally and posteriorly along ribs almost to posterior midline below scapula (location of intercostal incision depends on surgical site); used less frequently with availability of VATS techniques	Lateral with arms extended and axilla and head supported; knees and legs protected	First-rib resection; lobectomy	Similar to needs for lateral thoracotomy
Transsternal bilateral anterior thoracotomy ("clamshell"): Submammary incision extending from one anterior axillary line to other across sternum at fourth interspace	Supine	Bilateral lung transplant; emergency access to heart when sternal saw not available	Same as median sternotomy; requires transection of left and right IMA
Subxiphoid incision: Vertical midline incision from over xiphoid process to about 10 cm inferiorly (may divide lower portion of sternum to enhance exposure)	Supine	Pericardial drainage, pericardial biopsy, attachment of pacemaker electrodes, MAS	Same as median sternotomy
Thoracoabdominal incision: Low curvilinear incision on left side extended to anterior midline, continued vertically down abdomen	Anterior thoracotomy with chest at 45-degree angle to table; abdomen supine	Thoracoabdominal aneurysm	Same as anterolateral thoracotomy

CABG, Coronary artery bypass graft; *IMA,* internal mammary artery; *MAS,* minimal access surgery; *MIDCAB,* minimal access direct coronary artery bypass; *OPCAB,* off-pump coronary artery bypass; *VATS,* video-assisted thoracoscopic surgery.

Adapted from Bishop P: Position the patient. In Phippen ML et al, editors: *Competency for safe patient care during operative and invasive procedures,* Denver, 2009, Competency and Credentialing Institute; Walton-Geer PS: Prevention of pressure ulcers in the surgical patient, *AORN J* 89(3):538-548, 2009.

minimally invasive systems (Sarin et al, 2009; Sellke et al, 2005). Table 16-6 lists revascularization procedures that can be performed using a variety of on- or off-pump techniques. Advantages of the minimally invasive techniques, with or without CPB, include more cosmetic incisions, less perioperative bleeding, fewer surgical wound infections, and earlier postoperative ambulation. Previous disadvantages attributed to OPCAB (e.g., more technically challenging, prolonged operative time, and less complete revascularization) have been overcome, as depicted in a review of two randomized, controlled trials that showed similar outcomes, including health-related quality of life (Angelini et al, 2009). Procoagulant activity in the first 24 hours after OPCAB increases the risk of graft thrombosis. Therefore perioperative anticoagulation therapy should be "more aggressive" than that for conventional CABG, according to Shimokawa and colleagues (2009, p. 1419). In patients with myocardial infarction (MI), off-pump CABG surgery performed within 6 hours of the onset of symptoms showed better results than CABG with CPB (Fattouch et al, 2009).

Distal and proximal anastomotic devices have the potential to make it easier to perform bypass procedures in confined spaces on a beating heart, but many of these devices require further refinement. These new vascular connectors employ a variety of designs: grasping hooks that attach the vein to the aorta, magnets, U clips, and other coupling systems (Nasso et al, 2009). Another innovative proximal anastomotic technique consists of a clampless device that reduces the risk of disrupting aortic atherosclerotic plaque, which may be dislodged and embolize after the application of a partial occlusion clamp (Shimokawa et al, 2009).

Standard surgical treatment of CAD includes myocardial revascularization with CABG by use of the internal (thoracic) mammary artery (IMA), greater saphenous vein, radial artery, and other autogenous arterial and venous conduits. CABG often alleviates angina pectoris and prolongs life in patients with CAD of the left main and left anterior descending coronary arteries (Serruys et al, 2009; Patel et al, 2009; Li et al, 2009). The IMA demonstrates excellent long-term patency (Morrow and Gersh, 2008), and this has promoted the use of arterial conduits such as the radial artery (Collins et al, 2008), especially in diabetic patients (Singh et al, 2008); the gastroepiploic artery (Sasaki, 2008); and the inferior epigastric artery (Tavilla et al, 2004). The saphenous vein remains an effective conduit when multiple grafts are needed (Ozcan et al, 2008). Although the majority of saphenous vein grafts currently are harvested via the endoscopic technique (see #3 in the outline on p. 751), a large study of approximately 2900 patients

TABLE 16-6

Types of Myocardial Revascularization

Acronym	Procedure Name	Incision	Indication
MIDCAB	Minimally invasive direct coronary artery bypass (infrequent)	Left anterolateral thoracotomy	Single left anterior descending (LAD) and/or diagonal coronary artery anastomosis with left internal mammary artery (LIMA)
LATCAB	Lateral anterior thoracotomy coronary artery bypass	Anterolateral thoracotomy	Saphenous vein or radial artery from descending aorta to circumflex coronary artery system
OPCAB	Off-pump coronary artery bypass	Median sternotomy with full or limited skin incision	Multiple anastomoses
TECAB (also called ECABG)	Totally endoscopic coronary artery bypass; endoscopic coronary artery bypass graft (CABG)	Thoracic ports	Multiple anastomoses; on or off bypass
PACAB (also called port-access CAB)	Port-access coronary artery bypass	Thoracic ports	Multiple anastomoses; robot may or may not be used
Robotic CAB	Minimally invasive surgery (MIS) employing robotic assistance	Thoracic ports, small incisions	Multiple anastomoses
Robotic or nonrobotic LTMR	Laser transmyocardial revascularization	Thoracic ports, small incisions	Multiple anastomoses
Hybrid	Combined surgery and percutaneous coronary intervention (PCI)	Sternotomy (usually)	CABG: LAD and/or diagonal coronary artery; PCI: lateral and/or posterior coronary arteries

Modified from McCarthy P: Surgical management of heart failure. In Libby P et al, editors: *Braunwald's heart disease*, ed 8, Philadelphia, 2008, Saunders; Bridges CR et al: The Society of Thoracic Surgeons practice guideline series: transmyocardial laser revascularization, *Ann Thorac Surg* 77:1494-1502, 2004; Yuh DD et al: Totally endoscopic robot-assisted transmyocardial revascularization, *J Thorac Cardiovasc Surg* 130(1):120-124, 2005.

(Lopes et al, 2009) has shown less optimal outcomes with the endovascular technique. The increasing number of reoperations for CAD has also stimulated the use of alternative conduits (Box 16-4).

Dysrhythmias, and AF in particular, are common after CABG and can lead to hemodynamic compromise, systemic embolism, the need for extended anticoagulation therapy (with its attendant risk of bleeding complications), cardiac pacing, patient discomfort and anxiety, and increased cost and length of stay. Preoperative, intraoperative, or early postoperative administration of amiodarone is effective in reducing the incidence of postoperative AF (Gray and Sethna, 2008).

Increasing controversy over gender differences and their effect on outcomes after CABG has stimulated perioperative practice guidelines for CABG in women (Babb, 2009; Edwards et al, 2005; Puskas et al, 2007; Toumpoulis et al, 2006) (Evidence for Practice, p. 716). In particular, the guidelines focus on use of the IMA, glycemic control, avoidance of anemia and hypothyroid states, the questionable value of hormone replacement therapy, and off-pump CABG.

Other ischemia-related disorders (including heart failure) that can benefit from surgery include postinfarction ventricular septal defect (VSD), mitral regurgitation (MR), and certain ventricular (e.g., tachycardia) and supraventricular (e.g., AF) dysrhythmias.

BOX 16-4

Alternative Conduits for Use as Coronary Bypass Grafts

♦ Splenic artery
♦ Lesser saphenous vein
♦ Cephalic vein
♦ Basilic vein
♦ Greater saphenous vein allografts (homografts)
♦ Synthetic grafts (e.g., Dacron, PTFE)

PTFE, Polytetrafluoroethylene
Modified from Hsia TY et al: Coronary artery disease. In Conte JV et al, editors: *The Johns Hopkins manual of cardiac surgical care*, ed 2, St Louis, 2008, Mosby.

Coronary Artery Bypass Grafts with Arterial and Venous Conduits

Operative Procedure

Coronary artery instruments are added to the basic setup for cardiac surgery.

1. A median sternotomy is performed as described.
2. Conduit preparation:
   a. *IMA.* A special retractor, such as the one shown in Figure 16-15, elevates the sternum to expose the IMA. The

surgeon dissects the IMA from its retrosternal bed until the necessary length is obtained (Figure 16-46). The surgeon clamps the exposed artery, cuts the IMA caudal to the clamp, and confirms that blood flow through the IMA is adequate. The surgeon may inject papaverine (or another antispasmodic drug) into the IMA lumen with a blunt-tip needle and then occlude the tip of the IMA with a small bulldog clamp. The surgeon may wrap the pedicle with a papaverine-soaked sponge and store the vessel in the left (or right) pleural space until needed. The remaining clamped portion of the distal IMA is ligated with a tie to prevent backbleeding. Occasionally, both right and left IMAs are used. Heparin is given before arterial grafts are clamped and cut to prevent intraluminal thrombosis.

b. Endoscopic IMA dissection can be performed through thoracic ports (see Table 16-6) inserted into the left anterior thorax at the level of the fourth intercostal space. Ligation of arterial branches and venous tributaries is performed with hemostatic clips and electrocoagulation.

c. *Radial artery.* Generally the artery is taken from the patient's nondominant arm; adequate blood flow through the ulnar artery must be confirmed (commonly by Doppler). The artery may be removed endoscopically or through a longitudinal incision beginning 3 cm distal to the elbow crease lateral to the biceps tendon and ending 1 cm before the wrist crease (Figure 16-47). The artery is exposed and mobilized with a vessel loop and harvested as a free graft with adjacent veins and fatty tissue. The artery is ligated proximally and distally after systemic heparinization. Papaverine may be injected into the lumen to reduce spasm. The arm incision is closed and may be dressed and repositioned along the patient's side; additional drapes may be applied to maintain sterility of the field.

d. *Gastroepiploic artery.* When an additional arterial conduit is needed, the gastroepiploic artery may be used, although the required entry into the peritoneum to dissect the artery increases the risk of postoperative complications (Figure 16-48).

e. *Saphenous vein.* The necessary length of saphenous vein is harvested from one or both legs either with video-assisted endoscopic techniques or (less commonly) by a traditional open incision (Figure 16-49). Tributaries on the leg side are ligated, electrocoagulated, or clipped. After the saphenous vein is dissected free, it is removed and tributaries on the vein side are ligated. The distal end of the vein is identified to place the vein in a reversed position so that the semilunar valves do not interfere with the flow of blood. The vein is flushed with heparinized blood or saline and kept moist until needed.

3. With the endoscopic technique, saphenous vein harvesting is performed through one to three incisions over the vein at the knee and at the ankle and the groin if necessary. The vein is located under direct vision; the remaining length of vein is excised using a 5-mm angled endoscope and endoscopic scissors. An endoscopic clip applier and bipolar electrocoagulation can be used to seal tributaries on the leg side. Once the vein is removed, the vein tributaries are ligated with silk ties. To reduce postoperative tunnel dead

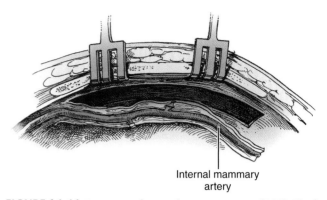

Internal mammary artery

FIGURE 16-46 Dissection of internal mammary artery (IMA). Bleeding from side branches is controlled by vascular clips on the IMA side and electrocoagulation on the sternal side. Dilute solution of papaverine is sprayed onto or into the lumen of the IMA to dilate the artery and reduce muscular spasm. The IMA pedicle is placed in the pleural cavity until needed for anastomosis.

space and minimize fluid accumulation, the leg is wrapped with a pressure bandage.

4. CPB with mild hypothermia is instituted. (If CABG is performed without CPB, the patient is not cooled. CPB standby is usually available.) Antegrade-retrograde cardioplegic solution is infused after the aorta is cross-clamped.

5. Coronary anastomoses using the saphenous vein, free arterial grafts, and in situ arterial grafts (e.g., IMA and gastroepiploic artery) are performed.

a. The affected coronary artery is identified, and a small incision is made into the artery. The graft conduit is beveled to approximate the incision (side-to-side jump grafts may be performed as well).

b. The anastomoses are made with fine cardiovascular sutures (Figure 16-50). Before each anastomosis is completed, the distal coronary artery may be probed to ensure patency.

6. Steps 5a and 5b are repeated for each subsequent anastomosis.

7. The distal anastomosis of the IMA to the coronary artery is done as described for the anastomosis of the saphenous vein graft to the coronary artery. No aortic (proximal) anastomosis is required because the IMA remains attached proximally to the subclavian artery. Because the IMA has demonstrated superior long-term patency—and the left anterior descending (LAD) coronary artery is a critical source of blood to the left ventricle—the IMA is commonly attached to the LAD coronary artery.

8. Aortic anastomoses:

a. Proximal aortic anastomoses may be performed with a partial occlusion clamp but more often the anastomoses are performed during a single aortic cross-clamping to avoid excessive manipulation of the aorta that could lead to intimal injury or dislodgment of atherosclerotic material. Increasingly, the aorta is assessed with TEE before the anastomoses are performed to identify proximal anastomotic sites that are relatively free of atherosclerotic plaque. After the proximal anastomoses are completed, the aortic cross-clamp is removed and the heart is defibrillated. Assessment of the aorta

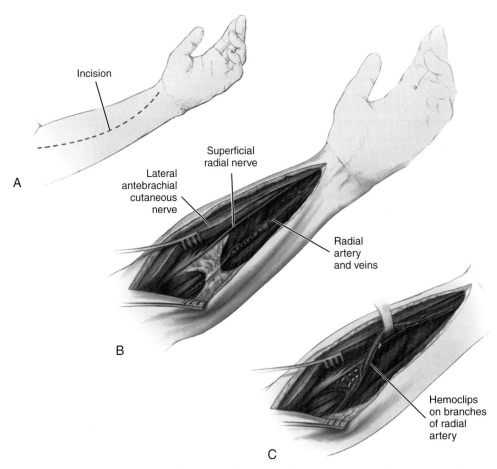

FIGURE 16-47 Dissection of radial artery. Before removal of the radial artery, Allen's test is performed to ensure that the ulnar artery will provide sufficient blood flow to the hand if the radial artery is excised: the radial and ulnar arteries are compressed to produce blanching of the hand. The ulnar artery is released while compression is maintained on the radial artery. The skin on the palm of the hand should immediately become red as blood flow is restored through the ulnar artery to the hand. **A,** Incision line. **B,** Deep forearm dissection exposes the radial artery and vein pedicle. **C,** Radial artery pedicle is mobilized, and the multiple side branches are clipped. The artery is removed and may be irrigated with a vasodilator. A continuous intravenous infusion of diltiazem helps to prevent vasoconstriction of the artery.

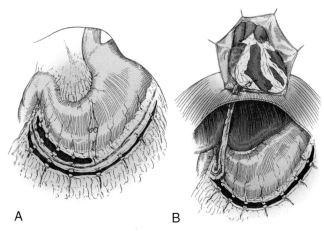

FIGURE 16-48 Right gastroepiploic artery mobilization. **A,** Branches to the stomach are divided with clamps and ties; omental branches may be divided with a staple gun. The gastroepiploic pedicle is isolated proximally to its origin from the gastroduodenal artery. **B,** The pedicle is brought up into the pericardium and anastomosed to the right coronary artery (shown here). The artery can also be grafted to the distal right and left anterior descending coronary arteries.

is especially helpful during *beating heart surgery* (usually through a median sternotomy) that requires proximal aortic anastomoses (with a saphenous vein or other free graft) to be completed while the heart is contracting. After identification of a suitable site (i.e., relatively free of plaque), the proximal anastomoses may be performed with a partial occlusion clamp. The aorta is partially occluded with an angled vascular clamp, and a small segment is resected (approximately the diameter of the vein graft). The aortotomy is made with a knife blade and the opening is enlarged with a punch (Figure 16-51).

b. The conduit is anastomosed, end to side, to the aorta with fine vascular sutures (Figure 16-52). The partial occlusion clamp (if used) is removed, so that the proximal portion of the vein graft can fill with blood. Needle aspiration of the vein graft is performed to prevent air from entering the coronary circulation.

c. When proximal anastomoses are performed during a single period of cross-clamping, air is aspirated from the grafts before the cross-clamp is removed.

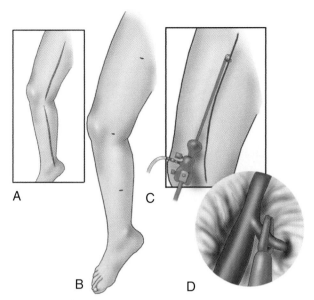

FIGURE 16-49 Excision of greater saphenous vein. **A,** Traditional open incision. **B,** Incision sites (ankle, knee, groin) for video-assisted, endoscopic vein harvesting. **C,** Endoscope inserted into medial knee incision and used to dissect the vein. **D,** Venous tributaries may be divided and electrocoagulated or clipped on the leg side; silk ties are commonly used on the vein side.

9. The aortic anastomoses of the vein grafts may be marked with radiopaque clips or rings for future identification.
10. Cardiopulmonary bypass is discontinued, and the sternum is closed.
11. Minimally invasive procedures:
    a. Minimally invasive direct coronary artery bypass (MIDCAB) may be performed, albeit less frequently, in patients with lesions (e.g., narrowings in the LAD and diagonal coronary arteries) that are easily accessible through an anterior thoracotomy. Beating heart procedures performed through a median sternotomy allow surgeons to access lateral and posterior arteries. When endovascular CPB and cardioplegic solution are used, more lateral and posterior arteries (e.g., obtuse marginal and right coronary arteries) may be grafted because ventricular fibrillation secondary to stimulation of the heart is obviated with induced cardioplegic arrest. A double-lumen endotracheal tube may be inserted so that the left lung can be hypoventilated to enhance visualization of the LAD (and the IMA) while the right lung is ventilated sufficiently to oxygenate pulmonary blood flow.
    b. With OPCAB, cardiac contraction may pose a technical difficulty for the surgeon in creating a precise anastomosis. Coronary stabilizers are used to reduce the motion of the heart in the vicinity of the anastomosis (Figure 16-53). These attachments fit onto the retractor, thereby freeing the surgeon's hands to suture the anastomosis. Left ventricular apical suction cups allow the apex to be retracted, thereby exposing lateral and posterior coronary arteries (see Figure 16-17). Pharmacologic cardiac motion reduction has been achieved with beta-blocker drugs and adenosine, but the newer stabilizers have reduced the need for these drugs. Bleeding from

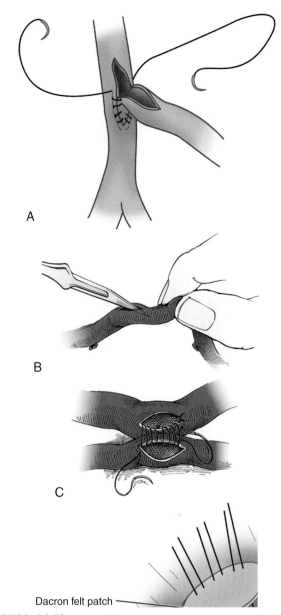

Dacron felt patch

FIGURE 16-50 **A,** End-to-side coronary anastomosis with bypass graft conduit. Side-to-side coronary anastomosis with bypass graft conduit. **B,** Arteriotomy made with #11 blade is shown. **C,** Double-ended suture used to create anastomosis. **D,** Completed anastomosis. Side-to-side anastomoses are used to make more than one attachment of a conduit to an artery, especially when there may be insufficient available conduit material.

the arteriotomy (because of the continued beating of the heart) obscures the field; a fine mist of humidified CO_2 gas sprayed over the anastomotic site and the use of elastic coronary artery tourniquets may be used to control bleeding.
    c. Port-access procedures (Figure 16-54) may be performed with a robot and the use of endovascular catheters (see Figure 16-45). Anastomoses are achieved with video-assisted thoracoscopic techniques. If better visualization is desired or required, the surgeon can convert to a median sternotomy.

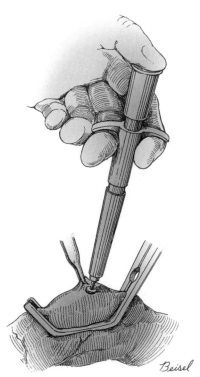

FIGURE 16-51 Proximal anastomosis of bypass graft. A partial occlusion clamp isolates the portion of the ascending aorta where the aortotomy is to be made with the punch.

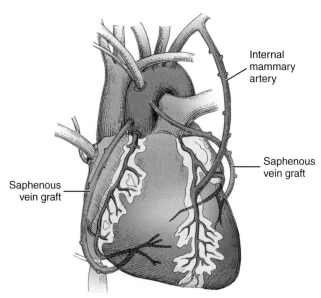

Internal mammary artery

Saphenous vein graft

Saphenous vein graft

FIGURE 16-52 Coronary artery bypass grafts with reversed saphenous vein and the left internal mammary artery.

Laser Transmyocardial Revascularization

Patients with chronic, severe angina who cannot be revascularized with either coronary bypass surgery or PCI may be appropriate candidates for laser transmyocardial revascularization (TMR) (Horvath and Zhou, 2007). Channels are created in the left ventricular wall with laser energy (e.g., CO_2, holmium:yttrium-aluminum-garnet [Ho:YAG]). Endoscopic,

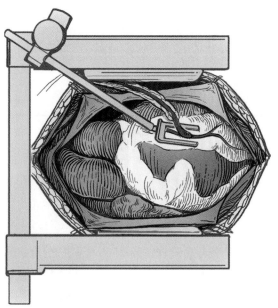

FIGURE 16-53 Coronary anastomotic site stabilizer used during beating heart bypass surgery. The horseshoe-shaped foot has a non-smooth surface to provide an atraumatic grip on the epicardium, reduce the movement of the beating heart, and isolate the target coronary artery site for anastomosis.

laser, robot-assisted TMR can further enhance the role of TMR as a surgical treatment or as an adjunct to PCI. Laser safety precautions should be followed.

Ventricular Aneurysmectomy

Left ventricular aneurysmectomy (LVA) is the excision of an aneurysmal portion of the left ventricle and reinforcement with synthetic patch material. LVA is a form of left ventricular reconstruction undertaken to optimize cardiac function. An aneurysm of the left ventricle occasionally develops after a severe myocardial infarction in which part of the myocardium is replaced by thin scar tissue that can rupture. The LV undergoes *remodeling* when the scar stretches as a result of the left ventricular pressure and forms an aneurysm (McCarthy, 2008). The aneurysm is usually adherent to the pericardium; it may not be possible to dissect it free until CPB has been established.

Procedural Considerations. The patient is placed in the supine position. The setup is the same as that described for open-heart surgery, with the addition of synthetic patch material, Teflon felt pledgets, and 0, 3-0, and 4-0 cardiovascular sutures. Occasionally, Teflon felt strips are required to bolster the suture lines. Patch closure of the ventriculotomy (endoaneurysmorrhaphy) is performed more often than the traditional excision, plication, and oversewing of the ventricular tissue. Patch closure better preserves the geometry of the left ventricle (McCarthy, 2008; Lundblad et al, 2009).

Operative Procedure
1. A median sternotomy is performed, and CPB is begun as previously described.
2. The scar tissue of the ventricle is excised, and any clot is carefully removed (Figure 16-55, *A* and *B*).

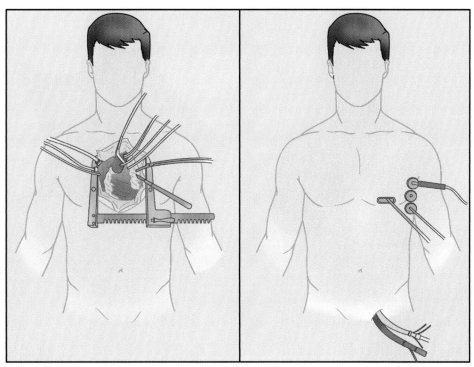

FIGURE 16-54 Traditional sternotomy *(left)* compared with minimally invasive incisions *(right)* that provide access to the heart and to the femoral artery and vein.

3. A circular cuff of scar tissue is left, through which a purse-string suture with felt pledgets is placed through the rim of the scar (Figure 16-55, *C*).
4. A patch of woven Dacron is sewn to the rim with interrupted sutures (Figure 16-55, *D*). A second (internal) patch of pericardium may be placed for hemostasis.
5. The edge of the patch is reinforced with a running suture (Figure 16-55, *E*).
6. The left ventricle may be vented with a catheter inserted into the right superior pulmonary vein; after the ventricle is deaired, the catheter is removed and closure of the incision completed.

Postinfarction Ventricular Septal Defect. Ventricular septal or free-wall rupture is a catastrophic complication of myocardial infarction, creating an acute left-to-right shunt and cardiac failure requiring early surgical repair. The defect is closed with a prosthetic patch and other materials commonly used for postinfarction ventricular aneurysm. Felt strips and plicating sutures may be used to reinforce the suture line (McCarthy, 2008).

SURGERY FOR HEART FAILURE

Early procedures to reconstruct the left ventricle, introduced by Batista and modified by Dor, were developed for patients with heart failure mainly caused by ischemic coronary disease and hypertension (McCarthy, 2008). The dilated, hypokinetic portions of the ventricle are excised and repaired to produce a more efficient pumping chamber. Techniques for ventricular reconstruction have expanded options for surgical treatment of heart failure. Additional interventions include mitral valve repair (see following section) for ischemic mitral regurgitation

(de Varennes et al, 2009), mechanical and biologic support, and cardiac transplantation (described later).

SURGERY FOR THE MITRAL VALVE

Mitral *stenosis* (MS) is a narrowing of the valve orifice such that it causes impedance to forward blood flow. It is often caused by rheumatic fever. The normal orifice area of the valve is about 5 cm². As the disease progresses, the mitral valve becomes a narrow slit in a fibrotic plaque, severely limiting blood flow into the left ventricle. MS causes a rise in pressure and dilation of the left atrium. This pressure is transmitted throughout the pulmonary vascular bed, with subsequent pulmonary hypertension, right ventricular hypertrophy, and possibly tricuspid valve regurgitation (Otto and Bonow, 2008). The major symptoms of MS are dyspnea, fatigue, and orthopnea. Late findings are severe pulmonary congestion and right ventricular failure. A characteristic diastolic murmur is heard, and AF is not unusual. Thromboembolism may result from stasis of blood in the left atrial appendage.

Mitral *regurgitation* (MR) occurs when the valve leaflets do not close properly or when the leaflets are perforated and blood escapes back into the left atrium during ventricular systole (Stout and Verrier, 2009). Common causes of MR are myxomatous degeneration and a secondary result of aortic valve stenosis. Other causes of MR are degenerative, ischemic, and dilated cardiomyopathy. During ventricular diastole, the blood regurgitated into the left atrium augments blood volume entering the left ventricle. MR may accompany MS or be attributable to leaflet tears, annular dilation, or elongated or ruptured chordae. Ischemic heart disease may produce papillary muscle dysfunction, which prevents sufficient anchoring of the leaf-

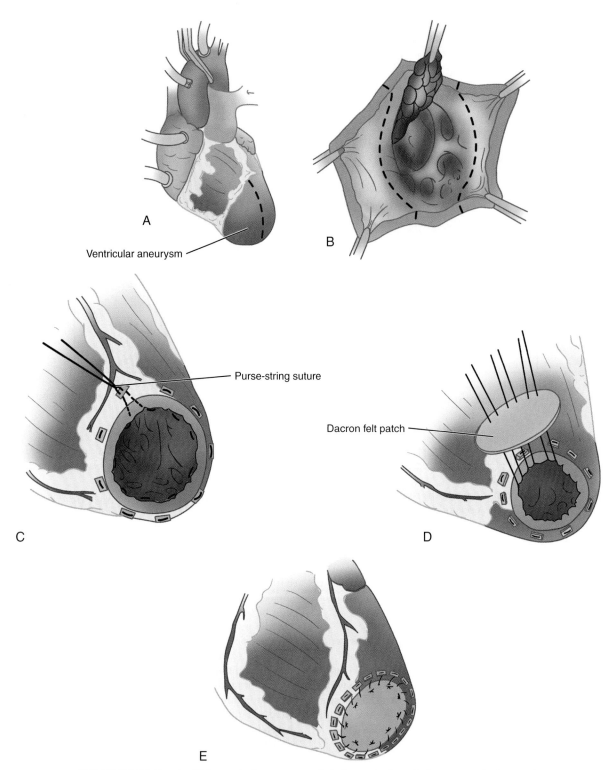

Ventricular aneurysm

Purse-string suture

Dacron felt patch

FIGURE 16-55 Repair of left ventricular aneurysm. **A,** Left ventricular apical aneurysm. **B,** Intracavitary clot is removed. **C,** Pledgetted sutures placed around the edge of the excised ventricular tissue. **D,** A patch is inserted. **E,** Completed repair.

lets in the closed position. Symptoms are primarily dyspnea on exertion and easy fatigability related to pulmonary congestion.

The surgeon's selection of the procedure (repair or replacement) is determined by the mitral valve anatomy, stage of disease, presence or absence of calcification, history of thromboembolism and dysrhythmia, the patient's ability to tolerate long-term anticoagulation therapy (required after insertion of a mechanical valve prosthesis), the patient's willingness to undergo reoperation if a bioprosthesis deteriorates, and additional associated pathologic defects (Kumar, 2008). Improvements in imaging capabilities with two-dimensional, three-dimensional, and color-flow Doppler echocardiography have enabled surgeons to diagnose more precisely and subsequently to identify the most appropriate reparative procedure (Lee and Bonow, 2008). Improved imaging has also fostered the development of a consistent nomenclature to describe specific segments of the mitral valve leaflet anatomy. Quill and colleagues (2009), building on the studies of Kumar and associates (1995) and the classic work of Carpentier (1983), have suggested dividing each mitral leaflet into an alpha-numeric system: (1) the *anterior* leaflet is divided into three sections that are designated from the lateral to the medial position (left to right): *A1* (lateral), *A2* (middle), and *A3* (medial); (2) the *posterior* leaflet is divided into three sections that are designated (left to right): *P1* (lateral), *P2* (middle), and *P3* (medial) (see mitral valve in Figure 16-6, *B*). The goal of this system is to provide consistent descriptions for planning, performing, and documenting the care for this highly variable, complex, and dynamic structure.

Consistency in description also promotes reproducibility of the reparative procedures performed to preserve the native valve. Mitral valve repair is widely employed because the complications associated with prosthetic replacement and anticoagulation therapy can be avoided. The technique selected must be tailored to the unique pathophysiologic findings; therefore the surgeon carefully evaluates the leaflets and related structures at the time of surgery before deciding which procedure to perform. Because there is a possibility that the valve may have to be replaced, instruments (and prostheses) for replacement as well as repairs should be available. Also included are atrial handheld or self-retaining retractors, obturators for sizing prosthetic rings and valves, sizer or prosthesis handles, and special sutures if requested. Bicaval cannulation often is used to enhance exposure of the operative field and to decompress the heart (see Figure 16-36). TEE is used to establish a cardiac functional baseline and to confirm efficacy of the repair both after the cross-clamp is removed and the heart resumes beating and after bypass is discontinued. TEE is also used intraoperatively to assess left ventricular function and to detect the presence of air (seen as white specks) within the cardiac chambers.

Mitral Valve Repairs

Open Commissurotomy of the Mitral Valve for Mitral Stenosis.
Open commissurotomy is the separation of fused, adherent leaflets of the mitral valve.

PROCEDURAL CONSIDERATIONS. The patient is placed in the supine position for a median sternotomy. The setup is the same as that described for open-heart procedures, with mitral valve instruments.

OPERATIVE PROCEDURE
1. A median sternotomy is performed, and bicaval cannulation is performed for CPB.
2. The left atrium is incised, and the valve is inspected; in some cases, a transseptal approach (right atrium to left atrium) may be used.
3. Fused leaflets are separated with vascular forceps and scissors or a knife (Figure 16-56). A dilator may be used to enlarge the mitral valve orifice.
4. The valve is again inspected for any resultant insufficiency.
5. An annuloplasty ring may be inserted to reinforce the repair.
6. The left atrium is closed with a continuous cardiovascular suture.

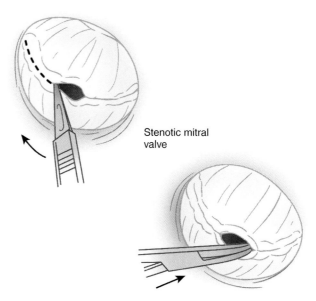

FIGURE 16-56 Mitral commissurotomy (see text).

Stenotic mitral valve

Mitral Annuloplasty for Mitral Regurgitation.
Mitral annuloplasty is the reduction of a dilated annulus by inserting a prosthetic ring. Although it has been assumed that only the posterior leaflet is subject to annular dilation, it has been demonstrated that the anterior portion can also be affected. Prostheses are available to repair the entire circumference of the annulus (see Figure 16-32, *A*) or only the posterior leaflet (see Figure 16-32, *B*). The techniques (and associated prostheses) introduced by Carpentier (1983) and others continue to expand.

OPERATIVE PROCEDURE
1. The left atrium is incised, and sump suctions are inserted into the atrial cavity to remove blood.
2. The annulus, leaflets, chordae, and the rest of the mitral complex are inspected.
3. If generalized annular dilation is present, an annuloplasty ring is inserted; a C-shaped ring may be used for dilation affecting the posterior leaflet (see Figure 16-32). An obturator is used to determine the appropriate-size ring (Figure 16-57, *A*). Interrupted sutures are placed around the circumference of the annulus and then into the ring (Figure 16-57, *B*). When the stitches are tied, the excess annular tissue of the posterior leaflet is evenly drawn up against the prosthesis (Figure 16-57, *C*).
4. The valve is inspected for competency; a bulb syringe filled with saline may be used to distend the ventricle and confirm the competence of the valve leaflets. The left atrium is closed.

Mitral Valvuloplasty Repairs for Mitral Regurgitation.
Mitral valvuloplasty is the repair of the valve leaflets or related structures. Selection of the appropriate repair for perforated or redundant valve leaflets or for shortened or elongated chordae tendineae requires careful assessment and evaluation of the abnormalities present. Historically most mitral valve repairs have been performed on the posterior leaflet, but a number of anterior leaflet repairs have been developed (see steps 5 to 8 in the following Operative Procedure).

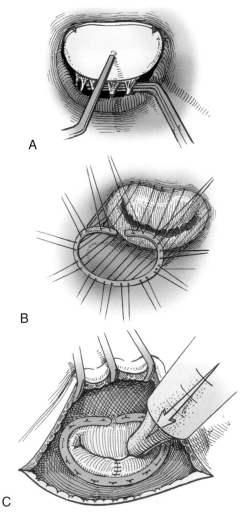

FIGURE 16-57 Mitral valve annuloplasty (see text).

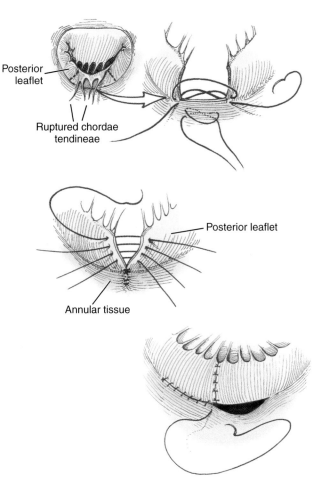

FIGURE 16-58 Quadrangular resection of nonsupported posterior leaflet tissue caused by ruptured chordae tendineae (see text). A similar technique can be used to resect *redundant* tissue causing mitral regurgitation.

OPERATIVE PROCEDURE

1. Perforated leaflets can be patched with pericardium.
2. Redundant, prolapsed *posterior* leaflet tissue can be resected (Figure 16-58). The cut edges of the posterior leaflet are sewn together, and the corresponding annular segment is plicated. An annuloplasty ring is inserted to reinforce the leaflet repair and reduce annular dilation.
3. Shortened, fused chordae tendineae can be lengthened and mobilized by their division into secondary chordae or by incising the tip of the papillary muscles.
4. Redundant tissue of elongated chordae may be implanted into the papillary muscle head or folded over itself and secured with a suture (rarely performed).
5. *Anterior* leaflet prolapse is a greater challenge and traditionally has been an indication for valve replacement. A small triangular resection of the anterior leaflet (reinforced with annuloplasty ring insertion) can be performed.
6. Elongated or ruptured chordae may be replaced with polytetrafluoroethylene (PTFE) suture (Figure 16-59).
7. A chordal flip procedure (Figure 16-60) can be used to reestablish chordal attachment to the *anterior* leaflet. A section of the posterior leaflet with attached chordae is cut, swung over to the anterior leaflet, and sewn onto the anterior leaflet. The remaining posterior leaflet defect is closed with suture (see step 2).

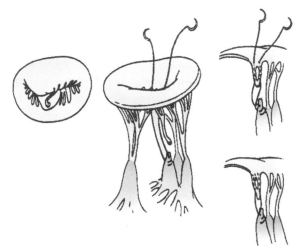

FIGURE 16-59 Chordal replacement with polytetrafluoroethylene (PTFE) (see text).

8. The edge-to-edge technique introduced by Alfieri and colleagues (2001) can be used to repair mitral valves with bileaflet prolapse (i.e., both the *anterior* and *posterior* leaflets are incompetent, producing severe MR). The free edges of the mitral leaflets are approximated, and a figure-of-eight suture (or percutaneously delivered clip) is placed in the central por-

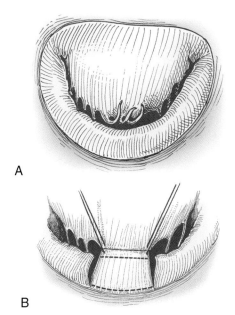

A

B

FIGURE 16-60 Chordal flip procedure. Although portions of the posterior leaflet can be resected with success, the same is not true of the anterior leaflet because the shape of the valve and the coaptation margin are altered. **A,** When there are ruptured chordae of the *anterior* leaflet of the mitral valve, the flip procedure can be used to reestablish chordal support for the anterior leaflet. **B,** A portion of normal posterior leaflet tissue with attached chordae is cut, swung over, and sewn onto the flail segment of the anterior leaflet.

tion of the apposed leaflets. This creates a double-orifice mitral valve that can significantly reduce MR and preserve the native valve (Mascagni et al, 2005). Frequently an annuloplasty ring supplements the Alfieri technique (Fedak et al, 2008).

Percutaneous mitral valve repair employing various devices and delivery methods is under investigation. The complex nature of the mitral valve apparatus poses particular challenges to avoid injury to the valve components or other cardiac structures (Fedak et al, 2008).

Mitral Valve Replacement

Mitral valve replacement (MVR) is the excision of the mitral valve leaflets and replacement with a mechanical or biologic prosthesis. Generally, the mural (posterior) leaflet and associated chordae and papillary muscles are retained to maintain left ventricular configuration (*geometry*), thereby enhancing postoperative ventricular function. If possible, the anterior leaflet is also retained if it does not interfere with prosthetic function and it is not too heavily calcified.

Median sternotomy is performed in most cases, but right thoracotomy incisions are useful in selected cases (e.g., reoperation, especially in patients with CABG IMA and vein grafts to the LV coronary circulation). Minimally invasive (and robotic) procedures on the mitral valve can also use right and left thoracotomy incisions or ports.

Procedural Considerations. Although the surgeon may intend to implant a specific type of prosthesis, patient-related factors (Box 16-5) or prosthetic valve complications (Box 16-6) may modify the plan (Oakley et al, 2008). A complete range of the surgeon's preferred valves should be available, as well as saline to rinse the glutaraldehyde storage solution (see Risk Reduction

---

Strategies box on p. 730) from biologic prostheses if they are used. Pledgetted sutures of alternating colors are used, and suture holders may be available additionally to keep the stitches in the correct order. Venting catheters and aspirating needles are used to remove air from the heart and ascending aorta. A small dental mirror may be used after a bioprosthesis has been implanted to ensure that sutures are not caught in the struts of the valve.

Operative Procedure. Double venous cannulation is used.

1. The aorta is cross-clamped, and cardioplegic solution is infused through the aortic root and/or retrograde through the coronary sinus.

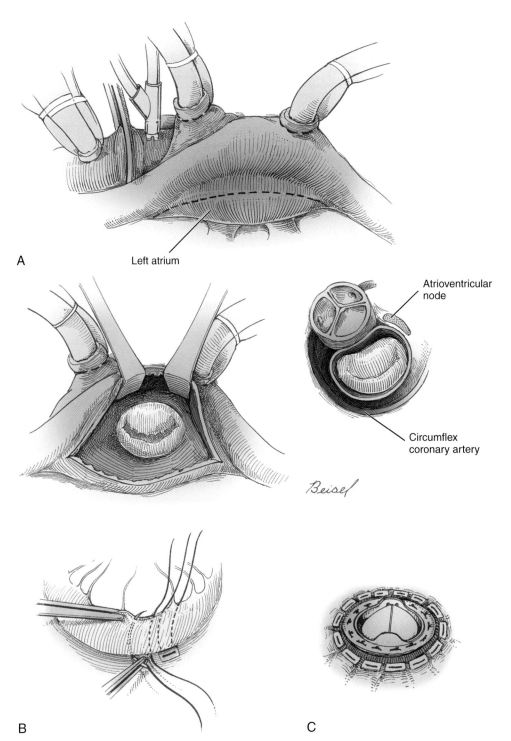

A Left atrium

Atrioventricular node

Circumflex coronary artery

Beisel

B   C

FIGURE 16-61 Mitral valve replacement. **A,** Line of incision and cannulation for bypass, anatomic relationship between mitral and aortic valves with location of conduction node, and exposure of valve. **B,** Placement of pledgetted double-armed sutures in native valve annulus. **C,** Completed valve replacement.

2. The left atrium is incised along the interatrial groove to expose the mitral valve (Figure 16-61, *A*).
3. The valve is assessed, and the anterior leaflet is excised. The posterior leaflet and occasionally the anterior leaflet are retained to enhance the ventricular configuration and postoperative function. Rongeurs may be used to debride heavy calcification; loose debris is removed. A margin of the valve

annulus is retained to insert fixation sutures to the prosthesis (Figure 16-61, *B*).
4. A valve sizer is used to determine the correct size of the prosthesis, which is delivered to the field.
5. Nonabsorbable cardiovascular sutures (15 to 20 or more) are placed in the annulus of the valve and then placed into the sewing ring of the prosthesis.

6. The sutures are held taut (and moistened with saline) as the prosthesis is guided into position and secured, and the sutures are tied and cut (Figure 16-61, *C*).
7. Continuous nonabsorbable sutures are used to partially close the atriotomy. The patient is placed in the Trendelenburg position, and the lungs are inflated to remove air from the pulmonary veins and atrium. Air is aspirated from the left ventricle through a hypodermic needle inserted into the LV apex or through the vent catheter, and the atrial closure is completed.

Endoscopic, video-assisted, robotic mitral valve surgery has progressed from a technical curiosity to an acceptable method (albeit with a significant learning curve) of intracardiac, telemanipulated valve repair. Both mitral valve repair and replacement have been performed with these techniques (Figure 16-62), as well as procedures to correct other intracardiac structural lesions (Chitwood, 2005; Chitwood et al, 2008).

SURGERY FOR THE TRICUSPID VALVE

Right-sided valve disease "deserves a little more respect" according to the title of a review by Bruce and Connolly (2009, p. 2726). The authors recommend more aggressive therapy in patients with both tricuspid and pulmonary valve disease before clinical deterioration occurs. Among the treatment options for tricuspid valve disease are suture annuloplasty, ring annuloplasty, and valve replacement with either a biologic or a mechanical prosthesis. Percutaneous approaches have been investigated in the experimental setting (Rogers and Bolling, 2009).

Like the mitral valve, the tricuspid annulus is saddle-shaped and techniques to repair the valve should consider this anatomic configuration for optimal repair (Rogers and Bolling, 2009). Annuloplasty ring insertion may be preferable to suture annuloplasty (Tang et al, 2006; Bruce and Connolly, 2009).

Tricuspid Valve Annuloplasty

Tricuspid valve annuloplasty reduces a dilated annulus with a suture technique (Rabago et al, 1980) or a prosthetic ring. Tricuspid valve regurgitation may be caused by bacterial or viral endocarditis, the presence of a pacemaker or defibrillator lead through the valve annulus, or the functional result of mitral valve disease. After mitral valve correction, tricuspid valve function may return to normal, although this theory has been questioned (Rogers and Bolling, 2009; Bruce and Connolly, 2009). Preoperatively, if the tricuspid annular dilation is diagnosed to be severe, ring repair (similar to mitral annuloplasty) or valve replacement may be performed. Caution is taken to avoid injury to the conduction tissue in the area of the AV node. A pulmonary artery catheter is usually not inserted preoperatively because it can interfere with the surgical field. A catheter may be inserted after the repair is completed.

Patients with significant tricuspid stenosis or regurgitation or failed tricuspid (suture or ring) annuloplasty may require insertion of a prosthetic biologic or mechanical valve (Bruce and Connolly, 2009). There are no specific tricuspid prosthetic valves; rather, a mitral prosthesis would be implanted.

Operative Procedure

1. Double venous cannulae are inserted so that they do not cross one another in the right atrium, and occluding tapes are tightened around the cavae and cannulae to prevent venous return from entering the right atrium and obscur-

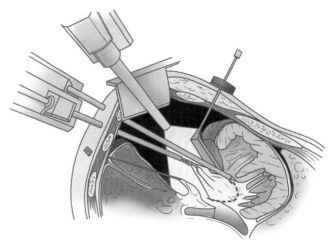

FIGURE 16-62 The 1-cm robotic instrument arms are placed through the chest wall. A transthoracic retractor arm elevates the interatrial septum toward the sternum. The three-dimensional camera is placed through a 4-cm incision, which also serves as a working port for the assistant.

ing the surgical site. A right-angled venous cannula may be placed into the superior vena cava to enhance exposure.
2. The right atrium is opened longitudinally to expose the tricuspid valve. Sump suctions are inserted to remove coronary sinus drainage.
3. In the DeVega (Rabago et al, 1980) suture annuloplasty technique (Figure 16-63), a double-armed, felt-pledgetted suture is placed in the valve annulus, beginning at the anteroseptal commissure and continued around to the level of the coronary sinus orifice. The remaining arm of suture is similarly placed. The suture is tied over a pledget with sufficient tension to reduce the annular area to the size desired.
4. In the ring annuloplasty technique, a prosthetic ring is inserted in a manner similar to that used for mitral valve annuloplasty (see Figure 16-57).
5. For valve replacement, the surgeon selects the desired prosthesis and inserts it in a manner similar to that for mitral valve replacement (see Figure 16-61).
6. Saline may be injected into the ventricle to test the competence of the repair, and TEE is also employed.
7. The right atrium is closed with nonabsorbable suture.

SURGERY FOR THE PULMONARY VALVE

Pulmonary valve surgery in the adult is unusual, although patients with genetic deformities or those who have undergone repair of congenital pulmonary valve or right ventricular outflow tract obstruction may present with significant pulmonary valve disease (Bruce and Connolly, 2009). Generally mild or moderate pulmonary stenosis (PS) produces few symptoms. For patients with severe PS, treatment options include valvulotomy or valve replacement via percutaneous or standard surgical techniques. Generally an aortic bioprosthesis or an allograft is inserted for valve replacement.

SURGERY FOR THE AORTIC VALVE

Aortic *stenosis* (AS) produces obstruction to left ventricular outflow. Whether caused by rheumatic fever, a congenital

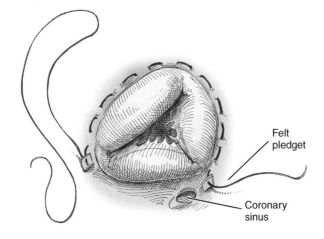

Felt
pledget

Coronary
sinus

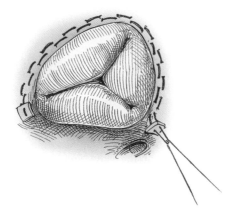

FIGURE 16-63 DeVega tricuspid valve suture annuloplasty.

bicuspid valve, or calcification, the fused valve leaflets present an increasing resistance to left ventricular outflow, thus increasing the pressure inside the left ventricle. Recent histopathologic and clinical data suggest that calcified AS is not a "degenerative" passive process but, rather, an active and possibly inflammatory disease process (Otto and Bonow, 2008).

To compensate for the increased pressure load, the ventricle hypertrophies so that it can generate sufficient pressure to eject blood through the narrowed opening. When disease is severe, large pressure gradients are often measured during cardiac catheterization, with differences in systolic pressures between the ventricle and the aorta reaching 50 mm Hg or more. In the early stages of the disease, a systolic ejection murmur may be heard, but patients are rarely symptomatic. Eventually, fatigue, exertional dyspnea, angina pectoris, syncope, and congestive heart failure may develop, presenting a grave prognosis. Although infrequent, sudden death may be the first sign of AS in asymptomatic patients who are not well monitored (Coglianes and Davidoff, 2009; Dal-Bianco et al, 2008).

In developing countries aortic *insufficiency (regurgitation)* is most often caused by rheumatic fever, and in developed countries it is usually caused by congenital anomalies (commonly a bicuspid aortic valve) (Otto and Bonow, 2008). Although *repair* of the aortic valve is challenging because of the precise closing mechanism of the valve leaflets, aortic valve repara-

tive techniques have been employed successfully in selected patients (Otto and Bonow, 2008). Total valve excision and replacement with a prosthesis or an allograft are commonly performed.

Interventional percutaneous and minimally invasive techniques have been developed. Transcatheter aortic valve implantation performed in the cardiac catheterization laboratory is increasingly employed as a treatment option; long-term data are not widely available, but the trend is toward more percutaneous interventions in high-risk patients (Webb et al, 2009). Mini-sternotomy incisions can be employed although objective advantages over conventional sternotomy have not been seen with this technique (Brown et al, 2009).

In addition to selection of access, other challenges include the choice and size of a prosthetic valve. Selection is based on achieving appropriate hemodynamic function in relation to body size. The small aortic root (e.g., less than 21 mm) presents challenges to provide an adequate cardiac output. In patients with a small aortic annulus and large body mass (referred to as *patient/prosthesis mismatch*), the surgeon selects a prosthesis that will provide flow adequate to meet the body's needs. The stentless aortic valve (see Figure 16-27, *B*) is frequently used because of the excellent hemodynamics (Cheng et al, 2009). Patch enlargement of the small aortic root is another option (Feindel, 2006; Sellke and Ruel, 2009) (described in the following Operative Procedure), and the patient's own pulmonary valve can be used as an autograft to replace the aortic valve; the pulmonary valve is then replaced with an allograft. Allografts may be used to replace the aortic valve as well.

Aortic Valve Replacement

The aortic valve is excised and replaced with a mechanical or biologic prosthesis or an aortic valve allograft or autograft.

Procedural Considerations
To the basic setup the following may be added:

◆ Aortic valve instruments
◆ Aortic valves, sizers, and holders
◆ Coronary sinus retrograde-infusion cannula and venting catheters
◆ Saline and three basins to rinse the glutaraldehyde storage solution from bioprostheses
◆ Saline bath to thaw frozen allografts

Operative Procedure
1. After the institution of CPB, a left ventricular vent is inserted through a stab wound into the right superior pulmonary vein and the tip is advanced into the left ventricle. A retrograde cardioplegia catheter is inserted into the coronary sinus (Figure 16-64, *A*).
2. The aorta is cross-clamped. If aortic insufficiency is present, the initial bolus of cardioplegic solution is infused retrogradely; subsequent cardioplegic infusions are also given retrogradely. Occasionally, direct coronary perfusion (Figure 16-64, *B*) is given if a retrograde catheter cannot be inserted; however, direct perfusion is avoided when possible (because of the risk of injuring the coronary endothelium). If aortic stenosis is present, the initial bolus of cardioplegic solution may be infused by needle through the aorta into the aortic root. Once the heart is arrested, the aorta is opened.

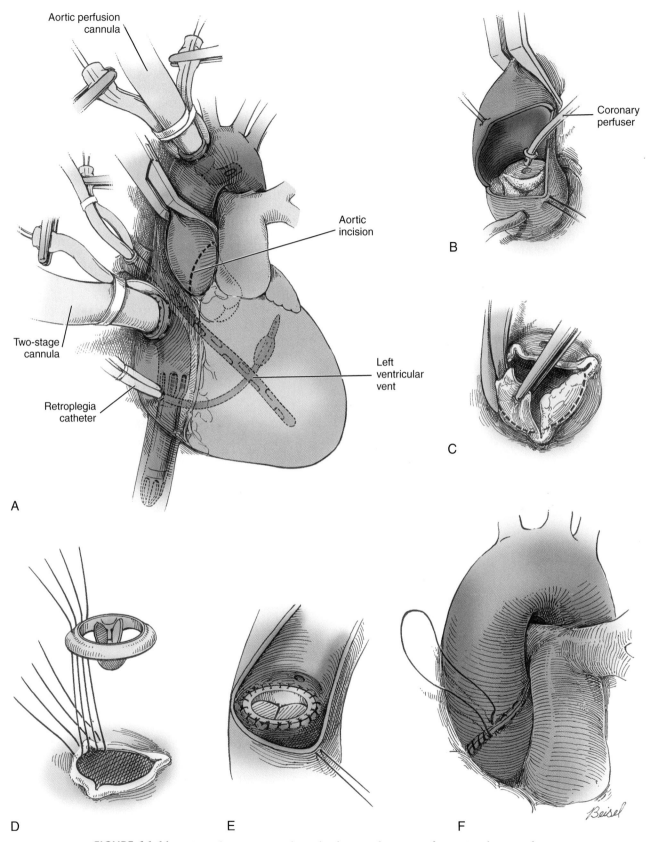

FIGURE 16-64 A, Cannulation, retrograde cardioplegia, and vent sites for aortic valve procedures. Note incision line. **B,** If retrograde cardioplegia is not used, handheld coronary ostial catheters can deliver antegrade cardioplegic solution. **C,** Diseased valve is completely excised. **D,** Sutures are placed in the valve annulus and the prosthetic sewing ring. **E,** Stitches are tied and cut. **F,** Closure of the aortic suture line.

3. The native valve is inspected. The valve is carefully excised to avoid injury to the annulus and underlying structures (Figure 16-64, *C*). Calcium is debrided from the annulus with scissors or rongeurs, or both. Narrow packing may be used in the left ventricle to confine small, loose, calcified fragments that could subsequently embolize. Instruments should frequently be wiped clean with a moist sponge.

4. The annulus is sized, the proper prosthesis is selected, and a prosthesis holder is attached.

5. a. If a biologic valve is selected, it is delivered to the field and rinsed in three saline baths according to the manufacturer's instructions (see Risk Reduction Strategies box on p. 730). Biologic valves should be kept moist with frequent saline rinsing; they should *not* be immersed in antibiotic solution.

   b. If an allograft is used, it is delivered to the field and thawed in saline baths according to protocol.

   c. If a mechanical valve is chosen, it should be protected from scratches or other injury.

6. a. The new valve is implanted (Figure 16-64, *D* and *E*) by use of a technique similar to that previously described for MVR.

   b. If the aortic annulus is too small to accept a prosthesis of adequate size, the annulus and proximal portion of the ascending aorta can be enlarged. A patch of bovine peri-cardium or Dacron graft can be placed longitudinally in the proximal anterior ascending aorta where the aortic annulus has been incised (Figure 16-65, *A* and *B*). The valve prosthesis is sutured to the natural annulus and then to the patch (Figure 16-65, *C*). The patch is sutured to the remaining edges of the aortotomy (Figure 16-65, *D*).

7. The aorta is closed with nonabsorbable sutures, and the cross-clamp is removed.

8. The left side of the heart is deaired (by vent, by moving the OR bed side to side, or by other maneuvers chosen by the surgeon). The patient is placed in the Trendelenburg's position, and the lungs are inflated. The heart is not allowed to eject blood until the surgeon is satisfied that no air remains within the left ventricle. TEE is used to identify residual air. The heart is defibrillated if it does not resume beating spontaneously.

9. Rewarming of the heart continues, the venting catheter or catheters are removed, and the chest is closed in the routine manner.

Combined Surgery

When CABG is to be performed with aortic valve replacement, the procedure usually is done in the following order:

1. The diseased valve is excised, the annulus is sized, and the prosthesis is selected.

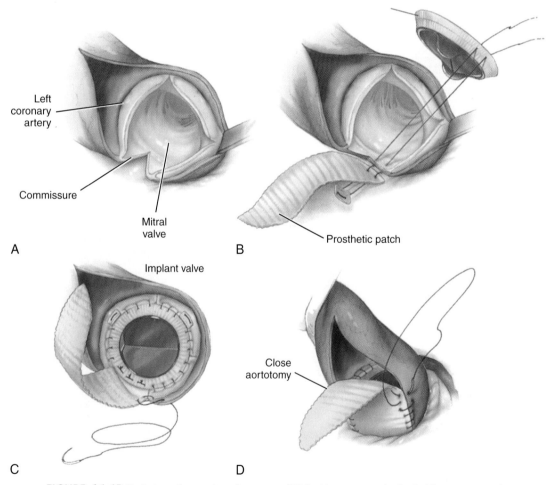

FIGURE 16-65 Technique for aortic enlargement (Nicks-Nuñez operation). **A,** The aortotomy is extended through the commissure separating the left and noncoronary cusps. **B,** A prosthetic patch is sewn into the cut portion of the aorta and into the prosthetic valve. **C,** The prosthetic valve is seated, and the stitches are tied and cut. **D,** The patch is incorporated into the aortotomy closure.

2. Distal coronary anastomoses are performed.
3. The prosthetic valve is inserted.
4. The aorta (or left atrium in MVR) is closed.
5. The proximal coronary anastomoses are inserted into the aorta, after which the aortic cross-clamp is removed.

Double Valve Replacement

When the *aortic and mitral valves are both replaced,* the valves are first excised and the annuli sized. Then the mitral valve prosthesis is first implanted, followed by the aortic valve. (If the aortic prosthesis is inserted first, the firm prosthetic aortic annular ring could cause cardiac injury and make insertion of a mitral prosthesis difficult.) The aorta is closed, and after sufficient deairing of the left ventricle, the left atrium is closed.

SURGERY FOR THE THORACIC AORTA

Thoracic aortic aneurysmectomy is excision of an aneurysmal portion of the ascending aorta, aortic arch, or descending thoracic aorta and replacement with a prosthetic graft, valve-graft conduit, or intra-aortic prosthesis. Collagen-impregnated grafts have significantly reduced interstitial bleeding and obviated the need for preclotting techniques.

Aneurysms may be caused by atherosclerosis, trauma, infection, or cystic medial degeneration (Isselbacher, 2008). *Athero-*

sclerosis affects large and medium arteries with tunica intima deposits of plaques containing cholesterol, lipoid material, and lipophages. Atherosclerosis generally affects the smaller arteries rather than the aorta. *Arteriosclerosis* is a condition characterized by loss of elasticity and by thickening and hardening of the arteries. Both conditions may lead to aneurysm formation within an artery.

Aortic *dissection* is a unique entity and is related to a tear in the tunica intima of the aorta that exposes underlying degenerative changes in the tunica media layer of the artery. Intraluminal blood flow penetrates and flows through the tear, resulting in subsequent dissection of the tunica media (Isselbacher, 2008). As blood passes between the layers of the wall, it forms a false channel; as the channel extends and enlarges, the blood flow can be obstructed through the aorta and its branches, or the aorta can rupture, causing severe hemorrhage (Figure 16-66, A).

Surgical intervention becomes necessary when presenting symptoms indicate a compromised circulation or danger of rupture; generally, medical management with hypotensive agents to reduce stress on the vessel is the preferred initial treatment until surgical repair can be performed.

Aneurysms can be characterized morphologically as follows: (1) saccular—a sac type of formation with a narrowed neck projecting from the side of the artery; (2) fusiform—a spindle-shaped formation with complete circumferential involvement of the artery. Dissections can be characterized in at least two systems according to type, origin, and extent of the lesion (Table 16-7).

Procedural Considerations

Several methods of surgical treatment are described in the classic study by Crawford (1990). In situations where ascending aortic aneurysm or aortic dissection produces annular dilation

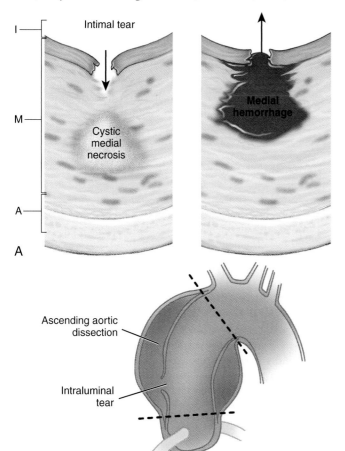

FIGURE 16-66 Aortic dissection. **A,** Proposed mechanism of the initiation of an aortic dissection (*A* = adventitia; *M* = media; *I* = intima). **B,** Intimal tear in the ascending aorta causing a dissection.

TABLE 16-7

Commonly Used Classification Systems to Describe Aortic Dissection

Type	Site of Origin and Extent of Aortic Involvement
DEBAKEY	
Type I	Originates in ascending aorta, propagates at least to aortic arch and often beyond it distally
Type II	Originates in and is confined to ascending aorta
Type III	Originates in descending aorta and extends distally down aorta or, rarely, retrograde into aortic arch and ascending aorta
STANFORD	
Type A	All dissections involving ascending aorta, regardless of site of origin
Type B	All dissections not involving ascending aorta
DESCRIPTIVE	
Proximal	Includes DeBakey types I and II or Stanford type A
Distal	Includes DeBakey type III or Stanford type B

Modified from Libby P et al: *Braunwald's heart disease,* ed 8, Philadelphia, 2008, Saunders.

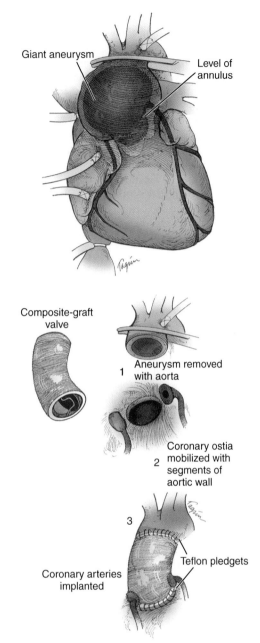

FIGURE 16-67 Bentall-DeBono procedure (see text).

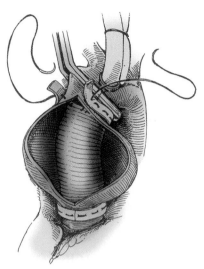

FIGURE 16-68 Resection and graft repair of ascending aortic aneurysm.

with subsequent aortic valve insufficiency, a modified Bentall-DeBono procedure with a composite graft-valve conduit and reimplantation of the coronary ostia may be performed to replace the aortic valve and the aneurysmal aorta (Quigley et al, 2008; Isselbacher, 2008) (Figure 16-67). Retrograde cardioplegia is usually employed to arrest the heart; if necessary, selective coronary infusion may be used. The Bentall-DeBono procedure necessitates reimplanting the right and left coronary ostia into the prosthetic graft; in patients with CAD, vein grafts may be inserted and anastomosed proximally to the prosthesis.

The type of CPB depends on the location of the aneurysm or dissection. Generally, the atrium can be cannulated for venous return and the femoral or axillary artery is used for arterial

inflow (because the weakened ascending aorta cannot be safely cannulated). Deep hypothermia with circulatory arrest and cerebroplegia may be needed to protect the heart and brain in particularly complex lesions of the aortic arch where placement of a cross-clamp is difficult. Cerebral oximetry may be used to monitor oxygenation of the brain.

Traditionally, during the open repair of descending thoracic aortic aneurysms, the heart is not arrested; it continues beating to perfuse the upper body. Femoral bypass may be instituted to perfuse the kidneys and lower extremities; however, normothermia usually is maintained. Hypothermic CPB can be used to repair complex descending and thoracoabdominal aneurysms to provide protection against paralysis and renal, cardiac, and visceral organ system failure. Increasingly, an endovascular stent (see Figure 16-22) is used for aneurysms and dissections (Svensson, 2009); the prosthesis is inserted through the femoral artery and guided under fluoroscopy to the area of the descending aortic aneurysm.

In complex lesions involving the ascending aorta, arch, and descending aorta, the ascending aorta and arch repair may be performed with an open technique. Subsequently, repair of the descending aorta may be performed with an endovascular graft (see Repair of Descending Thoracic Aortic Aneurysm, p. 768) (Isselbacher, 2008).

Repair of Ascending Thoracic Aortic Aneurysm or Dissection

Procedural Considerations. To the basic setup are added aneurysm instruments. Valve instruments, coronary instruments, and an array of tube grafts, valves, or valved conduits should be available. Bicaval cannulation for venous drainage is preferred, but if the cavae cannot be safely accessed, the femoral vein is used initially for venous drainage. Once the aneurysm is controlled, the femoral venous line can be Y-ed to a vena caval cannula.

Operative Procedure
1. The patient is positioned for a median sternotomy.
2. Cannulation for CPB is performed.
3. The sternum is opened, and the aneurysm is inspected.

4. The involvement of the aortic annulus is then considered.
   a. If the aortic annulus is not involved, the aneurysm is incised longitudinally and a woven graft is anastomosed proximally and distally to the healthy aorta (Figure 16-68). Felt strips incorporated into the anastomosis may be used to bolster friable tissue.
   b. If the aortic annulus is involved, the ascending aorta is incised to the annulus and the aneurysm may be excised. The leaflets are excised, and the annulus is measured. The proximal end of a valved conduit is inserted. An eye electrocoagulator is used to create openings in the graft at the location of the right and left coronary ostia, which are mobilized and anastomosed to the graft. (If the patient has concomitant CAD, saphenous vein grafts are inserted.) The distal end of the conduit is sutured to healthy aorta.
5. Bypass is discontinued, and all incisions are closed.

Repair of Aortic Arch Aneurysm

Procedural Considerations. Aneurysm instruments and woven grafts are available. If deep hypothermia is to be used, the patient's head may be covered with bags of ice at the beginning of the procedure to reduce cerebral oxygen demand. Precautionary measures (e.g., padding) to prevent frostbite are instituted. The location of the aneurysm will determine the positioning. Aneurysms of the proximal arch can be accessed through a median sternotomy; distal arch aneurysms may require a modified thoracotomy position to optimize exposure. Selective cerebral perfusion may be used during circulatory arrest to perfuse the brain. *Retrograde* cerebral perfusion is performed via the superior vena caval venous line that is Y-ed off the arterial line; arterial blood is slowly infused through the SVC line into the cerebral circulation while the distal aortic anastomosis is performed. *Antegrade* cerebral perfusion is achieved by infusing arterialized blood through one or more catheters into aortic arch vessels (i.e., brachiocephalic artery and left common carotid artery).

Operative Procedure

1. Cannulation of the right atrium and femoral or axillary artery is performed.
2. Once the patient is cooled to the desired temperature, the arch vessels are individually cross-clamped (Figure 16-69,

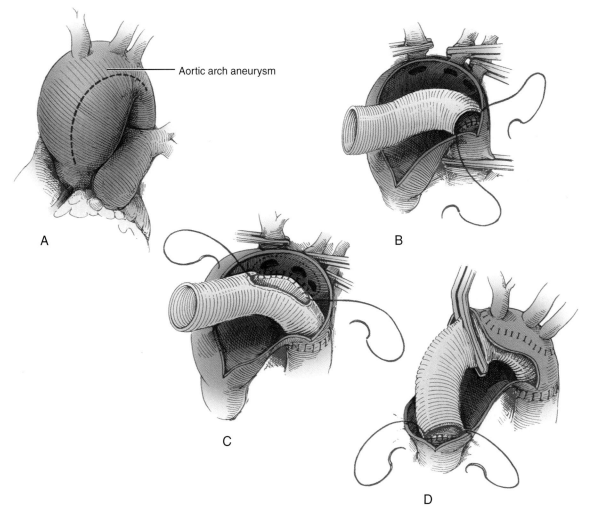

A — Aortic arch aneurysm

FIGURE 16-69 Repair of aortic arch aneurysm. **A,** Incision. **B,** Distal anastomosis. **C,** Anastomosis of graft to common origin of arch vessels. **D,** Proximal anastomosis.

A and *B*). (If circulatory arrest is indicated, cross-clamps are not used.) The aneurysm is incised, a tube graft (with or without side branches) is selected, and the anastomosis to the descending aorta is performed.

3. An opening is made into the side of the graft, and the graft is anastomosed to the common origin of the brachiocephalic, left carotid, and left subclavian vessels. Alternatively, when a graft with side branches is used, individual anastomoses to the head vessels are created. The graft is cross-clamped proximally to the arch and deaired (Figure 16-69, *C*).

4. The proximal aorta is anastomosed to the graft while the patient is rewarming. The graft is deaired, and the patient is weaned from bypass (Figure 16-69, *D*).

5. All incisions are closed.

Repair of Descending Thoracic Aortic Aneurysm

Procedural Considerations. Endovascular repair (see Figure 16-22) of descending aortic aneurysms and dissections has largely replaced the traditional open technique, although anatomic considerations may increase the difficulty of placing the straight endovascular tube graft into the angled portion of the proximal descending aorta (just distal to the left subclavian artery). Additionally, endovascular insertion requires nondiseased tissue for implantation of the device in the areas proximal and distal to the lesion (the "landing zones"); in patients with diffuse atherosclerotic disease or extensive dissection, viable tissue may not be present (Thompson and Bertling, 2009). It is not unusual to deploy more than one graft in order to cover the lesion. Endovascular instruments, guidewires, introducer sheaths, pigtail catheters, intravascular dye, dilators, catheters, an array of stent graft sizes, and deployment devices are required. The procedure is performed with fluoroscopy and is usually performed on an OR bed that allows imaging without extensive manipulation of the bed. Radiation precautions must be taken. The guidewires may be more than 6 feet in length so the scrub person should protect the sterility of the distal portion of the guidewire by anchoring the wire with towels or other sterile objects when not being used. The postoperative period is considerably shorter than that for a thoracotomy approach. Potential complications include bleeding and migration of the device (requiring adjustment and/or insertion of another device) (Thompson and Bertling, 2009).

For *open* repair, thoracotomy instruments and supplies are added to the basic setup; additional long aortic cross-clamps may be needed. Prosthetic grafts are available. The patient is positioned for a left posterolateral thoracotomy. Femoral vein–femoral artery bypass may be performed to perfuse the lower body. In this situation, the heart perfuses the upper body proximal to the aneurysm and normothermia is maintained.

If hypothermic CBP with circulatory arrest is employed, instruments and supplies per the surgeon's request should be available. Protective covering for the patient's head, face, and extremities may be required to avoid frostbite.

Operative Procedure—Endovascular Repair

1. One or both femoral arteries are accessed via a percutaneous (Seldinger) or cutdown technique. A hypodermic needle is inserted into the femoral artery. A guidewire is passed

through the needle and threaded into the aorta. Fluoroscopy may be used to image the aortic lumen and measure targeted segments of the aorta. The hypodermic needle is removed and a sheath inserted (through which the device will be inserted).

2. A delivery catheter housing the graft is inserted into the descending aorta.

3. A monitoring device may be inserted through the contralateral femoral artery to measure intraluminal pressures.

4. Under fluoroscopy, the graft is guided into position and deployed into the aorta (see Figure 16-22). The device self-expands; a balloon may be inflated against the inside of the graft to secure the prosthesis against the aortic lumen.

5. Fluoroscopy is used to image the aorta and to confirm exclusion of the aneurysm/dissection.

6. The deployment devices and other intraluminal catheters and wires are removed and the incision(s) is (are) closed.

Operative Procedure: Open Repair

1. Cannulation for femoral vein–femoral artery bypass is performed.

2. A thoracotomy incision is made, the aneurysm is exposed, and the surrounding structures are inspected. (Occasionally the surgeon makes two thoracotomy incisions for better access to and control of the aorta.) Renal involvement is assessed; if indicated, measures to protect the kidneys are instituted (e.g., local cooling).

3. Normothermic femoral bypass is initiated.

4. The aneurysm is incised longitudinally, and the aorta is sized.

5. A woven graft (Figure 16-70) is inserted, and the aneurysmal remnants are wrapped around the graft.

ASSISTED CIRCULATION

Mechanical circulatory support has been available for more than 35 years (Gemmato et al, 2005), expanding the treatment for heart failure into a rapidly growing specialty that

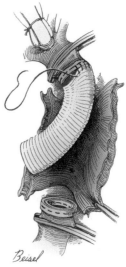

FIGURE 16-70 Resection and graft replacement for descending thoracic aortic aneurysm.

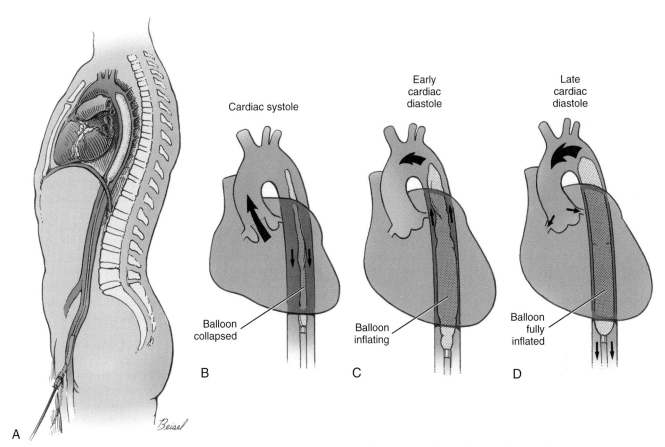

Cardiac systole

Early cardiac diastole

Late cardiac diastole

Balloon collapsed

Balloon inflating

Balloon fully inflated

B

C

D

A

FIGURE 16-71 Phases of balloon pumping. **A,** Balloon inflation occurs from closure of aortic valve to end of diastole. Inflation causes retrograde flow of blood in aorta, increasing coronary perfusion pressure without increasing myocardial work or oxygen demand. Inflation also causes antegrade flow, increasing mean arterial pressure, renal flow, and cerebral flow. **B,** Balloon deflation occurs from just before opening of aortic valve to closure of aortic valve. Deflation encourages antegrade flow, decreasing afterload or resistance to left ventricular ejection. Deflation also decreases oxygen required by left ventricle, shortens systolic ejection, and increases stroke volume. **C** and **D,** When the balloon reinflates, the cycle is repeated.

also includes coronary artery revascularization, left and right ventricular reconstruction, circulatory assist device implantation, and cardiac transplantation (McCarthy, 2008). Formerly, ventricular assist devices were reserved for those patients who could not be weaned from CPB after open-heart operations, or who had end-stage cardiomyopathy. Current indications and choices have expanded and a variety of active and passive devices are available to support the circulation for short-, intermediate-, and long-term support (Wilson et al, 2009). Selected ventricular assist devices have been approved for "destination" therapy, while other devices are indicated for patients awaiting a donor heart ("bridge-to-transplant" devices) (McCarthy, 2008; Naka and Rose, 2008; Miller et al, 2007).

Biologic assistance in the form of an autogenous muscle wrap (*cardiomyoplasty*) may be useful in some patients who may not be candidates for transplantation, but the procedure is used infrequently. The left latissimus dorsi muscle is dissected from the back and repositioned around the heart, where it is sewn around the ventricle. This (skeletal) muscle is then transformed into a continuously beating muscle by a cardiomyostimulator that paces the muscle with increasing fre-

quency, allowing the muscle to become fatigue-resistant. The muscle wrap squeezes the heart in synchronization with natural electrical impulses moving through the heart muscle.

Intra-Aortic Balloon Pump

The most widely used short-term device is the intra-aortic balloon pump (IABP). The IABP (Figure 16-71) employs the principle of counterpulsation to increase coronary blood flow and decrease afterload (i.e., the resistance the ventricle must overcome to open the aortic valve).

Operative Procedure

1. A flexible guidewire is passed through a percutaneous needle into the femoral artery. The needle is removed, and graduated dilators are inserted over the guidewire to dilate the overlying tissue and the artery wall.
2. The IABP catheter (with the furled balloon) is inserted into the artery and advanced to a position just distal to the left subclavian artery. The catheter can be marked at the proximal end with a silk tie to measure the distance the catheter should be inserted.
3. The balloon is unfurled and activated.

Ventricular Assist Device

VADs are designed to augment cardiac output from the left (LVAD), right (RVAD), or both (biventricular—BiVAD) ventricles and to decrease the workload of the heart by diverting blood from the ventricle or ventricles to an artificial pump that maintains systemic perfusion. Patients with an LVAD can become better transplant candidates because the LVAD enhances anabolism, ambulation, and improved organ function. LVADs are employed as a bridge to cardiac transplantation by supporting the circulation while a suitable donor heart can be found. Based on the results of the Randomized Evaluation of Mechanical Assistance for the Treatment of Congestive Heart Failure (REMATCH) trial (Lietz et al, 2009; Long et al, 2005; Park et al, 2005; Rose et al, 2001), the use of the HeartMate (vented electric) LVAD (see Thoratec HeartMate LVAD section) was approved by the U.S. Food and Drug Administration in November 2002 for *destination therapy/ permanent replacement* for the left ventricle. Although complications (e.g., bleeding, thromboembolism, infection, device failure) persist, they have been reduced with the newer VADs (Naka and Rose, 2008).

Among the increasing number of designs are the axial flow pump based on Archimedes' third-century screw pump that was used to raise well water for irrigation; the pump is inserted into the left ventricle to propel blood flow and the distal end is anastomosed to the descending aorta. Miniaturized centrifugal pumps, totally implantable pulsatile devices incorporating a transcutaneous energy transmission (and power regeneration) system, and artificial hearts (Naka and Rose, 2008) are some of the innovative responses for the treatment of heart failure.

Procedural Considerations. Insertion of an assist device may be indicated for patients who cannot be weaned from CPB with the use of IABP; device insertion also may be scheduled. Depending on the system, components of the system should be collected and prepared according to the manufacturer's instructions. Device components may include external centrifugal pumps, internal pneumatically (Figure 16-72) or electrically powered assist devices, or wholly implantable systems with transcutaneous, rechargeable power sources.

The LVAD device described in the following section is approved for support of the left ventricle when right ventricular function is normal. Prosthetic valves are incorporated into the circuit to maintain unidirectional blood flow. All VADs will differ and preparation should be specific to the device. In preparation for VAD insertion, perioperative nurses and surgical technologists are encouraged to discuss the type of VAD, insertion considerations, possible complications, and troubleshooting scenarios with the surgeon.

Operative Procedure
THORATEC HEARTMATE LVAD
1. A median sternotomy incision is made and extended to the umbilicus (Figure 16-72, *A*).
2. A preperitoneal pouch is made for placement of the assist device.
3. CPB is established, and the aorta is cross-clamped. The atrial septum is inspected for defects, which are closed if found.
4. A Dacron graft is anastomosed to the aorta (Figure 16-72, *B*).

5. The left ventricular apex is mobilized, and an opening is created in the apex (Figure 16-72, *C*).
6. A connector is inserted into the apex, and the flange is sewn to the surrounding left ventricular myocardium with pledgetted sutures. The inflow conduit is attached to the apical connector (Figure 16-72, *D* to *G*).
7. An opening is made into the diaphragm near the location of the apical connector and inflow conduit. The conduit is passed through the diaphragm and attached to the assist device.
8. The aortic graft is attached to the outflow conduit, which is connected to the assist device (Figure 16-72, *H* and *I*).
9. The driveline is tunneled to the left lower quadrant, where it exits through the skin. The driveline can be connected to the drive console or to a battery pack. Blood flows from the left ventricular apex, to the device, and back into the body through the aortic conduit (Figure 16-72, *J*).
10. CPB is discontinued, and incisions are closed.

To remove or replace the pump, the patient is returned to the OR, the sternotomy is reopened, the cannulae are removed, and the device is removed (or replaced).

Total Artificial Heart

The total artificial heart (TAH) continues to be refined and implanted in patients with end-stage biventricular failure. Complications associated with thromboembolism and infection have been reduced, but not eliminated, with technical and material refinements of VAD systems. Long-term right or left VADs have been increasingly employed as a bridge to cardiac transplantation by supporting the circulation until a suitable donor heart can be found (Naka and Rose, 2008).

Implantation of the first totally artificial heart by AbioCor—approved for implantation by the Food and Drug Administration (FDA) in 2006—was performed in June 2009 in a 76-year-old male who did not qualify for heart transplantation because of his age. The device employs two pumping chambers made of titanium and plastic. An internal rechargeable battery powers the device (Rothman, 2009). With greater emphasis on interventions for heart failure, surgical technologists can anticipate an increased demand for univentricular and biventricular mechanical support.

HEART AND HEART-LUNG TRANSPLANTATION

Heart Transplantation (Figure 16-73)

Orthotopic transplantation (replacing one heart with another) is most commonly performed; less commonly, heterotopic (piggyback) and combined heart-lung procedures are performed. Important considerations continue to be recipient and donor selection, the immune response, and infection control. Older recipients and donors (older than 65 years) have demonstrated acceptable morbidity and survival (McCarthy, 2008; Hunt, 2006).

Modification of the traditional transplantation technique (e.g., atrial-atrial anastomoses) has reduced some of the dysrhythmias and valvular dysfunction associated with the traditional method of transplantation. End-to-end anastomoses between the donor and recipient SVC and the donor and recipient IVC are created, producing a more physiologic atrial contribution to ventricular filling and less distortion of the mitral and tricuspid annuli (McCarthy, 2008; Blanche et al, 1997).

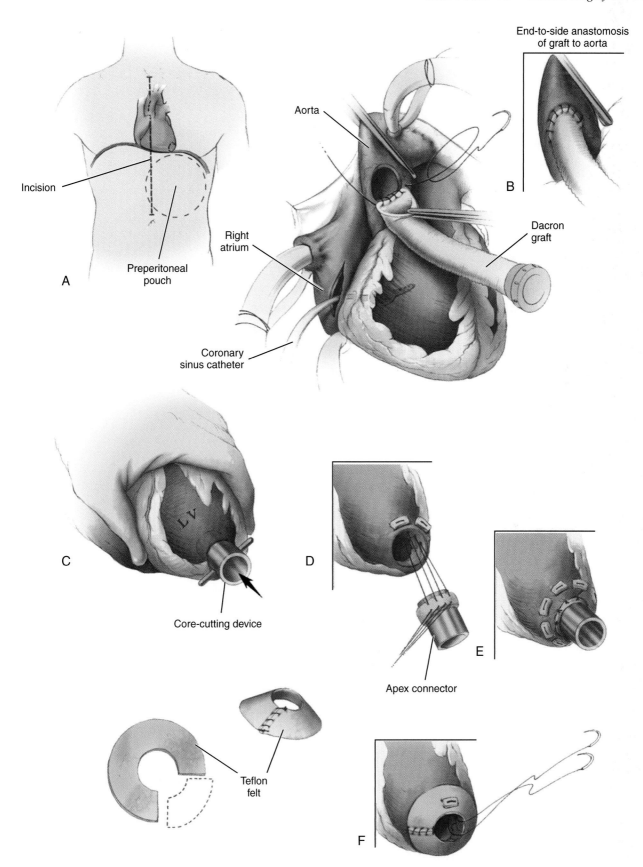

End-to-side anastomosis
of graft to aorta

Aorta

B

Dacron
graft

Incision

Right
atrium

Preperitoneal
pouch

A

Coronary
sinus catheter

C

Core-cutting device

D

E

Apex connector

Teflon
felt

F

FIGURE 16-72 Left ventricular assist device (see text).

Continued

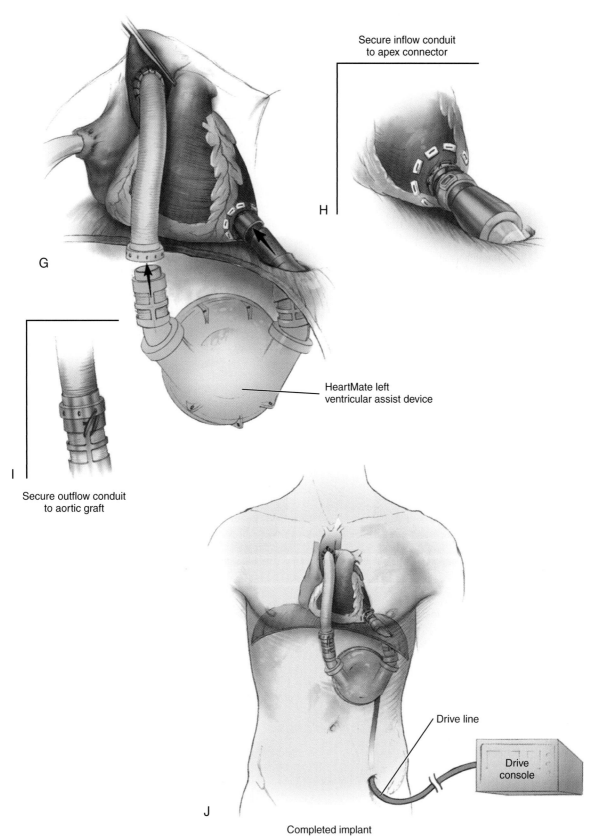

Secure inflow conduit
to apex connector

H

G

Secure outflow conduit
to aortic graft

I

HeartMate left
ventricular assist device

Drive line

Drive
console

J

Completed implant

FIGURE 16-72, cont'd Left ventricular assist device.

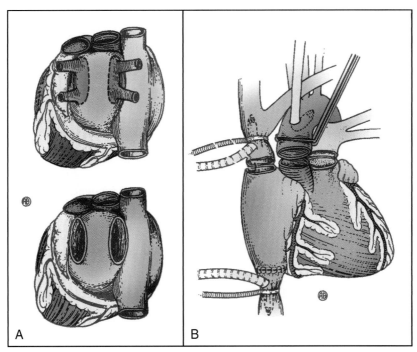

FIGURE 16-73 **A**, Heart transplantation with pulmonary venous anastomoses on right or left side, and caval anastomoses at the superior and inferior vena cavae. **B**, Aorta and pulmonary artery are joined last.

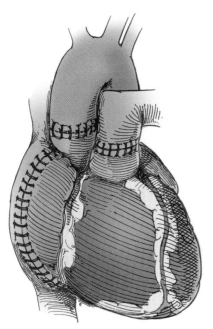

FIGURE 16-74 Traditional atrial anastomosis for heart transplantation.

Tricuspid suture or ring annuloplasty may be performed on the donor heart to minimize tricuspid insufficiency (Jeevanandam et al, 2004). Revised pulmonary venous connections produce fewer dysrhythmias. These changes also lead to less AV valve regurgitation. Pulmonary artery and aortic anastomoses are performed in the traditional manner.

Procedural Considerations. Individual instrument setups are necessary for the donor and the recipient.

Operative Procedure

DONOR HEART. The donor heart is exposed through a median sternotomy. The aorta, pulmonary artery, and venae cavae are dissected. The venae cavae are occluded, the left atrium is opened to decompress the ventricle, and the heart is rapidly cooled and arrested.

The heart is excised by incision of the SVC and the IVC, the left atrium, the aorta, and the pulmonary artery (Hunt, 2006). The donor heart is immediately placed into cold saline and transported to the site where it will be inserted into the recipient.

RECIPIENT HEART. The recipient is placed on bypass with cannulation of the IVC and the SVC; caval tapes are placed around the cavae. The patient is cooled to approximately 32° to 34° C (89.6° to 93.2° F), and the caval tapes are tightened. The pulmonary trunk and aorta are dissected immediately above their respective semilunar valves; the left atrium is incised to leave intact portions of the left atrial wall and the atrial septum of the recipient; and the right atrium is incised, retaining the SVC and IVC for anastomosis to the donor heart. The recipient heart is then removed.

The donor heart is placed in the pericardial well. The pulmonary anastomoses are performed (Figure 16-73, *A*). The SVC and IVC are anastomosed with running cardiovascular sutures (Figure 16-73, *B*). The donor and recipient aortas and pulmonary arteries are similarly joined. Air is removed from the left side of the heart. Before the pulmonary artery is sutured, all caval and atrial suture lines are carefully inspected for significant bleeding areas, and the cross-clamp is removed. Figure 16-74 illustrates the traditional (but less frequently anastomosed) right atrial suture line; aortic and pulmonary anastomoses are similar to the technique just described.

Defibrillation of the ventricles is usually effected with a single direct-current shock. A needle vent in the ascending aorta allows residual air to escape. The patient is then gradually weaned from the bypass. Cannulae are removed from the venae cavae and the aorta. The incisions are closed as described previously.

Heart-Lung Transplantation

Newer techniques for lung and heart-lung transplantation incorporate the bicaval anastomoses used for orthotopic heart transplantation and also employ a bibronchial anastomosis that reduces bleeding and enhances the integrity of the airway. To maximize the allocation of scarce donor organs, transplantation procedures for the lungs may use a single lung or bilateral lungs; heart-lung transplantation is infrequent (Cooper, 2004). Preservation of the *donor's* sinus node and the *recipient's* recurrent laryngeal, vagus, and phrenic nerves are important surgical considerations.

Operative Procedure. The recipient's diseased heart and lung(s) are excised separately or en bloc, with care taken not to injure the major nerves listed previously. The recipient's right atrium, SVC, and IVC are saved to create bicaval attachments to the donor heart. The bronchi are transected. The donor heart and lungs are brought onto the field. The right lung is placed in the right pleural space, and the left lung is positioned in the left pleural space. The bronchial and the bicaval anastomoses are performed, and rewarming is begun. The aortic anastomosis is performed, the aorta is deaired, and the cross-clamp is removed.

SURGERY FOR CONDUCTION DISTURBANCES

Disturbances of the conduction system affect the rate, rhythm, and effectiveness of the contracting heart. Surgical techniques have been developed to treat a variety of supraventricular dysrhythmias (e.g., atrial fibrillation [AF] and Wolff-Parkinson-White reentry tachycardia) and both ischemic and nonischemic ventricular tachydysrhythmias (e.g., ventricular tachycardia or fibrillation). Preprocedural electrophysiologic mapping of the patient's conduction pathways identifies and locates aberrant pathways, tachydysrhythmias, and the existence of additional pathways, as well as the effects of medications on a particular dysrhythmia. Indications for pacemaker implantation (including resynchronization therapy) and antitachycardia-antifibrillation devices have been expanded. Many (but not all) pacemaker and internal cardioverter defibrillator (ICD) insertions are currently performed in the electrophysiology (EP) laboratory or the cardiac catheterization suite. Ablation procedures for AF may be performed in the EP laboratory. Depending on the anticipated origin of the problem, the electrophysiologist inserts a catheter percutaneously into the femoral vein or artery and threads the catheter retrograde to the right or left atrium and ventricle. The electrophysiologist tests various areas of the heart in an attempt to reproduce the dysrhythmia and then ablates the area of the heart where the rhythm disturbance originates. Postoperative considerations are similar to those for atrial fibrillation surgery. Surgical correction is performed in the OR.

AF is the most common cardiac dysrhythmia, affecting more than 2 million adults in the United States (AHA, 2009b).

Atrial fibrillation is an abnormal heart rhythm that causes discomfort and stasis of blood in the atria. AF was considered a "benign" condition in the past, but the serious consequences associated with the dysrhythmia have made it the subject of intense study. AF interferes with the atrial kick (which contributes a significant amount of "preload") and the dysrhythmia can lead to insufficient cardiac output. Moreover, the stasis of blood within the atria promotes the formation of thrombus (clotting), which leads to cerebrovascular accident or pulmonary embolism.

Although *intermittent* AF commonly occurs after CABG, it is potentially preventable by treatment with amiodarone, beta-blockers, angiotensin-converting enzyme (ACE) inhibitors, and/or nonsteroidal antiinflammatory drugs. Treatment includes restoration of sinus rhythm (when possible), control of ventricular rate, and administration of anticoagulants. New techniques to treat *continuous* AF are based on research demonstrating that the pulmonary veins are an important source of the ectopic beats that can initiate paroxysms of AF (Haissaguerre et al, 1998). Surgical interventions for AF have expanded beyond Cox's original Maze procedures (Cox et al, 1991), in which extensive atrial incisions were sutured to create a maze through which electrical impulses were directed from the SA node to the AV node. The early research of Cox (Cox et al, 1991) demonstrated that electrical impulses are unable to cross incised and sutured tissue and consequently cannot regenerate the reentry circuits producing the dysrhythmia. Cox revised the cut-and-sew technique of the initial Maze procedures with a cryosurgical technique that ensures the creation of transmural lesions in the vicinity of the pulmonary veins and in other areas of the heart, generating impulses producing AF. This "mini-Maze" can be performed through a sternotomy or through a minimally invasive thoracic route and requires placement of fewer lesions in the left and right atria. Currently, the focus is on the selective ablation (with cryotherapy [Figure 16-75] or ultrasonic or radiofrequency [RF] energy sources) of tissues surrounding, for example, the pulmonary veins to reestablish normal conduction pathways.

Surgery for Atrial Fibrillation (The "Maze" Procedure)

Surgery for AF may also be performed through an open sternotomy or right mini-thoracotomy incisions. The appropriate supplies (including energy sources) should be available (Seifert et al, 2007). By creating small areas of scar tissue in the cardiac muscle, electrical impulses are forced to follow an alternative conduction path or "maze."

Operative Procedure—Sternotomy

1. The surgeon performs a midline sternotomy.
2. Cannulation of the superior and inferior venae cavae is performed for total cardiopulmonary bypass.
3. The ascending aorta is occluded, and cardioplegic solution is infused through the aortic root and into the coronary arteries.
4. A right atriotomy is performed, and the first set of lesions is ablated in the right atrium (Figure 16-76, *A*).
5. A left atriotomy is performed, and the left atrial lesions are ablated (Figure 16-76, *B*).
6. The atriotomies are closed, and the aorta is unclamped.

7. Cardiopulmonary bypass is discontinued, and the cannulae are removed.
8. Chest tubes and pacing wires are inserted, and the wound is closed.

Postoperative Considerations. Postoperatively, patients are monitored for heart rhythm problems. In patients treated for AF, it may take up to 3 months for the heart to resume beating in a normal manner. Additional postoperative considerations include monitoring for bleeding, infection, and other potential complications related to heart surgery.

Insertion of Permanent Pacemaker

A permanent pacemaker (pulse generator and electrodes) initiates atrial or ventricular contraction, or both. Complete heart block and bradydysrhythmias (i.e., slow heart rates) are the most common indications for pacemaker implantation. The development of multiprogrammable and physiologic pacemakers has made possible the treatment of many forms of dysrhythmias and neuroconductive disturbances as well as tachydysrhythmias. A temporary pacemaker may also be used for acute forms of heart block and dysrhythmias that occasionally occur during and after cardiac surgery (Hayes and Zipes, 2008).

Dual-site pacing of both the right and the left ventricle is another treatment for patients with dilated cardiomyopathy and heart failure. *Cardiac resynchronization therapy* (CRT) employs leads placed on the right atrium and the right ventricle. Left ventricular pacing is achieved with an electrode introduced transvenously into the coronary sinus and extended into the great cardiac vein (or a tributary) to a position in the left side of the heart; this electrode functions as the second ventricular lead. The three electrodes are connected to the pacemaker generator. Resynchronization improves the mechanical pumping action between the right and left ventricles and optimizes AV synchrony; as a result, hemodynamic function is improved in heart failure patients.

The *transvenous* or the *epicardial* approach may be used to place the electrodes. The transvenous route is most commonly used because it does not require a major thoracotomy or a general anesthetic and is therefore safer for high-risk patients. Permanent epicardial electrodes may be placed during cardiac operations when the chest is opened and the heart is exposed; however, if a permanent pacemaker is required, it is likely to be inserted transvenously during the postoperative period (pacing is achieved with the temporary electrodes placed during surgery). To avoid opening the sternum a subxiphoid approach may be used to place epicardial leads.

Insertion of Transvenous (Endocardial) Pacing Electrodes

Procedural Considerations. The patient is placed in the supine position. Continuous ECG monitoring is essential. A defibrillator and emergency drugs should be available because lethal dysrhythmias can occur during catheter insertion. The patient should be made as comfortable as possible because this procedure can sometimes be lengthy and is frequently performed using local or local standby anesthesia (monitored anesthesia care).

Fluoroscopy is required; thus either a portable image intensifier is needed or the procedure is done in the special studies

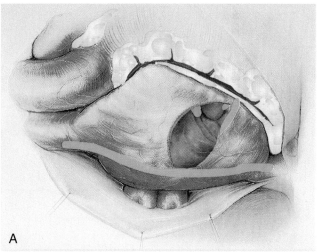

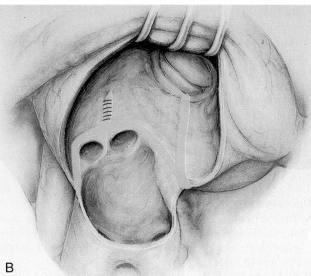

FIGURE 16-76 A, First lesion set for Maze procedure. **B,** Second lesion set for Maze procedure.

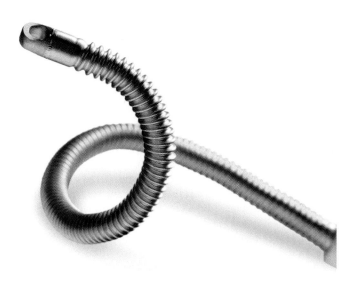

FIGURE 16-75 Articulated cryo probe for Maze procedure.

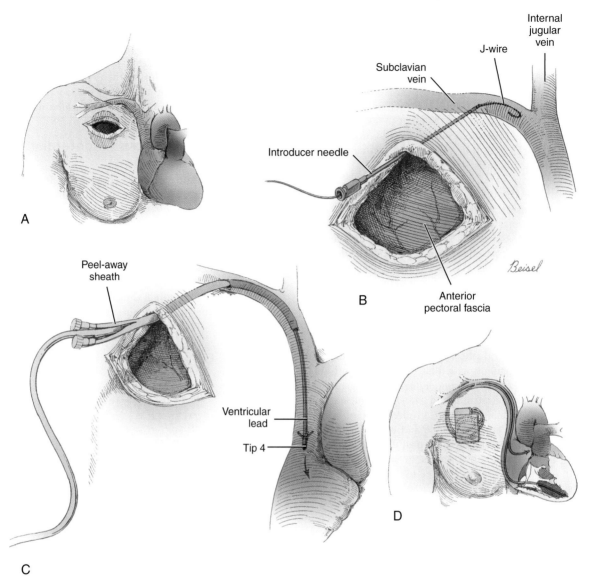

FIGURE 16-77 Insertion of transvenous pacemaker (see text).

section of the radiology or cardiac catheterization department. A minor set of instruments is used, plus the following:

◆ Vascular dissecting instruments
◆ Tunneling instrument
◆ Sterile pacemaker and electrodes
◆ Introducer set
◆ External pacemaker (for testing) or a pacing system analyzer (PSA)
◆ Alligator test cables
◆ Screwdriver and other accessory items as needed

Operative Procedure
1. The skin and subcutaneous tissue are infiltrated with a local anesthetic, and the patient is placed in the Trendelenburg position (to engorge the vein for easier access and to avoid air emboli).
2. A skin pocket is made close to the subclavian vein (Figure 16-77, *A*). The vessel may be encircled with a heavy suture.

3. A venotomy is performed with an introducer needle (Figure 16-77, *B*). A guidewire is threaded to the desired cardiac chamber, and the needle is removed. The pacing electrode is inserted through a peel-away dilator sheath, which is withdrawn after the lead insertion (Figure 16-77, *C*). The guidewire is withdrawn. A stylet is then inserted to help position the electrode.
4. The electrode is advanced under direct fluoroscopic vision into the right atrium, through the tricuspid valve, and into the right ventricle (Figure 16-77, *D*).
5. The surgeon attempts to entrap the tip of the electrode in the trabeculae carneae cordis of the right ventricular apex to stabilize it. Once the electrode is positioned and tested with alligator test cables and the pacing analyzer to confirm proper placement and function, the stylet is removed. If a dual-chamber pacemaker is inserted, the second lead is entrapped in the right atrial appendage (Figure 16-77, *D*).
6. The electrode or electrodes are brought down and attached to the pulse generator.

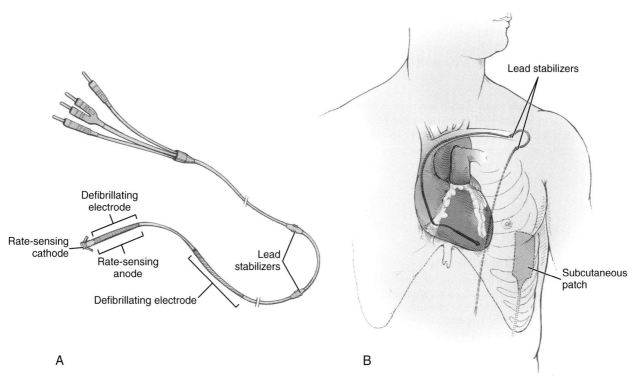

FIGURE 16-78 Nonthoracotomy internal cardioverter defibrillator (ICD) insertion. **A,** The lead system is composed of sensing and defibrillating electrodes in one unit and is inserted transvenously. **B,** The proximal end of the electrodes is tunneled to the abdomen (or the chest) and attached to the generator (not shown). The rate-sensing cathode at the tip relays information to the generator, which initiates an electrical shock by means of the defibrillating electrodes. A second (patch) electrode, placed subcutaneously on the left chest wall, may be necessary if the transvenous electrode alone cannot successfully defibrillate the patient during testing of the unit. If the nonthoracotomy system does not result in suitable defibrillation thresholds, a left thoracotomy or subxiphoid approach may be used to place sensing leads and defibrillation patches directly on the heart.

7. The pulse generator is placed into the pocket, and the incision may be irrigated with an antibiotic solution. If the pocket must be made farther away from the vein, a tunneling device may be used to thread the electrode to the pocket.
8. The incision is closed in layers with absorbable sutures.

Insertion of Myocardial (Epicardial) Pacing Electrodes

A subxiphoid left anterior thoracotomy approach or sternotomy approach can be used; the setup is the same as that described for placement of endocardial electrodes. The subxiphoid process and left upper quadrant area are infiltrated with the anesthetic agent. A small transverse incision is made below the xiphoid process and is extended down to the linea alba. A tunnel is created under the xiphoid process to the pericardium, which is incised to expose the heart. The pacing electrode, mounted on its carrier, is screwed into the ventricular myocardium, and the carrier is removed. The remainder of the procedure is the same as that described for insertion of the endocardial electrode.

For the sternotomy approach, the mediastinum is opened for a concomitant cardiac procedure and an area of myocardium is chosen for placement of the pacing electrodes. The electrode tips are either screwed into or sutured to the myocardium and are attached by an appropriate cable to an external

pulse generator or pacing analyzer for testing. The pocket and subcutaneous tunnel are created as described for insertion of the endocardial electrode.

Insertion of Implantable Cardioverter Defibrillator

Surgery or pharmacologic intervention may not prevent malignant ventricular dysrhythmias (ventricular fibrillation and ventricular tachycardia) in persons who survive sudden cardiac death. The ICD is an electronic device designed to monitor cardiac electrical activity and deliver prompt defibrillator shocks. The ICD differs from a pacemaker in that the former senses ventricular tachycardia or fibrillation and the latter senses asystole. Current models are capable of tiered therapy, whereby increasingly stronger impulses are delivered depending on the underlying dysrhythmias; some devices can also be used to terminate AF. These devices are capable of pacing as well as defibrillating (pacing cardioverter defibrillators [PCDs]). The ICD device consists of a generator and sensing and defibrillator electrodes (Figure 16-78). Many ICD electrodes currently employed consist of transvenous electrodes inserted into the generator much like a transvenous pacemaker system. Myocardial or thoracic subcutaneous patches may be added if the transvenous catheters alone do not adequately defibrillate the heart. Patients with previously applied defibrillator patches may present for removal of a patch or patches; surgical technologists should be prepared for emergency intervention if there is excessive bleeding or lethal dysrhythmia. EP studies are performed before and after insertion to diagnose the dysrhythmia and to evaluate device function, respectively.

The transvenous route with fluoroscopy is commonly employed, and insertion is similar to that described for transvenous pacemaker insertion (Figure 16-78, *B*). The free ends of the lead system are tunneled to the generator, which is implanted in a subcutaneous pocket in the chest wall. The device is tested, and the incisions are closed.

CARDIAC SURGERY SUMMARY

Cardiac surgery encompasses surgical procedures involving the heart and the circulation of blood in the body. The performance of a surgical procedure varies according to the preference of the surgeon; therefore supplies and equipment may differ among surgeons. However, care of the cardiac patient remains the same regardless of the surgeon. In every procedure, the surgical technologist should comprehend the surgeon's preferences and the importance of prepping, draping, and positioning, as well as the required instruments and equipment.

GERIATRIC CONSIDERATIONS

The Elderly Patient—Cardiac Surgery

Aging is a process that can be described in chronologic, physiologic, and functional terms. Human aging from a physiologic perspective has changed little in the past 300 years. In general, we age neither faster nor slower than we did in Colonial America. Chronologic age, the number of years a person has lived, is an easily identifiable measurement. Average/median life span, or life expectancy, is the age at which 50% of a given population survives. Maximum life span potential (MLSP) is the age of the longest-lived member or members of the population or species. The average life span of humans has increased dramatically, yet our MLSP has not changed substantially. Although the number of people living beyond their 90s has increased more recently, the MLSP, estimated at 125 years for women and somewhat less for men, has not changed significantly in recorded history. Chronologic age or MLSP may not be the most meaningful measurement of age, however. The youth-oriented culture of the United States tends to judge based on age and appearance. Nevertheless, many people who have lived a long time remain physiologically and functionally young, whereas others are chronologically young but physiologically and functionally old (Wold, 2008).

Cardiac disease can be considered as a progressive disorder on a continuum occurring in parallel with aging. The progressive biologic changes during aging that contribute to heart failure in the elderly are:
◆ Poor regulation of repair mechanisms
◆ Mitochondrial dysfunction
◆ Increased fibrosis
◆ Increased ventricular–arterial stiffening
◆ Left ventricular diastolic dysfunction (Jugdutt, 2010)

More than 55% of coronary artery bypass graft procedures are performed on patients older than 65 years. Several risk factors associated with increased mortality include emergency procedure, severe left ventricular dysfunction, mitral insufficiency requiring combined procedure, elevated preoperative creatinine level, chronic obstructive pulmonary disease (COPD), anemia, and prior vascular surgery. Factors associated with morbidity in the elderly population include obesity, diabetes mellitus, aortic stenosis, and cerebrovascular disease (Berger et al, 2008).

Symptoms associated with atypical presentation of coronary artery disease in older adults include:
◆ Shortness of breath
◆ Fatigue
◆ Syncope
◆ Confusion
◆ Abdominal or back pain (Meiner, 2011)

Modified from Berger DH et al: Surgery in the elderly. In Townsend CM et al: *Sabiston textbook of surgery*, ed 18, Philadelphia, 2008, Saunders; Jugdutt BI: *Heart failure in the elderly: Advances and challenges.* Expert review of cardiovascular therapy, 2010;8(5):695–715, available at www.medscape.com/viewarticle/723852. Accessed August 1, 2010; Meiner SE: *Gerontologic nursing*, ed 4, St Louis, 2011, Elsevier; Wold GH: *Basic geriatric nursing*, ed 4, St Louis, 2008, Mosby.

REVIEW QUESTIONS

1. The heart is a _____ chamber muscular pump that propels into the systematic and pulmonary circulatory system.
   a. two
   b. five
   c. four
   d. three

2. On pump, myocardial protection includes:
   a. hypothermia
   b. cardioplegia, invasive
   c. circulatory arrest
   d. all of the above

3. The diaphragm is positioned _____ the heart
   a. above
   b. below
   c. medial to
   d. lateral to

4. When dye is injected into the vascular system, the testing is considered:
   a. semi-invasive
   b. invasive
   c. noninvasive
   d. none of the above

5. The four valves in the heart include the:
   a. tricuspid, pulmonary, aortic, and mitral
   b. bicuspid, pulmonary, aortic, and mitral
   c. pericardium, pulmonary, brachial, and mitral
   d. atrial, auricular, tricuspid, and bicuspid

6. A median sternotomy is an incision:
   a. midline from over the xiphoid process
   b. along the center of the sternum
   c. from the sternal notch to the midpoint of the sternum
   d. along the costochondral junction

7. An OPCAB is this type of myocardial revascularization:
   a. minimally invasive direct coronary bypass
   b. off-pump coronary artery bypass
   c. port-access coronary artery bypass
   d. laser transmyocardial revascularization

8. A history of _____ or frequent tonsillitis as a child is significant because the infections and sequelae can lead to damage of cardiac valves.

9. _____ are placed on the tips of a hemostat to protect suture clamped by the hemostat.

10. Vascular clamps are designed to _____ blood flow partially or completely.

11. Internal mammary artery retractors expose the retrosternal artery bed by elevating the _____ border.

12. Femoral arterial blood pressure supplies include hypodermic needles, a _____, stopcocks, and pressure tubing.

13. True or false: A sternal saw will be necessary for some cardiac surgeries.

14. True or false: Patients with chronic severe angina may be candidates for transmyocardial revascularization.

15. True or false: Heterotopic and combined heart-lung transplants are performed more commonly than orthotopic transplants.

16. Define and briefly describe the following procedures:
    Coronary artery bypass grafts with arterial and venous conduits
    Mitral valve replacement
    Heart transplantation

Critical Thinking Question

Large operating rooms are necessary when performing cardiac surgery to accommodate bulky specialized equipment; in addition, multiple electrical outlets are necessary. What other features would be preferable in a cardiac surgical suite? What does a large operating room and multiple electrical outlets allow for in cardiac surgery?

REFERENCES

Alfieri O et al: The double-orifice technique in mitral valve repair: a simple solution for complex problems, *J Thorac Cardiovasc Surg* 122(4):674–681, 2001.

American College of Surgeons (ACS): Patient education, 2009a., available at www.facs.org/patienteducation/. Accessed June 30, 2009.

American College of Surgeons (ACS): Surgical organizations with patient education, 2009b, available at www.facs.org/patienteducation/proresources. html#sso. Accessed June 30, 2009.

American Heart Association (AHA) (2009a): For patients, available at www.americanheart.org/presenter.jhtml?identifier=1200000. Accessed June 30, 2009.

American Heart Association (AHA): Heart disease and stroke statistics—2009 update, 2009b, available at www.americanheart.org/presenter.jhtml?identifier=1200026. Accessed June 22, 2009, http://circ.aha journals.org/cgi/reprint/CIRCULATIONAHA.108.191261(Circulation) www.americanheart.org/downloadableheart/1240250946756LS-1982 %20Heart%20and%20Stroke%20Update.042009.pdf.

American Heart Association (AHA): Review of 1994 revisions to classification of functional capacity and objective assessment of patients with diseases of the heart, 2009c, available at www.americanheart.org/presenter. jhtml?identifier=1712. Accessed July 5, 2009.

American Society of Anesthesiologists (ASA): Patient education, cardiac surgery, 2009, available at www2.asahq.org/google/index.asp?q=cardiac+ surgery. Accessed June 30, 2009.

Angelini GD et al: Effects of on- and off-pump coronary artery surgery on graft patency, survival, and health-related quality of life: long-term follow-up of 2 randomized controlled trials, *J Thorac Cardiovasc Surg* 137(2):295–303, 2009.

Association of periOperative Registered Nurses (AORN): *The geriatric patient: AORN's age-specific competencies series*, Denver, 1997a, The Association.

Association of periOperative Registered Nurses (AORN): *The neonate, infant, and toddler patient: AORN's age-specific competencies series*, Denver, 1997b, The Association.

Association of periOperative Registered Nurses (AORN): *The premature infant patient: AORN's age-specific competencies series*, Denver, 1997c, The Association.

Association of periOperative Registered Nurses (AORN): *The preschool, school-age, and adolescent patient: AORN's age-specific competencies series*, Denver, 1997d, The Association.

Association of periOperative Registered Nurses (AORN): *Competencies for perioperative practice*, Denver, 2008, The Association.

Babb M: Clinical risk assessment: identifying patients at high risk for heart failure, *AORN J* 89(2):273–288, 2009.

Bickler PE et al: Effects of skin pigmentation on pulse oximeter accuracy at low saturation, *Anesthesiology* 102:715–719, 2005.

Bishop P: Position the patient. In Phippen ML et al, editors: *Competency for safe patient care during operative and invasive procedures*, Denver, 2009, Competency and Credentialing Institute.

Blanche C et al: Heart transplantation with bicaval and pulmonary venous anastomoses: a hemodynamic analysis of the first 117 patients, *J Cardiovasc Surg (Torino)* 38:561–566, 1997.

Brown ML et al: Ministernotomy versus conventional sternotomy for aortic valve replacement: a systematic review and meta-analysis, *J Thorac Cardiovasc Surg* 137(3):670–679, 2009.

Bruce CJ, Connolly HM: Right-sided valve disease deserves a little more RESPECT, *Circulation* 119:726–734, 2009.

Bujdoso PJ: Blanket warming: comfort and safety, *AORN J* 89(4):717–722, 2009.

Cameron DE et al: Aortic root replacement in 372 Marfan patients: evolution of operative repair over 300 years, *Ann Thorac Surg* 87:1344–1350, 2009.

Camp SL et al: Quality improvement program increases early tracheal extubation rate and decreases pulmonary complications and resource utilization after cardiac surgery, *J Card Surg* 24(4):414–423, 2009.

Campeau L: Grading of angina pectoris, *Circulation* 54:522, 1975.

Carapetis JR: Rheumatic heart disease in developing countries, *N Engl J Med* 357(5):439–441, 2007.

Carpentier A: Cardiac valve surgery: the French correction, *J Thorac Cardiovasc Surg* 86:323, 1983.

Cheng D et al: Stentless versus stented bioprosthetic aortic valves: a systematic review and meta-analysis of controlled trials, *Innovations* 4(2):61–73, 2009.

Cherry C et al: Ebstein's anomaly: a complex congenital heart defect, *AORN J* 89(6):1098–1110, 2009.

Chitwood WR: Current status of endoscopic and robotic mitral valve surgery (Supplement), *Ann Thorac Surg* 79:S2248–S2253, 2005.

Chitwood WR et al: Robotic mitral valve repairs in 300 patients: a single-center experience, *J Thorac Cardiovasc Surg* 136(2):436–441, 2008.

Clancy CM: Reducing central line-related bloodstream infections, *AORN J* 89(6):1123–1125, 2009.

Coglianese EE, Davidoff R: Predicting outcome in patients with asymptomatic aortic stenosis, *Circulation* 120:9–11, 2009.

Collins P et al: The radial artery versus saphenous vein patency (RSVP) trial investigators, *Circulation* 117:2859–2864, 2008.

Cooper DKC: The surgical anatomy of experimental and clinical thoracic organ transplantation, *Tex Heart Inst J* 31(1):61–68, 2004.

Cox JL et al: The surgical treatment of atrial fibrillation. III. Development of a definitive surgical procedure, *J Thorac Cardiovasc Surg* 101(4):569–583, 1991.

Crawford ES: The diagnosis and management of aortic dissection, *JAMA* 264(9):2537–2541, 1990.

Dal-Bianco JP et al: Management of asymptomatic severe aortic stenosis, *J Am Coll Cardiol* 52:1279–1292, 2008.

De Varennes B et al: Initial results of posterior leaflet extension for severe Type IIIb ischemic mitral regurgitation, *Circulation* 119:2837–2843, 2009.

Dickson VV, McMahon JP: Optimal patient education and counseling. In Moser DK, Riegel B, editors: *Cardiac nursing: a companion to Braunwald's heart disease*, St Louis, 2008, Saunders.

DiNardo JA, Zvara DA: *Anesthesia for cardiac surgery*, ed 3, Malden, MA, 2008, Blackwell Publishing.

Edmunds LH: Cardiopulmonary bypass after 50 years, *N Engl J Med* 351(16):1603–1606, 2004.

Edwards FH et al: Gender-specific practice guidelines for coronary artery bypass surgery: perioperative management, *Ann Thorac Surg* 79: 2189–2194, 2005.

Elliott P et al: Genetic loci associated with C-reactive protein levels and risk of coronary heart disease, *JAMA* 302(1):37–48, 2009.

Engelman R et al: Workforce on Evidence-Based Medicine, Society of Thoracic Surgeons. The Society of Thoracic Surgeons practice guideline series: antibiotic prophylaxis in cardiac surgery, part II: Antibiotic choice, *Ann Thorac Surg* 83(4):1569–1576, 2007.

Falk-Brynhildsen K, Nilsson U: Cardiac surgery patients' evaluation of the quality of theatre nurse postoperative follow-up visit, *Eur J Cardiovasc Nurs* 8(2):105–111, 2009.

Fang JC, O'Gara PT: The history and physical examination: an evidence-based approach. In Libby P et al, editors: *Braunwald's heart disease*, ed 8, Philadelphia, 2008, Saunders.

Fattouch K et al: Off-pump versus on-pump myocardial revascularization in patients with ST-segment elevation myocardial infarction: a randomized trial, *J Thorac Cardiovasc Surg* 137(3):650–657, 2009.

Fedak PWM et al: Evolving concepts and technologies in mitral valve repair, *Circulation* 117:963–974, 2008.

Feindel CM: Aortic root enlargement in the adult. In Cohn LD, editor: *Operative techniques in thoracic and cardiovascular surgery: a comparative atlas*, New York, 2006, Elsevier.

Frasure-Smith N, Lesperance F: Depression and anxiety as predictors of 2-year cardiac events in patients with stable coronary artery disease, *Arch Gen Psychiatry* 65(1):62–71, 2008.

Frumento RJ, Bennett-Guerrero E: Prime solutions for extracorporeal circulation. In Mongero LB, Beck JR, editors: *On bypass: advanced perfusion techniques*, Totowa, NJ, 2008, Humana Press.

Gardner TJ: Building a healthier world, free of cardiovascular diseases and stroke, *Circulation* 119:1838–1841, 2009.

Gemmato CJ et al: Thirty-five years of mechanical circulatory support at the Texas Heart Institute, *Tex Heart Inst J* 32(2):168–177, 2005.

Gourlay T, Qureshi T: Blood flow during cardiopulmonary bypass. In Mongero LB, Beck JR, editors: *On bypass: advanced perfusion techniques*, Totowa, NJ, 2008, Humana Press.

Gray RJ, Sethna DH: Medical management of the patient undergoing cardiac surgery. In Libby P et al, editors: *Braunwald's heart disease*, ed 8, Philadelphia, 2008, Saunders.

Groom RC et al: Detection and elimination of microemboli related to cardiopulmonary bypass, *Circulation Cardiovasc Qual Outcomes* 2:191–198, 2009.

Grundy SM: Is lowering low-density lipoprotein an effective strategy to reduce cardiac risk? Promise of low-density lipoprotein-lowering therapy for primary and secondary prevention, *Circulation* 117:569–573, 2008.

Haissaguerre M et al: Spontaneous initiation of atrial fibrillation by ectopic beats originating in the pulmonary veins, *N Engl J Med* 339(10):659–666, 1998.

Halpin LS, Barnett SD: Preoperative state of mind among patients undergoing CABG, *J Nurs Care Qual* 20(1):73–80, 2005.

Hayes DL, Zipes DL: Cardiac pacemakers and cardioverter-defibrillators. In Libby P et al, editors: *Braunwald's heart disease*, ed 8, Philadelphia, 2008, Saunders.

Hayman LL: Primary prevention in childhood. In Moser DK, Riegel B, editors: *Cardiac nursing: a companion to Braunwald's heart disease*, St Louis, 2008, Saunders.

Hill JA, Olson EN: Cardiac plasticity, *N Engl J Med* 358(13):1370–1380, 2008.

Hjortnaes J et al: Translating autologous heart valve tissue engineering from bench to bed (Abstract). Tissue Eng Part B Reviews. May 18. [Epub ahead of print], 2009. available at www.ncbi.nlm.nih.gov/pubmed/19450137?ordinalpos=8anditool=EntrezSystem2.PEntrez.Pubmed.Pubmed_ResultsPanel.Pubmed_DefaultReportPanel.Pubmed_RVDocSum. Accessed July 5, 2009.

Hlatky MA et al: Criteria for evaluation of novel markers of cardiovascular risk: a scientific statement from the American Heart Association, *Circulation* 119:2408–2416, 2009.

Horvath KA, Zhou Y: Transmyocardial laser revascularization and extravascular angiogenic techniques to increase myocardial blood flow. In

Cohn LH, editor: *Cardiac surgery in the adult*, ed 3, New York, 2007, McGraw-Hill.

Hu KK et al: Use of maximal sterile barriers during central venous catheter insertion: clinical and economic outcomes, *Clin Infect Dis 39*, November 15, 2004.

Hunt SA: Taking heart—cardiac transplantation past, present, and future, *N Engl J Med* 355:231–235, 2006.

Hussey LC et al: Risk factors for sternal wound infection in men versus women, *Am J Crit Care* 10(2):112–116, 2001.

Isselbacher EM: Diseases of the aorta. In Libby P et al, editors: *Braunwald's heart disease*, ed 8, Philadelphia, 2008, Saunders.

Jansens JL et al: Robotic hybrid procedure and triple-vessel disease, *J Card Surg* 24(4):449–450, 2009.

Jeevanandam V et al: A one-year comparison of prophylactic donor tricuspid annuloplasty in heart transplantation, *Ann Thorac Surg* 78:759–766, 2004.

Jin R et al: Is obesity a risk factor for mortality in coronary artery bypass surgery, *Circulation* 111:3359–3365, 2005.

Journal of the American Medical Association (JAMA): JAMA patient's page, 2009. Available at www.jama.com.

Kamstrupp PR et al: Genetically-elevated lipoprotein (a) and increased risk of myocardial infarction, *JAMA* 301:2331–2339, 2009.

Khonsari S et al: *Cardiac surgery: safeguards and pitfalls in operative technique*, ed 4, Philadelphia, 2008, Wolters Kluwer/ Lippincott Williams and Wilkins.

Kirtane AJ et al: Safety and efficacy of drug-eluting and bare metal stents: comprehensive meta-analysis of randomized trials and observational studies, *Circulation* 119:3198–3206, 2009.

Kokotsakis J et al: Right axillary artery cannulation: surgical management of the hostile ascending aorta, *Tex Heart Inst J* 32(2):189–193, 2005.

Korngold EC et al: Amino-terminal pro-B-type natriuretic peptide and high-sensitivity C-reactive protein as predictors of sudden cardiac death among women, *Circulation* 119:2868–2876, 2009.

Kouchoukos NT et al: *Kirklin/Barratt-Boyes cardiac surgery*, ed 3, Philadelphia, 2003, Churchill Livingstone, vol. I.

Kuchukarian N et al: Eleven-year experience in diagnosis and surgical therapy of right atrial masses, *J Card Surg* 22:39–42, 2007.

Kumar AS: *Techniques in valvular heart surgery*, New Delhi, India, 2008, CBS Publishers and Distributors.

Kumar N et al: A revised terminology for recording surgical findings of the mitral valve, *J Heart Valve Dis* 4:70–75, 1995, discussion 76–77.

Kutcher MA et al: Percutaneous coronary interventions in facilities without cardiac surgery on site: a report from the National Cardiovascular Data Registry (NCDR), *J Am Coll Cardiol* 54(1):16–24, 2009.

Lachman N et al: Pericardiectomy: a functional anatomical perspective for the choice of left anterolateral thoracotomy, *J Card Surg* 24(4):411–413, 2009.

Lamendola C: Insulin resistance, diabetes, and cardiovascular disease. In Moser DK, Riegel B, editors: *Cardiac nursing: a companion to Braunwald's heart disease*, St Louis, 2008, Saunders.

Lee TH, Bonow RO: Guidelines: management of valvular heart disease. In Libby P et al, editors: *Braunwald's heart disease*, ed 8, Philadelphia, 2008, Saunders.

Leeson A et al, editors: *Cardiac catheterization and coronary intervention (Oxford Specialist Handbooks)*, New York, 2008, Oxford University Press.

Li Y et al: Comparison of drug-eluting stents and coronary artery bypass surgery for the treatment of multivessel coronary disease: three-year follow-up results from a single institution, *Circulation* 119:2040–2050, 2009.

Libby P et al, editors: *Braunwald's heart disease*, ed 8, Philadelphia, 2008, Saunders.

Lietz K et al: Impact of center volume on outcomes of left ventricular assist device implantation as destination therapy: analysis of the Thoratec HeartMate Registry, 1998 to 2005, *Circ: Heart Fail* 2(1):3–10, 2009.

Long JW et al: Long-term destination therapy with the HeartMate XVE left ventricular assist device: improved outcomes since the REMATCH study, *Congestive Heart Failure* 11:133, 2005.

Lopes RD et al: Endoscopic versus open vein-graft harvesting in coronary-artery bypass surgery, *N Engl J Med* 361(3):235–244, 2009.

Lorenz RA et al: Perioperative blood glucose control during adult coronary artery bypass surgery, *AORN J* 81(1):126–150, 2005.

Lundblad R et al: Surgical repair of postinfarction ventricular septal rupture: risk factors of early and late death, *J Thorac Cardiovasc Surg* 137(4):862–868, 2009.

Lytle BW: Who are we—who we will be, *J Thorac Cardiovasc Surg* 135(5):965–975, 2008.

Mancini ME, Bubien RS: Care of patients with sudden cardiac death, cardiac arrest, and life-threatening dysrhythmias. In Moser DK, Riegel B, editors: *Cardiac nursing: a companion to Braunwald's heart disease*, St Louis, 2008, Mosby.

Mascagni R et al: Edge-to-edge technique to treat post-mitral valve repair systolic anterior motion and left ventricular outflow tract obstruction, *Ann Thorac Surg* 79:471–474, 2005.

McCarthy P: Surgical management of heart failure. In Libby P et al, editors: *Braunwald's heart disease*, ed 8, Philadelphia, 2008, Saunders.

McSweeney JC, Lefler LI: Women and cardiovascular disease. In Moser DK, Riegel B, editors: *Cardiac nursing: a companion to Braunwald's heart disease*, St Louis, 2008, Saunders.

Menasche P: Stem cell therapy for heart failure: are arrhythmias a real safety concern? *Circulation* 119:2735–2740, 2009.

Mentzer RM et al: Myocardial protection. In Cohn LH, editor: *Cardiac surgery in the adult*, ed 3, New York, 2007, McGraw Hill Medical.

Miller LW et al: Use of a continuous-flow device in patients awaiting heart transplantation, *N Engl J Med* 357:885–896, 2007.

Miller M, Beauman G: Preoperative assessment. In Conte JV et al: *The Johns Hopkins manual of cardiac surgical care*, ed 2, St Louis, 2008, Mosby.

Mirzaie M et al: A new storage solution for porcine aortic valves, *Ann Thorac Cardiovasc Surg* 13:102–109, 2007.

Mongero LB, Beck JR: *On bypass: advanced perfusion techniques*, Totowa, NJ, 2008, Humana Press.

Moons P et al: Care of adults with congenital heart disease. In Moser DK, Riegel B, editors: *Cardiac nursing: a companion to Braunwald's heart disease*, St Louis, 2008, Saunders.

Morrow DA, Gersh BJ: Chronic coronary artery disease. In Libby P et al, editors: *Braunwald's heart disease*, ed 8, Philadelphia, 2008, Saunders.

Mosca L et al: Evidence-based guidelines for cardiovascular disease prevention in women: 2007 update, *Circulation* 115:1481–1501, 2007.

Moser DK, Riegel B: Care of patients with acute coronary syndrome: ST segment elevation myocardial infarction. In Moser DK, Riegel B, editors: *Cardiac nursing: a companion to Braunwald's heart disease*, St Louis, 2008, Mosby.

Moss CJ, Moss R: Assist the anesthesia provider. In Phippen ML et al, editors: *Competency for safe patient care during operative and invasive procedures*, Denver, 2009, Competency and Credentialing Institute, 2009.

Naka Y, Rose EA: Assisted circulation in the treatment of heart failure. In Libby P et al, editors: *Braunwald's heart disease*, ed 8, Philadelphia, 2008, Saunders.

Nasso G et al: Arterial revascularization in primary coronary artery bypass grafting: direct comparison of 4 strategies—results of the Stand-n-Y mammary study, *J Thorac Cardiovasc Surg* 137(35):1093–1100, 2009.

Newby LK, Douglas PS: Cardiovascular disease in women. In Libby P et al, editors: *Braunwald's heart disease*, ed 8, Philadelphia, 2008, Saunders.

Oakley RE et al: Choice of prosthetic heart valve in today's practice, *Circulation* 117:253–256, 2008.

Otto CM, Bonow RO: Valvular heart disease. In Libby P et al, editors: *Braunwald's heart disease*, ed 8, Philadelphia, 2008, Saunders.

Ozcan AV et al: 30-year patency of saphenous vein graft in coronary bypass graft surgery (case report), *Ann Thorac Surg* 85(4):e23, 2008.

Pagana KD, Pagana TJ: *Mosby's diagnostic and laboratory test reference*, ed 9, St Louis, 2009, Mosby.

Park SJ et al: Left ventricular assist devices as destination therapy: a new look at survival, *J Thorac Cardiovasc Surg* 129(1):9–17, 2005.

Patel MR et al: ACCF/SCAI/STS/AATS/AHA/ASNC 2009 Appropriateness Criteria for Coronary Revascularization: A Report by the American College of Cardiology Foundation Appropriateness Criteria Task Force, Society for Cardiovascular Angiography and Interventions, Society of Thoracic Surgeons, American Association for Thoracic Surgery, American Heart Association, and the American Society of Nuclear Cardiology. Endorsed by the American Society of Echocardiography, the Heart Failure Society of America, and the Society of Cardiovascular Computed Tomography, *Journal of the American College of Cardiology* 53:530–553, doi:10.1016/j.jacc.2008.10.005 (Published online 5 January 2009), available at http://content.onlinejacc.org/cgi/content/full/j.jacc.2008.10.005. Accessed July 7, 2009.

Pear SM, Williamson TH: The RN first assistant: an expert resource for surgical site infection prevention, *AORN J* 89(6):1093–1097, 2009.

Pepper J et al: Stentless versus stented bioprosthetic aortic valves. A Consensus Statement of the International Society of Minimally Invasive Cardiothoracic Surgery (ISMICS) 2008, *Innovations* 4(2):49–60, 2009.

Petersen C, editor: *Perioperative nursing data set*, revised 2nd edition, Denver, 2007, Association of periOperative Registered Nurses, Inc.

Pradhan AD et al: Symptomatic peripheral arterial disease in women: nontraditional biomarkers of elevated risk, *Circulation* 117:823–831, 2008.

Pretre R, Turina MI: Deep hypothermic circulatory arrest. In Cohn LH, editor: *Cardiac surgery in the adult*, ed 3, New York, 2007, McGraw-Hill.

Puskas JD et al: Off-pump techniques benefit men and women and narrow the disparity in mortality after coronary bypass grafting, *Ann Thorac Surg* 84:1447–1456, 2007.

Quigley GD et al: Diseases of the aorta. In Conte JV et al: *The Johns Hopkins manual of cardiac surgical care*, ed 2, St Louis, 2008, Mosby.

Quill JL et al: Mitral leaflet anatomy revisited, *J Thorac Cardiovasc Surg* 137(5):1077–1081, 2009.

Rabago G et al: The new DeVega technique in tricuspid annuloplasty, *J Thorac Cardiovasc Surg* 21:231, 1980.

Rahimtoola SH: Choice of prosthetic heart valve for adult patients, *J Am Coll Cardiol* 41(6):893–904, 2003.

Rahimtoola SH: The year in valvular heart disease, *J Am Coll Cardiol* 43(3):491–504, 2004.

Rich MW: The impact of aging on cardiac function. In Moser DK, Riegel B, editors: *Cardiac nursing: a companion to Braunwald's heart disease*, St Louis, 2008, Saunders.

Rogers JH, Bolling SF: The tricuspid valve: current perspective and evolving management of tricuspid regurgitation, *Circulation* 119:2715–2718, 2009.

Rose E et al: Long-term use of a left ventricular assist device for end-stage heart failure: the Muenster experience, *N Engl J Med* 345:1435–1443, 2001.

Rothman C: Surgeons perform first artificial heart implant in New Jersey. The Star Ledger (New Jersey), Wednesday, June 24, 2009, available at www.nj.com/news/index.ssf/2009/06/first_artificial_heart_implant.html. Accessed July 9, 2009.

Ruz MEA, Lennie TA: Inflammation. In Moser DK, Riegel B, editors: *Cardiac nursing: a companion to Braunwald's heart disease*, St Louis, 2008, Saunders.

Salerno TA: Warm heart surgery: reflections on the history of its development, *J Cardiac Surg* 22:257–259, 2007.

Sarin EL et al: Off-pump coronary bypass grafting is associated with reduced operative mortality and in-hospital adverse events in patients with left main coronary artery disease, *Innovations* 4(2):80–85, 2009.

Sasaki H: The right gastroepiploic artery in coronary artery bypass grafting, *J Cardiac Surg* 23:398–407, 2008.

Savino JS, Cheung AT: Cardiac anesthesia. In Cohn LH, editor: *Cardiac surgery in the adult*, ed 3, New York, 2007, McGraw-Hill.

Schulze CJ et al: Phosphorylcholine-coated circuits improve preservation of platelet count and reduce expression of proinflammatory cytokines in CABG: a prospective randomized trial, *J Cardiac Surg* 24(4):363–368, 2009.

Seifert PC: Nurses in perioperative settings. In Moser DK, Riegel B, editors: *Cardiac nursing: a companion to Braunwald's heart disease*, St Louis, 2008, Saunders.

Seifert PC: Care of the cardiac surgical patient. In Drain CB, Odom-Forren J, editors: *Perianesthesia nursing: a critical care approach*, St Louis, 2009, Saunders.

Seifert PC, Collins J: Cardiac surgery. In Phippen ML et al, editors: *Competency for safe patient care during operative and invasive procedures*, Denver, 2009, Competency and Credentialing Institute.

Seifert PC et al: Surgery for atrial fibrillation, *AORN J* 86(1):23–40, 2007.

Sellke FW et al: Comparing on-pump and off-pump coronary artery bypass grafting: numerous studies but few conclusions: a scientific statement from the American Heart Association Council on Cardiovascular Surgery and Anesthesia in collaboration with the interdisciplinary working group on quality of care and outcomes research, *Circulation* 111:2858–2864, 2005.

Sellke F, Ruel M: *Atlas of cardiac surgical techniques: a volume in the surgical techniques atlas series*, Philadelphia, 2009, Saunders.

Serruys PW et al: Percutaneous coronary intervention versus coronary-artery bypass grafting for severe coronary artery disease, *N Engl J Med* 360(10):961–972, 2009.

Sethares K et al: Care of patients undergoing cardiac surgery. In Moser DK, Riegel B, editors: *Cardiac nursing: a companion to Braunwald's heart disease*, St Louis, 2008, Saunders.

Seymour GJ et al: Infection or inflammation: the link between periodontal and cardiovascular diseases, *Future Cardiology* 5(1):5-9, 2009, available at www.medscape.com/viewarticle/587591). Accessed April 3, 2009.

Shimokawa T et al: Intermediate-term patency of saphenous vein graft with a clampless hand-sewn proximal anastomosis device after off-pump coronary bypass grafting, *Ann Thorac Surg* 87:1416–1420, 2009.

Simmonds PK et al: Cardiovascular pharmacologic agents. In Conte JV et al: *The Johns Hopkins manual of cardiac surgical care*, ed 2, St Louis, 2008, Mosby.

Singh SK et al: The impact of diabetic status on coronary artery bypass graft patency: insights from the radial artery patency study, *Circulation* 118(suppl 1):S222–S225, 2008.

Smith PK: Treatment selection for coronary artery disease: the collision of a belief system with evidence, *Ann Thorac Surg* 87(5):1328–1331, 2009.

Sniecinski RM, Levy JH: The inflammatory response to cardiopulmonary bypass. In Mongero LB, Beck JR, editors: *On bypass: advanced perfusion techniques*, Totowa, NJ, 2008, Humana Press.

Society of Thoracic Surgeons (STS): STS patient information, available at www.sts.org/sections/patientinformation/. Accessed June 30, 2009.

Sommer RJ et al: Pathophysiology of congenital heart disease in the adult. Part I: Shunt lesions, *Circulation* 117:1090–1099, 2008a.

Sommer RJ et al: Pathophysiology of congenital heart disease in the adult. Part II: Simple obstructive lesions, *Circulation* 117:1228–1237, 2008b.

Sommer RJ et al: Pathophysiology of congenital heart disease in the adult. Part III: Complex congenital heart disease, *Circulation* 117:1340–1350, 2008c.

Starr A, Edwards ML: Mitral replacement: clinical experience with a ball-valve prosthesis, *Ann Surg* 154:726, 1961.

Stoney WS: *Pioneers of cardiac surgery*, Nashville, 2008, Vanderbilt University Press.

Stout KK, Verrier ED: Acute valvular regurgitation, *Circulation* 119:3232–3241, 2009.

Superko HR, King S: Is lowering low-density lipoprotein an effective strategy to reduce cardiac risk? Lipid management to reduce cardiovascular risk, *Circulation* 117:560–568, 2008.

Svenarud P et al: Effect of CO_2 insufflation on the number and behavior of air emboli in open-heart surgery, *Circulation* 109:1127–1132, 2004.

Svensson L: Aortic dissection endovascular stenting: less pain, survival gain? *Ann Thorac Surg* 87:1332–1333, 2009.

Tang GH et al: Tricuspid valve repair with an annuloplasty ring results in improved long-term outcomes, *Circulation* 114(suppl):I-577–I-581, 2006.

Tavilla G et al: Long-term follow-up of coronary artery bypass grafting in three-vessel disease using exclusively pedicled bilateral internal thoracic and right gastroepiploic arteries, *Ann Thorac Surg* 77:794–799, 2004.

The Criteria Committee of the New York Heart Association: *Nomenclature and criteria for diagnosis of diseases of the heart and great vessels*, ed 9, Boston, 1994, Little, Brown and Co, pp. 253-256.

Thompson J, Bertling G: Endovascular leaks: perioperative nursing implications, *AORN J* 89(5):839–846, 2009.

Tinkham MR: The endovascular approach to abdominal aortic aneurysm repair, *AORN J* 89(2):289–302, 2009.

Todd R, Phippen M: Cardiac catheterization and electrophysiology. In Phippen ML et al, editors: *Competency for safe patient care during operative and invasive procedures*, Denver, 2009, Competency and Credentialing Institute.

Toumpoulis IK et al: Assessment of independent predictors for long-term mortality between women and men after coronary artery bypass grafting: are women different from men? *J Thorac Cardiovasc Surg* 131:343–351, 2006, available at http://jtcs.ctsnetjournals.org/cgi/content/full/jtcs; 131/2/343. Accessed July 4, 2009.

Walton-Geer PS: Prevention of pressure ulcers in the surgical patient, *AORN J* 89(3):538–548, 2009.

Warziski MT et al: Obesity. In Moser DK, Riegel B, editors: *Cardiac nursing: a companion to Braunwald's heart disease*, St Louis, 2008, Saunders.

Webb JG et al: Transcatheter aortic valve implantation: impact on clinical and valve-related outcomes, *Circulation* 119:3009–3016, 2009.

Wilson SR et al: Evaluation for a ventricular assist device: selecting the appropriate candidate, *Circulation* 119:2225–2232, 2009.

Pediatric Surgery

Overview

Pediatrics is a specialty focused on the health and well-being of neonates, infants, children, and adolescents. The pediatric patient often needs surgery for congenital anomalies that threaten life or the child's ability to function. Trauma also impacts a child's health far more often than an adult's; injury is a common reason for surgical intervention. Pediatric surgery is

This chapter was originally written by Leigh Ann DiFusco, RN, MSN, CNOR, for the 14th edition of Alexander's Care of the Patient in Surgery *and has been revised by Sherri M. Alexander, CST, for this text.*

an area of practice unto its own because the pediatric patient is so very different from an adult. The field is even further subdivided into all the surgical specialties. It is important to recognize that the difference between pediatric care and adult care is not just a size issue; from birth onward, the body and organs exist in a continual state of development, and multiple physiologic changes occur with age. Major areas of distinction are the airway and pulmonary status, cardiovascular status, temperature regulation, metabolism, fluid management, and psychologic development. A thorough knowledge of these differences is integral to the provision of nursing care for the pediatric patient in the OR.

Advances in surgical interventions for children have been phenomenal in the last two decades for many reasons. The advancement of improved diagnostic and interventional technology, the development of new anesthetics and pharmacologic agents for pain management, and the creation of even smaller and more delicate instrumentation have revolutionized perioperative care of the pediatric population. Numerous pediatric surgeries that were once performed as open cavity procedures are now being done endoscopically with minimally invasive techniques, resulting in shorter hospital stays and faster recovery times. Improvements in the transport of critically ill children and the intensive care management of neonatal and pediatric patients as well as the development of new surgical procedures are also saving more lives yet presenting medical professionals with a new and unique set of problems as complex, medically fragile children are now surviving into adulthood.

Pediatric Surgical Anatomy

Airway/Pulmonary Status

Respiratory mechanics alter dramatically from infancy to adulthood, resulting from increases in airway size, transformations in the rigidity of airway and chest structures, and major changes in neuromuscular status. A proportionally large head, a short neck, and a large tongue in relation to jaw size create more of a challenge for airway management. The glottis is very anterior, moving from the level of the second cervical vertebra to the level of the third to fourth vertebrae in the adult. The epiglottis is floppy and more curved, and the vocal cords are slanted anteriorly. The airway forms an inverse cone with the narrowest portion at the cricoid cartilage until 8 years of age; endotracheal tube size is therefore very important, since a tube that passes easily through the glottis may be too tight at the subglottic area, compromising the child's airway in the immediate postoperative period because of swelling. The infant is an obligate nasal breather, and the chest wall of an infant is very compliant, leading to increased work of breathing with any type of airway compromise. Infants also have type 2 respiratory muscle fibers until age 2 years, which fatigue more easily than type 1 muscle fibers. Premature infants are at risk for postanesthetic apnea until 60 weeks after conception age. There is a depression in the CO_2 response curve in infants; compared to an adult, the respiratory rate does not increase as readily in response to a rising CO_2 level, although all ages undergo a CO_2 response depression related to inhalational agents and narcotics. One of the most important considerations is that children have a much smaller pulmonary functional residual capacity; a child becomes hypoxic more quickly if the airway is lost. Alveolar maturation is not complete until 8 years of age. Smaller airways have higher resistance; airway resistance decreases approximately 15 times from infancy to adulthood, again with a major change occurring around 8 years of age. It is important to note that smaller airways can become compromised with even a minor amount of swelling. Be aware that loose teeth are common in children aged 5 to 14 years; a dislodged tooth is a potential airway foreign-body risk.

Cardiovascular Status

The most dramatic changes in the cardiovascular system occur at birth with the transition from fetal circulation. Even in full-term infants, persistent transitional circulation may occur. Heart rate is the predominant determinant of cardiac output in infants and children; bradycardia drastically decreases cardiac output and requires swift intervention. There is a decreased cardiac compliance because of a lower proportion of muscle to connective tissue until age 1 to 2 years, making infants preload insensitive. Young children are predisposed to parasympathetic hypertonia (increased vagal tone), which can be induced by painful stimuli such as laryngoscopy, intubation, eye surgery, or abdominal retraction. Attention to blood loss in young patients is very important because the patient's total blood volume is very small. Blood volume in neonates is 80 to 90 ml/kg; at 1 to 6 years it is 70 to 75 ml/kg; and at age 6 years to adult it is 65 to 70 ml/kg. At birth, 70% to 90% of the hemoglobin is fetal hemoglobin with a high affinity for oxygen. It is normal for hemoglobin levels to fall at about 2 to 3 months of age (physiologic anemia) to a hematocrit level of 29% and a hemoglobin level of 10 mg/dl as the infant's body begins to produce its own blood cells. A cardiology evaluation is essential if a murmur is auscultated. A murmur can be from a patent foramen ovale, which normally closes at 3 to 12 months; a patent ductus arteriosus, which can be present for up to 2 months; a previously undetected cardiac anomaly; or an innocent flow murmur. The evaluation is critical because anesthetic agents cause vasodilation and potentiate cardiac dysrhythmias.

Temperature Regulation

Infants and young children are most at risk of hypothermia because of their increased body surface area/weight ratio and thin fat layer. Cold stress leads to increased oxygen consumption, resulting in hypoxia, respiratory depression, acidosis, hypoglycemia, and pulmonary vasoconstriction. Hypothermia alters drug metabolism, prolongs the action of neuromuscular blockers, and delays emergence from anesthesia. The child's temperature must be monitored continuously throughout the intraoperative experience. An axillary temperature probe is acceptable for short procedures in healthy children; an esophageal or rectal temperature probe provides more accurate monitoring of the child's temperature for longer procedures. Hyperthermia should also be avoided, because it leads to increased oxygen consumption and increased fluid losses.

It is vital to maintain normothermia in children, and the easiest way to do this is by exposing only the area on which surgery is being performed. Additional thermoregulatory interventions include altering the room temperature before the child enters the room, using a water-filled temperature-regulating blanket under the patient, or using a forced-air warming blanket over nonsurgical areas of the child. An overhead heater can be used during the anesthetic induction and patient preparation period immediately before prepping and draping. The anesthesia ventilation circuit can be heated and humidified, as can insufflated carbon dioxide during minimally invasive surgical procedures. For surgical procedures with large areas of exposure, warmed solutions should be available for use instead of room temperature solutions. Intravenous (IV) solutions can also be warmed before administration.

Metabolism

Infants have a higher basal metabolic rate than adults, and it is greatest at 18 months. Most importantly, children younger than age 2 years have immature liver function; pharmacologic response is altered, and there is slower hepatic clearance, decreased hepatic enzyme function, and decreased protein binding. Drug distribution is different in neonates and infants compared with older children and adults because of an increased percentage of total body weight and extracellular body fluid. Infants have an immature blood-brain barrier and decreased protein binding, which results in an increased sensitivity to sedatives, opioids, and hypnotics.

Fluid Management

Renal function at birth is immature, and the ability of the kidneys to concentrate urine is limited, so the infant is much more prone to dehydration. Complete maturation of renal function occurs at about 2 years. Compared to an adult, a child has a higher body water weight, a higher body surface area, and an increased metabolic rate, resulting in increased fluid requirements per kilogram of body weight. Despite these significant points, it is also important to remember that the body weight of the child, the length of time without fluids, and surgical losses are the primary factors in the calculations of the child's hydration needs.

PSYCHOLOGIC DEVELOPMENT

A child's comprehension of and responses to the environment are based on his or her developmental age. A key factor is that a child's developmental age does not necessarily match the chronologic age. Patient care should be tailored to the developmental age of the child to optimize the child's ability to understand the situation, to minimize the child's and family's stress and anxiety, and to facilitate the development of a trusting and supportive medical relationship. The types of fears are also related to the child's level of psychologic development.

Predictable stages mean predictable behaviors. The stages of growth have been described from a variety of different aspects; Dr. Jean Piaget described the stages by changes in cognition and the ability to think, and Dr. Erik Erikson based the stages on psychosocial and emotional needs. Their work provides an excellent guideline for assessing the pediatric patient's developmental level in order to use appropriate interventions (Table 17-1).

Surgical Technologist Considerations

The initial patient assessment provides information necessary to develop a plan of care specific to the needs of each particular pediatric patient related to age, developmental level, and diagnosis. The unique aspects of care of the pediatric surgical patient revolve around the fact that the child is constantly growing and changing.

Anticipating that pediatric patients will have anxiety about leaving their parents, the surgical technologist may need to be available to help the circulator when the patient is brought into the OR. The surgical technologist will need to have equipment, supplies, and instrumentation specific to the scheduled specific surgical procedure or unscheduled surgical procedure in pediatric surgery. It is also important to know the age and weight of the child. This information will guide selection of the correct instruments, supplies, and solutions used.

TABLE 17-1

Developmental Stages

Approximate Ages	Piaget's Stage	Erikson's Stage	Developmentally Based Fears
Infancy to 1 yr (Erikson) Infancy to 2 yr (Piaget)	Sensorimotor Uses senses and motor skills to understand world Develops memory; begins to imitate others	Trust vs. mistrust—develops belief that world can be counted on to meet basic needs Who to trust? Identifies strangers at 7-8 mo	Separation
Toddlerhood	Preoperational Use of symbols, creative play (can pretend) Is very egocentric	Autonomy vs. shame, doubt Develops free will; increasing control of their bodies Feels regret, sorrow for inappropriate behavior	Separation Forced dependence
Early childhood, preschool	Preoperational continues	Initiative vs. guilt Begins to explore, imagine Feels remorse for actions Thinking dominated by perceptions—distorted reasoning	Separation Body mutilation
Middle childhood, elementary school age (Erikson) Ages 7-11 yr (Piaget)	Concrete operations Uses symbols, logic, principles to solve problems Classifies, sorts everything	Industry vs. inferiority Beginning to understand time and unseen body functions Is cooperative; desires recognition for achievements	The unknown Body mutilation Inadequate performance
Adolescence, puberty	Formal operations Uses logical and abstract thinking Understands hypothetical concepts	Identity vs. role diffusion Peer group has increased importance Body image, clothing, activities help define identity	Altered body image Death

Modified from Taylor E: Providing developmentally based care for toddlers, *AORN J* 87(5):992-999, 2008; Taylor E: Providing developmentally based care for school-aged and adolescent patients, *AORN J* 90(2):261-269, 2009; *Stages of social-emotional development in children,* available at www.childdevelopmentinfo.com/development. Accessed August 23, 2009.

Pediatric patients differ dramatically from adult patients; therefore, the surgical technologist will need to anticipate the possible need for changes in instrumentation and sponge sizes as well as the temperature of irrigations and solutions. In some instances, the pediatric patient will have had several procedures, and this can lead to longer procedure time and the need for additional specialty instruments and supplies because of the buildup of scar tissue and adhesions. There may be a need for warming lights in addition to the heating blanket used to keep the child's temperature stable.

Multiple procedures may be done simultaneously on the pediatric patient. The surgical technologist will need to be prepared to have more than one sterile operative setup, or break down and re-establish the operative field several times. As with any surgical procedure, the principles of aseptic technique must be adhered to diligently. The pediatric patient with either congenital condition or traumatic injury is susceptible to infections.

When involved with pediatric surgery, it is imperative for the surgical technologist to have knowledge of the procedure being performed and the equipment to be used. Keeping current on the latest advancements in pediatric surgery will help ensure the most positive outcome for the patient.

Informed Consent. Informed consent from the parent or legal guardian of the pediatric patient is required unless the patient is an emancipated minor. An emancipated minor is one who is legally under the age of consent but is recognized as having the legal capacity to consent. Minors may become emancipated by pregnancy, marriage, high school graduation, independent living, and military service. It is important for children to develop a trusting relationship with medical professionals and that these older children are in agreement (within their developmental capabilities) with their family's decision regarding surgery.

Child Abuse and Neglect. The surgical team is obligated to screen all pediatric patients for abuse or neglect. Child abuse and neglect are defined as "physical or mental injury, sexual abuse or exploitation, negligent treatment or maltreatment" (Betz and Sowden, 2008). Child abuse is found in all segments of society, crossing cultural, ethnic, religious, socioeconomic, and professional groups. The surgical team is in a unique situation to assess for the presence of abuse because the patient will be disrobed in the OR. Box 17-1 lists the clinical manifestations of child abuse. Every state has a child abuse law that dictates legal responsibility for reporting abuse and suspicion

---

BOX 17-1

Clinical Manifestations of Child Abuse and Neglect

SKIN INJURIES
Skin injuries are the most common and easily recognized signs of maltreatment of children. Human bite marks appear as an ovoid area with tooth imprints, suck marks, or tongue thrust marks. Multiple bruises in inaccessible places are indications that the child has been abused. Bruises in different stages of healing may indicate repeated trauma. Bruises that take the shape of a recognized object are generally not accidental.

TRAUMATIC HAIR LOSS
Traumatic hair loss occurs when the child's hair is pulled or used to drag or jerk the child. The result of the pulling on the scalp can cause the blood vessels under the skin to break. An accumulation of blood can help differentiate between abusive and nonabusive loss of hair.

FALLS
If a child is reported to have experienced a routine fall but appears to have severe injuries, the inconsistency of the history with the trauma sustained indicates suspected child abuse.

EXTERNAL HEAD, FACIAL, AND ORAL INJURIES
Cuts, bleeding, redness, or swelling of the external ear canal; facial fractures; tears or scarring of the lip; oral, perioral, and/or pharyngeal lesions; loosened, discolored, or fractured teeth; dental caries; tongue lacerations; unexplained erythema or petechiae of the palate; and bilateral black eyes without trauma to the nose may all indicate abuse.

DELIBERATE OR UNEXPLAINED THERMAL INJURIES
Immersion burns, with a clear line of demarcation; multiple small circular burns, in varying stages of healing; iron burns (show iron pattern); diaper area burns; and rope burns suggest intentional harm.

SHAKEN BABY SYNDROME
A shaken baby may suffer only mild ocular or cerebral trauma. The infant may have a history of poor feeding, vomiting, lethargy, and/or irritability that occurs periodically for days or weeks before the initial healthcare consult. In 75% to 90% of the cases, unilateral or bilateral retinal hemorrhages are present but may be missed unless the child is examined by a pediatric ophthalmologist. Shaking produces an acceleration-deceleration (shearing) injury to the brain, causing stretching and breaking of blood vessels that results in subdural hemorrhage. Subdural hemorrhage may be most prominent in the interhemispheric fissure. However, cerebral edema may be the only finding. Serious insult to the central nervous system may result, without evidence of external injury.

UNEXPLAINED FRACTURES AND DISLOCATION
Posterior rib fractures in different stages of healing, spiral fractures, or dislocation from twisting of an extremity may provide evidence of nonaccidental injury in children.

SEXUAL ABUSE
Abrasions or bruising of the inner thighs and genitalia; scars, tearing, or distortion of the labia/hymen; anal lacerations or dilation; lacerations or irritation of external genitalia; repeated urinary tract infections; sexually transmitted disease; nonspecific vaginitis; pregnancy in young adolescent; penile discharge; and sexual promiscuity may provide evidence of sexual abuse.

NEGLECT
The symptoms of neglect reflect a lack of both physical and medical care. Manifestations include failure to thrive without a medical explanation, multiple cat or dog bites and scratches, feces and dirt in the skinfolds, severe diaper rash with the presence of ammonia burns, feeding disorders, and developmental delays.

Modified from Betz CL, Sowden LA: *Mosby's pediatric nursing reference,* ed 6, St Louis, 2008, Mosby.

RAPID RESPONSE TEAM

Cardiopulmonary arrest in hospitalized children is a rare event, but one that occurs in 0.19 to 2.45 of 1000 admissions. Comparable figures for adult cardiopulmonary arrest range from 2.6 to 6.5 per 1000 admissions. Rapid response teams (RRTs), common in facilities providing care to adults, have demonstrated effectiveness in preventing complications by initiating interventions when a patient begins to decline. The goal of RRTs is to interrupt the cascade of events that often results in cardiac arrest. Clinicians are generally familiar with the signs of impending cardiopulmonary arrest in adults. The origin of cardiopulmonary arrest in adults is generally cardiac related and is often preceded by hypotension. Despite the fact that some hospitalized children may suffer arrest attributable to dysrhythmia, airway obstruction, or other events, the majority of cardiopulmonary arrests in children are often related to respiratory failure. Children have greater reserves than adults and may not appear to be unstable as quickly as an adult. By the time a child exhibits signs of secondary cardiopulmonary arrest the period of hypoxemia has been longer, vital organs have been deprived of oxygen, and outcomes are generally worse. Clinicians must recognize the differences between adults and children to intervene appropriately when caring for pediatric patients.

The trend toward dedicated pediatric RRTs is increasing. In facilities where pediatric RRTs exist, staff that are credentialed with Basic Life Support (BLS) or Advanced Life Support (ALS) initiate resuscitation and emergency services within the scope of their certification and activate the RRT. Staff who are not certified in BLS or ALS must contact the RRT and remain with the victim until assistance arrives. Often, patient care areas with high acuity (such as the OR, pediatric intensive care unit [PICU], cancer intensive care unit [CICU], newborn infant center, emergency department, or cardiac catheterization lab) do not routinely use the RRT, except in those instances where a parent or visitor exhibits signs consistent with intervention. The OR also benefits from the close proximity of anesthesia and critical care attending physicians within the patient care areas. When critical incidents occur in the OR during times of limited resources (weekends, off-shifts, holidays), the staff have the option of activating the Code Team, rapid response team or communicating with the charge nurse in the PICU to mobilize additional clinical support in addition to in-house attending physicians, residents, and fellows already assigned to the OR.

Modified from Institute for Health Care Improvement: *Children count in the 100,000 Lives Campaign,* available at www.ihi.org/IHI/Topics/CriticalCare/IntensiveCare/ImprovementStories/ChildrenCountinthe100000LivesCampaign.htm. Accessed August 23, 2009; Children's Hospital of Philadelphia: *Administrative policy and procedure manual, A-4-19 Resuscitation and emergency services;* Tibballs J, van der Jagt EW: Medical emergency and rapid response teams, *Pediatr Clin North Am* 55:989-1010, 2008; Van Voorhis KT, Schade-Willis T: Implementing a pediatric rapid response system to improve quality and patient safety, *Pediatr Clin North Am* 56:919-933, 2009.

SURGICAL TECHNOLOGY PREFERENCE CARD

Keep in mind in pediatric surgery size matters. The weight and age of your patient will direct you in setting up for the procedure.

In pediatric surgery you may have more than one surgical team and additional healthcare personnel in the OR. Arrive in the room early to get acquainted with the room layout and equipment and supplies stored in the room. Discuss the position of the OR bed and surgical equipment with the surgical team, taking into consideration that additional equipment may be needed. Organizing equipment location before setting up sterile tables for the procedure allows a safe traffic pattern to be established. This helps ensure sterility of the field and facilitates effective communication between the circulator and scrub. It also provides space for other personnel involved in the surgical procedure.

Room Prep: Basic OR furniture in place, thermoregulatory devices, extra blankets, padding, positioning supplies to achieve optimal patient safety. Determine if a latex-free environment is required before opening or using any supplies containing latex.

Prep Solution: In room and warmed according to manufacturer's instructions
- Chlorhexidine gluconate (CHG)
- Iodine and iodophors (these may be diluted)
- Technicare
- Ivory soap
- Baby shampoo

Catheter: In room and correct size
- Catheter set and tray
  - Latex/rubber
  - PVC
  - Silicone
- Sizing
  - French
- Nonretaining
  - Red rubber (Robinson)
- Retaining
  - Foley
    - 2-way
    - 3-way
  - Mushroom/Pezzer/Malecot
  - T-tube
- Other urine collection devices applicable to pediatric patients

SURGICAL TECHNOLOGY PREFERENCE CARD—cont'd

PROCEDURE CHECKLIST

Instruments
◆ Standard major and minor instrument sets
◆ Open instruments if needed to convert from laparoscopic to open
◆ Anticipated additional instruments

Specialty Suture
◆ As per surgeon's preference—typically fine suture with small needles

Other Hemostatic Agents
◆ Mechanical
  • Staplers
  • Clip appliers and clips
  • Pressure
  • Ligatures
  • Bone wax
  • Pledgets
◆ Chemical
  • Absorbable gelatin
  • Collagen
  • Oxidized cellulose
  • Silver nitrate
  • Epinephrine
  • Thrombin
◆ Thermal
  • Electrosurgical unit
  • Harmonic scalpel
  • Argon beam coagulator
  • Laser

Additional Supplies: both sterile and nonsterile
◆ If the physician is requesting supplies, instruments, or equipment not normally used, check to be sure all have arrived to the room before opening any other sterile supplies
◆ Sponges
◆ Drapes
◆ Gowns and gloves for team members
◆ "Have ready" or "hold" supplies

Medications and Irrigation Solutions
◆ Warmed (follow manufacturer's recommendations for warming any medications or solutions)
◆ Appropriate-sized syringes, hypodermic needles, labels, and marking pen

Drains
◆ Correct size and type for planned surgery
  • Open—Not attached to a drainage system
    • Penrose
    • Cigarette
  • Closed—Attached to a closed reservoir for fluid collection
    • Hemovac
    • Jackson-Pratt
    • Autologous blood retrieval drainage system

Dressings
◆ As per surgeon's preference
◆ Cyanacrylate glue

Specimen Care
◆ Proper container for each specimen
◆ Labels for each specimen
◆ Proper solution for specimen type

Before opening for the procedure, the surgical technologist should:
◆ Arrange furniture
◆ Gather positioning devices
◆ Damp dust lights, furniture, and surfaces
◆ Verify functionality of equipment
◆ Place items to be opened in their appropriate places

When opening sterile supplies:
◆ Verify exposure to sterilization
◆ Use sterile technique
◆ Open bundles in appropriate locations
◆ Open additional supplies onto sterile field
◆ Open the room as close to the surgical start time as possible

Guidelines for Pediatric Ambulatory Surgery

Candidates for ambulatory surgery in a pediatric institution should:

◆ Be categorized as either class I or class II in accordance with the American Society of Anesthesiologists (ASA) guidelines; in some cases, patients who are categorized as class III may be eligible for ambulatory surgery with the approval of the medical director or attending surgeon
◆ Be older than 6 months of age

Procedures that are eligible for scheduling in ambulatory surgical settings should:

◆ Be no more than 4 hours in duration and have a total 4 hours of direct supervised recovery unless exceeded by patient condition demands that cannot be anticipated before surgery
◆ Be able to be performed using local or regional anesthetics, monitored anesthesia care (MAC), or general anesthetic with a duration of less than 4 hours
◆ Be able to be performed without the risk of extensive blood loss, major prolonged invasion of body cavities, or direct involvement of major blood vessels

Modified from Children's Hospital of Philadelphia: *Ambulatory surgery policy and procedure manual, 5.2.1 approved surgical procedures for ambulatory surgical centers; Ambulatory surgery policy and procedure manual, 2.1.1 patient selection criteria for the ambulatory surgery center.*

of abuse, and all healthcare providers are mandated reporters. Failure to report suspected child abuse could result in a fine or other punishment, according to individual statutes (Betz and Sowden, 2008).

Planning and Preparation

Assessment data, combined with information about the planned surgical procedure, enable the surgical technologist to anticipate requirements for surgical positioning, instrumentation, equipment and supplies, medications, and activities necessary for the provision of safe, competent care for the pediatric patient.

The presence of a parent during much of the preoperative period, including during anesthesia induction in the OR and after anesthesia emergence in the PACU, can help decrease anxiety for both young children and their families and facilitates family-centered care (Evidence for Practice).

Infants, reliant on family to meet their basic needs, are difficult to pacify when NPO for surgery. The facility should provide rocking chairs, pacifiers, warm blankets, and simple distractions such as music or toys. Preoperative teaching should include telling the family to provide fluids for the infant until the deadline for NPO status. Unnecessary delays should be avoided at all costs. Parents may need reassurance and support during the period immediately before surgery.

The toddler or preschooler fears parental separation and abandonment. Toddlers fear, among other things, strangers,

EVIDENCE FOR PRACTICE

Timely Postoperative Visitation

Parental visitation in the postanesthesia care unit (PACU) has been identified as a standard of care in some hospitals, but not all. In this study, researchers at a facility in Pennsylvania reviewed the literature to summarize the benefits of early parental visitation in the PACU, and then established a baseline within the unit. Through objective data collection and anecdotal reporting, they found that in 2004 only 44% of parents were reunited with children during the immediate postoperative phase. The team established a target goal of 75% parental visitation in the PACU within 6 months of initiating a quality improvement program.

Their quality improvement program consisted of a survey distributed to ambulatory surgery patients and families in April 2005 to ask families questions such as the following: Did they believe that their children were adequately prepared for the surgery? What aspects of care were most important to the family? What was the family's overall satisfaction with the ambulatory surgical experience? The results of the survey indicated that speaking with their child's surgeon after the procedure and being present with their child in the PACU as soon as possible after surgery were the top two priorities for family satisfaction.

The team decided to address barriers that prevented parental visitation in the PACU. Among the top concerns were the high acuity of patients upon arrival to the PACU; a change in efficiency related to phase I procedures and care; risks to patient safety because of negative reactions from parents related to laryngospasm, airway obstruction, and respiratory compromise; and increased risks to the safety of parents who were

unable to effectively cope with seeing their child during the immediate postoperative period.

The first step in garnering support for change was recognition from nursing leadership that the concerns shared by the nursing staff regarding the delivery of patient care balanced with parental visitation were real and valid. The team worked to help the nursing staff understand that they all owned the process, and accepted that resistance was more a result of a caring and committed staff. In order for timely postoperative visitation to occur, resources, adequate systems, and support from management were readily available. In addition, the practice was championed and clear expectations were shared with the staff.

Ultimately, change could only occur with multidisciplinary acceptance of the new practices. A team represented by various stakeholders in the surgical process, including members from a family advisory committee, was created to establish a foundation for work, review the current philosophy of care and key elements of family-centered care, and develop a theoretical framework for the group's work. Any staff member who provided direct patient care was educated about the quality improvement program, and before surgery all patients were provided with education and information regarding parental visitation in the PACU.

Their target goal was reached in January 2005 and has continued to increase. In January 2007, 90% of parents were reunited with their child within 30 minutes of the patient's arrival to the PACU.

Modified from Kamerling SN et al: Family centered care in the pediatric postanesthesia care unit: changing practice to promote parental visitation, *J Perianesth Nurs* 23(1):5-16, 2008.

the dark, and machines. They attribute lifelike qualities to inanimate objects, believing that the objects, like them, have feelings. Thus a blood pressure cuff that squeezes the child's arm may be perceived to be doing so because it is angry with the toddler. Toddlers may also believe that their body is held together by their skin; anything that violates the skin integrity is feared. For this reason, bandages are very important. Toddlers and preschoolers interact with the environment using their senses. To integrate this into the patient's care, give the toddler the opportunity to touch and play with objects that he or she will encounter. An example is to give the child a small anesthesia mask to put on his or her teddy bear. Sensory information should be provided in a soft, gentle voice (i.e., what the toddler will see, feel, touch, and hear). A security object is extremely comforting. The OR should be quiet; background noise should be controlled. Instruments that are frightening should be kept from view. To allow quick induction of anesthesia the toddler should be transferred into the surgical suite when the room and staff are completely prepared.

The school-age child may still perceive hospitalization or surgery as a punishment but can evaluate painful intrusive actions in terms of logical function (e.g., getting an IV line hurts, but then I can get medicine in it to make me feel better). Feelings of inadequacy may be associated with something the child thinks he or she should be expected to do or know. Fear of body injury or mutilation, loss of control, and fear of the unknown characterize this developmental stage. These children benefit from simple, concrete explanations in familiar terms; a book or other teaching aid can be helpful. The concepts of time and unseen body functions can now be incorporated in the explanations. The child should be allowed to make choices when possible (e.g., letting the child decide in which hand to place the IV line or which flavor to add to the anesthetic mask).

Adolescents may fear altered body image, peer rejection, disability, and loss of control or status. The fear of death is more prevalent in this age-group than any other, and adolescents may find explanations of monitoring and safety measures reassuring. They need as much privacy as possible, and their attempts to be independent should be respected (e.g., walking into the OR instead of being wheeled in on a stretcher if the patient has not been sedated). The adolescent may not wish to show any fear; questions might not be asked while the parents are present. Information and explanations should be provided as reasonably and truthfully as possible. If appropriate, some choices should be allowed, such as wearing underwear to the OR. Patient care procedures that violate privacy, such as hair removal, skin preparation, or insertion of an indwelling urinary catheter, should be conducted after the patient is anesthetized.

Key points in providing perioperative care to pediatric patients include remaining alongside the child until the child is anesthetized, keeping the room quiet during induction, accepting a child's need to express fear and fearful behaviors (e.g., crying), and using simple words without double meanings to explain care. Security objects should remain with the child until induction has been completed. A child's behavior during induction is likely to be the same during emergence; thus all attempts should be made to provide calm, reassuring care. Parents should be alerted to delays in the surgery schedule; in some instances, the child may be allowed to have fluids if the surgery is delayed by several hours.

Remaining with the child during induction, positioning, and prepping the surgical site; creating and maintaining a sterile field; collecting, documenting, and disposing specimens; and administering medications are all part of helping to provide a safe environment for the pediatric surgical patient.

Instrumentation. The same types of instruments used in adult surgery are used in pediatric surgery. However, pediatric instruments are usually shorter, have more delicate or less pronounced curves, and are smaller. A complete range of instrument sizes is necessary to make the appropriate size available to each child, since pediatric patients can range in size from less than 1 kg to more than 100 kg. Fewer instruments are normally required because incisions in children are shorter and shallower than those in adults. Use of basic instrument sets, grouped according to types of surgery performed (e.g., minor, major), facilitates instrument counts. These sets are easily adapted to the patient's needs as well as the surgeon's preferences and eliminate unnecessary instruments from the sterile field.

The following sets are examples of instrumentation used in pediatric surgery. The minor set is used for procedures such as inguinal hernia repair, head and neck procedures, and pyloromyotomy. The major set is used for major chest and abdominal procedures, such as tracheoesophageal fistula (TEF) and diaphragmatic hernia repair, omphalocele repair, bowel resection, and pull-through for Hirschsprung's disease. Smaller and larger instruments should be in separate, additional sets to be dispensed to the surgical field as determined by the patient's size.

In addition to basic instruments, the minor pediatric instrument set should include curved Knapp iris scissors, both sharp and blunt; a Jacobsen curved clamp for delicate dissection; straight and curved Halsted mosquito clamps; sharp and blunt Senn retractors (two of each); 0.5-mm Castroviejo forceps; single-toothed Adson forceps; 6-inch fine DeBakey forceps; a small Weitlaner retractor; an Andrews-Pynchon 9½-inch suction; sizes 7- and 9-French (7F, 9F) Frazier suctions; a Castroviejo locking needle holder; and two Webster needle holders. The major pediatric instrument set should include the components of the minor set, slightly longer (7- to 8-inch) basic instruments (scissors, forceps, needle holders), and the following: curved Schnidt forceps; fine Kelly clamps; Gemini right-angled clamps; Army-Navy, small Deaver, and Richardson retractors (two of each size); Gerald forceps; Singley ring forceps; a set of malleable retractors; a grooved director; and a Poole suction. Examples of pediatric instruments are shown in Figures 17-1 through 17-8.

Sutures. A variety of sutures are used with the pediatric population because of the wide range of patient size; size 0 to 7-0 are routinely stocked. Both absorbable and nonabsorbable sutures on cutting and tapered needles are employed. The most frequently used sizes are 3-0 to 5-0 with ½- and ⅜-circle needles. Staples, both pediatric and regular sizes, are occasionally used. Many skin incisions are closed with subcuticular techniques, over which adhesive strips or cyanoacrylate glue is then applied. The use of tape to apply dressings is done conservatively because of the delicate nature of children's skin; frequently, either a small transparent or an elastic net dressing is used to hold gauze dressings in place.

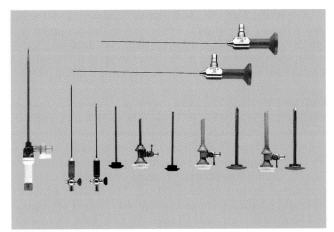

FIGURE 17-1 *Top to bottom:* 2 Stryker laparoscopic lens, 2.7 mm, 30 degree, 70 degree. *Left to right:* 1 3-mm Ethicon disposable needle; 2 Veress needles, 100 mm, 70 mm; 1 obturator, 3.5 mm, sharp; 1 3.5-mm × 40 mm cannula with port; 1 obturator, 3.5 mm, blunt; 1 5-mm × 40 mm cannula with port; 1 obturator, 5 mm, blunt; 1 5-mm × 50 mm cannula with port; and 1 obturator, 5 mm, sharp.

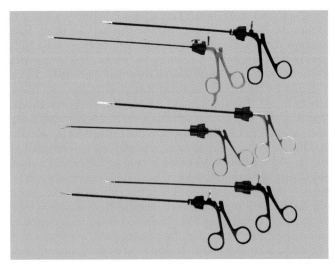

FIGURE 17-3 *Top to bottom:* 1 3.5-mm × 24 cm Hook scissors; 1 3.5-mm × 24 cm Babcock forceps; 1 3.5-mm × 24 cm Hunter bowel grasper; 1 3.5-mm × 24 cm grabber forceps; 1 3.5-mm × 24 cm monopolar Metzenbaum dissecting scissors; and 1 3.5-mm × 24 cm Maryland dissector.

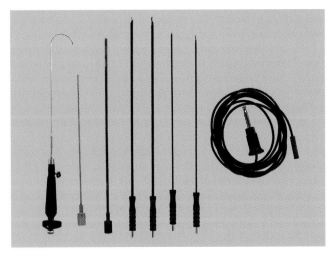

FIGURE 17-2 *Left to right:* Endoflex liver retractor; 1 3.5-mm suction/irrigator; 1 5-mm suction/irrigator, disposable; 1 spatula cautery, 5 mm, disposable; 1 hook cautery, 5 mm, disposable; 1 hook, 3.5 mm, disposable; 1 spatula 3.5 mm, disposable; and 1 monopolar cord.

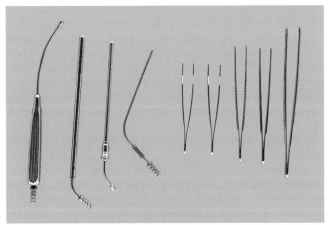

FIGURE 17-4 *Left to right:* 1 Andrew-Pynchon suction tube; 1 Poole suction tube, 16 Fr; 1 Poole suction tube with valve, 23 Fr; 1 Frazier suction tube, 8 Fr; 2 Adson tissue forceps, 1 with teeth (1 × 2), 1 without teeth; 2 Cushing tissue forceps, without teeth; and 1 Russian tissue forceps, medium.

Anesthetic Considerations. Anesthesia is approached differently in pediatric patients than it is in adults. The equipment and supplies are scaled down to match the size of the patient, and different anesthesia circuits and delivery systems may be used. The most common technique used in the pediatric population is a general inhalational anesthetic administered by facemask, laryngeal airway, or endotracheal tube. Selection of the endotracheal tube involves several considerations; the tube must be large enough to permit ventilation but small enough to minimize damage to the trachea while maintaining a seal to prevent aspiration. Pressure from the cuff can cause tracheal damage (Cote, 2005). Uncuffed endotracheal tubes are used in children up to 8 years of age. Table 17-2 provides a guide to choosing endotracheal tubes and laryngoscope blades for pediatric patients.

Microdrip IV tubing and burettes are commonly used to avoid the administration of excess fluids in pediatric patients under the age of 8 years, and only 500-ml bags of IV solution are used. The patient's IV line is usually started in the OR after induction with mask anesthesia, depending on the patient's diagnosis and medical history. Patients who require emergency surgery who have not been NPO; have increased intracranial pressure, an unusually difficult airway, or neuromuscular disease; or have been diagnosed with malignant hyperthermia require an IV placement before anesthesia induction. If the IV line is started before induction, measures should be taken to lessen the discomfort, such as an intradermal injection of 1% buffered lidocaine or saline at the site or the application of topical anesthetic creams. If possible, the surgical team should allow the child the option of sitting up or lying down during

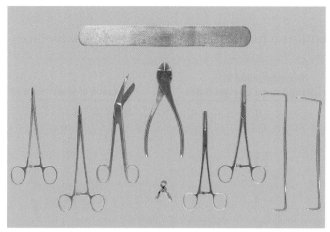

FIGURE 17-5 *Top:* 1 Ochsner malleable retractor, medium. *Bottom, left to right:* 1 Jarit sternal needle holder, 7 inch; 1 Jarit sternal needle holder, 8 inch; 1 bandage scissors, heavy; 1 wire cutter, heavy; 1 Edwards holding clip; 2 Jarit (Vorse) tubing occluding clamps; 2 Army-Navy retractors.

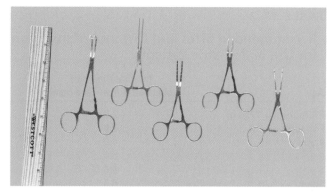

FIGURE 17-7 *Left to right:* 12-inch ruler showing the size of the neonatal vascular clamps. 1 Satinsky neonatal vascular clamp; 1 DeBakey neonatal vascular clamp, straight; 1 Cooley neonatal multipurpose clamp, angled; 1 Cooley neonatal peripheral vascular clamp, angled; and Cooley neonatal vascular clamp.

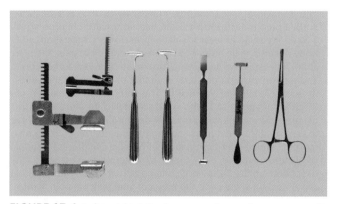

FIGURE 17-6 *Left to right:* 2 Cooley neonatal sternal retractors, pediatric, infant; 2 Doyen rib elevators and raspatories, right, left; 1 Alexander rib raspatory (periosteotome), double-ended, child; 1 Matson rib stripper and elevator, child; 1 Pennington hemostatic forceps.

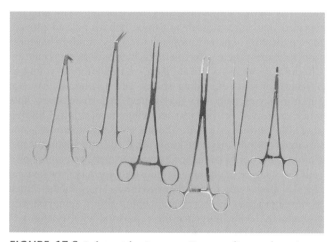

FIGURE 17-8 *Left to right:* 1 reverse Potts cardiovascular scissors; 1 Potts cardiovascular scissors; 2 DeBakey coarctation and peripheral vascular clamps, 9 inch, straight, angled; 1 Gerald tissue forceps without teeth, 7 inch; and 1 Ryder needle holder, 7 inch.

IV placement; if developmentally appropriate, hold the child's hand and tell the child about each step in the placement of an IV line.

Preoperative sedation is generally accomplished by the oral administration of midazolam. Midazolam is the most commonly used pediatric premedication in the United States and can be given orally, nasally, rectally, intramuscularly, or intravenously (Cote, 2005). Oral midazolam should be administered in a flavored base to mask the bitter taste. Relaxation is noted 15 to 45 minutes after administration; the child should be kept in a safe, observable environment after being medicated. Other agents used for premedication include fentanyl and, infrequently, ketamine.

Depending on institutional policy, a parent may be present during induction to comfort the child and decrease the child's anxiety. The circulator should provide the parent an explanation of how the OR will appear and who will be present in the OR, how the child's anesthesia induction will be performed, and how the child will appear as the anesthetic takes effect. An additional staff person, such as a parent services' provider

or child life therapist, should be present to escort the parent to and from the OR so that the circulator can focus on providing care for the patient once the child has been anesthetized.

Malignant hyperthermia (MH), although very rare, may be more prevalent in the pediatric population as a result of the administration of inhalational anesthetics and succinylcholine. In addition, physiologic conditions present in some pediatric patients are associated with a higher risk of MH. These conditions are myotonia congenita, Duchenne's muscular dystrophy, Becker's muscular dystrophy, osteogenesis imperfecta, arthrogryposis, kyphoscoliosis, and King-Denborough syndrome (Gronert, 2005). Careful assessment of family history is essential to identify patients at risk for developing MH.

Pain Management. In the past, many common fallacies existed about pain in the pediatric population. Some of these mistruths were that infants do not feel pain; children have better pain tolerance than adults; children cannot tell the healthcare provider where they hurt; children always tell the truth about pain; children become accustomed to pain or painful

TABLE 17-2

Recommended Sizes and Distance of Insertion of Endotracheal Tubes and Laryngoscope Blades for Use in Pediatric Patients

Age	Internal Diameter of Endotracheal Tube (mm)	Recommended Size of Laryngoscope Straight Blade	Distance of Insertion (cm)
Premature (<1250 g)	2.5	0	6-7
Full term	3.0	0-1	8-10
1 yr	4.0	1	11
2 yr	5.0	1-1.5	12
6 yr	5.5	1.5-2	15
10 yr	6.5	2-3	17
18 yr	7-8	3	19

Modified from Cote CJ: Pediatric anesthesia. In Miller RD, editor: *Miller's anesthesia*, vol 2, ed 6, Philadelphia, 2005, Churchill Livingstone.

procedures; and narcotics are more dangerous for children than they are for adults. Research into this important area has revealed that infants do demonstrate behavioral and physiologic indicators of pain. Compared to adults, children have less pain tolerance; their pain tolerance increases as they mature. Children are able to indicate pain, and children as young as 3 years can use pain-rating scales. Often children may not admit to having pain; they may believe that others know how much they hurt, or they fear receiving an injection. Children may also feel that pain and suffering are punishment for some misdeed, or they may not know what the word *pain* means. Children do not become accustomed to pain or painful procedures. They actually may demonstrate increased behavioral signs of pain with repeated procedures. Many factors, such as developmental level, culture, coping ability, temperament, and activity levels, influence the behavioral manifestations of pain exhibited by the patient. Narcotics are no more dangerous for children than they are for adults and are not excluded as a treatment modality. The evaluation of a pediatric patient's level of pain is performed using a variety of assessment tools (pain scales) that are based on the age and developmental level of the child. Often, these scales are tested for reliability and validity (Research Highlight). In infants and nonverbal children, evaluation is based on physiologic changes and observation of behaviors. Children with verbal skills are able to articulate pain. One assessment strategy to use with pediatric patients is the *QUESTT* method:

Question the child.
Use pain-rating scales.
Evaluate behavior and physiologic changes.
Secure the parents' involvement.
Take cause of pain into account.
Take action, and evaluate results.

Questioning the child provides the most reliable indicator of pain. Children may not be familiar with the word *pain* and may be more comfortable with words like "ouch," "hurt," or "owie." It may also be helpful to ask the child to point to where it hurts. The FACES pain scale uses cartoon faces with a variety of expressions ranging from happy to crying. The child selects the face that best describes his or her pain. The Oucher scale has a numeric component and a component similar to the FACES scale but uses actual photographs of children. The adolescent pediatric pain tool (APPT) is a line drawing of a

RESEARCH HIGHLIGHT

Behavioral Observational Pain Scale (BOPS)

The Behavioral Observational Pain Scale (BOPS) is a postoperative pain measurement scale geared toward children ages 1 to 7. The scale assesses facial expression, verbalization, and body position in an attempt to score the degree of pain felt by a child. A prospective study was conducted on a day-surgery unit and a neurosurgical postoperative unit to determine the validity and reliability of the BOPS. The sample size consisted of 76 children ages 1 to 7 who were scheduled for elective surgical procedures. The study was divided into interrater reliability (based on different nurses scoring patients on the BOPS), concurrent validity (comparing the BOPS to the Children's Hospital of Eastern Ontario Pain Scale to determine whether each described similar behaviors), and construct validity (assessing baseline pain scores and the effect of analgesic on pain scores at 15, 30, and 60 minutes after administration). The findings of this study indicated that there was extensive agreement between different nurses who scored patients on the BOPS. Positive correlation between the BOPS and the Children's Hospital of Eastern Ontario Pain Scales indicated that both tools described similar behaviors (p <.001). There was significance (p <.01) before the administration of analgesia and at 15, 30, and 60 minutes after medication administration; in addition, there was no significant difference (p <.01) between results recorded at 15 and 60 minutes. The BOPS allows for evaluation and documentation of pain scales in a manner that is reliable and consistent. The scoring system is simple, and can be easily incorporated into a postoperative unit. These findings indicate the potential for improved postoperative pain treatment when using the BOPS in children ages 1 to 7.

Modified from Hesselgard K et al: Validity and reliability of the Behavioural Observational Pain Scale for postoperative pain measurement in children 1-7 years of age, *Pediatr Crit Care Med* 8(2):102-108, 2007.

body; the child marks the drawing where he or she has pain. Other tools include Likert-type scales rating pain on a score of 0 (no pain) to 10 (worst pain) or incorporate several components of pain assessment (subjective and objective data).

Physiologic indicators of pain, such as increased blood pressure, respirations, and heart rate and restlessness, are the same for children as for adults but may not be as reliable, except in neonates and nonverbal children. These indicators may also reflect anxiety or fear and should not be the sole indicator used to determine pain. Children may also tug or hold painful areas or show preference to a painful extremity.

Parental involvement in pain management is important. Parents know their child's normal behavior and can provide input into the behaviors being exhibited in the perioperative setting. Parents should be queried about the child's previous experiences with pain and be taught the nonverbal behaviors that may indicate pain.

Effective pain management requires a willingness to use a variety of methods and modalities to achieve optimal results. Pharmacologic methods include the administration of analgesics, both narcotic and non-narcotic. Patient-controlled analgesia (PCA) is an option for children. Children as young as 4 years have the cognitive and physical capabilities to successfully use this modality with appropriate instruction and support (Wu, 2005). Nonpharmacologic methods include distraction, relaxation, guided imagery, behavioral contracting, and cutaneous stimulation. Nonpharmacologic methods should never be used as substitutes for appropriate medication administration but instead should be used to enhance the management of pain.

Surgical Interventions

As mentioned, children require surgery for congenital malformations, an acquired disease, or trauma. The field of pediatric surgery is further subdivided into all the specialties. Several surgical procedures that may be designated pediatric are presented in previous chapters of this text under particular specialty headings. The surgical interventions presented here represent procedures that are most commonly performed on children.

VASCULAR ACCESS

Vascular access in pediatric patients may be established intraoperatively for short-term (weeks) or long-term (months, years) use. Examples of short-term use include peripherally inserted central venous catheters (PICC lines) for antibiotic therapy. Central venous lines or implanted ports are placed for long-term access to provide parenteral nutrition, chemotherapy, bone marrow transplantation, or multiple IV access lines for the critically ill patient. Common complications of vascular access include infection; thrombosis; catheter occlusion; extravasation/migration; malposition/displacement; vascular stenosis; catheter fracture/embolization; surgical damage to nerves, lymphatics, vessels, or pleura; and poor cosmesis (Turner, 2005). The potential for central line–associated bloodstream infections (CLABSIs) has been recognized in many institutions throughout the country. The Risk Reduction Strategies box addresses ways in which the integrity of these lines can be preserved.

Central Venous Catheter Placement

The preferred site of placement is the external jugular vein. The internal jugular vein may be chosen if the external jugular vein has been used or is too small. From the cannulation site the catheter is tunneled under the skin about 5 to 10 cm. This is done to inhibit contamination of the bloodstream from frequent dressing changes. Subcutaneous ports

are placed in a similar fashion. In cases where the internal or external vein sites are unavailable, the catheter may be placed into the external iliac vein by way of a cutdown in the greater saphenous vein. In these cases the catheter is tunneled into the abdominal wall.

Procedural Considerations. The manufacturer's instructions for handling and preparing the catheter must be followed. The catheter must not contact lint, glove powder, or other foreign matter. Before insertion, the catheter is flushed and filled with heparinized saline (1 unit of heparin to 1 ml of saline) to prevent air bubbles from entering the circulatory system and to eliminate blood clots in the catheter lumen. Fluoroscopy is used to confirm proper placement of the catheter; lead shielding must be provided for patient and staff, with appropriate warning signs placed on room doors. The use of a lead shield for the patient should be documented in the perioperative record.

▶▶ RISK REDUCTION STRATEGIES

Preventing Central Line–Associated Bloodstream Infections (CLABSIs)

When patients with a central venous catheter are admitted into the OR for surgical procedures, staff may take the following precautions to prevent central line–associated bloodstream infections (CLABSIs):

◆ Make every effort not to access the central line for general purposes in the OR; use peripheral lines as much as possible.

◆ Practice hand hygiene before and after handling a central line.

◆ If a central line needs to be used in the OR, healthcare providers must perform a 10-second hub scrub that encompasses the threads of the catheter hub.

◆ If a central line dressing needs to be changed* in the OR, keep the following in mind:

• Don nonsterile exam gloves to remove the old dressing.

• Dried blood, crusty accumulations should be cleaned with an alcohol pad.

• ChloraPrep is the solution of choice in some hospitals for central line dressing changes.

• Establish a sterile field with prep solution and new dressing material.

• If using ChloraPrep, apply the solution using a "back and forth" motion as opposed to concentric circles. The "back and forth" motion creates more friction on the skin and helps to decrease the bacterial load.

• Scrub the area for 30 seconds (recommended time for some hospitals).[†]

• Allow the prep solution to dry.

• Don sterile gloves to apply transparent, semi-permeable dressing.[‡]

• Write the date on the dressing label and apply to the central line dressing site.

---

*Central line dressings are routinely changed every 7 days, unless there is a need to do so (e.g., soiled, bloody). Smartsites (Clave) are changed every 72 hours unless damaged.
[†]If the central line is in the femoral/groin area, scrub the site for 2 minutes.
[‡]SorbaView dressing is only recommended for those patients who have a contraindication (e.g., sensitivity, reaction) to Tegaderm dressings.
Modified from Children's' Hospital of Philadelphia Blood Stream Infection (BSI) Task Force, 2008-2009.

The child is appropriately positioned as dictated by the site chosen for cannulation, and organs are protected with a lead shield. The area is prepped and draped.

Operative Procedure—External Jugular Vein Site

1. The surgeon uses a needle and syringe to puncture the external jugular and aspirates to confirm blood flow.
2. The syringe is removed from the needle, and a guidewire is fed through the needle into the vein. An intraoperative x-ray is taken to confirm correct position.
3. Once the position is confirmed, the surgeon makes an incision over the insertion site. A silver probe or tendon passer is used to create a tunnel beneath the skin to the desired exit site of the catheter. A second incision is made over the tip of the probe or passer.
4. The implantable end of the catheter is attached to the end of the passer or probe and pulled through the subcutaneous tunnel. The catheter is cut to a desired length.
5. The needle is removed from the vein, leaving the guidewire in place. An obturator is placed over the guidewire, and the wire is removed. The catheter is placed through the obturator into the vein and an intraoperative x-ray is taken to confirm position.
6. The catheter is secured at the exit site on the chest wall with nonabsorbable sutures, flushed with a "super flush" of heparinized saline (10 units of heparin to 1 ml of saline in children younger than 12 months or 100 units of heparin to 1 ml of saline in children older than 12 months), and clamped.
7. An occlusive transparent dressing is placed over the catheter site. The catheter is coiled under this dressing to avoid tension on the line and accidental displacement.

MINIMALLY INVASIVE SURGERY

Improvements in instrumentation and the development of equipment in smaller sizes have resulted in the evolution of minimally invasive surgery (MIS) from that of a rapidly growing field to one of routine practice in the pediatric surgical arena. Much like the adult population, many traditional "open" pediatric surgical procedures are being replaced by MIS procedures. Because the field of pediatric MIS is relatively new, surgeons are at an advantage because they are able to combine virtual reality techniques and robotics with the most current technology and instrumentation (Harrington et al, 2008). Advantages of minimally invasive surgery include diminished postoperative pain, improved cosmetic results, decreased prevalence of adhesion formation, and accelerated recovery periods and shorter hospital stays.

Despite the technical congruence with adult MIS procedures, the pediatric populations undergoing these procedures have specific needs that must be satisfied in order to promote positive outcomes. Anesthesia providers must take the size and age of the patient into consideration because of the risk of physiologic compromise related to insufflation. Likewise, steps are taken intraoperatively to decrease the likelihood of intraabdominal injury, such as insertion of an appropriate size Foley catheter to decompress the bladder or application of thromboembolic hose or sleeves to prevent deep vein thrombosis.

Common pediatric MIS procedures for general surgery include diagnostic laparoscopy, pyloromyotomy, splenectomy, gastric fundoplication, and cholecystectomy. Thoracoscopic approaches may be used for correction of pectus excavatum, lung biopsy, sympathectomy, and closure of a patent ductus arteriosus (PDA). Procedures that are currently less common but increasing in prevalence include pancreatectomy for focal lesion, choledochal cyst excision, lobectomy for congenital cystic adenomatoid malformation (CCAM), and repair of congenital diaphragmatic hernia (CDH) and transcutaneous esophageal fistula (TEF). Minimally invasive procedures in other disciplines include (but are not limited to) ventriculoscopy, which can be used to view the ventricles of the brain; functional endoscopic sinus surgery (FESS); and nephrectomy and pyeloplasty, both of which may involve the use of a surgical robotic system.

Laparoscopic Pyloromyotomy for Pyloric Stenosis

Pyloric stenosis (Figure 17-9) is the most common cause of gastric outlet obstructions in children and is the most common condition requiring surgery in the newborn. Signs and symptoms of high gastrointestinal (GI) obstruction appear at 2 to 6 weeks of age. The first sign is bile-free projectile vomiting after feeding. The infant usually fails to gain weight adequately, and there may be a severe loss of body fluids and electrolyte imbalance, evidenced as hypochloremic, hypokalemic metabolic alkalosis. Once the diagnosis of hypertrophic pyloric stenosis is made, either through physical examination or by imaging techniques, surgical intervention is planned. Electrolyte imbalances must be corrected before surgery. The Fredet-Ramstedt pyloromyotomy for pyloric stenosis is an open procedure that involves the incision of the muscles of the pylorus to treat congenital hypertrophy of the pyloric sphincter that is obstructing the stomach. However, laparoscopic pyloromyotomy has replaced the open procedure as the standard for repair. The laparoscopic procedure is described in the following Operative Procedure.

Procedural Considerations. The stomach is emptied just before induction of anesthesia, and the nasogastric tube is removed to guard against reflux of gastric contents around the tube during induction. The patient is positioned transverse on the OR bed so that the operating surgeon stands at the patient's feet. A video monitor is positioned above the patient's head. The abdomen is prepped in the usual manner, and trocar sites are injected with a local anesthetic. The perioperative team must consider the location of the incision and position the patient in a fashion that facilitates maximum exposure of the surgical site. Appropriate-sized instrumentation and sterile supplies must be available, along with the appropriate imaging equipment. Insufflation flow rate should be set to the lowest acceptable level for achieving pneumoperitoneum and increased slowly.

Operative Procedure

1. The surgeon makes a small incision in the umbilicus and places a 3-mm or 5-mm trocar through it to accommodate the telescope. Insufflation tubing is attached to this trocar and the abdomen is insufflated (maximum pressure of 10 mm Hg).
2. Using a #11 blade, the surgeon makes a small stab incision laterally, slightly above the umbilicus on each side.
3. The 3-mm laparoscopic instruments are passed directly through the stab incisions.

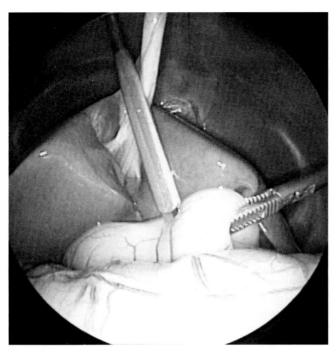

FIGURE 17-9 Pyloric stenosis.

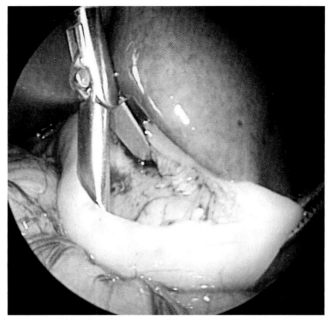

FIGURE 17-10 Laparoscopic pyloromyotomy.

4. The surgeon makes an incision in the serosa on the anterior wall of the pyloric mass from the duodenal junction proximally to a point proximal to the area of hypertrophied muscle using an arthroscopic knife and laparoscopic grasper. The circular muscle is spread with the 3-mm laparoscopic pyloric spreader on the submucosal base, so that all muscle fibers are completely divided (Figure 17-10).
5. The anesthesia provider injects 60 to 120 ml of air into the stomach through an orogastric (OG) tube to ensure that there are no air bubbles at the pyloric incision.
6. The umbilical incision is closed using absorbable suture and cyanoacrylate glue applied to each incision.

Laparoscopic Nissen Fundoplication

Nissen fundoplication is indicated for infants and children who experience severe gastroesophageal (GE) reflux. The cause of GE reflux in these patients is believed to be an inadequate anti–reflux barrier. The anti–reflux barrier normally consists of a combination of anatomic and physiologic factors, including sufficient amount and strength of muscle fibers located in the lower esophageal sphincter, adequate length of the abdominal esophagus, and a high-pressure zone in the lower esophagus. An incompetent anti–reflux barrier can result in life-threatening complications, including obstructive apnea, aspiration pneumonia, esophagitis, and failure to thrive. The goal of the Nissen fundoplication is to create a competent anti-reflux barrier. Nissen fundoplications can be performed using open or laparoscopic technique. There are several types of laparoscopic fundoplications. The traditional laparoscopic wrap is described in Chapter 2. The partial laparoscopic wrap (Toupet) is described below.

Procedural Considerations. The patient is positioned supine for induction of general anesthesia. The anesthesia provider inserts an OG tube, which serves as a stent for the wrap dur-

ing the procedure. Once the endotracheal tube location is confirmed and secured, the patient is moved to the foot of the OR bed and positioned in low lithotomy position using stirrups and protective padding. The operating surgeon stands in the area between the patient's legs. A video monitor is positioned above the patient's head. The abdomen is prepped in the usual manner, and trocar sites are injected with local anesthetic. The perioperative nurse must consider the location of the incision and position the patient in a fashion that facilitates maximum exposure of the surgical site. Appropriate-sized instrumentation and sterile supplies must be available, along with the appropriate imaging equipment. Insufflation flow rate should be set to the lowest acceptable level for achieving pneumoperitoneum and increased slowly.

Operative Procedure
1. Using a #15 blade the surgeon creates a tiny fasciotomy, places a trocar, and insufflates the abdomen with CO_2 gas. After insufflation, the abdomen is inspected for gross abnormality. Additional fasciotomies and trocars are placed to accommodate camera, telescope, and instrumentation.
2. A Colorado clamp is used to elevate the liver away from the stomach, and gastrohepatic connections are cut from the right crus. The crus is carefully dissected away from the esophagus, taking care to preserve the integrity of the peritoneum.
3. Any adhesions on the left side of the stomach are taken down in order to mobilize the fundus and provide access to the left crus.
4. The surgeon uses a blunt dissector to create a retroesophageal tunnel for the esophageal length. The hiatus is reapproximated and tightened using endoscopic suturing devices.
5. A 270-degree (Toupet) wrap is completed. Two sutures incorporate the esophagus, stomach, and crus at the 10 o'clock and 2 o'clock positions on the diaphragmatic hiatus. Four sutures create intraabdominal esophageal length

with stitches anchored at the gastroesophageal junction, giving the fundoplasty the appearance of a "hot dog in a bun" (Figure 17-11).

6. The OG tube is removed and a final barrel suture is placed at the posterior portion of the wrap to anchor it to the right crus and keep it from unwrapping.

7. The stomach is inspected again to rule out gross abnormality or injury and desufflated. Incisions are closed in layers using absorbable suture and sealed with cyanoacrylate glue.

Endoscopic Correction of Pectus Excavatum— Nuss Procedure

Pectus excavatum (funnel chest) is a visually obvious defect of the sternum, seen as a deep depression on the chest as a result of posterior displacement of the sternum (Figure 17-12). It is usually associated with kyphosis. The defect may be asymmetric, most often deeper on the right side, with sternal angulation. In a majority of cases, surgical treatment is cosmetic; impaired cardiorespiratory function is the underlying reason for surgical intervention in fewer cases. The procedure is most commonly performed in patients between 10 and 16 years of age, when children become embarrassed to undress in front of peers (Research Highlight). Rigid fixation has become a choice for correction of the defect, wherein a metal retaining strut is added to gain chest wall stability and prevent recurrence. This strut must be removed 2 to 4 years later (Nuss et al, 2005). Other treatments may cosmetically correct the situation over the short term but usually result in progressive retraction of the sternum.

Procedural Considerations. Adolescent endoscopic instrumentation is used along with a camera, telescopes, corresponding thoracic instrumentation, and a fixation rod. The patient is positioned supine with the arms positioned along the sides and the elbows flexed 90 degrees and propped so that they are anterior to the chest. The hands are propped so that they are anterior to the elbows. The upper chest is elevated on a soft roll or sheets. A Foley catheter may be placed, and the patient is prepped and draped in sterile fashion.

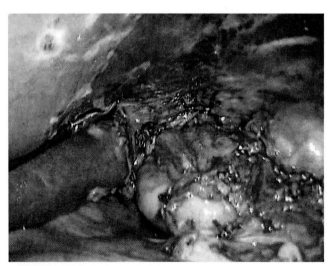

FIGURE 17-11 Laparoscopic Nissen fundoplication, 270-degree (Toupet) wrap.

Operative Procedure

1. The surgeon measures the patient's chest to determine the size of the stabilization bar to be used, and bends an aluminum template to the desired shape of the chest. A stainless-steel bar is bent to match the aluminum template using plate benders.

2. Two lateral chest incisions are made in-line with the deepest part of the pectus using a #15 blade and subcutaneous pockets are created.

3. A port is placed into the left chest through which gentle insufflation takes place.

4. An incision is made via the subcutaneous pocket in order to pass the Lorenz introducer. The introducer is positioned through one side of the chest, across the mediastinum, and out the other side guided by thoracoscopic visualization techniques.

5. A doubled tracheostomy tape is placed at the end hole of the Lorenz introducer and brought through the anterior mediastinal tunnel. The tracheostomy tape is then tied to the stainless-steel bar, which is brought through the chest using the same tunnel and flipped using a flipping device. Chest configuration is checked for correction, contour, and symmetry.

6. A side bar (strut) is placed on each side of the bar and a stainless-steel wire is wrapped around the main bar both medially and laterally. Two sutures are placed between the chest wall and the end holes of the side and main bars. The suture knots are buried within the holes and the thoracic cavity may be irrigated with antibiotic irrigation.

7. The wounds are closed in layers using absorbable suture and a chest x-ray is obtained postoperatively to rule out pneumothorax.

RESEARCH HIGHLIGHT

Pectus Excavatum Repair

Surgical repair of pectus excavatum is often dismissed as a strictly cosmetic intervention. However, correction of the defect may dramatically improve body image and physiologic and psychosocial functioning. In this study, 264 patients (ages 8 to 21) and 291 parents completed a pectus excavatum evaluation questionnaire during the immediate postoperative period. Responders rated questions on a scale of 1 to 4, with higher scores indicating less desirable outcomes.

A follow-up questionnaire was repeated at the 1-year mark (n = 247 patients and 274 parents). Although there was no correlation between the severity of the defect and preoperative psychosocial functioning, 97% of the patients felt that surgical repair of pectus excavatum improved the appearance of their chest, which resulted in improved perceptions of body image (score improved from 2.30 to 1.40). Parental survey results described an overall reduction of emotional (score improved from 1.81 to 1.24) and physical difficulties (score improved from 2.86 to 1.33) in the child and an increase in self-confidence (score improved from 2.14 to 1.32). These results indicate that both the physical as well as the psychosocial implications of pectus excavatum should be considered when evaluating candidates for surgery.

Modified from Kelly RE et al: Surgical repair of pectus excavatum markedly improves body image and perceived ability for physical activity: multicenter study, *Pediatrics* 22(6):1218-1222, 2008.

Video-Assisted Thoracoscopic Surgery for Patent Ductus Arteriosus (PDA)

Although thoracoscopy was first described in 1910 (Rao, 2009), the application of video-assisted thoracoscopic surgery (VATS) to the pediatric population for cardiovascular repairs did not occur until recently. The procedure requires thoracoscopic equipment and supplies, including 0-degree and 30-degree, 4.0-mm and 2.7-mm thoracoscopes, depending on the surgeon's preference and the patient's age and size. The endoscopic instruments, made smaller for the pediatric patient, include an electrocoagulation hook; Castroviejo type of scissors; graspers and right-angle clamps; fan lung retractors of varying sizes, either medium or medium-large; large endoscopic clip appliers; trocars with ports; and suction tip, preferably one that has a porthole to occlude when suction is required. Instrumentation for closure of PDA by thoracotomy is also set up in case the thoracoscopy fails or a complication arises and the chest needs to be opened emergently.

Procedural Considerations. Before the procedure, the television cameras are set up on either side of the OR bed. The patient is placed in a right lateral position.

Operative Procedure

1. Usually four small incisions are made along the line of the posterolateral thoracotomy incision and ports are introduced.
2. The surgeon inserts the thoracoscope. The first assistant holds the lung retractor while the second assistant holds the camera. Some institutions use a mechanical articulating arm.
3. A grasper is used to elevate the pleura overlying the aorta near the insertion of the PDA and pulmonary artery, and careful dissection is begun with electrocoagulation. Suction

is required to keep the area of dissection clear to enhance the surgeon's vision.

4. When the ductus has been clearly identified, a right-angle clamp may first be introduced and a tie applied to the duct. The clip applier is then inserted, and clips are applied.
5. Transesophageal or transthoracic echocardiography is usually performed by a cardiologist before closure of the porthole incisions to ensure closure of the ductus. Also, a chest tube will be inserted into the pleural space, the lungs are inflated, and the chest tube is removed; alternately, a chest tube may be left in place before porthole incision closures.

BARIATRIC SURGERY

More than 15% of children and adolescents are obese, a prevalence that has more than tripled in the past 2 decades. Obesity in adolescents is defined as having a body mass index (BMI; kg/m^2) greater than the 95th percentile for age and weight. Overweight or "at risk" for overweight has been defined as a BMI greater than the 85th percentile for age and weight (Inge et al, 2005). Risk factors that have been identified for pediatric obesity are low birth weight, bottle feeding, having a diabetic mother, and parental obesity (Inge et al, 2005).

Bariatric surgery is gaining popularity as a treatment option for obesity in some adolescents. The timing of the surgical procedure is critical. The patient must be physically mature. Skeletal maturation is generally complete by age 13 to 14 years in girls and age 15 to 16 years in boys. Bariatric surgery can be safely performed once the child has attained more than 95% of adult stature. Candidates undergo psychologic evaluation before surgery to ensure they are cognitively mature enough to participate in decision-making and to comply with postoperative regimens. Box 17-2 details desirable attributes of the adolescent bariatric surgery candidate.

Procedural Considerations

The bariatric procedure most commonly performed in adolescents is the laparoscopic Roux-en-Y gastric bypass. The adjust-

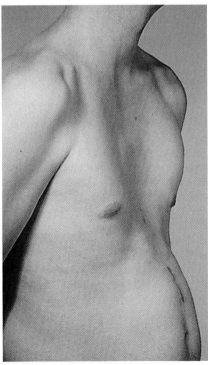

FIGURE 17-12 Pectus excavatum.

BOX 17-2

Characteristics of "Good" Adolescent Patients for Bariatric Surgery

◆ Patient is motivated and has good insight.
◆ Patient has realistic expectations.
◆ Family support and commitment are present.
◆ Family is compliant with healthcare commitments.
◆ Family and patient understand long-term lifestyle changes are needed.
◆ Patient and family agree to long-term follow-up.
◆ Decisional capacity is present.
◆ Well-documented and at least temporarily successful weight loss attempts have been made.
◆ No major psychiatric disorders that may complicate postoperative regimen adherence are present.
◆ No major conduct/behavioral problems are present.
◆ Patient has had no substance abuse in preceding years.
◆ Patient has no plans for pregnancy in upcoming 2 years.

From Inge TH et al: Bariatric surgical procedures in adolescence. In Ashcraft KW et al, editors: *Pediatric surgery,* ed 4, Philadelphia, 2005, Saunders.

able gastric band (i.e., lap band) has not been approved by the U.S. Food and Drug Administration for use in adolescents. The perioperative nurse and surgical technologist must plan carefully for this surgical intervention with an emphasis on obtaining the appropriate-sized transport vehicle and monitoring devices (e.g., larger blood pressure cuff, possibly longer electrocardiogram [ECG] leads to accommodate placement on a larger patient), an OR bed rated for the patient's weight, and appropriate-length instruments in case conversion to an open procedure is necessary. Obesity places this patient group at risk for deep vein thrombosis (DVT); the circulator should ensure that elastic stockings and sequential compression devices are available.

Operative Procedure

The operative procedure is described in Chapter 2.

GENERAL SURGERY: GASTROINTESTINAL PROCEDURES

Repair of Atresia of the Esophagus

Esophageal atresia is a congenital anomaly that may develop between the third and sixth weeks of fetal life. Several types are recognized, the most common being an upper segment of esophagus ending in a blind pouch and a lower segment of esophagus communicating by a fistula with the trachea (esophageal atresia with TEF). Ideally this defect is recognized in the first hours of life, but more often the diagnosis is made in the first 36 to 48 hours of life. Drooling, the need for frequent suctioning, and coughing or cyanosis during oral feeding are the most common presentations (Spitz, 2005). Prompt surgical intervention allows the child to breathe and eat without the danger of aspirating mucus, saliva, feedings, or stomach contents. Atresia of the esophagus is repaired through a right retropleural thoracotomy, with closure of the TEF and anastomosis of the segments of the esophagus.

Procedural Considerations. A bronchoscopy is done to promote accurate placement of the endotracheal tube before surgical repair. Additionally, a gastrostomy may be done first to decompress the air-distended stomach, thus facilitating chest movement and ventilation and preventing reflux of stomach contents into the trachea. The patient is then positioned for a right thoracotomy (sometimes rather posteriorly), prepped, and draped. The major instrument set and a thoracotomy set are required with the appropriate size of chest tube and infant chest drainage system.

Operative Procedure
1. The surgeon enters the chest through the fourth intercostal space. Removal of the rib is not necessary (Figure 17-13, *A*).
2. The pleura is gently dissected off the chest wall (Figure 17-13, *B*).
3. As the dissection proceeds posteriorly, the azygos vein is identified, which is reflected inferiorly after its highest intercostal branches are divided to expose the fistula beneath (Figure 17-13, *C*).
4. The surgeon passes an umbilical tape or vessel loop under the fistula to apply traction gently (Figure 17-13, *D*). Dissection of the mediastinum begins with the TEF and dis-

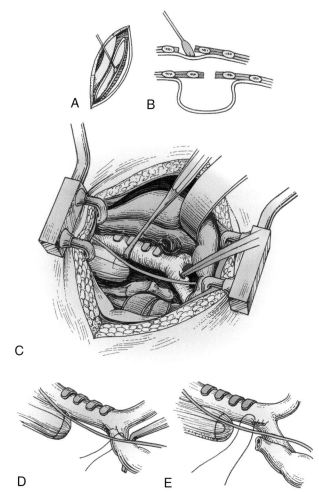

FIGURE 17-13 Repair of atresia of the esophagus. **A,** Incision at fourth intercostal space. **B,** Dissection of pleura off chest wall. **C,** Identification and division of azygos vein to expose fistula beneath. **D,** Traction applied to fistula. **E,** Transection of fistula leaving 3-mm cuff on trachea.

tal end of the esophagus. The vagus nerve is an important landmark for the distal end of the esophagus.
5. The fistula is clamped and transected, leaving a thin cuff of esophageal tissue on the tracheal side to allow closure of the trachea without narrowing it and compromising the lumen of the airway (Figure 17-13, *E*).
6. To close the fistula, three or four interrupted atraumatic sutures of 5-0 nonabsorbable suture are used.
7. The upper esophageal pouch is dissected; passage of a nasogastric tube by the anesthesia provider aids in its identification. The proximal pouch is identified and dissected as needed to allow it to reach the distal esophageal segment with minimal tension for anastomosis. At this point the surgeon decides whether to attempt primary anastomosis. If primary anastomosis is impossible, the distal esophagus is closed and tacked high on the prevertebral fascia. Infrequently the gap between the proximal and distal portions of esophagus is so long that esophageal replacement is required. In these cases the upper pouch is brought out to the neck in the form of a cervical esophagostomy.

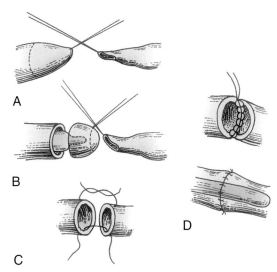

FIGURE 17-14 Primary repair of atresia of the esophagus: single-layer repair. **A,** Traction applied to proximal and distal portions of esophagus. **B,** Blind proximal pouch transected. **C,** Full-thickness bites of anterior and posterior borders. **D,** Repair completed with Replogle tube in place to allow adequate lumen of esophagus.

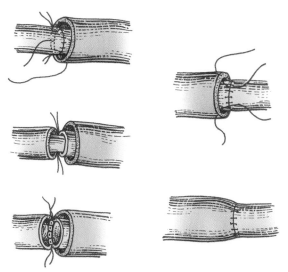

FIGURE 17-15 Haight anastomosis. Mucosal layer of proximal pouch sutured to full thickness of distal esophagus. Muscular sleeve of upper pouch pulled down over inner anastomosis and sutured to muscle of distal esophagus.

8. Primary anastomosis is performed with 5-0 or 6-0 nonabsorbable suture, taking full-thickness bites along anterior and posterior borders (Figure 17-14). Some surgeons prefer the Haight, or two-layer, anastomosis (Figure 17-15). The inner layer is composed of the upper pouch mucosa sutured to the full thickness of the distal esophagus. The muscular sleeve of the upper esophagus is then pulled down over the inner anastomosis and sutured to the muscular layer of the inferior esophagus. The incision is irrigated with saline.
9. Some surgeons place a 14F or 16F extrapleural chest tube near the anastomosis through a posterior stab wound. It is

secured with sutures to prevent it from putting direct pressure on the anastomosis.
10. Muscle layers and fascia are closed with nonabsorbable sutures.
11. Skin is closed with a continuous absorbable suture. The incision is approximated with cyanoacrylate glue or Mastisol and wound closure strips.
12. The extrapleural chest tube is water-sealed after ensuring that the number of centimeters of water and the suction-control chamber are appropriate for the size of the infant. A chest x-ray examination is performed.

When the child reaches 1 year of age, esophageal replacement is attempted through colon interposition or construction of a reverse gastric tube (Figure 17-16).

Gastrostomy

Gastrostomy is establishment of a temporary or permanent channel from the gastric lumen to the skin to permit gastric emptying, liquid feeding, or retrograde dilation of an esophageal stricture. The procedure may be completed as a separate procedure or be performed with other surgical procedures to facilitate care of the infant or child after surgery. A growing number of surgeons are inserting low-profile (e.g., button, Gastroport) devices upon initial creation of the gastrostomy, as these are preferred for children receiving long-term feedings through the device. Low-profile devices, which protrude slightly from the abdomen, are more cosmetically acceptable and allow more mobility for the child. A gastrostomy tube can be placed in the OR as an open or laparoscopic procedure, or it can be performed as a percutaneous procedure under fluoroscopy; both require the patient to receive a general anesthetic. The open surgical procedure is described in the following section.

Procedural Considerations. A minor instrument set is required, plus a gastrostomy feeding catheter (generally a 14F or 16F for infants, or an 18F, 20F, or 22F for older children) and a #11 knife blade on a knife handle. A variety of latex-free gastrostomy catheters are available.

Operative Procedure
1. The surgeon makes a short incision over the outer border of the left rectus muscle (Figure 17-17, *A*).
2. The subcutaneous tissues and rectus fascia are exposed with two small retractors (Figure 17-17, *B*).
3. The anterior rectus fascia is opened, and the rectus muscle is split for exposure of the posterior rectus sheath (Figure 17-17, *C*).
4. The peritoneum is opened for exposure of the liver edge and the greater curvature of the stomach (Figure 17-17, *D*).
5. The stomach is pulled out through the wound with Babcock forceps. A circular, nonabsorbable purse-string suture is placed: in the center of this a very small incision is made with the #11 blade through the gastric wall (Figure 17-17, *E*).
6. A second purse-string suture is placed outside the first one, and the same needle is then taken through the peritoneum and the posterior surface of the rectus fascia to place the stomach against the peritoneum and thus prevent leaks (Figure 17-17, *F* and *G*).

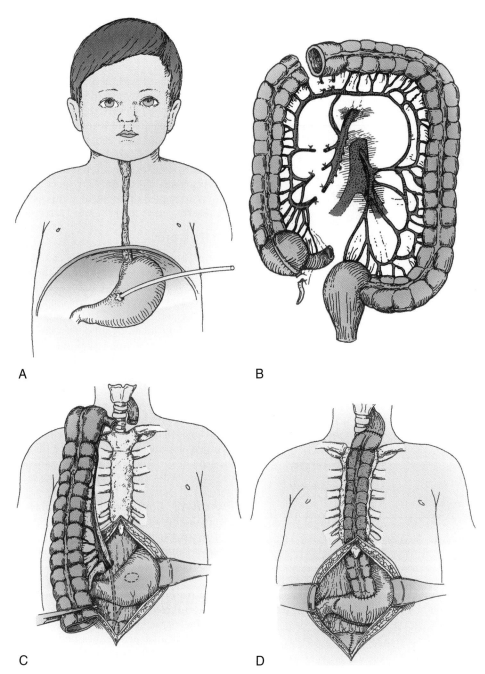

A

B

C

D

FIGURE 17-16 Esophageal replacement. **A,** Gastrostomy. **B,** Isolation of right colon and ileum. **C,** Colon pedicle prepared for anastomosis. **D,** Anastomosis.

7. The feeding catheter is inserted into the stomach through the small incision, and the purse-string suture is tied (Figure 17-17, *H*). Some surgeons may choose to use a dilator kit to assist with proper insertion of the tube. When inserting a gastrostomy tube with a balloon, sterile water and water-based lubricant should be used to avoid breakdown of the tube itself.

8. The catheter is then exteriorized through the skin by way of a small stab wound left, lateral to the skin incision (see Figure 17-17, *A*).

9. The stomach wall adjacent to the gastrostomy site is tacked to the undersurface of the peritoneum with interrupted nonabsorbable sutures.

10. Routine abdominal closure is performed. The gastrostomy tube is left open to straight drainage at the end of the surgical procedure.

Reduction of Intussusception

Intussusception is the telescopic invagination of a portion of intestine into an adjacent part, with mechanical and vascular impairment (Figure 17-18). It is relieved by reduction of invaginated bowel by the hydrostatic pressure of a barium enema or by laparotomy and manual manipulation. The highest incidence of intussusception occurs in infants between the ages of 5 and 9 months. More than half the cases occur within the first year of life, and only 10% to 25% of

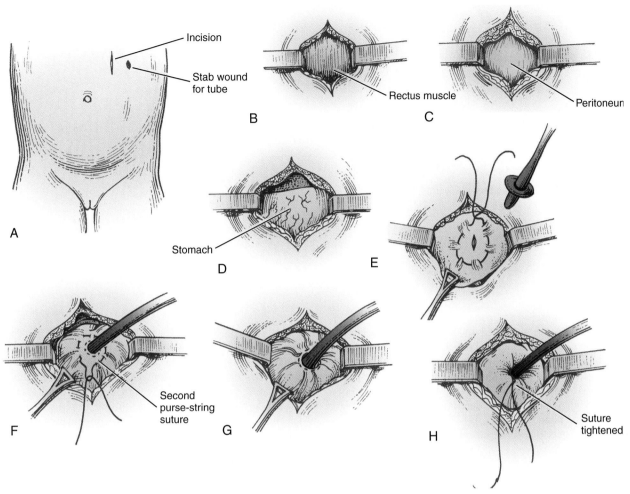

FIGURE 17-17 Gastrostomy. **A**, Incision. **B**, Rectus muscle exposed. **C**, Posterior rectus sheath exposed. **D**, Peritoneum opened. **E**, Purse-string suture placed. **F**, Second purse-string suture placed. **G**, Mushroom catheter inserted. **H**, Suture tightened.

cases occur after the age of 2 years (Fallat, 2005). The most common site for intussusception is the ileocecal junction. Intussusception in most children is idiopathic; in others, causes may include Meckel's diverticulum, polyps, or hematoma of the bowel. Early diagnosis and reduction are essential to bowel viability.

Procedural Considerations. The child is prepped for surgery as described previously. Reduction by barium enema is attempted only with the collaboration of the radiologist, surgeon, and pediatrician, with the OR team on standby. If reduction is unsuccessful, a surgical reduction by laparotomy or laparoscopy must be performed. The open procedure is described in the following Operative Procedure, and requires a major instrument set and pediatric bowel clamps.

Operative Procedure

1. The surgeon makes a right lower quadrant transverse or right paramedian incision and enters the peritoneum.
2. The cecum and ileum are identified; the intussusception is located and elevated with fingers.
3. If there is no evidence of bowel compromise, the bowel immediately distal to the intussusception is occluded with

one hand and stripped proximally with the other in an attempt to achieve manual reduction (Figure 17-19). If the serosa splits during attempted reduction or if the mass cannot be reduced, bowel resection is done.

4. The abdomen is closed in layers, and the wound is dressed.

Bowel Resection and Colostomy for Necrotizing Enterocolitis (NEC)

Necrotizing enterocolitis (NEC) is a condition that manifests with death of intestinal lining and sloughing of corresponding tissues. Its exact cause is unknown, but it is suspected that NEC may result from two mechanisms: decreased blood flow to the bowel, which prevents the bowel from secreting the protective mucus that protects the GI tract; or bacteria within the intestine (Medline Plus Medical Encyclopedia, 2007). NEC primarily affects premature newborns. When surgical intervention is needed, the patient undergoes a bowel resection and ostomy procedure. The type of ostomy created depends on the location of the necrotic bowel. The procedures for bowel resection and colostomy are described in the following sections.

Procedural Considerations. The major instrument set and pediatric bowel clamps are required. The infant is positioned

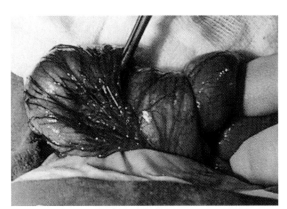

FIGURE 17-18 Operative view of intussusception.

supine, and routine prepping and draping of the abdomen are done.

Bowel Resection

Operative Procedure
1. An abdominal incision is made.
2. The intestines are explored to determine the location of the obstruction. The entire bowel must be examined to rule out multiple areas of involvement in infants with atresia or stenosis. If aganglionosis of the colon is suspected, sequential biopsy specimens are sent fresh immediately to the pathology laboratory to determine the segment of large bowel to be resected.
3. Resection is performed as indicated.

Colostomy

Operative Procedure
1. A transverse incision usually is preferred, and the abdomen is entered in the right upper quadrant for a transverse colostomy or the left lower quadrant for a sigmoid colostomy.
2. The loop of colon is freed of peritoneal attachments until it can be brought easily through the abdominal wall without tension.
3. The edges of the mesentery are then sutured to the parietal peritoneum, and the serosa of the colonic loop is sutured with fine absorbable suture materials to the peritoneum and fascia as well as to the skin.
4. The colostomy may be sutured immediately. Some surgeons prefer to close the skin under a colostomy loop; others prefer to suture mucosa directly to skin edges. This decision may depend on the location of the colostomy. An important point is that each layer must be securely attached to the serosa of the colon to prevent evisceration and prolapse. The posterior wall of a loop colostomy may be divided by electrosurgery several days after surgery.

Resection and Pull-Through for Hirschsprung's Disease (Reconstruction)

Hirschsprung's disease is characterized by the absence of ganglion cells in a distal portion of the bowel. The distal colon is more frequently involved, but the disease may encompass the entire colon, with a less favorable prognosis. The absence of ganglion cells results in a lack of peristalsis. The normal proximal colon becomes dilated with stool, since intestinal contents do not pass through the involved segment normally. The child presents with an abnormally distended abdomen. Barium enema reveals

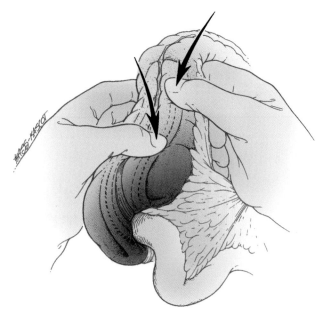

FIGURE 17-19 Manual reduction of intussusception.

proximal distention of the colon and then a transition zone where the bowel appears funnel-shaped, followed by the distal aganglionic segment, which is narrowed. The child is taken to the OR for a leveling colostomy. Multiple frozen-section biopsy specimens from the muscularis of the proximal portion of the colon are taken to determine the presence of ganglion cells. The colostomy is performed at the most distal portion of the colon that contains ganglion cells. Some surgeons prefer a routine right transverse colostomy at this time and delay frozen-section biopsy specimens until the time of the definitive procedure. Resection and pull-through for Hirschsprung's disease, the definitive surgical procedure, consists of the removal of the aganglionic portion of the bowel and anastomosis of the normal colon to the anus. The child is returned to the OR for the definitive repair at 1 year of age if clinical and nutritional status permit.

Several surgical techniques have been devised. The procedure may be done laparoscopically or by an open approach. The Soave procedure of endorectal pull-through employs internal bypass of the involved segment. The internal sphincter muscle of the anus is kept intact for continence.

Procedural Considerations. The child is prepped and draped from the nipples down to and including the buttocks, genitalia, perineal area, and upper thighs to permit positioning for the perineal stage without redraping. (Before prepping, the rectum may be irrigated with warm saline solution.) An indwelling catheter is inserted to keep the bladder empty during the operation. The major instrument set, a minor instrument set, and pediatric intestinal clamps are needed.

Operative Procedure
1. A left paramedian incision that includes the sigmoid colonic stoma, if present, is made.
2. The surgeon frees the stoma from the abdominal wall, and mobilizes the left portion of the colon. (If there is no sigmoid colonic stoma, the extent of aganglionic intestine is

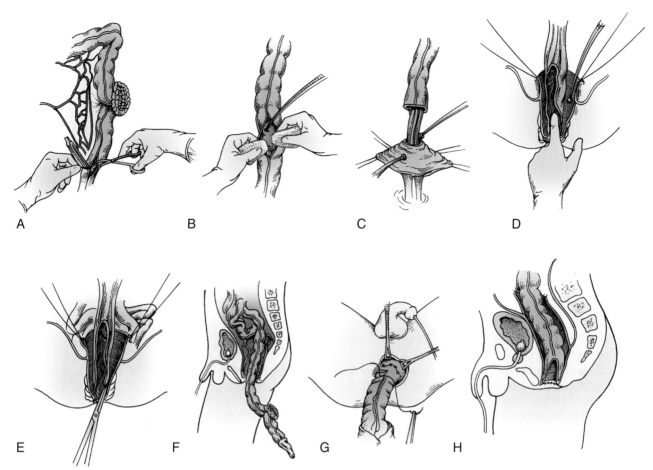

FIGURE 17-20 Pull-through for Hirschsprung's disease. **A,** Dissection of mucosal tube begun through longitudinal incision. **B,** Blunt dissection with sponges used to dissect entire circumference of tube. **C,** Muscular sleeve transected. **D,** Depth of dissection determined by insertion of finger into anus. **E,** Circumferential incision made. **F,** Mucosal tube and proximal portion of colon and stoma pulled through rectal muscular cuff. **G,** Anastomosis performed among all layers of colon and anal mucosa. **H,** Anastomosis completed.

established by biopsy and frozen section, and all involved colon is excised. If a stoma is present and the area has already been established as normal, the colon above it constitutes the proximal end of the resection.)

3. The mesocolon and the vessels of the intestine to be resected are divided close to the intestine, with care taken to preserve the blood supply to the rectum (Figure 17-20, *A*).

4. The mucosal tube is freed from the outer muscular layers by sharp dissection with Metzenbaum scissors and blunt dissection (Figure 17-20, *B*).

5. A muscular sleeve is transected, and 4-0 nonabsorbable traction sutures are placed on the distal edge (Figure 17-20, *C*). The mucosa is stripped down to the anus. The depth of the dissection may be checked by inserting a finger into the anus (Figure 17-20, *D*).

6. When the mucosa is adequately freed, the perineal phase is started and the perineal instrument table is used.

7. The anus is dilated and retracted with Allis forceps. A circumferential incision is made, and the mucosal stripping is completed (Figure 17-20, *E*).

8. The proximal portion of the intestine is pulled through the rectal muscular sleeve and out the anus (Figure 17-20, *F*). If the portion of colon to be resected is large, it is excised

abdominally before the proximal portion of the intestine is pulled through the anus.

9. Absorbable sutures are used to secure the seromuscular layers of the intussuscepted colon to the rectal muscular cuff. The colon is divided into axial or longitudinal quadrants, and an anastomosis is performed with 3-0 absorbable sutures (Figure 17-20, *G*).

10. Gowns and gloves are changed, and abdominal instruments are used. The abdominal phase of the operation is completed by approximating the proximal edge of the muscular cuff to the seromuscular layer of the colon with 4-0 nonabsorbable sutures (Figure 17-20, *H*). The abdomen is closed in the routine manner, without the use of drains.

Repair of Imperforate Anus

Congenital imperforate anus (Figure 17-21) presents in a variety of forms, classified as low, intermediate, and high lesions. Baby girls commonly have low lesions, and baby boys primarily exhibit high lesions. A covered anus and anovulvar fistula is an example of a low lesion. A high lesion consists of a blind rectal pouch, a "flat bottom," and a posterior urethral fistula or a fistula to the bladder. This type is the most prevalent and the most difficult to repair. An imperforate anus is repaired by

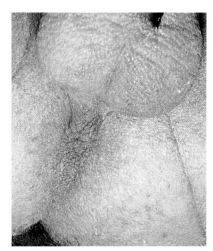

FIGURE 17-21 Imperforate anus.

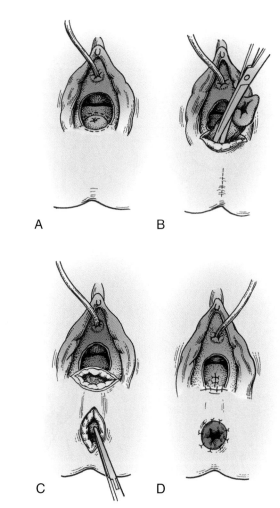

FIGURE 17-22 Anal transposition. **A,** Fistula excised by means of oval incision. **B,** Dissection of bowel from surrounding structures. **C,** Vertical midline incision at site of true anus; identification of external sphincter fibers; mobilized rectum pulled down through subcutaneous tissue to new location. **D,** External sphincter sutured to rectal mucosa; new anus constructed with interrupted sutures through all layers.

establishing colorectoanal continuity through the external anal sphincter and closure of fistulas, if present.

Repair of Low Imperforate Anus in a Girl—Anal Transposition

Procedural Considerations. The infant is placed in the lithotomy position. A Foley catheter is inserted, and the perineum is prepped and draped. The major instrument set is required, with the addition of both a nerve and a muscle stimulator. The anesthesia team must avoid the use of neuromuscular blocking agents for the nerve/muscle stimulator to work during the surgical procedure.

Operative Procedure

1. An electrical stimulator is applied to elicit muscle contractions and serve as a guide to the midline of the anus. The goal is to leave equal innervated tissue on both sides of the anus, so that the child can be continent of stool.
2. Stay sutures are placed in the fistula, and it is excised using an oval incision (Figure 17-22, *A*).
3. The surgeon dissects the bowel free from surrounding structures, taking care not to damage the vagina (Figure 17-22, *B*).
4. When the dissection is complete, a vertical midline incision is performed at the opening of the true anus and the fibers of the external sphincter are identified (Figure 17-22, *C*).
5. The mobilized rectum is pulled down through the subcutaneous tissue to its new location.
6. The end of the fistula is amputated. Using 4-0 nonabsorbable interrupted sutures, the surgeon sutures the external sphincter to the rectal serosa.
7. Using 4-0 absorbable suture, the surgeon constructs a new anus with interrupted sutures through all layers (Figure 17-22, *D*).
8. A drain may or may not be placed in the anterior incision before it is closed in layers with interrupted 4-0 absorbable sutures.
9. A Hegar dilator is used to calibrate the size of the new anus after closure.

Repair of High Imperforate Anus—Posterior Sagittal Anorectoplasty

When a high imperforate anal anomaly presents, surgical intervention is indicated within 24 to 48 hours of birth. A transverse or sigmoid colostomy is performed to irrigate the hiatal lumen and to remove meconium plugs while allowing proximal colon function. After the colostomy, further diagnostic studies, such as cystograms and vaginograms, are done. The posterior sagittal anorectoplasty (PSARP) is the definitive surgical procedure and is performed when the condition and size of the child permit—usually around 1 year of age.

The PSARP is a highly technical procedure that uses electrostimulation throughout and may require position changes.

Procedural Considerations. The child is placed in jackknife position with the hips flexed. Adequate padding must be placed under the hips to avoid compression injury to the femoral nerves. The major instrument set, nerve stimulator, and intestinal instruments are required.

Operative Procedure (Figure 17-23)

1. The surgeon uses the electrostimulator to locate the true anus, and makes a midsagittal incision through the skin from the midsacrum to the anterior border of the anal site.
2. Dissection continues through subcutaneous tissue until the external sphincter muscle layers are identified.

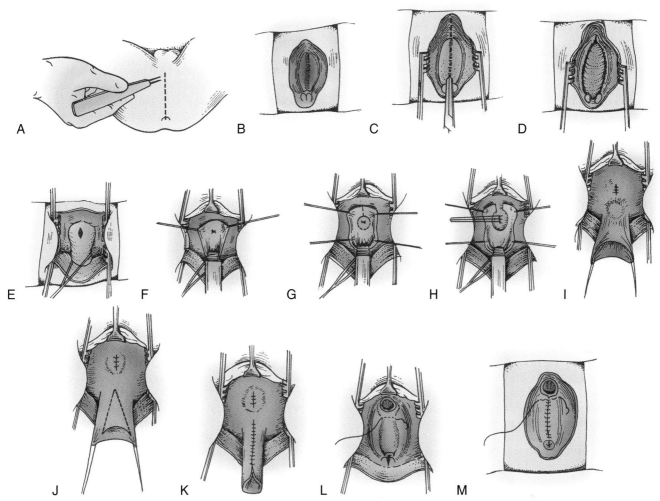

FIGURE 17-23 Posterior sagittal anorectoplasty. **A,** Line of incision and electrical stimulation to determine appropriate anal site. **B,** Midsagittal incision through coccyx and external sphincter fibers of anus, showing striated muscle complex deep to anal site; subcutaneous external sphincter extending about halfway to coccyx; superficial external sphincter inserting on coccyx; levator deeper in midline. **C,** Right-angled forceps beneath levator ani. **D,** All layers of striated muscle partially retracted laterally to expose visceral endopelvic fascia. **E,** Sagittal incision in terminal bowel after proximal dissection around rectum and placement of tape around rectum proximally. **F,** Retracted rectotomy showing fistula site. **G,** Semicircumferential incision through mucosa-submucosa for placement of first sutures to close fistula. **H,** Completed closure of fistula orifice. **I,** Stippled area where muscular bowel wall is left in place and clear area above where peritoneum may be encountered. **J,** Extent of anterior wedge resection for tapered repair of rectum (*dotted line*). **K,** Approximation of tapered edges of rectum. **L,** First and deepest suture for approximation of levators to establish beginning of canal. **M,** After reapproximation of levator ani to coccyx, interrupted sutures are placed in edges of superficial external sphincter muscle.

3. With electrostimulation, the surgeon dissects the fibers midsagittally, exactly in the midline.
4. A midsagittal split of the coccyx is performed, and the striated muscle complex found beneath the coccyx is incised sagittally, along with the visceral endopelvic fascia. Electrostimulation is used to aid in identifying muscle complexes.
5. Next, the surgeon identifies the rectal pouch and urethra, and incises the bowel vertically to expose the fistulas.
6. The fistula is closed in layers—first the mucosa with interrupted absorbable sutures and then the muscle layer with 5-0 nonabsorbable sutures.
7. The rectum is then mobilized and tapered to allow its placement within the muscle complexes. Tapering consists

of excising a wedge of bowel from either the ventral or the dorsal surface. The edges are approximated, and the mucosal layer is closed with 5-0 absorbable interrupted sutures. The muscularis layer is closed with interrupted 5-0 nonabsorbable sutures.
8. Again using electrostimulation, the tapered rectum is placed deep within the muscle complex. Then 5-0 nonabsorbable sutures are used to reconstruct the muscles. The seromuscular layer of the bowel is incorporated into these sutures to keep it securely positioned within the muscle complex.
9. The external sphincter muscles and coccyx are reapproximated.

10. Excess bowel is trimmed before it is secured to the skin edges of the anus.
11. The surgeon closes the skin with running absorbable subcuticular sutures.

In cases of very high rectal pouches and fistulas, an abdominal approach may be required. After the midsagittal incisions and dissections are completed, a rubber drain is placed through the pelvis with one end in the peritoneal cavity and the other through the center of the anus to the skin, where it is temporarily sutured. The child is then turned supine, and an abdominal incision is made. The rectal pouch is mobilized, and the fistula is closed. The bowel is tapered as described previously, and the terminal portion is attached to the rubber tube, which then is used to pull the rectum through the anal orifice. The bowel is sutured to the muscle complex, and reapproximation of the coccyx and external sphincter muscle is done as described earlier.

GENERAL SURGERY: HERNIAS

Umbilical Hernia Repair

Umbilical hernias are frequently seen in pediatric populations and are 10 times more common in African American children than in Caucasians (Garcia, 2005). These hernias are also common in premature infants and are corrected by repair of the defect where the intestine protrudes at the umbilicus. An umbilical hernia is always covered by skin. Small umbilical hernias may be left untreated. They usually close within a few months to 1 year. If surgical repair is required in a large fascial defect, it may be delayed until the child is at least 2 years of age; some surgeons delay repair until 5 years of age.

Procedural Considerations. Surgical correction of umbilical hernia may be an ambulatory surgical procedure. A general anesthetic is used. A minor instrument set is required. Several variations in technique have been used; an infraumbilical approach is most common, and its description follows.

Operative Procedure
1. An incision is made below the umbilicus through the skin and subcutaneous tissue.
2. Flaps of skin and subcutaneous tissue are mobilized and held back with small retractors to expose the rectus fascia and hernial protrusion.
3. The hernia sac, which is between the rectus muscle sheaths in the midline, is completely freed from all surrounding structures.
4. The hernia sac may be invaginated, dissected free and ligated, or excised.
5. The peritoneum is closed with interrupted suture, and each suture is tagged, and then closed all at once.
6. The two edges of the rectus fascia are approximated using interrupted 3-0 nonabsorbable sutures.
7. Subcuticular closure of the skin with a continuous fine absorbable suture is performed, and a pressure dressing is applied.

Inguinal Hernia Repair with Laparoscopic Exploration of Contralateral Side

An inguinal hernia is a protrusion into the inguinal canal of a sac that contains the intestine. The testis develops high on the posterior wall of the abdomen. It gradually descends into the scrotum. Before the testis enters the inguinal canal, the processus vaginalis projects downward but retains a communication with the peritoneal cavity. The upper part of the processus does not project downward; the remaining sac constitutes an indirect inguinal hernia. In a female child, a similar hernial sac is contiguous with the round ligament.

Procedural Considerations. A minor instrument set is used. A laparoscope may be used to visualize the contralateral side, as it is not uncommon for inguinal hernias to occur bilaterally. In these instances, a camera, insufflation tubing, 20-gauge intravenous catheter, 2.7-mm telescope, and light cord must be presented to the sterile field. The child is positioned supine, and routine prepping is done.

Operative Procedure
1. The surgeon makes an incision over the inguinal area in the direction of the skin crease.
2. The subcutaneous tissue is opened, and hemostats are placed on bleeding vessels, which are then ligated or electrocoagulated.
3. Right-angle retractors are placed inferiorly and medially.
4. The surgeon identifies the external ring, and uses small Metzenbaum scissors to free and clean the external oblique fascia.
5. Using a #15 blade, the surgeon opens the external oblique fascia and frees the upper flap. The lower flap is freed to expose the inguinal ligament.
6. Cord structures are opened at the upper end of the cord. Two forceps are used to grasp tissues at the same level and to separate them.
7. The hernia sac is grasped with a hemostat, and structures of the cord are peeled downward and away from the sac with forceps until the sac is freed. Care is taken to protect the spermatic cord and major vessels as the sac is freed.
8. After the sac is opened, the surgeon's index finger is inserted and the sac is pulled upward. The upward traction is maintained with two or three hemostats.
9. If laparoscopic exploration of the contralateral side is taking place, the 20-gauge intravenous catheter is inserted over the opposite inguinal area. The insufflation tube is connected, and CO_2 instilled. The contralateral side is explored using a 2.7-mm telescope.
10. The sac is ligated with 3-0 nonabsorbable suture, and excess sac is removed. Repair of the inguinal canal may be done with nonabsorbable sutures.
11. The subcutaneous tissue is closed with interrupted fine sutures; closure of the skin is with fine nonabsorbable subcuticular sutures. Cyanoacrylate glue or wound closure strips are applied.
12. If a bilateral hernia is diagnosed, steps 1-10 are repeated on the contralateral side.

Omphalocele and Gastroschisis Repair

An omphalocele is the protrusion of abdominal viscera outside the abdomen through a defect in the umbilical ring into a sac of amniotic membrane and peritoneum at the base of the umbilical cord. There is no skin covering (Figure 17-24). Gastroschisis is the protrusion of the viscera through a defect in the abdominal wall to the right of the umbilical cord. No amniotic membrane or peritoneum covers the defect.

Omphalocele occurs during the eleventh week of fetal life when the viscera fail to withdraw normally from the exocoelomic position to occupy the peritoneal cavity. The resulting

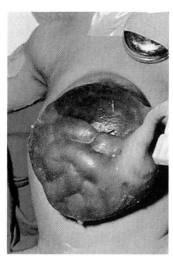

FIGURE 17-24 Newborn with giant omphalocele containing liver and intestine.

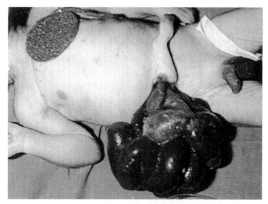

FIGURE 17-25 Gastroschisis. A large amount of small intestine has eviscerated through a defect to the right of a normal-appearing umbilical cord. No sac is visible, and the intestine is thickened, edematous, and ischemic in areas.

abdominal wall defect can vary in size from 2 to 15 cm. The sac may contain only a few loops of bowel, or nearly all the intestines and the liver and spleen. Associated anomalies can include disorders of the cardiac, musculoskeletal, genitourinary, and nervous systems, along with malrotation and abnormal fixation of the bowel. Gastroschisis, on the other hand, is generally not associated with major congenital defects other than intestinal atresia (Davis, 2007) (Figure 17-25).

Because the infant is at risk for hypothermia, hypoglycemia, shock, sepsis, and vascular injury to the bowel, immediate management after birth is necessary (Klein, 2005). Treatment consists of inserting a nasogastric tube to prevent distention and aspiration, and beginning IV access with fluid resuscitation and antibiotic therapy. Surgical intervention is necessary to prevent rupture of the sac, infection, or both. If intrauterine rupture of the sac has occurred, the newborn is kept warm, and the bowel is inspected for perforation and torsion. In certain cases, a petroleum gauze dressing may be applied to the defect, but care must be taken to keep it moist.

Omphaloceles and gastroschisis are repaired by placement of the viscera in the abdominal cavity, with reconstruction of the abdominal wall. Surgical procedures for omphaloceles may be primary (Shuster procedure) or staged (giant omphaloceles). Mesh may be used as a barrier to create tension that helps to push the internal organs into the abdominal cavity. In some cases of gastroschisis, a silo is applied to the defect. The silo is made of a flexible ring that sits inside the abdomen and its size is gradually decreased to facilitate movement of the organs back to the abdominal cavity. Silo material may be prepackaged and kept at the patient's bedside if the patient is unable to tolerate an immediate trip to the OR.

Procedural Considerations. Particular attention to maintaining body temperature is essential because of the massive exposed surface area from which body heat can be lost. The use of nitrous oxide as an anesthetic agent is avoided during this procedure because it causes increased gas in the intestine, which in turn makes the reduction of abdominal contents into the peritoneal cavity very difficult. Repeated rectal irrigation with warm saline to evacuate meconium from the bowel

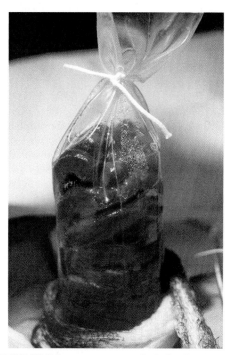

FIGURE 17-26 Operative view of silo for the intestines.

may be carried out before the abdominal prep to aid in bowel decompression.

The major instrument set is required. The infant is positioned supine; the abdomen, umbilical cord, and sac are gently prepped with a povidone-iodine solution.

Gastroschisis with Silo Placement

Procedural Considerations. A major instrument set is required. The patient is positioned supine for the procedure. The abdomen, umbilical cord, and sac are gently prepped with povidone-iodine.

Operative Procedure

1. The surgeon examines the bowel and measures the size of the defect to determine silo size. The silo is applied so that the flexible ring is positioned inside the abdomen (Figure 17-26).

2. The patient returns to the OR every 48 hours for a reduction of the silo, which is accomplished by decreasing the size of the ring to help guide the contents back into the abdominal cavity.

3. The height of bowel in the silo and length of reduction are measured with each procedure. When the amount of bowel remaining in the silo is 1 cm or less, the patient is transferred to the OR for closure of the defect.

4. The silo is trimmed and the spring-loaded ring is removed. The wound site and bowel are inspected and cleaned with surgical prep material.

5. The surgeon closes the defect using synthetic purse-string sutures or, if the defect is too large, using running sutures that begin at each end of the wound and meet in the middle to preserve the umbilical cord stump.

6. The inferior aspect of skin is wrapped around the stump and secured with absorbable suture. Any redundant skin is trimmed and the stump is ligated using nonabsorbable suture.

7. A subcutaneous drain may be left in place and a dry, sterile dressing is applied.

Omphalocele Repair

Procedural Considerations. The patient is positioned supine for the procedure and the abdomen is prepped as described for silo placement.

Operative Procedure

1. The surgeon dissects the amnion of the omphalocele circumferentially from the dermis.

2. The umbilical vein is identified and ligated with absorbable suture. Umbilical cord structures and arteries are dissected and ligated with absorbable suture, and then oversewn with nonabsorbable suture.

3. Organs connected to the omphalocele are dissected, reduced (if necessary), and mobilized, and the internal mucosal layer is closed with running nonabsorbable suture.

4. The outer muscular layer is closed with interrupted nonabsorbable suture, organs are returned to the peritoneal cavity, and fascia is closed with interrupted nonabsorbable suture.

5. If necessary, an umbilicoplasty may be performed using interrupted absorbable suture. Dry, sterile dressings are placed over the incision.

In certain cases in which the defect is of medium to large size, a primary closure may not be accomplished. In these situations a staged procedure is done using prosthetic reduction. In the first stage the infant is brought to the OR and positioned and prepped as previously described. Then the following steps are performed:

1. The sac is excised, and the umbilical vein and arteries are ligated.

2. A gastrostomy may be performed at this time.

3. A barrier is then created with Silastic mesh. The mesh is secured through all layers of the edge of the defect using a continuous locking nonabsorbable suture. The open end of the barrier is closed in the same manner.

4. The open end of the cylinder is closed with umbilical tape or, alternatively, attached to a specifically designed roller clamp.

5. The mesh barrier suture line and edge of the defect are wrapped with roller gauze dipped in an iodophor solution to prevent infection. The infant is transferred to an open Isolette, and the silo is suspended from the top of the Isolette.

Plastic wrap is applied to the barrier to prevent heat loss. The infant is then transported to the NICU, where daily reduction of abdominal contents is performed by adding a lower tie of umbilical tape or by adjusting the roller clamp. The abdominal viscera are gradually reduced over several days, taking care to avoid respiratory compromise from abdominal distention. When reduction has successfully approached skin level, the infant is returned to the OR for the final stage of repair.

6. The mesh barrier is removed, and the remaining abdominal contents are brought into the peritoneal cavity. The peritoneal fascia is closed with interrupted nonabsorbable sutures. The skin is closed with interrupted nonabsorbable suture. In an attempt to create the appearance of an umbilicus, a purse-string suture is used to close the inferior 2 cm of incision.

GENERAL SURGERY: ABDOMINAL PROCEDURES

Correction of Biliary Atresia—Hepatic Portoenterostomy (Kasai Procedure)

Biliary atresia is a congenital defect that results from nonpatent extrahepatic bile ducts. Bile is unable to drain from the liver to the small intestine, leading to eventual cirrhosis and death. The Kasai procedure is the construction of a bile drainage system by use of an intestinal conduit. This procedure is indicated in patients with extrahepatic biliary atresia who are younger than 3 months. All atretic segments of the existing bile ducts are removed. An intraoperative cholangiogram and frozen-section biopsy of the hepatic duct remnant are included in the surgical procedure.

Procedural Considerations. The infant is positioned supine over a radiographic plate, or fluoroscopy is used. Both a major instrument set and bowel clamps are required, as well as radiopaque dye and a 6F or 8F catheter for the cholangiography.

Operative Procedure

1. The surgeon makes a right upper quadrant incision and exposes the gallbladder.

2. A small catheter is placed into the gallbladder and secured with a purse-string suture. Radiopaque dye is instilled into the gallbladder, and an x-ray examination is done. The surgeon observes for free flow of the dye through the ducts and into the duodenum, which occasionally is seen. These patients are then categorized as having correctable biliary atresia. In such situations, a liver biopsy is performed and the incision is closed. The majority of patients with correctable biliary atresia demonstrate progressive improvement. More commonly, however, there is a very small amount of flow or none at all, for which the Kasai procedure is performed.

3. A thorough inspection of the intraabdominal organs is then done because of the high prevalence of associated anomalies.

4. The hepatoduodenal ligament is explored, and all drainage structures are ligated (Figure 17-27, *A*).

5. The hepatic duct remnant is identified and traced to the liver hilum. The remnant is transected as high as possible using frozen-section biopsy specimens as a guide. Frozen-section biopsy specimens are also obtained at the porta hepatis to denote the presence of ductules. Precise identification of this location is essential (Figure 17-27, *B*).

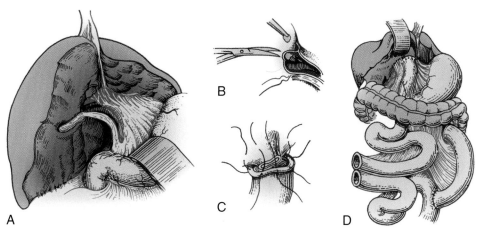

FIGURE 17-27 Kasai procedure. **A,** Exploration of hepatoduodenal ligament and ligation of drainage structures. **B,** Transection of hepatic duct remnant using frozen-section biopsy specimens as a guide. **C,** Anastomosis of jejunal conduit at porta hepatis. **D,** Exteriorization of conduit using double-barreled Roux-en-Y approach.

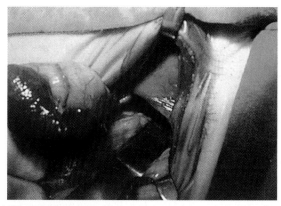

FIGURE 17-28 Defect in the posterolateral aspect of the left diaphragm (diaphragmatic hernia).

6. The proximal portion of the jejunum is generally used as the intestinal conduit. A meticulous anastomosis is performed at the porta hepatis as previously identified, using a single running layer of absorbable sutures (Figure 17-27, *C*).
7. The conduit is exteriorized with a double-barreled Roux-en-Y approach (Figure 17-27, *D*).
8. A liver biopsy is then performed.
9. A drain is placed, and the incision is closed in layers.

The procedure just described is one approach of many. Others include exteriorization of the jejunal conduit as a cutaneous jejunostomy and use of double Roux-en-Y loops, avoiding any need for an enterostomy. If none of these procedures is successful, the child may be a candidate for liver transplantation.

Repair of Congenital Diaphragmatic Hernia

A congenital diaphragmatic hernia (CDH) is repaired by replacement of the displaced viscera into the abdominal cavity with surgical correction of the diaphragm defect (Figure 17-28). The conventional surgical repair is through the abdomen, though some cases of CDH can be repaired using a thoracic approach. The concurrence of intraabdominal abnormalities is somewhat high in infants with diaphragmatic hernia; therefore treatment is facilitated with an abdominal approach. It is tech-

nically easier to extract the viscera from below than to push them out of the thorax. The abnormal intrathoracic intrusion of the abdominal viscera usually causes severe compromise of intrathoracic pulmonary and vascular activities. Therefore urgent restoration of more normal intrathoracic and intraabdominal relationships is the rule in these newborns. The lung may be hypoplastic because of prolonged compression in utero by the displaced abdominal viscera. A residual intrapleural space usually remains for a few days after surgery.

Procedural Considerations. Direct suturing of the margins of the defect is usually possible. Insertion of prosthetic Silastic sheeting is occasionally required and should be available. The major instrument set is required. The infant is positioned supine.

Operative Procedure
1. The surgeon makes a subcostal incision on the side of the defect, going through all muscle layers.
2. The abdominal viscera are withdrawn from the chest and held downward through the abdominal wound. Because abnormalities of abdominal viscera, such as malrotation, are associated with diaphragmatic hernia, the organs are carefully inspected at this time. If a malrotation is found, the surgeon may repair it if the clinical condition of the infant is amenable to the procedure.
3. The defect is then carefully inspected, including a search for a hernia sac, which is present in fewer than 5% of cases. If a sac is identified, it is excised.
4. The posterior and anterior rims of the diaphragm are identified, and primary closure is performed with mattress sutures of nonabsorbable material. If the rim of tissue is too small for mattress sutures, ample nonabsorbable sutures are used. Occasionally, reinforced Silastic sheeting may be needed if sufficient diaphragm is not available for primary closure.
5. The abdominal wall is then closed, followed by subcutaneous tissue and skin closure. If the musculature cannot accommodate the abdominal viscera, it is left open and the skin is closed to leave a ventral hernia. In severe cases, the patient may be given extracorporeal membrane oxygenation (ECMO) for

several days before repair of the defect. The infant is returned to the OR within 7 days for repair of the ventral hernia.

Pancreatectomy

Pancreatectomy is the treatment for several disorders, including congenital hyperinsulinism (HI) and pancreatitis. A pancreatectomy may be total, meaning that the entire pancreas is removed. In some cases, the common bile duct, spleen, gallbladder, and portions of the small intestine and stomach may be removed along with it. Pancreatectomies may also be partial—only the body and tail of the pancreas are removed. Pancreatectomy for congenital hyperinsulinism is described in the following Operative Procedure. Congenital hyperinsulinism is a condition in which the release of insulin is not properly regulated and insulin (beta) cells of the pancreas secrete too much insulin at the wrong time (Children's Hospital of Philadelphia [CHOP], 2009). Treatment of HI is focused on regulating blood glucose level to reduce the risk of brain damage. Surgical intervention is recommended when medical management of HI proves unsuccessful. The procedure for a total pancreatectomy for congenital hyperinsulinism is described in the following section.

Procedural Considerations. Multiple specimens are sent to the pathology laboratory for frozen-section analysis throughout the procedure in order to confirm the extent of the disease. The child is positioned supine with the hips elevated.

Operative Procedure

1. The surgeon makes a transverse supraumbilical incision using a #15 blade. The Denis Browne retractor is placed.
2. The body and tail of the pancreas are exposed for biopsy for analysis by frozen section.
3. The hepatic flexure of the colon and the duodenum are exposed for additional biopsy and frozen section.
4. If results indicate the need for total pancreatectomy (large nuclei in islet cells), the dissection is begun at the pancreatic tail, and then extended to the body and head.
5. A vessel loop is used to isolate the common bile duct and care is taken to preserve duodenal blood supply to the pancreatic head during dissection. Once the uncinate process is mobilized from behind the superior mesenteric vessels and the common bile duct is dissected away from its entry point into the duodenum, the pancreatic head is freed.
6. A pancreatectomy is performed and blood supply to the duodenum is evaluated. In the event that a pancreatic remnant remains, it is ligated using nonabsorbable interrupted horizontal mattress sutures. Omentum is tacked down to the dissected area, and the gallbladder is milked to evaluate patency and test for bile leak.
7. In certain cases, a gastrostomy tube may be placed.
8. The abdominal incision is closed in layers using nonabsorbable suture for fascia and absorbable sutures for subcutaneous and subcuticular tissue. The incision is dressed with Mastisol adhesive and wound closure strips.

GENERAL SURGERY: RESECTION OF TUMORS

Nearly two thirds of childhood cancers occur as solid tumor malignancies. As is always the case, the therapy administered depends on the type of tumor. Examination and judicious investigation of all unusual masses are imperative. Thorough diagnostic workup and prompt definitive treatment may result in cure, even if the tumor is malignant. Chemotherapy and radiation therapy are adjuncts to surgical excision of tumors.

Wilms' Tumor

Wilms' tumor, also known as *nephroblastoma,* is the most common intraabdominal childhood tumor. It presents as a painless mass whose enlargement may laterally distend the abdomen (Figure 17-29). The child may be asymptomatic or may have weight loss, malaise, or abdominal pain. Nephroblastomas may cause obstruction of the vena cava, hepatic veins, or renal veins.

Procedural Considerations. The child is positioned supine with a roll under the affected side. Both chest and abdomen are prepped. Infrequently the tumor extends into the inferior vena cava as well as the right atrium of the heart, and in such cases cardiopulmonary bypass (CPB) should be readily available. Lines are placed into the arms and neck to facilitate clamping of the inferior vena cava if needed. Separate sterile gloves and instruments should be available for inspection of the contralateral kidney. Careful attention should be given when handling tumor and lymph nodes to avoid tumor spillage.

Operative Procedure

If the tumor is operable, the following aspects are important:

1. The transabdominal approach, which may be extended to a combined transabdominal-transthoracic approach, is used to inspect abdominal contents and clamp the vessels of the renal pedicle before tumor dissection.
2. All suspicious lymph nodes are removed, placed into separate containers, and labeled. If no suspicious nodes are present, biopsy specimens are obtained of those in adjacent areas.
3. The opposite kidney is explored before dissection of the tumor.
4. The extent of the tumor can be marked with hemostatic clips to facilitate radiation therapy.
5. The entire primary tumor is removed if doing so does not place the patient in jeopardy.
6. Any residual tumor is marked with clips.
7. Because of its proximity to the kidney, the adrenal gland is usually removed.
8. The abdominal cavity and viscera are thoroughly inspected for evidence of tumor extension or metastases. Extensive surgery may include partial colectomy or partial resection of the diaphragm.

Neuroblastoma

Neuroblastoma is responsible for 6.9% of all childhood cancers and is the third most common childhood cancer after leukemia and brain and nervous system cancers (American Cancer Society [ACS], 2009). It arises from neural crest tissue and can develop anywhere sympathetic nerve tissue is found; the most common sites are the retroperitoneum and adrenal medulla. The mass is usually firm, irregular, and nontender. It is a silent tumor in its early stages and metastasizes rapidly, often to the lymphatics, liver, skin, bone marrow, lung, brain, or orbits.

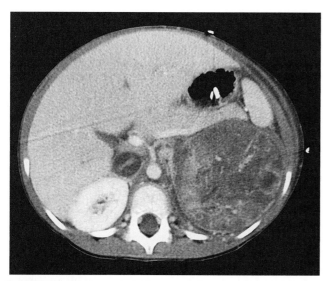

FIGURE 17-29 Computerized tomographic scan showing left-sided Wilms' tumor with compression of the inferior vena cava.

Treatment includes an operation to ligate the tumor's blood supply and remove as much of the tumor as possible, as well as chemotherapy and radiation.

Sacrococcygeal Teratoma

A sacrococcygeal teratoma is a tumor that originates early in embryonic cell division. The tumor consists of cell types from more than one embryonic germ layer. Teratomas range from benign, well-differentiated cystic lesions to solid, malignant lesions. They are the most common tumor in newborns, occurring in 1:35,000 to 1:40,000 births (Laberge et al, 2005). The sacrococcygeal area is the most common extragonadal site of teratoma, usually presenting as a large protuberance rising from that site (Figure 17-30). It may be irregular or symmetric, may vary in size, and may be pedunculated.

A sacrococcygeal teratoma is usually resectable but may undergo malignant changes if not removed early in life. Sacrococcygeal teratomas can be resected prenatally using fetal surgery techniques (see Chapter 5) or postnatally. Tumors resected in the newborn period show microscopic evidence of malignant cells, but surgical cures have been achieved. Early surgical resection is important because these tumors are not sensitive to irradiation and are only temporarily responsive to chemotherapy.

The tumor is in the area of the sacrum and coccyx but may extend into the pelvis or abdomen. Resection is usually feasible by placing the patient in the jackknife position and excising the tumor mass and coccyx en bloc. In cases where the tumor extends high into the pelvis, an abdominal incision may also be required.

GENITOURINARY SURGERY
Pediatric Cystoscopy

Pediatric cystoscopy is endoscopic examination of the lower urinary tract of pediatric patients. The major difference between adult and pediatric cystoscopy is the size of the instruments used and consideration of the small, delicate orifices of the pediatric patient. Indications for pediatric cystos-

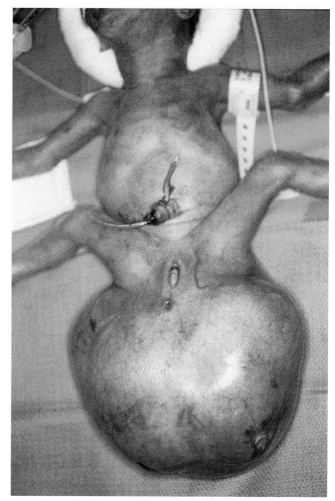

FIGURE 17-30 Infant with large sacrococcygeal teratoma.

copy include urinary tract infections, enuresis, urethral valves, vesicoureteral reflux, diverticula, bladder neck contractures, bladder tumors, and urinary tract obstructions. Pediatric cystoscopy may also be used in conjunction with Deflux injection for minimally invasive treatment of vesicoureteral reflux.

Procedural Considerations. The cystoscopy setup will have the same type of components as those for the adult cystoscopy patient, except that the size of the cystourethroscope system will be specific to the pediatric patient's needs.

Each pediatric cystourethroscope is designed to fit specific component parts and is very delicate. Therefore the surgical technologist must be familiar with the proper use of the system and handle the components carefully. The resectoscope loop is commonly used to resect urethral valves and occasionally bladder tumors. The cold knife may be used with the resectoscope to cut urethral strictures and occasionally to resect a urethral valve.

The most common type of anesthesia used for the pediatric patient is general anesthesia. After induction of anesthesia, the child is placed in a lithotomy or frog-leg position and prepped and draped according to established procedure.

Operative Procedure. The pediatric cystourethroscope is lubricated and inserted through the urethra into the bladder.

The light cord and irrigation tubing are attached to the telescope and cystoscope, and the examination is performed. Most commonly the interior of the bladder is viewed on a video monitor by means of a camera attached to the cystoscope.

Circumcision

Circumcision is the excision of the foreskin (prepuce) of the glans penis. Circumcision may be done for therapeutic reasons or for perceived prophylactic benefits; it may also be done for religious reasons, as is required in specific faiths. Provision should be made to observe the religious needs and preferences of the parents.

Therapeutic indications include correction of phimosis or paraphimosis or treatment of balanoposthitis. Phimosis is a condition in which the orifice of the prepuce is stenosed or too narrow to permit easy retraction behind the glans. Balanoposthitis is characterized by an inflamed glans and mucous membrane with purulent discharge and may require circumcision. Paraphimosis is a recurrent condition in which the prepuce cannot be reduced easily from a retracted position.

Procedural Considerations. Newborns are generally positioned on a specially constructed board that facilitates restraint by immobilizing the limbs and exposing the genitalia. Although it was once thought that circumcision caused infants little pain, the neonatal foreskin contains mature nerve endings that allow for the transmission of pain. Measures to ameliorate the pain of the procedure include local dorsal penile nerve block, a ring block with buffered lidocaine and bupivacaine, or the topical application of a eutectic mixture of local anesthesia (EMLA) cream. Older children require general anesthesia.

For infants, the setup includes fine plastic surgery instruments. A Gomco clamp of the appropriate size, a Plastibell, or the Hollister disposable circumcision device may be employed. The Hollister device includes sutures that are sealed in a sterile packet ready for use. The Plastibell technique uses a plastic ring and suture tied around the foreskin like a tourniquet. The excess tissue is trimmed, and in about 5 to 8 days the ring falls off. For older patients, the circumcision clamp is not needed, and only a plastic surgery instrument set is used. Petrolatum gauze for dressing should be available.

Operative Procedure *(Figure 17-31)*

1. If the prepuce is adherent, the surgeon may use a probe or hemostat to break up adhesions. The prepuce is clamped in the dorsal midline and incised toward the coronal mucosa margin, leaving about 5 cm of coronal mucosa intact. A similar procedure is performed ventrally. The two incisions are then joined circumferentially. Alternatively, a superficial circumferential incision is made in the skin with a scalpel at the level of the coronal sulcus and mucosa at the base of the glans. The redundant skin is undermined between the circumferential incisions and removed as a complete cuff.

2. Bleeding vessels are coagulated or clamped with mosquito hemostats and tied with fine absorbable ligatures. Before closure, the area may be cleansed with an appropriate antiseptic solution.

3. The raw edges of the skin incision are approximated to a coronal cuff of mucosal prepuce, generally with interrupted 4-0 or 5-0 absorbable sutures on fine plastic cutting or GI needles. The wound is usually dressed with petrolatum gauze or an antibiotic ointment. A penile block with bupiv-

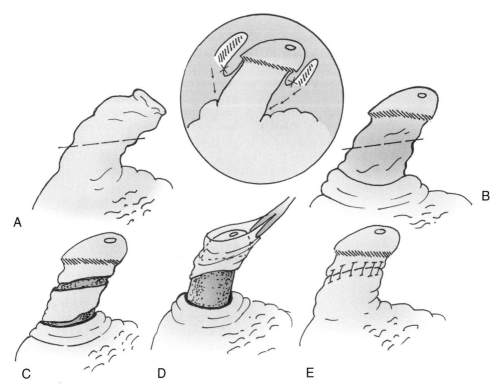

FIGURE 17-31 Circumcision. **A,** Initial incision made in the shaft. **B,** Second incision made in subcoronal sulcus. **C,** Amount of tissue to be removed. **D,** Removal of tissue. **E,** Shaft skin sutured to subcoronal skin.

acaine is often done for immediate postoperative pain, thus providing a more comfortable emergence from anesthesia.

Hypospadias Repair

Hypospadias is a developmental anomaly characterized by a urethral meatus that opens onto the ventral surface of the penis proximal to the end of the glans (Figure 17-32). There are varying degrees of hypospadias. The meatus may be on the ventral surface of the glans, on the corona, anywhere along the shaft, in the scrotum, or even in the perineum. The more proximal the opening, the greater the degree of chordee (downward curvature of the penis). Chordee is caused by fibrous bands that extend from the hypospadiac urethral meatus to the tip of the glans and represent the abnormally developed urethra and its investing layer of Buck's fascia, dartos, and skin. In some cases of clinical curvature, however, these fibrous bands may not be present. Although these curvatures are still termed *chordee,* they are not true fibrous chordee.

The principal methods of hypospadias repair are meatoplasty and glanuloplasty, orthoplasty (release of chordee, thereby straightening the penis), urethroplasty (reconstruction of the urethra), skin cover, and scrotoplasty. These may be done in one- or two-stage repairs depending on the extent of the condition. Recently efforts have increased to relocate the meatus to the apex of the glans, especially in the more extensive one-stage repair.

One complication of hypospadias repair is urethral fistula formation, which can be repaired without much difficulty. Correction of strictures is more troublesome.

Procedural Considerations. The patient (the majority are infants and young children) is placed in the supine position with legs apart. The urine may be diverted with a urethral catheter intraoperatively. The instrument setup varies according to the surgeon's preference. However, a minor set with fine plastic surgery instruments is generally required. Owens gauze, Elastomull, Coban, and Elastoplast, as well as adhesive tape, are generally required for the dressing, which is an important part of the hypospadias repair.

Meatoplasty and Glanuloplasty Incorporated (MAGPI) Procedure
OPERATIVE PROCEDURE
1. The surgeon makes a subcoronal circumferential incision about 8 mm proximal to the meatus and corona. The skin is

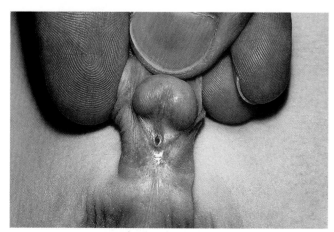

FIGURE 17-32 Hypospadias.

stripped back from the phallus by subcutaneous dissection (Figure 17-33).
2. A bridge of tissue between the meatus and glanular groove is made, with a transverse closure of the dorsal (upper) meatal edge to the distal glanular groove.
3. Three traction sutures are placed where the foreskin stops, at the apex of the ventral meatus (on the lower side) and lateral areas of the glans.
4. The edges of the glans are sutured together ventrally in a V configuration, and the redundant edges are excised. Vertical mattress sutures are used to approximate the glans beneath the meatus.
5. If foreskin is excessive, it may be trimmed, followed by a sleeve style of reapproximation of the penile skin. If a ventral skin defect is present, a rotational skin flap closure is used.
6. An indwelling catheter is placed, and the wound is dressed.

Orthoplasty. *Orthoplasty* is the proper designation for the plastic procedure performed to straighten the penis. *Chordee repair* is the more common term employed. In true fibrous chordee the penis is curved downward, with the meatus and glans in proximity to one another.

Artificial erection is achieved by injecting 0.9% preservative-free, injectable saline solution into the corpus cavernosum. Both corporal bodies fill, making it possible to determine the degree of curvature before and after the resection of the fibrous bands.

OPERATIVE PROCEDURE
1. The surgeon makes a circumferential incision around the corona and carries it distally to the urethral meatus and well below the glans cap (Figure 17-34, *A*). Dissection continues to the level of the tunica albuginea of the corpora cavernosa.
2. With proximal dissection the adherent fibrous plaque is freed, working in a side-to-side fashion. The urethra is

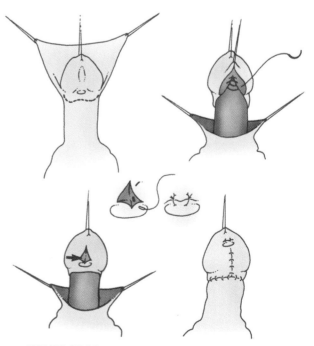

FIGURE 17-33 Meatal advancement and granuloplasty.

elevated from the corpora during this process (Figure 17-34, *B*).

3. The chordee generally surrounds the urethral meatus and often extends for some distance. It is important to free it completely along the entire penile shaft to the penoscrotal junction or, in severe cases, into the scrotum or perineum.

4. After release of the chordee, the glans penis is closed with 4-0 absorbable sutures in a circular manner (Figure 17-34, *C*).

5. If urethroplasty is either delayed or unnecessary, excess dorsal skin is excised (Figure 17-34, *D*) and the incision is closed along the dorsal midline with interrupted absorbable mattress sutures (Figure 17-34, *E*). The wound is dressed according to established protocol.

Urethroplasty. Many procedures are described for reconstruction of a urethra. They may be divided into three general groups: adjacent skin flaps, free skin grafts, and mobilized vascular flaps. There are also many combinations of these procedures. In all the procedures, some type of temporary urinary diversion, such as a perineal urethrostomy, may be used.

The procedural considerations are the same as those for chordee repair.

Adjacent Skin Flap. It is possible to tubularize skin adjacent to the meatus to create a neourethra in a one-stage repair. Transfer of dorsal skin to the ventrum will also provide graft material close to the meatus. However, this is generally done in two stages, and the vascularity of this thin rotational flap is less than optimum, with results that are prone to complication.

OPERATIVE PROCEDURE

1. The surgeon places traction sutures in the tip of the penis and in the glans wings for stabilization and exposure.

2. The distance between the glans tip and the lower edge of the meatus is measured. An outline of the proposed incision is drawn on the penile shaft (Figure 17-35, *A*). In a one-stage approach the distal length must be increased to compensate for the added penile length after chordee release.

3. An incision is made around the outlined flap and carried proximally to a point on the shaft that corresponds to the distance required to reach the glans tip. A flap width of 14 to

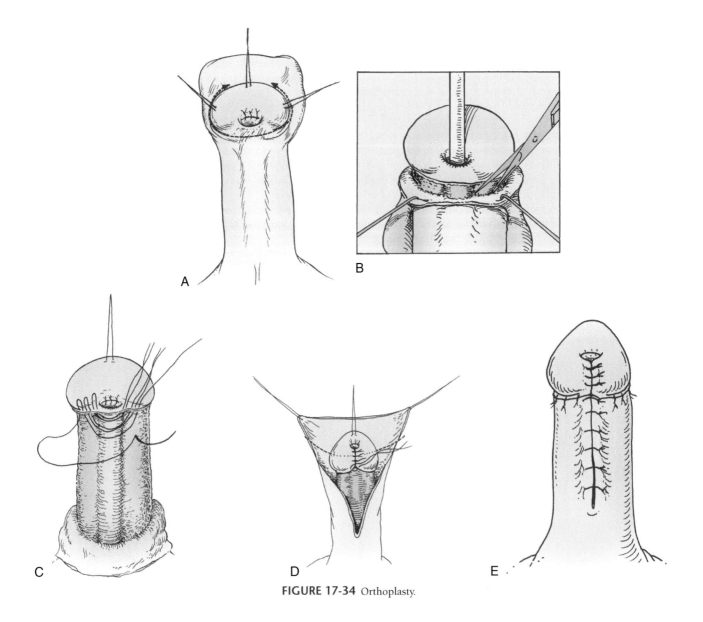

FIGURE 17-34 Orthoplasty.

16 mm is usually sufficient to ensure good circumference of the neourethra.

4. Once incised, the tube is rolled over an 8F or 10F catheter (Figure 17-35, *B*) with an inverted running stitch of 4-0 or 5-0 absorbable suture.

5. The glans penis is incised, and the glans wings are undermined and freed. The neourethra is carried to the distal portion of the glans and sutured in place (Figure 17-35, *C*).

6. The glans wings are sutured around the neourethra with absorbable interrupted mattress sutures. The redundant foreskin is split down the midline, and the flaps are transposed in a Z-plasty manner (Figure 17-35, *D*).

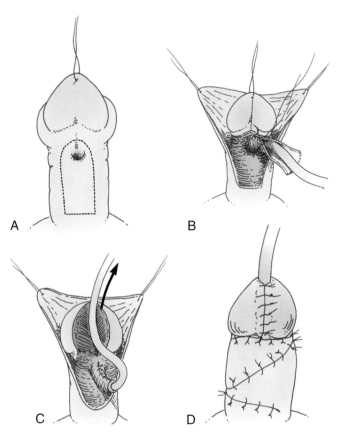

FIGURE 17-35 Urethroplasty with adjacent skin flap.

7. A dry, sterile pressure dressing is applied. The patient can often be discharged on the same day, without the need for an indwelling catheter.

Free Skin Graft. Free skin grafts should be of full thickness. Because the free graft must be revascularized, it is important that it have a perfect skin cover of dorsal preputial penile skin that is well vascularized. This type of graft is generally used with a one-stage hypospadias repair.

OPERATIVE PROCEDURE

1. A V-shaped incision is made on the glans, and the penile skin is mobilized after the chordee is released (Figure 17-36, *A*).

2. Glans wings are developed in a triangular fashion, and ventral preputial skin is used for the full-thickness free graft (Figure 17-36, *B*).

3. The graft is formed into a neourethra over a stenting catheter (Figure 17-36, *C*).

4. The graft is anastomosed proximal to the urethra with the suture line of the graft next to the corpora. The middle glans dart is fixed to the corpora (Figure 17-36, *D*).

5. A meatoplasty with the dorsal glans dart is accomplished.

6. Fine absorbable interrupted sutures are placed around the meatus and glans and along the dorsal penile shaft (Figure 17-36, *E*).

7. The wound is dressed according to established protocol.

Mobilized Vascularized Flaps. Vascularized flaps of preputial penile skin may be mobilized to the ventrum by leaving them attached to the outer surface of the prepuce or as an island flap. One modification is the transverse preputial island-flap neourethra with glans-channel positioning for the meatus. Preputial skin seems to be preferred because of its rich, reliable blood supply.

OPERATIVE PROCEDURE

1. The chordee is released (Figure 17-37, *A*).

2. Ventral preputial skin is dissected free and fanned out (Figure 17-37, *B*).

3. The rectangle of skin is rolled into the neourethra and measured (Figure 17-37, *C*).

4. The island flap is developed by dissection of the subcutaneous tissue from the dorsal penile skin (Figure 17-37, *D* and *E*).

5. A glans channel is created with fine scissors in a plane just above the corpora. The glans tissue is removed with the 14F

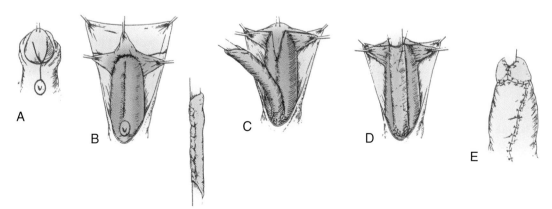

FIGURE 17-36 Urethroplasty with free graft.

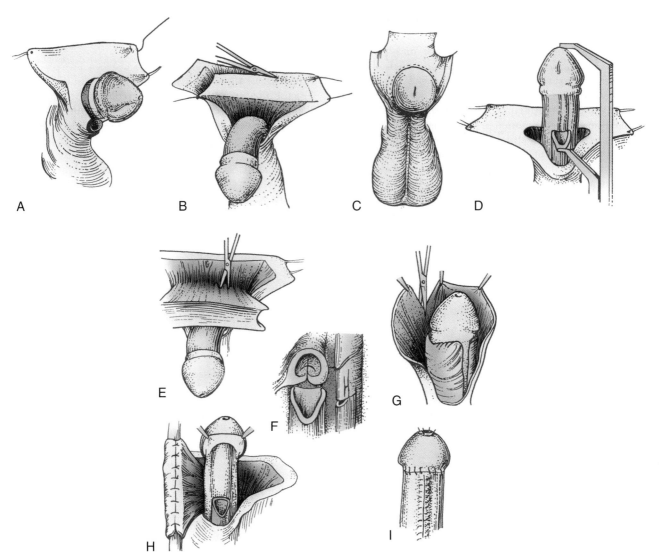

FIGURE 17-37 Urethroplasty, island flap.

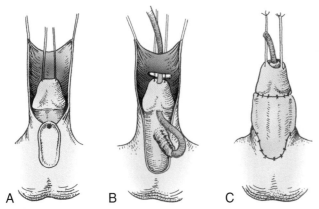

FIGURE 17-38 Skin cover procedure.

channel, and the island-flap urethra is spiraled to the ventrum (Figure 17-37, *F*).

6. The neourethra is anastomosed proximal to the urethra (Figure 17-37, *G*).

7. The neourethra is carried to the tip of the glans (Figure 17-37, *H*).

8. The dorsal penile flaps are transposed laterally to the midline, and excess skin is excised. Closure is with fine absorbable interrupted mattress sutures around the glans and down the penile shaft (Figure 17-37, *I*).

9. Dressings are applied according to established protocol.

Skin Cover. After orthoplasty and urethroplasty, the penis must be resurfaced with skin. Abundant excess dorsal foreskin is usually adequate to achieve the desired results.

OPERATIVE PROCEDURE

1. Preputial tissue is transposed through a small buttonhole opening in the midline (Figure 17-38, *A*).

2. The vasculature is spread laterally, and the glans penis is delivered through the hole (Figure 17-38, *B*).

3. The skin flap is then sutured with fine absorbable interrupted mattress sutures (Figure 17-38, *C*).

Epispadias Repair

An epispadias is a congenital anomaly characterized by a urethral opening on the dorsum of the penis. The surgical procedures employed in the correction of epispadias depend on the extent of the deformity. In mild, incomplete defects the repair is the same as a simple hypospadias repair. Complete deformity is always associated with urinary incontinence because of little or no development of the bladder neck; thus the operation is much more involved. The least severe forms of the exstrophy-epispadias complex are (1) balanic epispadias, in which the urethra opens on the dorsum of the glans, and (2) penile epispadias, in which the urethra opens on the shaft of the penis. The more severe variety, which occurs when the urethra opens on the proximal end of the shaft or in the penopubic position, is generally associated with severe dorsal chordee and urinary incontinence.

Procedural Considerations. The setup for an epispadias repair is the same as that described for hypospadias repair.

Operative Procedures
FIRST-STAGE EPISPADIAS REPAIR
1. The surgeon makes a vertical incision distal to the epispadial meatus and extends it circumferentially to the dorsal coronal margin.
2. The foreshortened dorsal urethral strip is lifted off the corpora cavernosa, and the ventral prepuce (foreskin) is rotated dorsally to cover the dorsal skin defect created by penile straightening.

SECOND-STAGE EPISPADIAS REPAIR
1. A vertical suprapubic incision is made to expose the anterior bladder wall and widened vesical neck. A wedge section of the anterolateral prostatic urethra is removed on either side so that when it is reconstructed, a more normal-caliber prostatic urethra is formed.
2. The roof of the membranous urethra is removed.
3. The prostatic urethra is closed, including muscle that is sutured together in the midline, with absorbable sutures. The bladder is closed so that an indwelling suprapubic catheter is left. The abdomen is closed in layers.
4. The anterior urethra is closed after an appropriate size of octagonal strip of dorsal penile skin is outlined.
5. The remainder of the repair—the creation of the urethra and its coverage with lateral penile skin—is the reverse procedure of a second-stage hypospadias repair.

Bladder Exstrophy Repair

Bladder exstrophy repair corrects a more severe form of epispadias, in which the anterior bladder wall as well as the roof of the urethra is absent. Bladder exstrophy is always accompanied by wide separation of the rectus muscles of the lower abdominal wall and by diastasis of the pubic bone with anterior displacement of the anus. Repair of bladder exstrophy requires an adequate size of bladder for ultimate continence to be achieved. It is preferable to perform this procedure in the neonatal period.

Procedural Considerations. The infant is placed in a supine position, and the abdomen and thighs are prepped and draped. Instruments are the same as those required for hypospadias repair.

Operative Procedure
1. The surgeon makes an incision around the exposed bladder medial to the paravesical neck mucosa. The incision is carried distally across the epispadial urethra distal to the verumontanum. The paravesical mucosa is preserved for urethral lengthening. The bladder is then freed from the rectus fascia and the peritoneum. The dorsal chordee is released, and the mobilized paravesical mucosa is apposed in the midline and sutured to the proximal end of the urethra just distal to the verumontanum.
2. The bladder wall is closed vertically in two layers with 3-0 absorbable sutures; a suprapubic tube is inserted for drainage.
3. The bladder neck is loosely reconstructed by approximating the interpubic ligament, which extends between the proximal end of the phallus and the pubic bone.
4. The symphysis pubis is approximated with a heavy nonabsorbable suture. During this step the assistant rotates the iliac bones anteriorly.

Hydrocelectomy

A hydrocele is an abnormal accumulation of fluid within the scrotum. The fluid is contained within the tunica vaginalis. Excessive secretion or accumulation of hydrocele fluid may be the result of infection or trauma. A hydrocelectomy is the excision of the tunica vaginalis of the testis to remove the enlarged, fluid-filled sac. In older patients, the procedure is performed through a scrotal incision.

Procedural Considerations. The patient is placed in the supine position. Preparation and draping of the patient include routine cleansing of the external genitalia and draping of the patient with a fenestrated sheet. A minor instrument set is required, plus a small drain; a 30-ml syringe with a 20-gauge, 2-inch aspirating needle; and a suspensory dressing.

Operative Procedure
1. The surgeon makes an anterolateral incision in the skin of the scrotum over the hydrocele mass with a #10 or #15 blade (Figure 17-39, *A*). Bleeding is controlled with the electrosurgical unit (ESU).
2. Small retractors may be placed, after which the fascial layers are incised to expose the tunica vaginalis (Figure 17-39, *B*). With fine scissors, forceps, and blunt dissection, the hydrocele is dissected free and delivered (Figure 17-39, *C*). The sac is opened, and the fluid contents are aspirated.
3. The sac is inverted so that it surrounds the testis, epididymis, and distal cord. Excess tunica vaginalis is excised, and the edges of the tunica are sutured with a continuous 4-0 absorbable suture behind the testicle (Figure 17-39, *D*). The testicle is "bottled" by the inverted tunica vaginalis, and this may then be returned to the sac.
4. A drain is placed within the scrotum and exteriorized through a stab wound in the most dependent portion of the scrotum. The scrotal incision is closed in layers with 3-0 and 4-0 absorbable sutures. A fluff compression dressing contained in a scrotal support (suspensory) helps reduce postoperative scrotal edema.

Orchiopexy

An orchiopexy is the surgical placement and fixation of the testicle in a normal anatomic position in the scrotal sac. If the testis fails to descend into the scrotum during gestation, it is considered undescended. An undescended testis becomes arrested somewhere along its normal path of descent. If it is palpable in a position other than its normal path of descent, its position is considered to be ectopic.

A retractile testis has fully descended into the scrotum but retracts out of the scrotum as a result of contraction of the

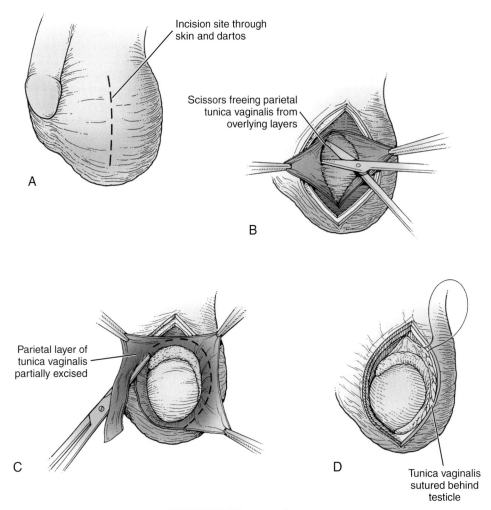

FIGURE 17-39 Hydrocelectomy.

cremaster muscle. Gentle manipulation allows replacement of the testis in the most dependent portion of the scrotum. Retractile testes require no surgical or hormonal treatment.

All testes that are undescended after 1 year, including those that are unresponsive to hormone injections, require surgical placement in the scrotum for optimum maturation. Laparoscopic exploration may also be used to determine position, existence, or size of a "hidden" testis.

Procedural Considerations. The setup is the same as that described for hydrocelectomy. Prepping and draping include the lower abdomen, genitalia, and thighs. Because this operation is usually performed on children, a setup containing small, delicate instruments and sutures is required.

Operative Procedure

1. An inguinal incision is generally employed for exploration of undescended testes (Figure 17-40, *A*). Most undescended testes are located in the superficial inguinal pouch or inguinal canal.
2. The external oblique aponeurosis is opened through the external inguinal ring to expose the inguinal canal; the gubernacular attachments of the undescended testis are dissected free as high as the internal inguinal ring or into the abdominal cavity (Figure 17-40, *B*).

3. All adhesions and the associated inguinal hernia sac are freed to lengthen the cord so that the testis is allowed to reach the scrotal cavity (Figure 17-40, *C*). The hernia sac is transected, twisted, and ligated with sutures.
4. To draw vessels into the inguinal canal, more proximal to the scrotum, the floor of the inguinal canal may have to be divided at the internal ring (Figure 17-40, *D*).
5. The lateral portion of the internal ring is closed to prevent herniation. A scrotal pocket is created, and the testis is anchored in a normal anatomic position within the scrotum with absorbable sutures (Figure 17-40, *E* to *K*).

Orchiopexy may be accomplished by several surgical methods. The dependent portion of the undescended testis may be sutured to the base of the scrotum with absorbable or nonabsorbable sutures exteriorized through the scrotal wall and tied over a peanut dissector or pledget. The most popular method is to anchor the testis into a dissected subdartos pouch. In this procedure, a small midtransverse scrotal incision is made and the skin and dartos muscle are dissected to create a pouch. The testis is then moved through a small hole in the dartos into the subdartos pouch and anchored in position by the traction suture. The overlying skin of the subdartos pouch is closed with fine absorbable suture material. The inguinal incision is repaired in layers with 3-0 absorbable sutures. The skin is

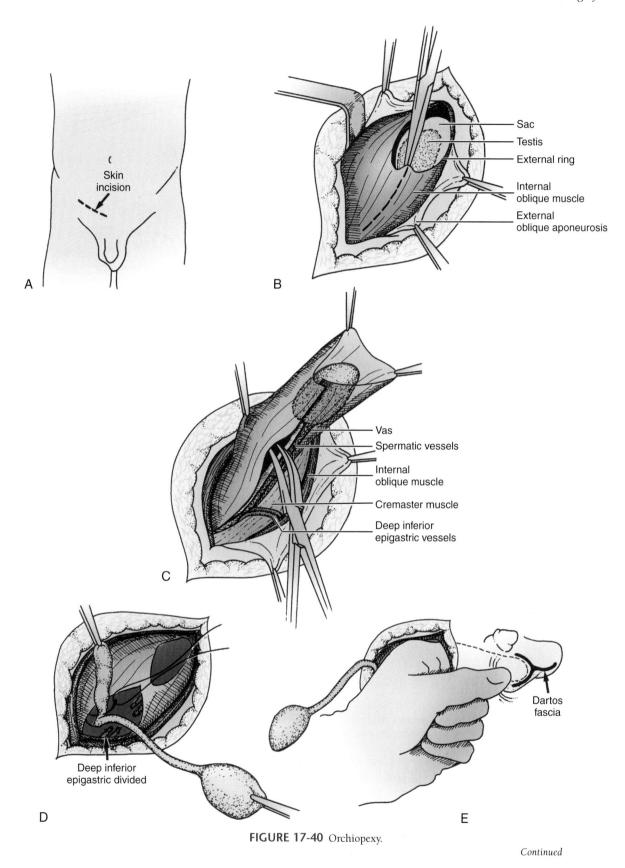

FIGURE 17-40 Orchiopexy.

Continued

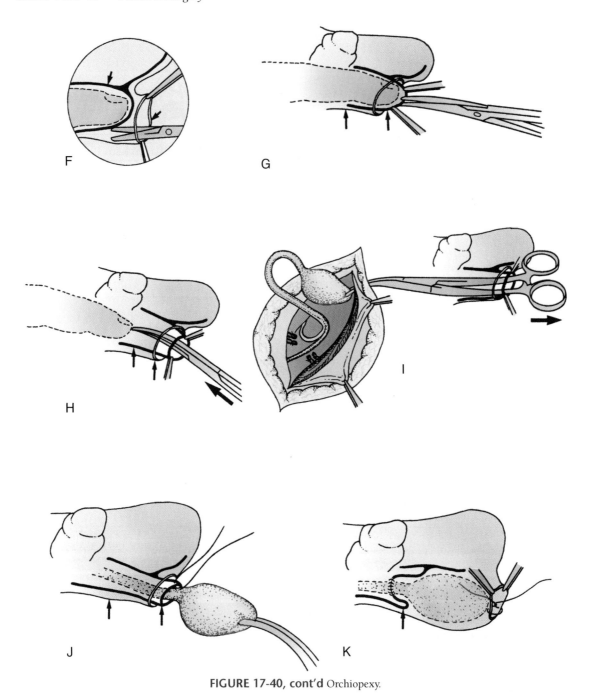

FIGURE 17-40, cont'd Orchiopexy.

closed with a subcuticular suture, and cyanoacrylate glue is used for dressing.

Vesicoureteral Reflux

Vesicoureteral reflux (VUR) is defined as the retrograde flow of urine from the bladder to the ureter and even to the kidney pelvis. Children are usually initially diagnosed with the occurrence of a febrile urinary tract infection (UTI). The workup for reflux will include a renal bladder ultrasound with prevoid and postvoid views as well as a voiding cystourethrogram (VCUG). The VCUG is used to grade the reflux, with grade I being the least and grade V being the most extensive reflux. Children with VUR are given prophylactic antibiotics and checked yearly. Children with unresolved reflux or breakthrough infections will probably require repair of the reflux. Currently there are two types of repair. For lower-grade reflux the most common approach is the minimally invasive approach of cystoscopy with injection of Deflux at the ureteral orifice into the bladder wall. If the reflux is more severe, the child may require reimplantation of the ureter into the bladder wall.

Procedural Considerations—Deflux. The setup for Deflux injection includes the same basic instrument setup as described for cystoscopy including a 10F offset cystoscope, light cord with a light source, cystoscopy fluid delivery tubing, Deflux needle, syringe of Deflux, and camera and monitor for the surgeon to view the procedure. The offset scope is the key to a good injection because the lens is offset at approximately a

45-degree angle and the port to insert the needle through the scope comes straight off the end of the scope. The patient is placed in dorsal lithotomy position for the procedure.

Operative Procedure

1. The pediatric offset cystourethroscope is lubricated and inserted through the urethra into the bladder. The light cord, camera, and irrigation tubing are attached to the cystoscope, a urine specimen for culture is obtained, and then an examination is performed.
2. The bladder is partially filled, to allow for visualization.
3. The irrigation fluid is jetted into the ureteral orifice, opening it wide (hydrodistention), and then the needle is introduced under the mucosa of the midureteral tunnel at the 6-o'clock position. The needle tip is positioned just under the urothelium and is advanced 4 to 5 mm in the submucosal plane of the ureter. Deflux is injected until a prominent bulge appears, and the orifice has assumed a volcano-like shape.
4. The needle is kept in position for 15 to 30 seconds after the injection to prevent extravasation of Deflux.
5. The needle is removed, the bladder is decompressed, the scope is removed, and the patient is returned to the supine position.

Procedural Considerations—Reimplantation of the Ureter.
Reimplantation of the ureter is indicated in children with high-grade VUR. The patient rarely requires a cystoscopy before the operative procedure. A Foley catheter will be placed intraoperatively. The patient is placed in the supine position.

Operative Procedure

1. The surgeon makes a Pfannenstiel incision.
2. The anterior rectus fascia is opened transversely, and then flaps are developed superiorly and inferiorly above the muscle using blunt dissection.
3. The rectus muscle is separated at the midline along the linea alba.
4. The bladder is exposed and then opened in the midline approximately 2 cm above the bladder neck. The bladder is decompressed and then packed with radiopaque sponges.
5. A Denis Browne retractor is placed, and the trigone is exposed.
6. The ureter is identified, and a 6F or 8F feeding tube is placed; then the ureter is dissected with minimal tissue handling and an absorbable stitch is used to tag the orifice. The ureter is then further dissected sharply with tenotomy scissors, completely freeing it from the bladder wall and allowing it to move freely.
7. The original ureteral orifice is then used to begin the dissection for a tunnel leading to the new outlet between the bladder mucosa and the detrusor muscle.
8. The suture tag is then passed through the tunnel, bringing the ureter to its new outlet.
9. The ureter is sutured in place with interrupted absorbable stitches circumferentially, and the feeding tube is removed from the ureter. If ureteral catheters are left in place, they are exteriorized through the bladder and skin and sutured in place.
10. The sponges are removed from the bladder.
11. The Denis Browne retractor is removed from the field.
12. The bladder is closed with a running absorbable suture (a suprapubic tube may be placed during the closure). A Penrose drain may be inserted and stitched in place with a nylon suture.
13. The fascia is closed with a running absorbable suture, and the skin is approximated with a running subcuticular closure. Cyanoacrylate glue is applied. If a drain is used, an absorbent wound dressing is applied and Montgomery straps are used in order to make dressing changes easier for the child, using twill tape to string in shoelace-like fashion to close the dressing.

OTORHINOLARYNGOLOGIC PROCEDURES

Foreign-Body Removal

In the normal course of exploration and play, children often ingest foreign objects or place objects in their noses or ears. Most foreign bodies that are ingested pass safely through the digestive tract without incident and do not need to be removed. If the foreign body is sharp, is caustic (i.e., batteries), or becomes lodged (Figure 17-41), it may need to be removed by esophagoscopy (see Chapter 10) or through an open procedure.

The external ear canal and nose are other areas of interest to curious children. Common objects placed in the nares and external ear canal are dried beans, buttons, plastic objects, metals, food, erasers, nuts, seeds, and button batteries. Items placed in the ear can cause bleeding and difficulty with hearing. A high index of suspicion should be raised in the child with unilateral rhinorrhea, nasal crusting, and air outflow obstruction because these symptoms are often caused by a nasal foreign body. Foreign bodies in the nose and ear may require removal in the OR setting with conscious sedation or a general anesthetic.

The most significant risk of foreign-body ingestion is aspiration. Children are more prone to aspiration than adults because their laryngeal sphincters are immature, they do not have molars to chew all foods adequately, and they often run, shout, and play with objects in their mouths. A study conducted at the Johns Hopkins Hospital tracked common aspirated items between 1939 and 1991 (History box). Today, children continue to present with the similar trends in terms of commonly aspirated food items—candy/gum, peanuts and other nuts, seeds, popcorn, hot dogs, vegetable matter, meat matter, and fish bones. The most commonly aspirated nonfood items are coins, toy parts, crayons, pen tops, tacks, nails, needles, pins, beads, and screws. Aspiration may produce a complete or partial airway obstruction (Figure 17-42). Foreign objects in the respiratory tree are removed by means of rigid or flexible bronchoscopy (see Chapter 14).

Tonsillectomy and Adenoidectomy

A tonsillectomy and adenoidectomy is indicated primarily either for relief of pharyngeal obstruction or for recurrent pharyngitis or tonsillitis.

Pharyngeal obstruction is revealed by a history of sleep-disordered breathing. Mouth breathing, snoring, pauses in breathing, restless sleep, waking at night, and enuresis may be related to obstruction. Daytime somnolence and an inability to concentrate may also be indicators of poor sleep quality. Tonsil size is graded on a scale of 1 to 4, with 1 being contained within the tonsillar fossa and 4 with the tonsils touching each other in the middle of the pharynx. Adenoids are not able to

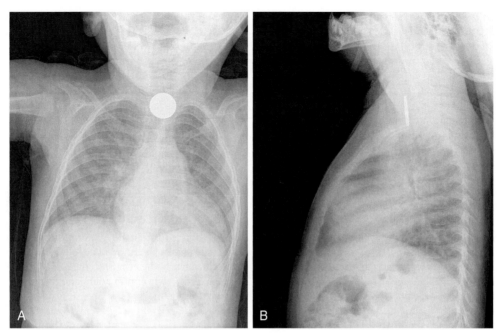

FIGURE 17-41 **A,** Anteroposterior view of coin trapped in esophagus. **B,** Lateral view.

be visualized through the mouth, but symptoms of adenoid enlargement can include mouth breathing, nasal congestion, rhinorrhea, and hyponasal speech. Flexible nasolaryngoscopy and lateral neck radiography can aid in diagnosis of nasopharyngeal obstruction.

Recurrent episodes of pharyngitis sufficient enough to warrant surgical removal should take into consideration the amount of time a child is absent from school, the amount of work time the parent misses, the number of days a child requires antibiotics, and the child's risk for poststreptococccal complications such as glomerulonephritis or mitral valve damage. Three episodes of β-hemolytic streptococcus pharyngitis or more than five episodes of streptococcal/non-streptococcal pharyngitis in the course of a 1-year period would generally merit surgical removal.

An additional reason for tonsillectomy would be a marked difference in tonsil size. Lymphoma on rare occasion may present in this fashion. Unusually enlarged tonsils in an immunosuppressed transplant recipient may also be indicative of post-transplant lymphoproliferative disorder.

Other indications include dysphagia from obstructing tonsils, halitosis from tonsilloliths, and recurrent adenoiditis contributing to sinusitis or otitis media.

A variety of surgical techniques are currently used for tonsillectomy and adenoidectomy. The technique most commonly used is electrosurgery for both (hot) dissection and hemostasis. Other techniques include cold dissection (adenoid curettage and #12 blade for tonsillectomy), radiofrequency, coblation, and laser.

Procedural Considerations. The patient is positioned supine. An oral endotracheal tube with a preformed bend, such as the Ring, Adair, or Elwin (RAE), is used to facilitate visualization of the surgical field. The neck is extended by placing a small roll under the shoulders. Typical draping includes a head drape and an impervious sheet over the patient; no prep is used. The following description is of a hot (electrocoagulation) dissection tonsillectomy with microdebrider dissection adenoidectomy.

Operative Procedure

1. The surgeon inserts a mouth gag retractor with a size-appropriate tongue blade, taking care to keep the tongue in midline position with the endotracheal tube protected by the blade.
2. The posterior and lateral walls of the pharynx are carefully inspected and palpated to detect abnormally positioned vessels.
3. The soft palate is palpated to detect a submucous cleft palate. A bifid uvula is often associated with this anomaly. If this is the case, complete removal of the adenoids can cause velopharyngeal insufficiency.
4. The tip of a 12F red rubber catheter is advanced through one of the nares, into the nasopharynx and out through the mouth. The catheter is gently stretched and the two ends are clamped snugly with a Kelly clamp near the upper lip to retract the soft palate forward.
5. The adenoids are visualized with a laryngeal mirror and removed under direct visualization using either a microdebrider or a suction electrocoagulator. Care is taken to preserve the torus tubarius surrounding the eustachian tube opening. If a microdebrider is used, the nasopharynx is then packed firmly with thoroughly moistened radiopaque tonsil sponges.
6. The superior pole of the first tonsil is grasped with an Allis clamp. A monopolar electrosurgery pencil with a guarded spatula tip is used to make mucosal cuts along the anterior tonsil pillar and superior edge of the fossa.
7. The tonsil is carefully dissected out, following the plane of the tonsillar capsule, while retracting the tonsil medially with the Allis clamp.
8. The final attachment of the inferior portion of the pharyngeal tonsil to the lingual tonsil is transected with the

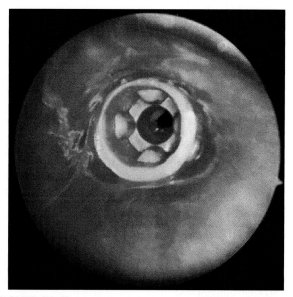

FIGURE 17-42 Foreign body causing partial airway obstruction.

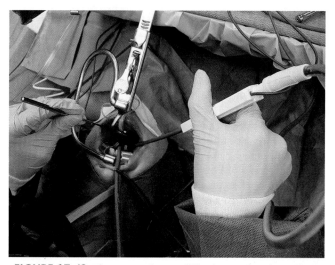

FIGURE 17-43 Electrocoagulation of bleeding in the adenoid bed.

electrocoagulator. Any vessels encountered during the dissection are electrocoagulated.

9. Monopolar suction electrocoagulation is used to attend to any residual bleeding or prominent bleeding vessels. A Hurd dissector is used to retract the anterior tonsillar pillar and improve exposure of the tonsillar fossa during hemostasis. The laryngeal mirror is used to help visualize the recessed superior pole of the tonsillar fossa.

10. This procedure is repeated for removal of the left tonsil.

11. The sponges packing the nasopharynx are then removed. Any areas of bleeding in the adenoid bed are electrocoagulated using the suction electrocoagulator and laryngeal mirror (Figure 17-43).

12. At this point, the mouth gag is released for a brief period, and then reopened. The nasopharynx and oropharynx are reinspected to ensure that there is no further bleeding from vessels that may have been compressed by the opened mouth gag.

13. The oropharynx may be irrigated with 50 to 60 ml of normal saline solution to evaluate for any additional signs of bleeding. The endotracheal tube cuff should be inflated or the anesthesia provider should maintain positive-pressure inflation during the irrigation to prevent inadvertent passage of the irrigation into the trachea.

14. The red rubber catheter is removed. The mouth gag retractor is carefully removed from the oral cavity to prevent inadvertent extubation of the patient.

15. Dentition, temporomandibular joint mobility, and perioral skin are reinspected for inadvertent surgical complications.

Excision of Branchial Cleft Cyst/Remnant/Sinus Tract

Congenital branchial cleft anomalies are remnants of the branchial arch apparatus that failed to disappear during early embryologic development. At approximately 5 weeks' gestation, the branchial arches are associated with an external cleft of ectodermal origin and an internal pouch of endodermal origin. Anomalies that remain from incomplete resolution can be in the form of a branchial cleft cyst, a sinus, or a fistula. The location of branchial cleft anomalies ranges from the preauricular area (type 1) to the lateral neck along the sternocleidomastoid muscle (types 2, 3, and 4). A cyst may not become apparent until later in childhood, typically during times of acute infection or possible abscess formation, and can occur anywhere along the course of a branchial sinus tract or fistulous tract. A sinus tract usually has an external opening to the neck, generally along the anterior border of the sternocleidomastoid muscle. A fistula has both an external opening and an internal opening; the internal opening is usually in the area of the pyriform sinus near the tonsil on that side. Excision of the branchial cleft anomaly is indicated if it is cystic in nature or if it has become infected. The infection must be treated before surgical excision; if an abscess is present an incision and drainage may be needed.

Procedural Considerations. Imaging studies (computed tomography [CT], magnetic resonance imaging [MRI]) are helpful to determine the presence of an associated tract. The patient will be positioned supine with a roll under the shoulders to slightly extend the neck. A surgical drain, such as a rubber band, is frequently placed. Antibiotics are usually given intraoperatively before surgical incision. Description of a branchial cyst (type 2) excision follows.

Operative Procedure

1. A transverse skin crease overlying the lesion and 1.5 cm below the margin of the mandible is selected. The surgeon injects the proposed incision line with 1% lidocaine with 1:100,000 epinephrine.
2. The surgeon makes the skin incision with a #15 blade through the skin and subcutaneous tissues.
3. The platysma muscle is divided with the ESU.
4. The tissues overlying the cyst are gently dissected with fine forceps and small scissors or a small gauze peanut.
5. The cyst is gently grasped with a Babcock clamp. Surrounding tissue is dissected free from the cyst using small scissors to spread between the cyst capsule and surrounding tissue and then to cut through fibrous attachments.
6. If a pedicle or fibrous tract is identified, it is followed as far cephalic as possible before it is clamped, cut, and tied with 3-0 absorbable suture.
7. A small rubber band drain is usually placed to prevent accumulation of fluid or blood in the dissected cavity. A safety pin or suture is attached to the distal end of the drain; the drain is removed within 24 hours.
8. The wound is closed in layers. The skin is closed with subcuticular sutures, and adhesive strips are applied to keep the wound edges approximated.

NEUROSURGICAL PROCEDURES

Neuropathologic conditions requiring surgical intervention can be found in any age group. The most common problems requiring neurosurgical procedures in infants and children include meningocele, myelomeningocele, encephalocele, craniosynostosis, hydrocephalus, brain tumors, and trauma. The surgical approach, instruments, and equipment required for brain tumors and trauma are relatively similar to those required for adults; consequently, the majority of these procedures are as described in Chapter 12.

Myelomeningocele/Meningocele

Myelomeningocele (Figure 17-44) is a form of spina bifida and is always associated with Chiari type II malformations. It occurs because of a congenital flaw in neural tube closure at approximately 8 to 12 days after conception. The failure of the neural tube to close correctly causes a defect in the posterior elements of the lumbar vertebrae, fascia, and dura, allowing the meninges, spinal cord, and nerve roots to protrude out in a sac or cyst through the skin. The exposed spinal cord is called the neural placode and is not properly developed; there is always some degree of paralysis and loss of sensation below the defect. The amount of disability depends on the vertebral level of the spina bifida and frequently includes loss of bladder and bowel function and hydrocephalus. Meningoceles are similar to myelomeningoceles but not as neurologically devastating: meninges and cerebrospinal fluid (CSF) protrude into the defect but not the spinal cord.

Procedural Considerations. Infants born with either of these defects need to be given broad-spectrum antibiotics immediately after birth and taken to the OR within 24 hours for closure of the defect. A very high percentage of children with this defect develop an allergy to latex; surgical closure and all subsequent surgical procedures should be performed in a latex-free environment.

Operative Procedure

1. The surgeon makes an elliptical incision around the defect with a #15 blade.
2. Metzenbaum scissors are used to remove the pearly epithelial tissue around the neural placode. Retention of the epithelial tissue can lead to formation of a postoperative epidermoid.
3. Using the Metzenbaum scissors, the surgeon performs blunt dissection following the nerve tissue on the ventral side of the placode down to the spinal canal.
4. The dura is then separated from the fascia with the Metzenbaum scissors.
5. Using 4-0 braided nylon suture, the surgeon closes the dura over the neural placode.
6. A #11 blade and Metzenbaum scissors are used to free the fascia from the muscle layer.
7. Braided nylon suture is used to close the fascial layer over the dura.
8. The muscle layer is then closed, followed by skin closure.

Craniectomy for Craniosynostosis

Craniosynostosis is the premature fusion of one or more cranial sutures. The condition can occur as part of a syndrome or as an isolated process. Craniosynostosis is characterized as "simple" when only one suture line is involved and "compound" when two or more suture lines are involved. The defect occurs in utero, and the exact etiology remains unknown. The purpose of the cranial sutures is to allow the calvaria to bend during the birth process and to allow the skull to expand to accommodate normal brain growth during infancy. The normal brain is finished growing by 2 years of age; at this time fusion of the cranial sutures normally begins. The fusion process is complete by 8 years of age.

Sagittal synostosis accounts for approximately 50% to 58% of all the synostoses with equal distribution between males and females (Sheth et al, 2008). The sagittal suture runs in the midline of the skull, connecting the anterior fontanelle to the posterior fontanelle. Premature closure of this fontanelle produces an elongation of the skull in the anteroposterior plane. Surgical intervention involves a linear strip craniectomy to excise the sagittal suture line from the anterior fontanelle to the lambdoidal suture line. Surgery is generally performed on the infant between 6 weeks and 6 months of age, with the best cosmetic results coming from the earlier repair. A craniectomy for sagittal synostosis is described.

Procedural Considerations. The infant is positioned supine using a cerebellar headrest. Additional measures need to be taken to maintain the infant's normal body temperature; room temperature should be elevated, and a forced air–warming blanket should be used. An overbed warmer should be used during anesthesia induction and IV placement.

Operative Procedure
1. A sinusoidal incision is made midway between the anterior and posterior fontanelles from ear to ear, just posterior to the pinna.
2. The scalp is elevated off the skull anteriorly and posteriorly to expose the anterior fontanelle, posterior fontanelle, and asterion. Care is used to leave the pericranium attached to the skull to minimize bleeding.
3. A burr hole is made on each side of the sagittal suture on the lambdoidal suture.
4. A craniotome is used to cut anteriorly to the anterior fontanelle on each side of the sagittal suture. A Leksell or Lempert rongeur is used to cut across the sagittal suture and connect the burr holes.
5. A Cobb periosteal elevator is used to carefully dissect the sagittal suture off the underlying dura.
6. A burr hole is placed at the asterion on each side. The craniotome is used to make a curvilinear cut just posterior to the coronal suture.
7. The parietal bone is then "greensticked" (fractured but leaving the periosteum intact) laterally.
8. The skin is then closed with 3-0 and 4-0 absorbable sutures.

Ventriculoatrial and Ventriculoperitoneal Shunts

Hydrocephalus is characterized by excess production of CSF or is associated with a blockage in the ventricular drainage system. Early intervention is indicated in infants to prevent cranial distortion caused by the increasing size of the ventricles (Figure 17-45).

The two most widely used pediatric surgical procedures to divert excessive CSF from the ventricles to other body cavities from which it can be absorbed are ventriculoatrial (ventriculocardiac) (Figure 17-46) and ventriculoperitoneal shunts. See Chapter 12 for complete information related to these two procedures.

ORTHOPEDIC PROCEDURES

Pediatric orthopedic surgery may encompass the following areas: spine disorders, sports medicine, cerebral palsy, mus-

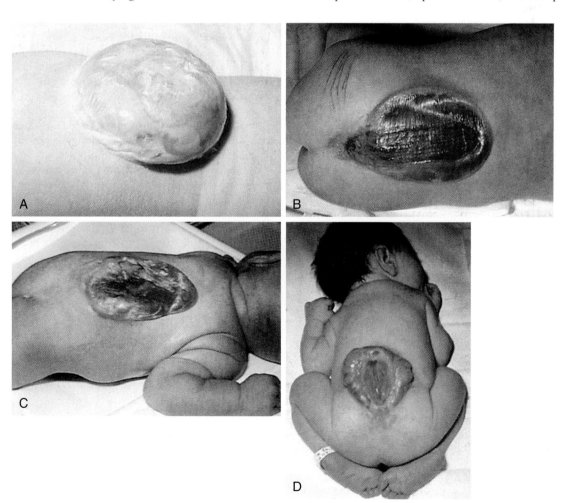

FIGURE 17-44 Examples of meningocele and myelomeningoceles. **A,** Meningocele. Lesion is covered by skin and meninges. **B,** Myelomeningocele. Neural component evident at central strip of lesion. **C,** Thoracolumbar myelomeningocele. **D,** Severe myelomeningocele. Neural tissue in center represents the open spinal canal.

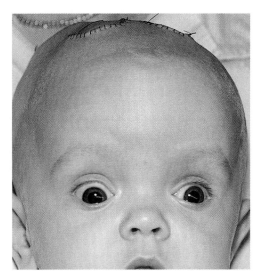

FIGURE 17-45 Infant with hydrocephalus.

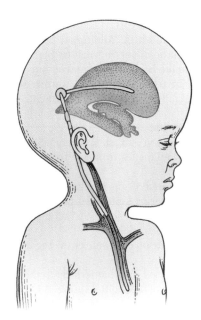

FIGURE 17-46 Placement of ventriculoatrial shunt.

culoskeletal tumors and injuries, foot and ankle disorders, limb length discrepancy, hip disorders, hand surgery, limb deficiency (amputations), thoracic insufficiency, and trauma. The majority of instrumentation, equipment, and procedural considerations are similar to those described in Chapter 11, Orthopedic Surgery. Nonetheless, there are treatment modalities and procedures that are more commonly performed in the pediatric population than in the adult population. Procedures for developmental dysplasia of the hip, abductor and adductor tenotomy, and variations of clubfoot will be described in this section.

Developmental Hip Dysplasia

Until recently, dislocation of the hip seen in newborns was referred to as "congenital dislocation of the hip" (CDH). The term *developmental dysplasia of the hip (DDH)* has replaced the former name to reflect the evolutionary nature of hip problems in the first few months of life. DDH is a progressive condition in which the hip structures fail to develop adequately. Because the pathologic process leading to hip dysplasia may not be present or identifiable at birth, periodic exams of every infant's hips are essential at each routine baby exam until the child is 1 year old. About 1% of infants have dislocated, dislocatable, or subluxatable hips. Sixty percent of DDH cases occur in females, and 60% of all cases involve only the left hip (Wilson et al, 2008). DDH encompasses the entire spectrum of abnormalities involving the growing hip, ranging from simple dysplasia to dysplasia with subluxation or dislocation of the hip joint. The goal of DDH management is to achieve and maintain a concentric reduction of the femoral head within the acetabulum, in order to provide the optimal environment for the normal development of both structures. When proper alignment is disrupted, soft tissue and bony changes cause contractures of the hip muscles, a shallow acetabulum, and possibly a deformed femoral head. Treatment of congenital dislocation of the hip varies depending on the age of the patient and the stability of the hip. A Pavlik harness is the most commonly used nonoperative device in infants. If the Pavlik harness fails, the infant is brought to the OR and anesthetized for a closed reduction of the hip (proper positioning of the femur head within the acetabulum) confirmed by intraoperative arthrogram and fluoroscopy, with application of a spica cast. Failure of closed reduction and immobilization necessitates an open reduction with an adductor tenotomy to allow adequate abduction to reduce the femoral head; after surgery, children younger than 2 years are then placed in a postreduction spica cast. For children older than 3 years the surgeon may need to perform a shortening varus femoral osteotomy (derotational osteotomy) to facilitate reduction of the femoral head into the acetabulum. In addition, if the acetabulum coverage is inadequate, a pelvic realignment (pelvic osteotomy) procedure may be necessary. Many of the pediatric orthopedic plating systems offer congenital dysplastic hip implants, which can be used in the reconstruction.

Procedural Considerations. The patient most often is in the lateral position for these procedures. An anterior incision is usually made for open reduction, whereas a lateral incision is made for the subtrochanteric femoral osteotomy. A soft tissue set and bone set (appropriate for age) are required as well as an oscillating saw, a wire driver, Steinmann pins, blade plate implants, and instrumentation.

Operative Procedure

DDH OPEN REDUCTION (Figure 17-47)
1. The hip joint is opened, and the soft tissue in the acetabulum is excised.
2. The femoral head is then reduced into the acetabulum and held by suturing of the capsule.
   DEROTATIONAL OSTEOTOMY. A derotational osteotomy is performed when the femoral head is improperly seated in the acetabulum.
1. The femur is placed in internal rotation and divided.
2. The distal fragment is rotated externally to place the knee and foot straight ahead.
3. If the patient is a young child, the osteotomy is frequently performed in the supracondylar region, and the patient is immobilized in a plaster spica cast.

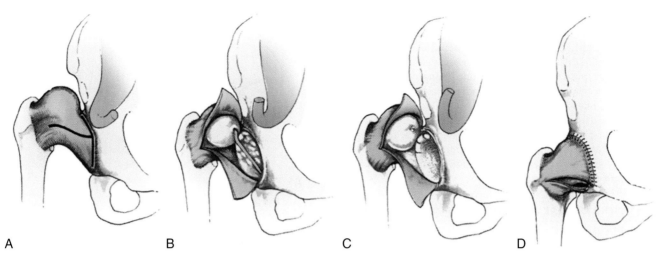

FIGURE 17-47 Repair of congenital hip disorder using open reduction. **A,** T-shaped incision of capsule. **B,** Capsulotomy of the hip and locating the true acetabulum. **C,** Removal of tissue from the depth of the acetabulum. **D,** Capsulorrhaphy.

4. For an older child, the osteotomy is frequently done in the subtrochanteric region and the osteotomized fragments are held with an osteotomy blade plate or an intermediate compression screw. Immobilization may not be necessary.

PELVIC OSTEOTOMY

1. A complete division of the wing of the ilium is made by an osteotomy from the sciatic notch to the anterior margin of the ilium, superior to the acetabulum.
2. The ilium is then wedged down to increase the depth of the acetabulum when the osteotomy site is opened and a bone graft is inserted.
3. Heavy suture is used to close the capsule, and a spica cast is applied for postoperative immobilization.

Tenotomy/Lengthening Procedures

Tenotomies and lengthening procedures are commonly recommended for children with cerebral palsy to treat contractures or because the spasticity of these muscles makes mobility and abduction and adduction of the extremities difficult (Wilson, 2008). These procedures may also be recommended as treatment for groin injuries where traditional medical treatment has failed. Once the tendons are cut, the affected extremity may be immobilized in a cast, brace, or splint to allow for healing and promote normal growth patterns. In other cases, a dressing may be applied without immobilization. The procedure may be performed open (as described here) or using percutaneous techniques.

Procedural Considerations. The patient is positioned supine for the procedure with the affected extremity or extremities draped free for prepping and draping.

Operative Procedure

1. The adductor longus, gracilis, and adductor brevis are lengthened through a medial groin incision to improve hip abduction.
2. The pectineus adductor brevis interval is exposed to locate the iliopsoas tendon. The iliopsoas tendon is divided to correct hip flexion contractures.

3. Wounds are irrigated and closed using absorbable suture. Cyanoacrylate glue dressing is applied to each incision line.

Clubfoot

Clubfoot is a complex deformity that is diagnosed prenatally through ultrasound or at birth. According to the American Academy of Orthopedic Surgeons (AAOS), clubfoot may occur unilaterally or bilaterally and may be idiopathic or one in a combination of other syndromes with associated anomalies (AAOS, 2007). The general characteristic for all cases includes inversion of the foot such that the anterior foot is located in the typical position of the posterior foot. Often, there is a deep crease in the midfoot. Each case of clubfoot differs in severity, but all require treatment. Treatment options include nonsurgical methods such as taping, bracing, physical therapy, or continuous passive motion exercise using a machine. When clubfoot is treated surgically, the following procedures are required: release of soft tissue and joint contractures, tendon lengthening, and temporary pin fixation of the joints in the foot. Many variations of surgical intervention exist, and one method is described in the following Operative Procedure.

Procedural Considerations. The patient is positioned supine for induction of anesthesia and surgical repair. A tourniquet is applied to the affected leg. The leg is prepped and draped free.

Operative Procedure

1. The surgeon makes an incision through the skin, subcutaneous tissue, and scar tissue posteriorly and medially on the affected foot with a #15 blade and dissects the tissue to locate the Achilles' tendon.
2. The Achilles' tendon is lengthened by tenotomy and scar tissue is removed.
3. The peroneal tendons are identified and lengthened by tenotomy, and dissection is carried around to the medial aspect of the foot.

4. The posterior subtalar capsule is identified and divided, and scar tissue is removed.

5. The posterior aspect of the ankle is identified, divided, and debrided of scar tissue. Dissection is carried around medially to the posterior tibialis tendon, taking care to isolate and protect the neurovascular bundle. The posterior tibialis tendon is released.

6. The medial aspect of the talonavicular joint is released. Foot flexion and rotation are verified and the surgical incision is irrigated and closed using absorbable dressings.

7. A bulky dressing and cast are applied to the affected foot and the tourniquet is deflated.

PLASTIC AND RECONSTRUCTIVE SURGERY

Cleft Lip Repair

The normal upper lip is composed of skin, underlying orbicularis oris muscle, and mucosa. Two skin ridges are situated near the midline of the central philtrum of the lip. The vermilion (red portion of the lip) peaks at the philtral ridge on each side and gently curves downward as it reaches the midline to form the Cupid's bow. A deficiency in tissue (skin, muscle, and mucosa) along one or both sides of the upper lip or, rarely, in the midline results in a cleft at the site of this deficiency. The deficiency of tissue present with a cleft lip results in distortion of the Cupid's bow, absence of one or both philtral ridges, and distortion of the lower portion of the nose. Cleft lip is usually associated with a notch or cleft of the underlying alveolus and a cleft of the palate.

Cleft lip repair is most often performed when the infant is about 3 months of age. Timing of the repair follows the "rule of 10": the infant is 10 weeks of age, weighs 10 pounds, and has a hemoglobin level of 10 g/dl. Early surgical correction aids in feeding and infant-parent bonding. Lip repair is directed toward rearrangement of existing tissues to approximate the normal lip as closely as possible. Some considerations may also be given to correcting the nasal deformity at the time of the cleft lip repair.

Procedural Considerations.
A plastic surgery local instrument set is required, plus the following special instruments: Brown lip clamps; calipers; a Foment retractor; Beaver blades, #64 and #65; and a Logan bow. The OR bed is usually reversed to create more knee room if the surgeon prefers to sit during the surgery. The patient is placed in the supine position, with the head at the edge of the OR bed. The face is prepped, and the head drape is used. The surgeon may stand or sit at the patient's side or just above the patient's head during the operation.

Operative Procedure
Many types of cleft lip repair are in common use, one of which is illustrated in Figure 17-48. The following steps are applicable to all lip repairs:

1. Normal landmarks are identified and marked or tattooed. Precise measurements, taken with calipers and a ruler, are made so that corresponding points can be marked along the cleft.

2. The lip may be infiltrated with epinephrine 1:200,000, or lip clamps may be used to aid hemostasis.

3. Incisions are made along the markings for the repair.

4. The abnormal musculature is dissected.

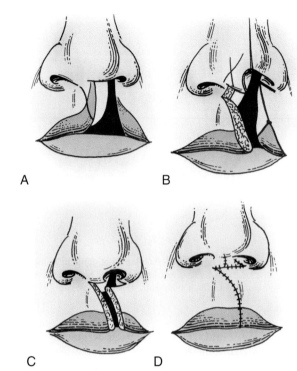

A   B

C   D

FIGURE 17-48 Rotation-advancement method to correct complete unilateral cleft of lip. **A,** Rotation incision marked so that Cupid's bow–philtral dimple component will rotate down into normal position; flap advances into columella to form nostril sill. **B,** Dimple component has dropped down; second flap has advanced into columella. **C,** Flap is being advanced into rotation gap, while skin-roll flap is interdigitated at mucocutaneous junction line. **D,** Scar is maneuvered into strategic position where it is hidden at nasal base and floor and at philtrum column; then it is interdigitated at mucocutaneous junction.

5. Additional dissection along the maxilla and nose may be performed.

6. Closure is done in three layers: muscle, skin, and mucosa. Adhesive strips may be used. A Logan bow is applied to the cheeks with tape strips, and elbow restraints are placed.

Cleft Palate Repair

The palate is composed of the bony or hard palate anteriorly and the soft palate posteriorly. The alveolus borders the hard palate. A separation or cleft of the palate occurs in the midline and may involve only the soft palate or both hard and soft palates. The alveolus may be cleft on one or both sides.

The major function of the soft palate is to aid in the production of normal speech sounds. An intact hard palate is necessary to prevent escape of air through the nose during speech and to prevent the egress of liquid and food from the nose.

Cleft palate repair is usually performed when the child is 6 months of age and should be achieved before the beginning of speech. Variable factors, including the child's weight and the possibility of other disease processes, can affect the timing of the surgery. The various operations used to achieve surgical closure of the palate all employ tissue adjacent to the cleft (in the form of flaps), which is shifted centrally to close the defect.

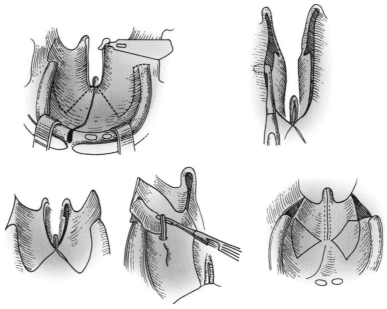

FIGURE 17-49 Closure of cleft of soft palate by V-Y (Wardill-Kilner) palatoplasty. A V-shaped incision is made on oral side of palate; mucoperiosteal flaps are elevated on oral and nasal sides, with preservation of blood vessels; Y-shaped closure (in three layers) closes cleft and lengthens palate.

Procedural Considerations. A basic plastic surgery instrument set is required, plus the following special instruments: Dingman mouth gag with assorted blades; Blair palate hook; palate knives; Blair palate elevators; and Fomon lower lateral scissors, short and long. The patient is placed in the supine position, with the head at the edge of the OR bed. The head drape is used. Many surgeons sit just above the patient's head and cradle the head on their lap (with the patient's neck hyperextended).

Operative Procedure
One of the most frequently used cleft palate repairs is illustrated in Figure 17-49. The following steps are common to all palate repairs:
1. The Dingman mouth gag is inserted. Maintenance of the position of the endotracheal tube is crucial at this point. The surgeon may also insert a throat pack to absorb blood that may drain into the throat.
2. The outlines of the palatal flaps are marked.
3. The palate is injected with 1% lidocaine with epinephrine 1:100,000 for hemostasis.
4. The flaps are incised and elevated.
5. Closure is in three layers: nasal mucosa, muscle, and palatal mucosa.
6. A large horizontal mattress traction suture is placed through the body of the tongue. If the patient experiences upper airway obstruction after extubation, traction is placed on this suture to pull the tongue forward, rather than insert an airway that might harm the palate repair. The throat pack is removed.

Pharyngeal Flap

When abnormal speech (velopharyngeal insufficiency) results despite a cleft palate repair, a secondary surgical procedure may be necessary to improve speech. Primarily an excess of air

escaping through the nose during speech characterizes typical "cleft palate speech." This hypernasality often results from insufficient bulk or movement of the muscles of the soft palate. To decrease or eliminate this problem, tissue from the pharynx, in the form of a pharyngeal flap, is added to the soft palate. This flap also reduces the size of the opening between the oropharynx and nasopharynx, thus decreasing or eliminating the nasal escape of air during speech.

A pharyngeal flap repair may be done at any age, but most are done before the patient is 14 years old. A pharyngeal flap also may be part of primary cleft palate repair.

Procedural Considerations. Positioning, draping, and instruments are the same as those described for cleft palate repair, with the addition of two 12F red rubber catheters.

Operative Procedure
1. The Dingman mouth gag is inserted. A throat pack may be inserted.
2. The surgeon injects the palate and posterior wall of the pharynx with 1% lidocaine with epinephrine 1:100,000 for hemostasis.
3. The palate is incised, and the pharyngeal flap is incised and elevated.
4. The pharyngeal wall donor site may be sutured or left open.
5. The pharyngeal flap is sutured to the palate, and the palate is closed.
6. A traction suture is placed through the body of the tongue. The throat pack is removed.

Total Ear Reconstruction

An absent external ear presents the surgical team with the objective of developing or restoring a part of the appearance that will help with self-esteem and confidence in daily interactions as well as enhance hearing, since the external ear funnels sound waves from the environment into the inner ear. Emotional support is a key aspect of the plan of care for these patients.

The external ear consists of skin, subcutaneous tissue, and cartilage. The surgical procedure to create an external ear involves the retrieval of rib cartilage, carving the cartilage, placing the newly fashioned ear on the side of the patient's head, and skin grafting and dressing of the operative sites, with continual assessment and reassessment of the preoperative sketches made of the patient's ear with relation to facial structure. This can be accomplished as a one-stage procedure or as a sequence of surgeries. For congenital defects, the ideal time for initiating the procedure is between 6 and 10 years of age. In the case of traumatic loss of the external ear (as from burns), the time is individually determined. The use of tissue expanders may be considered in some cases to stretch the skin surface required to cover the ear.

Procedural Considerations. A basic plastic surgery instrument set is required, with the addition of rib graft instrumentation for autologous rib cartilage retrieval in total ear reconstruction. A sterile Doppler probe with sterile conduction gel should be available for intraoperative use. Preoperative sketches of the ear are done with the use of unexposed x-ray film. Symmetric and anatomic landmarks are vital considerations in the patterns developed for the reconstruction. When the sketches are complete, the films are sterilized with care not to remove the markings made by the surgeon. The patient is supine with the arms tucked securely at the sides. Appropriate padding and protection of vulnerable neurovascular bundles and pressure sites are critical. Use of a sequential compression device and a forced air–warming unit over the lower half of the patient's body should be considered because of the anticipated length of the procedure. Before the skin prep, the surgeon will assess the vascular integrity of the temporoparietal flap with an unsterile Doppler probe and conduction gel and will mark the incision sites. Infiltration of the operative sites with local anesthetic with epinephrine 1:200,000 can be used for hemostasis. Epinephrine in higher concentrations (e.g., 1:100,000) is not recommended for use in the area of the flap because of the possible obliteration of the vascular complexes present. The patient's face, torso, and an additional site if a skin graft is anticipated. A standard head drape and a split drape (or U drape) for the patient's torso allow the team access to the auricular area and chest, respectively. Usually two instrument tables are used, with one designated for carving the rib cartilage. Because the procedure is lengthy (6 to 8 hours on average), rolling sitting stools should be provided for the team. Periodic progress of the procedure should be relayed to the patient's family members in the surgical waiting room.

Operative Procedure
1. The temporoparietal fascia flap is lifted, and a sterile Doppler probe and sterile conduction gel are used to assess the vascular integrity of the flap.
2. The chest wall is incised, and the rib cartilage segments are removed with care to preserve the perichondrium. This will encourage bone growth and help to prevent a chest wall defect. The assessment of intact pleura is critical before closure of the chest. Instillation of saline into the wound is

done; if bubbles appear, the pleura is not intact; a chest tube is then inserted and attached to a chest drainage system. If the integrity of the pleura is in question, an intraoperative chest x-ray film may be taken to assess for a pneumothorax. If the pleura is intact, closure of the wound is performed and injection of 0.25% bupivacaine to the intercostal incision area is performed.
3. While one team closes the chest, another team begins the process of carving the rib cartilage for the ear reconstruction. The previously marked radiographs are crucial aids for the artistic abilities of the surgeon, providing a blueprint for the sculpting phase of the procedure. Surgical wire is used to connect the carved pieces of rib cartilage as it is shaped to resemble the external ear.
4. A skin graft is taken, and the donor site is covered with a dressing of choice.
5. Hemostasis is maintained with the ESU, topical thrombin, and infiltration of local anesthetic with epinephrine.
6. The flap covers the sculpted ear, and the skin graft is used to cover any exposed areas (this is a technique used especially with burn patients who have less available skin for coverage).
7. Drains are placed and attached to closed-wound suction, or gauze stents wrapped with nonadherent gauze are sutured in place behind the ear. Soft, bulky dressings are applied to the ear and secured with a head wrap of rolled gauze. Standard dressings are applied to the chest wall.

Otoplasty

A congenital deformity in which the ear protrudes abnormally from the side of the head is generally the result of an absent or insufficiently pronounced antihelical fold of the external ear. The various methods of otoplasty are an attempt at correction by creating an antihelical fold that positions the ear more normally (Figure 17-50). Protruding ears may be unilateral or bilateral. An otoplasty is generally performed for children who are uncomfortable or self-conscious about the deformity, usually in the elementary school–age years.

Procedural Considerations. A plastic surgery instrument set is needed. The patient is placed supine on the OR bed, and a head drape is used, leaving both ears well exposed. The patient's head is turned with the affected ear up and with the lower ear well padded to avoid pressure injury.

Operative Procedure
1. The antihelical fold is created when the external ear is bent backward. The position of the antihelical fold is marked by placing 25-gauge or straight needles through the ear from anterior to posterior, applying methylene blue to the tips of the needles, and withdrawing them to mark the cartilage within.
2. An ellipse of skin is excised from the posterior surface of the ear after it has been infiltrated with 1% lidocaine with epinephrine 1:100,000.
3. The ear cartilage is usually incised near the antihelical fold, and the anterior surface of the cartilage is scored to allow it to bend backward.
4. Sutures are usually placed to hold the cartilage in its new position.
5. The skin incision is closed.

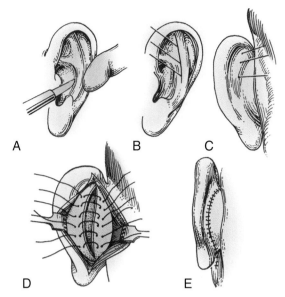

FIGURE 17-50 Otoplasty for correction of protruding ears. **A,** Antihelix defined by application of pressure to ear. **B,** Position of antihelical fold marked by the passage of straight needles through ear. **C,** Needle points visible along posterior surface of ear with ellipse of skin to be excised marked. **D,** Section of ear cartilage incised and scored or excised with sutures placed to hold cartilage back. **E,** Posterior ear incision sutured.

6. A drain may be placed to aid in the skin's adherence to the cartilage framework beneath.
7. A nonadherent dressing, such as petroleum gauze or cotton coated with Polysporin antibiotic ointment, is usually placed in front of and behind the ear, followed by fluffed gauze and a bulky dressing made of rolled gauze to exert moderate compression on the ear.

Repair of Syndactyly

Syndactyly refers to a congenital webbing of the digits of the hands or feet. It is occasionally seen in association with other abnormalities, such as extra fingers or toes (polydactyly), or with bony abnormalities. In syndactyly with normal digits, most commonly seen, a web of skin joins adjacent fingers (Figure 17-51) but each finger has its own tendons, vessels, nerves, and bony phalanges. Although the skin web may appear loose, a deficiency in skin is always present when surgical separation is performed. Plans for taking a skin graft (usually full thickness) should always be made. Surgical separation of syndactyly is performed at any time, usually after approximately 12 months of age.

Toe syndactyly is less often treated surgically than finger syndactyly because proper function of the foot does not require fine movements of individual toes. Although the setup and description that follow are for the repair of finger syndactyly, they can also be applied to the repair of toe syndactyly.

Procedural Considerations. A plastic surgery local instrument set is required, plus a sterile marking pen, sterilized unexposed x-ray film, a pediatric pneumatic tourniquet, and an Esmarch bandage. The patient is placed supine on the OR bed with the affected arm extended on a hand table. A hand drape is used, and the affected hand and wrist are prepped

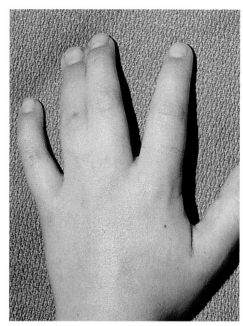

FIGURE 17-51 Syndactyly involving third and fourth fingers.

and draped as well as both inguinal areas (donor sites for full-thickness skin grafts). Some surgeons prefer to use the wrist or forearm as donor sites.

Operative Procedure

1. The skin is incised and small flaps at the sides of fingers and in the web are elevated.
2. After the flaps have been sutured into position, patterns of areas of absent skin on the sides of fingers are made and transferred to the skin-graft donor site.
3. The skin graft is taken; if a full-thickness skin graft is used, it must be defatted before the graft is sutured in place.
4. Skin grafts are sutured to fingers.
5. Stent dressings are placed over the skin grafts. The entire hand is immobilized in a bulky dressing or in a long arm cast.

Orbital-Craniofacial Surgery

Some congenital anomalies involve the orbital-craniofacial skeleton. These include hypertelorism, in which the distance between the orbits is increased as seen in Crouzon's disease and Apert's syndrome. Crouzon's disease (Figure 17-52) is characterized by premature closure of the cranial sutures, resulting in an abnormally shaped skull, exophthalmos and hypertelorism, parrot's beak nose, and maxillary hypoplasia. Apert's syndrome (Figure 17-53) includes the same craniofacial deformities as Crouzon's disease and also syndactyly or other hand anomalies. Recent advances in plastic surgery make surgical correction of some of these deformities possible.

Binocular vision is normal in humans. It involves the coordinated use of both eyes to obtain a single mental impression of objects. Binocular vision is usually absent in craniofacial anomalies because of the increased distance between the orbits. The purposes of orbital-craniofacial surgery are to provide the patient with binocular vision by moving the orbits closer together and to provide the patient with a more accept-

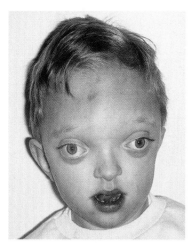

FIGURE 17-52 Crouzon's disease.

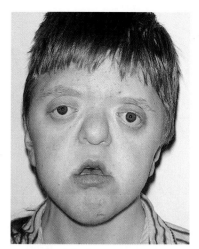

FIGURE 17-53 Apert's syndrome.

able appearance by moving the bones of the orbital-craniofacial skeleton into a more normal position. Correction of the deformity seen in Crouzon's disease and Apert's syndrome involves a surgically created Le Fort III maxillary fracture.

Although an extracranial approach may be used, an intracranial approach is used in most cases; therefore a neurosurgeon and a plastic surgeon perform these operations through a bifrontal (coronal) craniotomy. A tracheostomy may be done before the start of the procedure. Bone grafts from hips or ribs are necessary to augment areas of bone deficit, which result from movement of the craniofacial skeleton.

Procedural Considerations. These operations are usually performed on children. They are very extensive procedures, often lasting 12 to 14 hours. Blood loss is considerable. Postoperative complications, such as cerebral edema or meningitis, can be formidable. The surgical team must pay particular attention to the following important details: (1) insertion of a Foley catheter into the patient's bladder before the operation is started, (2) positioning of the patient on the OR bed so that all bony prominences are well padded, and (3) availability of accurate means for measuring blood loss. Use of a sequential compression device and forced air–warming units should also be anticipated.

A basic plastic surgery instrument set, craniectomy instruments and supplies (see Chapter 12), plastic hand instrumentation, and tracheostomy instruments and supplies are required. A high-speed drill, saws, and general orthopedic instrumentation are also needed. A separate setup is necessary for obtaining the bone graft.

The patient is positioned, prepped, and draped as described for bifrontal craniotomy (see Chapter 12). The entire face is left exposed, however, and may temporarily be covered with a plastic drape until the portion of the operation requiring access to the face is reached. The bone-graft donor site is also prepped and draped so that both iliac crests and the lower ribs are exposed.

Operative Procedure

1. Tracheostomy, if required, is performed first, followed by application of arch bars (when indicated as in Crouzon's disease and Apert's syndrome).

2. The bifrontal craniotomy with craniectomy is performed.
3. Bilateral orbital osteotomies (Figure 17-54, *A*) into the anterior cranial fossa are performed. Bilateral conjunctival (lower eyelid) and labiogingival sulcus incisions (for Crouzon's disease and Apert's syndrome) are made for orbital and maxillary osteotomies.
4. The bones of the orbital-craniofacial region are now moved (Figure 17-54, *B*), based on measurement of the intercanthal distance (in hypertelorism) or occlusion of the teeth (in Crouzon's disease and Apert's syndrome).
5. Bone grafts may be taken from the calvaria, ribs, or hips to augment areas of bone deficit, which result from movement of the craniofacial skeleton.
6. Bone grafts are fixed in place with interosseous wires and by means of intermaxillary fixation applied to arch bars (for Crouzon's disease and Apert's syndrome) (Figure 17-54, *C*). Rigid plate-and-screw fixation is another option.
7. The craniotomy, conjunctival, intraoral, and bone-graft donor site incisions are closed and dressings applied.

Pediatric Ophthalmic Surgery

Although the anatomy of the eye remains the same (refer to Chapter 9), children experience different eye conditions from adults that are specifically related to vision development in the brain. Vision develops in the brain until approximately 9 years of age. It is affected by eyes that are not straight or do not focus correctly. Therefore it is imperative that any vision problems are detected and corrected early.

Pediatric ophthalmologists participate in specific programs of study that focus on examination and care of childhood vision problems and structural disorders of the eye. Their scope of practice includes not only examination and treatment, such as vision testing and treatment of eye infections, but also surgical management of disorders such as congenital nasolacrimal duct obstruction, pediatric cataracts, ptosis, strabismus, pediatric glaucoma, and eye injuries (American Association for Pediatric Ophthalmology and Strabismus [AAPOS], 2005). It is not uncommon for pediatric ophthalmology to be subdivided into specialty categories. The field of oculoplastics was first identified in 1966. Oculoplastics encompasses the merging of plastic surgery and ophthalmology in attempt to treat or repair the oculo-orbital region of the

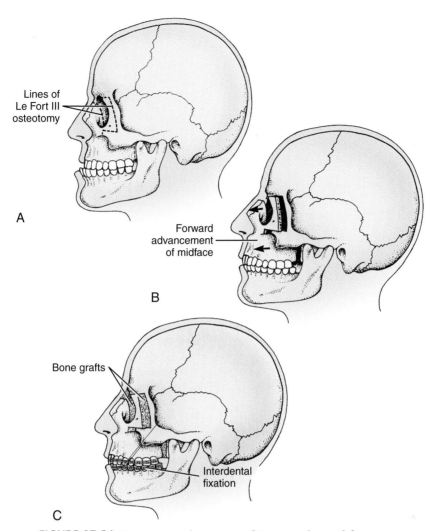

FIGURE 17-54 Steps in surgical correction of Crouzon's disease deformities.

face, be it structural (drainage problems) or cosmetic in nature (Whitaker, 2002). Surgeons may also focus their practice on corneal disorders, retinal disorders, or neuro-ophthalmology.

Eye Muscle Surgery for Strabismus (Figure 17-55). Any misalignment of the eyes is called strabismus. Strabismus is further subdivided into the categories listed in Box 17-3. Strabismus occurs as a result of poorly controlled neuromuscular eye movements. Any child can suffer from strabismus, but disorders that affect the brain (cerebral palsy, hydrocephalus, Down syndrome, brain tumors) are associated with an increased prevalence of the disorder. Additionally, strabismus may occur in conjunction with traumatic brain, nerve, or ocular injury.

The goal for treatment of strabismus is to straighten the eyes so that binocular vision functions appropriately. Nonsurgical treatments may include eyeglasses and eye exercises. Surgery may be recommended to change the alignment of the eyes relative to each other by strengthening, weakening, or repositioning the eye muscles. If a child presents with strabismus in addition to another eye disorder (e.g., ambylopia, cataract, or ptosis), the other condition will be treated before corrective surgery.

Skin incisions are not necessary to repair strabismus. Instead, the surgeon will use a lid speculum to retract the eyelid

and incise the conjunctiva to expose the muscles. Box 17-4 differentiates between the methods of muscle repair. The repaired muscles are sutured using a standard knot or adjustable suture. Adjustable sutures consist of temporary knots (bow or slip) placed in an accessible position so that eye alignment can be altered approximately 24 hours after surgery. The lateral rectus recession and lateral rectus resection procedures are described below.

PROCEDURAL CONSIDERATIONS. The patient receives a general anesthetic, and the full face above the nose is prepped with half-strength Betadine. Both eyes are prepped so that the repair can be measured against the contralateral eye for symmetry.

OPERATIVE PROCEDURE—LATERAL RECTUS RECESSION
1. A lid speculum is placed in the affected eye and the unaffected eye is taped closed.
2. The infratemporal limbus is grasped using Moody locking forceps and the eye is rotated superonasally.
3. A conjunctival fornix incision is made posterior to the limbus in the infratemporal quadrant.
4. Tendons and episclera are dissected until bare sclera is reached, and the lateral rectus is isolated with a Green muscle hook.

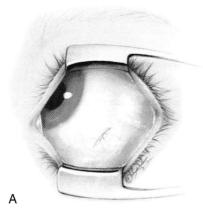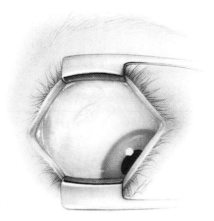

A   B

FIGURE 17-55 Forniceal incisions for strabismus surgery. All six muscles can be isolated from these two incisions. **A,** Inferotemporal incision: isolates the lateral rectus, inferior rectus, and inferior oblique muscles. **B,** Superonasal incision: isolates the medial rectus, superior rectus, and superior oblique muscles.

BOX 17-3

Types of Strabismus

◆ Esotropia: Inward turning of one or both eyes
◆ Exotropia: Outward turning of one or both eyes
◆ Hypertropia: One eye higher than the other
◆ Hypotropia: One eye lower than the other

BOX 17-4

Methods of Muscle Repair

RECESSION
◆ Is a weakening procedure.
◆ Alters the attachment site of the eye muscle on the eyeball.
◆ Muscle is cut from the surface of the eye and reattached at a point further back from the front of the eye.

RESECTION
◆ Is a strengthening procedure.
◆ Extraocular muscle is reattached to the eyeball at its original site.
◆ A section of the muscle is removed and a stitch is placed in the muscle at the intended new attachment site.
◆ The segment of muscle between the stitch and the eyeball is removed.
◆ The shortened muscle is reattached to the eye.

---

5. A suture is passed through the original insertion of the lateral rectus muscle and locked on superior and inferior aspects. The muscle is then cut from its insertion on the globe using Aebli scissors.
6. Calipers are used to mark a location posterior to the insertion point, and suture is passed through the sclera using "crossed swords" technique.
7. The muscle is pulled up firmly to the globe and tied into position. The location is measured again using calipers.
8. Conjunctiva is closed using plain gut suture.

9. The surface of the eye may be covered in neomycin/polymyxin/dexamethasone and tetracaine ointment.

OPERATIVE PROCEDURE—LATERAL RECTUS RESECTION
1. A lid speculum is placed in the affected eye and the unaffected eye is taped closed.
2. The infratemporal limbus is grasped using Moody locking forceps and the eye is rotated superonasally.
3. A conjunctival fornix incision is made posterior to the limbus in the infratemporal quadrant.
4. Tendons and episclera are dissected until bare sclera is reached, and the lateral rectus is isolated with a Green muscle hook.
5. A suture is passed through the original insertion of the lateral rectus muscle and locked on superior and inferior aspects. The central sutures are tied together and a resection clamp is placed anteriorly.
6. The muscle is cut anterior to the resection clamp, and the remaining muscle stump is cut from its original insertion point.
7. The suture needles are passed through the original insertion in a perpendicular fashion and tied together.
8. The muscle is pulled up firmly to the globe and tied into position.
9. Conjunctiva is closed using plain gut suture.
10. The surface of the eye may be covered in neomycin/polymyxin/dexamethasone and tetracaine ointment.

Ptosis (Blepharoptosis) Surgery. Defined as a droopy eyelid, ptosis is either congenital or acquired. Congenital ptosis (Figure 17-56) is usually a result of a deficit in the levator palpebri muscle in the upper eyelid. Acquired ptosis occurs as a result of neurologic conditions that affect the nerves of the eye (myasthenia gravis, Horner's syndrome, third nerve paralysis). It can also manifest in conjunction with movement disorders, resulting in double vision. Ptosis may also result from orbital tumors.

Ptosis is treated with corrective lenses if amblyopia with astigmatism is present. Surgery is indicated for cases in which the droopy eyelid is blocking normal vision or causes the child to position their head with the chin up in attempt to compensate for the block in vision. The goal of surgery is

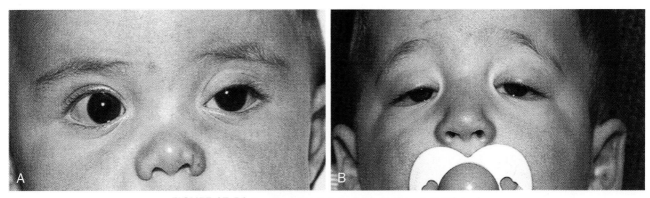

FIGURE 17-56 Simple congenital ptosis. **A,** Unilateral. **B,** Bilateral.

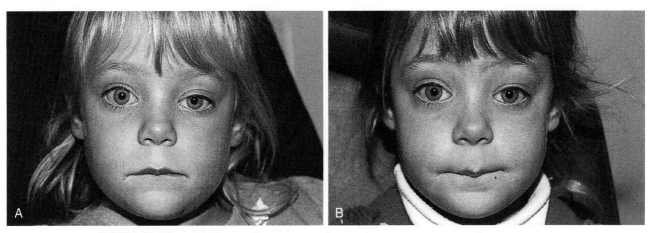

FIGURE 17-57 Modified Fasenella-Servat procedure. **A,** Preoperative. **B,** Six months postoperative.

to create as perfect of an anatomic result as possible by elevating the position of the lid, creating a lid fold, and preserving the contour and symmetry of both lids (Figure 17-57). The Fasenella-Servat procedure is indicated for mild congenital ptosis (less than 2 mm of lid droop) with good levator function. Variations of this procedure are favored over other types of repair, including Werb's procedure (Heher and Katowitz, 2002).

PROCEDURAL CONSIDERATIONS. The patient is positioned supine with the head on a gel ring. The eyes are prepped with half-strength povidone-iodine (1:1 povidone-iodine and normal saline solution). The patient is draped to expose both eyes for comparison during the procedure. Ointment is applied to the contralateral eye, and the eye is taped shut for protective purposes during surgery.

OPERATIVE PROCEDURE

1. A scleral shell is placed into the affected eye to protect the globe.
2. The upper lid is everted and two curved hemostats are placed at the upper tarsal border and adjusted so that the tips are centrally located (Figure 17-58, *A*).
3. Traction sutures are passed through the tissue at the nasal and temporal end, approximately 3 mm below the clamps (Figure 17-58, *B*).
4. The tissue between the two clamps and traction sutures is excised using a #15 blade (Figure 17-58, *C*) or sharp scissors (Figure 17-58, *D*).

5. A nylon suture is passed through the end of the lid crease out through the apex of the incision and run in a "serpentine" fashion. The suture reconnects the conjunctiva and Müller's muscle to the cut edge of the tarsus (Figure 17-58, *E* to *G*).
6. At the opposite end of the incision, the suture is passed through the apex of the incision and out through the crease, and then buried beneath the conjunctival surface (Figure 17-58, *H* and *I*).
7. The traction sutures are removed and the lid is returned to its normal position. A lid plate is used to smooth the incision line by pressing directly on the skin surface to flatten the tissues against the plate (Figure 17-58, *J*).
8. The nylon suture is tied snugly over the skin and remains in place approximately 1 week following surgery to allow for lid adjustment (Figure 17-58, *K*).
9. The scleral shell is removed and antibiotic ointment is applied to the eye and suture line. A dressing may be applied to the surgical site.

Cataract Surgery. Cataracts occur in approximately 3 out of 10,000 children and are primarily classified as nuclear, lamellar, or traumatic in nature (AAPOS, 2005) (Box 17-5). If a cataract causes significant vision loss, it must be removed as soon as possible. An intraocular lens may be used in order to replace the focusing power once the natural lens is surgically removed. Criteria for placement of an intraocular lens specify

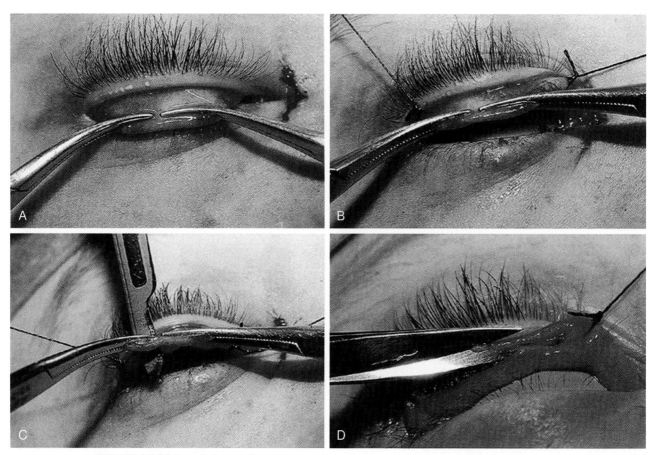

FIGURE 17-58 Modified Fasenella-Servat procedure. **A,** Hemostats at upper tarsal border. **B,** Passage of traction sutures. **C,** Excision of tissue using blade. **D,** Excision of tissue using sharp scissors.

that the child must be 1 year of age or older, as these devices have not been approved by the U.S. Food and Drug Administration for younger populations. In these instances, other options include wearing glasses or contact lenses to correct the deficit.

Corneal Surgery. The cornea is only about 0.5 mm thick, and consists of many layers. The stroma is the thickest part of the cornea. Diseases of the cornea include, but are not limited to, allergies, conjunctivitis (pink eye), corneal infections, dry eye, herpes zoster (shingles), ocular herpes, pterygium, and Stevens-Johnson syndrome. In some cases, corneal surgery or a corneal transplant is necessary, particularly when high pressure from glaucoma allows fluid to accumulate in the stroma. Once this occurs, it may lead to a cloudy cornea.

Trabeculotomy for Glaucoma. The pathophysiology of glaucoma is markedly different for infants and children than in adults, and its occurrence is rare, occurring in approximately 1 in 10,000 births (AAPOS, 2005). Pediatric glaucoma is categorized according to age of onset (Table 17-3). Cases of glaucoma are classified as primary (without specific identifiable cause) or secondary (occurring in conjunction with another disorder, medication use, or eye trauma). Children with glaucoma could have other eye abnormalities in addition to the glaucoma, including opacities of the cornea (Peters' anomaly, for example).

Pediatric glaucoma is treated by a combination of medical and surgical intervention, as the goal of treatment is more

---

BOX 17-5

Types of Cataracts

- Nuclear: Cloudiness in the center part of the lens
- Lamellar: Cloudiness between the nuclear and cortical layers of the lens
- Traumatic: Results from blunt or penetrating force that damages the lens

---

than simply lowering intraocular pressure. Children diagnosed with congenital or infantile glaucoma often develop myopia and require glasses. There is also an increased occurrence of strabismus and amblyopia in children with glaucoma. Extreme cases may result in vision loss, supporting the need for early diagnosis and management of the disorder.

Pediatric glaucoma is commonly evaluated by examining the child under anesthesia (EUA). At this time, the ophthalmologist will measure intraocular pressure, corneal length, axial diameter, and refractive error and assess corneal clarity and the optic nerve. If the intraocular pressure is elevated, it can be treated medically or surgically. The majority of primary pediatric glaucoma cases are treated surgically.

The most common surgical approaches are trabeculotomy with goniometry. These procedures open the drainage canal

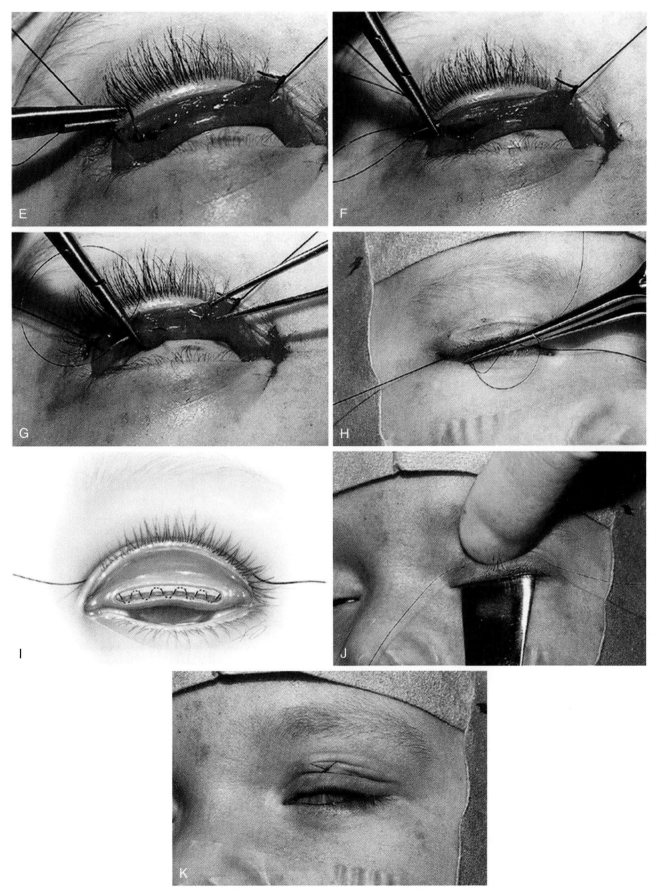

FIGURE 17-58, cont'd E-G, Reconnection of conjunctiva and Müller's muscle to edge of tarsus. **H** and **I,** Suture passed through apex of incision and out through crease. **J,** Smoothing incision line with lid plate. **K,** Nylon suture allows for lid adjustment.

TABLE 17-3

Categories of Glaucoma

Category	Age at Presentation	Symptoms at Presentation
Congenital	Glaucoma present at birth	Excessive tearing Light sensitivity Large, cloudy cornea Dull-appearing iris
Infantile	Glaucoma presents between 1 and 24 months of age	Excessive tearing Light sensitivity Large, cloudy cornea Dull-appearing iris
Juvenile	Glaucoma presents after 36 months of age	No obvious symptoms; presents similar to adult-onset glaucoma

and facilitate aqueous drainage. Other options, such as trabeculotomy with tube placement, create a bypass route to shunt aqueous drainage. Laser procedures are also effective in some cases of glaucoma. Successful management of the disease typically requires multiple examinations and procedures.

Retinal Disorders. Retinal diseases include retinopathy of prematurity (ROP). ROP is one of the most common causes of visual loss in childhood and can lead to lifelong vision impairment and blindness. The most effective proven treatments for ROP are laser therapy or cryotherapy. Both laser treatments and cryotherapy are performed only on infants with advanced ROP. Severe cases (stage V) of this disorder are treated with scleral buckle and posterior vitrectomy (see Chapter 9).

TRAUMA

When caring for the pediatric trauma patient in surgery, the perioperative team must possess additional knowledge in order to develop a detailed plan of action that effectively drives the delivery of safe patient care. The urgency of injury will dictate the timeliness of surgical intervention—in some instances, pediatric trauma patients may require transfer to a level I trauma center. The criteria for transfer are outlined in Box 17-6. The OR team should be prepared to administer care to any type of injury in a safe and effective manner that is appropriate across all age levels.

Trauma is the leading cause of death in children from 1 to 14 years of age. Each year, another 100,000 children experience disability from trauma. Several factors, such as age, gender, behavior, and environment, influence the risk of traumatic injury. For instance, infants and toddlers are more prone to falls resulting in severe injury, which may be related to the pliable nature of their skeletal system. If broken bones are present, a severe force of injury must be assumed. Older children and adolescents are at higher risk for bicycle-related and motor vehicle–related injuries. In this age group, blunt injuries resulting from motor vehicle accidents or direct blows (as with contact sports or child abuse) along with falls are the most common mechanisms of injury (Cooper, 2005). It is not uncommon for pediatric traumatic injuries to occur in the home environment, stressing the importance of community awareness and education as it relates to trauma prevention.

BOX 17-6

Trauma Transfer Criteria for Pediatric Patients Less Than or Equal to Age 14

CONSIDER TRANSFER TO PEDIATRIC TRAUMA CENTER
- Nonoperative management of solid organ injury
- Assessment of any of the following "negative points" on the pediatric trauma scale:
  - Weight less than 10 kg
  - Unstable airway
  - Blood pressure less than 50 mm Hg (systolic)
  - Coma
  - Major open, penetrating wound
  - Open, multiple fractures
- Injury severity score greater than 9
- Victim or nonaccidental injury that requires intervention from child protective team or other resources
- Anticipated complexity of care exceeds the capabilities of local resources at adult trauma center

TRANSFER TO PEDIATRIC TRAUMA CENTER
- Persistent physiologic demise
- Traumatic brain injury
- Intubation and mechanical ventilation with no expectation to wean within 24 hours
- Children with special needs or other co-morbid conditions

Modified from Pennsylvania Trauma Systems Foundation: *Adult trauma center accreditation, Appendix C: Transfer guidelines: adult trauma centers (level I, II, and III) to pediatric trauma centers,* 2009.

Some of the most significant prevention strategies focus on car seat safety as a means of preventing injury from motor vehicle accidents (Patient Safety).

Throughout the pediatric population, neurologic injuries are the most common cause of traumatic death in children; their head is proportionately larger in relation to their body mass and especially vulnerable to injury. Table 17-4 gives a guideline for using the Glasgow Coma Scale for infants and children. Because children have a much smaller reserve than adults, once a decline in vital functions is noted, demise is rapid. Information about commonly used medications in pediatric resuscitation is noted in the Surgical Pharmacology box.

IV access is often difficult in the pediatric patient, and an intraosseous line may be inserted by emergency rescue personnel before arrival at the hospital or in the emergency department (ED). These lines are inserted by use of an intraosseous needle or bone marrow aspiration needle and are placed slightly below the knee on the anterior aspect of the tibia at a 90-degree angle (Figure 17-59). Stabilization of the line may be difficult, but the line can remain for up to 24 hours and provides rapid access when other routes are too time-consuming or difficult to access. Fluid resuscitation levels for children experiencing hemorrhage, as well as types and dosages of medications, are based on body weight, since weight provides a better mechanism of accuracy when calculating dosage.

Because of the nature of the trauma, exact body weight may be unable to be obtained. In these instances, body weight can be estimated using Broselow tapes or palmar methods. The body size of the patient determines the type of instrumentation required. Pediatric trauma instrument sets, including vascular clamps and retractors, and suture supplies should be available and organized in a fashion that promotes easy and timely

PATIENT SAFETY

Child Passenger Safety

The number one killer of children ages 3 to 14 is motor vehicle crashes. Parents and caregivers should be encouraged to follow these steps to reduce the risk of injury or death for children who ride in motor vehicles:

INFANTS
◆ Ride in rear-facing car seats until 1 year old and 20 pounds.
◆ Check the weight requirements of the car seat against the infant's height and weight—keep track of these measurements with each visit to the pediatrician.
◆ Harnesses should be even with or below the infant's shoulders and worn tightly. You should not be able to pinch extra webbing at the shoulder.
◆ Adjust the chest clip to armpit level.
◆ Recline the seat no more than 45 degrees.

TODDLERS
◆ Use a forward-facing seat until the harness no longer fits the child. Most children will outgrow the seat between ages 4 and 5.
◆ Check the weight requirements of the car seat against the child's height and weight—keep track of these measurements with each visit to the pediatrician.
◆ Harnesses should be even with or below the child's shoulders and worn tightly. You should not be able to pinch extra webbing at the shoulder.
◆ Adjust the chest clip to armpit level.
◆ If possible, use a top tether. Tethers limit the forward motion of the head in a crash.

BOOSTERS
◆ Booster seats are used in conjunction with the vehicle lap and shoulder belts for children who do not meet the size requirements for standard seat belts. Normal seat belts begin to fit children between the ages of 8 and 12.
◆ Boosters should be used in the back seat only.
◆ The weight range for booster seats is between 40 and 100 pounds.
◆ Use the lap and shoulder belts every time a child is in a booster seat. Never use only the lap belt, and make sure that the seat belt is properly buckled.

SAFETY BELTS
◆ Safety belts fit properly when the knees bend over the edge of the seat, the lap belt rests on the upper legs or hips, and the shoulder belt rests on the shoulder or collarbone.
◆ Never put the shoulder belt under a child's arm or behind a child's back.
◆ Ensure that children sit upright when wearing seat belts. Avoid leaning against windows, slouching, or lying down.

Modified from Safe Kids USA: *Child passenger safety,* 2006, available at www.usa.safekids.org/skbu/cps/index.html. Accessed February 21, 2009.

access when urgent situations arise. Creative problem solving may be required of the surgical team in adaptation of feeding tubes, drains, and other equipment.

Maintenance of body temperature is of utmost concern in the pediatric population, and undue skin exposure should be avoided. Fluids for irrigation and IV infusion may be warmed, depending on the preferences of the surgeon and the status of the child. Whenever possible, room temperature is elevated. Warming blankets and head coverings (stockinettes) may be

TABLE 17-4
Pediatric Modification of Glasgow Coma Scale

Glasgow Coma Scale	Pediatric Modification
EYE OPENING	
Birth to 1 year	12 months or older
4 Spontaneously	4 Spontaneously
3 To shout	3 To verbal command
2 To pain	2 To pain
1 No response	1 No response
BEST MOTOR RESPONSE	
Birth to 1 year	12 months or older
5 Localizes pain	6 Obeys command
4 Flexion, withdrawal	5 Localizes pain
3 Flexion, abnormal	4 Flexion, withdrawal
2 Extension, rigidity	3 Flexion, abnormal
1 No response	2 Extension, rigidity
	1 No response

BEST VERBAL RESPONSE

Birth to 2 years	2-5 years	Older than 5 years
5 Cries appropriately, coos	5 Appropriate words, phrases	5 Oriented and converses
4 Cries	4 Inappropriate words	4 Disoriented, converses
3 Inappropriate crying	3 Cries, screams	3 Inappropriate words
2 Grunts	2 Grunts	2 Incomprehensible sounds
1 No response	1 No response	1 No response

Modified from Emergency Nurses Association (ENA): *Trauma nursing core course,* ed 6, Des Plaines, Ill, 2007.

used to prevent heat loss; this is especially critical with children who have sustained burns.

Traumas are graded based on the severity of injury (Table 17-5). The surgical team should attempt to obtain a trauma history from ED personnel or the family if the patient comes directly to the OR. Initial vital signs should be obtained and compared with those obtained during prehospital care or in the ED; Table 17-6 presents normal vital sign ranges for infants and children. Box 17-7 gives a formula for blood pressure estimation. During traumatic events, it is imperative to consider the well-being of patients, families, and caregivers. The surgical team plays an integral role in preparing those associated with the child for outcomes associated with trauma surgery and may help facilitate consults from the departments of child life, social work, and clergy.

Airway and breathing are part of the primary survey for pediatric trauma victims. Anatomic variations of the upper airway related to age must be considered. Airway patency must be assessed and secured. Initial assessment for all pediatric trauma patients may best be obtained by application of the head tilt–chin lift or jaw-thrust method, depending on the age of the child and the nature of the injury. When the integrity of the spinal cord is questionable, in-line cervical traction should be applied. Collars and stabilizing devices must remain in place until cervical fracture has been ruled out and the spine "cleared," or declared free of injury by a radiologist.

SURGICAL PHARMACOLOGY

Medications Used in Pediatric Resuscitation

The surgical team must always be prepared in the event of a cardiac event in the pediatric patient. The information contained in this list provides several commonly used medications, usual dosage, and mode of action.

Drug	Dosage	Action
Epinephrine HCI	Intravenous/intraosseous (IV/IO): 0.01 mg/kg (1:10,000) Endotracheal (ET): 0.1 mg/kg (1:1000) Repeat doses = 0.1 ml/kg (1:1000)	Adrenergic; acts on both alpha- and beta-receptor sites, especially heart and vascular and other smooth muscle
Sodium bicarbonate	IV/IO: 1-2 mEq/kg	Alkalinizer, buffers pH
Atropine sulfate	20 mcg/kg dose Minimum dose: 100 mcg Maximum single dose: infants and children, 0.5 mg; adolescents, 1.0 mg	Anticholinergic-parasympatholytic; increases cardiac output, heart rate by blocking vagal stimulation in heart
Calcium chloride	20 mg/kg IV 10.2 mg/kg May repeat dose every 10 min	Electrolyte replacement; needed for maintenance of normal cardiac activity
Lidocaine HCI	0.5-1 mg/kg dose	Antidysrhythmic, inhibits nerve impulses from sensory nerves
Amiodarone	IV: 5 mg/kg over 30 min followed by continuous infusion starting at 5 mcg/kg/min; may increase to maximum 10 mcg/kg/min	Antidysrhythmic agent, inhibits adrenergic stimulation; prolongs action potential and refractory period in myocardial tissues; decreases atrioventricular (AV) conduction and sinus node function
Adenosine	First dose: 100 mcg/kg (maximum dose 6 mg) Second dose: 200 mcg/kg (maximum dose 12 mg) Follow with 2- to 3-ml normal saline flush	Antidysrhythmic, for supraventricular tachycardia (SVT) Causes temporary block through AV node and interrupts reentry circuits
Naloxone (Narcan)	0.01-0.1 mg/kg/dose (<5 years/20 kg) (>5 years/20 kg = 2 mg)	Reverses respiratory arrest caused by excessive opiate administration
Magnesium sulfate	IV/IO: 25-50 mg/kg	Inhibits calcium channels and causes smooth muscle relaxation
IV INFUSIONS		
Epinephrine HCI infusion	0.1-1 mcg/kg/min	Adrenergic—see above
Dopamine HCI infusion	1-20 mcg/kg/min (maximum dose 50 mcg/min)	Agonist; acts on alpha receptors, causing vasoconstriction Increases cardiac output
Dobutamine HCI infusion	2.5-15 mcg/kg/min	Adrenergic direct-acting beta$_1$-agonist Increases contractility and heart rate
Lidocaine HCI infusion	20-50 mcg/kg/min	Antidysrhythmic Increases electrical stimulation threshold of heart

Modified from Lexi-Comp ONLINE, available at www.crlonline.com/crlsql/servlet/crlonline. Accessed May 21, 2009.

Airway equipment sizes may be selected based on age as well as whether the child is breathing spontaneously and whether the child is unconscious. An assessment of relevant systems will be performed on stabilization of the pediatric airway, and surgery will progress as planned.

SURGERY FOR CONGENITAL HEART DISEASE

Congenital heart disease (CHD) occurs in approximately 5 to 8 of every 1000 live births. Structural abnormalities of the heart and great vessels result in an embryologic failure in septation, malalignment, failure to develop, and/or failure to progress.

The etiology of CHD varies, although certain factors are associated with increased prevalence. For example, risk of CHD is increased secondary to environmental factors: rubella during the first 8 weeks of gestation may result in patent ductus arteriosus and pulmonary artery stenosis (along with other syndromes). Other risk factors include maternal chronic illnesses such as diabetes or poorly controlled phenylketonuria (PKU), alcohol consumption, and exposure to environmental toxins. The incidence of CHD is increased also in certain chromosomal

TABLE 17-5

Trauma Grading

	Physiologic Considerations	Anatomic Considerations
Level I: Life-threatening injuries, unstable vital signs	Respiratory distress Intubated before transport Unstable airway Cardiac arrest Glasgow Coma Score (GCS) ≤8 Unstable vital signs Lateralizing neurologic signs or worsening neurologic exam Any signs of shock Severe uncontrolled hemorrhage Systolic blood pressure <80 mm Hg that does not respond to fluid resuscitation	Airway compromise Major vascular injury Crush injury Above-elbow or above-knee amputation with high probability of surgical intervention Penetrating injury to abdomen, chest, head, neck, or groin Burns >25% total body surface area Spinal cord injury with neurologic signs or symptoms and unstable vertebral fractures
Level II: Potentially life-threatening injuries, vital signs stable at present	GCS ≥9 and ≤13 Hypotension before transport, resolved during transport	Blunt abdominal trauma with abnormal exam Blunt chest trauma with ≥2 rib fractures Significant penetrating trauma to upper extremities or distal to groin Significant crush or amputation distal to elbow or knee with high probability of operative intervention

Modified from Children's Hospital of Philadelphia: *2008-2009 Trauma program resident/fellow manual.*

defects; for example, atrial septal defects are seen in children with trisomy 21 (Down syndrome). In addition, an increased prevalence is seen in small-for-gestational-age (SGA) babies and in children who have a positive family history of CHD (that is, those families with a sibling or parent who has CHD).

Congenital cardiac abnormalities are classified as cyanotic or acyanotic as well as by their effect on pulmonary blood flow (Box 17-8). Of the acyanotic lesions, there are those that increase pulmonary blood flow, such as patent ductus arteriosus (PDA), atrial septal defect (ASD), ventricular septal defect (VSD), and atrioventricular canal defects (AVCs). With these abnormalities, blood flows from the high-pressure left side of the heart to the low-pressure right side of the heart because of an abnormal connection either between the septum or in the great arteries. The resultant increase in pulmonary blood flow causes the right side of the heart and lungs to become overloaded. Congestive heart failure (CHF) may develop, pulmonary vascular resistance may increase, and the pulmonary vessel walls may thicken; and if left untreated, the condition may become irreversible.

Acyanotic obstructive lesions, such as aortic stenosis, pulmonary stenosis, or coarctation of the aorta, increase the workload of the chamber that pumps against the obstruction (increases afterload). Cardiomegaly and ventricular hypertrophy may be seen in response to the increased workload, and if the obstruction is severe, heart failure may ensue.

The presence of cyanosis implies that one of the following conditions is present: right-sided heart obstruction with blood traveling right to left without passing through the lungs; mixing of venous and arterial blood within the heart or great vessels; or incorrect positioning of the great vessels. The degree of cyanosis depends on pulmonary blood flow and intracardiac mixing of blood through a shunt. This classification of lesions includes, but is not limited to, tetralogy of Fallot (TOF), pulmonary atresia with intact ventricular septum (PA/IVS), tricus-

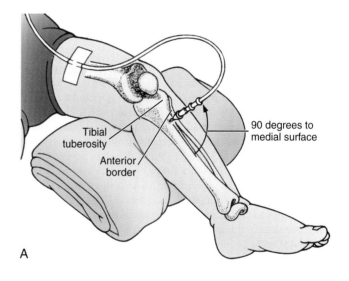

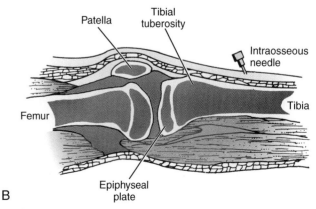

FIGURE 17-59 **A,** Intraosseous infusion technique. **B,** Insertion.

TABLE 17-6

Pediatric Vital Signs

Age	Heart Rate (beats/min)	Respirations (breaths/min)	Systolic Blood Pressure (mm Hg)
Newborn	100-150	30-55	50-70
Infants to 2 years	80-120	25-40	70-88
2-6 years	70-110	20-30	88-94
6-10 years	60-95	16-22	94-102
10-16 years	60-85	12-20	80-111

From Ball JW, Bindler RC: *2008 Pediatric nursing: caring for children,* Upper Saddle River, NJ, 2008, Pearson Prentice-Hall.

BOX 17-7

Estimating Blood Pressure for the Pediatric Patient

Systolic BP (mm Hg) = (2 × age in years) + 80
Diastolic BP (mm Hg) = ⅔ Systolic BP

pid atresia (TA), transposition of the great arteries (TGA), total anomalous pulmonary venous return (TAPVR), and hypoplastic left heart syndrome (HLHS). Treatment goals for these lesions include managing pulmonary blood flow and/or arterial oxygen saturation.

Repair of Atrial Septal Defect

Congenital defects in the atrial septum occur in approximately 10% of CHD cases (Melek, 2006). The classification within this group of defects is based on anatomic location and associated abnormalities (Figure 17-60). The ostium secundum defect is located in the superior and central portions of the septum. The ostium primum defect is located in the lower portion of the atrial septum and is associated with other defects in the atrioventricular canal, usually with a cleft of the mitral valve or occasionally of the tricuspid valve. An accompanying VSD may also be present. The sinus venosus defect is located at the right atrium–superior vena cava junction and is associated with partial anomalous pulmonary venous return.

An ASD results in a left-to-right atrial shunt whose direction and magnitude are determined by the size of the defect and relative resistance to flow into the ventricles and great vessels (Figure 17-61). ASDs are often tolerated well with no symptoms during childhood, especially if the defect is small. However, if the defect is large or of the ostium primum type, with a pronounced shunting of blood, the workload of the right side of the heart is increased. On assessment, there is a characteristic systolic pulmonary murmur at the second intercostal space at the left sternal border, and a fixed splitting of the second heart sound may also be heard. The right side of the heart and the pulmonary artery and its branches become enlarged. The vascularity of the lung field is increased, with resulting pulmonary hypertension and subsequent failure of the right side of the heart. At this point the shunt may reverse. The initial symptoms may include fatigue, retardation of normal weight gain, and increased susceptibility to respiratory tract infections. Later signs and symptoms include those of failure of the right side of the heart and cyanosis with a reverse

BOX 17-8

Classification of Congenital Cardiac Defects

ACYANOTIC WITH INCREASED PULMONARY BLOOD FLOW
◆ Patent ductus arteriosus
◆ Atrial septal defect
◆ Ventricular septal defect
◆ Atrioventricular septal defect

ACYANOTIC OBSTRUCTIVE LESIONS
◆ Coarctation of the aorta
◆ Aortic stenosis
◆ Pulmonary stenosis

CYANOTIC WITH DECREASED PULMONARY BLOOD FLOW
◆ Tricuspid atresia
◆ Tetralogy of Fallot
◆ Pulmonary atresia with intact ventricular septum

CYANOTIC WITH INCREASED PULMONARY BLOOD FLOW
◆ Total anomalous pulmonary venous connection (return)
◆ Truncus arteriosus
◆ Hypoplastic left heart syndrome

CYANOTIC WITH VARIABLE PULMONARY BLOOD FLOW
◆ Transposition of the great arteries
◆ Double-outlet right ventricle
◆ Double-outlet left ventricle
◆ Single ventricle

shunt. Asymptomatic children whose ASD is left unrepaired until adulthood may develop right atrial and right ventricular hypertrophy, atrial dysrhythmias, CHF, embolic events, and pulmonary vascular disease. The defect is common in children with Down syndrome.

Procedural Considerations. ASDs are closed, under direct vision, by a simple suture technique (primary closure) or by insertion of a synthetic prosthetic patch or pericardial patch.

The child is placed in the supine position for a median sternotomy or in a right anterior oblique position for an anterolateral thoracotomy. The instrument setup is the same as that described for basic open-heart surgery (see Chapter 16), with consideration given to the age and size of the child; intracardiac patch material, 2 × 2 inches or larger, may also be required.

Operative Procedure (Figure 17-62)
1. A median sternotomy incision is performed, and cardiopulmonary bypass (CPB) is instituted. (Infrequently, a right anterolateral incision is performed.) Many bypass strategies can be employed. With bicaval cannulation, the child remains on bypass during the repair and blood is directed away from the right atrium through cannulae in the superior and inferior venae cavae. Occasionally, with this method the cannulae may obstruct the view of the ASD. With single venous cannulation, a cannula is placed into the right atrium and the child remains on bypass during the repair. With this technique, the venous line is clamped immediately before the right atrium is incised and pump suctions are placed into the inferior and superior venae cavae during ASD closure. Deep hypothermic circulatory arrest is sometimes used in more complicated repairs, such as ostium primum ASD or

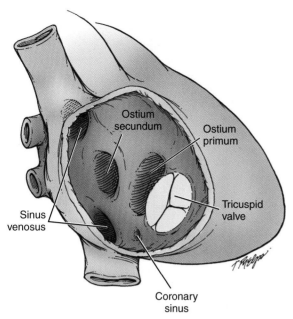

FIGURE 17-60 Various types of atrial septal defects (ASDs) viewed through the right atrium (ostium secundum, ostium primum, sinus venosus). An unroofed coronary sinus may also act as an ASD.

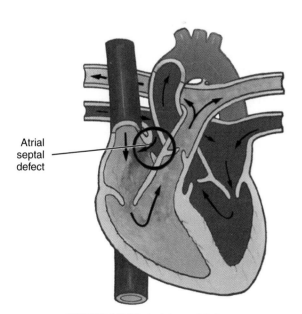

FIGURE 17-61 Atrial septal defect.

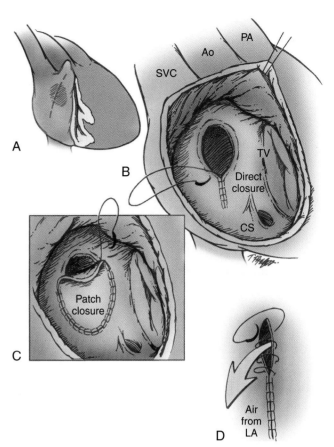

FIGURE 17-62 Surgical procedure for atrial septal defect (ASD) closure. **A,** Incision through right atriotomy. Direct suture closure, **B,** and patch closure, **C,** of secundum ASD. **D,** Deairing of the left atrium. *Ao,* Aorta; *CS,* conduction system; *LA,* left atrium; *PA,* pulmonary artery; *SVC,* superior vena cava; *TV,* tricuspid valve.

Repair of Ventricular Septal Defect

One of the most common congenital cardiac anomalies, VSDs (Figure 17-63) occur in approximately 2% to 7% of live births, with as many as 60% closing spontaneously (Ramaswamy et al, 2009). Most VSDs are small with little physiologic importance. As with ASDs, the classification of VSDs depends on location and associated lesions (Figure 17-64). Perimembranous VSDs (also called *conoventricular, subaortic, infracristal,* or *membranous*) are most commonly found. These defects occur directly adjacent to the membranous septum and the fibrous trigone of the heart where the aortic, mitral, and tricuspid valves are in fibrous continuity. The tricuspid valve tissue sometimes forms an aneurysm of the membranous septum, which may be a mechanism of defect closure for this type of defect. Subpulmonary VSDs (also referred to as *supracristal, infundibular, intracristal, outlet, conoseptal,* or *conal*) are located above the crista supraventricularis within the outlet septum and border the semilunar valves. Muscular-type VSDs can be located anywhere in the muscular septum, including apical, anterior, or posterior, or in the midseptum inlet and outlet. Malalignment-type VSDs are created by a malalignment between the infundibular septum and the trabecular muscular septum. Canal-type or inlet defects are located posteriorly within the area confined by the tricuspid valve septal leaflet papillary muscles. The defect borders the tricuspid valve annulus.

sinus venosus defects associated with anomalous pulmonary venous return.

2. The right atrium is incised, and the pathologic defect is determined.

3. The defect is closed with a continuous suture, or a patch of pericardium or prosthetic material may be used. By filling the atrium with blood before the atriotomy is completely closed, the surgeon can express air from the atrium. For the ostium primum defect with a cleft mitral valve, repair of the cleft is accomplished by approximation, with use of interrupted (possibly pledgetted) sutures.

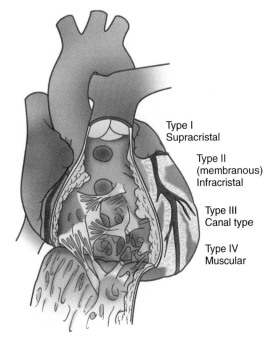

FIGURE 17-63 Ventricular septal defects: anatomic classification.

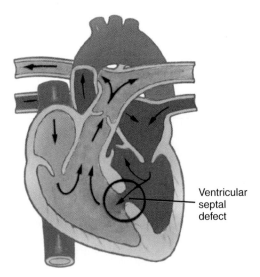

FIGURE 17-65 Ventricular septal defect.

The hemodynamics depend on the size and location of the defect as well as the pulmonary vascular resistance (PVR) and systemic vascular resistance (SVR). Newborns are often asymptomatic until the PVR decreases—then a left-to-right shunt occurs, and the corresponding murmur is auscultated. Small defects with moderate shunt and increased pulmonary blood flow but not increased pulmonary pressure may not produce any symptoms. A large VSD, however, may produce high pulmonary flow under high pressure and contribute to CHF. In this case the patient is at risk of developing pulmonary hypertension (Figure 17-65). Surgical closure of the defect should be performed to prevent increased pulmonary hypertension. If PVR further increases and rises above SVR, shunt reversal (Eisenmenger's syndrome, or shunting from right to left) and cyanosis may occur.

Operative Procedure. Under direct vision, a congenital defect in the ventricular septum (Figure 17-66) is closed by a simple suture technique or, in most instances, by insertion of a synthetic prosthetic or pericardial patch.

1. A median sternotomy is performed, and CPB is instituted.
2. The location of the defect determines the location of the incision. For membranous and canal defects, an incision is usually made in the right atrium, the atrium is retracted, and the VSD is identified by use of a pump suction through the tricuspid valve into the right ventricle. For supracristal VSDs, an incision is usually made in the pulmonary artery and may be extended into the right ventricle. A muscular VSD may require a ventriculotomy.
3. A patch is most frequently used to close the defect. To place the patch, a continuous 6-0 or 5-0 nonabsorbable suture on a small needle or an interrupted suture with or without pledgets may be used. Rarely is the defect closed primarily.
4. CPB is discontinued, and the sternum is closed.

Correction of Tetralogy of Fallot

TOF, described initially in the early nineteenth century, includes the association of four anatomic findings: VSD, subpulmonic stenosis, aortic override of the ventricular septum, and right

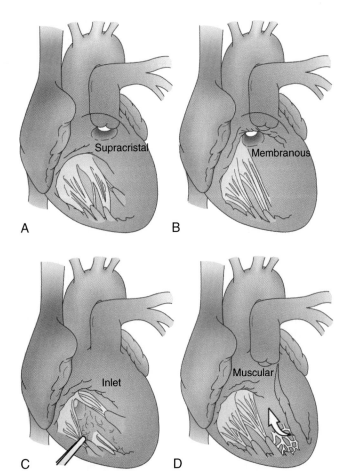

FIGURE 17-64 Various types of ventricular septal defects viewed within the right ventricle. **A,** Infundibular (supracristal). **B,** Membranous. **C,** Inlet (AV canal). **D,** Muscular (trabecular).

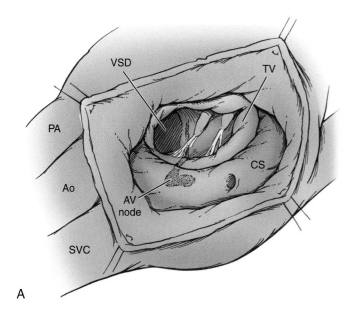

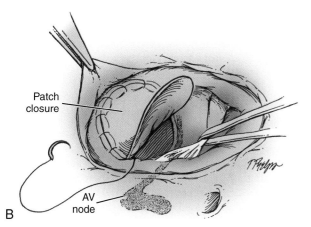

FIGURE 17-66 Ventricular septal defect *(VSD)* closure through the tricuspid valve *(TV)*. **A,** Open site. **B,** Partial closure. *Ao,* Aorta; *AV,* atrioventricular; *CS,* conduction system; *PA,* pulmonary artery; *SVC,* superior vena cava.

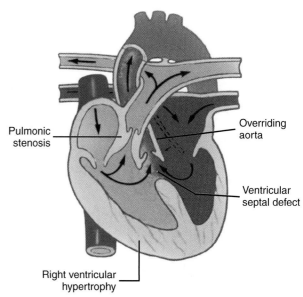

FIGURE 17-67 Tetralogy of Fallot.

ventricular hypertrophy (RVH) (Figure 17-67). Occurring in approximately 10% of congenital heart defects, TOF is actually the result of a single anatomic abnormality: anterior malalignment of the infundibular septum with the muscular septum (Davis, 2007).

The preoperative hemodynamics or physiology depends mainly on the degree of pulmonary stenosis. In patients with minimal obstruction to pulmonary blood flow, the physiology is similar to that of a VSD with left-to-right shunting. These patients will have pulmonary overcirculation and symptoms of CHF. Occasionally labeled as "pink tets," these patients have little to no right-to-left shunting and do not exhibit cyanosis.

At the other end of the spectrum of this particular type of heart defect are children with severe pulmonary stenosis, who may have significant right-to-left shunting at the VSD level and exhibit hypoxemia with oxygen saturations in the 60% to 80% range. Cyanosis, as seen in the superficial vessels of the skin, is the result of shunting unoxygenated blood into the systemic circulation. Other clinical manifestations may include episodes of acute dyspnea with cyanosis, retarded growth, clubbing of

extremities, reduced exercise tolerance, and increased prevalence of "tet," or hypercyanotic spells. A systolic murmur and secondary polycythemia are usually present in the cyanotic child. Echocardiography is performed to confirm the diagnosis of TOF; occasionally a cardiac catheterization and angiography may be necessary in delineating other anatomic abnormalities, such as with the coronary arteries, before surgical repair.

The selection of a palliative or corrective procedure is based on the age and general condition of the child and the severity of the pulmonary stenosis. The treatment of choice is primary repair; contraindications for primary repair include anomalous origin of the anterior descending coronary artery and presence of pulmonary atresia. Complete or primary repair consists of closure of the VSD and repair of the pulmonic stenosis under direct vision.

Procedural Considerations. The child is placed on the OR bed in a supine position. The setup is the same as that described for open-heart surgery, with consideration given to the child's age and size. Additional items to be added to the basic open-heart setup include the following: intracardiac patch, 2 × 2 inch; outflow cardiac patch, 2 × 2 inch; and a felt or Gore-Tex patch, 4 × 4 inch.

Operative Procedure
1. A median sternotomy is performed, and CPB with hypothermia is instituted.
2. A vertical ventriculotomy over the infundibular area may be performed (Figure 17-68, *A*).
3. The VSD is identified. Closure requires an intracardiac patch in almost all instances. This can be of a synthetic material or a piece of pericardium.
4. Interrupted or continuous cardiovascular sutures are placed in the septum with caution because of the danger of suturing a branch of the neuroconductive system.
5. The hypertrophied infundibular muscle is excised, as completely as possible, from the right ventricular outflow tract. If the pulmonic valve is stenosed, the fused commissures are incised.

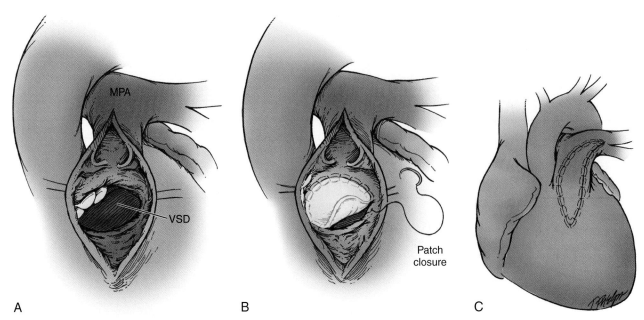

A   B   C

FIGURE 17-68 **A,** The most common ventricular incision used for repair of tetralogy of Fallot is vertical so that it can be extended as shown from the right ventricle across the pulmonary valve annulus and onto the main pulmonary artery *(MPA)*. It is possible to gain adequate exposure to the ventricular septal defect *(VSD)* by extending the incision a short distance beyond the infundibular septum. This "limited ventriculotomy" may help preserve late right ventricular function yet enable adequate enlargement of the hypoplastic area in the right ventricular outflow tract. **B,** The VSD is closed with a prosthetic patch. Right ventricular outflow obstruction is relieved when the outflow tract is enlarged with a patch as shown. **C,** In some cases it may be necessary to extend the incision onto the left pulmonary artery and to taper the patch at its most distal extent.

6. An estimate is made about whether the right ventricle can be closed primarily or if a patch is necessary. If the pulmonic stenosis cannot be relieved adequately by valvulotomy and infundibulectomy, an outflow patch of synthetic material or pulmonary homograft tissue may be needed to enlarge the outflow tract (Figure 17-68, *B*). If the pulmonary artery or valve annulus is quite small, it may be necessary to extend the patch across the valve ring to the proximal portion of the pulmonary artery (Figure 17-68, *C*).

7. CPB is discontinued, and the sternum is closed.

Closure of Patent Ductus Arteriosus

PDA occurs because of persistence of the fetal ductus arteriosus, which connects the pulmonary artery to the aorta. The condition is common in premature infants. In fetal life, blood bypasses the lungs, traveling directly to the systemic circulation through the PDA. This vessel normally closes shortly after birth as a result of the onset of respiration causing an increase in PaO_2 level and the release of circulating humoral substances. However, if this does not occur, the ductus arteriosus remains open (Figure 17-69), creating a shunt from the aorta through the ductus into the pulmonary circulation. This increases the workload of the heart and causes subsequent enlargement and hypertrophy of the left atrium and ventricle. However, when persistent patency of the ductus is associated with other malformations such as TOF and extreme stenosis of the pulmonary orifice, it is a means of maintaining life. Surgery is not performed if the PDA is serving in a compensatory capacity.

Many children have few symptoms because of the small size of the shunt. A frequent clinical sign associated with this condition is a harsh, continuous murmur. Because the blood passing through the shunt is oxygenated, there is no cyanosis, clubbing, or reduction in peripheral arterial oxygen saturation. However, growth is retarded in children who have a large ductus. Other signs and symptoms may include dyspnea, frequent upper respiratory tract infections, palpitations, limited exercise tolerance, and cardiac failure.

Procedural Considerations. Closure of the PDA is achieved by suture ligation or by division of the ductus. For newborns, the surgeon and anesthesia provider may elect to perform this procedure in the intensive care nursery bed because the operation is a short one. However, after the newborn period, the surgery is done in the OR. The child is placed in a right lateral position. The setup is the same as that described for open-heart surgery, but with special patent ductus clamps and without items for CPB. Generally a left posterolateral approach is used; in some cases, however, a left anterolateral approach is used.

Operative Procedure

1. The incision is carried through the muscles over the fourth interspace. The chest wall is entered through the third or fourth intercostal space, with use of items as described for thoracotomy (see Chapter 14). The wound edges are protected and retracted with a Finochietto rib spreader.

2. The pleura is incised with Metzenbaum scissors, and the left lung is protected and retracted with a moist pack and a malleable retractor.

3. The mediastinal pleura is opened between the phrenic and vagus nerves over the region of the ductus. The pleura is

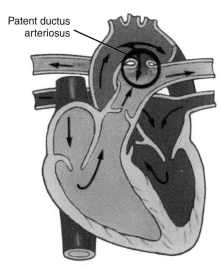

FIGURE 17-69 Patent ductus arteriosus.

retracted by insertion of stay sutures. The recurrent laryngeal nerve is identified and protected. The aortic arch and pulmonary artery are dissected with fine scissors and dry dissectors. Fine arterial branches are divided and ligated with curved Crile or mosquito hemostats and nonabsorbable ligatures and cardiac suture ligatures.

4. The parietal pleura overlying the ductus is dissected with fine vascular forceps and scissors. Stay sutures may be inserted to facilitate retraction.
5. The adventitial layer of the ductus is dissected free. A small portion of the obscure posterior ductus is carefully freed to admit a right-angle clamp.
6. The final step is performed in one of the following ways:
   a. For the suture-ligation method (Figure 17-70, *A*), two ligatures are placed around the ductus—one near the aorta and the other near the pulmonary artery side, both of which are tied in place. Between these two ligatures, two transfixion sutures may be inserted.
   b. For the division of the ductus method, the patent ductus clamps are applied as close to the aorta and pulmonary artery as possible. The ductus is divided halfway through and partially sutured with mattress cardiovascular sutures and continued back over the free edge with an over-and-over whip suture (Figure 17-70, *B*). After both openings are sutured, a sponge is held on the area for compression while the patent ductus clamps are removed.
   c. In premature infants, only a hemoclip may be applied to the ductus because of the friable nature of the ductal tissue. The mediastinal pleura is closed with interrupted sutures. The lung is reexpanded, and a chest catheter may be inserted to establish closed drainage. In newborns, reexpansion of the lung may be accomplished by gradual withdrawal of a catheter during closure; no chest drainage tube is required unless there is oozing. The chest wall is closed in layers, and dressings are applied.

Repair of Hypoplastic Left Heart Syndrome

Hypoplastic left heart syndrome (HLHS) (Figure 17-71) is one of the most common forms of single ventricle malformation. HLHS describes a range of congenital cardiac malformations

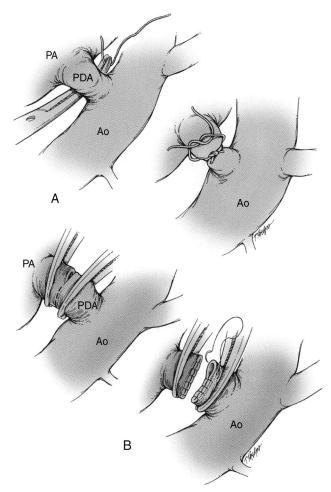

FIGURE 17-70 Surgical correction of patent ductus arteriosus (*PDA*). **A,** Ligation of ductus arteriosus. **B,** Division of ductus arteriosus. *Ao,* Aorta; *PA,* pulmonary artery.

that have in common underdevelopment of the left-sided heart structures, which include aortic valve atresia and stenosis with associated hypoplasia or absence of the left ventricle. The ascending aorta and arch are usually only a few millimeters in diameter and are functionally a branch of the ductus arteriosus–thoracic aorta continuum, with blood flowing retrograde through the aortic arch and into the small ascending aorta to the coronary arteries. Mitral valve atresia or stenosis also is present.

Survival in the newborn period depends on a PDA to maintain systemic circulation; therefore these infants are maintained on an infusion of prostaglandin E_1 (PGE_1) to maintain ductal patency before surgical intervention.

Newborns with HLHS typically present with cyanosis, respiratory distress, and variable degrees of circulatory collapse during the first few days of life. If left untreated, a majority of these neonates will die within the first month of life; without surgical intervention, HLHS is fatal.

It was not until the development of the Fontan procedure— a surgical correction for another form of single ventricle malformation (tricuspid atresia)—that long-term survival in patients with HLHS was considered possible. However, because of the neonate's high PVR, the Fontan procedure is not a surgi-

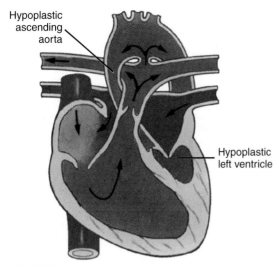

Hypoplastic ascending aorta

Hypoplastic left ventricle

FIGURE 17-71 Hypoplastic left-sided heart syndrome.

cal option in the newborn period. A palliative repair (stage I) was developed in the late 1970s by Norwood to prepare the heart for the Fontan procedure.

Two surgical options for patients with HLHS exist: a series of reconstructive procedures or heart transplantation. The series of reconstructive procedures usually involves three stages. Stage I is performed during the newborn period. The goals of stage I are to (1) maintain systemic perfusion, (2) preserve the function of the only ventricle, and (3) allow normal maturation of the pulmonary ventricle. The first goal is met by creating an unobstructed communication between the right ventricle and the systemic circulation. This is accomplished by transecting the main pulmonary artery and creating a neoaorta from the main pulmonary artery, native aorta, and pulmonary homograft tissue. The other two goals are met by creating a right modified Blalock-Taussig (BT) shunt and a nonrestrictive interatrial communication. These measures allow for adequate pulmonary blood flow and for the PVR to decrease as the child grows while the volume interposed on the single ventricle is limited.

The modified Fontan procedure was initially performed on a child at approximately 18 months of age. However, since 1989 a staged approach to the Fontan procedure has been undertaken to minimize the effect of rapid changes in ventricular configuration and diastolic function that can be associated with a primary Fontan procedure and its accompanying postoperative complications. In the stage II procedure (hemi-Fontan or the bidirectional Glenn shunt), superior vena cava (SVC) blood flow is directed to the lungs and inferior vena cava (IVC) blood flow continues to flow to the right ventricle. The third and final stage, the modified Fontan procedure, separates the systemic and pulmonary circulations.

Procedural Considerations. Additional items for the open-heart setup include the following:

◆ Stage I: polytetrafluoroethylene (PTFE) tube graft, 3.5 or 4 mm, and pulmonary homograft tissue
◆ Stage II: oscillating saw and pulmonary homograft tissue
◆ Stage III: oscillating saw and PTFE tube graft, 10 mm; a higher-than-usual supply of blood should be available

Operative Procedure
STAGE I (NORWOOD PROCEDURE) (Figure 17-72)
1. A median sternotomy is performed. The aortic cannula is placed into the main pulmonary artery rather than the diminutive aorta, and the venous cannula is placed into the right atrium. CPB is instituted, and the right and left pulmonary arteries are immediately occluded with tourniquets to force the blood through the ductus arteriosus to the systemic circulation.
2. When deep hypothermic circulatory arrest is about to be instituted, the innominate and left carotid arteries are occluded with tourniquets. The venous and aortic cannulae are removed.
3. The septum primum is excised through the venous cannulation site; occasionally a right atriotomy is necessary to facilitate the atrial septectomy.
4. The main pulmonary artery is transected immediately before the bifurcation of the right and left pulmonary arteries.
5. The distal pulmonary artery is closed with a small patch of homograft tissue.
6. The ductus arteriosus is then exposed and closed using a 2-0 nonabsorbable tie. The tie is left long to better expose the thoracic aorta. The ductus is transected.
7. At the point where the ductus was attached to the aorta, the thoracic aorta is opened 1 to 2 cm, and the aortic arch and ascending aorta are opened to a point adjacent to the main pulmonary artery.
8. A gusset of homograft tissue is joined to the aorta starting at the thoracic end, and the pulmonary artery is incorporated at the proximal end of the ascending aorta. A continuous monofilament stitch is used. Occasionally interrupted sutures are used to attach the main pulmonary artery to the aorta.
9. To perform a right BT shunt, the innominate artery is cross-clamped and incised and a 3.5- or 4-mm PTFE tube graft is interposed.
10. CPB is instituted, and the pulmonary end of the shunt is performed by incising the pulmonary artery and interposing the distal end of the tube graft.
11. Immediately after the shunt is completed, the shunt is occluded with a bulldog clamp until termination of bypass.

STAGE II (HEMI-FONTAN PROCEDURE) (Figure 17-73)
1. Because these patients have had previous surgery, an oscillating saw is used for the median sternotomy.
2. The aorta, right atrium, and right BT shunt are exposed.
3. CPB is instituted, and the shunt is immediately occluded with a clip.
4. The branch pulmonary arteries are exposed.
5. Depending on the surgeon's preference, deep hypothermic circulatory arrest may be instituted.
6. An incision is made in the confluence of the pulmonary arteries, extending to the pericardial reflections.
7. An incision is made in the dome of the right atrium, extending to the SVC.
8. The pulmonary artery is then anastomosed to the SVC–right atrial junction.
9. The pulmonary arteries are augmented with a gusset of homograft tissue. In the hemi-Fontan procedure, part of the homograft tissue is incorporated intraatrially as a dam between the common atrium and the vena cava–pulmonary artery anastomosis. In the Glenn shunt, there is no intraatrial incorporation.

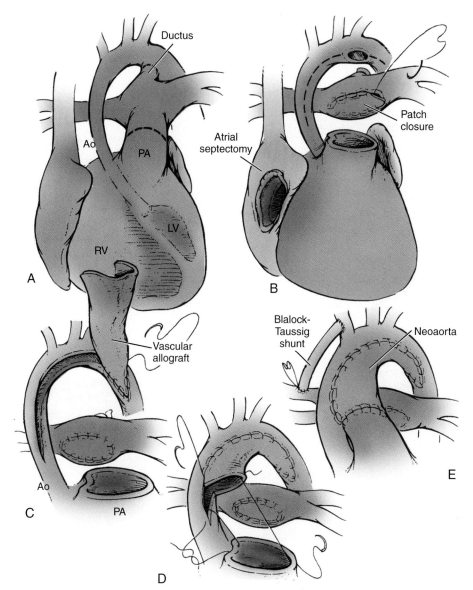

FIGURE 17-72 Stage I Norwood procedure. **A,** Transection points of the main pulmonary artery (*PA*) and ductus arteriosus. **B,** Atrial septectomy to avoid pulmonary venous hypertension. Patch closure of the distal main PA. Division and ligation of the ductus arteriosus. **C** and **D,** Construction of a "neo-aorta" with use of the proximal main PA, diminutive ascending aorta, and vascular allograft. **E,** Pulmonary blood flow supplied by a right modified Blalock-Taussig shunt connecting the right subclavian artery to the right PA. *Ao,* Aorta; *LV,* left ventricle; *RV,* right ventricle.

10. CPB is reinstituted until the patient is normothermic. CPB is then discontinued, and chest closure is completed.

STAGE III (MODIFIED FONTAN PROCEDURE)
(Figure 17-74)

1. A median sternotomy is performed with an oscillating saw.
2. The aorta and right atrium are exposed.
3. CPB is instituted.
4. Deep hypothermic circulatory arrest may be used.
5. A lateral incision is made in the right atrium.
6. A 10-mm PTFE tube graft is cut in half lengthwise and is placed intraatrially by suturing the inferior end of the graft around the orifice of the IVC and up the right lateral free wall of the right atrium to the superior dome of the right atrium. This creates a tunnel in which the inferior blood

flow is directed to the pulmonary arteries. The superior vena cava blood flow was directed to the pulmonary arteries during the stage II repair. (The surgeon may perform variations on this procedure, such as excluding a hepatic vein or performing a fenestrated Fontan by making a series of small openings in the PTFE tube graft or a single 4-mm opening with an aortic punch in the graft material.)

7. The atria are closed, and CPB is reinstituted until the patient is normothermic. CPB is then discontinued, and chest closure is completed.

Extracorporeal Membrane Oxygenation

Extracorporeal membrane oxygenation (ECMO) is a therapy used on pediatric patients who have reversible pulmonary or

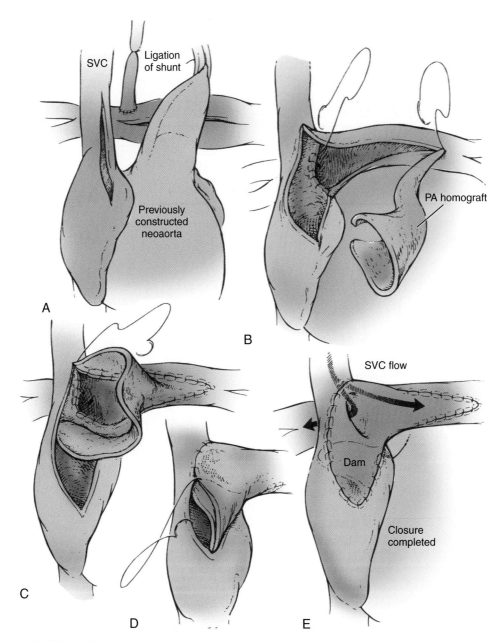

FIGURE 17-73 Hemi-Fontan procedure in a patient with hypoplastic left-sided heart syndrome. **A** and **B**, Ligation of the systemic-to-pulmonary artery shunt and side-to-side anastomosis of the superior vena cava *(SVC)* to the confluence of the pulmonary artery *(PA)* with allograft augmentation. **C** to **E**, Placement of a dam to close the junction of the atrium with the SVC so that saturated pulmonary venous blood mixes in the common atrium with desaturated blood draining from the inferior vena cava. Pulmonary blood flow is supplied exclusively through the SVC.

cardiac disease. Many patients are neonates with respiratory disease syndrome (RDS), persistent pulmonary hypertension (PPH), meconium aspiration (MA), or congenital diaphragmatic hernia (CDH) requiring adequate tissue oxygenation and waste removal from the body. In the cardiac patient, it may also be used as a bridge to heart or lung transplantation until donor organs are available. To perform ECMO, a facility must have an established ECMO service.

Most of the time children are placed on ECMO in the ICU. For venoarterial ECMO the surgical approach is usu-ally through the right carotid artery and internal jugular vein. For the cardiac patient after surgical repair, cannulation of the carotid artery and jugular vein provides good venous drainage of the right atrium, and the incision site is remote from the sternotomy wound. However, the surgeon may choose to reopen the sternum on postoperative patients and cannulate the aorta and right atrium. In the OR, for a patient who cannot be successfully weaned from bypass after surgery, the patient's bypass circuit may be switched to an ECMO circuit and the patient may be transferred on ECMO to the ICU.

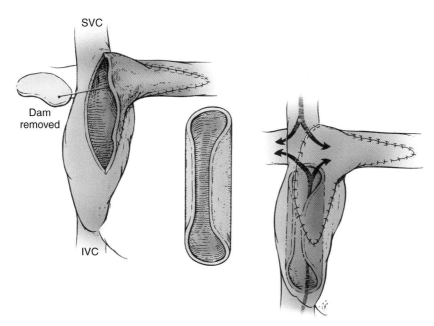

FIGURE 17-74 Conversion of hemi-Fontan to completion of Fontan. Excision of the dam between the right atrium and the superior vena cava–pulmonary artery anastomosis. Inferior vena cava flow is directed to the inlet of the superior vena cava–pulmonary artery anastomosis by a baffle. *IVC,* Inferior vena cava; *SVC,* superior vena cava.

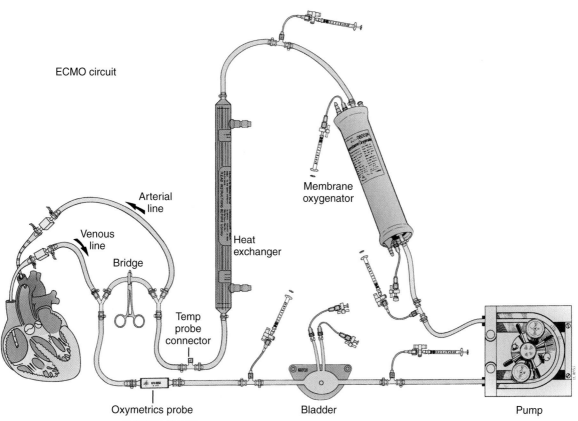

FIGURE 17-75 Extracorporeal membrane oxygenation (ECMO) circuit.

Procedural Considerations. An area by the patient's bedside should be provided for the ECMO pump, surgical table and instrumentation, electrosurgical unit (ESU), surgeon's headlight, and defibrillator with external and sterile internal paddles. A wall suction outlet should be available. Appropriate surgical attire should be provided for everyone involved with the procedure, and traffic should be limited.

Operative Procedure

FOR NECK CANNULATION. A shoulder roll is placed under the patient, and the neck and chest to the nipple line are prepped and draped. The ears should also be exposed and prepped for use as reference points.

1. An incision is made in the neck, and the right common carotid artery and right internal jugular vein are exposed for venoarterial ECMO.
2. The surgeon may cannulate the vessels through a purse-string suture and then reconstruct these vessels at the time of decannulation.
3. After insertion of the arterial and venous cannulae, the clamped cannulae are connected to the ECMO circuit. All the air is eliminated (Figure 17-75).
4. The cannulae are secured to the skin. The neck incision is closed and dressed. The surgical instruments are kept sterile until proper positioning of the venous and arterial cannulae is confirmed by x-ray examination.

FOR MEDIAN STERNOTOMY CANNULATION. The patient is prepped from neck to umbilicus and draped.

1. The patient has usually had a prior sternotomy incision, and so the sternum is opened with wire cutters.
2. A chest retractor is inserted, and purse-string sutures for cannulation are placed in the aorta and right atrium.
3. The aorta and venous cannulae are inserted and clamped.
4. The clamped cannulae are connected to the ECMO circuit. All the air is eliminated.
5. The sternum is left open to prevent kinking of the cannulae and ECMO pump tubing. The wound is closed with a synthetic patch sutured to the skin. An antibiotic ointment may be applied and an "Open Chest" sign placed on top of the outer dressing to serve as a warning related to potential chest compressions.

PEDIATRIC SURGERY SUMMARY

It is imperative to know the anatomy and physiology of the surgical area when dealing with pediatric procedures. A prepared surgical technologist will be able to anticipate the unforeseen as well as be adequately prepared for the scheduled operation. Planning ahead will greatly help the surgical team work cohesively to provide the best care possible for the pediatric patient. It is important to fully understand all aspects of positioning, surgical equipment, supplies, and instrumentation.

REVIEW QUESTIONS

1. The Nissen fundoplication is performed to:
   a. reduce a hernia
   b. treat GERD
   c. repair a defect in the diaphragm
   d. all of the above

2. An epispadias is a congenital anomaly characterized by a uretheral opening:
   a. on the ventral surface of the penis
   b. on the chordee
   c. on the dorsum of the penis
   d. none of the above

3. The hypertropia type of strabismus is:
   a. inward turning of one or both eyes
   b. outward turning of one or both eyes
   c. one eye higher than the other
   d. one eye lower than the other

4. Trauma is the leading cause of death in children from 1 to 14 years of age. Several factors influence the risk of trauma, including:
   a. age
   b. behavior
   c. gender
   d. all of the above

5. True or false: A warming light is never used in pediatric surgeries.

6. True or false: Children feel more anxiety entering surgery than their parents.

7. True or false: For laparotomy and laparoscopic procedures, the patient is usually placed in the supine position.

8. True or false: Hirschsprung's disease is characterized by the absence of ganglion cells in the distal portion of the bowel.

9. True or false: ECMO is a therapy used on pediatric patients who have reversible pulmonary or cardiac disease.

10. True or false: It is not commonly recommended to do tenotomies and lengthening on children with cerebral palsy.

11. Define and briefly describe the following surgical procedures:
    Umbilical hernia repair
    Tonsillectomy and adenoidectomy
    Cleft lip and cleft palate repair

Critical Thinking Questions

1. The surgical technologist is preparing for a pediatric trauma procedure. What details will help the surgical technologist deliver the most efficient care?

2. The surgical team is obligated to screen all pediatric patients for abuse and neglect. Abuse can be defined as "physical or mental injury, sexual abuse or exploitation, negligent treatment or maltreatment." What does the surgical technologist need to keep in mind as the patient is screened for abuse?

REFERENCES

American Academy of Orthopedic Surgeons (AAOS): Children's clubfoot: treatment with casting or operation, 2007, available at http://orthoinfo.aaos.org/topic.cfm?topic=A00296. Accessed May 18, 2009.

American Association for Pediatric Ophthalmology and Strabismus (AAPOS): Frequently asked questions, 2005, available at www.aapos.org/displaycommon.cfm?an=1& subarticlenbr=231. Accessed February 24, 2009

American Cancer Society (ACS): *Cancer facts and figures 2009*, Atlanta, 2009, The Society.

Betz CL, Sowden LA: *Mosby's pediatric nursing reference*, ed 6, St Louis, 2008, Mosby.

Children's Hospital of Philadelphia (CHOP): *Congenital Hyperinsulinism Center*, available at www.chop.edu/consumer/jsp/division/generic.jsp?id=71065. Accessed May 15, 2009.

Cooper A: Early assessment and management of trauma. In Ashcraft KW et al, editors: *Pediatric surgery*, ed 4, Philadelphia, 2005, Saunders.

Cote CJ: Pediatric anesthesia. In Miller RD, editor: *Miller's anesthesia*, ed 6, vol 2, Philadelphia, 2005, Churchill Livingstone.

Davis GT: Hemolytic disorders and congenital abnormalities. In Lowdermilk DL et al, editors: *Maternity and women's health care*, ed 9, St Louis, 2007, Mosby.

Fallat ME: Intussusception. In Ashcraft KW et al, editors: *Pediatric surgery*, ed 4, Philadelphia, 2005, Saunders.

Garcia VF: Umbilical and other abdominal wall hernias. In Ashcraft KW et al, editors: *Pediatric surgery*, ed 4, Philadelphia, 2005, Saunders.

Gronert GA et al: Malignant hyperthermia. In Miller RD, editor: *Miller's anesthesia*, ed 6, vol 2, Philadelphia, 2005, Churchill Livingstone.

Harrington S et al: Pediatric laparoscopy, *AORN J* 88(2):211–236, 2008.

Heher KL, Katowitz JA: Pediatric ptosis. In Katowitz JA, editor: *Pediatric oculoplastic surgery*, New York, 2002, Springer.

Inge TH et al: Bariatric surgical procedures in adolescence. In Ashcraft KW et al, editors: *Pediatric surgery*, ed 4, Philadelphia, 2005, Saunders.

Klein MD: Congenital abdominal wall defects. In Ashcraft KW et al, editors: *Pediatric surgery*, ed 4, Philadelphia, 2005, Saunders.

Laberge JM et al: Teratomas, dermoids and other soft tissue tumors. In Ashcraft KW et al, editors: *Pediatric surgery*, ed 4, Philadelphia, 2005, Saunders.

Melek BH: Atrial septal defect, 2006, available at www.emedicine.com/MED/topic3519.htm. Accessed August 22, 2009.

Medline Plus Medical Encyclopedia: Necrotizing enterocolitis, 2007, available at www.nlm.nih.gov/MEDLINEPLUS/ency/article/001148.htm. Accessed May 21, 2009.

Nuss D et al: Congenital chest wall deformities. In Ashcraft KW et al, editors: *Pediatric surgery*, ed 4, Philadelphia, 2005, Saunders.

Ramaswamy P et al: Ventricular septal defect, general concepts, 2009, available at www.emedicine.com/PED/topic2402.htm. Accessed August 22, 2009.

Rao PS: Tricuspid atresia, 2009, available at www.emedicine.com/PED/topic 2550.htm. Accessed August 22, 2009.

Sheth RD et al: Craniosynostosis, 2008, available at: http://emedicine.medscape.com/article/1175957-overview. Accessed August 22, 2009.

Spitz L: Esophageal atresia and tracheoesophageal malformations. In Ashcraft KW et al, editors: *Pediatric surgery*, ed 4, Philadelphia, 2005, Saunders.

Turner CS: Vascular access. In Ashcraft KW et al, editors: *Pediatric surgery*, ed 4, Philadelphia, 2005, Saunders.

Whitaker L: Foreword. In Katowitz JA, editor: *Pediatric oculoplastic surgery*, New York, 2002, Springer.

Wilson D: The child with neuromuscular or muscular dysfunction. In Hockenberry MJ, Wilson D, editors: *Wong's essentials of pediatric nursing*, ed 8, St Louis, 2008, Mosby.

Wilson D et al: The child with musculoskeletal or articular dysfunction. In Hockenberry MJ, Wilson D, editors: *Wong's essentials of pediatric nursing*, ed 8, St Louis, 2008, Mosby.

Wu CL: Pain management. In Miller RD, editor: *Miller's anesthesia*, ed 6, vol 2 Philadelphia, 2005, Churchill Livingstone.

CHAPTER 18

Trauma Surgery

This chapter was originally written by Diane Catherine Saullo, RN, MSN, CNOR, BC, for the 14th edition of Alexander's Care of the Patient in Surgery and has been revised by Sherri M. Alexander, CST, for this text.

LEARNING OBJECTIVES

After studying this chapter the reader will be able to:
- Identify common surgical procedures and interventions in trauma surgery
- Understand positioning, prepping, and draping of the surgical trauma patient
- Identify common instrumentation, sterile supplies, implants, suture, and medication used in trauma surgery pertaining to each specialty
- Describe appropriate Mayo stand setup

CHAPTER OUTLINE

Overview

Trauma is ranked as one of the foremost public health issues in the United States today. Unintentional injury related to trauma is the fifth leading cause of death today and the leading cause of death for persons aged 1 to 44 years (Barclay, 2009). Trauma is the leading nonobstetric cause of maternal mortality and is associated with fetal mortality directly related to the severity of maternal injury (Cusick and Tibbles, 2007). Whether the injury is a result of a motor vehicle collision, violence, crime, or work-related injury, trauma occurs unplanned and without warning. The unpredictable nature of trauma poses a major challenge to the surgical technologist and the patient care team.

The potential for injury has existed since the beginning of humanity. Most of the major advances in care of critically injured patients have been accomplished through experience in the military. Clearly, the shorter the response time, the greater the survival rate for casualties. This was demonstrated by the success of the mobile army surgical hospitals (MASH) during the Korean conflict and again during the Vietnam conflict; MASH brought the necessary supplies, equipment, and personnel closer to the battlefields and, consequently, improved patient outcomes.

Eventually this concept was applied to the civilian population and is now commonly referred to as the "golden hour" of trauma care. More specifically, the golden hour refers to the time immediately after the injury when rapid and definitive interventions can be most effective in the reduction of morbidity and mortality. The golden hour starts at the scene, where prehospital personnel determine the severity of injury, initiate medical treatment, and identify the most appropriate facility to which to transport the patient. Traumatic deaths may occur in three phases, or time frames. The first occurs immediately after the injury. This accounts for approximately 50% of the deaths from trauma and is usually a result of lacerations to the heart or aorta or brainstem injury. These patients rarely survive transport to the hospital and die at the scene. The second phase occurs within the first 1 to 2 hours after the injury, representing approximately 30% of total fatalities. These patients have injuries to the spleen, liver, lung, or other organs that result in significant blood loss. This is the group in which definitive trauma care (i.e., appropriate and aggressive resuscitation with adequate volume replacement) may have the most significant effect (the golden hour). The third phase occurs days to weeks after the injury, often during the intensive care phase, and is usually caused by complications or a failure of multiple organ systems.

The wars in Iraq and Afghanistan have resulted in some changes in the way traumatic injuries are managed; the military has not set up convalescence centers as in Vietnam and Desert Storm. Rather, the doctrine of "essential care in theater" is followed. Physicians and nurses have been trained to provide immediate care, keeping in mind the treatment resources that will be available at the next level of care. Soldiers with upper body injuries are surviving because of body armor. However, there is no protection for upper extremities; therefore there are many amputations being performed, including above-elbow and shoulder disarticulations. The new philosophy is to stress continuity of care with the goal of returning the soldier to the highest possible level of function.

Time is of the essence in providing definitive care to the critically injured person. A significant number of patient deaths can be prevented if rapid transport is provided from the scene to a facility equipped to provide resuscitation and treatment in an efficient and timely manner. This concept is reflected in the national development of the Emergency Medical Services (EMS) system. Facilities and resources are allocated and coordinated to provide specific interventions for a group of patients. For example, facilities that meet certain criteria to accommodate the specialized needs of the critically injured patient are designated as *trauma centers*. Communities establish transfer and triage protocols that allow for a trauma patient to reach the appropriate facility with the least out-of-hospital time possible. This may be accomplished by a helicopter with a specially trained flight crew or by the use of ground transport with an Advanced Life Support (ALS) ambulance team (Figure 18-1).

Trauma centers (TC) are classified based on the scope of services and resources that are available. A level I TC is capable of providing total care for every type of injury. Accepting this designation commits the TC to providing qualified personnel and equipment necessary for rapid diagnosis and treatment on a 24-hour basis. A level II TC provides comprehensive care for all injuries but lacks some of the specialized clinicians and resources required for the level I designation. A level II facility may provide surgical intervention if the critical nature of the injury dictates immediate intervention before transfer to a level I facility. A level III facility provides prompt evaluation, resuscitation, emergency surgery, and stabilization, as needed, before transfer to a higher-level facility. The American College of Surgeons (ACS) recommends that in level II and III centers, an OR team is readily available at all times. Depending on the population served and the volume of urgent cases, this requirement may be met with on-call staff. A level IV trauma center has the ability to provide advanced trauma life support before patient transfer. These facilities may be located in rural areas with limited access and may be a clinic or a hospital.

Although the risk for death is 25% lower for a severe injury treated in a level I TC (Barclay, 2009), not all patients require the services of a level I TC and so may be transported to the closest emergency department for care. New guidelines and recommendations for triage, first developed as a position statement by the ACS in 1986, have been published (Barclay, 2009). Known as the "Decision Scheme," this algorithm guides EMS personnel through the following four decision points: physiologic parameters, anatomic param-

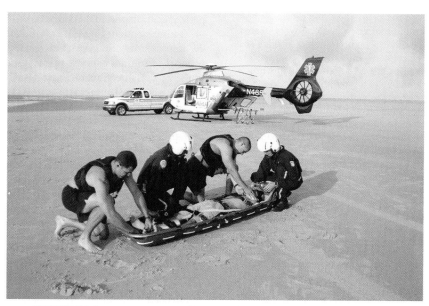

FIGURE 18-1 New Hanover Health Network EMS Air Link rescue at the beach.

HISTORY

Triage Development

The origin of the term "triage" is sketchy but the earliest use was seen in the late 1700s and is attributed to Baron Dominique Jean Larrey. He said, "Those who are dangerously wounded should receive the first attention, without regard to rank or distinction."

Triage was further developed during the Civil War. The injured were separated into immediate treatment versus delayed treatment versus no treatment. Amputation was the most common life-saving procedure performed; gunshot wounds to the abdomen were often ignored because of high mortality and lack of resources. A more formal triage system was developed in World War I and was advanced in World War II. Air-medical transport was first used in the Korean War.

Field triage criteria for civilian injuries refer to the decisions of prehospital personnel about where to transport the injured. Before the 1970s the injured were simply transported to the nearest facility with little prehospital intervention. In 1976 the American College of Surgeons (ACS) established the designation of "trauma centers" and set standards of personnel, facility, and processes to provide optimal care of the injured. Prehospital triage in the 1970s and early 1980s was based on anatomic, physiologic, and mechanistic domains. The establishment of specialized trauma centers led to one of the first triage protocols for trauma patients in 1987, developed by the ACS and known as the *Optimal Resources' Guide.*

With the establishment of both specialized trauma centers and triage guidelines, the problems of overtriage and undertriage became evident, which included diagnostic and treatment delays or errors, increased morbidity and mortality, and missed injuries. In 1990 the ACS revised the field triage decision scheme to include, among other things, use of the Revised and Pediatric Trauma Scores. The 1990 revisions included mechanism of injury criteria related to vehicular deformity and motorcycle criteria and established a four-step versus the previous three-step process. The dictum of the ACS guidelines became, "when in doubt take to a trauma center." The guidelines were revised in 1993 and included changes in the Glasgow Coma Scale and the addition of automobile-bicycle collision criteria; the 1999 revisions changed the triage process within the trauma system so patients who met specific physiologic or anatomic criteria were taken to the highest level of care available.

Opportunities for further development of triage criteria include:

◆ Standardization of the criteria used to define overtriage and undertriage
◆ Improved balance between transport distance and severity of injury
◆ Incorporation of automated vehicular telemetry information to determine severity of injury

Modified from Mackersie RC: History of trauma field triage development and the American College of Surgeons criteria, *Prehosp Emerg Care* 10(3):287-294, 2006.

RESEARCH HIGHLIGHT

Impact of Airbags

Seat belts were introduced in motor vehicles more than 40 years ago and have been refined during that time. After mandatory use legislation, seat belt use increased and there was an associated decrease in crash fatalities by up to 50%. Today, it is clear that seat belts reduce injuries and save lives.

Airbag use has increased in the last 15 years, and while published data are limited, indications are that airbags are associated with less severe injury (based on a study of second-generation depowered airbags). One study showed an almost 50% decrease in injuries to the brain, face, and cervical spine. Another study demonstrated that airbags alone were associated with a decrease in fatalities; a combination of airbags and seat belts had a greater protective effect. Other studies concluded that airbags are associated with an increase in extremity injury and are more effective at higher speeds.

Using the trauma registry, the authors conducted a study looking at motor vehicle collision victims admitted over an 11-year period, for a total of 14,390 patients. The patients were divided into four groups: unrestrained (n = 7881), airbag only (n = 692), seat belt only (n = 4909), or airbag and seat belt (n = 908). Although separate use of airbags and seat belt was associated with reduced injury, a larger association was seen when both airbags and seat belts were used. The conclusion states that seat belts, with or without airbags, are associated with decreased in-hospital mortality and a change in injury pattern, as well as reduced injury severity and hospital resource use.

From Williams RF et al: Impact of airbags on a level 1 trauma center: injury patterns, infectious morbidity, and hospital costs, *J Am Coll Surg* 206(5):962-969, 2008.

eters, mechanism of injury (MOI), and other special considerations. Personnel review physiologic parameters. Patients with a Glasgow Coma Scale score less than 14, systolic blood pressure less than 90 mm Hg, or respiratory rate less than 10 breaths per minute or greater than 29 breaths per minute should be transported to the highest level facility available. The anatomic parameters include specific types of injuries, such as penetrating injuries of the neck or torso, flail chest, or proximal long bone fracture; these patients are also transported to the highest level facility available. The MOI and other special considerations, such as age or prior medical history, are also reviewed to determine to what level facility the patient is transported (History box).

Trauma patients require immediate access to the OR 24 hours per day, 365 days per year. A sudden influx of a large number of trauma patients to a trauma center may necessitate triage or classification of those less seriously injured as less urgent, allowing immediate access for the critically injured patients. The elective surgery schedule may need to be interrupted to expedite care for the trauma patient or patients. Scheduling policies and procedures are established collaboratively by the departments of surgery, trauma, anesthesia, and perioperative nursing services. Consequently, the perioperative nurse and surgical technologist need to be familiar with supplies and equipment located in the OR designated for trauma or in the ORs that are used most frequently for these patients.

Surgical Technologist Considerations

When dealing with the unpredictable timing, it is often the on-call perioperative team who cares for the injured patient requiring surgery. In contrast to an elective surgical procedure, the team may know very little about the trauma patient. The surgical team may be working with reduced preparation before the patient enters the operating room. Speed and efficiency will be the key to the successful outcome of the trauma patient.

An experienced surgical technologist will have the clinical knowledge to prepare for unexpected complications, such as increased hemorrhage, multiple surgical teams, and a large number of equipment and supplies. The ability to prioritize and work calmly and collaboratively with the team enhances the level of patient care.

After the type of traumatic injury has been identified, the surgical technologist will select the appropriate equipment and supplies. Blunt trauma can present a greater risk to the patient than penetrating trauma. Because it is more difficult to identify and treat blunt trauma, the surgical technologist will need to have specific instruments to gain quick access to the site of the injury.

If it is blunt trauma to the abdomen, a laparotomy set of instruments and supplies is appropriate. Understanding that there will be a need for multiple sponges, suture, and ties, as well as having the appropriate electrosurgical equipment available, is key. Blunt trauma to the head will require the surgical technologist to be prepared for either burr holes or a craniotomy. The surgeon will need to quickly relieve the pressure on the brain; the ability to set up the specialized power equipment is paramount for the surgical technologist.

In penetrating trauma, there may be injuries to surrounding anatomic structures, which most often include the liver, spleen, intestines, and vascular system. The surgical technologist may need to secure lasers, anastomotic stapling devices, specialty instruments, and suture or vascular grafts to be prepared to effectively assist the surgeon.

The skin prep for traumatic injuries will vary depending on the location of the injury and the preference of the surgeon. Assisting to open and set up the sterile prep will facilitate a more expeditious start time. If there is debris present in the wound, the prep may need to include a sterile scrub brush or powerized irrigation equipment. While removing the debris, it is crucial to use caution to prevent further injury.

Results of diagnostic studies including x-ray films, CT scans, and MRIs, as well as lab values, are beneficial to the perioperative team, because these results can help guide the correct selection of instruments, supplies, and equipment.

With the knowledge that there may be several healthcare providers or multiple teams working on the patient simultaneously, room setup and traffic flow become extremely important to ensuring sterility in the room.

Understanding it will be difficult to regulate body temperature in the trauma patient, appropriate warming devices and fluids need to be readily available. Complicating this will be dealing with hypothermia and thermal injuries; these present the perioperative team with additional steps to ensure optimal patient outcomes.

Biomechanics in Trauma

Mechanisms of Injury	Phases of Injury
	Examples
Vehicle of transfer of energy from environment to human host	Falls
	Motor vehicle crashes
	Bullets
	Stabbing instruments
	Blasts/bombs
	External Forces
DECELERATION FORCES	
Decrease in speed of a moving object or person	Victim strikes steering column
	Victim impacts ground
ACCELERATION FORCES	
Increase in speed of a moving object or person	Pedestrian thrown when struck by moving vehicle
BLAST FORCES	
Heat, light, pressure	Bomb explosion
Low- and high-velocity missiles	Bullets
	Stabbing instruments
	Internal Forces
Human body's response to kinetic energy load	Stress
	Cells separate, stretch, compress, or shear
	Strain
	Tissue damage or deformation from stress
	Types of Injuries
Describing for clinical and diagnostic purpose	Blunt vs penetrating
	Closed vs. open
	Primary vs secondary
	Direct vs. indirect

Modified from Emergency Nurses Association (ENA): *Trauma nursing core course*, ed 6, Des Plaines, Ill, 2007, Author.

Stress debriefing is very important to the entire perioperative team. Most surgical interventions are of the curative nature, while trauma can result in less than optimal outcomes for the patient, including death. Learning to openly discuss the feelings and emotions this particular type of surgery evokes is an important part of becoming a successful trauma team member.

It is imperative for healthcare providers to care for themselves as well as their patients.

Assessment

The resuscitative process begins with arrival of emergency personnel on the scene and ends when the patient has been

---

SURGICAL TECHNOLOGY PREFERENCE CARD

This serves as a tool to assist the surgical technologist in the scrub role when preparing for trauma surgery. In contrast to an elective surgical procedure, the team may know very little about the trauma patient. The surgical team often works with reduced preparation time before the patient enters the operating room.

An experienced surgical technologist will have the clinical knowledge to prepare for unexpected complications, such as increased hemorrhage, multiple surgical teams, and a large number of equipment and supplies. The ability to prioritize and work calmly and collaboratively with the team enhances the level of patient care.

Understanding the room layout before setting up for the procedure allows the traffic pattern in the room to be maximized. This step can help ensure sterility of the field and facilitate effective communication of additional requests for supplies between circulator and scrub, as well as provide efficient space for other healthcare providers involved in the trauma procedure.

Room Prep: Basic OR furniture in place, thermoregulatory devices, extra blankets, padding, positioning supplies to achieve optimal patient safety

Prep Solution: In room
- Chlorhexidine gluconate (CHG)
- Iodine and iodophors

Catheter: In room and correct size
- Catheter set and tray
  - Latex/rubber
  - Silicone
  - Temperature sensing
- Sizing
  - French
- Retaining
  - Foley
    - 2-way
    - 3-way
  - Mushroom/Pezzer/Malecot
  - T-tube
- Other urine collection devices

PROCEDURE CHECKLIST

Instruments
- Standard sets
- As indicated for the area of the injury, can include:
  - Abdominal set
  - Chest set
  - Craniotomy set
  - Orthopedic set
  - Fracture fixation set
  - Maxillofacial fracture set
  - Plastic and reconstructive set
- Anticipated additional instruments
  - Bowel clamps
  - Bookwalter or other self-retaining retractor
  - Anastomotic stapling devices

Suture
- As per surgeon's preference

Other Hemostatic Agents
- Mechanical
  - Staplers
  - Clip appliers and clips
  - Pressure
  - Ligatures
  - Pledgets

- ◆ Chemical
  - Absorbable gelatin
  - Collagen
  - Oxidized cellulose
  - Silver nitrate
  - Epinephrine
  - Thrombin
- ◆ Thermal
  - Electrosurgical unit
  - Harmonic scalpel
  - Argon beam coagulator
  - Bipolar

Additional Supplies and Equipment: both sterile and nonsterile
- ◆ If the physician is requesting supplies, instruments, or equipment not normally used, check to be sure all have arrived to the room before opening
- ◆ Sponges/abdominal packing (damage control surgery)
- ◆ Drapes
- ◆ Gowns and gloves for team members
- ◆ Autologous blood salvage unit
- ◆ Sequential compression device (SCD)
- ◆ "Have ready" or "hold" supplies

Medications and Irrigation Solutions
- ◆ Warmed, if needed (follow manufacturer's recommendations when warming all solutions)
- ◆ Appropriate-sized syringes, hypodermic needles, labels, and a marking pen

Drains and Dressings
- ◆ Correct size and type for planned surgery
  - Open—Not attached to a drainage system
    - Penrose
    - Cigarette
  - Closed—Attached to closed reservoir for fluid collection
    - Hemovac
    - Jackson-Pratt
    - Autologous blood retrieval drainage system
- ◆ Anchoring methods
  - Suture
    - Nonabsorbable
    - Cutting needle
  - Tape

Dressings
- ◆ As per surgeon's preference and procedure performed

Specimen Care
- ◆ Proper container for each specimen
  - Permanent
  - Stones
  - Body fluids or washings
  - Cultures
  - Foreign bodies
- ◆ Labels for each specimen
- ◆ Proper solution for specimen type

Before opening for the procedure, the surgical technologist should:
- ◆ Arrange furniture
- ◆ Gather positioning devices
- ◆ Verify functionality of equipment
- ◆ Place items to be opened in their appropriate places

When opening sterile supplies:
- ◆ Verify exposure to sterilization
- ◆ Use sterile technique
- ◆ Open bundles in appropriate locations
- ◆ Open additional supplies onto sterile field
- ◆ Open all sterile supplies and equipment as quickly as possible

stabilized, received definitive care, and undergone a complete and thorough physical examination to determine all injuries sustained. When the patient arrives in the ED, the trauma team initiates a primary assessment. This is a logical, orderly process of patient assessment for potential life threats. These assessment activities are based on established protocols for advanced trauma life support (ATLS). The mnemonic "ABCDE" is used, representing assessment of the following:

◆ Airway (with cervical spine precautions)
◆ Breathing
◆ Circulation
◆ Disability (brief neurologic examination)
◆ Exposure (to reveal all life-threatening injuries) and environmental control (thermoregulation)

Airway interventions may include manual maneuvers (chin-lift, jaw-thrust), insertion of oral or nasopharyngeal airways, or intubation. The trauma team may also perform emergent procedures, such as tracheotomy or needle cricothyrotomy, to secure the patient's airway. Pulse oximetry and capnography monitoring are used. If cervical spine precautions were not implemented before arrival at the hospital, the team initiates them before performing any other procedures on the patient. A trauma team member can stabilize the head and neck, if necessary, until a cervical collar is placed. Once placed, the team does not remove it until a cervical radiograph clears the neck of injury.

During this time, the surgeon or ED physician and trauma team identify and correct life threats that are present before progressing to the next part of the examination. A patient requiring immediate surgery is transported to the OR, undergoes surgical intervention, and then is transferred to the postanesthesia care unit (PACU) or intensive care unit (ICU), depending on his or her condition. On the other hand, a patient may have a penetrating wound with evisceration of abdominal contents. However, correcting the obvious defect, which is currently not life-threatening, is postponed until the trauma team is assured that the patient has a patent airway and an effective breathing pattern and cervical spine precautions have been implemented. An evisceration needs to be corrected, but an inadequate airway is an immediate life threat and assumes priority.

Depending on the patient's injury, the surgeon may order an arterial blood gas (ABG) measurement. This test provides an accurate assessment of the ventilatory status of the patient and also evaluates resuscitative airway and breathing interventions (Table 18-1). Metabolic acidosis or a large base deficit (pH <7.35 or >7.45), with all other causes ruled out, may indicate internal bleeding.

After the trauma team completes the primary assessment and corrects any immediate life threats, they perform a secondary assessment. The purpose of the secondary assessment is to identify all injuries present. Sometimes the secondary assessment may be completed by the perioperative team, the PACU nurse, or the critical care nurse. This assessment is a more in-depth, head-to-toe evaluation of the patient. Inspection, palpation, percussion, and auscultation are used in the complete head-to-toe assessment to reveal any deformities, open injuries, tenderness, or swelling. The assessment begins at the head and face and then moves to the neck (including the spine), the chest, the abdomen, and the pelvis. The four extremities are next; distal pulses, motor function, and sensation are assessed. The final check is the back; the patient is carefully log-rolled to the side for a full visual and tactile assessment (Evidence for Practice).

The patient's vital signs, including a rectal or tympanic temperature, unless contraindicated, are obtained. Often during resuscitation, a Foley catheter is inserted to monitor urine output and fluid resuscitation efforts. The circulator should inspect the urinary meatus for the presence of blood before inserting the catheter. If blood is noted, the circulator notifies the surgeon and does not insert the catheter. The patient may have a ruptured bladder or a urethral injury, either of which is commonly associated with a fracture of the pelvis. The surgeon may wish to perform a retrograde urethrogram to examine the bladder and urethra for the presence of tears or disruption. After catheter insertion, urine is obtained for a urinalysis and urine drug screen. The identification of specific drugs in the urine may assist in further diagnosis and treatment. The urine will also be tested to determine the presence of red blood cells (RBCs) (Box 18-1). Depending on the amount of hematuria present, a renal con-

Mechanisms of Blast Injuries

Category	Areas Affected	Types of Injuries
Primary: Caused by blast itself	Gas-filled organs most susceptible:	
	◆ Eye	Rupture of globe
	◆ Middle ear/tympanic membrane	Rupture and permanent deafness possible
	◆ Lungs	Pneumothorax, alveolar rupture, air embolus
	◆ GI tract	Abdominal hemorrhage, contusions, rupture
	◆ Central nervous system	Diffuse cerebral hemorrhage, cerebral air embolism, concussion syndrome (injury without physical signs)
Secondary: Caused by debris and projectiles	Any body part	Varies depending on size of projectiles: penetrating or blunt injury
Tertiary: Caused by victim being thrown against stationary objects	Any body part	Similar to those seen in motor vehicle crashes: fractures, traumatic amputations, closed/open brain injury
Quaternary: Exacerbation or complications of existing conditions	Any body part	Burns, crush injuries, inhalation of dust or toxic gases causing exacerbation of asthma or COPD, angina

Modified from Emergency Nurses Association (ENA): *Trauma nursing core course,* ed 6, Des Plaines, Ill, 2007, Author.

tusion or other renal injury may be present. In addition, a nasogastric tube may be inserted at this time.

The circulator obtains a brief history from the family or significant others when possible. This history is referred to as the "AMPLE" history and may be obtained even after the patient is transferred to the OR by the ED personnel. The history includes the following:

- Allergies
- Medications
- Past medical history
- Last meal, last menstrual period (if appropriate)

- Events or environment leading to the accident or injury

If the history is obtained after the initiation of surgery, it is important to communicate it to the surgeon and the anesthesia providers.

Routine Laboratory Tests. Laboratory values aid the trauma team in evaluating the patient's status. Appropriate laboratory tests include a minimum of a complete blood count (CBC), hemoglobin and hematocrit (H&H) value, blood alcohol level (BAL), and a blood type and screen; other tests may be requested during evaluation. The results of the laboratory stud-

---

TABLE 18-1

Laboratory Values: Arterial Blood Gases (ABGs)

NORMAL VALUES

Pao_2	Pressure of oxygen in arterial blood	80-100 mm Hg
$Paco_2$	Pressure of carbon dioxide in arterial blood; measurement of how well lungs are discarding carbon dioxide (CO_2 level is controlled by lungs)	34-45 mm Hg
pH	Acidity or alkalinity of arterial blood; measurement of hydrogen ion concentration	7.35-7.45
HCO_3^-	Amount of bicarbonate in arterial blood; controlled by kidneys	21-28 mEq/L
O_2 saturation	Percentage of hemoglobin that is carrying oxygen	95-100%

ABNORMAL VALUES | | **POSSIBLE CAUSE**

Pao_2	<50 mm Hg	Hypoxia
$Paco_2$	>45 mm Hg	Hypoventilation/CO_2 retention by lungs
pH	<7.35	Acidosis
	>7.45	Alkalosis
HCO_3^-	<22 mEq/L	Renal excretion of too much bicarbonate
	>26 mEq/L	Renal retention of too much bicarbonate

Modified from Pagana KD, Pagana TJ: *Mosby's diagnostic and laboratory test references,* ed 9, St Louis, 2009, Mosby.

Decision Scheme Recommendations*

Steps	Transition	Recommendations
Step 1		Transport to TC for any of the following: GCS <14, systolic BP <90 mm Hg, respiratory rate <10 or >29 breaths/min
	1 to 2	These patients have potentially serious injuries and should be transported to highest level TC available
Step 2		Transport to TC for any of the following: penetrating injuries of head, neck, torso, and extremities proximal to elbow and knee; flail chest; 2 or more proximal long bone fractures; crushed, degloved, or mangled extremity; amputation proximal to wrist and ankle; pelvic fracture; open or depressed skull fracture; paralysis
	2 to 3	If yes to any criteria, transport to highest level TC available; if patient does not meet step 2 criteria, proceed to step 3
Step 3		Transport to TC for any of the following: falls >20 feet for adults, >10 feet or 2-3 times child's height; motor vehicle crash with partial or complete ejection of occupant; auto vs pedestrian/bicyclist thrown; motorcycle crash at speed >20 mph
	3 to 4	If yes to any criteria, transport to closest TC
Step 4		Consider transport to TC for the following: age >55 or <15, anticoagulation and bleeding disorders, burns, time-sensitive extremity injury, end-stage renal disease requiring dialysis, pregnancy, or provider judgment

*The Decision Scheme is an essential component of the trauma system, guiding EMS providers in transporting injured patients to the most appropriate facility, ensuring proper treatment, and thus reducing death and disability.
BP, Blood pressure; *GCS,* Glasgow Coma Scale; *TC,* trauma center.
Modified from Barclay L: *Guidelines issued for field triage of injured patients,* Medscape Medical News, 2009, available at www.medscape.com/viewarticle/587447. Accessed February 16, 2009.

BOX 18-1

Laboratory Values: Urinalysis (UA)*

NORMAL VALUES		ABNORMAL VALUES		In Trauma, May Indicate
Color	Amber yellow	Color	Dark or red	Presence of blood
Appearance	Clear	Appearance	Dark or red	Presence of blood
Specific gravity	1.005-1.030	Specific gravity	>1.030	Fluid volume deficit
pH	4.6-8.0	pH	Alkaline: >8.0	Alkalosis
Protein	Negative		Acidic: <4.6	Acidosis
Glucose	Negative	Glucose	Present	Diabetes
Ketones	Negative			Increased intracranial pressure
Microscopic findings		Protein	Present	Renal failure
◆ RBCs	0-2/high-power field (hpf)	Ketones	Present	Diabetes
◆ WBCs	0-4/hpf			Diarrhea and vomiting
◆ Epithelial cells	Few	Microscopic findings		
◆ Casts	0	◆ RBCs	>3/hpf	Kidney, ureteral, bladder trauma
◆ Crystals	0	◆ WBCs	>4/hpf	Urinary tract infection
◆ Bacteria	0	◆ Epithelial cells	↑	Renal tubular necrosis
◆ Yeast	0	◆ Casts	↑	Glomerular capsule trauma
		◆ Bacteria		Abnormalities not usually seen in early trauma

*A urinalysis is done to check for injury to the genitourinary system and for the presence of specific diseases.
Modified from Pagana KD, Pagana TJ: *Mosby's diagnostic and laboratory test references,* ed 9, St Louis, 2009, Mosby.

ies should be reviewed and communicated as appropriate (Box 18-2). An abnormal level of RBCs may signify dehydration, hypovolemia, or fluid overload (dilutional). An elevated white blood cell (WBC) count, indicating the presence of infection, may be related to inflammation, tissue necrosis, or immunocompromise. H&H values are also important to note. Caution is advised in evaluating an H&H drawn in the ED. The time delay between bleeding and a drop in the H&H value can be significant. It is only after hemodilution occurs (from shock compensation or crystalloid replacement) that hematocrit level drops. Frequently, abnormal values in the patient with blunt trauma alert the team to the possibility of internal bleeding.

BAL also assists the trauma team in their evaluation. If the patient's level is significantly high, the physical examination and response may be unreliable. In addition, the neurologic status of patients with high BALs is very difficult to assess. Abnormal clotting studies are of obvious significance in trauma patients. These results may be attributable to anticoagulant medication the patient is taking or the effects of profound hypothermia. Clotting times may also be prolonged in the presence of excessive alcohol ingestion or the use of anabolic steroids. Clotting times may decrease with the use of antihistamines and diuretics.

A blood type and screen shortens the time needed by the blood bank to obtain a crossmatch, if needed later. Most trauma centers have several units of type O–negative blood (universal donor) available in the event that a blood transfusion is required before a type and crossmatch (T&C) can be performed. Because of regional shortages of O-negative blood, O-positive blood can be used in male patients and adult female patients of non-childbearing age. Initially, trauma patients are fluid-resuscitated with warmed crystalloid solutions, such

as lactated Ringer's solution or normal saline solution. If the patient's blood pressure responds, the diagnostic examination continues. However, if the hypotension returns, blood transfusions may be initiated and the patient may be transported immediately to the OR for exploratory surgery.

Many trauma centers are implementing massive transfusion policies (MTP) for the clinical management of patients experiencing massive hemorrhage and to coordinate interdisciplinary and interdepartmental resources. Nessen and colleagues (2008) define massive transfusion as the replacement of one or more blood volumes within a 24-hour period, or 50% of estimated blood volume in 3 hours or less. This volume is approximately equal to the transfusion of 10 units of RBCs. Current research (Malone et al, 2006) suggests that improved patient outcomes are associated with the use of packed RBC/plasma/platelet ratios of 1:1:1. This simple ratio not only is easy to use but also has the benefit of administration of higher plasma and platelet volumes.

Diagnostic Procedures

RADIOLOGY. Depending on the trauma center protocol, a blunt trauma radiographic series may be part of the resuscitative phase. This minimally includes a lateral view of the cervical spine and an anteroposterior (AP) view of the chest. In addition, the patient also undergoes lateral thoracic and lumbar spine films and an AP view of the pelvis. Any area with deformity, swelling, or pain may also be examined by x-ray. Trauma patients are always treated as if they have a cervical spine injury until proven otherwise. When reviewing the cervical spine films for cervical spine injury clearance, the clinician should consider any existing factors that place the patient at high risk

EVIDENCE FOR PRACTICE

Assessing Neurovascular Status in Patients with Musculoskeletal Trauma

Trauma patients frequently present to the OR with fractures or other musculoskeletal injuries. A thorough assessment of the patient's neurovascular status is imperative to establish a baseline for nursing and surgical interventions.

ASSESSMENT TECHNIQUE	NORMAL FINDINGS
SKIN COLOR Inspect the skin distal to the injury.	There is no change in pigmentation compared with other parts of the body.
SKIN TEMPERATURE Palpate the area distal to the injury (the dorsum of the hands is the most sensitive to temperature).	The skin is warm.
MOVEMENT Ask the patient to move the affected area or the area distal to the injury (active motion). Move the area distal to the injury (passive motion).	The patient can move without discomfort. There is no difference in comfort compared with active movement.
SENSATION Ask the patient if numbness or tingling is present (paresthesia). Palpate with a paper clip (especially in the web space between the first and second toes or the web space between the thumb and forefinger).	There is no numbness or tingling. There is no difference in sensation in the affected and unaffected extremities. (Loss of sensation in these areas indicates perineal nerve or median nerve damage.)
PULSES Palpate the pulses distal to the injury.	Pulses are strong and easily palpated; there is no difference between the affected and unaffected extremities.
CAPILLARY REFILL (LEAST RELIABLE) Press the nailbeds distal to the injury until blanching occurs (or the skin near the nail if nails are thick and brittle).	Blood return (to usual color) is within 3 sec (5 sec for older people).
PAIN Ask the patient about the location, nature, and frequency of the pain.	Pain is usually localized and is often described as stabbing or throbbing. (Pain out of proportion to the injury and unrelieved by analgesics may indicate compartment syndrome.)

Modified from Murray CA: Interventions for clients with musculoskeletal trauma. In Ignatavicius DD, Workman ML, editors: *Medical-surgical nursing: patient-centered collaborative care*, ed 6, St Louis, 2010, Saunders.

for spine injury. These include age older than 65 years, a dangerous MOI, and paresthesias in the extremities. Patients with penetrating trauma injuries usually are transferred immediately to the OR for exploratory laparotomy.

If the resources are available, the trauma center protocol may also include a computerized tomography (CT) scan as a diagnostic or screening tool. Depending on the MOI, such as a fall, CT scans of the head and abdomen may be performed. Because injuries in blunt trauma are very difficult to diagnose, the CT scan is frequently done before patient transfer to the OR. A high index of suspicion is maintained for other injuries until proven otherwise. Bowel injuries may be missed during initial scanning. A CT scan of the brain revealing an injury incompatible with life may alter the course of definitive treatment for a patient.

A CT-angiogram may be indicated in diagnosis of vascular injuries. If the patient is hemodynamically stable, this test is of great value in determining the extent of the injury. It is particularly beneficial in the diagnosis of a ruptured thoracic aorta, in which extravasation of the dye at the area of aortic fixation to the chest wall is noted. Other uses include evaluation of penetrating wounds, especially in the extremity. Vessel injury can be noted and the need for surgical intervention determined.

OTHER DIAGNOSTIC TESTS. Cardiac monitoring is another component of the initial phase of trauma care and is particularly important in blunt trauma. Early detection of ventricular dysrhythmias may indicate a myocardial contusion, or bruising of the heart. An electrocardiogram (ECG) is obtained when indicated by the mechanism of injury or the patient's symptoms. Undiagnosed heart disease, as evidenced by an abnormal ECG, is noteworthy in a patient requiring operative intervention.

Focused assessment with sonography in trauma (FAST), used in the United States since the 1990s, may assist with diagnosis in difficult situations. FAST is a portable, noninvasive scan that can be used to determine the presence of free fluid in the chest or abdomen. The typical FAST scan consists of chest, pelvic, and four abdominal scans. The chest scan examines right and left chest views and can determine the presence of pericardial fluid. The upper right abdominal scan evaluates the hepatorenal area, the first area that shows the presence of air. The left upper scan examines the splenorenal area. The left and right paracolic gutters are also scanned. The pelvic scan assesses for free fluid near the bladder. FAST is also used in pregnant patients with blunt abdominal trauma; it is both faster and safer

BOX 18-2

Laboratory Values: Blood and Serum Electrolytes

RED BLOOD CELLS (ERYTHROCYTES)
RBC values vary, depending on age, gender, and geographic location (in relation to sea level) of the patient.

Normal Values

Children
Newborn	4.8-7.1 million/μl
2-8 wk	4-6 million/μl
2-6 mo	3.5-5.5 million/μl
6-12 mo	3.5-5.2 million/μl
1-6 yr	4-5.5 million/μl
6-18 yr	4-5.5 million/μl

Adults/Elderly
Male	4.7-6.1 million/μl
Female	4.2-5.4 million/μl
Pregnant female	Decreased

Abnormal Value	Probable Cause
↑	Dehydration
↓	Hypovolemia
	Fluid overload (dilutional)

WHITE BLOOD CELLS (LEUKOCYTES)
A WBC count is obtained to identify the presence of an infection.

Normal Value
5000-10,000/μl (elevated in pregnancy)

Abnormal Value	Probable Cause
>10,900/μl	Infection/inflammation
	Tissue necrosis
	Immunocompromise

HEMATOCRIT (HCT)
A hematocrit value is obtained to determine the percentage of RBCs in whole blood.

Normal Values

Children
Newborn	44%-64%
2-8 wk	39%-59%
2-6 mo	35%-50%
6-12 mo	29%-43%
1-6 yr	30%-40%
6-18 yr	3%-44%

Adult
Male	42%-52%
Female	37%-47%
Pregnant female	>33%

Abnormal Values in Trauma
↓	Hemodilution
	◆ From compensated hypovolemia
	◆ From excessive volume replacement
↑	Hemoconcentration

Note: When blood is lost acutely, the amount of hematocrit lost is in the same ratio as that of whole blood. Therefore the percentage of hematocrit in a whole blood sample would remain normal. It is only after hemodilution occurs (from shock compensation or crystalloid replacement) that the hematocrit value drops.

HEMOGLOBIN (HGB)
A hemoglobin value is obtained to measure the amount of hemoglobin in whole blood. The amount of hemoglobin determines the oxygen-carrying capacity of blood.

Normal Values

Children
Newborn	14-24 g/dl
0-2 wk	12-20 g/dl
2-6 mo	10-17 g/dl
1-6 yr	9.5-14 g/dl

Adult
Male	14-18 g/dl
Female	12-16 g/dl
Pregnant female	>11 g/dl
Elderly	Values slightly decreased

Note: When whole blood is lost acutely, the amount of hemoglobin that is lost is proportionate. It is only after hemodilution occurs (as a result of shock compensation or crystalloid volume replacement) that hemoglobin level drops.

PLATELETS (THROMBOCYTES)
A platelet count is obtained to test the amount of platelet function. Platelets play an essential role in coagulation. Particularly in vascular trauma, platelets are essential to hemostasis.

Normal Values
Newborn	150,000-300,000/μl
Infant	200,000-475,000/μl
Child	150,000-400,000/μl
Adult/elderly	150,000-400,000/μl

Abnormal Values	Probable Cause
↑	Splenectomy
	Living at high altitude
	Hemorrhage
↓	Disseminated intravascular coagulation

COAGULATION STUDIES: PROTHROMBIN TIME (PT, PRO TIME)
A prothrombin time is evaluated in trauma patients to measure clotting time (caused by factors I [fibrinogen], II [prothrombin], V, VII, and X). This is important in determining the blood's ability to clot.

Normal Value
11.0-12.5 sec

Abnormal Value	Probable Cause
↑	Deficiency of factors I (fibrinogen), II (prothrombin), V, VII, and X; 2.5× normal values means that there is a bleeding tendency.

Note: Clotting times may be prolonged in the presence of excessive alcohol ingestion or the use of anabolic steroids. Clotting times may decrease with the use of antihistamines and diuretics.

BOX 18-2

Laboratory Values: Blood and Serum Electrolytes—cont'd

COAGULATION STUDIES: ACTIVATED PARTIAL THROMBOPLASTIN TIME (APTT)

An APTT is obtained to screen for problems with intrinsic clotting factors (except factors VII and XIII). It can be used also to monitor the effectiveness of anticoagulation with heparin. This laboratory test measures the amount of time it takes for fibrin to form a clot. In the trauma patient it is used to determine the patient's tendency to bleed.

Normal Value
30-40 sec for the clot to form (after the clinical reagent is added)

Abnormal Value in Trauma	Possible Cause
>40 sec	Intrinsic factor deficiency

NOTE: Be sure to fill the laboratory tube completely because the tube contains anticoagulant and the ratio of blood to anticoagulant may be altered if the tube is not filled correctly, causing an inaccurate prolonged clotting time.

SERUM ELECTROLYTES: SODIUM (Na+)

Sodium is one of the two major extracellular cations. It is the major cause of osmotic pressure in extracellular fluid. Sodium also plays a major part in both acid-base balance and neuromuscular function.

Normal Value
136-145 mEq/L

Abnormal Values	Possible Cause
>145 mEq/L (hypernatremia)	↓ Fluid intake/fluid loss
	↑ Sodium intake
>136 mEq/L	↓ Sodium intake
	↑ Sodium loss

SERUM ELECTROLYTES: POTASSIUM (K+)

Because potassium is one of the two major cellular cations, it is essential for the maintenance of cellular osmosis. It plays a major role in the electrical conductivity of both cardiac and skeletal muscle. In addition, potassium plays a major role in both acid-base balance and kidney function.

Normal Value
3.5-5 mEq/L

Abnormal Values	Possible Cause
>5 mEq/L (hyperkalemia)	Major burns
	Renal failure
	Major crush injuries
<3.5 mEq/L (hypokalemia)	Hypovolemia

SERUM ELECTROLYTES: CHLORIDE (Cl−)

Measurement of serum chloride concentration is important for the assessment of acid-base status. Chloride is a major extracellular anion that plays a role in the maintenance of oncotic pressure and thus blood volume and arterial pressure.

Normal Value
98-106 mEq/L

Abnormal Values	Possible Cause
>106 mEq/L (hyperchloremia)	Dehydration
	Renal failure
	Central nervous system (CNS) trauma with central neurogenic breathing
<98 mEq/L (hypochloremia)	Excess vomiting
	Excess gastric suctioning

Modified from Pagana KD, Pagana TJ: *Mosby's diagnostic and laboratory test references,* ed 9, St Louis, 2009, Mosby.

than a computerized tomography (CT) scan, which is contraindicated in the pregnant patient because of the use of iodinated contrast medium and ionizing radiation (Cunningham, 2008).

Although FAST is useful in diagnosing free fluid, it cannot determine damage to solid organs; therefore it complements rather than replaces other imaging scans. Diagnostic peritoneal lavage (DPL) may be performed to determine the presence of abdominal injury. This tool is of particular benefit when evaluation of the abdomen is difficult, such as when the patient is intoxicated, unconscious, or hemodynamically unstable. DPL can be performed in the ED, OR, PACU, or ICU. Nonetheless, retroperitoneal blood may be missed with a DPL, whereas the FAST approach may be quicker and visualize more structures, even pericardium; it is also less expensive and noninvasive. Thus FAST may be used with patients who are unstable and need a quick approach without the risk of a false-positive tap (Table 18-2).

Internal compartment pressures may be measured with an injury to the extremity as well as to the abdomen. Swelling of the muscles below the fascia covering may compromise circulation and result in the eventual loss of the extremity because of tissue necrosis. This is known as *compartment syndrome*. There are multiple compartments in the lower extremity that may be affected (Figure 18-2). Surgeons may measure compartment

pressures with a manometer/stopcock/syringe or a commercial compartment pressure–measuring device. Normal compartmental pressures are less than 20 mm Hg. Pressures more than 30 mm Hg require a fasciotomy. Symptoms include severe pain, paresthesia, and a decrease in motor movement in the involved extremity, especially on passive movement (Table 18-3).

Massive intestinal edema may occur with trauma patients, causing compromise to internal organs and development of a different type of compartment syndrome. Abdominal compartment syndrome, also called abdominal hypertension, is characterized by increased intraabdominal pressure. Increased intraabdominal pressure (IAP) can have a negative impact on the respiratory, splanchnic, and cerebral functions. It contributes to sepsis or multiple organ failure seen in many trauma patients. Normal IAP is approximately 5 to 7 mm Hg; elevation to 25 mm Hg is often seen in patients with septic shock and correlates with high mortality (Vegar-Brozovic et al, 2008). IAP is graded from I to IV based on a 12 to >25 mm Hg scale. Adverse effects on organ function may be manifested as decreased cardiac output, oliguria, and hypoxia. Elevated intrathoracic pressure reduces left ventricular compliance, causing limitations in effective ventilation, often requiring ventilator support. Elevated IAP may cause an increase in intracranial pressure related to obstruction of cerebral venous blood out-

TABLE 18-2

Comparison of DPL, FAST, and CT Scans

Diagnostic Peritoneal Lavage (DPL) Documents Bleeding	Focused Assessment with Sonography in Trauma (FAST) Documents Fluid	Computed Tomography (CT Scan) Documents Organ Injury
ADVANTAGES		
Early diagnosis	Early diagnosis	Most specific to injury
Performed rapidly	Noninvasive	92% sensitive
98% sensitive	Performed rapidly	98% accurate
Detects bowel injury	86-97% accurate	
	Repeatable	
DISADVANTAGES		
Invasive	Operator dependent	Increased cost and time
Low specificity	Bowel gas and subcutaneous air distortion	Misses diaphragm, bowel, and some pancreatic injuries
Misses diaphragmatic and retroperitoneal injuries	Misses diaphragm, bowel, and pancreatic injuries	

Modified from Emergency Nurses Association (ENA): *Trauma nursing core course,* ed 6, Des Plaines, Ill, 2007, Author.

flow and increased intrathoracic and central venous pressure. Delay in treatment of IAP may lead to brain deterioration and damage.

Management involves a decompressive laparotomy. After a decompression, wound management is a priority. The swelling may render the abdomen difficult or impossible to close. If the abdomen is closed, intraabdominal pressure may rise to a level greater than 25 cm of H_2O, at which point it may lead to significant organ dysfunction (Kulaylat and Dayton, 2008). Intraabdominal pressure monitoring is accomplished with the use of a nasogastric tube in the stomach or a Foley catheter in the bladder. Simple water-column manometry is done at 2- to 4-hour intervals, although it is possible to connect a pressure transducer to a Foley catheter by way of the sampling port (Figure 18-3). By establishing a water column of urine in the Foley catheter with a clamp distal to the port, a pressure gradient is established. After zero-balancing the transducer, an 18-gauge needle is placed on the end of the pressure tubing and inserted into the sampling port. Using the pressure tubing and a 60-ml syringe, 50 to 60 ml of normal saline is then instilled into the Foley. On instillation of the saline, the waveform on the monitor is correlated to the existing bladder pressure. Normal intraabdominal pressure is zero or subatmospheric. A pressure of more than 25 cm of H_2O is considered diagnostic of abdominal compartment syndrome (Kulaylat and Dayton, 2008). Postoperatively, these patients are susceptible to fluid and heat loss. Continuous hemodynamic monitoring is essential in the critical care phase of treatment.

Admission Assessment. The perioperative team may not obtain information concerning the trauma patient until the patient arrives in the OR for surgical intervention. If the patient's condition permits, the perioperative team should obtain a brief, precise report from the ED that contains the following information: MOI, an AMPLE history (if available), condition on arrival (e.g., level of consciousness), availability of and prior administration of blood or blood products, spine clearance, injuries present, and any other pertinent information (e.g., family present, completion of secondary assessment). If the injury is life- or limb-threatening, implied

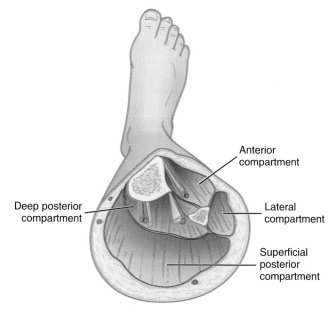

FIGURE 18-2 Compartments of the lower leg.

surgical consent is assumed (i.e., if the patient were able, consent would be given).

Additional data are collected as the patient is transported to the OR. The status of the airway, as well as breathing patterns and circulatory condition, can be observed. The ED record also provides information concerning amount and type of intravenous (IV) fluid received, vital signs, core temperature, and laboratory and other diagnostic examinations performed. A quick visual and physical survey of the patient when the circulator is preparing the patient for the procedure enables identification of other sites of injury that might require attention (Patient Safety).

The patient's psychologic status can also be assessed. If the patient is conscious, the perioperative team is challenged to allay fear and anxiety. The trauma patient has endured a

TABLE 18-3

Signs and Symptoms Associated with Compartmental Syndromes

Compartment	Location of Sensory Changes	Movement Weakened	Painful Passive Movement	Location of Pain or Tenseness
LOWER LEG				
Anterior	First web space	Toe extension	Toe flexion	Along lateral side of anterior tibia
Lateral	Dorsum (top) of foot	Foot eversion	Foot inversion	Lateral lower leg
Superficial posterior	None	Foot plantar flexion	Foot dorsiflexion	Calf
Deep posterior	Sole of foot	Toe flexion	Toe extension	Deep calf—palpable between Achilles' tendon and medial malleoli
FOREARM				
Volar	Volar (palmar) aspect of fingers	Wrist and finger flexion	Wrist and finger extension	Volar forearm
Dorsal	None	Wrist and finger extension	Wrist and finger flexion	Dorsal forearm
HAND				
Intraosseous	None	Finger adduction and abduction	Finger adduction and abduction	Between metacarpals on dorsum of hand

Modified from Matsen FA: *Compartmental syndromes,* available at www.orthop.washington.edu/faculty/matsen/compartmental. Accessed May 14, 2009.

very frightening experience and is in need of support. The circulator is often the best member of the surgical team to communicate with the patient and explain the interventions occurring before anesthesia induction. A touch or hand-hold is an important aspect of this communication process, demonstrating the circulator's caring behaviors and offering comfort.

Planning

Because of the unexpected nature of trauma, planning perioperative care is of the utmost importance. Equipment, instruments, and supplies that have a high probability of use must be immediately available. Autologous blood salvage units should also be considered during patient care preparation, because blood salvage will be done if not contraindicated by the nature of the injury.

Implementation

Multiple Operative Procedures. Depending on the severity of the injuries, the multiple trauma patient may require many surgical interventions. Some of these procedures may be performed simultaneously. This is determined through a collaborative effort among the surgeons, anesthesia provider, and perioperative team. If a patient has sustained severe head and abdominal trauma, a surgeon will need to place an intracranial pressure (ICP) monitoring device. However, the abdominal exploration is also emergently indicated. Consequently, the severe condition of the patient may require performance of both of these procedures at the same time

Multiple procedures, either simultaneously or in succession, require a great deal of preparation by the perioperative nurse, surgical technologist, and the trauma team. The order of procedures is determined by the presence or absence of life threats. The usual order of priority is chest, abdomen, head, and extremities. However, this priority is determined for each individual patient's situation and adjusted accordingly. Performance

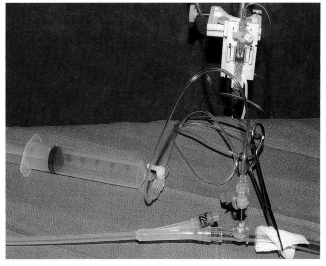

FIGURE 18-3 Setup for measuring abdominal compartment syndrome using a two-way Foley catheter and a pressure monitoring system.

of simultaneous procedures is preferable when physically possible. Anesthesia time is decreased for the critically ill patient, and definitive surgical interventions are accomplished more rapidly.

Increased Risk for Infection. Many trauma patients have wounds that are contaminated with roadside debris, dirt, grass, or automobile parts. Others have a perforated full stomach, and food particles are released into the peritoneum, increasing the risk of peritonitis. Consequently, many patients are at high risk for infection. Sterile technique may be compromised secondary only to immediate life threat. Pouring an antimicrobial solution across the surgical site may be the only surgical skin prep undertaken when an immediate life threat exists. The use of antimicrobial prophylaxis shortly before skin incision has become the standard of care for surgical procedures.

Wounds may need to be grossly decontaminated before the surgical skin prep. Sterile scrub brushes or a mechanical irrigation-under-pressure device may be used preoperatively and intraoperatively. Care must be exercised to remove as much contamination as possible, without creating further damage to the wound or body part. Perioperative personnel must wear personal protective equipment (PPE) during irrigation under pressure to prevent splashes and contamination from the lavage system. Traffic in the OR should be limited to essential personnel. Increased traffic in the room increases chances for contamination in an already compromised patient, as well as potentially interferes with the delivery of expedient care.

Procedure Preparation. Most level I trauma centers have a designated trauma OR that contains all equipment and supplies potentially needed for trauma patients. Many hospitals maintain an emergency abdominal procedure set, craniotomy procedure set, and chest procedure set either obtainable in the OR's sterile supply area or immediately available in the central supply department. This streamlines preparation for the surgical procedure and allows for the possibility of rapid preparation in those instances where the patient bypasses the emergency department on arrival and is transported directly to the OR.

Once the perioperative staff is notified of the surgical procedure, OR determination is made in consultation with the anesthesia provider and surgeon. Considerations include the following:

◆ Equipment required by the surgeon or surgeons to perform the surgical procedure
◆ Room availability
◆ Room size (to accommodate equipment, staff, and multiple procedures)
◆ Need for additional staff

◆ Capability for autologous blood salvage
◆ Availability of emergency procedure supplies (including power equipment)
◆ Selection of OR bed

Additional diagnostic procedures are often required during multiple trauma procedures. A fluoroscopic electric OR bed provides increased flexibility in patient management. The bed can be rotated on its base to facilitate two teams operating at once. The fluoroscopic capabilities allow for additional radiographs and arteriograms as needed. The bed should easily transform into different positions, such as lithotomy or lateral rotation. If a fluoroscopic bed is not available, arrangements must be made in advance to perform diagnostic radiologic procedures intraoperatively.

Before transfer of the patient to the OR bed, the perioperative team must ascertain if the spinal column has been cleared by the surgeon or attending physician as free from injury. If the spine has not been cleared, the surgeon must be consulted before removal of the patient from the backboard. Safe transfer of the patient from the transport vehicle to the OR bed can be accomplished using the log-rolling technique.

Positioning of the patient is based on the surgical approach. Ascertaining the type and location of the wound (anterior or posterior) and type of operative procedure dictates the patient's position. For example, an aortic injury may be approached through a thoracotomy or a median sternotomy incision. The thoracotomy requires lateral positioning devices, and the sternotomy necessitates a supine position.

If several procedures are being performed, positioning may change intraoperatively. Changing the anesthetized patient's position is accomplished under the supervision of the anesthesia provider, with particular attention to maintenance of the airway. The patient is moved slowly, allowing for assessment of

---

▼ PATIENT SAFETY

▽ Missed Injuries

The definition of a missed injury in trauma varies but is generally described as an injury not identified during the primary or secondary surveys or more than 24 hours after admission. Pfeifer and Pape (2008) identified patients with head injuries or a Glasgow Coma Scale score of 8 or less to be more likely to have a missed injury or delayed diagnosis. The literature review showed that the majority of errors occurred in the emergency department, intensive care unit, or OR. The injuries in the review were classified as minor, major, or life-threatening, with approximately 27% to 66% of missed injuries considered major and clinically significant (Pfeifer and Pape, 2008). The study also concluded that missed injuries result in significantly longer hospital stays and longer intensive care unit stays. Ekeh and colleagues (2008) studied diagnostic difficulties with blunt bowel and mesenteric injuries (BBMI) that cause delayed diagnoses even with computerized tomography (CT) scan, diagnostic peritoneal lavage, or FAST. They conclude that missed injuries are common in BBMI even with multislice CT capability.

Pfeifer and Pape (2008) reported that factors contributing to missed injuries include omission of radiographs of the specific

area of injury, misinterpreted x-rays, clinical inexperience, assessment errors, interrupted diagnoses, and neighboring injuries. Howard and colleagues (2006) included patient-specific factors such as altered level of consciousness, intoxication, or sedation to the possible cause of missed injuries. Howard and colleagues stated that the most commonly missed injuries were extremity fractures; they recommended increased focus on unconscious and/or intubated patients during the primary and secondary surveys. Howard and colleagues (2006) proposed the use of the tertiary survey to decrease the incidence of missed injuries. The tertiary survey, which includes a head-to-toe examination and review of all laboratory and radiologic studies, should be performed within 24 hours of admission. The conclusions of both studies call for adoption of the tertiary survey as the standard of care for all patients admitted to a level II trauma center. An unexpected outcome of the study by Howard and colleagues was the development of a culture of shared responsibility; nurses and therapists discovered injuries during their interactions with patients.

Modified from Ekeh AP et al: Diagnosis of blunt intestinal and mesenteric injury in the era of multidetector CT technology—are results better? *J Trauma* 65(2): 354-359, 2008; Howard J et al: Reducing missed injuries at a level II trauma center, *J Trauma Nurs* 13(3):89-95, 2006; Pfeifer R, Pape HC: Missed injuries in trauma patients: a literature review, *Patient Saf Surg,* 2008, available at www.pssjournal.com/content/2/1/20. Accessed May 16, 2009.

vital sign changes in response to the position movement. All precautions regarding positioning are reexecuted, with special attention given to the electrosurgical grounding pad. This pad may loosen during patient repositioning and require replacement to ensure adequate pad contact.

When the trauma patient is transferred to the OR, the extent of injury is not always known. The circulator should prep the patient from the suprasternal notch to the midthigh. This allows for rapid access to the chest to clamp the aorta should massive hemorrhage control be indicated; it also allows for exposure of the femoral arteries for potential cannulation and access to the thigh for harvesting a saphenous vein.

Established policies for counting sponges, instruments, and sharps should address surgical procedures of an emergent nature within the institution. Every attempt is made to verify appropriate numbers of counted items without compromising the timeliness of intervention in a life-threatening situation. If a preprocedural count is not performed, the circulator must document the occurrence and rationale used in accordance with established hospital policies and procedures. Some institutions require an x-ray examination postoperatively to examine the patient for the presence of a retained object. If counted sponges are intentionally left in the patient (e.g., in a damage control procedure at a level II, III, or IV center before transfer to a level I facility), the number and type of sponges left in the wound should be documented on the perioperative nursing record (AORN, 2009). The operative dictation by the surgeon should also verify the presence of retained sponges, their type, and their number. This allows for accurate counts in subsequent procedures and prevents the potential for an inadvertent retained sponge.

In the presence of clotting difficulties or specific types of organ injuries with continuous oozing of blood, the surgeon may elect to pack the surgical site with laparotomy sponges and close the patient as a temporary measure. After a period of 24 to 48 hours, the patient returns to the OR for removal of the laparotomy sponges and primary closure if possible. In such instances the perioperative nurse must document and record accurately the number of sponges used for packing, as just noted. When the sponges are removed, the exact number is verified and the sponges are isolated and contained in accordance with established hospital policy and procedure.

Autotransfusion. Considering the high blood loss associated with traumatic injuries, autotransfusion has become a vital asset in trauma care. Preoperative blood loss that is associated with an isolated hemothorax is collected in a designated chest-drainage device for reinfusion within 4 hours to avoid bacterial contamination. Intraoperative blood loss is collected, filtered, and reinfused to the patient. This provides immediate volume replacement, decreases the amount of bank blood used, and reduces the possibility of transfusion reactions or risk of transfusion with bloodborne pathogens.

The autologous blood salvage unit requires specialized training for operation. Institutional policies vary regarding appropriate personnel designated for operation of the equipment. Capabilities for autotransfusion should be considered during procedure preparation, since additional qualified personnel may be required.

During autologous blood salvage the surgical technologist squeezes out additional blood and fluid from saturated sponges before discarding them from the surgical field. The blood salvage suction is used whenever possible to maximize the amount of blood salvaged. However, care must be taken to ensure that the blood collected in the salvage unit is free from contamination. For instance, if the abdomen is contaminated with free food particles or colonic perforation is present, the blood cannot be used. Similarly, once antibiotic irrigation is initiated, the blood salvage unit is not used.

Evidence Preservation. If the injury to the patient is a result of a violent crime, the team must give special attention to preservation of evidence during the course of patient care. Physical evidence (e.g., bullets, bags of powder, weapons, pills, and other foreign objects), trace evidence (e.g., hair and fibers), biologic evidence (e.g., body fluids and blood), and clothing are considered types of evidence to be preserved. Specific procedures on handling of evidence may differ by institution and law enforcement agencies.

Clothing must be handled properly. When clothing is removed from the patient, the person removing it should cut along the seams or around the bullet or stab wound holes. The shape of the hole may help identify the weapon used. Clothing is placed in paper bags, labeled appropriately, and given to law enforcement personnel. Plastic bags trap moisture and may facilitate growth of mold, which could destroy evidence. The transport vehicle sheet should also be handled in a similar manner, since evidence may be present. The nurse must ensure that descriptions of wound appearances, body markings consistent with gang or cult activity, and statements from the patient are accurately recorded.

The chain of custody for all evidence, including clothing, is followed. This process allows for identification of all people handling the evidence. Documentation must verify that the evidence has been in secure possession at all times. Records should be kept of all evidence discovered, including its site of origin and when and to whom the evidence was given. A system of documentation using receipts or a specific form should be established to ensure appropriate compliance.

Gunpowder residues, tissue, hair, or other valuable information may be present on the hands of a trauma patient. This evidence can be preserved by placing the patient's hands in a paper bag and securing it with tape. Washing the hands should be avoided until evidence is collected, or until directed to do so by the police.

Bullets and retained implements offer valuable evidence and may assist in identifying the assailant. The weapon firing the bullet and the bullet itself can be matched by the specific grooves and markings placed on the bullet when the gun was fired. Most bullets are composed of soft lead, and handling with metal instruments can interfere with the markings. Therefore the surgeon should avoid using metal instruments to handle bullets. Some of the newer exploding types of bullets can present a risk to perioperative team members during wound exploration. Care should be exercised to avoid sterile glove tears, since these types of bullets are extremely sharp. Once a bullet is removed, the surgical technologist should place it in dry, clean gauze in a plastic specimen container and pass it off the sterile field to the perioperative nurse. Using the chain-of-custody procedures, the perioperative nurse should label the container appropriately and dispose of the bullet according to established institutional policies.

Deep Vein Thrombosis Prophylaxis. Because of the prolonged immobilization anticipated for the trauma patient, along with the frequency of orthopedic or lower extremity surgery, trauma patients are at high risk for developing venous thromboembolic events (VTE). Placement of a sequential compression device (SCD) preoperatively is ideal. These pneumatic compression devices assist in decreasing the possibility of deep vein thrombosis (DVT), and their effect is optimized when applied before surgical intervention. Preoperative placement is subject to the physician's preference; clinical research regarding similar devices and demonstrated product effectiveness is ongoing. The incidence of DVT and pulmonary embolism (PE) in trauma patients varies widely according to current literature. Meier and colleagues (2007) conducted a meta-analysis of trauma literature that estimated 11.8% of trauma patients develop a DVT and 1.5% develop a PE. The incidences are higher where there is severe head injury, pelvic fracture, and older age.

Currently, in patients with traumatic brain injury, the only recommended prophylaxis is SCD because of concerns with the use of heparin leading to bleeding complications. Subsequently, an inferior vena cava filter (VCF) may be inserted in high-risk patients to prevent pulmonary embolus. Risk factors for PE include prolonged immobility, multiple pelvic and lower extremity fractures, previous history of PE, severe head trauma, and incomplete spinal cord injury with paralysis. VCFs have success rates of 98% in preventing PE from lower extremity DVT (Meier et al, 2007). However, the placement of a VCF is associated with inferior vena cava obstruction and recurrent DVT. Contraindication to pharmacologic prophylaxis is generally limited to a short period after the initial trauma, and long-term vena cava filtration is rarely necessary (Research Highlight).

Anesthesia Implications. Depending on institutional protocol, the anesthesia team may be directly involved in resuscitation of the trauma patient immediately after arrival at the ED.

The anesthesia provider maintains the airway and intubates the patient if necessary. A critically injured patient may be transferred directly to the OR, whereas some interventions may be performed in the ED of a trauma center. These interventions vary from insertion of an ICP monitor to an emergent exploratory thoracotomy.

However, if diagnostic evaluation can be accomplished without intubation and sedation, the patient may be conscious upon arrival in the OR. A trauma patient is assumed to have a full stomach; thus these patients are at high risk for aspiration and resultant pneumonia. Under the direction of the anesthesia provider, the perioperative nurse applies cricoid pressure (Sellick maneuver) (Figure 18-4). This pressure is maintained over the cricoid area until the cuff on the endotracheal (ET) tube is inflated and tube placement verified by the anesthesia provider. This type of intubation is often referred to as a "crash induction."

In addition, the patient may require intubation for protection of the airway before radiologic examination of the cervical spine. If the cervical spine is not cleared or if the radiographic screening examination is not performed before intubation, ET intubation is done while cervical spine precautions (i.e., inline intubation) are maintained. The anesthesia provider may decide to use rapid-sequence intubation (RSI). RSI involves administration of 100% oxygen, an analgesic, and a neuromuscular relaxant; application of cricoid pressure; and insertion of a cuffed ET tube. Etomidate (Amidate) is the most commonly used induction agent (Emergency Nurses Association, 2007). It acts in about 1 minute and lasts about 5 minutes. It is often used in trauma patients because it does not cause an increase in ICP or worsening of hypotension. Succinylcholine (Anectine) is the most frequently used neuromuscular relaxant. The perioperative nurse can facilitate RSI by ensuring availability of all intubation and resuscitation equipment, assisting with monitoring devices, and confirming correct ET-tube placement (Box 18-3).

In injuries of the face where midface fractures are present, nasal intubation and nasogastric tube placement are avoided. Tube placement in the brain through a fracture of the cribriform plate is a well-known complication. To avoid this, oral

---

RESEARCH HIGHLIGHT

Early Placement of Optional Vena Cava Filters

Trauma patients are at increased risk for developing thromboembolic events such as deep vein thrombosis. Standard anticoagulant therapy may not be suitable for certain traumas, such as brain injuries. In this study, investigators evaluated 34 patients who had a prophylactic vena cava filter (VCF) implanted. Those included in the study were high-risk patients with contraindications to pharmacologic prophylaxis for more than 5 days because of traumatic brain injury. The OptEase VCF was used on all patients and was placed infrarenally. Of the patients, 27 (or 84%) had their filters retrieved with no related mortality. Five (16%) patients had VCFs that were permanently implanted. One patient developed early inferior vena cava occlusion and DVT occurred 14 days after VCF placement. One patient developed symptomatic pulmonary embolus 5 days after VCF retrieval. The researchers concluded that early VCF placement may benefit patients in whom pharmacologic intervention is contraindicated.

Modified from Meier C et al: Early placement of optional vena cava filter in high-risk patients with traumatic brain injury, *Eur J Trauma Emerg Surg* 33(4): 407-413, 2007.

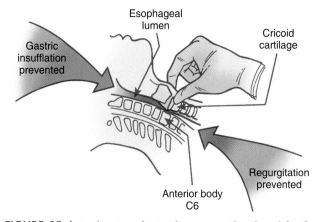

FIGURE 18-4 Application of cricoid pressure. Thumb and forefinger are used to depress cricoid cartilage, causing it to impinge on the lumen of esophagus and sealing it closed against the anterior body of C6. As a result, gastric insufflation secondary to positive-pressure ventilation (bag-valve-mask apparatus) from above, as well as regurgitation of stomach contents from below, is largely prevented. *C6,* Sixth cervical vertebra.

ET intubation is the technique of choice. The anesthesia provider places an oral gastric tube to achieve stomach decompression. An oral intubation on a conscious patient is often necessary because anesthetics and muscle relaxants can result in the loss of any remaining airway in the presence of facial trauma.

Large-bore IV access used with rapid-infusion fluid warmers may be employed in the ED. These fluid warmers can deliver high volumes of crystalloid solution at body temperature. Use of the fluid warmer may continue during the intraoperative phase to facilitate volume replacement and help maintain normothermia. A number of factors may influence a trauma patient's response to fluid loss. These factors include age, severity of injury, type and location of injury, time lapse from injury to treatment, prehospital fluid therapy, prehospital use of a pneumatic antishock garment, and medications taken for chronic conditions. Fluid resuscitation should be initiated when early signs of blood loss are suspected. A classification system can be useful in determining the needs of the patient (Table 18-4).

Pregnancy. The normal physiologic changes that occur during pregnancy increase the challenge of evaluation and treatment when these individuals are victims of trauma. Cusick and Tibbles (2007) note that while the incidence of trauma in pregnant patients is low, it is still the leading cause of obstetric mortality. A trend noticed in this study identified more severe abdominal injuries and less severe head injuries in the pregnant patient. It is most important to remember that two patients are being treated. The key to resuscitation of the fetus is to resuscitate the mother. One of the first physiologic changes to note is that the pregnant trauma patient has a much larger circulatory volume (Table 18-5). The cardiac output may be increased by as much as 40%. Oxygen requirements are increased. Heart rate increases over the pre-pregnant state. The usual clinical indicators of hypovolemic shock are unreliable in the pregnant trauma patient (Table 18-6). The team must assume that the pregnant trauma victim is in shock until proven otherwise. Early aggressive treatment is essential. The uterus is enlarged and no longer a pelvic organ, and it elevates the bladder out of the pelvis as well. Supine position for the pregnant patient can result in a decrease in cardiac output as a result of compression of the inferior vena cava. If the patient is close to term, cardiac output can be reduced by as much as 30% as a result of compression on the inferior vena cava. Consequently, patients who are 20 weeks or more into their pregnancy should be placed in the left lateral decubitus position to avoid a hypotensive episode and maintain blood flow to the uterus and placenta. If this is not possible, man-

BOX 18-3

Rapid-Sequence Intubation Steps

Preparation	Assist anesthesia care provider as needed. Ensure all equipment is available.
Preoxygenation	Administer 100% oxygen.
Pretreatment	Assist anesthesia care provider in medication administration, as indicated (atropine, lidocaine, etomidate).
Paralysis with induction	Anesthesia is induced (midazolam, fentanyl), patient loses consciousness, and neuromuscular agent is administered (succinylcholine).
Protection and positioning	Use Sellick maneuver to provide cricoid pressure. Must be applied continuously and until anesthesia care provider asks to have pressure released to avoid aspiration.
Placement with proof	Inflate cuff; check placement with exhaled carbon dioxide detector and by listening to lungs with stethoscope.
Postintubation management	Secure tube, verify ventilator settings, and monitor per routine.

Modified from Emergency Nurses Association (ENA): *Trauma nursing core course,* ed 6, Des Plaines, Ill, 2007, Author.

TABLE 18-4

Estimated Fluid and Blood Losses Based on Patient's Initial Presentation*

	Class I	Class II	Class III	Class IV
Blood loss (ml)	Up to 750	750-1500	1500-2000	>2000
Blood loss (% blood volume)	Up to 15%	15%-30%	30%-40%	>40%
Pulse rate (beats/min)	<100	>100	>120	>140
Blood pressure	Normal	Normal	Decreased	Decreased
Pulse pressure	Normal or increased	Decreased	Decreased	Decreased
Respiratory rate (breaths/min)	14-20	20-30	30-40	>35
Urine output (ml/hr)	>30	20-30	5-15	Negligible
Central nervous system (CNS)/ mental status	Slightly anxious	Mildly anxious	Anxious, confused	Confused, lethargic
Fluid replacement (3:1 rule)	Crystalloid	Crystalloid	Crystalloid and blood	Crystalloid and blood

*The guidelines are for a 70-kg man. They are based on the 3:1 rule. This rule derives from the empiric observation that most patients in hemorrhagic shock require as much as 300 ml of electrolyte solution for each 100 ml of blood loss. Applied blindly, these guidelines can result in excessive or inadequate fluid administration. For example, a patient with a crush injury to the extremity may have hypotension out of proportion to his or her blood loss and require fluids in excess of the 3:1 guidelines. In contrast, a patient whose ongoing blood loss is being replaced by blood transfusion requires less than 3:1. The use of bolus therapy with careful monitoring of the patient's response can moderate these extremes.
Modified from American College of Surgeons: *ATLS program for doctors,* ed 7, Chicago, Ill, 2004, Author; Boswell SA, Scalea TM: Initial management of traumatic shock. In McQuillan KA et al, editors: *Trauma nursing: from resuscitation through rehabilitation,* ed 4, St Louis, 2009, Saunders.

TABLE 18-5

Maternal Adaptation During Pregnancy and Relation to Trauma

System	Alteration	Clinical Responses
Respiratory	↑ Oxygen consumption	↑ Risk of acidosis
	↑ Tidal volume	↑ Risk of respiratory mismanagement
	↓ Functional residual capacity	↓ Blood-buffering capacity
	Chronic compensated alkalosis	
	↓ $Paco_2$	
	↓ Serum bicarbonate	
Cardiovascular	↑ Circulating volume, 1600 ml	Can lose 1000 ml of blood
	↑ Cardiac output	No signs of shock until blood loss >30% of total volume
	↑ Heart rate	↓ Placental perfusion in supine position
	↓ Systemic vascular resistance (SVR)	Point of maximal impulse, fourth intercostal space
	↓ Arterial blood pressure	Heart displaced upward to left
Renal	↑ Renal plasma flow	↑ Risk of stasis, infection
	Dilation of ureters and urethra	↑ Risk of bladder rupture
	Bladder displaced forward	
Gastrointestinal	↓ Gastric motility	↑ Risk of aspiration
	↑ Hydrochloric acid production	Passive regurgitation of stomach acids if head lower than stomach
	↓ Competency of gastroesophageal sphincter	
Reproductive	↑ Blood flow to organs	Source of ↑ blood loss
	Uterine enlargement	Vena caval compression in supine position
Musculoskeletal	Displacement of abdominal viscera	↑ Risk of injury, altered rebound response; altered pain referral
	Pelvic venous congestion	↑ Risk of pelvic fracture
	Cartilage softened	Center of gravity changed
Hematologic	Fetal head in pelvis	↑ Risk of fetal injury
	↑ Clotting factors	↑ Risk of thrombus formation
	↓ Fibrinolytic activity	

Modified from Dorman KF: Obstetric critical care. In Lowdermilk DL, Perry SE, editors: *Maternity & women's health care,* ed 9, St Louis, 2007, Mosby.

TABLE 18-6

Signs of Hypovolemic Shock in Pregnancy

	Circulating Blood Volume Deficit	
	Early (20%)	Late (25%)
Pulse rate	<100 beats/min	>100 beats/min
Respiratory rate	12-20 breaths/min	>20 breaths/min
Blood pressure	Normal	Hypotensive
Skin perfusion	Warm, dry skin	Cool, ashen skin
Capillary refill time	<2 sec	>2 sec
Level of consciousness	Alert	Agitated, lethargic
Urine output	>30-50 ml/hr	<30-50 ml/hr
Fetal heart rate (normally 120-160 beats/min)	High, low, late decelerations	High, low, absent, late decelerations

ual displacement of the uterus by lateral abdominal pressure should be attempted. As a result of the physiologic changes just described, the pregnant patient is at risk for aspiration. Rapid-sequence induction, along with the Sellick maneuver, is the preferred method for intubation.

Ultrasound studies are conducted to determine viability of the fetus when possible. In the event of a ruptured uterus, a cesarean delivery and hysterectomy may be required if the fetus is viable. Neonatal resuscitation is of the utmost importance immediately on delivery of the fetus.

Pregnant patients requiring surgery also need fetal assessment performed intraoperatively. Any fetal movement should be noted. In addition, fetal monitoring is continuous. This includes fetal heart rate and uterine contractions. Fetal monitoring provides information on the condition of the fetus and the response to uterine contractions, if present. Fetal heart rate can usually be obtained after 10 weeks of gestation. Abnormalities in fetal heart rate can be an early sign of maternal compromise because the pregnant uterus is viewed as a nonessential peripheral organ in states of hypovolemic shock. The study by Cusick and Tibbles (2007) also noted that the presence of disseminated intravascular coagulation (DIC) was associated with fetal mortality. Personnel qualified in the interpretation of fetal heart rate patterns must be present. This expertise may be provided by the obstetric nursing staff.

Perimortem (postmortem) cesarean delivery may be performed in the event of the sudden death of the mother and the presence of a viable fetus.

Pediatric Trauma Patients. Special considerations related to the care of infants and children who have sustained a trauma are described in Chapter 17. Table 17-4 details a modified Glasgow Coma Scale for children.

▶▶ RISK REDUCTION STRATEGIES

Special Considerations for the Bariatric Trauma Patient

Bariatric trauma patients (e.g., those weighing more than 350 pounds) present special challenges to the surgical team. Morbidly obese trauma patients have an eight times greater risk of dying from their injuries than patients who are of normal body weight (Szczensiak, 2009). Several strategies must be developed to reduce risk to the patient and the healthcare team. The facility should be cognizant of the needs of bariatric patients and have policies and protocols established to facilitate effective and safe care.

Once the OR is notified of the arrival of a bariatric trauma patient, the perioperative nurse and surgical technologist must consider the planned procedure and the availability of necessary equipment, including a bariatric OR bed, foot board, and side extensions as well as long surgical instruments. A large blood pressure cuff will also be necessary for accurate blood pressure monitoring so that hemodynamic changes are quickly observed and treated.

As with all trauma patients, airway maintenance is a prime consideration. The bariatric patient often has a history of sleep apnea and is unable to lie flat for any length of time. The nurse should pad the head of the OR bed so that the patient's head is elevated as much as possible. In addition, the nurse should be prepared to assist the anesthesia care provider with intubation and also ensure that the difficult airway cart is available. The bariatric trauma patient is at increased risk for aspiration. The nurse can assist with airway protection by performing the Sellick maneuver at the anesthesia provider's direction.

Protection from positioning injury is a critical risk reduction strategy that the surgical team should provide for the bariatric patient. Whenever feasible, it is best to have the patient move from the transport vehicle to the OR bed; if not, adequate personnel should be available to assist with the transfer and positioning so that both the patient and the surgical team can avoid injury. The increased adipose tissue of the bariatric patient does not protect the patient from pressure sores; the surgical team must pad all bony prominences and pressure points well. Pillows collapse easily under a heavy load, so foam supports should be used. Shear injury can easily occur; therefore the surgical team must check the patient's position and remove blankets or other materials under the patient if they are preventing a smooth surface.

All trauma patients are at increased risk for DVT. Bariatric patients have an even greater risk for developing this complication. The surgical team should obtain the appropriate size of stockings and compression sleeves; these must be placed carefully, without any folds.

Skin breakdown, tissue injury, and dermatitis between the obese patient's layers of adipose tissue are very common. The perioperative nurse must retract skin folds while prepping to ensure the area is clean and well-prepped. If a limb is to be prepped, help should be obtained; another person or a sling may be used. Because one leg is 16% of body weight, it may weigh as much as 62 pounds; if not held securely, the weight of the limb can cause knee or ankle dislocation.

Care must also be taken in the placement of the ESU dispersive pad. Because of the increased amount of adipose tissue, the surgical team may consider applying two dispersive pads to prevent the concentration of electrical current in a single area.

The bariatric trauma patient is at increased risk for retention of foreign bodies related to the size of the abdominal and other cavities. The perioperative nurse and surgical technologist must scrupulously count all sponges and instruments on the surgical field.

Modified from Bell S: Current issues and challenges in the management of bariatric patients, *J Wound Ostomy Continence Nurs* 32(6):386-391, 2005; Ide P et al: Perioperative nursing care of the bariatric surgical patient, *AORN J* 88(1):30-58, 2008; Muir M, Archer-Heese G: Essentials of a bariatric patient handling program, *Online J Issues Nurs* 14(1), 2009; Szczensiak SL: Trauma in the bariatric patient. In McQuillan KA et al, editors: *Trauma nursing: from resuscitation through rehabilitation*, ed 4, St Louis, 2009, Saunders.

Elderly Trauma Patients. As the number of adults older than 65 years continues to grow, so does the number of elderly patients requiring surgical intervention related to trauma. The physiologic effects of aging combined with the preinjury health status of many elderly patients significantly affect their ability to respond to initial treatment for traumatic injuries and subsequent surgical intervention. Consequently, the mortality for elderly trauma patients is significantly higher than that in younger patients with the same level of injury. Preexisting medical conditions, medication use, decreased physiologic reserves, and the physical and psychologic stress experienced during surgical interventions place elderly trauma victims at increased risk for perioperative complications (Plummer, 2009).

Bariatric Trauma Patients. There has been a notable increase in admissions of bariatric patients in all healthcare facilities. Bariatric medicine is defined as the care of the extremely obese patient, as measured by body mass index (BMI). The World Health Organization (WHO) defines obese as a BMI greater than 30 and severely obese as a BMI greater than 40 (Muir and Archer-Heese, 2009). The obese patient often has several co-morbid conditions, including cardiac disease, hypertension, respiratory disease, diabetes, osteoarthritis, and stress incontinence. Because of their size and their decreased self-esteem the needs of bariatric patients are different from those of other patients. Societal prejudice against obesity is well established. Studies show that healthcare providers are often less attentive to the needs of the obese patient and are often worried about the possibility of personal injury related to positioning the patient. Sharma (2005) states that diagnosis can be very difficult in the absence of routine symptoms; CT and MRI scans are often not possible because of the limitations of the equipment. The use of ultrasonography may be limited because of distortion caused by the thickness of the abdominal wall. There are many strategies that the surgical team may use to decrease risk for this patient group (Risk Reduction Strategies).

Invasive Emergency Department Interventions. If a patient has shown a very recent deterioration of vital signs, either en route to the hospital or on arrival at the ED, the surgeon may elect to perform an emergency thoracotomy in the ED. A left-sided approach is usually performed because this allows rapid access to the heart for external cardiac massage and exposure of the great vessels for clamping in the event of severe blood loss (Figure 18-5). The incision can be extended

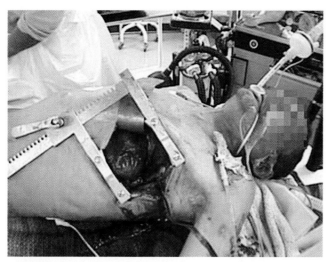

FIGURE 18-5 Emergency exploratory thoracotomy performed in the emergency department.

to the right side by cutting across the sternum. This procedure can be used to gain control in hemorrhage of the great vessels, to access the heart, or, in a grave situation, as a final effort to save a life. The procedure is used more often in penetrating injuries where a laceration to a ventricle or other potentially treatable, life-threatening injury may be present.

In some facilities, perioperative nurses may assist the rapid response team in this role (Rapid Response Team box). Rapid access to the heart and great vessels is the goal. The patient is then transported to the OR for additional interventions once hemorrhage is controlled.

In a similar fashion, an exploratory laparotomy can be initiated in the ED to control abdominal hemorrhage, especially when a splenic rupture is suspected and the patient is severely compromised.

If all other techniques of airway access are unsuccessful, the surgeon performs a cricothyrotomy. The surgeon makes a vertical incision through the skin, and incises the cricothyroid membrane. An ET or tracheostomy tube can be inserted through the membrane to create an airway. In the event a tube is not immediately available, a large-bore needle can be inserted into the membrane and the catheter left in place. This provides a temporary airway access measure but is inadequate to effectively ventilate the patient without a jet oscillating ventilator.

Successive Surgical Interventions. Often the multiple trauma patient requires a multitude of surgical procedures— either specialty-related or as a stepwise progression in the primary treatment of the initial injury. Initially the trauma patient is critically ill and requires intensive care facilities. When surgery is scheduled, the perioperative team may need additional assistance in transport of the patient as transport monitoring of the ECG, arterial line, and blood pressure is performed. Oxygen administration and mechanical ventilation with an Ambu bag are necessary for the intubated patient. Acalculous cholecystitis is often a secondary complication of the trauma patient's postoperative course that requires cholecystectomy. Fixation of initially undiscovered fractures, debridements, secondary wound closures, flap constructions, and other reconstructive procedures make up the majority of follow-up procedures. Depending on the patient's condition, some procedures may be performed after discharge on an outpatient basis.

Postoperative Management

If the patient sustained numerous injuries and remains critically injured, the PACU may be bypassed and the patient may be transferred directly to the ICU. The perioperative nurse should accompany the patient, along with the anesthesia provider, to the ICU. At this point, family members may have been contacted or are present, allowing more specific medical history information to be obtained. However, the mechanism of injury and events surrounding the trauma are still significant. A high index of suspicion remains during postoperative care of the patient sustaining multiple injuries. Attention can be diverted from a less significant injury in the presence of a highly visible or obvious trauma. Once the obvious trauma undergoes intervention, pain or discomfort from other injuries becomes more apparent. In the care of a patient with neurologic deficit, physical assessment and continued evaluation are essential because patient self-report is nonexistent.

The circulator should also report the status of progress in the secondary assessment. Any additional laboratory work or interventions that have yet to be completed should be discussed. It is imperative in a thorough examination to view the back of the patient in an effort to locate all injuries.

Additional diagnostic procedures may be required after completion of the surgical procedure if the patient's condition is stable. The perioperative nurse may be requested to accompany the patient to the diagnostic department with the anesthesia provider. In addition, respiratory care personnel may assist in patient transport and maintenance of the airway.

End-of-Life Care

Unfortunately, some accidental injuries result in death. Many facilities have a chaplain or social worker available to assist family members during this time of crisis. These caregivers assist in the initial family contact and provide immediate support. Providing end-of-life care for patients and family is relevant, even in trauma situations. Trauma is different in that the patient and family do not have a prior relationship with the healthcare team. This makes it difficult for the team to know and/or understand the wishes and values of the patient and family. Jacobs and colleagues (2005) believed that there was a need to develop guidelines for end-of-life care that incorporates aspects of trauma into a model. The American Trauma Society (ATS) sponsored a Trauma Leadership Forum (TLF) to identify specific problems related to trauma and end-of-life issues. A result of one of the forums was TELOS (Trauma End-of-Life Optimum Support), the primary goal of which is to standardize care given to trauma victims and their families from incident through the dying process. Healthcare professionals are obligated to support healthy survival as well as peaceful dying. According to Jacobs and colleagues (2005), "Even if the healing for certain patients is death, the dying process leading to ultimate healing, ought to be supported with compassion, care, comfort, and respect." This standard prompts the healthcare team, from the ED through the OR, to support the patient and family with honesty and truthfulness.

RAPID RESPONSE TEAM

The Ohio State University Medical Center (OSUMC) conducted a 2-week trial of the in-house "stat" nurse position. Nurses accepted into this position need prior experience in critical care with a demonstrated ability for critical thinking. At OSUMC the role of the stat nurse includes assisting with patient transport to and from diagnostic tests, helping nurses perform difficult intravenous starts, responding to cardiac arrest and trauma calls, assisting with procedural sedation, and serving as a clinical resource for staff. The stat nurse, typically a non–emergency department (ED) professional, rarely takes the lead in patient care but rather acts as an assistant to the ED nurse. In a trauma situation, the stat nurse serves as an extra hand by setting up needed equipment, transporting blood specimens to the laboratory, and comforting family members as needed. The ability to provide an experienced critical care nurse in the trauma setting has had a positive impact on both patient care and staff morale.

Modified from Sinclair TD: The role of the rapid response nurse: hospital wide and in trauma resuscitations, *J Trauma Nurs* 13(4):175-177, 2006.

Critical Incident–Stress Debriefing

When the end result of a traumatic injury is death, it can be particularly difficult for the perioperative team, since most surgical interventions are of a curative or restorative nature. In many emergency medical systems, a critical incident–stress debriefing team exists. It is composed of mental health professionals and specially trained volunteers who are also professionals and peers in the healthcare field. Police officers, firefighters, paramedics, ED nurses, and ICU nurses may also be on the team. In the event of a particularly tragic death of a patient, the team can be contacted, and a meeting with that patient's care providers is arranged. The benefit of this team is enhanced when intervention is timely for the care providers. Opportunity for them to discuss their feelings and emotions is provided and encouraged as each provider discusses feelings related to personal participation in the care of the patient. Gray and Litz (2005) emphasize that critical incident–stress debriefing teams enhance coping mechanisms and can provide a healthy professional growth from what may otherwise be considered a tragedy.

Surgical Interventions

DAMAGE CONTROL SURGERY

Damage control surgery is a well-recognized surgical strategy that sacrifices complete, immediate repair to adequately address the physiologic impact of trauma and surgery. Damage control surgery is a series of operations performed to accomplish definitive repair of abdominal injuries with consideration of the patient's physiologic tolerance. The focus is on control of hemorrhage and contamination to stop bleeding and control any intestinal, biliary, or urinary leak into the abdominal cavity. Indications for the potential need for damage control surgery include hemodynamic instability, hemorrhagic shock, coagulopathy, hypotension, tachycardia, tachypnea, inaccessible major anatomic injury, concomitant major injury, and altered mental status.

Abdominal packing is the foundation principle of damage control surgery, first reported in the early twentieth century. Later reports detailed survival of patients with severe liver injuries that were packed. In 1981 a report described operative management that included initial abandonment of laparotomy, use of intraabdominal packing, correction of coagulopathy and metabolic acidosis, and later reoperation for definitive repair (Germanos et al, 2008). The term "damage control" was first used in 1993 along with a detailed approach. The components are stop bleeding, close perforations; continue resuscitation, emphasizing correction of coagulopathy, acidosis, and hypothermia; plan reoperation for definitive repair.

There are five decision-making stages for damage control.

◆ *Stage 1*—Patient selection and decision to perform damage control: The emphasis is on early recognition for potential damage control surgery, including rapid transport to the hospital and early decisions related to control of hemorrhage.

◆ *Stage 2*—Operation and intraoperative reassessment of laparotomy: This consists of control of hemorrhage and contamination with rapid packing and temporary abdominal closure.

◆ *Stage 3*—Physiologic restoration in the intensive care unit: The focus here is restoration of physiologic status, which may include rewarming and fluid replacement.

◆ *Stage 4*—Return to OR for definitive procedures: The focus is on removal of packing, repair of injuries, and closure. Indications for emergency reoperation include massive ongoing bleeding, evidence of bowel leak or ischemic organ, and presence of abdominal compartment syndrome.

◆ *Stage 5*—Abdominal wall closure/reconstruction: It is not always possible to close the abdominal wall in stage 4, necessitating further repair.

INJURIES OF THE HEAD AND SPINAL COLUMN

Trauma to the head is responsible for half of all trauma deaths. Brain injury occurs either as a direct result of the trauma to the tissue or as a complication. Often, forces of energy from the impact are tolerated by the rigid skull, but the soft tissue of the brain is traumatized, resulting in the formation of subdural (Figure 18-6), epidural, or intracerebral hematomas. Blood clots are classified by their location in the brain and range from mild to life-threatening. A clot under the skull but on top of the dura is an epidural hematoma, which often results from a tear in an artery under the skull. A clot under the skull and dura but outside the brain is a subdural hematoma, often resulting from a tear in a vein or from a cut on the brain itself. An injury to the brain itself, a contusion, is an intracerebral hematoma, a result of a skull fracture or other blood clot causing swelling inside the brain. In addition, cerebral swelling can result in herniation of the brain despite treatment (Figure 18-7).

A baseline neurologic examination is extremely important. The pupils are examined, and the presence or absence of posturing is noted. The Glasgow Coma Scale provides a universally accepted mechanism to assess the baseline data for the trauma

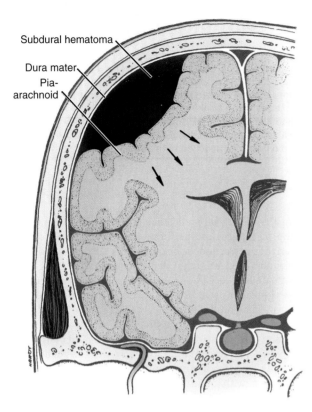

FIGURE 18-6 Subdural hematoma causing increased intracranial pressure with shifting of tissue.

team. However, in the presence of alcohol or drug intoxication or chemical paralysis, the scale cannot be used. For patients with a score of 8 or less, intubation with controlled ventilation is the immediate treatment of choice. In the highly combative patient, intubation may also be performed to allow adequate assessment of the extent of injury.

Previously, ICP hyperventilation was routinely used to decrease ICP in the initial management of patients with neurologic deterioration. No studies have shown improved outcomes for these patients, and other methods of assessment have shown that hyperventilation can cause significant constriction of cerebral vessels and may reduce cerebral blood flow to an ischemic level. One study has shown long-term improvement when hyperventilation was not used. Occasionally, hyperventilation may be necessary with persistently high ICP unresponsive to other treatment modalities.

An osmotic diuretic, such as mannitol, can be used in the treatment of ICP. Osmotic effects take place in 15 to 30 minutes (Hodgson and Kizior, 2009) and instigate an osmotic gradient to extract water from neurons. Osmotic diuretics such as mannitol have proven benefits in lowering ICP without reducing cerebral blood flow. They are given by bolus administration to create an acute reduction phase in ICP. These agents are excreted in the urine and cause a rise in serum and urine osmolality. Patients with serum osmolalities higher than 320 mOsm/kg (Kulaylat and Dayton, 2008) are at risk of acute tubular necrosis. Hypovolemia should be avoided with the infusion of isotonic fluids as necessary. Because such agents act quickly, fluid intake and output and the potential for fluid and electrolyte imbalances mandate close hemodynamic monitoring (Surgical Pharmacology). Elevating the head of the bed 30 degrees and keeping the patient's head midline (to promote venous drainage) can also be beneficial.

Skull fractures usually do not require operative intervention when there is no displacement and the fracture is linear.

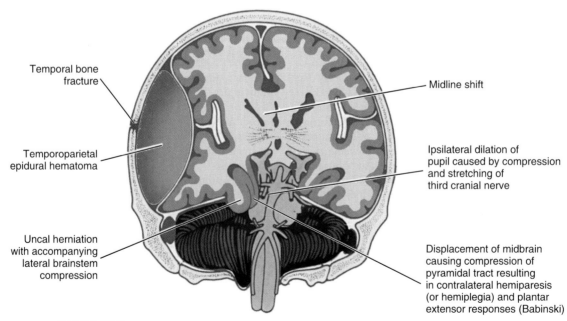

FIGURE 18-7 Cross section showing herniation of lower portion of temporal lobe (uncus) through tentorium caused by temporoparietal epidural hematoma. Herniation may occur also in cerebellum. Note mass effect and midline shift.

Depressed fractures or the presence of bone in the brain frequently requires elevation and debridement (Figure 18-8). Hematoma evacuation is based on its location as well as the size and number of hematomas present. Before performing a craniotomy or drilling a burr hole, the CT scan, the neurologic status of the patient, the morbidity or mortality associated with the procedure, and the presence of other injuries or underlying medical problems, if known, are evaluated. An ICP monitor may be placed in the patient who is at risk for increased ICP. Chapter 12 discusses neurosurgical procedures.

The patient with a cervical spine injury at or near C3 to C5 is at great risk for respiratory difficulties because this is the area of diaphragmatic innervation. There is also the possibility of swelling above the area of injury, and the surgical team should be alert for the potential of respiratory distress even if it is not initially present. A 24- to 48-hour dose of methylprednisolone (Solu-Medrol), calculated by body weight, is considered to decrease initial cord swelling.

The standard indicators of possible cord injury are absence of rectal tone and bradycardia in the presence of hypotension. The body's normal response is to increase heart rate in the presence of decreased blood flow or hypotension. These responses are not present in injury of the spinal cord, and vagal control results in bradycardia.

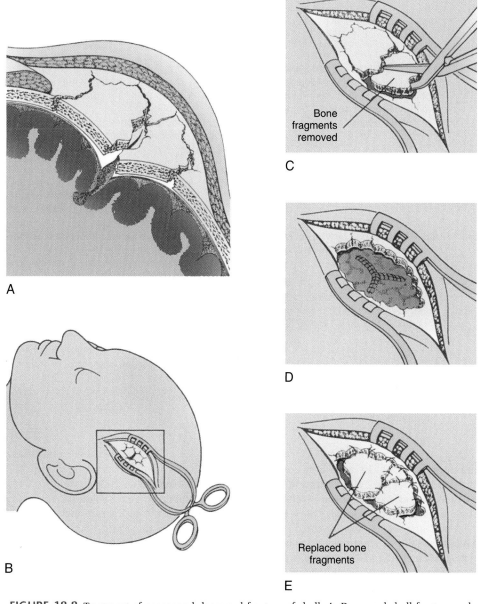

FIGURE 18-8 Treatment of compound depressed fracture of skull. **A**, Depressed skull fracture and scalp injury. **B**, Incision to expose fracture and remove the portion of the scalp that is devitalized. **C**, Removal of impacted bone by burr hole to locate and identify normal dura, followed by resection of bone fragments. **D**, Watertight closure of dura after brain debridement. **E**, Replacement and fixation of bone fragments.

SURGICAL PHARMACOLOGY

Commonly Used Medications and Head Trauma

Trauma patients may have situations arise with the diagnosis of head trauma that require immediate attention at the scene, in the emergency department, and in the OR and ICU. With injury to the brain, swelling may occur quickly, requiring a host of aggressive decisions to manage increasing intracranial pressure (ICP). Increased ICP may result in changes in the patient's stability that make survival a priority, including instituting mechanical ventilation, monitoring intraventricular stability, and administering medications necessary to maintain hemodynamic stability. Familiarity with the medications frequently used with head trauma patients is vital.

Medication	Usual Dosage	Rationale for Use
BENZODIAZEPINES		
Midazolam (Versed)	0.05-0.1 mg/kg IV, may be repeated prn, not to exceed 6 mg for infants or 10 mg for children	Use for sedation with patients having increased ICP, especially if on mechanical ventilation Adverse reactions can occur if patient not ventilated
Lorazepam (Ativan)	*Adult:* 4 mg/kg IV over 2-5 min, repeat in 10-15 min prn, not to exceed 8 mg/12 hr *Pediatric:* 0.05-0.1 mg/kg IV over 2-5 min, may be repeated in 10-15 min	Long-acting benzodiazepine; used as anticonvulsant for immediate control of seizure activity
ANTICONVULSANTS		
Phenytoin (Dilantin)	*Adult:* Loading dose for status epilepticus: 15-20 mg/kg IV once or in divided doses, followed by 100-150 mg dose at 30-min intervals *Pediatric:* Loading dose 15-20 mg/kg IV once or in divided doses	Prophylactic measure for patients at increased risk for seizure activity following head trauma May act on motor cortex to inhibit spread of seizure activity Preferred to phenobarbital because it does not cause as much CNS depression
DIURETICS		
Furosemide (Lasix)	*Adult:* 20-80 mg IV; may increase dose, not to exceed 600 mg/day *Pediatric:* 1-2 mg/kg IV every 6-12 hr	Loop diuretic helpful in decreasing ICP Influences CSF formation by affecting sodium-water movement across blood-brain barrier and shows preferential excretion of water over solute in distal tubule
Mannitol (Osmitrol)	*Adult:* 1.5-2 g/kg IV as 20% solution over 30 min *Pediatric:* 0.5-1 g/kg IV initial dose; 0.25-0.5 mg/kg IV every 4-6 hr	Osmotic diuretic that lowers blood viscosity and produces cerebral vasoconstriction with normal cerebral blood flow; ICP decrease occurs subsequent to decrease in cerebral blood volume
BARBITURATES		
Thiopental (Pentothal sodium)	*Adult:* 75-250 mg/kg IV; repeat prn *Pediatric:* Induction 4-7 mg/kg IV	Use as an adjunct in management of elevated ICP Facilitates transmission of impulses from thalamus to cortex of brain, resulting in imbalance in central inhibitory and facilitatory mechanisms
Phenobarbital (Luminal)	*Adult:* 300-800 mg followed by 120-240 mg/kg IV at 20-min intervals until seizures controlled or total dose of 1-2 g administered *Pediatric:* Loading dose 15-20 mg/kg IV in single or divided doses	Adjunct for seizure control in patients with head trauma

Injuries involving the spinal cord can range from complete transection, without hope of recovery, to a contusion of the cord. Fractures or dislocation of a vertebra can result in the protrusion of small pieces into the spinal canal. This is known as a *burst fracture.* Several vertebrae may be fractured or have fractured components. Generally, in compression fractures, if the loss of vertebral height is more than 20%, surgical treatment may be indicated. Spinal bracing can be considered an option if the compression is less than 20% and no neurologic signs or symptoms are present. Cerebral arteriography may be used to screen patients with cervical vertebral fractures for blunt vertebral artery injuries (BVIs). Patients who sustain blunt trauma with unilateral headache or posterior neck pain, particularly if it is sharp, sudden, and severe, should be screened for BVIs

and treated with anticoagulant therapy if not contraindicated (Inamasu and Guiot, 2006).

Treatment of spinal column fractures can involve surgery. Stabilization of the fracture may be necessary, depending on the severity of the injury. For cervical spine fractures, traction may be used initially to reduce the fracture, followed by surgical intervention as soon as the patient's condition permits. Internal fixation devices are discussed in Chapter 11.

INJURIES OF THE FACE

Motor vehicle crashes account for about 60% of maxillofacial injuries. Mandibular fractures alone are highly associated with assault as the MOI. In the patient who presents with facial

SURGICAL PHARMACOLOGY

Commonly Used Medications and Head Trauma—cont'd

Medication	Usual Dosage	Rationale for Use
NEUROMUSCULAR BLOCKERS		
Vecuronium (Norcuron)	*Adult:* 0.1 mg/kg IV *Pediatric:* Loading dose 0.08-0.1 mg/kg IV	Therapy directed at controlling ICP with multiple medications, including neuromuscular blockers Used as adjunct to sedative or hypnotic agent Facilitates endotracheal intubation and mechanical ventilation
Cisatracurium (Nimbex)	*Adult:* 0.10-0.2 mg/kg bolus; maintain at 2.5-3 mcg/kg/min *Pediatric:* 1 yr-23 mo: 0.15 mg/kg over 5-10 sec 2 yr-12 yr: .1-.15 mg/kg over 5-10 sec Infusion 3 mcg/kg/min; may titrate to 2 mcg/kg/min	Used for control of refractory ICP, mechanical ventilation, and ease of endotracheal intubation Used as adjunct to sedative or hypnotic agent
SEDATIVE/HYPNOTIC/ AMNESIC		
Propofol (Diprivan)	100-200 mcg/kg/min *For general anesthesia:* *Adult:* 5 mcg/kg/min IV infusion for 5 min; titrate in 5-10 mcg/kg/min increments for desired sedation. Maintain at 5-50 mcg/kg/min or possibly higher	Sedation for mechanically ventilated patient; titrated to achieve desired level of sedation Short-acting agent used for induction of general anesthesia; provides no analgesia

Modified from Association of periOperative Registered Nurses: *AORN drug information handbook for perioperative nursing,* Denver, 2006, AORN Lexi-Comp; Hodgson BB, Kizior RJ: *Saunder's nursing drug handbook,* St Louis, 2009, Saunders.

injury, the airway must be secured. This requires ensuring patency and removing any items that pose the threat of aspiration. If a midface fracture is present, the anesthesia provider avoids nasogastric tube placement and nasotracheal intubation. A tracheostomy may need to be performed before initiation of the operative procedure. Control of scalp or facial hemorrhage can be achieved through a pressure dressing until surgical intervention is possible, since exsanguinations can occur. Treatment of the fracture may be delayed until the immediate life threats have been successfully managed. Goals of operative intervention are to reduce and immobilize the fracture, prevent infection, and restore facial cosmesis and function.

Facial fractures can be categorized into Le Fort I, II, or III (Figure 18-9). A Le Fort I fracture is the most common maxillary fracture. It involves a horizontal interruption of the anterior and lateral wall of the maxillary sinus. Le Fort II is a pyramidal fracture along the maxilla and lacrimal bones and through the infraorbital rim. Le Fort III is otherwise known as *craniofacial disjunction.* The midface is completely disengaged from the cranial base, resulting from a fracture across the frontomaxillary sutures. Specific information regarding these injuries is in Chapter 13.

INJURIES OF THE EYE

Injuries to the eye can result from blunt or penetrating types of trauma. Penetrating objects in the globe are stabilized and not removed until the patient is in the OR. These injuries threaten loss of vision because of the injury itself, inflammation, or infection. Blunt injury to the eye can result in hematomas and accompanying fractures. A blow-out fracture is the result of a blunt force to the eye that pushes soft tissue through the thin bony orbital floor. The patient has recession of the eye into the

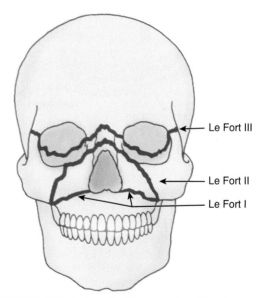

FIGURE 18-9 Le Fort classification of maxillary fractures.

orbit and loses the ability to gaze upward. Surgical repair is often indicated. Chapter 9 discusses ophthalmic procedures.

INJURIES OF THE NECK

Injury to the neck and soft tissue structures is most commonly a result of penetrating trauma. The neck can be divided into three zones with respect to injury and consequence. Zone I is the base of the neck below the clavicles. Anatomic structures located in this region are the great vessels and aortic arch, innominate veins, trachea, esophagus, and lungs. Zone II is the area in the middle of the neck between the clavicles and the mandible. Structures located in this area include the carotid artery, internal jugular vein, trachea, and esophagus. Zone III is located between the angle of the mandible and the base of the skull. The primary target of evaluation in these injuries is vascular structures.

Zone II injuries may necessitate an otorhinolaryngology specialist. Penetrating injuries to the larynx and trachea can be primarily repaired. Blunt force to the larynx can result in a fracture and impose immediate airway obstruction. These patients require immediate tracheotomy followed by repair of the fracture when it is unstable or displaced. Chapter 10 provides specific information concerning otorhinolaryngologic procedures.

INJURIES OF THE CHEST AND HEART

Trauma to the chest area is the primary cause of death in approximately 25% of trauma victims. Blunt trauma is most often associated with high-speed motor vehicle crashes. Penetrating traumas may be associated with violent crimes. Penetrating injuries at or immediately below the nipple line or level of the scapular tips are evaluated for both chest and abdominal involvement. Diaphragmatic injury is also a possibility.

Deceleration injury, such as that occurring from a fall or from striking the steering wheel in a motor vehicle crash, may cause contusions of the chest wall, fractures of the ribs or sternum, contusions of the heart or lungs, or rupture of the aorta

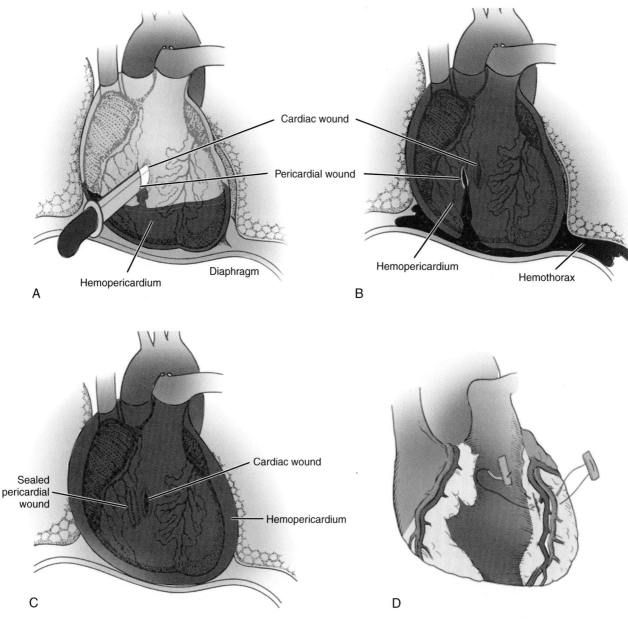

FIGURE 18-10 A, Cardiac injury with pericardial disruption. **B,** Bleeding from heart through pericardial tear into pleural space. **C,** Self-sealing of pericardial wound resulting in pericardial tamponade. **D,** Sutured cardiac wound with the use of pledgets.

and other major vessels. Rib fractures are also associated with a hemothorax or pneumothorax. A flail-chest segment may result when two or more adjacent ribs are broken in two or more places. This results in paradoxical chest wall movement as a result of loss of bony support; that is, the affected segment of the chest wall will move in the opposite direction. If respiratory distress and diminished breath sounds are present, a chest tube is indicated immediately; an autotransfusion chest drainage device is also considered. Chest tube output must be closely monitored intraoperatively because accumulation of 1000 to 1500 ml of blood is an indication for chest exploration. Penetrating wounds, as a result of either gunshot or stab injuries, may cause hemothorax and pneumothorax as well. Lacerations or perforation of the lung, heart, great vessels, trachea, esophagus, and bronchus is possible.

Myocardial contusion usually involves the right ventricle and can be evidenced by dysrhythmias on patient arrival or shortly thereafter. The patient is monitored on a telemetry unit, and surgical intervention is not required. Rupture of a heart valve can occur, depending on the timing of the contusion in relation to the phase of the cardiac cycle. If valve rupture has occurred, surgical repair is necessary. Heart sounds should be evaluated during the secondary assessment to document the presence or absence of murmurs. Heart valve rupture can occur as a late complication of myocardial contusion. Pericardiocentesis is performed for signs and symptoms of pericardial tamponade (Figure 18-10), which include jugular venous distention, muffled heart sounds, and a narrowing pulse pressure. Patients may present to the OR for a pericardial window either emergently or during the recovery phase.

An emergency thoracotomy may be indicated in the patient with penetrating trauma to the chest in full arrest or pulseless electrical activity on ECG. If a laceration to the heart is suspected and the patient is rapidly deteriorating, a thoracotomy may be performed in the ED. The laceration may be primarily repaired and the patient transferred to the OR for irrigation, wound debridement, and closure. Otherwise, surgical intervention is initiated in the OR. Wounds located across the mediastinum accompanied by hemodynamic instability, massive penetrating lung injuries, and disruption of the trachea, bronchus, or esophagus also require surgical intervention. Rupture of the thoracic aorta is another injury requiring surgical intervention and includes the use of extracorporeal bypass. This injury is an obvious life threat but may be difficult to diagnose. An arch aortogram is indicated in trauma patients who may have sustained such an injury. Rupture of the thoracic arch is associated with first rib or sternal fractures. Chapters 14 and 16 provide additional information about associated surgical procedures in thoracic and cardiac surgery, respectively.

INJURIES OF THE ABDOMEN

The spleen is the most common organ injured in blunt trauma, and the liver, because of its large size, is the most common organ injured in penetrating trauma. Historically, initial efforts were aimed at performing splenectomy with splenic injury. However, because of the role of the spleen in the body's defense against infection, the surgeon makes every effort to control hemorrhage in the spleen and avoid its removal. Treatment is determined by the condition of the spleen and of the patient. Injury to the spleen occurs with deceleration injuries, resulting in fracture of the organ because of its multiple fixation points. Splenic injury may be associated with fractures of the left tenth through twelfth ribs. The patient may exhibit left shoulder pain (Kehr's sign), upper left quadrant tenderness, abdominal wall muscle rigidity, spasm or involuntary guarding, and/or signs and symptoms of hemorrhage and hypovolemic shock. Splenic injuries (Table 18-7) range from laceration of the capsule to ruptured subcapsular hematomas or parenchymal laceration. The most serious injury is a severely fractured spleen or vascular tear, producing massive blood loss and splenic ischemia. Rupture of the spleen can be immediate or delayed. Splenic lacerations may be treated nonoperatively by close monitoring and bed rest or operatively for lacerations of a more severe nature. The surgeon creates a midline incision, which allows for exposure of all abdominal contents. Topical hemostatic agents are also used with success, as well as suturing and the argon laser in some instances. In some cases, angiographic embolization may be attempted. A laceration involving the splenic hilum or complete shattering of the organ usually results in splenectomy.

The severity of hepatic injury ranges from controlled hematoma to severe vascular injury of the hepatic veins or

TABLE 18-7

Splenic Injury Scale

Grade	Type of Injury	Description of Injury
I	Hematoma	Subcapsular: <10% of surface area
	Laceration	Capsular tear: <1 cm parenchymal depth
II	Hematoma	Subcapsular: 10%-50% of surface area; intraparenchymal: <5 cm in diameter
	Laceration	Capsular tear: 1-3 cm; parenchymal depth that does not involve a trabecular vessel
III	Hematoma	Subcapsular: >50% of surface area or expanding; ruptured subcapsular or parenchymal hematoma; intraparenchymal hematoma; >5 cm or expanding
	Laceration	>3 cm parenchymal depth or involving parenchymal vessels
IV	Laceration	Laceration involving segmental or hilar vessels, producing major devascularization (>25% of spleen)
V	Laceration	Completely shattered spleen
	Vascular	Hilar vascular injury that devascularizes spleen

Modified from Hoyt DB et al: Management of acute trauma. In Townsend CM et al, editors: *Sabiston textbook of surgery,* ed 18, Philadelphia, 2008, Saunders.

TABLE 18-8

Liver Injury Scale

Grade	Type of Injury	Description of Injury
I	Hematoma	Subcapsular: <10% of surface area
	Laceration	Capsular tear: <1 cm parenchymal depth
II	Hematoma	Subcapsular: 10%-50% of surface area; intraparenchymal: <10 cm in diameter
	Laceration	Capsular tear: 1-3 cm parenchymal depth; <10 cm in length
III	Hematoma	Subcapsular: >50% surface area of ruptured subcapsular or parenchymal hematoma; intraparenchymal hematoma: <10 cm or expanding
	Laceration	>3 cm parenchymal depth
IV	Laceration	Parenchymal disruption involving 25%-75% of hepatic lobe or 1-3 of 8 Couinaud segments
V	Laceration	Parenchymal disruption involving >75% of hepatic lobe or >3 of 8 Couinaud segments within a single lobe
	Vascular	Juxtahepatic venous injuries (i.e., retrohepatic vena cava/central major hepatic veins)
VI	Vascular	Hepatic avulsion

Modified from Hoyt DB et al: Management of acute trauma. In Townsend CM et al, editors: *Sabiston textbook of surgery,* ed 18, Philadelphia, 2008, Saunders.

hepatic avulsion (Table 18-8). Because liver tissue is so friable and has an extensive blood supply as well as blood storage capacity, hepatic injuries often result in profuse hemorrhage and require surgical control of bleeding. The patient usually exhibits upper quadrant pain, abdominal wall muscle rigidity, involuntary guarding, rebound tenderness, hypoactive or absent bowel sounds, and signs of hemorrhage or hypovolemic shock. Nonoperative treatment is indicated in minor capsular and subcapsular injuries. This can be accomplished with bed rest and close monitoring. Topical hemostatic agents and suturing are used in management of minor injuries. Fibrin glue is also used in some institutions as a topical hemostatic agent. More severe injuries with active expanding hematomas or lobe disruption require surgical exploration and may necessitate hepatic resection or ligation of associated vasculature. With massive hemorrhage, control of bleeding is the primary concern. Packing with laparotomy sponges may be indicated, along with manual compression of the organ if intraoperative hypotension becomes severe. A pressure dressing may be applied and the wound closed temporarily until associated coagulopathies, hypothermia, and hemodynamic instability can be corrected. The patient is usually returned to the OR within 24 to 72 hours postoperatively or when his or her condition permits further exploration and removal of the sponges.

Injuries to the gastrointestinal system are also associated with abdominal trauma. Bowel injuries may be missed on abdominal CT scan during the initial diagnostic period. The small bowel is frequently injured because deceleration may lead to shearing, which causes avulsion or tearing. The most commonly affected areas of the small bowel are areas relatively fixed or looped. Associated with any perforation of the gastrointestinal tract is a chance for peritonitis and sepsis or compartment syndrome from increased pressure. Crystalloid resuscitation and capillary leakage contribute to tissue swelling. The resulting abdominal edema creates a pressurized compartment that must be explored to render relief to the compromised organs.

If the abdomen is difficult to close, alternative wound closure techniques may be used to prevent the occurrence of abdominal compartment syndrome. One such method is to use

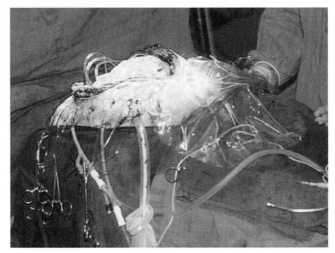

FIGURE 18-11 Alternative technique using plastic for temporary closure of the abdomen.

a silo-bag closure, in which heavy plastic is trimmed to fit and sutured to skin edges (Figure 18-11). A sterile absorbent drape may also be placed inside the abdomen to absorb fluid.

In the event of a penetrating injury, the trajectory of the missile or the implement is examined, and organs within the area are considered potentially injured. Exploration is indicated, and the components of the gastrointestinal system are thoroughly examined for any perforations, contusion, hemorrhage, or compromise of vasculature, such as a mesenteric hematoma. Once the injury is identified, suturing, stapling, or segmental excision may be indicated. Chapter 2 discusses gastrointestinal surgery and Chapter 3 addresses surgery of the liver, biliary tract, pancreas, and spleen.

Diagnostic laparoscopy is frequently used for direct visualization of abdominal organs to decrease the need for open abdominal exploration. This procedure allows the surgeon to effectively evaluate the presence of any injury and develop an appropriate plan of treatment in the stable patient. However, there is some concern that bowel injuries may not always be

TABLE 18-9

Renal Injury Scale

Grade	Type of Injury	Description of Injury
I	Contusion	Normal urinalysis except possible microscopic or gross hematuria
	Hematoma	Subcapsular, no parenchymal laceration
II	Hematoma	Perirenal, confined to renal retroperitoneum
	Laceration	>1 cm depth of renal cortex
III	Laceration	>1 cm parenchymal depth of renal cortex
IV	Laceration	Extends through cortex, medulla, and collecting system
	Vascular	Involves main renal artery or vein
V	Vascular	Completely shattered kidney
		Includes avulsion of renal hilum, which devascularizes kidney

Modified from Emergency Nurses Association (ENA): *Trauma nursing core course*, ed 6, Des Plaines, Ill, 2007, Author.

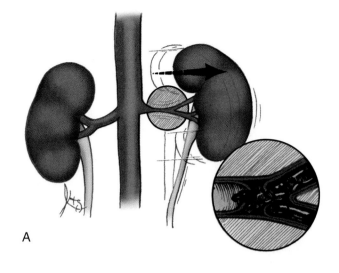

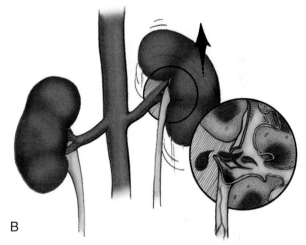

FIGURE 18-12 Renal injuries. Acceleration-deceleration injury may produce disruption of the (**A**) renal artery and the (**B**) ureteropelvic junction.

identified. Some therapeutic interventions may also be performed through the laparoscope so that the more invasive open approach is avoided. Increased intraabdominal pressure required in laparoscopic insufflation may create an adverse ventilatory effect. In the presence of abdominal vein injury with low pressures, CO_2 could leak into the vasculature and result in CO_2 emboli to the heart or lungs. Tension pneumothorax may be created in patients with a diaphragmatic injury. Consequently, indications for these procedures in the trauma setting continue to be evaluated.

INJURIES OF THE GENITOURINARY SYSTEM

Laceration of the kidney is closely associated with fracture of the ribs and transverse vertebral processes (Table 18-9). Because the kidney is retroperitoneal, the presence of bleeding may not be observed on diagnostic peritoneal lavage. Renal contusions often produce hematuria. Gross clots may also be seen in more serious injury, but it should be noted that hematuria is not present in a complete avulsion injury. Management of renal contusions can be nonoperative with monitoring of hematuria. Lacerations involving the collecting system, severe crush injuries, or pedicle injuries necessitate surgical intervention (Figure 18-12). Nephrectomy may be indicated with severe injury of the pedicle or massive hemorrhage.

Rupture of the bladder and urethral injury are most often associated with pelvic fractures. Both blunt trauma and penetrating trauma are causative factors. The type of bladder injury is a direct result of the amount of urine present in the bladder at the time of injury. Blunt forces applied to a full bladder result in an intraperitoneal rupture. This type of rupture is closely associated with alcohol consumption because of alcohol's diuretic effect. Pelvic fracture is associated with an extraperitoneal bladder rupture. Most often these patients present with gross hematuria. A small extraperitoneal rupture may be managed by urinary catheter drainage. A large extraperitoneal rupture and intraperitoneal rupture require surgical intervention.

A suprapubic cystostomy tube may be placed, and the bladder is repaired. Pelvic fracture reduction and fixation are also performed.

Urethral injuries require exploration and primary repair. These types of injuries are more common in the male because the male urethra is longer and less protected than the female urethra (Figure 18-13). A fall or straddle type of injury is usually responsible. This injury is detected by the presence of blood at the urinary meatus. In these instances an indwelling urethral catheter should not be inserted. Blood at the urinary meatus may indicate a tear in the anterior urethra. A retrograde urethrogram may be performed to evaluate for extravasation of urine and potential injury. Suspicion of a pelvic fracture raises the index of suspicion of a concomitant urethral injury. Chapter 6 provides additional information on urologic procedures.

SKELETAL INJURIES

Trauma to the skeletal system usually results in contusion or fracture. After stabilization of the patient, radiographs are

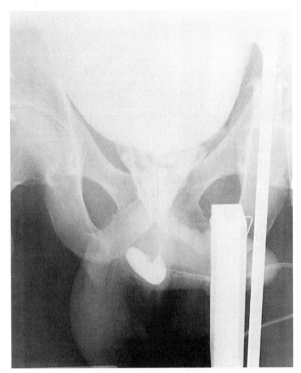

FIGURE 18-13 Complete urethral injury as demonstrated on urethrogram.

taken of any body part that is distorted, edematous, painful, or highly suspicious for fracture or dislocation. Treatment of fractures is aimed at restoring function with a minimum of complications. Immobilization of fractures can be accomplished by casting, bracing, splinting, application of traction, or hardware fixation. Femur fractures in particular can be associated with a high risk of hemorrhage and require traction before surgical repair. Closed and open reductions, application of internal and external fixators, and some types of traction may be performed in the OR. The surgical technologist involved in care of the trauma patient must have a working knowledge of orthopedics. Fractures must be repaired in a timely manner to avoid untoward complications; however, immediate life threats are corrected first. Open fractures are at an increased risk of infection. Chapter 11 contains information on the surgical procedures used in fracture management.

Pelvic fractures may pose an additional challenge to the perioperative team. Fractures within the pelvic ring are associated with significant internal blood loss and shock. Systemic peripheral vascular resistance is increased. A method to quickly minimize or tamponade blood loss in severe pelvic fractures is the application of a pneumatic antishock garment (PASG) or PASG trousers to provide stabilization of the fracture and reduce associated hemorrhage. The use of PASG trousers may be effective in patients who are 20 to 40 minutes away from the hospital and have unstable pelvic fractures and decompensated shock (Salomone et al, 2005). If a pneumatic garment is applied, the patient may be transported to the OR with the trousers still inflated. The perioperative nurse must be familiar with deflation procedures. The attending anesthesia provider directs deflation in collaboration with the surgeon. Blood pressure and other vital signs are closely monitored. The abdominal compartment is deflated first. Deflation continues

slowly while IV fluids are infused to maintain blood pressure. A 5 mm Hg drop in blood pressure requires fluid resuscitation of approximately 200 ml before deflation of the next compartment. If the patient remains stable, each leg compartment is deflated slowly, one at a time.

Some trauma centers apply external fixator devices in the ED during initial resuscitation. A pelvic C-clamp, sheet wrap, or a commercially available support binder may be used for initial stabilization of pelvic fractures. Severe hemorrhage associated with the fracture may be controlled by arterial embolization performed in the radiology department if surgical intervention for fracture fixation must be delayed.

Soft tissue injuries of an extremity are subject to compartment syndrome. This is a result of swelling of the soft tissues and muscles encased in the fascia. With a significant amount of swelling, pain is increased and the surrounding circulation may be compromised. The patient may experience a decrease in motor and sensory function. This injury must be treated surgically by a fasciotomy. Incising the fascia allows space for tissue swelling. Several days later, the patient returns to the OR for closure, which may require skin grafting for complete coverage.

HYPOTHERMIA

When trauma is involved, hypothermia often begins at the time of injury, related to heat loss through conduction and convection. A core body temperature of 32° C (89.6° F) is associated with a nearly 100% mortality rate (Moore, 2008). Moore (2008) reviewed a study designed to determine if trauma nurses check the patient's temperature during the secondary assessment. Only 40% of the patients had their temperature checked and of these 33% were hypothermic. Starting hypothermia prevention at the trauma scene and continuing measures to prevent hypothermia throughout surgery and into the ICU continue to be the recommended best practice.

For purposes of definition, generalized hypothermia is considered to be present when the core temperature is below 36° C (96.8° F). Hypothermia can be classified into three types. *Mild hypothermia* is a core temperature between 32° and 36° C (89.6° and 96.8° F). These patients may appear gray and are cool to the touch. Some alterations in level of consciousness can be present. If the patient's clothing is wet, the surgical team should remove it and cover the patient with warm blankets. Treatment is aimed at passive rewarming of the patient by means of warm ambient room temperature, warm fluids, and infrared radiant energy lights. *Moderate hypothermia* is characterized as core temperatures between 30° and 32° C (86° and 89.6° F). Warmed fluids are given by IV line and also by gastric or peritoneal lavage. In addition, a warming blanket, such as a forced air–warming device, may be used. Immersion in a Hubbard tank filled with warm water has also been successful. An irritable myocardium may cause dysrhythmias to be present. Shivering may or may not be present. If the patient is intubated, warmed, humidified gases can be administered. *Severe hypothermia* is diagnosed in the patient with a temperature below 30° C (86° F). The heart rate and the respiratory rate are greatly decreased. This patient is comatose, often appears deceased, and requires active rewarming processes. It is advisable to warm the core first to avoid complications associated with rewarming. This can best be accomplished by using cardiopulmonary bypass (CPB), which directly warms internal vital organs, including the heart. The patient should be handled gently during transfers to avoid further tissue injury and stimulation of an irritable myocardium.

In the trauma patient, hypothermia may be potentiated by hypovolemia, hypotension, and shock. Cold hemoglobin cannot release oxygen to tissue as readily as normothermic hemoglobin and decreased circulating volume related to hemorrhage reduces oxygen delivery to the tissues. The combination of hypothermia, acidosis, and coagulopathy is known as the trauma triad of death (Solheim, 2008). The three parts of the triad have a complex relationship; each may be influenced by the other and often results in high mortality if not interrupted. In hypoperfusion, cells burn glucose for energy (lactic acidosis), which increases total blood acidity (metabolic acidosis). Hypoperfusion may also halt the coagulation cascade (coagulopathy), thus triggering the triad. Hypothermia also affects other body systems already compromised by the trauma. At a core temperature of less than 30° C (86° F), atrial fibrillation is common; when the core temperature is below 25° C, the heart automatically converts to ventricular fibrillation (Moore, 2008). Cerebral blood flow is highly sensitive to hypothermia and the patient may appear to be dead. Resuscitation measures are ceased if the patient is rewarmed to at least 35° C (97° F) and cardiac functions remain nonexistent.

THERMAL INJURIES

Heat and cold exposure injuries require prompt initial management in the ED setting. Some institutions transfer pediatric burn patients and severely burned adult patients to a burn center for treatment once the patients' conditions are stabilized. In addition to treatment of the site of injury to decrease further tissue damage, fluid management is of the utmost importance in these patients. After hemodynamic stabilization of the patient, burn and frostbite wounds usually require a series of procedures. These patients may have multiple surgical debridement procedures before skin grafting and cosmetic interventions. Restoration of function is important. Circumferential burns may restrict the neurovascular structures during eschar formation. Chest burns with eschar may restrict movement of the chest wall and ventilatory function. An escharotomy (incision of the eschar) may be performed to alleviate the constriction. If necessary, this procedure may be performed at the bedside and the perioperative team may be asked to assist.

ORGAN AND TISSUE PROCUREMENT

As previously noted, trauma primarily affects young people. In the event that resuscitation efforts or surgical interventions are not successful, the patient may be declared dead. Depending on the cause of death and preexisting medical conditions, the patient may be an organ-donor candidate. Both federal and state laws mandate that local organ-procurement facilities are notified of potential donors and that families are informed that organ donation exists as an option. Organ-donation agencies can be contacted early and will assist in assessing the potential donor, as well as providing a protocol for donor management once the patient is declared dead. Brain death criteria for organ donation began around 1968, attributed to the Harvard Ad Hoc Committee on Brain Death. Most organ donations in this country are from patients who experience brain death. In 1980 the Uniform

Declaration of Death Act offered an additional option: cardiopulmonary death, defined as irreversible cessation of circulatory and respiratory function. This may present an ethical dilemma to some team members. With brain death, the physician declares the patient dead in the intensive care unit (ICU) and the family is offered an opportunity to say good-bye. The patient arrives in the OR on a ventilator, which is deactivated when the organs have been retrieved. In cardiopulmonary death, the physician accompanies the patient to the OR, the ventilator is deactivated, the staff wait for cessation of circulatory and respiratory function, and death is declared at that time (Saver, 2007). Definitions of brain and cardiopulmonary death are not uniform throughout the United States. The perioperative team should be familiar with the state's definitions of brain and cardiopulmonary death and the institution's criteria for the declaration.

Once a patient is declared dead and becomes a potential organ donor, the patient's family does not incur any financial costs acquired from that point. The patient is not disfigured in any way that will interfere with bereavement rituals.

A transplantation coordinator assists in managing the organ-donor patient in the ICU setting until the procurement teams arrive. The surgical technologist must prepare for the organ-procurement procedure. The harvesting of organs and tissue may take several hours and additional members of the perioperative team. Different organ-procurement agencies will provide a surgical team, but additional scrub and circulating personnel are needed. The transplantation coordinators actively seek tissue and organ recipients during the harvest procedure. Most organ-transplantation agencies contact the institution and provide follow-up information regarding the ultimate success of the transplantation procedures and information about the recipients.

The heart is removed first, followed by the lungs, pancreas, liver, and kidneys. Tissue dissection is performed in such a manner as to allow for optimal organ transplantation. Sterile technique remains important. In addition, traffic control is of concern during these procedures. Traffic should be limited to essential personnel. Bone, skin, and corneas can also be removed. Some procurement agencies remove bone and corneas in the morgue rather than in the OR.

TRAUMA SURGERY SUMMARY

To review, as with any surgical service, in trauma surgery it is imperative to know the anatomy and physiology of the surgical area. In trauma surgery there may be more than one area being operated on. A prepared surgical technologist needs to anticipate the unexpected; because there is little time for advanced planning with trauma patients, the surgical team must work cohesively and efficiently to provide the best care possible for the trauma patient.

It is important to know and fully understand all aspects of positioning, surgical equipment, supplies, and instrumentation, taking into consideration the severity and location of the injuries. The surgical technologist should understand the procedural considerations of several operative procedures because most trauma patients present with multiple injuries.

As trauma patients present a challenge with body temperature, being prepared with the proper warming units, blankets, and fluid warmers will help facilitate a better outcome for the trauma patient.

REVIEW QUESTIONS

1. In the trauma patient, airway intervention may include:
   a. manual maneuvers
   b. oral/nasopharyngeal airways
   c. intubation
   d. all of the above

2. Swelling of the muscles below the fascia covering may compromise circulation and result in the eventual loss of the extremity. This condition is known as:
   a. blunt trauma
   b. compartment syndrome
   c. penetrating trauma
   d. thermal trauma

3. Diagnostic procedures utilized in trauma patients include:
   a. computerized tomography
   b. standard x-ray
   c. cardiac monitoring
   d. all of the above

4. Motor vehicle accidents account for about _____ of maxillofacial injuries.
   a. 20%
   b. 70%
   c. 60%
   d. 30%

5. Myocardial contusions usually involve the:
   a. right ventricle
   b. right atrium
   c. left ventricle
   d. left atrium

6. An emergency thoracotomy may be indicated in the patient with:
   a. penetrating trauma to the chest
   b. compression fractures
   c. myocardial contusion
   d. cardiac arrest

7. The most common organ injured in blunt trauma is the:
   a. liver
   b. heart
   c. spleen
   d. brain

8. The small bowel is frequently injured because deceleration may lead to shearing, which causes:
   a. contusions
   b. avulsions or tearing
   c. rupture
   d. none of the above

9. Rupture of the bladder and urethral injury are most often associated with:
   a. vertebral fractures
   b. pelvic fractures
   c. high femur fractures
   d. none of the above

10. When trauma is involved, _____ often begins at the time of injury due to heat loss through conduction and convection.
    a. hypothermia
    b. hyperthermia
    c. seizures
    d. respiratory distress

11. Briefly describe special considerations surgical technologists should plan for in the following areas of trauma surgery:
    Injuries of the head and spinal column
    Injuries of the chest and heart
    Skeletal injuries

Critical Thinking Question

Trauma patients are at a greater risk for infection. Discuss the reasons for this and the steps taken to control the infection risk.

REFERENCES

Association of periOperative Registered Nurses (AORN): Counts-sponges, sharps and instruments recommended practice. In *Perioperative standards and recommended practices*, Denver, 2009, The Association.

Barclay L: *Guidelines issued for field triage of injured patients*, 2009, Medscape Medical News, available at www.medscape.com/viewarticle/587447. Accessed February 16, 2009.

Cunningham AR: FAST scan: ultrasound's role in trauma, *Radiol Technol* 79(5):455–457, 2008.

Cusick SS, Tibbles CD: Trauma in pregnancy, *Emerg Med Clin North Am* 25:861–872, 2007.

Emergency Nurses Association: *Trauma nursing core course*, 6th ed, Des Plaines, Ill, 2007, Author.

Germanos S et al: Damage control surgery in the abdomen: an approach for the management of severely injured patients, *Int J Surg* 6:246–252, 2008.

Gray MJ, Litz BT: Behavioral interventions for recent trauma: empirically informed practice guidelines, *Behav Modif* 29(1):189–215, 2005.

Hodgson BB, Kizior RJ: *Saunder's nursing drug handbook*, St Louis, 2009, Saunders.

Inamasu J, Guiot BH: Vertebral artery injury after blunt cervical trauma: an update, *Surg Neurol* 65(3):238–245, 2006.

Jacobs LM et al: A plan to improve end-of-life care for trauma victims and their families, *J Trauma Nurs* 12(3):73–76, 2005.

Kulaylat MN, Dayton MT: Surgical complications. In Townsend CM et al, editors: *Sabiston textbook of surgery*, ed 18, Philadelphia, 2008, Saunders.

Malone D et al: Massive transfusion practices around the globe and a suggestion for a common mass transfusion protocol, *J Trauma* 60 (6 Suppl):S91–S96, 2006.

Meier C et al: Early placement of optional vena cava filter in high-risk patients with traumatic brain injury, *EurJ Trauma Emerg Surg* 33(4):407–413, 2007.

Moore K: Hypothermia in trauma, *J Trauma Nurs* 15(2):62–64, 2008.

Muir M, Archer-Heese G: Essentials of a bariatric patient handling program, *Online Journal of Issues in Nursing* 14(1), 2009.

Nessen S et al: Acute resuscitation and critical care: massive blood transfusion in patient with hemoperitoneum. In Nessen S et al: *War surgery in Afghanistan and Iraq: a series of cases*, 2003-2007, USA, 2008, Department of the Army.

Plummer E: Trauma in the elderly. In McQuillan KA et al, editors: *Trauma nursing: from resuscitation through rehabilitation*, ed 4, St Louis, 2009, Saunders.

Salomone JP et al: Opinions of trauma practitioners regarding prehospital interventions for critically injured patients, *J Trauma* 58(3):509–515, 2005.

Saver C: Being prepared for donation after cardiac death, *OR Manager* 23(10):18–21, 2007.

Sharma AM: Managing weighty issues on lean evidence: the challenges of bariatric medicine, *CMAJ* 172(1):30–31, 2005.

Solheim J: *The trauma triad of death: hypothermia, acidosis, and coagulopathy*, 2008, available at www.ena.org/conferences/annual/2008/handouts/218-c.pdf. Accessed March 15, 2009.

Vegar-Brozovic V et al: Intra-abdominal hypertension: pulmonary and cerebral complications, *Transplant Proc* 40:1190–1192, 2008.

Illustration Credits

CHAPTER 2

2-4, 2-5, 2-33, 2-34, 2-35, 2-38, 2-39, From Thompson JC: *Atlas of surgery of the stomach, duodenum, and small bowel,* St Louis, 1992, Mosby; 2-7, 2-32, 2-46, 2-47, 2-48, 2-49, 2-50, 2-51, 2-52, 2-53, From Bauer JJ: *Colorectal surgery illustrated,* St Louis, 1993, Mosby; 2-8, 2-9, 2-10, 2-11, 2-12, 2-13, 2-14, 2-15, 2-16, 2-17, 2-18, 2-19, 2-20, 2-21, 2-22, 2-23, 2-24, 2-25, From Tighe SM: *Instrumentation for the operating room,* ed 7, St Louis, 2007, Mosby; 2-27, Adapted from Thibodeau GA, Patton KT: *Anthony's textbook of anatomy and physiology,* ed 18, St Louis, 2007, Mosby; 2-40, Courtesy Inamed Health, Inc, Santa Barbara, CA. In Townsend CM et al: *Sabiston textbook of surgery: the biological basis of modern surgical practice,* ed 17, Philadelphia, 2004, Saunders; 2-41, 2-42, 2-43, From Townsend CM et al: *Sabiston textbook of surgery: the biological basis of modern surgical practice,* ed 18, Philadelphia, 2007, Saunders; 2-44, 2-45, From Marceau P et al: Malabsorptive obesity surgery, *Surgical Clinics of North America* 81:1113-1127, 2001. In Townsend CM et al: *Sabiston textbook of surgery: the biological basis of modern surgical practice,* ed 17, Philadelphia, 2004, Saunders.

CHAPTER 3

3-6, From Townsend CM et al: *Sabiston textbook of surgery,* ed 16, Philadelphia, 2001, Saunders; 3-7, 3-8, 3-9, 3-10, 3-11, 3-12, 3-13, 3-14, 3-17, From Tighe SM: *Instrumentation for the operating room,* ed 7, St Louis, 2007, Mosby; 3-21, From Zuidema G, editor: *Shackelford's surgery of the alimentary tract,* ed 3, Philadelphia, 1996, Saunders; 3-27, Modified from Moody FG, editor: *Surgical treatment of digestive disease,* ed 2, St Louis, 1990, Mosby; 3-28, From Motoyama EK, Davis PJ: *Smith's anesthesia for infants and children,* ed 7, St Louis, 2006, Mosby; 3-29, 3-30, 3-31, Copyright © 1990 Lahey Clinic, Burlington, MA; 3-32, From Anscher NL et al (1984): In Simmons RL et al, editors: *Manual of vascular access, organ donation, and transplantation,* New York, 1984, Springer-Verlag.

CHAPTER 4

4-1, From Ignatavicius DD, Workman ML: *Medical-surgical nursing: patient-centered collaborative care,* ed 6, St Louis, 2010, Mosby; 4-2, From Harkreader H, Hogan MA, Thobaben M: *Fundamentals of nursing: caring and clinical judgment,* ed 3, St Louis, 2007, Mosby; 4-13, From Seidel HM et al: *Mosby's guide to physical examination,* ed 6, St Louis, 2006, Mosby; 4-15, From Schumpelick V: *Atlas of hernia surgery,* Toronto, 1990, BC Decker; 4-17, From Liechty RD, Soper RT: *Synopsis of surgery,* St Louis, 1985, Mosby.

CHAPTER 5

5-1, 5-22B, 5-23B, From Seidel HM et al: *Mosby's guide to physical examination,* ed 6, St Louis, 2006, Mosby; 5-2, 5-8, 5-38, From Lowdermilk DL, Perry SE: *Maternity and women's health care,* ed 9, St Louis, 2007, Mosby; 5-7, 5-9, 5-10, 5-33, 5-50, From Hacker NF, Gambone JC, Hobel CJ: *Hacker & Moore's essentials of obstetrics and gynecology,* ed 5, Philadelphia, 2010, Saunders; 5-11, 5-12, 5-13, 5-14, 5-15, 5-16, 5-17, 5-18, 5-19, From Tighe SM: *Instrumentation for the operating room,* ed 7, St Louis, 2007, Mosby; 5-24, Redrawn from Symmonds RE: Relaxation of pelvic supports. In Katz VL et al: *Comprehensive gynecology,* ed 5, Philadelphia, 2007, Mosby; 5-20, 5-52, From Townsend CM et al: *Sabiston textbook of surgery: the biological basis of modern surgical practice,* ed 18, Philadelphia, 2008, Saunders; 5-21, 5-37, From Ignatavicius DD, Workman ML: *Medical-surgical nursing: patient-centered collaborative care,* ed 6, St Louis, 2010, Mosby; 5-25, 5-26, 5-41, Katz VL et al: *Comprehensive gynecology,* ed 5, St Louis, 2007, Mosby; 5-32, 5-36, 5-46, 5-54, From Ball TL: *Gynecologic surgery and urology,* ed 2, St Louis, 1963, Mosby. Daisy Stillwell, medical illustrator; 5-35, Courtesy Dr. Henry J Norris, Orlando, FL. From Robboy SJ et al: *Robboy's pathology of the female reproductive tract,* ed 2, London, 2009, Churchill Livingstone;

5-37, From Lowdermilk DL, Perry SE: *Maternity and women's health care,* ed 8, St Louis, 2004, Mosby; 5-39, From Emond RT: *Colour atlas of infectious diseases,* ed 4, St Louis, 2003, Mosby; 5-42, 5-53, From Hacker NF, Moore JG, Gambone JC: *Essentials of obstetrics and gynecology,* ed 4, Philadelphia, 2004, Saunders; 5-43, 5-44, 5-45, From Edwards SK et al: Surgery in the pregnant patient, *Current Problems in Surgery* 38(4):213-292, 2001; 5-48, 5-55, 5-56, From Nichols DH: *Gynecologic and obstetric surgery,* St Louis, 1993, Mosby; 5-57, 5-58, 5-59, Courtesy Conceptus Inc; 5-62, From Holcomb GW, Murphy JP: *Pediatric surgery,* ed 5, Philadelphia, 2010, Saunders; 5-63, From Cortes RA, Farmer DL: Recent advances in fetal surgery, *Seminars in Perinatology* 28(3), 2004; 5-64, From Adzick NS et al: Successful fetal surgery for spina bifida, *The Lancet* 352(9141):1675-1676, 1998; 5-65, 5-66, Courtesy Marjorie Pyle, RNC, Lifecircle, Costa Mesa, CA. In Lowdermilk DL, Perry SE: *Maternity and women's health care,* ed 9, St Louis, 2007, Mosby.

CHAPTER 6

6-1, 6-6, 6-7, Modified from Seidel HM et al: *Mosby's guide to physical examination,* ed 6, St Louis, 2006, Mosby; 6-3, 6-24, 6-34, 6-39, 6-41, 6-49, 6-58, 6-59, 6-75, 6-89, From Nagle GM: *Genitourinary surgery,* St Louis, 1997, Mosby; 6-8, 6-9, 6-10, 6-11, 6-12, 6-13, 6-14, 6-15, 6-16, 6-29, 6-30B, 6-87, From Tighe SM: *Instrumentation for the operating room,* ed 7, St Louis, 2007, Mosby; 6-17, 6-73, Courtesy Bard Urological, Covington, GA; 6-19, 6-21, Courtesy Jeffrey Rosenblum, MD; 6-22, Courtesy CR Bard, Urological Division, Covington, GA. In Nagle GM: *Genitourinary surgery,* St Louis, 1997, Mosby; 6-23, 6-26, 6-40, 6-71, From Williamson MR, Smith AY: *Fundamentals of uroradiology,* Philadelphia, 2000, Saunders; 6-25, 6-42, 6-69, 6-70, Courtesy Gyrus-ACMI, Southborough, MA; 6-27, Courtesy Circon Corp, Santa Barbara, CA. In Nagle GM: *Genitourinary surgery,* St Louis, 1997, Mosby; 6-33, 6-36, 6-37, 6-81A, Courtesy American Medical Systems, Minnetonka, MN; 6-35, 6-51, 6-52, 6-53, 6-60, 6-61, 6-79, 6-80, 6-81B, 6-88, 6-90, From Droller MJ: *Surgical management of urologic disease,* St Louis, 1992, Mosby; 6-46, 6-47, Courtesy Ethicon, Inc, Somerville, NJ; 6-50, 6-56, Courtesy Omni-Tract Surgical, St Paul, MN; 6-63, Courtesy Intuitive Surgical, Inc.; 6-64, 6-65, From Wein AJ et al: *Campbell-Walsh urology,* ed 9, Philadelphia, 2007, Saunders; 6-67, Courtesy Gyrus-ACMI, Southborough, Mass.; 6-72, 6-74, From Raz S: *Atlas of transvaginal surgery,* ed 2, Philadelphia, 2002, Saunders; 6-82, 6-83, 6-85, From Gillenwater JY et al: *Adult and pediatric urology,* ed 3, vol 2, St Louis, 1996, Mosby; 6-84, From Gray M: *Genitourinary disorders,* St Louis, 1992, Mosby; 6-86, Copyright © Karl Storz Endoscopy America, Inc.

CHAPTER 7

7-1, 7-2, From Thibodeau GA, Patton, KT: *Anatomy and physiology,* ed 6, St Louis, 2007, Mosby; 7-3, From Wein RO, Weber RS: Parathyroid surgery, *Neuroimaging Clinics of North America* 18(3):554-555, 2008; 7-4, From Fakhran S et al: Parathyroid imaging, *Neuroimaging Clinics of North America* 18(3):538, 2008; 7-5, From Kukora JS et al: Thyroid nodule. In Cameron JL, editor: *Current surgical therapy,* ed 7, St Louis, 2001, Mosby; 7-6, 7-7, 7-8, 7-9, 7-10, From Dhingra JK, Raval T: Minimally invasive surgery of the thyroid, eMedicine.com, June 13, 2008, WebMD; 7-11, From Healy J, Hodge J: *Surgical anatomy,* ed 2, Philadelphia, 1990, BC Decker.

CHAPTER 8

8-1, 8-2, 8-3, From Isaacs JH: *Textbook of breast disease,* St Louis, 1992, Mosby; 8-4, From Townsend CM: *Sabiston textbook of surgery,* ed 16, Philadelphia, 2001, Saunders; 8-5, Courtesy Wende W. Logan, MD, Rochester, NY, and the Breast Clinic of Rochester; 8-6, Courtesy of Mammotome; 8-7A, Don Bliss, artist, National Cancer Institute (NCI), www.cancer.gov; 8-7B, From Ignatavicius DD, Workman ML: *Medical-surgical nursing:*

critical thinking for collaborative care, ed 5, St Louis, 2006, Mosby; **8-8,** From Townsend CM et al: *Sabiston textbook of surgery: the biological basis of modern surgical practice,* ed 18, Philadelphia, 2008, Saunders; **8-9,** From Ignatavicius DD, Workman ML: *Medical-surgical nursing: patient-centered collaborative care,* vol. 2, ed 6, St Louis, 2010, Mosby; **8-10,** From Ignatavicius DD, Workman ML: *Medical-surgical nursing: critical thinking for collaborative care,* ed 4, Philadelphia, 2002, Saunders; **8-11, 8-12, 8-13,** From Tighe SM: Instrumentation for the operating room, ed 7, St Louis, 2007, Mosby; **8-14,** Redrawn from Zollinger RM: *Atlas of surgical operations,* ed 6, New York, 1988, MacMillan.

CHAPTER 9

9-1, 9-8, 9-25, 9-38, 9-39, 9-45, Courtesy National Eye Institute, National Institutes of Health; **9-2,** From Seidel HM et al: *Mosby's guide to physical examination,* ed 6, St Louis, 2006, Mosby; **9-3,** From Thompson JM et al: *Mosby's clinical nursing,* ed 5, St Louis, 2002, Mosby; **9-4,** From Monahan FD et al: *Phipps' medical-surgical nursing: health and illness perspectives,* ed 8, St Louis, 2007, Mosby; **9-11, 9-12, 9-13, 9-14, 9-15, 9-16, 9-17, 9-18, 9-19, 9-20,** From Tighe SM: Instrumentation for the operating room, ed 7, St Louis, 2007, Mosby; **9-22,** Courtesy Don Mikes, Vice-President, Global Marketing, Moria, Inc., Doylestown, PA; **9-26,** Courtesy June Nichols, Board Certified Ocularist, Diplomate, American Society of Ocularists; **9-27,** From Swartz MH: *Textbook of physical diagnosis,* ed 6, Philadelphia, 2010, Saunders; **9-30, 9-32, 9-33, 9-34,** From Tenzel RR: *Textbook of ophthalmology,* vol 4. *Orbit and oculoplastics,* London, 1993, Gower; **9-31,** From Ignatavicius DD, Workman ML: *Medical-surgical nursing: critical thinking for collaborative care,* ed 5, St Louis, 2006, Mosby; **9-37,** From Wilson TS: *LASIK surgery, AORN J* 71(5):977-978, 2000; **9-41, 9-42, 9-43,** From Lindquist TD, Lindstrom RL: *Ophthalmic surgery: looseleaf and update service,* St Louis, 1990, Mosby; **9-44B,** Courtesy of Jason Malecka, President of IOP; **9-48, 9-49,** From Federman JL et al: *Retina and vitreous,* London, 1994, Mosby; **9-50,** From Ryan SJ et al: *Retina,* vol 3, ed 4, St Louis, 2006, Mosby.

CHAPTER 10

10-1, 10-2, 10-38, 10-40, From Ignatavicius DD, Workman ML: *Medical-surgical nursing: critical thinking for collaborative care,* ed 5, St Louis, 2006, Mosby; **10-3,** From DeWeese DD et al: *Otolaryngology: head and neck surgery,* ed 7, St Louis, 1988, Mosby; **10-5, 10-23A and C,** From Saunders WH et al: *Nursing care in eye, ear, nose, and throat disorders,* ed 4, St Louis, 1979, Mosby; **10-7,** From Seidel HM et al: *Mosby's guide to physical examination,* ed 6, St Louis, 2006, Mosby; **10-8,** From Huether SE, McCance KL: *Understanding pathophysiology,* ed 4, St Louis, 2008, Mosby; **10-9,** From Marino LB: *Cancer nursing,* St Louis, 1981, Mosby; **10-10, 10-22, 10-23B, 10-27,** From Myers EN: *Operative otolaryngology: head and neck surgery,* vol. 1 & 2, ed 2, St Louis, 2008, Saunders; **10-11, 10-34, 10-44, 10-45, 10-46, 10-58, 10-59,** From Cummings CW et al: *Otolaryngology: head and neck surgery,* ed 3, St Louis, 1993, Mosby; **10-13,** Courtesy NIM-Response, a registered trademark of Medtronic, Inc.; **10-15, 10-16, 10-17, 10-18, 10-19, 10-20, 10-21,** From Tighe SM: *Instrumentation for the operating room,* ed 7, St Louis, 2007, Mosby; **10-24,** Courtesy Richard A. Buckingham, MD, Clinical Professor, Otolaryngology, Abraham Lincoln School of Medicine, University of Illinois, Chicago. In Seidel HM et al: *Mosby's guide to physical examination,* ed 6, St Louis, 2006, Mosby; **10-28, 10-29,** Courtesy Cochlear, Ltd; **10-30, 10-31, 10-32,** Courtesy Cochlear, Ltd.; **10-33, 10-41, 10-56,** From DeWeese DD, Saunders WH: *Textbook of otolaryngology,* ed 6, St Louis, 1982, Mosby; **10-37,** From Schuller DE, Schleuning AJ: *Otolaryngology: head and neck surgery,* ed 8, St Louis, 1994, Mosby; **10-38,** From Thawley SE, Garrett H: Endoscopic sinus surgery; an outpatient procedure that minimizes tissue removal, *AORN J* 47:902, 1988. Copyright © AORN, Inc, Denver, CO; **10-48,** From Lewis SM et al: *Medical-surgical nursing: assessment and management of clinical problems,* ed 7, St Louis, 2007, Mosby; **10-49,** From Luckmann J: *Medical-surgical nursing,* ed 3, Philadelphia, 1987, Saunders; **10-51,** From Shah JP, Patel SG: *Head and neck surgery and oncology,* ed 3, London, 2003, Mosby Ltd.

CHAPTER 11

11-1, 11-2, 11-4, 11-5, 11-6, 11-8, 11-9, From Thibodeau GA, Patton KT: *Anatomy and physiology,* ed 7, St Louis, 2010, Mosby; **11-3,** Redrawn from Lewis RC: *Primary care orthopedics,* New York, 1988, Churchill Livingstone; **11-7A, 11-12, 11-13, 11-100,** From Thibodeau GA, Patton KT: *Anatomy and physiology,* ed 3, St Louis, 1996, Mosby; **11-11, 11-19, 11-43, 11-76, 11-80,** Courtesy Zimmer, Inc, Warsaw, IN; **11-15,** Courtesy

Innomed, Savannah, GA; **11-16, 11-65,** Courtesy Acufex Microsurgical, Inc, Mansfield, MA; **11-17,** Courtesy MIZUHO OSI, Union City, CA; **11-18, 11-27, 11-30, 11-39, 11-41, 11-50, 11-61, 11-82, 11-84,** From Gregory B: *Orthopaedic surgery,* St Louis, 1994, Mosby; **11-20, 11-54,** Courtesy Zimmer Traction Handbook, 1989, Zimmer, Inc., Warsaw, IN; **11-22,** From Mourad LA: *Orthopedic disorders,* St Louis, 1991, Mosby; **11-24, 11-86, 11-87, 11-88, 11-89, 11-92,** Courtesy ConMed Linvatec, Utica, NY; **11-25,** From Monahan FD et al: *Phipps' medical-surgical nursing,* ed 8, St Louis, 2007, Mosby; **11-26,** Courtesy EBI/Biomed, Parsippany, NJ; **11-28, 11-33, 11-52, 11-53,** From Gustilo RB et al: *Fractures and dislocations,* vol 2, St Louis, 1993, Mosby; **11-29, 11-31, 11-40, 11-66, 11-103, 11-104,** Courtesy Synthes, Inc., West Chester, PA. Copyright Synthes, Inc. or its affiliates; **11-32,** Courtesy Prototech AS, Bergen, Norway; **11-34,** Courtesy LTI Medica and the UpJohn Co. Illustration by Beverly Kessler, 1982, Learning Technology, Inc; **11-35, 11-45, 11-56,** From Canale ST, Beaty JH: *Campbell's operative orthopaedics,* ed 11, St Louis, 2008, Mosby; **11-36,** Courtesy Biomet, Inc, Warsaw, IN; **11-38,** Redrawn from Rockwood CA et al: *Fractures in adults,* ed 2, Philadelphia, 1984, Lippincott; **11-42,** Redrawn from Neer CS: *J Bone Joint Surg* 52-A:1007, 1970; **11-46, 11-48,** From Crenshaw AH: *Campbell's operative orthopaedics,* ed 8, St Louis, 1992, Mosby; **11-47,** Reproduced with permission from Knight RA: The management of fractures about the elbow in adults, in Raney RB (ed): *Instructional Course Lectures 14.* Rosemont, IL, American Academy of Orthopaedic Surgeons, 1957, pp 123-141; **11-49, 11-68,** From Muller ME et al: *Manual of internal fixation: techniques recommended by AO-ASIF group,* ed 3, Berlin, 1990, Springer-Verlag; **11-51,** Redrawn from Sprague HH, Howard FM: *Contemporary Orthopedics* 16:18, 1988; **11-55,** Courtesy OsteoMed, Addison, TX; **11-57,** Courtesy Exactech, Inc, Gainesville, FL; **11-58,** From Gustilo RB: *The fracture classification manual,* St Louis, 1991, Mosby; **11-59,** Redrawn from Muller ME et al: *The comprehensive classification of fractures of long bones,* Berlin, 1990, Springer-Verlag; **11-60,** Redrawn from Schatzker J et al: *Clinical Orthopedics* 138:94, 1979; **11-62,** From DePuy ACE Medical Co, El Segundo, CA; **11-63, 11-71, 11-72, 11-73, 11-75, 11-77, 11-81,** Courtesy Stryker, Kalamazoo, MI; **11-64,** Redrawn from Cox JS: *Am J Sports Med* 4:72, 1976; **11-67,** From Canale ST: *Campbell's operative orthopaedics,* ed 9, St Louis, 1998, Mosby; **11-69,** From Richards V: *Surgery for general practice,* St Louis, 1956, Mosby; **11-73, 11-75, 11-81,** Courtesy Howmedica, Inc, Rutherford, NJ; **11-78,** Redrawn from Gristina AG, Webb LX: *Proximal humeral and monospherical glenoid replacement: surgical technique,* Rutherford, NJ, 1983, Howmedica, Inc; **11-79,** Courtesy Smith & Nephew, Memphis; **11-83,** Courtesy College of Southern Idaho, Twin Falls; **11-85,** From Tighe SM: *Instrumentation for the operating room,* ed 7, St Louis, 2007, Mosby; **11-89, 11-90,** From Shahriaree H: *O'Connor's textbook of arthroscopic surgery,* Philadelphia, 1984, Lippincott Williams and Wilkins; **11-92,** Courtesy Johnson & Johnson; **11-96,** Courtesy Smith & Nephew Dyonics, Andover, MA; **11-97,** Courtesy David Greg Anderson, MD; **11-98,** From Kim DH et al: *Surgical anatomy and techniques to the spine,* St Louis, 2006, Saunders; **11-99,** Courtesy NuVasive, Inc, San Diego; **11-101,** From Bradford DS et al: *Moe's textbook of scoliosis and other spinal deformities,* ed 2, Philadelphia, 1987, Saunders; **11-102,** Courtesy Medtronic Sofamor Danek, Memphis; **11-105, 11-106,** Reprinted with permission from Synthes Spine LP; **11-107,** From Ortiz A: Vertebral body reconstruction: review and update on vertebroplasty and kyphoplasty, *Appl Radiol* 37(12): 10-24, 2008.

CHAPTER 12

12-1, 12-35, From Thibodeau GA, Patton KT: *Structure and function of the body,* ed 13, St Louis, 2008, Mosby; **12-2, 12-3, 12-4, 12-6,** From Thibodeau GA, Patton KT: *Anatomy and physiology,* ed 3, St Louis, 1996, Mosby; **12-5,** Photograph by Sarah-Jane Smith. Artwork modified from Lumley JSP: *Surface anatomy,* ed 3, Edinburgh, 2002, Churchill Livingstone. In Standring S: *Gray's anatomy,* ed 40, Edinburgh, 2008, Churchill Livingstone; **12-7, 12-9, 12-10, 12-12, 12-37,** From Conway-Rutkowski BL: *Carini and Owens' neurological and neurosurgical nursing,* ed 8, St Louis, 1982, Mosby; **12-8, 12-21, 12-22, 12-30,** From Anthony CP, Thibodeau GA: *Textbook of anatomy and physiology,* ed 11, St Louis, 1983, Mosby; **12-11,** Photograph by Kevin Fitzpatrick on behalf of GKT School of Medicine, London. In Standring S: *Gray's anatomy,* ed 40, Edinburgh, 2008, Churchill Livingstone; **12-13, 12-14, 12-15, 12-16, 12-17, 12-18, 12-23, 12-24, 12-39, 12-40, 12-62, 12-65, 12-66, 12-67, 12-68,** Courtesy William J. Nelson, MD; **12-19,** Modified from Thibodeau GA, Patton KT: *Anatomy and physiology,* ed 5, St Louis, 2003, Mosby; **12-20,** From Nolte J: *The human brain: an introduction to its fundamental anatomy,* ed 2, St Louis, 1988, Mosby; **12-25, 12-41, 12-42, 12-44, 12-56, 12-57, 12-58, 12-59, 12-60, 12-63, 12-69,**

12-72, From Rengachary SS, Ellenbogen RG: *Principles of neurosurgery,* ed 2, Edinburgh, 2005, Mosby Ltd; **12-26, 12-27, 12-28,** From Rengachary SS, Wilkins RH: *Principles of neurosurgery,* London, 1994, Wolfe/Mosby Europe Ltd; **12-29,** From Thibodeau GA, Patton KT: *Anatomy and physiology,* ed 7, St Louis, 2010, Mosby; **12-31,** From Standring S: *Gray's anatomy,* ed 40, Edinburgh, 2008, Churchill Livingstone; **12-32, 12-33,** From Mettler FA: *Neuroanatomy,* ed 2, St Louis, 1948, Mosby; **12-43,** Provided by Shaun Gallagher, GKT School of Medicine, London; photograph by Sarah-Jane Smith. In Standring S: *Gray's anatomy,* ed 40, Edinburgh, 2008, Churchill Livingstone; **12-45,** Courtesy Dr Justin Lee, Chelsea and Westminster Hospital, London. In Standring S: *Gray's anatomy,* ed 40, Edinburgh, 2008, Churchill Livingstone; **12-46,** Courtesy Integra LifeSciences Corp, Plainsboro, NJ; **12-48,** From Barker E: *Neuroscience nursing,* St Louis, 1994, Mosby; **12-50,** Courtesy ConMed Linvatec, Utica, NY; **12-51,** Courtesy Midas Rex, a registered trademark of Medtronic, Inc.; **12-53, 12-54, 12-55, 12-61A,** Courtesy Codman & Shurtleff, Inc, Randolph, MA; **12-61B,** Courtesy Holco Instrument Corp, New York; **12-61C,** Courtesy Omni-Tract Surgical, St. Paul, Minn.; **12-64,** From Sachs E: *Diagnosis and treatment of brain tumors and the care of the neurosurgical patient,* ed 2, St Louis, 1949, Mosby; **12-70, 12-71,** From Carini E, Owens G: *Neurological and neurosurgical nursing,* ed 6, St Louis, 1974, Mosby.

CHAPTER 13
13-1, From Townsend CM et al, editors: *Sabiston textbook of surgery,* ed 18, Philadelphia, 2008, Saunders; **13-2, 13-6, 13-14, 13-23, 13-24, 13-30, 13-38, 13-43, 13-44,** From Fortunato N, McCullough SM: *Plastic and reconstructive surgery,* St Louis, 1998, Mosby; **13-3, 13-4, 13-5, 13-7,** From Tighe SM: *Instrumentation for the operating room,* ed 7, St Louis, 2007, Mosby; **13-8,** Courtesy Carl Zeiss, Oberkochen, Germany; **13-9, 13-10, 13-20, 13-21, 13-25, 13-28,** Courtesy Ramasamy Kalimuthu, MD, FACS, Oak Lawn, IL; **13-11, 13-13,** From Thibodeau GA, Patton KT: *The human body in health and disease,* ed 5, St Louis, 2010, Mosby; **13-12, 13-16,** From Ignatavicius DD, Workman ML: *Medical-surgical nursing: patient-centered collaborative care,* ed 6, St Louis, 2010, Mosby; **13-19,** Courtesy Inamed Aesthetics, Santa Barbara, CA; **13-26,** From Weinzweig N, Weinzweig J: *The mutilated hand,* St Louis, 2005, Mosby; **13-29,** From Fonseca RJ et al: *Oral and maxillofacial trauma,* ed 3, Philadelphia, 2005, Saunders; **13-31, 13-37,** From Kaminer MS et al: *Atlas of cosmetic surgery,* ed 2, St Louis, 2009, Saunders; **13-39,** From Capella JF: Body lift, *Clinics in Plastic Surgery* 35(1):28, 2008; **13-40,** From Aly A et al: Brachioplasty in the massive weight loss patient, *Clinics in Plastic Surgery* 35(1):146, 2008; **13-41,** From Cram A, Aly A: Thigh reduction in the massive weight loss patient, *Clinics in Plastic Surgery* 35(1): 170, 2008; **13-45,** From Wilkinson TS: *Atlas of liposuction,* Philadelphia, 2005, Saunders.

CHAPTER 14
14-4, From Schottelius BA, Schottelius DD: *Textbook of physiology,* ed 18, St Louis, 1978, Mosby; **14-5,** From Townsend CM et al: *Sabiston textbook of surgery,* ed 16, Philadelphia, 2001, Saunders; **14-7, 14-8, 14-9,** From Tighe SM: Instrumentation for the operating room, ed 7, St Louis, 2007, Mosby; **14-10,** Courtesy Teleflex Medical, Research Triangle Park, NC; **14-11,** From Baumgartner FJ: Surgical approaches and techniques in the management of severe hyperhidrosis, *Thoracic Surgery Clinics* 18(2):167-181, 2009; **14-12,** From Kernstine KH et al: Robotic lobectomy, *Operative Techniques in Thoracic and Cardiovascular Surgery,* 13(3):204.e1-204.e23, 2009; **14-13,** From Damjanov I, Linder J, editors: *Anderson's pathology,* ed 10, St Louis, 1996, Mosby; **14-14, 14-20,** From McCance KL, Huether SE: *Pathophysiology—the biologic basis for disease in adults and children,* ed 6, St Louis, 2010, Mosby; **14-23,** From Sellke F et al: *Sabiston & Spencer surgery of the chest,* ed 7, Philadelphia, 2005, Saunders.

CHAPTER 15
15-1, 15-4, From Patton KT, Thibodeau GA: *Anatomy and physiology,* ed 7, St Louis, 2010, Mosby; **15-2,** From Thibodeau GA, Patton KT: *Anatomy and physiology,* ed 5, St Louis, 2003, Mosby; **15-3,** From Kumar et al: *Robbins and Cotran pathologic basis of disease,* ed 8, St Louis, 2010, Saunders; **15-5,** From Dettenmeier PA: *Radiographic assessment for nurses,* St Louis, 1995, Mosby; **15-8, 15-9, 15-10, 15-11, 15-13,** From Tighe SM: Instrumentation for the operating room, ed 7, St Louis, 2007, Mosby; **15-14,** From Haimovici H: *Vascular surgery: principles and technique,* ed 4, Oxford, 1995, Blackwell Science; **15-16, 15-19,** From Hershey FB, Calman CH: *Atlas of vascular surgery,* ed 3, St Louis, 1973, Mosby; **15-17, 15-18,** From MacVittie BA: *Vascular surgery,* St Louis, 1998, Mosby; **15-23, 15-25, 15-26,** From Wilson

SE: *Vascular access: principles and practice,* ed 3, St Louis, 1996, Mosby; **15-24,** From Calne R, Pollard SG: *Operative surgery,* London, 1992, Gower; **15-27, 15-28,** From Townsend CM et al: *Sabiston textbook of surgery,* ed 18, Philadelphia, 2010, Saunders.

CHAPTER 16
16-1A, 16-6A, From Thibodeau GA, Patton KT: *Anatomy and physiology,* ed 5, St Louis, 2003, Mosby; **16-2, 16-6B and C,** From Seifert PC: *Cardiac surgery,* St Louis, 1994, Mosby. Drawings by Peter Stone; **16-4,** From Levy MN, Pappano AJ: *Cardiovascular physiology,* ed 9, St Louis, 2007, Mosby; **16-5,** From Thompson JM et al: *Mosby's clinical nursing,* ed 5, St Louis, 2002, Mosby; **16-8, 16-11,** From Canobbio M: *Cardiovascular disorders,* St Louis, 1990, Mosby; **16-9A, 16-33, 16-52,** From Braunwald E et al, editors: *Heart disease,* ed 6, Philadelphia, 2001, Saunders; **16-9B, 16-32B and C, 16-40A,** From Seifert PC: *Cardiac surgery,* St Louis, 1994, Mosby; **16-10,** Courtesy Edward A Lefrak, MD, Annandale, VA; **16-12,** From Kinney M, Packa D: *Andreoli's comprehensive cardiac care,* ed 7, St Louis, 1995, Mosby; **16-13,** From Tighe SM: *Instrumentation for the operating room,* ed 7, St Louis, 2007, Mosby; **16-14,** Courtesy Scanlan International, St Paul; **16-15,** Courtesy Rultract, Inc, Cleveland; **16-16,** Courtesy Telefex Medical, Research Triangle Park, NC; **16-17, 16-49, 16-66,** From Zipes DP et al: *Braunwald's heart disease: a textbook of cardiovascular medicine,* ed 7, Philadelphia, 2005, Saunders; **16-18,** Courtesy Hewlett-Packard Co, Medical Products Group, Andover, MA; **16-19, 16-34, 16-36, 16-37, 16-41, 16-43, 16-46, 16-50, 16-55, 16-56, 16-57, 16-59, 16-60, 16-61, 16-63, 16-64, 16-65, 16-67, 16-68, 16-69, 16-70, 16-71, 16-73, 16-74, 16-77,** From Waldhausen JA et al: *Surgery of the chest,* ed 6, St Louis, 1996, Mosby; **16-20, 16-21,** Courtesy Meadox Medicals, a division of Boston Scientific Co; **16-22,** Courtesy WL Gore & Associates, Inc, Flagstaff, AZ; **16-23,** Courtesy St Jude Medical, Inc, St Paul; **16-24,** Courtesy Sulzer Carbomedics, Inc, Austin, TX; **16-25, 16-28, 16-32A,** Courtesy Baxter Healthcare Corp, Edwards CVS division, Santa Ana, CA; **16-26, 16-27, 16-31, 16-44, 16-72,** Copyright Medtronic, Inc, Minneapolis; **16-75, 16-76,** Courtesy ATS Medical, Minneapolis, MN; **16-29, 16-30,** Courtesy CryoLife, Inc, Marietta, GA; **16-35,** Courtesy Bard Cardiopulmonary GTC, Haverhill, MA; **16-38,** From Buxton B et al: *Ischemic heart disease surgical management,* London, 1999, Mosby; **16-39,** Courtesy Stockert Instrumente, Gmbh, Munich; Courtesy US distributor: COBE CV, division of Sorin Biomedica, Arvada, CO; **16-45, 16-54,** Courtesy Heartport, Inc., Redwood City, CA; **16-47,** From Doty DB: *Cardiac surgery: operative technique,* St Louis, 1997, Mosby; **16-48,** From Lytle BW et al: Coronary artery bypass grafting with the right gastroepiploic artery, *J Thorac Cardiovasc Surg* 976:826, 1989; **16-53,** Courtesy Heartport, Inc, Redwood City, CA; **16-59,** From David TE et al: Long-term results of mitral valve repair, *J Thorac Cardiovasc Surg* 115(6): 1279-1286, 1998.

CHAPTER 17
17-1, 17-2, 17-3, 17-4, 17-5, 17-6, 17-7, 17-8, From Tighe SM: *Instrumentation for the operating room,* ed 7, St Louis, 2007, Mosby; **17-9, 17-10, 17-11, 17-43,** From Children's Hospital of Philadelphia, Philadelphia, PA; **17-12,** From Swartz MH: *Textbook of physical diagnosis: history and examination,* ed 6, Philadelphia, 2010, Saunders; **17-13, 17-14, 17-15, 17-22, 17-27,** From Coran AG et al: *Surgery of the neonate,* Boston, 1978, Little, Brown; **17-16, 17-19, 17-29, 17-31, 17-33, 17-40, 17-41, 17-75,** From Holcomb GW, Murphy JP: *Pediatric surgery,* ed 5, Philadelphia, 2010, Saunders; **17-17,** Modified from Gross RE: *An atlas of children's surgery,* Philadelphia, 1970, Saunders; **17-18, 17-24, 17-25, 17-28, 17-44,** From Spitz L et al: *A colour atlas of paediatric surgical diagnosis,* London, 1990, Mosby Ltd; **17-20,** Modified from Boley SJ: An endorectal pull-through operation with primary anastomosis for Hirschsprung's disease, *Surgery, Gynecology and Obstetrics* 127(2):253, 1986; **17-21,** From Chessell G et al: *Diagnostic picture tests in clinical medicine,* vol 2, St Louis, 1984, Mosby; **17-23,** From DeVries PA: Posterior sagittal anorectoplasty. In Holmann von Kap S, editor: *Anorektale Fehlbildungen,* Stuttgart, 1984, Gustav Fischer-Verlag; **17-26,** Courtesy Dr David Clark, NeoPIX, Albany, NY; **17-30,** From Townsend CM et al: *Sabiston textbook of surgery,* ed 18, Philadelphia, 2008, Saunders; **17-32,** Courtesy H Gil Rushton, MD, Children's National Medical Center, Washington, DC. In Hockenberry MJ, Wilson D: *Wong's nursing care of infants and children,* ed 8, St Louis, 2007, Mosby; **17-34, 17-35, 17-39,** Modified from Droller MJ: *Surgical management of urologic disease,* St Louis, 1992, Mosby; **17-36,** From Devine CJ, Jr: Chordee and hypospadias. In Glenn JF, Boyce WH, editors: *Urologic surgery,* ed 3, Philadelphia, 1983, Lippincott; **17-42,** From Fuhrman BP, Zimmerman J: *Pediatric criti-*

cal care, ed 3, Philadelphia, 2006, Mosby; **17-45,** Courtesy Albert Biglan, MD, Children's Hospital of Pittsburgh. In Zitelli BJ, Davis HW: *Atlas of pediatric physical diagnosis,* ed 5, St Louis, 2007, Mosby; **17-46,** From Neurosurgery wound closure, Ethicon, Inc; **17-51, 17-52, 17-53,** From Zitelli BJ, Davis HW: *Atlas of pediatric physical diagnosis,* ed 5, St Louis, 2007, Mosby; **17-54,** Courtesy Emory University School of Medicine, Atlanta; **17-55, 17-56, 17-57, 17-58,** Katowitz JA, editor: *Pediatric oculoplastic surgery,* Philadelphia, 2002, Springer; **17-59A,** Redrawn from Chameides L: *Pediatric advanced life support,* Dallas, 1988, American Heart Association; **17-59B,** From Barkin RM, Rosen P: *Emergency pediatrics: a guide to ambulatory care,* ed 3, St Louis, 1990, Mosby; **17-60, 17-62, 17-64, 17-66, 17-70,** From Nichols DG, Cameron DE: *Critical heart disease in infants and children,* ed 2, St Louis, 2006, Mosby; **17-61, 17-65, 17-67, 17-69, 17-71,** From Hockenberry MJ, Wilson D: *Wong's nursing care of infants and children,* ed 8, St Louis, 2007, Mosby; **17-63,** From Cooley DA, Norman JC: *Techniques in cardiac surgery,* Houston, 1975, Texas Medical Press; **17-68, 17-72, 17-73, 17-74,** From Nichols DG et al: *Critical heart disease in infants and children,* St Louis, 1994, Mosby.

CHAPTER 18

18-1, Courtesy New Hanover Health Network EMS Air Link, EMS, Emergency Medical Services, Wilmington, NC; **18-4,** From Grande CM: *Textbook of trauma anesthesia and critical care,* St Louis, 1993, Mosby; **18-5,** From Brohi K: www.trauma.org, available at www.trauma.org/index.php/search/image_results/3af7210b6a3eb8cf1bb9b55839a3070d/. Accessed December 2009; **18-6,** From Cosgriff H, Jr, Anderson DL: *The practice of emergency care,* ed 2, Philadelphia, Lippincott; **18-7,** Redrawn from Kintzel KC: *Advanced concepts in clinical nursing,* ed 2, Philadelphia, 1997, Lippincott; **18-8,** Redrawn from Becker DP et al: Diagnosis and treatment of head injury. In Youman JR, editor: *Neurological surgery,* ed 3, Philadelphia, 1990, Saunders; **18-9, 18-10,** From Neff JA, Kidd PS: *Trauma nursing: the art and science,* St Louis, 1993, Mosby; **18-11,** Courtesy Haim Paran, MD; **18-12,** From McQuillan KA et al: *Trauma nursing,* ed 4, St Louis, 2009, Saunders; **18-13,** From Townsend CM et al: *Sabiston textbook of surgery,* ed 18, Philadelphia, 2008, Saunders.

Index

Page numbers followed by *f* indicate figures; *t,* tables; *b,* boxes.